TEXTBOOK OF NUTRITIONAL MEDICINE

Also by Melvyn R. Werbach

SourceBooks of Clinical Research

Botanical Influences on Illness (Michael T. Murray, co-author)

Foundations of Nutritional Medicine

Nutritional Influences on Illness

Nutritional Influences on Mental Illness

Healing Through Nutrition:
A Natural Approach to Treating 50 Common Illnesses with Diet and Nutrients

Third Line Medicine:
Modern Treatment for Persistent Symptoms

Textbook of Nutritional Medicine

Melvyn R. Werbach, M.D.
Assistant Clinical Professor
School of Medicine, UCLA
Los Angeles, California

with Jeffrey Moss, D.D.S., C.N.S., C.C.N.

THIRD LINE PRESS, INC.
Tarzana, California

Information presented in this book changes rapidly and is subject to differing interpretations. It is up to you to check it thoroughly before relying on it. Neither the author nor the publisher makes any guarantees regarding the outcome of the uses to which this book is put.

The treatment of illness should be supervised by a physician or other licensed health professional. Information presented herein does not contain treatment recommendations for the public.

Printed in the United States of America

ISBN 0-9618550-9-6

Library of Congress Catalog Card Number: 99-073820

To my wife, Gail, and my sons, Kevin and Adam,
for their love and support that made this book possible,
To Jeff Moss, whose insights and assistance were invaluable,
To my mentors who taught and inspired me, and
To the investigators whose pursuit of knowledge
is summarized in these pages.

Melvyn R. Werbach

To my parents and family, who gave me the opportunity,
To George Eversaul, who opened my eyes,
To Harry Eidenier, Jr., who shined the light that led me out of darkness,
To Mel Werbach, who allowed me to be part of this project,
and, most of all,
To my wife Joanne and daughter Jennie,
who have given and continue to give me purpose.

Jeffrey Moss

TEXTBOOK OF NUTRITIONAL MEDICINE

TABLE OF CONTENTS

PART THREE: APPENDICES

INTRODUCTION

My professional interest in nutritional medicine developed during my years as director of psychiatric services and clinical biofeedback at the UCLA Pain Control Unit, part of the Department of Anesthesiology, UCLA Hospital and Clinics in Los Angeles, California.

While trained as a psychiatrist, I had developed a special interest in finding methods of helping the many patients who fail to respond to standard treatments. I had already developed expertise in relaxation training procedures and was brought to the Unit to develop a program utilizing biofeedback instruments for selected chronic pain patients which would attempt to teach them to achieve pain relief by calming their bodies.

During those years I also functioned as a patient manager. It was my responsibility to evaluate patients who had failed for years to achieve pain relief from a variety of procedures, usually including drugs and often including surgery, and to suggest individualized treatment programs utilizing the relatively safe and gentle procedures that we offered but to which they had not been previously exposed.

I found these patients to be remarkably similar to others with chronic physical complaints who I was seeing in my private practice. It was clear that, while their medical diagnoses were helpful, the diagnosis itself rarely suggested the treatment; it was only one of a number of factors that needed to be considered. My background and experience had already sharpened my acumen in discerning psychological and physiological factors.

As my experience grew, it became increasingly clear that nutritional status was another one of those factors, and reactivity to foods and environmental chemicals was yet another. (My first book, *Third Line Medicine: Modern Treatment for Persistent Symptoms*, was born of my desire to share the insights I had gained into the deficiencies of the contemporary medical model.)

What particularly intrigued me about nutrition and environmental sensitivities was the failure of so many clinicians to recognize their importance. As a medical student at Tufts University School of Medicine, I received only a few hours of training in nutrition, and that was a year *before* I began to treat patients. In fact, I remember one of my professors stating categorically that, in industrialized societies, nutritional deficiencies only occur in severe alcoholics.

After graduation from medical school, I took a year of internship in internal medicine and then completed the equivalent of three years of residency in psychiatry. Those years added little to my knowledge of the relationship between nutrition and illness.

The staff on the Pain Control Unit worked closely together to blend their individual expertise into a unified program. We taught each other how we believed our respective fields related to the pain experience, and then saw for ourselves through interaction with our patients the efficacy of many different approaches to the treatment of chronic pain.

As I gradually became aware of the relevance of foods and nutrients to illness, I became eager to apply my new knowledge in my private practice and began to incorporate questions about nutrition into my patient evaluations. Later, I began to do laboratory testing in order to gather additional information.

Despite my growing appreciation of nutritional factors, I found that I was hampered in my attempts to quickly review the scientific literature concerning the many illnesses that burdened my patients. There was no central place to turn to for information. It was a large enough task to review the literature on one illness, and an overwhelming task to do so for the numerous illnesses, most of which poorly defined, that my patients brought to the practice.

My first attempt at organization consisted of a series of 3" by 5" cards, each labeled with a different medical diagnosis. Whenever I found a reference to a relationship between a nutrient and that disorder, I would list that nutrient on the card. That way, when I wished to consider nutritional factors in a particular disorder, I already knew which nutrients to review.

My lists grew longer and longer; yet it became increasingly clear that they were very inadequate for my needs. I began, instead, to write notes summarizing the nutritional factors for each disorder as I learned about them along with references to the literature so that I could readily go back to them; later I began to type those notes. That system, too, proved to be very inadequate.

One day, while looking at my growing stack of note pages, I realized that, if I was having so much difficulty practicing science-oriented nutritional medicine, then my colleagues who were attempting to do the same must be having the same difficulties. It was then that I decided to develop my materials into books, so that all of us could improve the quality of care that we offered by having better access to the rapidly expanding nutritional literature.

In the years since, I have written, or co-authored, several "sourcebooks" that organize and provide abstracts from the major literature on nutritional medicine. These include a general book *(Nutritional Influences on Illness)*, a book on nutritional psychiatry *(Nutritional Influences on Mental Illness)*, a book on medicinal herbs *(Botanical Influences on Illness)*, and a book summarizing some of the essential information needed in daily practice *(Foundations of Nutritional Medicine)*.

I designed these books so that clinicians could quickly access the major studies in order to gain an appreciation of the knowledge - and the controversies - of the developing field of nutritional medicine. I intentionally avoided taking any position; I let the literature speak for itself, warts and all.

I believe these books, which have continued to evolve with each edition, have helped to fill the gap. What still was missing, however, was a textbook. In contrast to the sourcebooks, which seek to display the highlights of the literature, a textbook should seek to synthesize current knowledge and to provide rational tools for applying that knowledge in clinical practice.

Perhaps nutritional medicine was too young a field to warrant a textbook in the past. In my judgment, the field has now matured to the point that a suitable textbook is vitally needed.

I hope this book will fulfill that need.

Melvyn R. Werbach, M.D.
Tarzana, California

PART ONE

GENERAL EVALUATION AND TREATMENT

NUTRITION AND INTEGRATIVE MEDICINE

INTRODUCTION

As you will see in the forthcoming chapters, a voluminous amount of literature exists documenting the impact of nutrients in relationship to various disease states. However, to what extent can the results that are obtained in research studies be directly extrapolated to the clinical setting? Much of the promotional material on nutritional supplements certainly seems to suggest that everybody could benefit from taking supplements of almost every conceivable nutrient.

Of course, if you take the time to read the studies, researchers readily admit that this is rarely the case, for even those that find a particular nutrient to be highly effective will usually show that a significant percentage of the study group did not respond positively, demonstrating that not everyone in a particular diagnostic group responds the same when supplemented with a nutrient.

We will explain in this chapter some of the reasons why we believe this occurs, and suggest measures that can be taken to give nutritional therapeutics a higher chance of success, no matter how difficult the case.

Integrative Medicine - A Comprehensive Paradigm

During the last few years, a more comprehensive approach to determining nutritional requirements has arisen that comes closer to accurately identifying the needs of today's chronically ill patient. This method takes what we already know about clinical nutrition and places it into a different perspective, a perspective that maintains that no physiologic process, including one relating to nutrition, can be fully understood when examined as an isolated entity. The true significance of nutritional factors can only be comprehended when considered in conjunction with the physiologic processes which are, in turn, impacted by those factors.

Is it necessary to know the many physiologic interrelationships of nutritional factors in order to successfully employ nutrition clinically? For treating many patients, direct application of the information in ensuing chapters that are organized according to specific illnesses will be enough. However, for treating other chronically ill patients who "have been everywhere and tried everything," an understanding of the integrative principles discussed below may be necessary.

Of the many names this comprehensive approach has been given, we prefer "integrative medicine." Although nutrition is only one aspect of a comprehensive integrative approach, we did not choose "integrative nutrition" because the integrative model is more than just nutritional evaluation and treatment; it represents a different way of looking at patients.

In terms of evaluating the needs of the chronically ill patient, integrative medicine assumes that they are suffering due to a variety of causes that are working together in sometimes intricate ways to create the clinical picture. For decades, modern medicine has employed a "single cause, single cure" approach to disease which, as can be seen from the massive amount of studies on the effects of single nutrients on illness, has largely been adopted by clinical nutrition as well. Unfortunately, while this philosophy of health care was quite successful in the days when infection and gross nutrient deficiency were common, it is yielding diminishing returns now.

A discussion of the broad range of factors - including, for example, physical fitness and mental health - which are encompassed in the concept of integrative medicine is well beyond the scope of this text. Instead, we will limit ourselves to the most common nutritionally-relevant causes of chronic illness. These can be divided into five broad categories:

> **I. NEUROENDOCRINE IMBALANCE** - This category primarily includes the stress response and its numerous downstream effects on endocrine function.

II. IMPROPER NUTRITION - Micronutrient imbalances need to be considered when evaluating the chronic patient. Also, we will demonstrate that another aspect of nutritional imbalance, *macronutrient* imbalance, is epidemic yet much less appreciated in the chronically ill population.

III. CHEMICAL AND/OR HEAVY METAL TOXICITY - The evidence that environmental toxins are playing a major role in creating chronic illness is compelling. Research will be presented demonstrating how the ultimate clinical toxicity of xenobiotics can vary greatly in different individuals.

IV. COMPROMISED MUCOSAL BARRIERS - Improper function of the gastrointestinal tract can be a major cause of chronic illness due to poor digestive capacity, suboptimal absorption, and/or increased absorption of toxic substances, no matter whether their origin is exogenous or endogenous. We will show that factors such as poor diet, elevated stress hormones, and dysbiotic organisms can work together to make a major contribution to much of the chronic illness that exists today.

V. GENETICS - This area has traditionally received little attention because genes were believed to be impermeable to environmental influences. Exciting new research is suggesting, however, that genetic expression is quite responsive to external surroundings. Furthermore, this research demonstrates that nutrients have a powerful impact on both gene expression and the function of DNA repair mechanisms.

According to this proposed model, in order to properly address the needs of the chronic patient, the following points must be kept in mind:

- *These major causes of chronic illness rarely work in isolation to create ill health.* Rather, they interact in often intricate ways to create the clinical picture.

- *All five causes may be of etiologic importance.* This represents a key difference between a disease-oriented model and the integrative model. Using the integrative approach, diagnostic procedures continue beyond simply putting together sufficient data to fit the patient with a disease label. Instead, they continue until the causative factors can be reasonably determined.

What follows next is an in-depth exploration of each of the above-mentioned causes of chronic illness. Even though there is some extrapolation, the voluminous amount of research will demonstrate that utilization of an integrative model is a necessity for practitioners wish to optimally address our increasingly sophisticated understanding of the complicated nature of illness.

I. NEUROENDOCRINE IMBALANCE

This aspect of the integrative approach is being mentioned first, not because it is more important than the others, but because it appears to be the aspect that is most often ignored by both clinicians and researchers when considering chronic illness. Furthermore, it is virtually omnipresent in the population of chronic patients. While neuroendocrine imbalance can take many forms in the chronically ill, only one form, the *stress response*, will be discussed here. The reason for this is two-fold. First, the stress response, as will be demonstrated, can have a major impact on clinical findings. Secondly, many other endocrine abnormalities that are commonly thought as being "stand alone" illnesses in chronically ailing patients can, very often, be downstream effects of the stress response.

The stress response is actually composed of two interrelated systems. The first, the *catecholamine-mediated* system, is controlled by two primary hormones, epinephrine and norepinephrine. This system, commonly known as the sympathetic or "fight or flight" system, prepares the body to act. The second, the *hypothalamic-pituitary-adrenal axis*, is mediated primarily by cortisol which mobilizes energy *(Michelson;McCance)*.

A paramount goal of the stress response is to maintain glucose levels *(Ober)*. When functioning correctly, the stress response is quite efficient at maintaining serum glucose levels that optimize health. However, when the system malfunctions, it will err by promoting an elevation of glucose levels rather than risking the potential disaster of a low glucose supply *(Ober)*. In this instance, the stress response becomes a potent destructive, catabolic force mediated by a vicious circle of elevated glucocorticoids, insulin hypersecretion and insulin resistance *(McEwen)*.

Whether the stress response will be adaptive or maladaptive depends upon its ability to shut itself down when the danger has passed *(MeEwen)*. The ability to successfully shut down depends on a receptor-mediated negative-feedback loop which can be neutralized with great effectiveness by chronically elevated cortisol *(Meaney)*.

Why would cortisol be elevated? Consider the following list of potential inducers of cortisol secretion, most of which may be encountered by patients on an almost daily basis *(McCance)*:

infection
noise
decreased oxygen supply
pain
malnutrition
heat
cold
trauma
prolonged exertion
radiation
obesity
old age
drugs
disease
surgery
medical treatment
responses to life events

The last inducer, namely responses to life events, is included because stressors do not even require a physical presence to induce cortisol secretion. Simply the perception of stress is a powerful inducer *(LeDoux)*.

The vast importance of a maladaptive stress response is demonstrated by the following list of ailments which the response is believed able to induce or exacerbate *(McCance)*:

Cardiovascular system
- Coronary artery disease
- High blood pressure
- Stroke

Musculoskeletal system
- Tension headaches
- Muscle contraction
- Backache

Connective tissues
- Rheumatoid arthritis and related connective tissue disorders

Pulmonary system
- Asthma
- Hay fever

Immune system
- Immunodepression
- Autoimmune disease

Gastrointestinal system
- Ulcer
- Irritable bowel syndrome
- Diarrhea
- Nausea and vomiting
- Ulcerative colitis

Genitourinary system
- Diuresis
- Impotence
- Frigidity

Skin
- Eczema
- Acne

Endocrine system
- Diabetes mellitus
- Amenorrhea

Central nervous system
- Fatigue and lethargy
- Overeating
- Depression
- Insomnia

Why does the stress response contain biochemical mechanisms that are so destructive when functioning in a maladaptive manner? This question can best be answered by using the analogy of the proverbial caveman and saber-toothed tiger. The stress response is an ancient set of responses designed to help early humans escape danger. Furthermore, like most other physiologic pathways, it exists in contemporary humans in a form that is largely the same as that which was found in ancestral populations.

Consider the following key aspects of the stress response and note that, while they seem primarily destructive in the context of modern society, they were quite helpful in promoting the survival of the caveman:

Elevation of Serum Glucose

The caveman had to first decide that danger existed and then determine the best course of action with extreme rapidity. This activity requires proper brain function, a process that requires glucose. Second, he or she had to make an appropriate physical action. This requires increased cardiovascular tone and respiration - which is also fueled by glucose.

Where would this glucose come from? The first thought might be glucose storage depots. However, the human species is unable to store glucose with the exception of small amounts in the form of glycogen. Another possibility would be to eat a glucose-producing food such as an apple before starting the escape process, but taking the time to do so would be a fatal error in this instance. Therefore, since glucose cannot be stored to any meaningful extent, and since taking time to eat is inherently self-destructive, something in the caveman must be converted to glucose almost instantaneously in order to assure escape.

Since fat is stored in large quantities in adipose tissue, it would be the logical choice of a substance to be converted. Fat, however, cannot be converted to glucose *(Coffee)*. This leaves protein as the only substance that exists in adequate quantities to fuel the escape process by its conversion to glucose. Thus, in the stress response, protein catabolism is greatly increased while the resulting amino acids are converted to sugar in the process of gluconeogenesis *(Matthews DE)*.

Gluconeogenesis

The major sources of protein for catabolism are muscle and gut *(Leverve)*. While these sources are less than ideal, they make sense because the stress response is a biochemical compromise during which the body uses whatever resources are available in order to gain an advantage over immediate danger. Thus, during physiologic stress, *long-term health is sacrificed in order to assure short-term survival.*

While gluconeogenesis primarily involves the conversion of protein to glucose, it also includes other, less dominant glucose-forming pathways. One of these, which again may compromise long-term health, is *enhanced conversion of pyruvate to lactate (Mizock)*. Under ideal circumstances, pyruvate is converted to acetyl CoA which in turn is converted to ATP via the Krebs cycle. The stress response, however, takes advantage of the ability of lactate to be converted to glucose in a process known as the Cori cycle *(Mizock)*. While this results in a higher production of glucose, lactate - a muscle irritant - is increased, and energy-efficient aerobic metabolism is sacrificed in favor of energy-inefficient anaerobic, glycolytic metabolism. This process, which has been called *the futile cycling of carbohydrate (Fish)*, may help to explain why fatigue and achy muscles are so common in chronically ill patients.

Increased lipolysis is a third aspect of gluconeogenesis that provides approximately 20% of the glucose production during stress *(Mizock)*. Fats are composed of fatty acids attached to a backbone of glycerol, and glycerol can be converted to glucose. Moreover, some fat can still be converted to ATP via the Krebs cycle, and ATP fuels the engine of gluconeogenesis by promoting the activity of three key gluconeogenic enzymes *(Salway)*.

This aspect of stress metabolism may seem like a blessing for overweight individuals. Unfortunately, like most other aspects of the stress response, it is another metabolic compromise of long-term health that occurs in order to assure short-term survival. For, in the long term, the fat loss is far from uniform and often causes increased visceral fat accumulation *(Bjornstorp)*.

Insulin Resistance

Another aspect of stress-induced glucose production is one of the most important. For the caveman to successfully escape the saber-toothed tiger, it is not enough to just produce more glucose. A mechanism must also exist that assures the glucose is preferentially directed to the systems that are most vital to the escape process. This is accomplished by producing a state of *insulin resistance (Matthews DE)*.

The function of insulin is to facilitate entry of glucose into insulin-sensitive tissues. By creating a state of insulin resistance, the stress response assures that glucose will only be used by tissues that can utilize glucose without the aid of insulin, namely those that are most vital to the escape process - such as the brain *(Little)*. Thus insulin resistance may merely be another compromise of long-term health to assure short-term survival *(Clark)*.

Suppression of Nonessential Functions

To successfully escape the saber-toothed tiger, the caveman must funnel tremendous amounts of energy to key systems in an extremely rapid manner. Therefore, many functions considered to be nonessential or even detrimental to the escape process are down-regulated. These functions include the following:

- Sleep - Because of the serious danger caused by fatigue, sleep-inducing mechanisms are suppressed *(Michelson)*.

- Feeding - If the caveman instinctively responded to hunger pangs and stopped to eat an apple during the escape process, the caveman would become the tiger's meal. Therefore, this both non-essential and, in terms of escape, counterproductive behavior is suppressed *(Michelson)*. Suppression is accomplished by decreasing both splanchnic circulation *(Matuschak)* and vagus nerve stimulation *(Stratakis)*. In turn, decreased vagus nerve stimulation causes decreased gastric motility and increased colonic motility, all of which serve to suppress the desire to feed.

- Reproduction - Engaging in reproductive behavior during escape is also counterproductive. Therefore, elevated cortisol suppresses the production of all major reproductive hormones *(Stratakis)*.

- Growth - As the anabolic processes necessary for growth are irrelevant for escape, production of both growth hormone and insulin-like growth factor-1 (IGF-1) are down-regulated by cortisol *(Stratakis)*.

Modification of Metabolic Rate and Immune Function

As might be expected, the tremendous demands of the stress response lead to an overall increase in metabolic rate *(Matthews DE)*. However, this increase comes at a tremendous cost, for the process is catabolic in nature, leading to the loss of many vital tissues, particularly those that are protein-based. In fact, the process has been described as "autocanibalism" *(Fish)*.

To help counterbalance the loss of protein caused by the hypermetabolic state, the body employs an ingenious device during the stress response. Thyroid function is down-regulated *(LoPresti)*. This process is often called *euthyroid sick syndrome (LoPresti)* because all major diagnostic indicators of thyroid function (TSH, T_3, T_4) will demonstrate low thyroid function even though the thyroid gland itself demonstrates no physical evidence of ill-health. (This raises the question of whether hypothyroidism, a common disorder in our society, could be better treated by optimizing stress physiology than by hormone replacement.)

One well-known result of chronically elevated glucocorticoid levels is suppression of immunity. However, during the stress response, the effects of cortisol are not uniform *(McCance)*. Specifically, mediators of systemic immunity such as immunoglobulins, lymphocytes, eosinophils, kinins, prostaglandins, and histamines are suppressed, at least initially. In contrast, the quantity of the primary mediator of local immunity, polymorphonuclear leukocytes, is increased.

Why might this occur? Again, consider the analogy of the caveman and the saber-toothed tiger. What if, while running, the caveman was injuring by tripping over a log or was actually bitten by the tiger but was still able to escape and continue running? In such a situation, it is important to have a mechanism in place that would quickly halt the bleeding and also be able to prevent infection - both of which can be accomplished by increasing polymorphonuclear lymphocytes. In contrast, the development of effects of systemic inflammation, i.e., fever, malaise, achy muscles, would be counterproductive. Therefore, production of mediators of systemic immunity such as lymphocytes, eosinophils, kinins, prostaglandins, and histamines is suppressed.

Unfortunately, this down-regulating effect is somewhat short-lived. Eventually, prolonged inflammation - as is seen with autoimmune conditions such as rheumatoid arthritis - can lead to glucocorticoid resistance by reducing glucocorticoid receptor-binding affinity *(Torpy)*. The result is a heightened proinflammatory response, primarily through increased cytokine production *(Moldawer)*.

Maintenance of Blood Volume

Another important function of the stress response is the maintenance of proper blood volume. Consider again our troubled friend, the caveman. In order to facilitate escape, increased levels of blood must get to key organs such as the heart and lungs. Furthermore, in case of an injury that is not incapacitating, mechanisms must exist to prevent fatal blood loss.

To accomplish this, elevated cortisol signals an increase in production of the mineralocorticoids aldosterone and antidiuretic hormone *(Fish)*. This, in turn, alters renal filtration mechanics so that sodium and bicarbonate are retained and increased levels of potassium and magnesium *(Fish;Quamme)* are excreted. The net result is water retention, which enables maintenance of blood volume. (Could essential hypertension be nothing more than an out-of-control stress response?)

Nutrient Depletion

Several important nutrients undergo significant depletion during the stress response. These include:

- Magnesium and potassium - Both are significantly depleted due to losses in the urine *(Fish;Quamme)*.
- Glutamine - Due to its conversion to alanine and glucose during stress-mediated gluconeogenesis *(Bucci)*, glutamine can be depleted by up to 50%. Furthermore, the ability to restore glutamine levels after stress-mediated loss can be quite slow *(Bucci)*.
- Carnitine - Due to the increased rate of lipolysis during stress, carnitine levels can be significantly depleted *(Bahl)*.
- Vitamin C, Zinc and Coenzyme Q_{10} - Due to hypermetabolism, higher levels of these nutrients may be required *(DiPasquale)*.

Clinical Implications

Why would a process that is so destructive exist at all? Perhaps the answer is that the world of the caveman was primarily benevolent; thus the stress response was only activated occasionally. Eventually the caveman would escape the saber-toothed tiger, allowing him or her to eat, sleep, repair, and reproduce. By contrast, how many of today's chronically ill patients never escape the "saber-toothed tigers" that are chasing them, at least from a standpoint of their perception? How many of your patients view the world as a fundamentally hostile place where even seemingly innocuous situations are viewed as dangerous or, at minimum, highly suspicious?

Given that the stress response can be initiated by a perception of danger even though no actual danger exists, and given that "stressed out" has become a popular expression in modern society, the answers to these questions are self-evident. When a person's perception of the world is transformed from primarily benevolent to primarily hostile, the development of illness is fostered for, when the stress response operates ceaselessly, it is also transformed. The short-term advantages it yields are eventually lost so that what remains is only its destructive capacity.

To comprehend the formidable destructive force of an excessive stress response, consider the following list of chronic conditions that it may promote:

Obesity - Elevated cortisol and associated insulin resistance have been highly correlated with visceral fat accumulation *(Bjornstorp)*. This combination of findings is often referred to as the metabolic syndrome or "Syndrome X" *(Bjornstorp;Reaven)*. In females, besides its direct adverse effects on health, "Syndrome X" may cause other, downstream, hormonal imbalances, as they can produce significant quantities of testosterone and estradiol in adipose tissue *(Kopelman)*. In males, by contrast, obesity is correlated with *decreases* in testosterone production *(Bjornstorp)*.

Diabetes mellitus - Given that the primary goal of the stress response is to raise serum glucose and cause hyperinsulinemia and insulin resistance, and since the stress response often appears to be working overtime for inhabitants of modern industrialized societies, it is not surprising that the incidence of diabetes is on the rise *(Clark)*.

Cardiovascular disease including high blood pressure and elevations in blood fats - Recall the statement above that prolonged elevations of glucocorticoids will cause hyperinsulinemia and insulin resistance. These two factors are part of the "Syndrome X" complex, which has been strongly correlated with the incidence of cardiovascular disease *(Reaven)*.

Infectious disease - Prolonged stress will, in a predictable manner, increase susceptibility to both bacterial and viral infections due to its effects on the immune response *(Solomon)*.

Gastrointestinal illness – A prolonged stress response can stimulate colonic transit and fecal excretion. It can also lower pain thresholds for visceral sensation in patients with functional gastrointestinal disorders *(Stratakis)*.

Increased gastrointestinal permeability ("leaky gut") - Sustained activation of the catecholamine (sympathoadrenal) branch of the stress response can result in diversion of splanchnic flow and lead to a compromised gut mucosal barrier *(Matuschak)*.

Inflammatory (autoimmune) illness - Since cortisol suppresses the inflammatory response, one may think that individuals under high stress should never develop autoimmune diseases such as lupus or rheumatoid arthritis. However, long-term exposure to excess cortisol can actually have proinflammatory effects because of delayed and heightened cytokine production *(Moldawer)*. This may be because tissues exposed to excessive levels of glucocorticoids can become glucocorticoid-resistant *(Torpy)*. Another possibility is the effect of glucocorticoids on the enzyme phospholipase

A_2, the enzyme that is responsible for the formation of arachidonic acid-derived proinflammatory prostaglandins.

Increased effects of mind-altering drugs - Repeated stress can increase the behavioral response to drugs such as cocaine and amphetamines *(Sorg)*. Conversely, acute cocaine ingestion increases plasma cortisol levels *(Sorg)* while tricyclic antidepressants can up-regulate the activity of corticosteroid receptors *(Torpy)*. Thus, stress can magnify the effects of drugs, and drugs can magnify the effects of stress.

Infertility – Due to the effects on hypothalamic/pituitary activity, stress hormones decrease gonadal production of both male and female reproductive hormones *(Stratakis)*.

Growth failure - Chronic stress is associated with decreases of both growth hormone and prolactin *(Stratakis;Torpy)*.

Hypothyroidism - Cortisol negatively impacts on TSH production and conversion of T_4 to T_3 *(Stratakis)*.

Osteoporosis - Increased cortisol can lead to mobilization of calcium from bone and increases in urinary calcium *(Brown)*.

Poor wound repair - Chronic cortisol excess retards proliferation of fibroblasts and function at the site of inflammation, resulting in poor wound healing *(McCance)*.

Amenorrhea - Overexercise or psychological stress can result in amenorrhea *(Stout)*.

Impaired detoxification - Some people are believed to be "pathologic detoxifiers" in that laboratory testing shows that phase I (cytochrome P450) enzymes are elevated while phase II enzymes are depressed *(Bland)*. *(See the next section for a description of phase I and II detoxication pathways.)* The up-regulation of phase I may primarily be due to increased exposure to toxins, as is seen with alcohol *(Bland)*. Cortisol, however, can also up-regulate phase I enzymes *(Michelson)*.

Brain damage - Prolonged glucocorticoid secretion may lead to deficits in memory and cognition because of neurotoxic effects on the hippocampus *(O'Brien)*. This has been clinically linked with both depression and Alzheimer's disease *(Nasman)*. Furthermore, the neurotoxic effects of glucocorticoids may cause further promotion of an out-of-control stress response by adversely affecting negative feedback mechanisms *(Duman)*.

Aphthous stomatitis (canker sores) – There is a positive correlation between salivary cortisol levels and the incidence of recurrent aphthous stomatitis *(McCartan)*.

Chronic fatigue syndrome - Several authors have noted that disturbances of the hypothalamic-pituitary-adrenal axis as occurs during prolonged stress can have a major etiologic impact on the incidence of this disorder *(Demitrack)*.

Modulation of gene expression - Genetic expression can be modulated by stress-induced adrenal glucocorticoids *(Duman)*. While the genetic expression of many substances is modified by glucocorticoids, two which are of particular interest are phospholipase A_2, the major enzyme involved in the production of arachidonic acid-derived proinflammatory prostaglandins, and serotonin, a major central nervous system neuromodulator associated with sleep and depression.

Salivary cortisol measurements, which are available from several laboratories, can provide evidence to assist in the determination of an overactive stress response. Not only is this test convenient and inexpensive, it has been recognized as being one of the best, if not the best, method of measuring diurnal changes in *free* cortisol, the only form of cortisol that has significant metabolic activity *(Allolio;Bantle)*.

In order to treat an out-of control stress response, psychophysiologic approaches such as relaxation training should be considered, and the intake of both macronutrients and micronutrients should be optimized. In the next section, we will discuss the importance of optimizing nutrient intake.

II. IMPROPER NUTRITION

A. MACRONUTRIENT IMBALANCES

With so much current emphasis on *micronutrient* intake, imbalances on *macronutrient* intake are frequently neglected, yet imbalances in macronutrient intake are a major problem in our society and a potent factor in the etiology of many of the most prevalent chronic illnesses.

Macronutrient imbalances can be divided into two broad categories, namely quantitative and qualitative imbalances:

1. *Quantitative* Imbalances -

Energy (calories)

Excess caloric intake promotes chronic illness. A common assumption is that reducing fat calories and replacing them with an equal number of carbohydrate calories can successfully address obesity and other related metabolic disorders. Recent research, however, has shown that excess caloric intake is an independent risk factor for chronic illness *(VanItallie)*.

While gross starvation is rare in industrialized countries, suboptimal caloric intake is a serious concern for some patient populations. Besides poverty, causes include the anorexia of chronic illness, depression and old age, the overpopularity of low calorie, fad diets, and the increasingly common practice of skipping meals.

Protein

Excessive protein ingestion can lead to such negative sequelae as loss of bone mass *(Einhorn)* and exacerbation of renal dysfunction *(Reaich)*. Insufficient protein intake is involved in numerous health problems ranging from growth retardation *(Berdanier,1995)* to decreased phase I (cytochrome P-450) detoxication capacity *(Yang)*.

Fat

Numerous studies have demonstrated the dangers of a high fat diet *(Van Gaal)*, a reality which appears, judging from the increased availability of low fat foods and low fat diets, to be quite well accepted by the public. Other research, however, which has been much less publicized, emphasizes that ingesting a diet too *low* in fat has its own dangers *(Simopoulos)*.

Carbohydrate

Despite the importance of appropriate intakes of fats and proteins, the evidence is that excessive carbohydrate intake - especially excessive intake of refined and simple carbohydrates - clearly take precedence in regard to their effects upon the health of most chronically ill patients. This important issue has been discussed at length both in the professional literature *(Chwals;Heller,1994;Jones;Reiser)* and in the popular press *(Atkins;Eades;Heller,1991;Sears)*. The impact of excessive carbohydrate intake on endocrine function is of particular concern *(Eades;Heller,1991;Sears)* as it leads to hyperinsulinemia and, eventually, to insulin resistance *(Heller,1994)*. Hyperinsulinemia can lead, in turn, to inappropriate drops of blood glucose, leading to stimulation of the stress hormones, epinephrine and cortisol *(Cryer)*.

In regard to making the diagnosis of hyperinsulinemia/insulin resistance, a history of carbohydrate cravings is suspicious *(Heller)* and has been reported to be associated with elevated cortisol levels *(Bjornstorp)*. Serum insulin levels, while important to measure, can be misleading due to lack of proper determination of laboratory ranges *(Heller)*. Moreover, the glucose tolerance test often has little value *(Cryer)*.

Excessive carbohydrate intake can be a potent exacerbating factor in many of the stress-related chronic conditions outlined above including the development of obesity, now considered by many to be occurring in epidemic proportions *(Coulston)*. We noted earlier how prolonged stress causes depletion of several important nutrients. Efforts to replete these nutrients will have limited success until the factors that caused and maintain the state of nutrient depletion, such as excessive carbohydrate intake, have been corrected.

Long-term ingestion of a very-low-carbohydrate diet can have detrimental effects. First, it causes *ketosis*, a condition which can have several negative effects on acid-base chemistry *(Abrumrad)*. Efforts to lose weight via a ketotic diet will be hampered by the inevitable down-regulation of lipolysis that occurs during long-term ketosis *(Abrumrad)*. Second, pyruvate, a major end product of glucose metabolism, acts though the anaplerotic pathways as a key precursor to oxaloacetate, an integral component of the Krebs cycle. Thus, with long-term ingestion of a diet that contains little or no carbohydrate, the ability to produce energy via aerobic metabolism will be impaired since pyruvate and oxaloacetate production will also be impaired. Because of these considerations, a minimum of 400 kcal per day of carbohydrate should be ingested to maintain optimal health *(Abumrad)*.

2. *Qualitative* Imbalances - The idea that specific proteins, fats, or carbohydrates are not necessarily interchangable with one another has been frequently ignored by both clinicians and the public. This is indeed unfortunate, since emerging literature strongly suggests the importance of addressing the *quality* of dietary macronutrients.

Proteins

Traditional dogma was that the value of a protein is determined solely by its amino acid content. The rationale for this tenet was the idea that proteins, at least in the healthy gastrointestinal tract, are totally digested to single amino acids and then absorbed as such. Numerous investigators have demonstrated that, in reality the reverse is true. Most protein is absorbed not as single amino acids but as partially digested peptide linkages of various lengths *(Roberts)*. Furthermore, these peptide linkages can have metabolic properties vastly different that what might be suggested by the individual amino acids making up the respective peptides *(Roberts)*.

For example, glutathione, a tripeptide made of glycine, glutamic acid, and cysteine, has the primary properties of acting as an antioxidant and a participant in detoxication pathways. Neither of these roles would be suggested by examining the roles of the amino acids that make up glutathione singly. Therefore, glutathione possesses metabolic properties as a tripeptide that are independent of the properties exhibited by the individual amino acids that comprise glutathione. Many other dietary peptide linkages of varying lengths can, in a similar fashion, exert powerful effects on immune function, endocrine status, and numerous other pathways *(Roberts)*.

Therefore, when determining protein nutriture for patients, both amino acid and peptide content should be considered. This is particularly important when therapeutic foods are prescribed. For example, the optimal form of glutamine supplementation is considered to be alanyl-glutamine dipeptide *(Furst)*. Evidence also suggests that whether a patient will respond favorably to soy, rice, or whey oral solutions depends, to a great extent, on which contains the peptides most optimally suited to that patient's needs *(Roberts)*. Moreover, the increasing evidence that oral peptides can influence metabolic activity provides a strong rationale for the use of oral glandular preparations *(Lewis)*.

Of course, while this issue of peptide nutriture is important, it by no means discounts the relevance of the individual amino acids when evaluating the needs of the chronically ill patient. Of particular importance are the sulfur amino acids, most notably the essential amino acid methionine. In the chronically ill patient and others under excessive physiologic stress, sulfur needs increase due to the importance of sulfur in key pathways such as protein crosslinking and the sulfation and glutathione-mediated detoxication pathways *(Klaassen)*.

Conventional thinking has suggested that sulfur deficiency is not a concern in industrialized countries because of the high consumption of red meat, which is high in the sulfurized amino acid methionine. However, under stress, the ability to convert methionine to cysteine (a key metabolic intermediate in the production of glutathione and taurine) is inhibited *(Young)*. Therefore, alternative sources of sulfur need to be considered when formulating therapeutic diets. (While soy is popular as an alternative protein source, it is notably low in methionine *[Holt])*. Thus, to gain proper sulfur nutriture, non-protein sources such as garlic, cruciferous vegetables, and supplementation may need to be considered for the chronically ill patient.

Due to increased demands placed by stress physiology, the need for certain non-essential amino acids may rise to the point that optimal amounts can only be obtained through an enhanced diet or nutritional supplementation. This is particularly an issue in regard to glutamine which, as noted above, is substantially depleted during stress.

Carnitine is another important amino acid whose nutriture during chronic stress is of concern, as fatty acids cannot gain entrance into the mitochondria and, hence, participate in oxidative metabolism, without carnitine. Endogenous carnitine levels can be significantly depleted by the high rates of lipolysis and fatty acid oxidation that occur during the stress response *(Bahl)*.

Fats

Society is paying a high price in terms of overall health because of the strong edicts about eliminating fats from the diet in a blanket fashion. True, certain fats are being ingested to excess. However, just as true is the fact that some of the essential fatty acids are not being ingested in adequate quantities. As will be seen in the main body of this text under the specific disease constellations, the connection between the type of fat ingested and chronic illness is well documented.

Carbohydrates

The same can be said for carbohydrates. Therefore, it is important that, as the message that excess carbohydrate intake is unhealthy continues to gain exposure, practitioners emphasize to patients the importance of high-quality carbohydrates in proper balance with healthy proteins and fats to gaining and maintaining optimal health.

Generally, the quality of the carbohydrate decreases in parallel with the amount of processing the food has undergone. Therefore, while fresh, raw, high fiber foods ingested in moderate amounts provide - both quantitatively and qualitatively - carbohydrates that promote health, the same cannot be said of refined carbohydrates. Refined carbohydrates pose a metabolic danger for two reasons:

1. *Refinement increases and concentrates the content of simple carbohydrates in most foods; thus absorption of the carbohydrate fraction will be more rapid in refined foods as opposed to foods in their fresh, raw state (Jenkins).* This is true whether the food consists of candy bars and soda or the so-called "healthy" carbohydrates, such as pasta and fruit juice.

   This rapid absorption causes several downstream metabolic compromises, including accentuated increases in blood glucose, insulin, and, ultimately, the stress hormones epinephrine and cortisol due to accelerated drops in blood glucose that inevitably follow hyperinsulinemia *(Cryer)*. Of course, repeated stimulation of stress physiology in this fashion, as stated by Selye's concept of the General Adaptation Syndrome *(McCance)*, is just as capable of creating the clinical conditions listed above as any other form of stress. Because the rate of carbohydrate absorption appears to be a key predictor of negative sequelae to health *(Heller)*, it may be wise to advise those patients who will not avoid refined carbohydrates to ingest snack foods containing quality protein, i.e., almonds, pecans, walnuts, etc. This is because amino acids, due to competitive inhibition at gastrointestinal binding sites, can effectively slow carbohydrate absorption *(Esposito)*.

2. *Sucrose and fructose have adverse effects beyond those relating to rapid absorption.* Since the detrimental effects of sucrose have been extensively examined and publicized, they will not be discussed here. The detrimental effects of fructose, however, are less well appreciated, especially as it has a reputation of being non-insulinogenic *(Reiser)* and, therefore, a safe carbohydrate. Moreover, fructose consumption, particularly by children, has risen dramatically over the last few years primarily due to well-meaning but misinformed parents who have been ill-advised that it can be substituted for sucrose without concern. What are the dangers of fructose consumption?

   - While it is true that fructose is often non-insulinogenic, it can exacerbate pre-existing hyperinsulinemia *(Reiser)*. Because of the high prevalence of hyperinsulinemia/insulin resistance in our society *(Reaven)*, fructose should rightly be considered insulinogenic and therefore just as detrimental to health as any other refined carbohydrate for most chronically ill patients.

   - Fructose can be an effective instigator of weight gain *(Simopoulos)* and other maladies related to hyperinsulinemia/insulin resistance-mediated stress physiology.

   - Fructose can, because of its incomplete absorption, contribute to the occurrence of osmotic diarrhea and irritable bowel syndrome *(Earnest)*. While food sources containing refined, concentrated forms of fructose (high fructose corn syrup, etc.) are the major concern, anecdotal reports suggest that excessive intake of fruit may instigate many of the adverse findings mentioned above in certain susceptible individuals.

Of course, a discussion on improper nutrition from an integrative standpoint would not be complete without a brief mention of water, one of the most ignored essential nutrient deficiencies. During stress physiology, intracellular dehydration is a significant intermediate step in many of the subsequent metabolic adversities that follow, particularly in relation to glutamine and insulin metabolism *(DiPasqale)*. Therefore, adequate fluid intake *(Batmanghelidj)* should be the cornerstone of any therapeutic program for the chronically ill patient.

B. MICRONUTRIENT IMBALANCES

Much of this text concerns the treatment of illness by correcting micronutrient imbalances. However, since the vast bulk of the treatment-oriented literature in nutritional medicine is directed towards the healing of specific illnesses according to the customary clustering of signs and symptoms that constitute formalized "diseases," we have chosen to follow that model in those chapters. Here we will discuss here some of the major *integrative* concepts, concepts which often span numerous disease categories.

1. Antioxidants

In 1955, Denham Harman speculated that free radical reactions may be a factor causing the progressive cellular damage that results in the diseases and death that accompany advancing age *(Harman)*. His studies, along with those of many others, have subsequently provided impressive evidence to substantiate his hypothesis.

A free radical is a molecule that contains an unpaired electron which makes it highly reactive and unstable. In order to stabilize itself, a free radical will seek out and grab an electron from a stable molecule. Since that molecule now has an unpaired electron, it becomes a new free radical. Thus, a chain reaction takes place which continues until two unpaired electrons pair up together, or until the lone electron is deactivated.

Let us briefly review some of the most important free radicals and reactive oxygen species. The *superoxide* radical is formed when a single electron is added to molecular oxygen. The addition of another electron and two hydrogen ions yields *hydrogen peroxide* which, while not a free radical, is a powerful oxidizing agent. Combining hydrogen peroxide with the superoxide radical produces the *hydroxyl* radical, the most active of all free radicals.

Singlet oxygen is a reactive, highly energized, unstable oxygen species. It contains a pair of electrons and therefore is not truly a free radical. Since these two electrons exist in an unstable conformation in the molecule, the potential exists for this molecule to participate in reactions that generate free radicals such as the superoxide radical. Singlet oxygen can be deactivated or "quenched" which dissipates energy contained in the molecule, depriving it of the energy to engage in superoxide-producing reactions.

The body is exposed to higher levels of free radicals and has difficulty in controlling free radical reactions when there is:

- Exposure to environmental pollutants (such as ozone and nitrogen dioxide), radiation or herbicides
- Inflammatory disease
- Low antioxidant status

Free radicals can attack, infiltrate and injure vital cell structures. For example, due to the actions of free radicals, peroxides are formed from unsaturated fatty acids, releasing free radicals and the consequent destructive chain reaction leading to peroxidation (i.e. auto-oxidation) of lipids in cell membranes. As another example, free radicals can damage the nucleic acid in cell nuclei, and even cause DNA breakage.

We now have evidence that free radical reactions foster the development of numerous degenerative diseases. Here are some examples:

Alzheimer's Disease: Free radical damage may cause progressive brain cell loss.
Atherosclerosis: Free radicals may, for example, transform LDL cholesterol to the toxic cholesterol epoxide which can penetrate the arterial endothelium to initiate atherogenesis *(Gey)*.
Autoimmune Disease: Free radical damage may help to explain tissue destruction.
Cancer: Free radicals may convert cholesterol and other organic chemicals into carcinogens. They both instigate and promote DNA mutations that trigger carcinogenesis.
Cataracts: Oxidative reaction to sunlight produces free radicals that may make the lenses of the eye prone to cataracts.
Cerebrovascular Accidents: Brain damage may result from free radical reactions upon the return of blood flow following temporary disruption.
Inflammatory Diseases: Superoxide radicals are generated which play an important role.
Myocardial Infarction: Myocardial damage may occur upon the return of blood flow following its interruption due to the transformation of oxygen into hydrogen peroxide by free radicals. Hydrogen peroxide then converts myoglobin into a toxic enzyme-like substance which causes tissue damage *(Simpson)*.
Parkinson's Disease: Free radical damage may cause progressive brain cell loss.

Antioxidant Defenses

A large number of substances have antioxidant effects. Three of the most important nutrient-derived antioxidants are:

Vitamin C, a water-soluble vitamin, helps guard the body against harmful reactions occurring within the cell and is the most important of the plasma antioxidants in defending against peroxy radicals formed in the plasma. It quenches singlet oxygen, stabilizes the hydroxyl free radical, and stabilizes the superoxide free radical.

Vitamin E, like beta carotene, is a fat-soluble vitamin located in the hydrophobic cellular membrane. It protects against peroxidation of cell membranes by free radicals by trapping lipid peroxides and thus stopping the chain reaction. Vitamin E also quenches singlet oxygen, stabilizes the hydroxyl free radical, and protects against ozone-induced free radical damage.

Beta-carotene which is lipid soluble and located in the hydrophobic cellular membrane, is the most efficient singlet oxygen quencher - although questions remain about its importance as an antioxidant in humans.

Also, we are equipped with endogenous antioxidant enzymes, such as *glutathione peroxidase*, which contains selenium, works in conjunction with vitamin E and converts lipid peroxides to harmless hydroxy acids. Another example is *superoxide dismutase*, which contains copper and zinc, reacts with superoxide molecules to form hydrogen peroxide which is then decomposed by *catalase* into water and oxygen. Another class of endogenous antioxidants are the metal-binding proteins, such as *ferritin, lactoferrin, albumin* and *ceruloplasmin*. They sequester free iron and copper ions which are capable of catalyzing oxidative reactions.

It is important to realize that antioxidants work closely together in the body, so that the efficacy of any one antioxidant may be influenced by the adequacy of others. For example, we know that the oxidative modification of low-density lipoprotein is an important factor in atherogenesis. In a study of antioxidant defenses against this process, vitamin C was found to be the first line of defense. Once it was dissipated, vitamin E became protective. When vitamin E was dissipated, carotenoids such as lycopene and lutein stepped it, and finally beta-carotene served as the very last defense *(Esterbauer)*. Once the full complement of antioxidants has been dissipated, lipid peroxidation proceeds very rapidly.

In foods, antioxidants are found together. This is often not the case with nutritional supplements. Recently, the disappointing results of two major studies involving beta-carotene supplementation surprised many who had been impressed by the repeated association between beta-carotene intake from foods and protection from degenerative diseases in epidemiological studies. While there were undoubtedly many reasons why beta-carotene was ineffective, the fact that foods rich in beta-carotene are also rich in other synergistic antioxidants has to be part of the explanation.

Therefore, in order to combat the deleterious effects of free radicals, a high intake of fruits and vegetables should always be recommended first. If you wish to recommend supplemental antioxidants, suggest a preparation that contains a variety of antioxidants, including vitamin C, mixed tocopherols, selenium and mixed carotenoids.

Despite their potential for destruction, free radicals are also essential for life. They are a normal byproduct of cellular respiration, a process that uses oxygen to liberate energy and dispose of harmful substances. Free radicals destroy cells that need to be destroyed to protect the body from them, and superoxide and hydroxyl radicals are used by phagocytes in the respiratory burst to destroy microbial invaders. Such beneficial effects may help to explain the apparent efficacy of therapies that supply oxidizing agents such as ozone or hydrogen peroxide to treat infections and other illnesses.

Although much remains to be understood about free radicals, it appears that their contradictory effects are explained by the concept of balance. Ideally, pro-oxidant and antioxidant factors should be in balance; it is only when free radical oxidation is excessive that degenerative disease is promoted.

2. Essential Fatty Acid Imbalance

While early investigators examined the effects of polyunsaturated fatty acids as a group, more recent research has focused on the effects of each of the two groups of essential fatty acids, the omega-3 and the omega-6 families, both consisting of polyunsaturates. The essential fatty acids and serve as precursors to the prostaglandins, the prostacyclins, the thromboxanes, and the leukotrienes. These are hormone-like substances that have important influences on immune function, smooth muscle function, platelet aggregation and inflammation.

Omega-3 Fatty Acids

α-linolenic acid → EPA → 3 series prostaglandins
└→ DHA

Omega-6 Fatty Acids

cis-linoleic acid → GLA → DGLA → 1 series prostaglandins

Much of the interest in the role of essential fatty acids in degenerative diseases stems from the observation that Greenland Eskimos eating their traditional diet which is particularly high in the omega-3 fatty acids are relatively protected against atherosclerosis, thrombosis, rheumatoid arthritis as well as other diseases. Also, a number of other degenerative diseases are associated with abnormalities in the distribution of essential fatty acids, including hypertension, diabetes mellitus and the autoimmune diseases.

The rate-limiting enzyme in the metabolism of both linoleic acid and alpha-linolenic acid is *delta-6-desaturase*. This important enzyme is inhibited by:

Age (over 40)
High carbohydrate diet
High cholesterol, high fat diet
Glucose
Alcohol
Trans fatty acids
Copper
Deficiencies of:
- Magnesium
- Zinc
- Vitamin B_6 (?)

Also of particular importance is the conversion of DGLA to PGE_1, a step that requires niacin and vitamin C.

The Western diet is notoriously deficient in the omega-3 fatty acids. Significant quantities of alpha-linolenic acid are not found in most available dietary oils, and the fatty cold-water fish which are excellent sources of eicosapentaenoic acid are usually eaten too infrequently.

In regard to the omega-6 family, available dietary oils are usually rich in linoleic acid; however, much of the dietary linoleic acid may be in the *trans* form which actually inhibits essential fatty acid metabolism *(Kinsella)*. For the reasons we have discussed, delta-6-desaturase activity may become insufficient leading to a relative deficiency of DGLA and of the compounds from which it is derived. Thus, for some people, a supplementary source of gamma linolenic acid such as evening primrose oil could be needed to bypass the metabolic block. Finally, the high meat and egg content of the diet supplies large quantities of arachidonic acid, the precursor to the proinflammatory prostaglandins, leukotrienes and thromboxanes.

Available evidence suggests that a balance between the omega-3 and omega-6 fatty acids in the diet may help to prevent degenerative diseases. For example, if either linoleic acid (omega-6) or alpha-linolenic acid (omega-3) is administered in high levels, it inhibits the metabolism of the other *(Holman)*. More of a balance could be achieved if cold-water fish replaced meat and eggs as a major protein source, and if linseed oil, which is high in alpha-linolenic acid became a common dietary oil. When there is reason to believe that delta-6-desaturase activity is impaired, supplementation with both fish oils that are high in eicosapentaenoic acid and with plant oils that are high in gamma linolenic acid may be indicated.

3. Homocysteine Accumulation

A number of years ago, Kilmer McCully, formerly professor of pathology at Harvard Medical School, theorized that the initial arterial damage which eventually leads to the development of atherosclerotic plaques may be caused by the accumulation of the amino acid homocysteine *(McCully)*. Since then, the evidence has been growing that his hypothesis was correct, and abnormal homocysteine metabolism causing the plasma concentration of homocysteine to rise is gaining acceptance as an independent risk factor for atherosclerosis *(Stampfer, 1992)*.

There now are numerous studies that suggest such a conclusion, including a study in which baboons who were injected with homocystine, the oxidized disulfide of homocysteine, intravenously developed arteriosclerotic lesions *(Harker)*. Recently, *JAMA* published a meta-analysis of the research and concluded that, because of consistency across studies by different investigators using different methods in different populations, homocysteine can be considered to be causal in the pathogenesis of vascular disease, and each 5-mmol/L increment in total homocysteine levels elevates coronary artery disease risk by as much as cholesterol increases of 0.5 mmol/L (30 mg/dL) *(Boushey)*.

The mechanism by which homocysteine does its damage is still under investigation. There are 3 major theories:

1. Homocysteine has a direct toxic effect on the endothelial cells that line the vessel walls. This may either impair their ability to dilate and contract or else it may impair their ability to prevent thromboses from forming at the vessel walls.
2. Homocysteine may stimulate coagulation through a direct thrombogenic effect.
3. Homocysteine may stimulate smooth muscle cell proliferation *(Stampfer, 1995)*.

Homozygous homocystinuria is an autosomal recessive trait that is marked by raised serum homocysteine concentrations as well has increased urinary excretion. It is extremely rare. However, as is true with other autosomal-recessive genetic disorders, a milder form of the biochemical abnormality exists in heterozygotes *(Vogel)*.

Roughly 1 out of 70 people will test positive for heterozygous homocystinuria, making it a common genetic disorder. Unfortunately this disorder is rarely diagnosed, even though it has been shown to be associated with premature occlusive arterial disease *(Boers)*.

It is interesting that genetic influences appear to have the opposite effect for patients with Down's Syndrome. Victims of this genetic syndrome rarely develop atherosclerosis, and scientists have long questioned why they are protected against this degenerative disease. As it turns out, when they are given a methionine load, their plasma homocysteine levels are not just normal, but below those of normal controls *(Brattström, 1987; Chadefaux)*.

While a genetic abnormality predisposes a person to develop homocystinuria, most people with elevated serum homocysteine levels are not genetically predisposed, but developed this serious metabolic disorder because their nutritional needs were not being adequately met by their diet, which caused them to develop at least a marginal deficiency of the vitamins that are needed to detoxify homocysteine. Clinicians commonly fail to realize how common this disorder is among patients with atherosclerosis; to be specific, it has been estimated that between 20 and 40 percent of these patients suffer from an inability to adequately detoxify homocysteine *(Ubbink, 1993)*.

Homocysteine is metabolized by one of three routes, depending upon the needs of the organism: transsulfuration, remethylation or hydrolysis.

- Transsulfuration: Homocysteine can be converted into the non-toxic cystathionine through the action of the enzyme cystathionine beta-synthase. Cystathionine is then converted to cysteine, a major sulfur amino acid, by cystathionase. (Both these enzymes require vitamin B_6 as coenzyme.)
- Remethylation: Homocysteine can be remethylated to convert it back to methionine.
- Hydrolysis: When both cysteine and methionine levels are adequate, homocysteine can be hydrolyzed by either of 2 routes to 2-oxobutyrate, splitting off ammonia and hydrogen sulfide.

The accumulation of homocysteine is strongly influenced by nutritional factors - even in people without a genetic predisposition to homocystinuria. The remethylation of homocysteine to methionine requires either folic acid and vitamin B_{12} or betaine, while vitamin B_6, in the form of pyridoxal-5-phosphate, is required for the conversion of homocysteine to cystathionine.

Moreover, marginal B vitamin nutriture may impair homocysteine metabolism and thereby provoke homocysteine accumulation. For example, when a group of 44 apparently healthy men with moderately elevated homocysteine levels was compared to a group of men with normal plasma homocysteine levels, they were found to have significantly lower levels of vitamin B_6, vitamin B_{12} and folic acid *(Ubbink, 1993)*. Current thinking is that inadequate folate intake is the main determinant of the destructive effects of homocysteine *(Stampfer, 1995)*.

In evaluating patients for elevated homocysteine, their levels should be measured twice. First, a baseline level should be taken. They should then be given a dose of methionine to challenge the ability of their metabolic pathways to detoxify homocysteine, after which the homocysteine level should be measured again.

Treatment

Since homocysteine can be detoxified by 3 different metabolic pathways. this serious metabolic disorder is remarkably easy to treat nutritionally.

1. Supplementation with folic acid at a dosage of 5 mg daily for 4 weeks has been found to significantly reduce homocysteine levels in homocystinuric patients both before and after methionine loading despite normal folic acid levels, suggesting that excess folate enhances the remethylation of homocysteine to methionine *(Brattström, 1985)*.

2. Both human and animal studies have demonstrated that methionine loading in the presence of vitamin B_6 deficiency leads to homocysteine accumulation. Also, one of the specific abnormalities that are found in genetically-determined homocystinuria is a deficiency of cystathionine beta-synthase, the enzyme that detoxifies homocysteine by converting it into cystathionine. For about half of the members of this group, high supplementary doses of vitamin B_6 will push the reaction forward, markedly reducing or even eliminating the biochemical abnormalities *(Mudd)*. Responsiveness to vitamin B_6 among those with this specific genetic disorder is also genetically determined since all affected siblings will be either B_6-responsive or B_6-unresponsive.

3. Vitamin B_{12} deficiency, even in the absence of deficiency symptoms, is frequently associated with increased homocysteine levels which return to normal with B_{12} supplementation *(Kuzminski)*.

4. When added to the other relevant nutrients, betaine may normalize amino acid metabolism in those patients with cystathionine beta-synthase deficiency whose homocystinuria is unresponsive to vitamin B_6 *(Wilcken)*.

Earlier we noted that marginal folate deficiency is believed to be the major cause of disordered homocysteine metabolism. Conversely, if we were to choose a single nutrient to supplement, folic acid may be the most effective, since a recent study found that supplementation with the combination of the 3 B-vitamins did not lower plasma homocysteine any further than supplementation with folic acid alone *(Ubbink, 1994)*.

Moreover, supplementation with 1 to 2 mg of folate daily, besides being safe, is usually adequate to normalize homocysteine levels even if the problem is not due to folate insufficiency *(Stampfer, 1995)*. Further studies should clarify whether a sub-group of patients is more effectively treated by a combination formula.

Dr. McCully blames the Western diet for promoting homocysteine accumulation and its consequences. He points out that, not only does modern food processing destroy vitamin B_6, but animal protein has 2 to 3 times as much methionine as plant protein by weight and is lower in B_6. (This may be a reason why vegetarian diets are associated with a lower risk of coronary heart disease.)

Currently in process are the long-term prospective randomized double-blind studies needed to provide definitive scientific verification that lowering elevated plasma homocysteine levels will retard the progression of atherosclerosis. In light of all the evidence that has already been accumulated, we can be optimistic that these studies will turn out to be positive.

4. Marginal Nutrient Deficiencies

We have already noted in this section how marginal deficiencies can promote illness by reducing defenses against oxidant stress, by unbalancing prostanoid metabolism and by reducing homocysteine detoxification. There are numerous other adverse effects of marginal deficiencies upon homeostatic defense mechanisms. For example, earlier we noted that the stress response causes magnesium loss. Conversely, a marginal magnesium deficiency will promote an exaggerated stress response *(Buist)*, and may increase the toxicity of heavy metals such as aluminum *(Nielsen)*, cadmium and lead *(Guiet-Bara)*.

We refer you to the next chapter for a detailed discussion of the extremely important, yet commonly overlooked, contribution of marginal nutritional deficiencies to illness.

III. CHEMICAL AND/OR HEAVY METAL TOXICITY

Of the five causes of chronic illness under discussion, chemical and metal toxicity may be the one that most effectively demonstrates the need for an integrative approach to chronic illness. This is because the metabolic pathways that involve detoxication of chemicals and metals affect and/or are affected by endocrine imbalance, nutritional needs, compromised mucosal barriers and gene expression.

Toxicity is viewed by many as primarily due to an increasingly hostile environment that has been created by the industrial revolution. With this idea in mind, some clinicians advise patients to cleanse their bodies as best as possible and then isolate themselves from the myriad of pollutants that permeate our society. Such an extreme measure is not necessary or even possible for the vast majority of patients. Even the simple recommendation to eat organically raised food is not always feasible for patients to follow.

The results of several studies suggests that the exclusive, one-to-one association between environmental illnesses and increasing levels of man-made toxins is far from being conclusively proven *(Ames)* - although some studies do show a compelling link *(Neumann)*. When viewed from an integrative perspective, environmental illness is not merely an issue of the total toxic load a patient has to bear. As a result of forest fires and volcanoes, many of the atmospheric pollutants that are in the headlines today (such as sulfur compounds) have actually been present for millions of years. Other sources of toxins that have challenged mankind through the ages are snake venoms and plant poisons *(Vermeulen)*. Thus, the industrial revolution did not introduce atmospheric pollution to mankind, it only increased it.

Because our environment is, and has always been, potentially threatening, life forms usually possess a marvelous array of complementary and overlapping detoxication mechanisms. As we will demonstrate, it is the dynamic relationship between toxic load and endogenous detoxication capacity that determines whether patients will present symptoms associated with environmental illness. While minimizing the toxic load, insofar as it is not unduly burdensome, is certainly advisable, the emphasis in treatment should be on improving detoxication capacity.

Health is more than just biochemical purity. As with stress physiology, optimal health is also highly dependent on the ability to continue to fully participate with family, friends, and co-workers in the experience of living. By using an integrative approach of optimizing detoxication capacity while simultaneously reducing the toxic load, we have the greatest chance of restoring total health in the environmentally sensitive patient.

The Two Phases of Detoxification

Detoxication capacity actually involves many different, overlapping pathways. For example, as will be discussed in the next section, the healthy gastrointestinal tract acts as a detoxifier by minimizing the growth of endotoxin-producing dysbiotic microflora. However, the brunt of the responsibility for detoxication falls upon the following two-stage process, primarily located in the liver:

1. *Phase I (cytochrome P-450)* - Phase I consists of several dozen cytochrome P-450 isoenzymes, each being specific for certain families of substances. (These enzymes have been given names that begin with CYP followed by a number, a letter, and then another number, for example CYP1A2.) The chief role of cytochrome P-450 enzymes is to convert fat-soluble compounds to substances that are more water-soluble *(Hodgson)*. This process is vital to proper detoxication since the body generally finds it metabolically difficult to effectively eliminate fat-soluble substances *(Hodgson)*.

2. *Phase II (conjugation)* - Phase II enzymes include a comparatively small group of compounds that are designed to take the intermediate created by the Phase I process and convert it to a substance that can safely be eliminated through the kidneys (smaller molecular weight substances) or bile (larger molecular weight substances) *(Matthews HB)*. Enzymes in this group fall into the major categories of glutathione conjugation, glucuronidation, sulfation, glycination, methylation, and acetylation *(Parkinson)*.

Information about levels of phase I and phase II enzymes for individual patients is available. Challenge tests have been developed where fairly innocuous xenobiotics are ingested by the patient (usually caffeine, aspirin, and/or acetaminophen) and then their metabolites are measured in either saliva or urine. By examining the concentrations of these metabolites, levels of the phase I and/or phase II enzymes that were involved in the production of their can be extrapolated with a fair degree of accuracy *(Great Smokies)*. While the level of accuracy of these challenge tests has been disputed *(Seaman)*, anecdotal reports suggest that the results obtained can yield clinical benefits.

Proper nutrition is vital to both phase I and phase II processes. It has been well documented that most major vitamins and minerals plus optimal amounts of protein, fats, and carbohydrates are required for phase I and II pathways to operate at maximal efficiency *(Gibson)*. To compound the problem, certain substances, including some found in the average Westernized diet, can up-regulate phase I and II enzymes. For example, substances found in cooked red meats are known to be linked with carcinomas in several sites because they up-regulate expression of cytochrome P450 1A2 which, in turn, transforms the food-derived compounds to carcinogens *(Sinha)*.

Trying to solve a patient's toxicity problems with an all-purpose detoxication supplement will often not be enough to restore optimal health, however, even though detoxication issues may be part of that patient's clinical picture, as it may also be necessary to address neuroendocrine, mucosal function, and genetics. These other factors are relevant because:

1. *Like cortisol, levels of detoxication enzymes go through predictable patterns when challenged by a xenobiotic on a long-term basis.*

   Analogous to Selye's alarm phase of stress *(McCance)*, levels of detoxication enzymes tend to rise or be "induced" *(Liska)*. This point is significant for several reasons:
   - Often, in the process of creating a water-soluble intermediate, CYP enzymes will also create, because of this increased water solubility, an intermediate that is more toxic than the parent compound *(Levi)*. An example is when acetaminophen is ingested with alcohol (ethanol). Since ethanol is a potent inducer of CYP enzymes *(Ronis)*, it induces a CYP enzyme that converts acetaminophen to a highly hepatotoxic intermediate *(Cohen)*.
   - A byproduct of CYP physiology is the potent free radical superoxide *(Vermeulen)*. Therefore, induction of CYP enzymes will yield increased amounts of superoxide, which can be damaging for many tissues.
   - Induction of a CYP enzyme can have unexpected results. Because all CYP enzymes have the ability to transform multiple xenobiotics *(Liska)*, a CYP enzyme that has been induced in order to more efficiently detoxify one compound, e.g., ethanol, may, in the process, react with another compound, e.g., acetaminophen, to create accelerated toxicity. Since xenobiotics that are quite innocuous with isolated exposure can become potent toxins when exposure occurs in association with other, similarly innocuous substances, and since most human exposures occur in multiples *(Gibson)*, the results of research that examines toxicity of individual compounds may be completely misleading in the clinical setting.

   Because the supply of these enzymes is finite (in part, due to their dependence on an adequate nutrient supply), long-term exposure of phase I and II enzymes to xenobiotics will cause eventual depletion *(Gibson)*. While this can happen to both groups of enzymes, the phase II enzymes are particularly important from a clinical standpoint. "Pathologic detoxifiers" may demonstrate an elevation of phase I enzymes along with a depression of phase II enzymes *(Bland)*. In this case, the intermediates produced by CYP enzymes cannot be efficiently eliminated by the phase II enzymes. The result is the development of clinical symptoms.

2. *Endogenously produced hormones such as cortisol, testosterone, and estrogen are metabolized through this same two-phase process (Gibson).*

   Due to lack of knowledge of this important aspect of hormone physiology, hormonal problems tend to be regarded as issues of over- or underproduction. In fact, phase I and phase II metabolism, along with the enterohepatic circulation (see below), is just as important in determining functional hormone levels as is production *(Belanger;Goldin)*. For example:
   - Induction of certain CYP enzymes by certain pharmaceuticals can cause increased loss of triiodothyronine (T_3) *(Utiger)*.
   - Increased reuptake of conjugated estrogen via the enterohepatic circulation can affect cancer risk *(Adlercreutz)*.
   - Decreased reuptake of conjugated estrogen via the enterohepatic circulation can reduce circulating levels enough to affect reproductive function *(Chipman)*.

3. *Enterohepatic circulation plays a vital role in determining functional levels of both xenobiotics and hormones.*

Enterohepatic circulation refers to a process whereby conjugated xenobiotics and hormones that have been excreted from the liver via the bile into the small intestine are deconjugated or reactivated in the large intestine and then reabsorbed *(Chipman)*. This deconjugation is accomplished by gut microflora, whose role in the process will be elucidated in the next section. Like many other physiologic pathways, the enterohepatic circulation can be a double-edged sword:

- When deconjugation and reuptake are too *high*, a large percentage of the toxins and hormones that have been eliminated via phase I and II pathways may be reabsorbed, exacerbating toxin accumulation and creating potential hormonal excesses *(Gibson;Goldin)*.
- When deconjugation and reuptake are too *low*, more of the conjugated toxins will be eliminated. However, levels of circulating reproductive hormones may be low *(Chipman)*.

4. *Rates of production of both phase I and II enzymes are genetically determined.* (See the section on genetics below.)

Because of the intimate relationship between hormone and xenobiotic detoxication, the following are examples of potential biochemical scenarios that could be clinically relevant:

- Since cortisol up-regulates CYP enzymes (see above), excessive stress could cause increased formation of toxic intermediates from certain xenobiotics. Furthermore, since excessive simple carbohydrate has a similar effect on cortisol production, the same could be said about high carbohydrate intake.

- If prior long-term exposure to xenobiotics had caused depletion of phase II enzymes in a patient whose enzymes were already genetically low, e.g., Gilbert's disease *(Parkinson)*, elevated levels of reproductive hormones could result, not because of too much production, but because of a decrease in eliminative capacity. As was suggested above, a similar scenario could occur if malfunctioning enterohepatic circulation was causing increased uptake. These elevated levels of reproductive hormones, in turn, could have an impact on hormone-sensitive pathology.

- With an up-regulation of detoxication enzymes caused by substances such as ethanol, excessive amounts of reproductive hormones might be eliminated. When combined with a low-functioning enterohepatic circulation, the resultant low hormone levels could adversely affect reproduction.

- Hypothyroid function, as suggested above, could result from increased elimination of T_3 caused by xenobiotic-induced up-regulation of detoxication enzymes.

Detoxification is an integrative process affecting and being affected by neuroendocrine function, diet, mucosal function, and genetics. It thus makes little biochemical sense to attempt to correct phase I and II detoxication without attempting to optimize other contributory factors to the clinical presentation. However, once these basics are addressed, research suggests that several phytonutrients have a clinically significant ability to modulate phase I and II enzyme levels. Examples are green tea *(Milner)*, grapefruit juice (naringin) *(Milner)*, garlic *(Wang)*, curcumin *(Piper)*, and cruciferous vegetables such as broccoli (sulfonophenes) *(Milner)*. Each substance mentioned is, however, fairly specific in regard to the enzymes it affects and whether the effect is one of elevation or depression. Thus, as already noted, it is advisable to first assess enzyme levels through laboratory testing.

IV. COMPROMISED MUCOSAL BARRIERS

Nutritional therapy of digestive dysfunction has traditionally focused on what goes on intraluminally. It therefore tended to be limited to replacement regimens (hydrochloric acid, digestive enzymes, bile salts, etc.), herbs and nutrients that address peristalsis and transit time (psyllium and other fibers), probiotics (*L. acidophilus* and *bifidobacteria*), and various antimicrobial substances. The use of these supplements and their rationale has been well delineated elsewhere *(Murray)* and will not be discussed here. What will be discussed, though, are two issues that consider the intestine from an integrative perspective:

1. The importance of the condition of the mucosa.
2. The nature of the relationship between the mucosa and gut microflora.

Feed the Gut Lining

Typically, nutritionists and supplement formulators have viewed the intestinal mucosa as merely a barrier through which nutrients must pass in order to get to the "important" areas. Therefore, the focus is on finding forms of micronutrients that can "outwit" the mucosa and gain absorption rates that are much higher than physiologic amounts. What is lost with this approach, though, is the fact that well-functioning mucosa has great powers of discrimination that allow it to determine proper absorption rates. It has a wonderful ability to sense, not only which substances should pass through, but how much of each should pass through, given the constantly fluctuating biochemical and physiologic needs of the tissues inside.

With the notable exceptions of iodine and vitamins A and K *(Bender)*, absorption rarely approaches 100% of the ingested nutrients *(Groff;Jackson)*. Furthermore, absorption rates can and do decrease as the ability of the mucosa to function optimally declines, a fact exemplified most prominently by the research on calcium absorption and aging *(Linder)*. What, then, is the best solution to assure absorption that can maintain optimal health? From an integrative perspective, the best solution may go beyond approaches such as replacement therapy and the introduction of exotic mineral chelates that can yield supraphysiologic absorption rates. It would seem that if the health of the mucosa itself could be improved, the need for therapeutic agents could be reduced both in terms of quantity and duration.

While the idea of healing the gut lining as a therapeutic goal may be somewhat new to many nutritional practitioners, it is well known among critical care practitioners since, following significant stressors such as burns, trauma, or surgery, the condition of the mucosal barrier can rapidly deteriorate *(Steele)*. This is due primarily to stress physiology (see above). Moreover, several studies have noted that, when parenteral feeding is utilized, an even more profound decline in gut integrity occurs *(Mainous)*. This occurs for two reasons:

1. While the cells comprising the gastrointestinal mucosa can gain nutriture from both the luminal contents and the systemic vasculature, the presence of a vast array of nutrients within the lumen is absolutely essential for proper mucosal function *(Rombeau)*. Furthermore, luminal sources of nutrients appear to take precedence over systemic sources in terms of maintaining gut integrity *(Scheppach)*.
2. The cells of the gut lining turn over every 2 to 3 days *(Alverdy,1994a)*. Therefore, lack of nutriture can cause a decline of gut integrity in a fairly short period of time.

Because of these facts, enteral nutrients are supplied in critical care nutrition that are specifically designed to feed mucosal cells. These nutrients include glutamine, arginine, fish oil, and nucleotides (RNA) *(Gardiner)*. Moreover, emerging research is demonstrating that factors such as stress, poor diet, and suboptimal calorie intake also affects gut health in patients not requiring hospital care. This has been particularly well demonstrated in inflammatory bowel disease *(Bennett;Jeejeebhoy)*, a malady common to many chronically ill patients.

The Role of Gut Microflora

Butyrate, a short-chain fatty acid, is another extremely important "nutrient" that is required for optimal gut health, specifically the health of the colonocyte *(Scheppach)*. (The word nutrient was in quotation marks because the colonic supply of butyrate, instead of coming from the diet, is produced by certain microorganisms residing in the colon.)

Within the colon billions of microorganisms of several different species reside, many of which are absolutely crucial to proper health of the colonocyte *(Grimble;MacFarlane)*. The relationship between the colon and its resident microflora is incredibly complex:

- The many different species of microflora are opportunistic.

  Which species survives and thrives is very much dependent on the type of food supply and specifics of the colon environment such as pH *(Freter)*. Thus, the overall makeup of the gut microflora is very dependent upon environmental variables.

- Many organisms promote optimal colon health.

  This is accomplished primarily through the byproducts produced by the bacteria, such as the above-mentioned butyrate, which either act as a fuel source for the colon cell or contribute, by affecting such factors as pH, to the overall colon environment *(Grimble;Hill)*.

- Many organisms produce byproducts that promote illness either locally or systemically.

  Many species produce substances such as endotoxin which can cause harm locally by increasing gut permeability and, if absorbed, can adversely affect several organ systems *(VanDeventer)*.

- The opportunistic nature of gut microflora largely determines whether probiotic organisms or pathogens ultimately prevail.

  In this microbial world of survival of the fittest, food supply and factors such as pH are important determinants of who wins and loses this constant life and death struggle *(Freter)*. Therefore, whether the overall microfloral population promotes or detracts from optimal health largely depends on which organisms find any particular environment most favorable.

  For example, if the diet is high in simple sugars that pass undigested into the large intestine, *Candida albicans* and other fungal forms may increase in numbers. Symptoms occasionally follow because certain strains of candida can produce ethanol-like compounds by what is known as the autobrewery syndrome *(Hunnisett)*. Another example is a diet high in sulfur compounds, which causes a proliferation of organisms that produce hydrogen sulfide gas, a known colonic irritant *(Pitcher)*. Conversely, a diet high in fiber tends to promote the growth of beneficial organisms such as *L. acidophilus* and *Bifidobacteria*.

With the above facts in mind, consider these clinical aspects of colonic microflora from an integrative perspective:

- The administration of natural antimicrobial substances that are designed to eliminate specific gut pathogens is of limited value.

  While natural antimicrobial therapies have earned a well-deserved niche in the clinical repertoire of the nutritionally-oriented practitioner, their long-term benefit may be quite limited if optimization of the colonic environment is not simultaneously addressed.

  The lesson taught by 60 years of antibiotics should not be ignored by those who employ naturally occurring antimicrobial therapies. Gut microflora are incredibly resilient and adaptive organisms *(Alverdy,1994b)*. No matter what antimicrobial therapy is employed, a small population of the organisms under attack will survive and repopulate to former levels if the initial environmental conditions that led to their proliferation in the first place are not changed. Furthermore, stress physiology plays an important role, as sustained sympathoadrenal stimulation causes a decrease in circulation to the gut lining, causing an increase in permeability *(Matuschak)*.

  Therefore, the integrative practitioner is concerned, not only with the pathogen, but also with the relationship between the pathogen and its environment. The question of therapy, then, becomes "How can I change the colonic environment through diet, stress modification, etc., so that (1) the pathogen cannot thrive as effectively or (2) other probiotic organisms grow to the point that the pathogen is overwhelmed."

- Certain species of gut microflora produce deconjugating enzymes such as β-glucuronidase that play an instrumental role in the enterohepatic circulation *(Chipman)*.

  Recall from above that the enterohepatic circulation, the reabsorption and recirculation of hormones and xenobiotic agents, plays an integral role in determining overall toxic load and hormonal status. Enzymes such as β-glucuronidase that are produced by certain species of gut microflora are the major determinants of the vitality of this process. Furthermore, diet plays a tremendous role in determining levels of these enzymes in the colon, primarily by regulating growth of the organisms that produce the enzymes *(Rowland)*.

  For example, a diet high in red meat can cause a proliferation of β-glucuronidase-producing organisms *(Rowland)*. In terms of toxic load, this would be a distinct disadvantage. However, in terms of maintaining optimal levels of reproductive hormones, this type of diet might be desired. Conversely, a diet high in soy and fiber appears to decrease production of deconjugating enzymes, thereby decreasing enterohepatic circulation *(Goldin)*.

As with the other factors mentioned above, optimal gut health cannot be attained by approaching the situation from a singular viewpoint. Rather, the condition of the mucosal barrier is dependent not only on its symbiotic relationship with gut microflora but with all the other factors mentioned above, i.e., stress, diet, and toxicology. In addition, gut health is also directly dependent on genetics, the subject of the next section. The most well known example of this connection is celiac disease, where a genetically determined sensitivity to gluten can cause tremendous destruction to the gut lining as well as adverse consequences to other organ systems *(Connon)*.

Diagnostics and treatment

Stool analysis *(Golan)* and urinary organic acids *(Lord)* can be extremely helpful in determining both the nutritional needs of the gut lining as well as microbial status. Treatment modalities, though, are many and varied and, thus, beyond the scope of this chapter, although much of the information contained in the chapter on irritable bowel syndrome is applicable.

V. GENETICS

Compared to the other 4 causes of chronic illness, an awareness of genetic factors currently has less to offer, both diagnostically and therapeutically, to the practice of integrative medicine. However, this in no way diminishes its importance, as genetics represents the future in terms of what will be accomplished in the field in this next century. Why the future? As will be demonstrated, much of the research that will be discussed in this section consists of experiments on animals for which there has yet been little extrapolation clinically. What we currently lack is the ability to conveniently detect aberrant genetic expression as well as the knowledge of how to effectively modulate gene activity with diet and supplementation in any single patient. We believe, however, that clinically applicable techniques will soon be developed that will allow practitioners of integrative medicine to determine where suboptimal genetic expression exists and then, sometimes, to apply nutritional modalities that will correct these suboptimal tendencies.

Traditionally, genetics has not been a subject of great interest in the clinical setting because it was accepted as fact that little could be done to alter genetic makeup or expression. However, within the last few years, an extensive body of research has demonstrated that genes are quite responsive to environmental factors. For example, on the negative side it is well known that several xenobiotics have significant mutagenic properties *(Pitot)* while, on the positive side, a recent study suggests that dietary supplementation of carotenoids, nicotinamide, and zinc can enhance DNA repair mechanisms *(Sheng)*. However, most of the research, from the perspective of the causative factors discussed above, has been in the area of genetic expression. Following is an overview of these integrative relationships.

Stress

As previously discussed, stress physiology can affect gene expression *(Duman)*.

Chemical and Metal toxicity

Several studies have demonstrated that the production of the enzymes involved in both phase I and phase II of detoxification are genetically determined *(Burchell;Hong)*. Furthermore, there appears to be significant variation in the levels of the various enzymes in different populations *(Ladona;Lamba)*. These findings suggest that a xenobiotic which is innocuous to one patient because of a robust supply of the specific phase I or phase II enzymes could be toxic to another patient because of low genetically-induced production of the same enzymes.

In fact, recognition of the importance of this variable to the proper use of pharmaceuticals has led to the development of the field of pharmacogenetics *(Weber)*. Inability to properly detoxify due to the presence of significant amounts of xenobiotic substances combined with genetically-induced low levels of certain phase I and II enzymes can cause potentially mutagenic substances to accumulate, possibly leading to carcinogenesis *(Sinha)*.

Concerning metal toxicity, zinc is known to up-regulate the genetic expression of metallothionein, a protein that both assures that concentrations of essential metals do not become excessive and assists in the detoxification of cadmium *(Heuchel;Sullivan)*.

Compromised Mucosal Barriers

An example of the possible interrelationship between diet, genetic expression, and mucosal health is the recent suggestion that, in conditions such as Crohn's disease, elemental diets decrease inflammation by altering the expression of genes in the epithelium that influence inflammation *(Sanderson).*

Other Nutrient-gene Interactions

The emerging research seems to indicate that modulation of genetics by nutrition is a ubiquitous phenomenon that is constantly shaping our lives from birth to death. Thus, it appears that management of genetic expression by the clinical nutritionist has been occurring as long as recommendations about diet and supplementation have been made. As radical as the idea seems, clinical nutritionists, without being aware, are treat genetic expression on a regular basis. While this idea is exciting, what is truly exciting is that the rate of advancement in this area also suggests that clinical tools will be developed in the 21st century that will allow clinicians to be more knowledgeable about the nutrient-gene interactions that they are already implementing. This, in turn, will give them the ability to improve the human condition in ways that have been deemed impossible in the past.

Nutrition can profoundly affect genetic expression virtually from the moment of birth. Biological mechanisms appear to exist to 'memorize' the metabolic effects of early nutritional environments. Epidemiological evidence for this relationship has been found in research on body mass index, cardiovascular disease, blood pressure, and type 2 diabetes *(Waterland).* Moreover, when foods interact with certain receptor sites in the enterocyte, genetic expression is directed in two important ways. First, digestive enzyme production is modulated so that optimal processing of the food can occur. Second, certain of the foods will induce genetic expression of cytokines and other signaling molecules that are, in turn, released into the circulation yielding sometimes widespread systemic effects *(Sanderson).*

What are some of the specific factors involved in this interplay between nutrition and enterocyte gene expression? One is *lactoferrin*, which is found significant quantities in breast milk. Beyond its well-known function of delivering iron to the intestinal epithelium, lactoferrin may enter these cells and modulate genetic programming. Depending on the degree of iron saturation of the lactoferrin molecule, lactoferrin has been demonstrated to affect cell proliferation and production of enzymes such as sucrase and alkaline phosphatase *(Sanderson).*

Another factor is *the mucosal immune system*. One of the primary roles of the intestinal lining is to absorb vital nutrients while, at the same time, acting as a barrier to the external world. It is the mucosal immune system, composed of secretory IgA and other immunoregulators, that informs the enterocyte what is acceptable for entry and what must be excluded from the inner workings of the body. As would be expected of such a system, genetic expression of the various factors that constitute mucosal immunity can be highly variable, with the response being largely determined by the specific chemistry of whatever enters the gut lumen. For example, consider the following:

- Butyrate, which is produced by intestinal microflora in varying quantities depending upon the types and amounts of fiber ingested, affects production of the cytokine IL-8 which, in turn, acts as a chemotactic factor drawing neutrophils to the gastrointestinal tract during inflammation.

- Butyrate affects the function of insulin-like growth factor I (IGF-1). This factor, which is commonly known for its role in control of body growth, is also involved in lymphocyte proliferation. Specifically, butyrate influences IGF-1 receptor sites in the intestine, thus playing a key role in the proliferation of the mucosal immune system. Glutamine also plays a similar role.

Specific nutrients have also been examined in the literature in terms of their effects on gene expression:

Macronutrients

Fat has been a favorite subject among genetic researchers for years. The role of polyunsaturated fatty acids (PUFA) in the regulation of gene expression has been extensively studied in regard to the repression of gene expression in lipogenic tissues as well as modulation in non-lipogenic tissues such as the immune system *(Iritani;Sessler).*

Important research on this topic is in the field of cancer research. An example of the relevance of genetics in regard to the relationship between PUFA intake and cancer was shown in an experiment with rodents. *Ras* proteins, which serve as connectors between signals generated in the plasma membrane and nuclear effectors, can be transformed to oncoproteins (proteins involved in cancer formation in tissues such as the colon, pancreas, and lung) via transformation by the enzyme farnesyl protein transferase (FPTase). Corn oil appeared to enhance expression of FPTase while fish oil suppressed it, suggesting that changing PUFA intake may have important implications in oncology.

Currently, several laboratories are trying to create FPTase inhibitors as potential anti-cancer agents. The nutritional approach to FPTase modulation using fish oil has two advantages over synthetic approaches. First, synthetic FPTase inhibitors demonstrate toxic side effects while fish oil exhibits none. Second, fish oil only demonstrates partial blockade of the enzyme. This is important because some *ras* proteins are necessary for optimal function. It is only when *ras* protein formation becomes excessive that carcinogenic changes appear to occur *(Singh)*.

Non-insulin-dependent diabetes mellitus (NIDDM) is another of the illnesses for which the nutritional modification of genetic expression may have important implications. Proper function of insulin is closely tied to the ability to produce adequate amounts of ATP. In turn, the ability to produce ATP is very much dependent on oxidative phosphorylation (OXPHOS) in the mitochondrion. One of the controlling factors for optimal function of OXPHOS is membrane fluidity, which is directly correlated with the amount of PUFAs present in the membrane. Mice fed a diet high in hydrogenated coconut oil and sucrose demonstrated decreased ability to produce ATP, a mutation in mitochondrial DNA, and increased incidence of NIDDM. Therefore, a diet low in PUFAs can potentially lead to detrimental changes in genetic expression of OXPHOS pathways which, ultimately, can lead to NIDDM *(Berdanier,1996)*.

Fat is not the only macronutrient relevant to gene expression. As we noted previously, excess carbohydrate intake can be quite detrimental to many physiologic processes due to its effect on cortisol and insulin metabolism. However, these detrimental effects do not end with endocrine manifestations, as several researchers have found a link between excess carbohydrate intake and adverse gene expression. Carbohydrates regulate expression of genes for both glycolytic and lipogenic enzymes *(Girard;Towle)*. Therefore, it is not surprising that animals fed a high-carbohydrate, low-fat diet had a dramatic induction of the enzymes involved in fatty acid and triacylglycerol synthesis. The investigators suggest that loss of control of these enzymes may be involved with diseases such as diabetes, obesity, hyperlipidemia, and cancer *(Sul)*.

Micronutrients

As with fatty acids, the relationship between vitamins and gene expression has generated many studies. What follows is a small sampling.

Characteristic chromosomal defects have been identified in malignant cells of most tumors *(Yunis,1983)*. One of these defects consists of sites on the chromosome that are particularly vulnerable to breakage when stressed, for example, by environmental mutagens and by certain nutritional deficiencies. Folic acid deficiency, which is well-known to promote the development of aplastic anemia, cancerous tumors and leukemia, is one of these deficiencies.

Folic acid plays an important role in DNA synthesis, repair and methylation *(Heimburger,1992)*. Tissue folate deficiency may provoke chromosomal breakage at a fragile site, while folate supplements may interfere with the detection of constitutive fragile sites *(Yunis,1984)*. This appears to be the mechanism by which tissue folate deficiency can provoke premalignant changes. An intriguing *in vitro* study examined chromosome fragility in cells grown in low-folate cultures. As expected, red cell folate levels were directly related to chromosome fragility. Cigarette smokers, known to be at high risk for lung cancer, also had a higher proportion of cells with chromosome aberrations; this was attributed to their lower red cell folate levels as compared to non-smokers *(Chen A)*.

In addition to solid cancers, fragile chromosome sites have so far been identified in serious hematologic diseases such as leukemia and aplastic anemia *(Marinello;Prasad)*. They have also been identified in the fragile X syndrome, the most important X-linked etiology of mental retardation and developmental disability currently known *(Reiss)*. Affected males frequently manifest behaviors from the autistic spectrum while females have difficulties in social interaction.

The relationship between folic acid nutriture and chromosomal aberrations has important treatment implications. Case reports have appeared in the literature suggesting that supplementation with folic acid may nullify or decrease the expression of abnormal cells while also improving the clinical picture. For example, a family with folic acid deficiency due to a genetic defect of cellular folate uptake was found to have 34 cases of proven or suspected serious hematologic diseases, including 5 cases of acute leukemia.

The high occurrence of hematologic disorders in folate deficiency suggested that they may have been the result of chromosomal breakage at a fragile site. Moreover, aplastic anemia in a family member went into remission following folate supplementation *(Branda)*. Also, boys, but not adult men, with fragile X syndrome showed improvement in their behavior as well as in their motor ability after receiving folate supplements. Concurrently, their fragile X positive cells became rarer or disappeared *(Gustavson)*.

The impact of not only folic acid, but also of vitamin B_{12}, on the genetic expression of homocysteine metabolism were investigated in a randomized double-blind study of young adults. The frequency of micronuclei was used as a marker for genetic damage. Within the study group that received supplementation with folic acid and vitamin B_{12}, there was a significant reduction in micronuclei in those with baseline micronucleus frequencies in the high 50th percentile. Likewise, there were significant reductions in serum homocysteine levels in those with baseline homocysteine levels in the high 50th percentile. These findings not only suggest the efficacy of folic acid and vitamin B_{12} in reducing chromosomal damage, but also suggest that elevated plasma homocysteine may be a risk factor for such damage *(Fenech)*.

Similarly, humans with genetically induced elevations in homocysteine due to polymorphism of the methylenetetrahydrofolate reductase gene were more susceptible to colon cancer formation when ingesting a diet low in folate and methionine and high in alcohol *(Chen J)*. Finally, it has been noted, *in vitro*, that folate deficiency induces genetically programmed cell death (apoptosis) in human hepatoma cells *(Huang)*.

Vitamin A has been shown to up-regulate gene expression of an enzyme *in vitro (Nikawa)*. In research that may have significant relevance to management of autoimmune conditions such as rheumatoid arthritis and asthma, ascorbic acid deficiency has been shown to correlate with gene expression of key factors (α_1-acid glycoprotein, haptoglobulin, interleukin-6) in the acute phase response, an important component in the activation of the immune system *(Ikeda)*.

Mineral nutriture is also relevant to gene expression. Earlier we noted the important role of zinc. Selenium appears to play an equally important role. For example, selenium is known to be required for formation of glutathione peroxidase. The basis for this relationship is that selenium regulates mRNA levels for this important antioxidant enzyme through posttranscriptional processes *(Larsen)*.

Another very interesting relationship between selenium and genetic expression involves changes in virulence of coxsackievirus B3. Normally this virus is quite benign. However, when mice infected with a myocarditic strain of coxsackievirus B3 had increased oxidative stress due to deficiencies of selenium and vitamin E, the virus became virulent and caused heart damage, a change which was found to be due to an alteration in nucleotide sequence to that which resembles the one found in virulent strains *(Beck)*.

Diagnosis and Treatment of Nutrition-gene Interactions

Studies have demonstrated how antioxidants and other micronutrients can prevent DNA damage *(Sheng)* and, as noted above, reduce breakage at fragile chromosomal sites *(Gustavson)*. Otherwise, unfortunately, little information is available to aid the clinician in applying studies on nutrition and gene expression to the routine outpatient setting. However, judging from the scope of recent investigations, it seems quite likely that diagnostic procedures will become more feasible in the near future so that our increasing knowledge of nutrient-gene interactions can be translated into treatments designed for the individual patient.

CONCLUSION

The several hundred pages of text that follow these introductory chapters demonstrate how the modification of nutritional factors can have a powerful impact on both the incidence and course of many, if not most, of the broad range of illnesses encompassed within specific diagnostic criteria. However, for many chronically ill patients, especially those whose disorder is not readily characterized by a conventional medical diagnosis, the nature and proper treatment of their illness can only be well understood when the integrative principles we have discussed are recognized and applied in a logical fashion.

REFERENCES

Abumrad NN et al. Energy metabolism, in Fischer JE, ed., Nutrition and Metabolism in the Surgical Patient. Little, Brown and Co., Boston, 1996, pp. 112-127

Adlercreutz H. Evolution, nutrition, intestinal microflora, and prevention of cancer: A hypothesis. Proc Soc Exp Biol Med Vol. 217, No. 3, pp. 241-246, March, 1998

Allolio B et al. Measurement of salivary cortisol in internal medicine – a significant improvement in the assessment of adrenocortical function, in Kirschbaum C et al, eds., Assessment of Hormones and Drugs in Saliva in Biobehavioral Research. Hogrefe & Huber Publ., Seattle, 1992, pp. 67-76

Alverdy JC & Faber EM. Nutrition and Immunity, in Zaloga GP ed., Nutrition in Critical Care. Mosby, St. Louis, 1994a, pp. 545-556

Alverdy JC et al. Causes and consequences of bacterial adherence to mucosal epithelia during critical illness. New Horizons: The Science and Practice of Acute Medicine Vol. 2, No. 2, pp. 264-272, May, 1994b

Ames BN &K Gold LS. Environmental pollution, pesticides, and the prevention of cancer: misconceptions. FASEB J Vol. 11, No. 13, pp. 1041-52, November, 1997

Atkins RC. Dr. Atkins' Diet Revolution. Bantam Books, New York, 1972

Bahl JJ & Bressler R. The pharmacology of carnitine. Ann Rev Pharmacol Toxicol Vol. 27, pp. 257-77, 1987

Bantle JP. The adrenal cortex, in Niewoehner CB, ed. Endocrine Pathophysiology. Fence Creek Publ., Madison, CT, 1998, pp. 61-76

Batmanghelidj F. Your Body's Many Cries for Water, Second Edition. Global Health Solutions, Inc., Falls Church, VA, 1995

Beck MA & Levander OA. Dietary oxidative stress and the potentiation of viral infection. Ann Rev Nutr Vol. 18, pp. 93-116, 1998

Belanger A et al. Characterization and regulation of UDP-glucuronosyltransferases in steroid target tissues. J Steroid Biochem Molec Med Vol. 65, No. 1-6, pp. 301-310, 1998

Bender DA. Nutritional Biochemistry of the Vitamins. Cambridge University Press, Cambridge, 1992

Bennett EJ et al. Level of chronic life stress predicts clinical outcome in irritable bowel syndrome. Gut Vol. 43, No. 2, pp. 256-261, August, 1998

Berdanier CD. Advanced Nutrition: Macronutrients. CRC Press, Boca Raton, 1995

Berdanier CD. Diabetes mellitus: a mitochondrial genomic error?, in Berdanier CD, ed. Nutrients and Gene Expression: Clinical Aspects. CRC Press, Boca Raton, 1996, pp. 141-164

Bjornstorp P. The etiology of the metabolic syndrome, in Bray GA et al, eds. Handbook of Obesity. Marcel Dekker, Inc., New York, 1998, pp. 573-600

Bland J. Toxicity related symptoms, in Advancement in Clinical Nutrition-1994 Seminar Series. HealthComm, Inc., Gig Harbor, WA, 1994

Boers GH. Hyperhomocysteinemia as a risk factor for arterial and venous disease. A review of evidence and relevance. Thromb Haemost 78(1):520-2, 1997

Boushey CJ et al. A quantitative assessment of plasma homocysteine as a risk factor for vascular disease: Probable benefits of increasing folic acid intakes. JAMA 274(13):1049-57, 1995

Branda RF et al. Folate-induced remission in aplastic anemia with familial defect of cellular folate uptake. N Engl J Med 298:469-75, 1978

Brattström LE et al. Folic acid responsive postmenopausal homocysteinemia. Metabolism 34(11):1073-77, 1985

Brattström L et al. Does Down syndrome support homocysteine theory of arteriosclerosis? Letter to the Editor. Lancet i:391, 1987

Brown SE. Better Bones, Better Body. Keats, New Canaan, CT, 1996, p. 167

Bucci LR. Nutrition Applied to Injury Rehabilitation and Sports Medicine. CRC Press, Boca Raton, 1997

Buist RA. Anxiety neurosis: The lactate connection. Int Clin Nutr Rev 5:1-4, 1985

Burchell B & Coughtrie MWH. Genetic and environmental factors associated with variation of human xenobiotic glucuronidation and sulfation. Environ Health Perspect Vol. 5, Suppl 4, pp. 739-747, 1997

Chadefaux B et al. Is absence of atheroma in Down syndrome due to decreased homocysteine levels? Letter. Lancet ii:741, 1988

Chen AT et al. Increased chromosome fragility as a consequence of blood folate levels, smoking status, and coffee consumption. Environ Mol Mutagen 13(4):319-24, 1989

Chen J et al. MTHFR polymorphism, methyl-replete diets and the risk of colorectal carcinoma and adenoma among U.S. men and women: An example of gene-environment interactions in colorectal tumorigenesis. J Nutr Vol. 129, No. 2S, pp. 560S-564S, February, 1999

Chipman JK & Coleman R. Mechanism and consequences of enterohepatic circulation, in Hill MJ, ed. Role of Gut Bacteria in Human Toxicology and Pharmacology. Taylor & Francis, Bristol, PA, 1995, pp. 245-260

Chwals WJ. Overfeeding the critically ill child: Fact or fantasy? New Horizons: The Science and Practice of Acute Medicine Vol. 2, No. 2, pp. 147-155, May, 1994

Clark CM. How should we respond to the worldwide diabetes epidemic? Diabetes Care Vol. 21, No. 4, pp. 475-6, April, 1998

Coffee CJ. Metabolism, First Edition. Fence Creek Publ., Madison, CT, 1998, pp. 101-109

Cohen SD et al. Acetaminophen-induced hepatotoxicity, in Plaa GL & Hewitt WR eds., Toxicology of the Liver, Second Edition. Taylor & Francis, Washington, DC, 1998, pp. 159-186

Connon JJ. Celiac disease, in Shils ME et al eds. Modern Nutrition in Health and Disease, Eighth Edition. Williams & Wilkins, Baltimore, 1994, pp. 1060-65

Coulston AM. Obesity as an epidemic: Facing the challenge. J Am Diet Assoc Vol. 98, No. 10, Suppl. 2, pp. S6-S8, October, 1998

Cryer PE. Hypoglycemia: Pathophysiology, Diagnosis, and Treatment. Oxford University Press, New York, 1997

Demitrack MA. Neuroendocrine correlates of chronic fatigue syndrome: A brief review J Psychiatr Res Vol. 31, No. 1, pp. 69-82, Jan/Feb, 1997

DiPasquale M. Amino Acids and Proteins for the Athlete: The Anabolic Edge. CRC Press, Boca Raton, 1997

Duman RS. Regulation of intracellular signal transduction and gene expression by stress, in Friedman MJ et al, eds. Neurobiological and Clinical Consequences of Stress. Lippincott-Raven, Philadelphia, 1995, pp. 27-43

Eades MR & Eades MD. Protein Power. Bantam Books, New York, 1996

Einhorn TA. Dietary protein and bone calcium metabolism, in Simmons DJ ed. Nutrition and Bone Development. Oxford University Press, New York, 1990, pp. 223-236

Earnest DL. Physiologic consequences of surgical treatment for inflammatory bowel disease, in Kirsner JB and Shorter RG, eds. Inflammatory Bowel Disease, fourth edition. Williams & Wilkins, Baltimore, 1995, pp. 923-960

Esposito G. Intestinal permeability of water-soluble nonelectrolytes: sugars, amino acids, peptides, in Csaky TZ et al, Pharmacology of Intestinal Permeation I. Springer-Verlag, Berlin, 1984, pp. 567-611

Esterbauer H et al. The role of lipid peroxidation and antioxidants in oxidative modification of LDL Free Rad Biol Med 13:341-90, 1992

Fenech M et al. Folate, vitamin B12, homocysteine status and DNA damage in young Australian adults. Carcinogenesis Vol. 19, No. 7, pp. 1163-1171, July, 1998

Fish JA, Friedman JM. Metabolic Stress, in Matarese LE & Gottschlich MM eds. Contemporary Nutrition Support Practice: A Clinical Guide. Saunders Co., Philadelphia, 1998, pp. 539-546

Freter R. Mechanisms that control the microflora in the large intestine, in Hentjes DJ, ed. Human Intestinal Microflora in Health and Disease. Academic Press, New York, 1983, pp. 33-50

Furst P & Stehle P. Glutamine and glutamine-containing dipeptides, in Cynober LA, ed. Amino Acid Metabolism and Therapy in Health and Nutritional Disease. CRC Press, Boca Raton, 1995, pp. 373-384

Gardiner KR et al. Novel substrates to maintain gut integrity. Nutr Res Rev Vol. 8, pp. 43-66, 1995

Gey KF. On the antioxidant hypothesis with regard to arteriosclerosis. Bibithca Nutr Dieta 3(1):53-91, 1986

Gibson GG & Skett P. Introduction to Drug Metabolism, Second Edition. Blackie Academic & Professional, London, 1994, pp. 133-156

Girard J et al. Mechanisms by which carbohydrates regulate expression of genes for glycolytic and lipogenic enzymes. Ann Rev Nutr Vol. 17, pp. 325-52, 1997

Golan R. Optimal Wellness. Ballantine Books, New York, 1995

Goldin BR & Gorbach SL. Impact of anaerobic bowel flora on metabolism of endogenous and exogenous compounds, in Finegold SM & George WL, eds. Anaerobic Infections in Humans. Academic Press, New York, 1989, pp. 691-714

Great Smokies Diagnostic Laboratory. Detoxification Profile Application Guide. Asheville, NC, 1997

Grimble GK. Essential and conditionally essential nutrients in clinical nutrition, in Kinney JM & Tucker HN eds. Organ Metabolism and Nutrition: Ideas for Future Critical Care. Raven Press, New York, 1994, pp. 267-300

Groff JL et al. Advanced Nutrition and Human Metabolism, Second Edition. West Publ. Co., Minneapolis/St. Paul, 1995

Guiet-Bara A et al. Magnesium: a competitive inhibitor of lead and cadmium. Ultrastructural studies of the human amniotic epithelial cell. Magnes Res 3(1):31-6, 1990

Gustavson KH et al. Effect of folic acid treatment in the fragile X syndrome. Clin Genet 27(5):463-67, 1985

Harker LA et al. Homocystine-induced arteriosclerosis. The role of endothelial cell injury and platelet response in its genesis. J Clin Invest 58(3):731-41, 1976

Harman D. Aging: A Theory Based on Free Radical and Radiation Chemistry. Berkeley, CA, U. of California Press, July, 1955

Heimburger DC. Localized deficiencies of folic acid in aerodigestive tissues. Ann N Y Acad Sci 669:87-96, 1992

Heller RF & Heller RF. Personal Communication

Heller RF & Heller RF. The Carbohydrate Addict's Diet. Dutton Books, New York, 1991

Heller RF & Heller RF. Hyperinsulinemic obesity and carbohydrate addiction: the missing link is the carbohydrate frequency factor. Med. Hypotheses Vol. 42, pp. 307-312, 1994

Heuchel R et al. Transcriptional regulation by heavy metals, exemplified at the metallothionein genes, in Baeuerle PA, ed. Inducible Gene Expression, Vol. 1. Birkhauser, Boston, 1995, pp. 206-240

Hill MJ. The normal gut bacterial flora, in Hill MJ ed. Role of Gut Bacteria in Human Toxicology and Pharmacology. Taylor & Francis, Bristol, PA, 1995, pp. 3-17

Hodgson E & Levi PE. Metabolism of toxicants: Phase I reactions, in Hodgson E & Levi PE, eds. Introduction to Biochemical Toxicology, Second Edition. Appleton & Lange, Norwalk, CT, 1994, pp. 75-112

Holman RT. Nutritional and metabolic interrelationships between fatty acids. Fed Proc 23:1062-67, 1964

Holt S. Soya for Health: The Definitive Medical Guide. Mary Ann Liebert, Inc., Larchmont, NY, 1996

Hong JY & Yang CS. Genetic polymorphism of cytochrome P450 as a biomarker of susceptibility to environmental toxicity. Environ Health Perspect Vol. 5, Suppl 4, pp. 759-762, 1997

Huang RFS et al. Folate deficiency induces a cell cycle-specific apoptosis in HepG2 cells. J Nutr, Vol. 129, No. 1, pp. 25-31, January, 1999

Hunniset A et al. Gut fermentation (or the "auto-brewery") syndrome: A new clinical test with initial observations and discussion of clinical and biochemical implications. J Nutr Med Vol. 1, pp. 33-38, 1990

Ikeda S et al. Ascorbic acid deficiency changes hepatic gene expression of acute phase proteins in scurvy-prone ODS rats. J Nutr Vol. 128, No. 5, pp. 832-838, May, 1998

Iritani N et al. Lipogenic enzyme gene expression is quickly suppressed in rats by a small amount of exogenous polyunsaturated fatty acids. J Nutr Vol. 128, No. 6, pp. 967-972, June, 1998

Jackson MJ et al eds. Assessment of the bioavailability of micronutrients, in Eur J Clin Nutr Vol. 51, Suppl 1, January, 1997

Jeejeebhoy KN. Nutritional aspects of inflammatory bowel disease, in Kirsner JB & Shorter RG, eds. Inflammatory Bowel Disease, Fourth Edition. Williams & Wilkins, Baltimore, 1995, pp. 734-749

Jenkins DJA et al. Diet factors affecting nutrient absorption and metabolism, in Shils ME et al, eds., Modern Nutrition in Health and Disease, Eighth Edition. Williams & Wilkins, Baltimore, 1994, pp. 583-602

Jones TW. Enhanced adrenomedullary response and increased susceptibility to neuroglycopenia: Mechanisms underlying the adverse effects of sugar ingestion in healthy children. J Pediatr Vol. 126, pp. 171-7, 1995

Kinsella JE et al. Metabolism of *trans* fatty acids with emphasis on the effect of *trans,trans*-octadecadienoate on lipid composition, essential fatty acid, and prostaglandins: an overview. Am J Clin Nutr 34:2307-18, 1981

Klaassen CD & Boles JW. The importance of 3'-phosphoadenosine 5'-phosphosulfate (PAPS) in the regulation of sulfation FASEB J Vol. 11, pp. 404-418, 1997

Kopelman PG. Endocrine determinants of obesity, in Bray GA et al. Handbook of Obesity. Marcel Dekker, Inc., New York, 1998, pp. 475-489

Kuzminski AM et al. Effective treatment of cobalamin deficiency with oral cobalamin. Blood 92(4):1191-8, 1998

Ladona MG et al. CYP2D6 genotypes in Spanish women with breast cancer. Cancer Lett Vol. 99, No. 1, pp. 23-28, January, 1996

Lamba JK et al. Genetic polymorphism of the hepatic cytochrome P450 2C19 in North Indian subjects. Clin Pharmacol Ther Vol. 63, No. 4, pp. 422-427, April, 1998

Larsen PR & Berry MJ. Nutritional and hormonal regulation of thyroid hormone deiodinases. Ann Rev Nutr Vol. 15, pp. 323-52, 1995

LeDoux JE. Setting "stress" into motion: Brain mechanisms of stimulus evaluation, in Friedman MJ et al, eds. Neurobiological and Clinical Consequences of Stress. Lippincott-Raven, Philadelphia, 1995, pp. 125-134

Leverve XM. Amino acid metabolism and gluconeogenesis, in Cynober LA, ed. Amino Acid Metabolism and Therapy in Health and Nutritional Disease. CRC Press, Boca Raton, 1995, pp. 45-56

Levi PE. Reactive metabolites and toxicity, in Hodgson E & Levi PE eds. Introduction to Biochemical Toxicology, Second Edition. Appleton & Lange, Norwalk, CT, 1994, pp. 219-240

Lewis AE & Schoen AM. Glandular therapy, cell therapy, and oral tolerance, in Schoen AM & Wynn SG, eds. Complementary and Alternative Veterinary Medicine: Principles and Practice. Mosby, St. Louis, 1998, pp. 81-92

Linder MC. Nutrition and metabolism of the major minerals, in Linder MC, ed. Nutritional Biochemistry and Metabolism with Clinical Applications, Second Edition. Elsevier, New York, 1991, pp. 191-214

Liska DJ. The detoxification enzyme systems. Alt Med Rev Vol. 3, No. 3, pp. 187-198, June, 1998

Little RA & Carlson GL. Insulin resistance and tissue fuels, in Kinney JM and Tucker HN, eds. Organ Metabolism and Nutrition: Ideas for Future Critical Care. Raven Press, New York, 1994, pp. 49-68

LoPresti JS & Nicoloff JT. Thyroid response to critical illness, in Ober KP ed. Endocrinology of Critical Disease. Humana Press, Totowa, NJ, 1997, pp. 155-173

Lord RS & Bralley A. Clinical applications of testing for organic acids in urine. Nutr Perspectives: J Am Council Nutr, Am Chiro Assoc Vol. 21, No. 4, pp. 23-31, January, 1999

MacFarlane GT & Gibson GR. Microbiological aspects of the production of short-chain fatty acids in the large bowel, in Cummings JH et al eds. Physiological and clinical aspects of short-chain fatty acids. Cambridge University Press, Cambridge, 1995, pp. 87-106

Mainous MR et al. Nutritional support of the gut: How and why. New Horizons: The Science and Practice of Acute Medicine Vol. 2, No. 2, pp. 193-201, May, 1994

Marinello MJ et al. Double minute chromosomes in human leukemia. Letter to the Editor. N Engl J Med 704-05, 1980

Matthews DE and Battezzati A. Substrate Kinetics and Catabolic Hormones, in Kinney JM and Tucker HN, eds. Organ Metabolism and Nutrition: Ideas for Future Critical Care. Raven Press, New York, 1994, pp. 1-22

Matthews HB. Excretion and elimination of toxicants and their metabolites, in Hodgson E & Levi PE eds. Introduction to Biochemical Toxicology, Second Edition. Appleton & Lange, Norwalk, CT, 1994, pp. 177-192

Matuschak GM. Liver-lung interactions in critical illness. New Horizons: The Science and Practice of Acute Medicine Vol. 2, No. 4, pp. 488-504, November, 1994

McCance KL and Shelby J. Stress and Disease, in McCance KL and Huether SE, eds. Pathophysiology: The Biological Basis for Disease in Adults and Children, Second Edition. Mosby, St. Louis, 1994, pp. 299-322

McCartan BE et al. Salivary cortisol and anxiety in recurrent aphthous stomatitis. J Oral Pathol Med, Vol. 25, No. 7, pp. 357-59, August, 1996

McCully KS. Vascular pathology of homocysteinemia: implications for the pathogenesis of arteriosclerosis. Am J Pathol 56(1):111-28, 1969

McEwen BS. Adrenal steroid actions on brain: Dissecting the fine line between protection and damage, in Neurobiological and Clinical Consequences of Stress. Lippincott-Raven, Philadelphia, 1995, pp. 135-147

Meaney MJ et al. Early environment and the development of individual differences in the hypothalamic-pituitary-adrenal stress response, in Pfeffer CR, ed., Severe Stress and Mental Disturbance in Children. American Psychiatric Press, Washington, D.C., 1996, pp. 85-130

Michelson D et al. Mediation of the stress response by the hypothalamic-pituitary-adrenal axis, in Friedman MJ et al, eds., Neurobiological and Clinical Consequences of Stress. Lippincott-Raven, Philadelphia, 1995, pp. 225-238

Milner JA. Nonnutritive components in foods as modifiers of the cancer process, in Bendich A & Deckelbaum R, eds. Preventive Nutrition: The Comprehensive Guide for Health Professionals. Humana Press, Totowa, NJ, 1997, pp. 135-152

Mizock BA. Alterations in carbohydrate metabolism during stress: A Review of the literature. Am J Med 98:75, 1995

Moldawer LL & Lowry SF. Interactions among inflammatory cytokines and the classic macroendocrine system in sepsis and inflammation, in Kinney JM & Tucker HN, eds. Organ Metabolism and Nutrition: Ideas for Future Critical Care. Raven Press, New York, 1994, pp. 119-136.

Mudd SH. Homocystinuria, in JB Wyngaarden & LH Smith Jr, Eds. Cecil: Textbook of Medicine. 18th Edition. Philadelphia, W.B. Saunders, 1988:1160-61.

Murray M & Pizzorno J. Encyclopedia of Natural Medicine, Second Edition. Prima Publishing, Rocklin, CA, 1998

Nasman B et al. Blunted adrenocorticotrophin and increased adrenal steroid response to human corticotrophin-releasing hormone in Alzheimer's disease. Biol Psychiatry Vol. 39, No. 5, March 1, 1996

Neumann DA & Kimmel CA, eds. Human Variability in Response to Chemical Exposures. CRC Press, Boca Raton, 1998

Nielsen FH et al. Dietary magnesium, manganese and boron affect the response of rats to high dietary aluminum. Magnesium 7(3):133-47, 1988

Nikawa T et al. Vitamin A up-regulates expression of bone-type alkaline phosphatase in a rat small intestinal crypt line and fetal rat small intestine. J Nutr, Vol. 128, No. 11, pp. 1869-77, November, 1998

Ober KP. Alterations in fuel metabolism in critical illness, in Ober KP, ed. Endocrinology of CriticalDisease. Humana Press, Totowa NJ, 1997, pp. 211-232

O'Brien JT. The 'glucocorticoid cascade' hypothesis in man. Br J Psychiatry Vol. 170, pp. 199-201, March, 1997

Parkinson A. Biotransformation of Xenobiotics, in Klaassen CD, ed. Casarett & Doull's Toxicology: The Basic Science of Poisons, Fifth Edition. McGraw-Hill, New York, 1996, pp. 113-186

Piper JT et al. Mechanisms of anticarcinogenic properties of curcumin: the effect of curcumin on glutathione linked detoxification enzymes on rat liver. Int J Biochem Cell Biol Vol. 30, No. 4, pp. 445-456, April, 1998

Pitcher MCL & Cummings JH. Hydrogen sulphide: a bacterial toxin in ulcerative colitis? Gut Vol. 39, No. 1, pp. 1-4, July, 1996

Pitot HC III & Dragan YP. Chemical carcinogenesis, in Klaassen CD ed., Casarett & Doull's Toxicology: The Basic Science of Poisons, Fifth Edition. McGraw Hill, New York, 1996, pp. 201-267

Prasad VS et al. Folate deficiency induced chromosomal lesions in cancer patients. Indian J Exp Biol 26(1):72-3, 1988

Quamme GA. Renal magnesium handling: New insights in understanding old problems. Kidney Int Vol. 52, No. 5, pp. 1180-1195, 1997

Reaich D & Maroni BJ. Protein and amino acid metabolism in renal disease and renal failure, in Kopple JD & Massry SG, eds. Nutritional Management of Renal Disease. Williams & Wilkins, Baltimore, 1997, pp. 1-34

Reaven GM. Syndrome X: Past, Present, and Future, in Draznin B & Rizza Robert eds. Clinical Research in Diabetes and Obesity, Vol. II. Humana Press, Totowa, NJ, 1997, pp. 357-382

Reiser S et al. An insulinogenic effect of oral fructose in humans during postprandial hyperglycemia. Am J Clin Nutr Vol. 45, pp. 580-7, 1987

Reiss AL, Freund L. Fragile X syndrome. Biol Psychiatry 27(2):223-40, 1990

Roberts PR. Dietary bioactive peptides. New Horizons: The Science and Practice of Acute Medicine. Vol. 2, No. 2, pp. 237-243, May, 1994

Rombeau JL & Lew JI. Intestinal Fuels: Implications for improvement of intestinal growth and function, in Fischer JE ed. Nutrition and Metabolism in the Surgical Patient, Second Edition. Little, Brown & Co., Boston, 1996, pp. 385-410

Ronis MJJ et al. The CYP2E subfamily, in Ioannides C, ed. Cytochromes P450: Metabolic and Toxicological Aspects. CRC Press, Boca Raton, 1996, pp. 211-239

Rowland I. Nutrition and gut microflora metabolism, in Rowland IR, ed. Nutrition, Toxicity, and Cancer. CRC Press, Boca Raton, 1991, pp. 113-136

Salway JG. Metabolism at a Glance. Blackwell Science, Ltd., Osney Mead, Oxford, 1994, p. 70

Sanderson IR. Dietary regulation of genes expressed in the developing intestinal epithelium. Am J Clin Nutr Vol. 68, No. 5, pp. 999-1005, November, 1998

Scheppach W. Effects of short chain fatty acids on gut morphology and function. Gut, Vol. 35, Suppl. 1, pp. S35-38, 1994

Seaman DR. Clinical Nutrition for Pain, Inflammation and Tissue Healing. NutrAnalysis, Inc., Hendersonville, NC, 1998

Sears B. Enter the Zone. Regan Books, New York, 1995

Sessler AM & Ntambi JM. Polyunsaturated fatty acid regulation of gene expression. J Nutr, Vol. 128, No. 6, pp. 923-923, June, 1998

Sheng Y et al. DNA repair enhancement by a combined supplement of carotenoids, nicotinamide, and zinc. Cancer Detection and Prevention Vol. 22, No. 4, pp. 284-292, 1998

Simopoulos AP. Evolutionary aspects of diet: Fatty acids, insulin resistance, and obesity, in VanItallie TB and Simopoulos AP, eds. Obesity: New Directions in Assessment and Management. The Charles Press, Philadelphia, 1995, pp. 241-261

Simpson P, Lucchesi B. Free radicals and myocardial ischaemia and reperfusion damage. J Lab Clin Med 110(1):13-30, 1987

Singh J et al. Dietary fish oil inhibits the expression of farnesyl protein transferase and colon tumor development in rodents. Carcinogenesis Vol. 19, No. 6, pp. 985-989, June, 1998

Sinha R & Caporaso N. Diet, genetic susceptibility and human cancer etiology. J Nutr, Vol. 129, No. 2S, pp. 556S-559S, February, 1999

Solomon GF. Clinical and social implications of stress-induced neuroendocrine-immune interactions, in Buckingham JC et al, eds. Stress, Stress Hormones and the Immune System. John Wiley and Sons, New York, 1997, pp. 385-402

Sorg BA & Kalivas PW. Stress and neuronal sensitization, in Friedman MJ et al, eds. Neurobiological and Clinical Consequences of Stress. Lippincott-Raven, Philadelphia, 1995, pp. 83-102

Stampfer MJ et al. A prospective study of plasma homocyst(e)ine and risk of myocardial infarction in US physicians. JAMA 268(7):877-81, 1992

Stampfer MJ, Malinow MR. Can lowering homocysteine reduce cardiovascular risk? Editorial. N Engl J Med 332(5):328-9, 1995

Steele KW. Gastrointestinal physiology and the gastrointestinal tract as a central organ in the hypermetabolic response to injury, in Borlase BC et al eds. Enteral Nutrition. Chapman & Hall, New York, 1994, pp. 3-14

Stout SC et al. Neuropeptides and stress: Preclinical findings and implications for pathophysiology, in Friedman MJ et al eds. Neurobiological and Clinical Consequences of Stress. Lippincott-Raven, Philadelphia, 1995, pp. 103-123

Stratakis CA & Chrousos GP. Neuroendocrinology and pathophysiology of the stress system. Ann N Y Acad Sci Vol. 771, pp. 1-18, 1995

Sul HS & Wang D. Nutrition and hormonal regulation of enzymes in fat synthesis: Studies of fatty acid synthase and mitochondrial glycerol-3-phosphate acyltransferase gene transcription. Ann Rev Nutr Vol. 18, pp. 331-51, 1998

Sullivan VK et al, Metallothionein expression is increased in monocytes and erythrocytes of young men during zinc supplementation. J Nutr Vol. 128, No. 4, pp. 707-713, April, 1998

Torpy DJ & Chrousos GP. General adaptation syndrome: An overview, in Ober KP, ed. Endocrinology of Critical Disease. Humana Press, Totowa, NJ, 1997, pp. 1-24

Towle HC et al. Regulation of the expression of lipogenic enzyme genes by carbohydrate. Ann Rev Nutr Vol. 17, pp. 405-33, 1997

Ubbink JB et al. Vitamin B-12, vitamin B-6, and folate nutritional status in men with hyperhomocysteinemia. Am J Clin Nutr 57:47-53, 1993

Ubbink JB et al. Vitamin requirements for the treatment of hyperhomocysteinemia in humans. J Nutr 124:1927-33, 1994

Utiger RD. The thyroid: physiology, thyrotoxicosis, hypothyroidism, and the painful thyroid, in Felig P et al, Endocrinology and Metabolism, Third Edition. McGraw-Hill, Inc., New York, 1995, pp. 435-519

VanDeventer SJH et al. Intestinal Endotoxaemia, Gastroenterology Vol. 94, No. 3, pp. 825-831, May, 1988

Van Gaal LF. Dietary treatment of obesity, in Bray GA et al. Handbook of Obesity. Marcel Dekker, Inc., New York, 1998, pp. 875-890

VanItallie TB & Simopoulos AP. Obesity: New Directions in Assessment and Management. The Charles Press, Philadelphia, 1995

Vermeulen NPE. Role of metabolism in chemical toxicity, in Ioannides C, ed. Cytochromes P450: Metabolic and Toxicological Aspects. CRC Press, Boca Raton, 1996, pp. 29-53

Vogel F. Clinical consequences of heterozygosity for autosomal-recessive diseases. Clin Genet 25(5):381-415, 1984

Wang EJ et al. Protective effects of garlic and related organosulfur compounds on acetaminophen-induced hepatotoxicity in mice. Toxicol App. Pharmacol Vol. 136, No. 1, pp. 146-154, January, 1996

Waterland RA & Garza C. Potential mechanisms of metabolic imprinting that lead to chronic disease. Am J Clin Nutr Vol. 69, No. 2, pp. 179-197, February, 1999

Weber WW. Pharmacogenetics. Oxford University Press, New York, 1997

Wilcken DE et al. Homocystinuria due to cystathionine beta-synthase deficiency: The effects of betaine treatment in pyridoxine-responsive patients. Metabolism 34(12):1115-21, 1985

Yang CS & Yoo JSH. Nutrition and hepatic Xenobiotic metabolism, in Rowland IR, ed. Nutrition, Toxicity, and Cancer. CRC Press, Boca Raton, 1991, pp. 53-92

Young VR & El-Khoury AE. The notion of the nutritional essentiality of amino acids, revisited, with a note on the indispensable amino acid requirements in adults, in Cynober LA, ed. Amino Acid Metabolism and Therapy in Health and Nutritional Disease. CRC Press, Boca Raton, 1995, pp. 191-232

Yunis JJ. The chromosomal basis of human neoplasia. Science 221:227-36, 1983

Yunis JJ, Soreng AL. Constitutive fragile sites and cancer. Science 226:1199-204, 1984

COMMON NUTRITIONAL DEFICIENCY SYNDROMES

"The clinical recognition of vitamin deficiency states is no longer confined to the diagnosis of the classical picture. Knowledge must be extended to the recognition of the 'Forme Frustes' by a greater appreciation of how the specific vitamin functions in maintaining nutritional balance under normal and pathologic conditions."

Rohmer P, Bezsnoff N. Investigations into the pathogenesis of scorbutic dystrophy. Arch Dis Child 10:319-26, 1935

Basic clinical nutrition textbooks provide detailed information on the classic presentations of severe nutritional deficiencies. While these are important to learn, severe deficiencies are rarely seen in prosperous societies. This chapter will focus instead on teaching the reader to recognize syndromes due to *marginal* nutritional deficiencies as, compared to severe deficiencies, marginal deficiencies are widespread. Moreover, they commonly go undiagnosed by uninformed health practitioners.

For heuristic reasons, we will discuss separately each of the nutritional deficiency syndromes that practitioners are most likely to see. It is more likely, however, that marginal nutritional deficiencies will coexist; thus evidence of one suggests a thorough evaluation for the existence of others.

As our knowledge of nutritional medicine has developed, there has been increasing recognition that marginal nutrient deficiencies may promote the development of an enormous variety of illnesses. The mechanisms are many. There may be, for example, adverse effects on antioxidants, immunologic competence, gene expression, neurotransmitters, or prostanoids. While these issues are of considerable importance, they are commonly unappreciated when the focus is on diagnosing and treating a specific disease.

Patients' histories will provide important diagnostic clues. Identify the major complaints that convinced the patient to seek professional help and then ask for the history of these complaints from inception until the present. Clues can often be found by asking what factors seem to influence these complaints - such as stress, particular foods, or the phase of the menstrual cycle. Ask yourself if any of these symptoms, or a combination of them, could be due to a nutritional deficiency. For example, a history of diminished taste and smell should cause you to suspect a zinc deficiency.

The history of other illnesses, including allergies and food sensitivities, should be included. A family history is valuable, as an illness in a close relative may increase the risk of that illness appearing in the patient. Evaluate the diet and the use of nutritional supplements, paying particular attention to any relationship between nutrient intake and the presenting complaints.

Information on the current diet, as well as a dietary history, are essential. Include the use of alcoholic and caffeinated beverages. Ask about food cravings, a symptom that suggests food sensitivities. Bloating after meals is particularly suspicious of a deficiency of hydrochloric acid.

Is there a history of weight loss with abdominal cramping, bloating or abnormal bowel movements? These symptoms can be due to abnormal gut microbial ecology. The importance of normal intestinal flora is frequently unrecognized. Disturbed bowel microbial ecology can cause a number of clinical problems, including the maldigestion and malabsorption of nutrients, resulting in malnutrition. Among their many functions, intestinal bacteria normally help synthesize members of the B vitamin family and vitamin K, as well as metabolize bile acids, sterols and antibiotics. Large intestinal microflora salvage energy from carbohydrate not digested in the upper intestines through fermentation and absorption of the resulting short-chain fatty acids *(Cummings)*.

Record all use of nutritional supplements and ask if ingestion of any of these supplements has had a noticeable effect. All drugs, including illegal drugs and tobacco, should be listed and their interactions with nutrients should be looked up.

The physical examination is also an important part of a nutritional evaluation. Within each section of this chapter, we will discuss the important physical signs that provide diagnostic clues. Marginal nutritional deficiencies can also affect brain function, so a brief mental status examination is also suggested.

Laboratory testing may be needed to complete the evaluation. (We will discuss the various laboratory testing procedures in the next chapter.)

MALNUTRITION

Malnutrition is a progressive series of metabolic, functional and body compositional changes due to inadequate nutrient intake to satisfy metabolic needs. While malnutrition can result from poverty, in industrialized countries it is commonly due to illness. The primary illness may be emotional, such as a failure to consume adequate nourishment as a manifestation of depression, or it may be physical. Physical illness causes malnutrition a number of ways. Anorexia (lack of appetite) is common. There may be difficulty achieving an adequate dietary intake due, for example, to problems with chewing or swallowing. Once ingested, impairment of gastrointestinal processes may reduce nutrient absorption, or absorbed nutrients may be unable to ensure normal metabolism due to other interfering factors.

Despite a close relationship between malnutrition and the course of the illness *(Hernández Plasencia)*, the diagnosis is often missed in clinical settings:

"Between 25 and 50% of patients admitted to an acute medical service are malnourished. Physicians are often unaware which patients are admitted at nutritional risk and make no attempt to arrest further nutritional decline until a dramatic deterioration has occurred (Roubenoff)."

When evaluating patients, be suspicious of malnutrition if the patient belongs to any of the high risk groups. Beside the poor, they include infants and young children who are not thriving, adolescents undergoing rapid growth spurts, pregnant and lactating women, and the elderly. Another group at increased risk consists of those on special diets for any reason. Illnesses such as chronic diseases of the gastrointestinal tract, liver and biliary tract, or kidneys, cancer or AIDS increase risk, as do drug treatments that impair nutrition as well as alcoholism and drug addiction.

Ask if dietary intake has been reduced (other than for reduction of obesity) over the previous weeks or months. If so, compare the current dietary intake to the usual one. Ask if there are significant gastrointestinal symptoms (anorexia, nausea, vomiting, diarrhea) on a daily basis for longer than the past 2 weeks. Ascertain if there has been an involuntary weight loss of at least 5% (the history of at least a 10% loss is definitely significant) in the 6 months prior to examination, especially if weight has not recently stabilized or increased. Evaluate the patient's energy level and functional capacity.

Measure the patient's height and weight and compare those measurements with a standard chart of ideal body weights. Look for loss of subcutaneous fat, particularly in the triceps region of the arms, the midaxillary line at the costal margin, the interosseous and palmar areas of the hand, and the deltoid regions of the shoulder. See if there is loss of fullness or areas where the skin fits too loosely over the deeper tissues - but be aware that this sign may be seen in well nourished elderly patients. Note if the skin has become dry and flaky, or appears waxy.

Examine for muscle wasting (loss of bulk and tone), especially in the quadriceps femoris and the deltoids. (The loss of subcutaneous tissue in the shoulders gives a 'squared off' appearance.) Finally, inspect for edema (loss of fluid from the intravascular to extravascular space). Press the ankle or sacrum. If there is edema, you will feel fluid move out of the subcutaneous tissue and then observe 'pitting' (persistent depression of the area pressed for more than 5 seconds) *(Detsky)*.

MARGINAL NUTRIENT DEFICIENCIES

Brin has described the marginal degree of vitamin deficiency as consisting of three stages. In the *preliminary* stage, although the clinical presentation is entirely normal, there is a gradual depletion of vitamin stores and reduced excretion. The patient with the *biochemical* stage presents with low energy. Laboratory testing now shows evidence of impaired vitamin biochemistry in addition to a further reduction of excretion.

In the *physiological* stage, the patient complains of additional non-specific symptoms such anorexia (appetite loss), malaise, insomnia and irritability, and the laboratory abnormalities increase. All three stages of marginal deficiency precede the *clinical* stage. If there is a classic deficiency syndrome, it only now becomes manifest *(Brin,1964)*.

Although 'latent scurvy' was described more than half a century ago, a recent study on vitamin C depletion demonstrates the far-reaching effects of marginal deficiencies. Non-scorbutic subjects with subnormal vitamin C status were placed on a diet low in vitamin C for 3 weeks and then gradually repleted. Both blood histamine and plasma free carnitine levels were found to be inversely related to vitamin C status, providing evidence that metabolic changes independent of collagen metabolism occur prior to the manifestation of scurvy *(Johnston,1996a)*.

It is now recognized that, besides vitamins, marginal deficiencies of other essential nutrients may follow a similar clinical course.

I. MARGINAL WATER-SOLUBLE VITAMIN DEFICIENCIES

The first indication of a marginal deficiency of the water-soluble vitamins is the gradual development of nonspecific symptoms. These were well-described by Spies *et al* half a century ago:

"Persons with early or subclinical deficiencies of the water-soluble vitamins have frequently been described as neurasthenic. Their complaints are extremely numerous and vague and limited to no particular portion of the body. Their appetite is poor, and they have lost weight and strength. Indigestion and dyspepsia are almost universal, and there frequently is some vague type of burning sensation in the epigastrium which most of the patients refer to as 'heartburn.'

The majority of the patients are constipated or have attacks of diarrhea and abdominal cramps. Many describe vague burning, itching and crawling sensations over the skin. The state that they are 'nervous', that their 'nerves are on edge' and that they are irritable, apprehensive, depressed and unable to sleep. Crying spells, flights of ideas, distractibility, mild mental confusion and forgetfulness are common complaints (Spies)."

This early stage is marked by impairments in biochemical processes, so the more sensitive laboratory tests will uncover evidence of deficiency. As body structure remains normal, more specific signs and symptoms, which bear evidence that structural abnormalities are developing, appear later as the deficiency worsens *(Brin,1978)*.

While there are differences in the effects of deficiencies of each of the water-soluble vitamins, in affluent societies low vitamin intakes tend to cluster together as they often result from a diet that is high in alcohol or other nutrient-poor foods *(van der Beek)*. Therefore nutritional assessment should not be limited to a single vitamin.

VITAMIN B COMPLEX

Interactions of the B-complex vitamins are essential for metabolic and catabolic reactions *(Sauberlich)*; thus a deficiency of one may affect the adequacy of the others.

In marginal deficiencies of folic acid, niacin, riboflavin, vitamin B_6 and vitamin B_{12}, there are two common physical features that suggest the diagnosis. The first is *angular stomatitis*. At the corners of the mouth, the mucocutaneous junctions are inflamed and fissures may form. Often one side is more affected than the other.

Certain tongue abnormalities constitute the other common physical feature. Early the tongue may be inflamed, bright red and sore (*acute glossitis*). Often, however, it is bluish or cyanotic, small and glistening due to atrophy of the filiform papillae causing the tissue covering the underlying capillary bed to be abnormally translucent (*atrophic glossitis*) *(Friedman)*. Assuming that the abnormal color is not due to a low blood oxygen level (hypoxemia) or to severe anemia, this particular finding means that there is an 80% chance of either a niacin or riboflavin deficiency *(Leevy)*. (Occasionally the tongue in niacin or riboflavin deficiency is black in color.)

A *vitamin dependency* is a state of impaired cellular metabolism which exists when a defect impairs the coupling of the coenzyme form of the vitamin to the apoenzyme, a step that is necessary in order to activate the enzyme. This may be due either to chemical interference with the availability of the coenzyme, or to a genetic defect in one or more of the enzymes involved in a reaction. Vitamin dependency has been shown to occur with three of the B vitamins, namely vitamin B_6, vitamin B_{12} and biotin. In this case, even an intake which is normally adequate will fail to protect against deficiency. The solution is to provide massive doses of the vitamin to push the reaction forward in order to correct the metabolic imbalance.

FOLIC ACID

The most common vitamin deficiency, a large national survey found that the average American consumed only about 60% of the recommended amount of folic acid *(Subar)*, while 11% of the population had deficient serum folate levels *(Senti)*. Other causes of deficiency include the exclusive ingestion of foods that are boiled for a long time, goat's milk as the sole source of infant nutrition, diseases of the small bowel, genetically determined inadequacy of enzymes involved in folate metabolism, thyrotoxicosis, mixed connective tissue disease and hepatic or renal failure.

The macrocytic (large cell) anemia of folate deficiency is well known, but the neuropsychiatric features of marginal deficiency are often missed. Depression is the most frequent symptom, and between 15 and 38 percent of adults diagnosed with depressive disorders will be found to have borderline low or deficient serum or red blood cell folate levels *(Alpert)*. Apathy, irritability and forgetfulness may be part of the picture. If the deficiency worsens, confusion or psychosis may occur. This metabolic encephalopathy is reflected in the electroencephalogram (EEG) which shows a pattern of diffuse, cortical dysrhythmia with an excess of slow-wave activity *(Runcie)*.

NIACIN

Perhaps one-third of the population consumes less than the recommended allowance for niacin *(Nutrition Monitoring)*. Pellagra, the classic niacin deficiency syndrome which is now rare in developed countries, presents with the "three Ds" of dermatitis, diarrhea and dementia.

In a borderline deficiency, any of these three signs may be present in a mild form. A slight periorificial (around the body openings) dermatitis may exist. If the patient has been exposed to the sun, the dermatitis may also cover exposed areas. The skin may be dry and atrophic and hyperpigmentation of the hands and the back of the neck may occur. Anorexia is common, and stools may be loose. A depression that is marked by high levels of anxiety may be present along with irritability. Weakness is a frequent complaint and there may be a slight tremor.

RIBOFLAVIN

This deficiency is especially common among the poor and the elderly, although it is possible that it is not uncommon in other population groups *(Southon)*. In addition to poor dietary habits, riboflavin deficiency may result from the use of drugs and from disorders such as endocrine abnormalities that interfere with its utilization.

Since riboflavin coenzymes are involved in the metabolism of 3 other B vitamins (folic acid, niacin and vitamin B_6) as well as vitamin K, a riboflavin deficiency may have adverse consequences for numerous other enzyme systems in addition to those directly requiring the vitamin as a coenzyme.

An isolated riboflavin deficiency is rarely seen, and the clinical manifestations are non-specific and typical of B vitamin deficiencies. Early features may include weakness, fatigue, mouth pain and tenderness, conjunctivitis and mental or emotional difficulties.

THIAMINE

While inadequate intake is the main cause of thiamine deficiency in underdeveloped countries, alcoholism, which results in malabsorption of the vitamin, is the most common cause in industrialized nations. Moreover, most of the nervous system abnormalities found in alcoholics is due to inadequate thiamine nutriture. Malabsorption for causes other than alcoholism can also cause deficiency. Among the various age groups, deficiency is most likely among children and the elderly *(Werbach)*.

Beriberi is the classic disease of severe thiamine deficiency, with manifestations focused on the neurological and cardiovascular systems. Marginal deficiencies, which are believed to be fairly common in developed countries, commonly cause non-specific symptoms such as tiredness, weakness, anorexia (lack of appetite) and headache. The symptom of "burning feet" is an early, and therefore relatively common, complaint suggesting a developing peripheral neuropathy; however, it also occurs in peripheral neuropathy due to other B vitamin deficiencies. In contrast to most of the other B vitamin deficiencies, thiamine deficiency is not associated with abnormalities of the corners of the lips (angular stomatitis) or of the tongue.

For people with subclinical thiamine deficiency, supplementation has been shown under double-blind conditions to significantly enhance the quality of life and decrease systolic blood pressure, with a trend towards improvements in sleep and energy *(Wilkinson)*.

VITAMIN B_6

Typically, vitamin B_6 intake averages 50% to 75% below the recommended levels *(Rall)*. Marginal deficiency is common. For example, in a group of British middle-class adolescents, it was found to be marginally deficient in 27% of the girls and 50% of the boys *(Southon)*. It is marginally deficient in about 50% of pregnant women *(Heller)* and, even if they have supposedly adequate dietary intakes and oral supplementation, the elderly are often deficient *(Frank)*. A periorificial (around the body openings) rash resembling seborrheic dermatitis and conjunctivitis are common features.

Vitamin B_6 deficiency usually occurs along with other B vitamin deficiencies. Because riboflavin is required for the metabolism of vitamin B_6, a concurrent deficiency of riboflavin will add to the seriousness of the resulting disorder *(Leklem)*.

VITAMIN B_{12}

Deficiency of this vitamin is primarily due to malabsorption. Therefore, while it is not terribly common in the general population, it should be kept in mind when there is reason to believe that a patient may have a problem with vitamin B_{12} absorption. Malabsorption may be secondary to gastric disorders (such as inadequate secretion of hydrochloric acid or intrinsic factor), intestinal disorders (such as inadequate exocrine pancreatic secretion, malabsorption syndromes, or alteration of the vitamin-intrinsic factor complex fixation to the ileal wall) or to congenital diseases.

The elderly, for example, are prone to vitamin B_{12} deficiency due to an increasing incidence of atrophic gastritis (in which they cannot absorb the vitamin when it is protein-bound in food but can absorb it from supplements) and pernicious anemia (in which they cannot absorb the vitamin from either source). Estimates of the prevalence of cobalamin deficiency in this group have varied from 3% to 42%, depending upon the population group studied and the method used *(Van Goor)*. In fact, low serum cobalamin levels are among the most common abnormalities in the elderly *(Carmel)*. Vegans (total vegetarians) are another group that is prone to develop a deficiency, in this case because of their dietary habits.

Early diagnosis of vitamin B_{12} deficiency is particularly important as the deficiency causes lesions in the ileal mucosal cells *(Pena)*. By reducing the vitamin's absorption, these lesions intensify the development of further deficiency. Eventually, with complete exhaustion of body reserves, the full clinical picture develops and diagnosis becomes relatively simple.

Paresthesias ("pins and needles" sensations) and ataxia (incoordination) are common initial symptoms of vitamin B_{12} deficiency; changes in mental function may also be noted. Up to 90% of B_{12}-deficient patients have some neurological problem and, in many, it is the only clinical manifestation of deficiency *(Green)*. Other early manifestations include weakness or fatigue, indigestion, diarrhea, or depression.

Commonly, however, there are no obvious clinical signs of deficiency, yet 50 to 75 percent of all low cobalamin concentrations are accompanied by metabolic evidence of deficiency. Moreover, in nearly every case, those metabolic changes respond to cobalamin therapy *(Carmel)*.

VITAMIN C

While scurvy, the classical vitamin C deficiency disease, is rare in developed countries, marginal deficiency of vitamin C appears to be common, especially among certain groups. Roughly one-quarter of the population in the United States appears to be at least marginally vitamin C-deficient *(Pao)*. Groups at high risk include those eating "junk food" diets, the elderly (who often eat poorly), the indigent, alcohol and drug abusers, smokers, and patients with chronic illness, on dialysis, or who avoid "acid" foods that cause gastrointestinal symptoms (such as heartburn) *(G Block)*.

Studies have shown that a marginal deficiency too subtle to be picked up on a physical exam can still have adverse effects on immunocompetence, antioxidant defenses *(Jacob)* and wound healing *(Ingalls)*. As with other marginal deficiencies of water-soluble vitamins, the earliest symptoms of vitamin C deficiency are non-specific and include complaints of malaise, lethargy, weakness, fatigue and irritability *(Levine)*.

Fortunately, the Rumpel-Leede test can uncover a marginal deficiency of the vitamin. Due to capillary fragility, the spontaneous development of petechiae (tiny hemorrhages into the skin) is an early sign of scurvy, but is not seen when the deficiency is only marginal. However, if the patient is marginally deficient, a blood pressure cuff placed around the upper arm and inflated for about a minute will cause petechiae to appear on the forearm *(Johnston, 1996b)*.

II. MARGINAL FAT-SOLUBLE VITAMIN DEFICIENCIES

VITAMIN A

Not only is vitamin A deficiency a major public health problem in many of the less industrialized nations of the world, but three major American national surveys have found that 20% or more of the population surveyed was consuming less than 70% of the Recommended Dietary Allowance *(Bendich)*, a level generally acknowledged as placing people at risk of developing a deficiency. Children are particularly vulnerable, with over 100 million children worldwide suffering from the effects of a marginal deficiency of the vitamin *(Underwood)*. Among adults, lactating women are the most prone to becoming marginally deficient.

Night blindness and xerophthalmia (excessive dryness of the cornea and conjunctiva) are common clinical signs of overt vitamin A deficiency. Children may have Bitot's spots, foamy white accumulations of sloughed cells that appear on the temporal (outer) quadrant of the conjunctiva. The skin may show follicular hyperkeratosis (phrynoderma; "toad skin") in which spinous papules appear at the tips of the hair follicles against a background of dry, rough skin.

These classic signs are usually lacking when the deficiency is only marginal. Instead, increased proneness to infection is the major manifestation. It should be suspected in patients with protein-calorie malnutrition, a low fat intake, lipid malabsorption syndromes or febrile diseases.

VITAMIN D

More than 40% of the population above age 50 may be vitamin D-deficient *(Holick)*. Since this vitamin is needed for the proper utilization of calcium, a marginal deficiency may promote the development osteoporosis or osteomalacia no matter how much calcium there is in the diet. While osteomalacia is relatively rare, perhaps 10% of the population suffers from osteoporosis and is therefore particularly liable to sustain bone fractures. Vitamin D is made from a precursor when ultraviolet light (UV-B) penetrates into the skin. It is estimated that at least 75% of vitamin D supplies come from this photochemical conversion; thus people who have little exposure to sunlight are more likely to become deficient.

VITAMIN E

The intake of this vitamin is often below recommended levels in Westernized countries; moreover intake has been shown to be related to biochemical markers of vitamin E nutriture *(Hercberg)*. Evidence of deficiency of the vitamin, however, is usually related to the presence of a fat malabsorption syndrome.

While atrophic glossitis is classically associated with B vitamin deficiencies, it has recently been found to be even more closely associated with marginal vitamin E deficiency *(Drinka)*. The majority of these vitamin E-deficient patients will be found to have multiple nutritional deficiencies

Although not recognized until recently, deficiency of this vitamin eventually causes a neurologic disorder. Typically, there is loss of deep tendon reflexes, impaired vibratory and position sensation, alterations in balance and coordination, ophthalmoplegia (impaired movement of the eyes), muscle weakness, and visual field disturbances. Due to their developing nervous systems, children with congenital malabsorptive disorders are particularly vulnerable to develop the neurologic syndrome; adults require 5 to

10 years of deficiency before neurologic abnormalities may appear.

VITAMIN K

For a substantial portion of the population of the developed countries, the intake of vitamin K may be inadequate for healthy bone metabolism *(Vermeer)*. Subclinical deficiency is particularly common in the newborn and in women who are pregnant or postmenopausal *(C Block;Ferland)*.

Because of the vitamin's role in coagulation, deficiency classically interferes with blood clotting. In adults, vitamin K-responsive hemorrhaging is most commonly seen when antibiotics are given to patients who already have a low dietary intake of the vitamin *(Alperin)*. Lipid malabsorption syndromes may also be responsible.

III. MARGINAL MINERAL DEFICIENCIES

CALCIUM

As roughly half of the population of developed countries consumes an inadequate amount of calcium *(McCarron)*, chronic marginal calcium deficiency is widespread. Its effects take many years to manifest themselves; however, the consequences of long-term marginal deficiency can be quite serious. Adequate calcium intake is particularly important for adolescent girls to help them achieve an optimal peak bone mass, and in women who are pregnant or nursing. Its importance in preventing osteoporosis in older people is well known. Periodontal disease, when due to loss of the underlying alveolar bone, appears to be part of the same process. As dietary calcium is also important in preventing the development of hypertension *(McCarron)*, the calcium intake of any patient presenting with elevated blood pressure should be investigated.

CHROMIUM

Normal dietary chromium intake in the United States and other westernized countries is roughly 50-60% of the minimal Estimated Safe and Adequate Daily Dietary Intake of 50 mcg established by the National Research Council (US) *(Anderson)*. The primary importance of adequate chromium nutriture is to assist in the function of insulin; thus, unless they had advanced diabetes mellitus, people with marginal chromium deficiencies will not present with any physical findings. Only laboratory testing can establish the diagnosis.

IRON

Chronic iron deficiency is believed to be the most prevalent worldwide nutritional deficiency, affecting more than a quarter of the world's population *(Werbach)*. Since adequate iron nutriture is neccssary in order for normal work, or exercise, capacity, iron-deficient patients commonly complain of a lack of energy to perform their usual tasks.

Iron deficiency is the most frequent cause of anemia, the presence of which is marked by pallor - particularly in the nail beds and tongue. In addition to fatigue and pallor, patients with iron deficiency anemia often complain of coldness and paresthesias ("pins and needles") in the hands and feet, palpitations, and dyspnea (shortness of breath) on exertion. Even if no anemia is found, patients suffering from insufficient energy to perform their usual tasks may still be iron-deficient, suggesting that the easy fatigability is not simply due to anemia. Angular stomatitis (sores at the corners of the lips) and glossitis (sore tongue) may occur; both are identical to the findings seen in many B vitamin deficiencies.

Advanced iron deficiency is associated with koilonychia. This is a process that starts with thinning and flattening of the nail beds. Eventually, they take on an indented, spoon-shaped appearance. There may also be dysphagia (difficulty swallowing) and other gastrointestinal complaints *(Finch)*.

MAGNESIUM

Chronic primary magnesium deficit, which is estimated to be present in 15 to 20% of the population, is the most common form of magnesium deficiency *(Durlach)*. Its classic presentation is one of nervous hyperexcitability which can manifest itself with any of a large number of peripheral and autonomic signs along with centrally-mediated (psychological) symptoms. Central symptoms include anxiety, emotional lability, fatigue, headaches, insomnia, lightheadedness, dizziness, nervous "fits," globus hystericus (sensation of a lump in the throat) and shortness of breath.

Cardiac symptoms are not uncommon and include symptoms of idiopathic mitral valve prolapse, palpitations, extrasystoles and dysrhythmias. Muscle symptoms, primarily painful cramping and involuntary fasciculations (twitches), are a frequent manifestation. In the hands and feet, there may be acroparesthesias ("pins and needles" sensations in the hands and feet) as well as Raynaud's syndrome (vasospasm causing the digits to turn a reddish-purple and to feel cold, numb and sometimes painful).

Since these symptoms are non-specific, testing to elicit specific signs is particularly revealing. Many of the symptoms, such as hyperventilation and muscle cramping (spasmophilia) can be characterized as suggestive of latent tetany; therefore tests that elicit evidence of tetany are especially revealing. Of these, the Chvostek's sign is most important; Durlach has found that, when elicited as he suggests, it is positive in 85% of patients. With a small reflex hammer, tap the soft parts of the cheek at the center of a line running from the ear lobe to the side of the mouth. Avoid taping the zygomatic arch (the part of the skull that protrudes beneath the eye), as this can produce a lightning-like contraction in normal people. Any degree of involuntary muscle contraction is considered positive *(Durlach)*.

For a more complete examination, the heart should be evaluated for clicks and murmurs and both an echocardiogram and an electromyogram should be performed.

ZINC

While, due to the lack of definitive indicators of zinc status, the exact figures are unknown, mild deficiency appears to be common *(Sanstead)*. High risk groups include vegetarians as well as children, adolescents, pregnant women, and the elderly *(Werbach)*.

Many of the manifestations of a mild zinc deficiency are too non-specific to suggest a diagnosis, although a combination of them should arouse suspicion. These include retarded growth and development in children, pregnancy complications, impotence and infertility, suppressed immune function, poor healing, peripherally-located skin lesions (especially eczema and seborrheic dermatitis), anorexia (lack of appetite), emotional disorders and tremors.

Fortunately, there are certain characteristics of mild zinc deficiency that can point to the correct diagnosis. The most specific, although also the least validated, is the presence of leukonychia (white spots or bands on the nails) that are not due to direct trauma. Because the data are so limited, we will review it in some detail. Leukonychia was first described by Muerhcke in 1956 as an indication of low serum albumin levels due to loss of this protein in the urine *(Muerhcke)*. Two decades later, Pfeiffer noted that patients with normal serum protein levels can have similar spots. These he found to be due to zinc deficiency, as zinc supplementation caused the small spots to resolve and the large ones to not reappear after they grew out. He noted that, since 70% of serum zinc is protein-bound, patients who lose albumin in the urine are also likely to be zinc-deficient; thus his observation was consistent with the earlier report *(Pfeiffer)*.

Bakan subsequently studied 494 university students to see if the presence of leukonychia was related to typical subjective symptoms of zinc deficiency, namely right-left confusion, sleep time and drowsiness. Students with leukonychia had a greater likelihood of right-left confusion, longer sleep times and a trend toward more drowsiness *(Bakan)*.

Another finding that suggests zinc deficiency is a loss of taste acuity (hypogeusia), a finding that is noted for almost everyone who is zinc-deficient. Taste and smell disorders are estimated to afflict about 15 million people in the United States alone, and one authority estimates that at least one-third of people with diminished sense of taste (which is strongly affected by the sense of smell) are zinc-deficient *(Henkin)*.

Finally, there may be a failure of dark adaptation (difficulty seeing in the dark). While this symptom is closely related to vitamin A deficiency, zinc is required for proper utilization of the vitamin.; thus patients who fail to respond to vitamin A are often zinc-deficient.

IV. MARGINAL ESSENTIAL FATTY ACID DEFICIENCY

Essential fatty acid deficiency is associated with increased thirst and frequent urination, dry, rough skin with perifollicular hyperkeratoses ('goose flesh'; spinous papules at the tips of the hair follicles), dry hair, dandruff, and brittle nails. Although nutritionally-oriented clinicians believe that marginal EFA deficiency is not uncommon, its prevalence in the general population is unknown. However, there is evidence that, among children with attention-deficit hyperactivity disorder, those who show manifestations of classic EFA deficiency also demonstrate significantly reduced plasma concentrations *(Stevens)*; future research may determine if this finding extends to a larger population.

REFERENCES

Alperin JB. Coagulopathy caused by vitamin K deficiency in critically ill, hospitalized patients. JAMA 256:1916-19, 1987

Alpert JE, Fava M. Nutrition and depression: the role of folate. Nutr Rev 55(5):145-9, 1997

Anderson RA. Chromium and its role in lean body mass and weight reduction. Nutr Rep 11(6), 1993

Bakan P. Confusion, lethargy and leukonychia. J Orthomol Med 5:198-202, 1990

Bendich A, Langseth L. Safety of vitamin A. Am J Clin Nutr 49:358-71, 1989

Block CA et al. Mother-infant prothrombin precursor status at birth. J Pediatr Gastroenterol Nutr 3(1):101-3, 1984

Block G et al. Vitamin C: A new look. Ann Intern Med 114(10):909-10, 1991

Brin M, Bauernfeind JC. Vitamin needs of the elderly. Postgrad Med 63(3):155-9, 1978

Brin M. Erythrocyte as a biopsy tissue in the functional evaluation of thiamin status. JAMA 187:762, 1964

Carmel R. Cobalamin, the stomach, and aging. Am J Clin Nutr 66:750-9, 1997

Cummings JH, MacFarlane GT. Role of intestinal bacteria in nutrient metabolism. Clin Nutr 16:3-11, 1997

Detsky AS et al. The rational clinical examination: Is this patient malnourished? JAMA 271(1):54-8, 1994

Drinka PJ et al. Nutritional correlates of atrophic glossitis: possible role of vitamin E in papillary atrophy. J Am Coll Nutr 12(1):14-20, 1993

Durlach J et al. Magnesium and therapeutics. Magnes Res 7(3-4):313-28, 1994

Ferland G. Subclinical vitamin K deficiency: recent developments. Nutr Rep 12(1), January, 1994

Finch CA. Editorial: Evaluation of iron status. JAMA 251(15):2004, 1984

Frank O et al. Superiority of periodic intramuscular vitamins over daily oral vitamins in maintaining normal vitamin titers in a geriatric population. Am J Clin Nutr 30:630, 1977

Friedman PJ, Hodges RE. Tongue colour and B-vitamin deficiencies. Letter. Lancet i:1159-60, 1977

Green R - interviewed in Helwick C. Red cell is inadequate as red flag for low B-12. Medical World News, November 1991:33.

Hercberg S et al. Vitamin status of a healthy French population: dietary intakes and biochemical markers. Int J Vitam Nutr Res 64(3):220-32, 1994

Heller S et al. Vitamin B6 status in pregnancy. Am J Clin Nutr 26(12):1339-48, 1973

Henkin, Robert, director of the Center for Molecular Nutrition and Sensory Disorders, Georgetown University Medical Center, Washington, DC - quoted in Yates J. Zinc for good taste. Prevention August, 1980:86-90

Hernández Plasencia D et al. Subjective nutritional assessment and short-term prognosis. J Nutr Med 2:151-63, 1991

Holick, Michael F, director of the Vitamin D, Skin and Bone Research Laboratory, Boston University Medical Center - interviewed by B Liebman in Vitamin D deficiency: the silent epidemic. Nutrition Action Healthletter October, 1997:3-6.

Horrobin DF. Nutritional and medical importance of gamma-linolenic acid. Prog Lipid Res 31(2):163-94, 1992

Ingalls TH, Warren HA. Asymptomatic scurvy. N Engl J Med 217(11):443-6, 1937

Jacob RA et al. Immunocompetence and oxidant defense during ascorbate depletion of healthy men. Am J Clin Nutr 54:1302S-1309S, 1991

Johnston CS et al. Vitamin C depletion is associated with alterations in blood histamine and plasma free carnitine in adults. J Am Coll Nutr 15(6):586-91, 1996a

Johnston CS. Capillary fragility as a functional measure of vitamin C status. Abstract. J Am Coll Nutr 15(5):536, 1996b

Leevy CM et al. Am J Clin Nutr 16:339, 1964

Leklem JE. Vitamin B-6, in EE Ziegler, LJ Filer JR, Eds. Present Knowledge in Nutrition. Seventh Edition. Washington, DC, ILSI Press, 1996:174-83

Levine M, Contry-Contilena C, Wang Y, et al. Vitamin C pharmacokinetics in healthy volunteers: evidence for a recommended dietary allowance. Proc Natl Acad Sci U S A 93(8):3704-9, 1996

McCarron DA, Hatton D. Dietary calcium and lower blood pressure. We can all benefit. Editorial. JAMA 275(14):1128-9, 1996

Muerhcke RC. The fingernails in hypoalbuminuria: A new physical sign. Br Med J 195:1327-8, 1956

Nutrition Monitoring in the United States: A Progress Report form the Joint Nutrition Monitoring Evaluation Committee. DHHS Publication No. (PHS)86-1255. Washington, DC: US Gov't Printing Office, 1986

Pao EM, Mickle SJ. Problem nutrients in the United States. Food Technol 35:58 62,64,66-9,79, 1981

Pena As et al. Small intestinal mucosal abnormalities and disaccharidase activity in pernicious anaemia. Br J Haematol 23:313, 1972

Pfeiffer CC, Jenney EH. Fingernail white spots: possible zinc deficiency. Letter. JAMA 228(2):157, 1974

Rall L, Meydani S. Vitamin B6 and immune competence. Nutr Rev 51:217-25, 1993

Roubenoff R et al. Malnutrition among hospitalized patients. A problem of physician awareness. Arch Intern Med 147(8):1462-5, 1987

Runcie J. Folate deficiency in the elderly, in MI Botez, EH Reynolds, Eds. Folic Acid in Neurology, Psychiatry and Internal Medicine. New York, Raven Press, 1979

Sanstead HH. Zinc deficiency. A public health problem? Am J Dis Child 145(8):853-9, 1991

Sauberlich HE. Interactions of thiamin, riboflavin, and other B-vitamins. Ann N Y Acad Sci 355:80-97, 1980

Schoenemann HM et al. Consequences of severe copper deficiency are independent of dietary carbohydrate in young pigs. Am J Clin Nutr 52:147-54, 1990

Schultz BM, Freedman ML. Iron deficiency in the elderly. Baillieres Clin Haematol 1(2):291-313, 1987

Senti FR, Pilch SM. Analysis of folate data from the Second National Health and Nutrition Examination Survey. J Nutr 115:1398-1402, 1985

Southon S et al. Micronutrient undernutrition in British schoolchildren. Proc Nutr Soc 52:155-63, 1993

Spies TD et al. Pellagra, beriberi and riboflavin deficiency in human beings. JAMA 113(10):931-7, 1939

Stevens LJ et al. Essential fatty acid metabolism in boys with attention-deficit hyperactivity disorder. Am J Clin Nutr 62:761-8, 1995

Stevens LJ et al. Omega-3 fatty acids in boys with behavior, learning, and health problems. Physiol Behav 59(4-5):915-20, 1996

Subar AF et al. Folate intake and food sources in the US population. Am J Clin Nutr 50:508-16, 1989

Underwood BA. Vitamin A in human nutrition: public health considerations, in MB Sporn, AB Roberts, DS Goodman, Eds. The Retinoids: Biology, Chemistry and Medicine, 2nd edition. New York, Raven Press, 1994:211-27

van der Beek EJ et al. Combinations of low thiamine, riboflavin, vitamin B6 and vitamin C intake among Dutch adults. (Dutch Nutrition Surveillance System) J Am Coll Nutr 13(4):383-91, 1994

Van Goor LP et al. Review: cobalamin deficiency and mental impairment in elderly people. Age Ageing 24:536-42, 1995

Vermeer C et al. Effects of vitamin K on bone mass and bone metabolism. J Nutr 126:2287S-1191S, 1996

Werbach MR. Foundations of Nutritional Medicine. Chapter Two: Common nutritional deficiencies. Tarzana, CA, Third Line Press Inc., 1997

Wilkinson TJ, Hanger HC, Elmslie J, et al. The response to treatment of subclinical thiamine deficiency in the elderly. Am J Clin Nutr 66:925-8, 1997

LABORATORY TESTING IN NUTRITIONAL MEDICINE

MALNUTRITION

A number of laboratory studies have been used in the nutritional assessment of malnutrition; however, they are unlikely to uncover marginal malnutrition. Although **plasma or serum albumin** is a popular measure, sick patients may have low levels for several other reasons, such as inflammatory processes, gut losses due to gastrointestinal or cardiac disease, and renal losses due to kidney disease. Moreover, even when malnutrition is chronic, this measure is often normal because of compensatory mechanisms.

Typical laboratory findings include serum albumin of less than 3.5 g/dL, serum prealbumin concentration less than 10 mg/dL, total lymphocyte count less than 1,200 mm^3, and an anemia of chronic disease *(Ehrenpreis)*.

HYDROCHLORIC ACID DEFICIENCY

Since measuring **gastric acidity** directly by gastric intubation is uncomfortable for the patient, other methods have been devised. Analysis can be done using the Heidelberger pH capsule gastrointestinal radio transmitter or even with a simple, inexpensive gelatin capsule containing specially treated cotton floss (Gastro-Test®, Diagnos-Techs, USA, 206-251-0596; Diagnos-Techs-Biocare, Ltd., UK 21-433-3727).

Even when it is absent in the fasting state, acid production following the entry of food is often normal; thus testing must be performed after the patient is given a potent parietal cell stimulus *(Rappaport)*.

Basal **serum gastrin** measurement may also be helpful, as somewhat increased levels can be found in conditions associated with achlorhydria if the antrum is not severely affected - such as atrophic gastritis and pernicious anemia *(Ravel)*.

SPECIFIC NUTRIENT ABNORMALITIES

Calcium

Ionized calcium measures unbound serum calcium. It is a useful measure of calcium balance when it is low; however, normal levels do not rule out a negative calcium balance *(Albanese)*.

Hair calcium must be interpreted with caution, as a negative calcium balance may be accompanied by elevated hair levels. (This combination suggests that possibility of a nutritionally-induced secondary hyperparathyroidism related to a low calcium, high phosphorus diet *(Bland,1979)*.) Moreover, grey hair is naturally lower in calcium *(Cranton)*.

Chromium

Functional testing methods are currently the most dependable means of assessing chromium nutriture. If, for example, the diet can be strictly controlled for an adequate period of time, then **improvement of impaired glucose tolerance in response to chromium supplementation** will prove that chromium nutriture was deficient *(Glinsmann)*. Functional testing can also be performed by examining **the effect of glucose loading (usually 100 g) upon the serum chromium concentration**. When chromium nutriture is deficient, serum chromium may drop one hour after the glucose load; thus, following chromium supplementation, a reduction in this response compared to baseline suggests improved chromium status *(Lui)*.

Since the majority of absorbed chromium is excreted in the urine *(Anderson)*, **urinary chromium** is a reasonable measure of chromium absorption. **Hair chromium** may be of some value in indicating inadequate tissue chromium nutriture (Hunt), although it is believed to be unreliable except for severe deficiencies *(Hambridge)*. Neither **serum chromium** *(Sauberlich)* nor **whole blood chromium** *(Mertz)* is a useful measure of tissue stores.

Copper

Sensitive indicators of copper status include **platelet copper** *(Milne)* or **total erythrocyte copper** *(Halloran)*, as well as the activity of **erythrocyte superoxide dismutase** *(Hill)*, or **glutathione peroxidase** *(Milne)*, or of **platelet cytochrome c oxidase** *(Milne)*.

Serum *(Klevay)* and **plasma** (Milne) **copper**, as well as **whole blood copper** *(Kiem)* and **ceruloplasmin** *(Hill)*, are not useful indicators of copper nutriture, and **hair copper** may be deceptive *(Werbach)*.

When an increased body copper burden is suspected, as in Wilson's disease, a **D-penicillamine challenge test** will confirm the diagnosis *(Walshe)*.

Fatty Acids

The measurement of **fatty acids in the total phospholipid fraction of plasma and erythrocytes**, while probably the most practical method of assessing fatty acid nutriture, suffers from the lack of long-term prospective studies of apparently healthy populations. Such studies would uncover sub-groups whose levels may be contributing to illnesses that only later will appear *(Horrobin)*.

Folic Acid

Severe folate deficiency is accompanied by a macrocytic anemia, although the size of erythrocytes may be entirely normal in lesser degrees of depletion *(Craig)*. **Serum folate** tends to reflect dietary intake over the past few weeks, while **erythrocyte folate** is much less sensitive to short-term variations in folate balance *(Herbert,1987)*. However, folate depletion in erythrocytes occurs only in the later stages of folic acid deficiency and is usually accompanied by megaloblastic anemia; thus patients with both acquired and inherited folate deficiency may remain moderately deficient for months or years, taking in just enough folate to prevent low red cell folate concentrations and frank anemia *(Botez)*. Therefore, both erythrocyte and serum folate studies should be performed.

Moreover, when evaluating for folate deficiency, **serum vitamin B_{12}** levels should be measured as, when both vitamins are low, deficiency of either may be primary. This is because megaloblastic intestinal cells may not absorb properly, causing a secondary deficiency of the other vitamin *(Skelton)*. Moreover, a low erythrocyte folate level may occur in primary vitamin B_{12} deficiency, because vitamin B_{12} is necessary to keep methylfolate in red cells *(Skelton)*.

A **microbiological assay** is the preferred procedure for measuring total folic acid activity in serum, blood and tissues. Although a number of commercial radioassay kits are available for measuring folic acid levels in serum and erythrocytes, some uncertainties exist about the validity of the folate values obtained *(Piyathilake)*.

Urinary formiminoglutamic acid (FIGLU) excretion is another commonly used test for folate deficiency. However, FIGLU also rises in vitamin B_{12} deficiency and in liver disease, and thus high FIGLU excretion is not specific for the diagnosis *(Herbert,1962)*.

The determination of **hypersegmentation of neutrophils** is yet another useful measure of folate deficiency. Like FIGLU, however, hypersegmentation also occurs in vitamin B_{12} deficiency. Moreover, it is unreliable during pregnancy *(Sauberlich)*. In folate deficiency, the ratio of neutrophils with 5 or more 'lobes' to those with 4 'lobes' ranges from 31.5% to 116% *(Bills)*.

Iron

The best widely-available test (besides bone marrow aspiration) is a functional one, namely **whether iron supplementation results in a significant rise in circulating hemoglobin** *(Fairbanks)*. Another informative functional assay, which is capable of diagnosing mild deficiency, is the **change in plasma iron following iron supplementation** *(Crosby)*. Since iron deficiency may be manifest by a hypochromic, microcytic anemia, a standard **erythrocyte count** with measurement of the **erythrocyte indices** is a valuable screening procedure.

Among the indices, an increased **red cell distribution width** (RDW) reflects iron deficiency which has existed long enough to affect erythropoiesis and is usually an earlier marker than a low mean corpuscular volume (MCV) *(Bessman)*. While measurement of **hemoglobin** also reveals evidence of iron-deficiency anemia, it reflects only a late stage in the development of iron deficiency *(Tershakovec)*.

Ferritin is an important iron storage protein which is an indicator of total body iron storage; however, iron status is not necessarily proportional to serum ferritin levels *(Nuviala)*. **Transferrin saturation** is based on the ratio between serum iron and total iron binding capacity. As a measure of the level of mobilized, circulating iron, a low value (<16%) is diagnostic of iron-deficient erythropoiesis. However, it is not always the best indicator of low iron status, especially in children, and may only become abnormal after iron stores have been completely exhausted *(Finch)*. Even in confirmed cases, it can occasionally be normal *(Herbert,1992)*.

Serum iron is a poor measure of iron nutriture as iron may be deficient despite the normal serum iron levels *(Finch)*. **Hair iron** is poor measure of body stores; disturbed iron metabolism, as in malnutrition, will cause it to become elevated *(Weber)*.

Magnesium

With the exception of magnesium deficiency due to urinary losses, a **magnesium challenge test** is usually the best available method of assessing body stores. A baseline urine is obtained and magnesium chloride or magnesium sulfate 0.2 meq/kg body weight is given intravenously over a 4 hour period. A second urine is begun at challenge and continued over a 24 hour period. Deficiency is defined as less than 80% excretion of the amount of challenged magnesium *(JE Jones)*.

Sublingual epithelial cell magnesium has been shown to correlate with tissue magnesium in atrial biopsy specimens *(Haigney)*. However myocardial magnesium may fail to correlate with skeletal magnesium *(Ralston)*, thus limiting the ability of the test to suggest the adequacy of total body stores.

The recent development of an ion-selective electrode has made the measurement of **ionized magnesium** possible. However, variations in ionized magnesium in a given type of cell do not necessarily mean that similar changes exist in other cells or in the magnesium pool. As functional and organic disorders may alter the distribution of the ion in the analyzed cell, this measure cannot reliably indicate body magnesium nutriture *(Millart)*.

Unfortunately, the various blood magnesium parameters (such as **plasma, serum, erythrocyte and leukocyte magnesium**) may fail to correlate with one another *(Ralston)* or with **24-hour urinary excretion** *(Yang)*. This, of course, limits their utility in assessing body nutriture. Of the various blood parameters, white blood cell measures (such as **lymphocytes, mononuclear cells** or **total leukocytes**) appear to be better correlated with total body stores *(Werbach)*. As only 1% of body magnesium is extracellular, it is not surprising that serum magnesium is a very poor indicator of magnesium nutriture *(Werbach)*. Hair magnesium is also of limited value as it tends to become elevated when magnesium is being lost from bones and is lower in grey hair *(Cranton)*.

Manganese

Both **whole blood manganese** *(Keen)* and **lymphocyte manganese** *(Matsuda)* are considered to be reliable indicators of tissue manganese levels, and **serum manganese** is responsive to moderate manganese supplementation *(Davis)*. **Hair manganese** is also a reliable indicator of manganese status so long as the norms are adjusting for grey hair *(Guillard)*.

Niacin

Attempts to diagnose deficiency by measuring nicotinic acid in body fluids have proved disappointing; measurements of metabolites have been more meaningful *(Jacob)*.

The **urinary excretion of both N^1-methyl-nicotinamide and 1-methol-5-carboxylamide-2-pyridone**, the two major urinary metabolites, is a reasonably good measure of niacin status *(Jacob)*. **Erythrocyte nicotinamide adenine nucleotide** (NAD) also appears to be a sensitive indicator of niacin nutriture, and a ratio of erythrocyte NAD to erythrocyte nicotinamide nucleotide phosphate (NADP) below 1.0 may identify subjects at risk of developing a niacin deficiency *(Fu)*.

Pantothenic Acid

Blood pantothenic acid responds less readily to intake than **urinary pantothenic acid** although, in general, blood pantothenic acid levels decrease in subjects given a pantothenic acid-deficient diet *(Fry)*.

Phosphorus

A primary dietary phosphorus deficiency is not known to occur in humans. **Plasma/serum phosphorus** is mainly controlled by renal excretion and thus is not a useful measure of phosphorus nutriture. However, a low value suggests, not only a number of non-nutrition-related medical disorders (particularly primary hyperparathyroidism), but also malabsorption or vitamin D deficiency. Calcium and phosphorus have a reciprocal relationship so usually, when one rises, the other falls.

Hair phosphorus has little or no relationship to phosphorus metabolism in the body or to dietary phosphorus intake *(Passwater).*

Potassium

Erythrocyte potassium (or **whole blood potassium**) is superior to **serum or plasma potassium** as an index of cellular potassium stores *(Bahemuka).*

Hair potassium does not reflect dietary intake or body stores *(Passwater).*

Riboflavin

The procedure most commonly used to evaluate riboflavin nutriture is the measurement of **erythrocyte glutathione reductase (EGR) activity** and the **stimulation of EGR activity by the addition of flavin adenine dinucleotide in vitro**. Besides riboflavin status, several other factors may influence the findings. Certain nutrient deficiencies, such as thiamine, nicotinic acid and vitamin B_6, may reduce EGR activity, and both the age of the subject and the age of the red cell may influence it. Also, drugs may affect EGR activity directly, by reducing the life span of the red cell or by interfering with the assay procedure *(Roe).*

Blood riboflavin measures have not been good measure of riboflavin status due to difficulties in achieving accurate measurements. However, new analytical procedures may improve their validity. **Urinary riboflavin excretion** depends recent intake, but also upon nitrogen balance and kidney function *(Heller).*

Selenium

The definitive test for selenium deficiency remains **the response to selenium supplementation** *(Neve).* Of the available tests, **blood glutathione peroxidase** is one that has been shown to be a sensitive index of selenium nutriture *(Ganther).*

Hair selenium is also of value. It is correlated with selenium intake as well as with selenium concentrations in the liver, lung and renal cortex. However, the use of selenium-containing shampoos will falsely elevate hair selenium levels *(Werbach).*

Toenail selenium, while unaffected by dietary intake in the prior 3 months, is a reasonable measure of intake over the past 6 to 12 months *(Longnecker).* **Blood selenium** is of limited usefulness as, while it responds quickly to dietary intake *(Tarp)*, it tends to stay in the normal range except at the extremes of tissue selenium levels *(Lane).* **Urinary selenium**, although inadequate as an indicator of tissue nutriture, may be useful to confirm the results of blood selenium testing *(Valentine).*

Sodium

Serum sodium is commonly used as a measure of sodium nutriture. The principal cation of the extracellular fluid, any change in serum sodium is associated with a fluid shift into or out of the cell. Serum levels, however, do not reflect total body sodium content *(Webb).*

Hair sodium does not reflect dietary intake or body stores *(Passwater).*

Thiamine

The most commonly used procedure for assessing thiamine nutriture has been the measurement of **erythrocyte transketolase activity** and its **stimulation in vitro by the addition of thiamine pyrophosphate (the thiamine pyrophosphate effect)**. Because of the limitations of these two tests *(Werbach),* both should be performed together, along with an assessment of thiamine intake.

If available, the **erythrocyte thiamine diphosphate** level may be superior to the measurement of erythrocyte transketolase activity *(Baines).*

Vitamin A

While low concentrations of **plasma or serum retinol** are suggestive of frank deficiency, more subtle tests are needed to identify the presence of a marginal deficiency *(Werbach).* Of these, the **modified relative-dose-response test** is proving to be highly reliable, while **isotope dilution assay methods** (which measure total body reserves) are currently being refined *(Olson).*

Vitamin B_6

Pyridoxal-5'phosphate (PLP) and **pyridoxal** (PL), its hydrolysis product and the ultimate transport form of B_6, are the predominant vitamin B_6 vitamers in the circulation; measurement of both (preferably in the *erythrocytes* rather than in the *plasma*) is recommended *(Vermaak)*. The **urinary pyridoxic acid** level may give additional information to that obtained from a combination of pyridoxal phosphate and pyridoxal plasma levels, for example during pregnancy when plasma pyridoxal phosphate is decreased while plasma pyridoxal is increased *(Rogers)*.

The **activities of enzymes that are vitamin B_6-dependent** (such as transaminases) are of some value in assessing nutriture. However, they have a number of limitations *(Werbach)*.

Xanthurenic acid and kynurenine excretion after a tryptophan load most likely represents an aberrant reaction to the load and has no documented clinical significance. In addition, pregnancy and contraceptive pills may render the test abnormal due to inhibition of kynureninase by estrogens *(Baker)*.

Vitamin B_{12}

The diagnosis of vitamin B_{12} deficiency is often missed by routine laboratory tests, as many practitioners are unaware that the vitamin may be deficient despite normal **serum vitamin B_{12}** levels and the absence of a megaloblastic (large cell) anemia *(Delva)*. Moreover, serum vitamin B_{12} levels are often normal when cerebrospinal fluid vitamin B_{12} is deficient *(van Tiggelen)*. Most low serum cobalamin levels are not due to vitamin B_{12} deficiency but to gastric dysfunction in which protein-bound cobalamin is not digested; this can be corrected with oral administration of crystal cobalamin concentrate *(Yulin)*.

One reason why serum, as well as intracellular, vitamin B_{12} may be misleading relates to the binding of the newly absorbed vitamin to transcobalamin II, a transport protein, to form **holotranscobalamin II**; thus this measure indicates the earliest stage of a negative B_{12} balance that is measurable from the serum *(Herbert,1994)*. In the elderly, a decline of this transport protein results in higher serum B_{12} levels but lower intracellular B_{12} levels *(Yulin)*; therefore, although >150 pmol/L is usually considered as normal, older individuals with serum vitamin B_{12} of 150-250 pmol/L may also have a tissue B_{12} deficiency *(Metz)*.

Another problem with serum vitamin B_{12} assays is that it is commonly due using radioisotope dilution techniques, resulting in values that may be falsely increased due to the presence of inactive cobalamin analogues *(Cohen)*. The solution is to employ instead a **microbiological assay**, since the microorganism whose growth is measured following feeding of the patient's serum will be unaffected by the inactive analogues *(Lee D)*.

If patients have hematological, neuropsychiatric or gastrointestinal disorders suggestive of cobalamin deficiency even though their serum cobalamin levels are normal, intracellular cobalamin deficiency can be diagnosed by testing for elevated **serum methylmalonic acid** and **homocysteine** levels *(Stabler)*. The serum methylmalonic acid assay appears especially useful in evaluating vitamin B_{12} status in hepatic disease as serum vitamin B_{12} may be increased *(Hagelskjaer)*.

Moreover, when evaluating for vitamin B_{12} deficiency, **serum folate** levels should be measured as, when both vitamins are low, deficiency of either may be primary. This is because megaloblastic intestinal cells may not absorb properly, causing a secondary deficiency of the other vitamin *(Skelton)*. Moreover, a low **erythrocyte folate** level may occur in primary vitamin B_{12} deficiency, because vitamin B_{12} is necessary to keep methylfolate in red cells *(Skelton)*.

The **Schilling test** is a popular test of B_{12} absorption although, because it only tests absorption of free vitamin B_{12}, the test is often normal despite malabsorption of vitamin B_{12} from food resulting in low serum B_{12} levels *(Carmel)*.

The determination of **hypersegmentation of neutrophils** is a useful measure of vitamin B_{12} deficiency, and may sometimes uncover a deficiency which failed to depress serum vitamin B_{12} *(Bunting)*. However, it is unreliable during pregnancy and fails to distinguish between vitamin B_{12} and folate deficiencies *(Sauberlich)*.

Vitamin C

There is to date no satisfactory assay technique for ascorbic acid status. In addition to physiologic status, many other factors influence the levels present at any particular time *(Lee W)*. Once collected, ascorbic acid readily oxidizes to dehydroascorbic acid; however, this can be prevented by acidifying the specimen immediately upon collection.

Urinary ascorbic acid excretion declines to undetectable levels during vitamin C depletion *(Hodges)*. By itself it is an inadequate measure of body reserves; however, it serves as the basis of an **ascorbic acid saturation test** in which a 24-hour urine is collected and analyzed prior to and following oral supplementation of 1 gram of ascorbic acid daily. Urinary ascorbic acid will rise until saturation is achieved. Normally, this should take one to two days; however, in borderline to frank scurvy, it takes 7 to 10 day to achieve saturation *(Milner)*.

Among the blood vitamin C assays, **leukocyte ascorbic acid** is one of the better choices. As it responds less readily than serum ascorbic acid to recent dietary intake, it is probably more closely related to tissue stores *(Burr)*. It is unreliable, however, as it may be normal despite other evidence of vitamin C deficiency *(AJ Thomas)*. While serum or plasma ascorbic acid is not a particularly sensitive measure of vitamin C nutriture, low levels suggest inadequate intake and diminished reserves *(Sauberlich)*. Whole blood and erythrocyte ascorbic acid are even less sensitive indicators *(Sauberlich)*.

A **lingual ascorbic acid** test has been developed as a simple screening test for reduced tissue nutriture. A small amount of a dark blue chemical (N-2,6 dichlorphenolinodolphenol) is placed on the tongue, preferably under fasting conditions. The faster the color vanishes, the greater the tissue vitamin C concentration. While the results are consistent and significantly correlated with intradermal ascorbate levels *(Cheraskin)*, they are unrelated to either changes in vitamin C intake or with plasma or leukocyte concentrations *(Leggott)*, making the value of test controversial.

Vitamin D

The diagnosis of inadequate tissue stores is made by testing the **plasma 25-hydroxyvitamin D** level, preferably in the middle of the winter when the lack of sunshine makes a deficiency more likely. Measurement of **plasma 1,25-dihydroxyvitamin D**, the activated form of the vitamin, provides an index of current biological action; however, it should be interpreted in the light of concurrent mineral nutriture and physiological state *(Stanbury)*.

Vitamin E

While **adipose tissue vitamin E** is one of the best markers of vitamin E intake *(Kardinaal)*, **platelet tocopherol** appears to be the best blood measure *(Lehmann)*.

Since the vitamin is not associated with a protein carrier in the blood, but travels with the different lipoprotein fractions, **plasma and serum vitamin E** are closely correlated with total serum triglycerides *(Farrell)*. Therefore, when these levels are being measured, **tocopherol to triglyceride serum ratios** should be calculated to more accurately assess tocopherol status. The normal range of this ratio is 35 to 120 *(Bland, 1984)*.

Vitamin K

Subclinical deficiency, which may be substantial enough to cause adverse changes in bone metabolism, does not usually affect blood clotting parameters. An example is **prothrombin time** which can still be normal when the **prothrombin concentration** is only 50% of normal *(Ferland)*.

Plasma phylloquinone is considered to be a sensitive measure of vitamin K nutriture *(Sokoll)*. Vitamin K acts as a cofactor in a reaction that converts specific glutamic acid residues present in vitamin D-dependent proteins to gamma-carboxyglutamic acid. When the vitamin is even mildly deficient, abnormal, des-gamma-carboxy forms of these proteins referred to as PIVKA (protein induced by vitamin K deficiency or antagonism) are secreted in the plasma. **PIKVA concentration**, using a highly sensitive immunological method, is an excellent measure of vitamin K nutriture *(Blanchard)*. **Undercarboxylated osteocalcin** is yet another sensitive measure for evaluating vitamin K status *(Sokoll)*.

Zinc

Patients with **serum zinc** above 7.6 μmol/L (50 μg/dL) are considered unlikely to develop symptoms due to zinc deficiency (Alpers). However, as there is no adequate laboratory test *(Thompson)*, the best way to determine whether an abnormality is due to a borderline or mild zinc deficiency is to perform a therapeutic trial.

Since **serum**, **salivary**, **urinary** and **hair zinc** are poorly correlated, a **zinc tolerance test** is perhaps the best available method of determining body zinc nutriture. After a fast, a baseline plasma level is drawn, and an oral loading dose of zinc sulfate 220 mg (50 mg elemental zinc) is given. Two hours later, plasma zinc is redrawn. A two or threefold increase in plasma zinc is indicative of zinc inadequacy *(Capel)*.

Of the various blood parameters, measures of zinc in **leukocytes** *(RB Jones)* and **platelets** *(Prasad,1988)* are more sensitive than in **plasma, serum** or **erythrocytes** *(Prasad,1985)*. **Sweat zinc** is also a sensitive index of zinc status *(Davies)*. While depressed **hair zinc** reliably indicates depletion (unless there is external contamination), normal or even high values do not rule out low body stores *(Davies)*.

A simple **zinc taste test** has been developed which suggests that there will be a favorable response to zinc supplementation uses a test solution made by dissolving zinc sulfate 1 gm in 1 liter of distilled water (0.1% solution). If the subject tasting 5 to 10 ml notes either no taste or a dry and furry taste developing after a few minutes, zinc supplementation is suggested. Adequate zinc nutriture is suggested by an immediate taste which may be strong and unpleasant *(Bryce-Smith)*. This test, however, has not been well-validated and, in its present form, appears to be of limited value *(Nichols)*.

Other tests that appear to be of some value include measurement of **neutrophil alkaline phosphatase activity** *(Prasad,1985)*, the enzyme **5'-nucleotidase** *(Bales)*, and **erythrocyte metallothionein** *(EA Thomas)*.

OTHER LABORATORY TESTS

Any of a wide variety laboratory studies can be valuable in evaluating a particular patient. So many tests are available that they need to be chosen carefully. Certainly, tests measuring the functioning of the various body systems are sometimes indicated; these are well discussed in standard medical texts. Stool analysis and tests for intestinal permeability and liver detoxification should also be considered for patients presenting with nonspecific complaints and an inconclusive physical examination.

REFERENCES

Albanese A. Bone Loss: Causes, Detection and Therapy. New York, Alan R. Liss, Inc., 1977

Alpers DH. Zinc and deficiencies of taste and smell. Questions and Answers. JAMA 272(16):1233-4, 1994

Anderson RA, Kozlovsky AS. Chromium intake, absorption and excretion of subjects consuming self-selected diets. Am J Clin Nutr 41:1177-83, 1985

Bahemuka M, Hodkinson HM. Red-blood-cell potassium as a practical index of potassium status in elderly patients. Age Ageing 5:24, 1976

Baines M, Davies G. The evaluation of erythrocyte thiamine diphosphate as an indicator of thiamine status in man, and its comparison with erythrocyte transketolase activity measurements. Ann Clin Biochem 25:698-705, 1988

Baker H. Analysis of vitamin status. J Med Soc N J 80:633-6, 1983

Bales CW et al. Marginal zinc deficiency in older adults: responsiveness of zinc status indicators. J Am Coll Nutr 13(5):455-62, 1994

Bessman JD, McClure S. Red cell distribution width in alcohol abuse and iron deficiency anemia. JAMA 267(8):1070-1, 1992

Bills T, Spatz L. Neutrophilic hypersegmentation as an indication of incipient folic acid deficiency. Am J Clin Pathol 68(2):263, 1977

Blanchard RA et al. Acquired vitamin K-dependent carboxylation deficiency in liver disease. N Engl J Med 30(5)5:242-8, 1981

Bland J, Prestbo E. Vitamin E: Comparative absorption studies. Int Clin Nutr Rev 4(2):82-6, 1984

Bland J. dietary calcium, phosphorus and their relationships to bone formation and parathyroid activity. J John Bastyr College of Naturopathic Medicine 1:3-7, 1979

Botez MI et al. Neurologic disorders responsive to folic acid therapy. Can Med Assoc J 115:217-22, 1976

Bryce-Smith D, Simpson RID. Anorexia, depression, and zinc deficiency. Lancet ii:1162, 1984

Bunting RW, Pachas WN. Neutrophil hypersegmentation may unmask vitamin B 12 deficiency in patients with normal serum B12 levels. J Am Geriatr Soc 45(5):657-8, 1997

Burr ML et al. Plasma and leukocyte ascorbic acid levels in the elderly. Am J Clin Nutr 27:144, 1974

Capel ID et al. The assessment of zinc status by the zinc tolerance test in various groups of patients. Clin Biochem 15(5):257-60, 1982

Carmel R et al. Food-cobalamin malabsorption occurs frequently in patients with unexplained low serum cobalamin levels. Arch Intern Med 148:1715-19, 1988

Cheraskin E. Vitamin C and stomatology: a mouthful of evidence. J Orthomol Med 6(3-4):147-54, 1991

Cohen KL, Donaldson RM Jr. Unreliability of radiodilution assays as screening tests for cobalamin (vitamin B12) deficiency. JAMA October 24, 1980, pp. 1942-5

Craig GM et al. Masked vitamin B12 and folate deficiency in the elderly. Br J Nutr 54(3):613-19, 1985

Cranton EM. Update on hair element analysis in clinical medicine. J Holistic Med. 7(2):120-34, 1985

Crosby WH, O'Neill-Cutting MA. A small dose iron tolerance test as an indicator of mild iron deficiency. JAMA 251(15):1986-7, 1984

Davies S. Assessment of zinc status. Int Clin Nutr Rev 4(3):122-9, 1984

Davis CD, Greger JL. Longitudinal changes of manganese-dependent superoxide dismutase and other indexes of manganese and iron status in women. Am J Clin Nutr 55:747-52, 1992

Delva MD. Vitamin B12 replacement. To B12 or not to B12? Can Fam Physician 43:917-22, 1997

Ehrenpreis ED et al. A practical guide to the recognition of nutritional deficiencies. Comp Ther 23(3):218-22, 1997

Fairbanks VF. Laboratory testing for iron status. Hosp Pract 26(suppl 3):17-24, 1991

Farrell PM, Biere JG. Megavitamin E supplementation in man. Am J Clin Nutr 28(12):1381-6, 1975

Ferland G. Subclinical vitamin K deficiency: recent developments. Nutr Rep 12(1), January, 1994

Finch CA. Editorial: Evaluation of iron status. JAMA 251(15):2004, 1984

Fry PC et al. Metabolic response to a pantothenic acid deficient diet in humans. J Nutr Sci Vitaminol 22:339-46, 1976

Fu CS et al. Biochemical markers for assessment of niacin status in young men: levels of erythrocyte niacin coenzymes and plasma tryptophan. J Nutr 119(12):1949-55, 1989

Gans DA, Harper AE. Thiamine status of incarcerated and nonincarcerated adolescent males: dietary intake and thiamin pyrophosphate response. Am J Clin Nutr 53:1471-5, 1991

Ganther HE et al. Selenium and glutathione peroxidase in health and disease - a review, in AS Prasad, D Overleas, Eds. Trace Elements in Human Health and Disease, Volume II. New York, Academic Press, 1976:165

Glinsmann WH et al. Plasma chromium after glucose administration. Science 152:1243-5, 1966

Guillard O et al. Manganese concentration in the hair of greying ('salt and pepper') men reconsidered. Clin Chem 31(7):1251, 1985

Hagelskjaer L, Rasmussen K. Methylmalonic acid concentration in serum not affected by hepatic disease. Clin Chem 38(4):493-5, 1992

Haigney MCP et al. Noninvasive measurement of tissue magnesium and correlation with cardiac levels. Circulation 92(8):2190-7, 1995

Halloran SP, in DF Williams, Ed. Copper In Systemic Aspects Of Biocompatability, Vol. 1. Boca Raton FL, CDC Press, 1981:211

Hambridge KM. Chromium nutrition in man. Am J Clin Nutr 27:505-14, 1974

Heller S et al. Riboflavin status in pregnancy. Am J Clin Nutr 27:1225-30, 1974

Herbert V. Staging vitamin B-12 (cobalamin) status in vegetarians. Am J Clin Nutr 59(suppl):1213S-22S, 1994

Herbert V. Everyone should be tested for iron disorders. J Am Diet Assoc 92(12):1502-9, 1992

Herbert V. Making sense of laboratory test of folate status: folate requirements to sustain normality. Am J Hematol 26:199-207, 1987

Herbert V. Experimental nutritional folate deficiency in man. Trans Assoc Am Phys 75:307-20, 1962

Hill G, Edes TE. Diabetes and carbohydrates: The copper connection. JAMA 257(19):2593, 1987

Horrobin DF. Nutritional and medical importance of gamma-linolenic acid. Prog Lipid Res 31(2):163-94, 1992

Jacob RA et al. Biochemical markers for assessment of niacin status in young men: urinary and blood levels of niacin metabolites. J Nutr 119(4):591-8, 1989

Jones JE et al. Magnesium requirements in adults. Med J Clin Nutr 20:632-5, 1967

Jones RB et al. The relationship between leukocyte and muscle zinc in health and disease. Clin Sci 60:237-9, 1981

Kardinaal A et al. Relations between antioxidant vitamins in adipose-tissue, plasma, and diet. Am J Epidemiol 141(5):440-50, 1995

Keen CL et al. Whole blood manganese as an indicator of body manganese. N Engl J Med 308:1230, 1983

Kiem J et al. Sampling and sample preparation of platelets for trace element analysis in nuclear activation techniques in the life sciences, 1978. IAEA, Vienna, 1979:143

Klevay LM. Re: serum copper and the risk of acute myocardial infarction: a prospective population study in men in eastern Finland. Letter. Am J Epidemiol 135(7):832-4, 1992

Lane HW et al. Blood selenium and glutathione peroxidase levels and dietary selenium of free living and institutionalized elderly subjects. Proc Soc Exp Biol Med 173(1):87-95, 1985

Lee DSC, Griffiths BW. B-12 assay methods. Clin Biochem 18:261-6, 1985

Lee W et al. Ascorbic acid status: Biochemical and clinical considerations. Am J Clin Nutr 48:286-90, 1988

Leggott PJ et al. Response of lingual ascorbic acid test and salivary ascorbate levels to changes in ascorbic acid intake. J Dent Res 65(2):131-4, 1986

Lehmann J et al. Vitamin E and relationships among tocopherols in human plasma, platelets, lymphocytes, and red blood cells. Am J Clin Nutr 47:470-4, 1988

Longnecker MP et al. A 1-y trial of the effect of high-selenium bread on selenium concentrations in blood and toenails. Am J Clin Nutr 57:408-13, 1993

Lui VJK, Morris S. Relative chromium response as an indicator of chromium status. Am J Clin Nutr 31:972-6, 1978

Matsuda A et al. Quantifying manganese in lymphocytes to assess manganese nutritional status. Clin Chem 35(9):1939-41, 1989

Mertz W. Chromium occurrence and function in biological systems. Physiol Rev 49(2):163-239, 1969

Metz J et al. The significant of subnormal serum vitamin B12 concentration in older people: a case control study. J Am Geriatr Soc 44(11):1355-61, 1996

Millart H et al. Red blood cell magnesium concentrations: analytical problems and significance. Magnes Res 8(1):65-76, 1995

Milne DB, Nielsen FH. Effects of a diet low in copper on copper-status indicators in postmenopausal women. Am J Clin Nutr 63:358-64, 1996

Milner G. Br J Psychiatry 109:294-9, 1963

Neve J et al. Selenium deficiency. Clin Endocrinol Metab 14(3):629-56, 1985

Nichols J et al. Postnatal depression and zinc status - a preliminary study. J Nutr Med 3:35-42, 1992

Nuviala RJ, Lapieza MG. Disparity between diet and serum ferritin in elite sportswomen. Nutr Res 17:451-61, 1997

Olson JA. Vitamin A, in EE Ziegler, LJ Filer Jr, Eds. Present Knowledge in Nutrition, 7th edition. Washington, DC, ILSI Press, 1996

Passwater RA, Cranton EM. Trace Elements, Hair Analysis and Nutrition. New Canaan, Connecticut, Keats Publishing, 1983:61

Piyathilake CJ et al. Comparison of microbiological assay with radio assay for the determination of tissue folates. Abstract. Am J Clin Nutr 66:212, 1997

Prasad AS. Zinc in growth and development and spectrum of human zinc deficiency. J Am Coll Nutr 7(5):377-84, 1988

Prasad AS. Laboratory diagnosis of zinc deficiency. J Am Coll Nutr 4(6):591-8, 1985

Ralston MA et al. Magnesium content of serum, circulating mononuclear cells, skeletal muscle, and myocardium in congestive heart failure. Circulation 80(3):573-80, 1989

Rappaport EM. Achlorhydria: Associated symptoms and response to hydrochloric acid. N Engl J Med 252(19):802-5, 1955

Ravel R. Clinical Laboratory Medicine. Third Edition. Chicago, Year Book Medical Publishers, 1978:399

Roe DA. Diet and Drug Interactions. New York, Van Nostrand Reinhold, 1989:141

Rogers K, Mohan C. Vitamin B6 metabolism and diabetes. Biochem Med Metab Biol 52:10-17, 1994

Sauberlich HE et al. Laboratory Tests For The Assessment Of Nutritional Status. Florida, CRC Press, 1984

Skelton WP III, Skelton NK. Deficiency of vitamins A, B, and C. Something to watch for. Postgrad Med 87(4):293-310, 1990

Sokoll LJ, Sadowski JA. Comparison of biochemical indexes for assessing vitamin K nutritional status in a healthy adult population. Am J Clin Nutr 63:566-73, 1996

Stabler SP et al. The use of homocysteine and other metabolites in the specific diagnosis of vitamin B-12 deficiency. J Nutr 126(4 Suppl):1266S-71272S, 1996

Stanbury SW. Vitamin D: metamorphosis from nutrient to hormonal system. Proc Nutr Soc 40:179-86, 1981

Tershakovec AM, Weller SC. Iron status of inner-city elementary school children: lack of correlation between anemia and iron deficiency. Am J Clin Nutr 54:1071-6, 1991

Thomas AJ et al. Is leucocyte ascorbic acid an unreliable estimate of vitamin C deficiency? Age Ageing 13(4):243-7, 1984

Thomas EA et al. Erythrocyte metallothionein response to dietary zinc in humans. J Nutr 122:2408-14, 1992

Thompson RP. Assessment of zinc status. Proc Nutr Soc 50(1):19-28, 1991

Valentine JL et al. Selenium levels in human blood, urine and hair in response to exposure via drinking water. Environ Res 17:347-55, 1978

van Tiggelen CJ et al. Assessment of vitamin B12 status in CSF. Letter. Am J Psychiatry 141(1):136-7, 1984

Vermaak WJH et al. Vitamin B-6 nutrition status and cigarette smoking. Am J Clin Nutr 51:1958-61, 1990

Walshe JM. The discovery of the therapeutic use of D-penicillamine. J Rheumatol (Suppl 7) 8:3-8, 1981

Webb WL, Gehi M. Electrolyte and fluid imbalance: neuropsychiatric manifestations. Psychosomatics 22(3):199-203, 1981

Weber CW et al. Trace elements in the hair of healthy and malnourished children. J Trop Pediatr 36(5):230-4, 1990

Werbach MR. Foundations of Nutritional Medicine. Chapter Nine: Laboratory methods for nutritional evaluation. Tarzana, CA, Third Line Press Inc., 1997

Yang XY et al. Blood and urine magnesium parameters compared. Abstract. J Am Coll Nutr 8(5):462, 1989

Yulin Y et al. Decline of serum cobalamin levels with increasing age among geriatric outpatients. Arch Fam Med 3:918-22, 1994

OVERVIEW OF THE CLINICAL USE OF NUTRITIONAL SUPPLEMENTS

In recent decades, advances in the discovery, isolation and synthesis of vitamins, minerals, amino acids, fatty acids and other nutrients have resulted in the availability of numerous substances provided in various formulations designed to supplement the diet in order to improve health, prevent illness and promote healing.

When should these supplements be recommended to patients? The answer to the question is highly controversial in the light of blanket statements against the use of nutritional supplements that have been made by major mainstream professional organizations. We believe such blanket statements to be unwarranted, and will try to give you enough background on the issue to put it in what we believe to be a reasonable perspective.

While there are unique considerations concerning the therapeutic indications for each nutrient, there are certain general issues that need to be addressed before health practitioners can make informed decisions. In order to properly address these issues, we will arbitrarily divide the general field of nutritional medicine into two parts: nutrient repletion and nutrient pharmacotherapy.

NUTRIENT REPLETION

Nutrient repletion consists of identifying nutritional deficiencies, prescribing appropriate foods and dietary supplements to attempt to correct those deficiencies, and monitoring progress. Some of these deficiencies are due to hunger, defined as a condition where health is threatened because a person repeatedly fails to consume adequate nutrients.

Hunger is not a problem that is confined to developing countries. In the United States today, for example, hunger remains a problem of great magnitude. In 1985, a national task force led by the director of Tufts University's Center on Hunger, Poverty and Nutrition Policy estimated that 20 million Americans suffered from hunger. In 1992, a follow-up study found that this figure had risen to 30 million, a 50% increase in just seven years *(AMA News)*. If the population of the United States is 250 million, then twelve percent of the population is liable to be nutritionally deficient.

Analyses of the adequacy of the diet for health usually use the Recommended Dietary Allowances as a measure of nutrient adequacy. These standards (RDAs) have been developed by the Food and Nutrition Board of the National Research Council (U.S.) as *"the levels of intake of essential nutrients that, on the basis of scientific knowledge, are judged by the Food and Nutrition Board to be adequate to meet the known nutrient needs of practically all healthy persons (RDA)."*

RDA levels are intentionally set high in order to provide a large margin of safety above the level of nutrient intake at which the earliest evidence of a deficiency begins to appear. For this reason, an intake of less than 70% of the RDA is often used as a measure below which a person is considered to be at risk of developing a deficiency of that nutrient.

When this measure is used as a cutoff point to analyze the data collected by the large surveys of food consumption by Americans, the results suggest that micronutrient deficiency are common. For example, analysis of data from the USDA Nationwide Food Consumption Survey, conducted between 1977 and 1978, showed that up to half of all individuals surveyed may be at least marginally deficient in vitamin B_6, almost one-third may be at least marginally deficient in vitamin A, and one-quarter may be at least marginally deficient in vitamin C *(Pao)*.

These data should not be taken as proof of widespread micronutrient deficiencies as the actual prevalence of micronutrient deficiencies in the survey populations was not studied and the methodology used in large dietary surveys tends to have many flaws *(NRC)*. Moreover, cutoff points are misleading since a sizable percentage of the people surveyed actually require either a higher or lower intake of specific nutrients to meet their needs *(NRC)*.

Micronutrient deficiencies are likely to be particularly common for several sub-groups of the population who have repeatedly been shown to be at greater risk of becoming nutritionally deficient either because of increased needs or because of reduced intake. In addition to the poor, they include adolescents, moderate to heavy consumers of alcohol, cigarette smokers, drug users, diabetics, women who are pregnant, lactating or on oral contraceptives, dieters, vegans, the chronically ill, the elderly and people with certain genetic disorders.

For example, analysis of data from the First Health and Nutrition Examination Survey conducted by the National Center for Health statistics between 1971 and 1972 showed that 40% of elderly people failed to consume two-thirds of the RDA for vitamin C, 28% failed to consume two-thirds of the RDA for calcium, 26% for vitamin A and 24% for iron *(Norton)*. Examination and testing of people taken from these sub-populations has tended to confirm the suggestion of nutritional surveys that deficiencies are indeed common. As an example, in the United States, roughly five to ten percent of people over 60 years of age have clinical findings associated with vitamin deficiency *(Bowman)*.

Gross malnutrition, advanced disease and genetic factors may foster the development of severe nutrient deficiencies. These present with numerous signs and symptoms, many of which are traceable to structural lesions and even to organ failure. Frequently, however, nutrient deficiencies are only marginal; in this case, there may be no evidence of organic pathology, yet the deficiencies may adversely affect the body's ability to maintain health in the face of biological and psychological stressors *(Brin)*.

Most of the evidence for the adverse effects of marginal nutrient deficiencies has come from studies of vitamins. Numerous biological changes are now known to be associated with marginal deficiencies, including fetal abnormalities, interference with the production or composition of breast milk, growth retardation, increased susceptibility to infection, altered response to dietary constituents and the promotion of degenerative tissue changes *(Thurnham)*. Neuropsychological symptoms such as lethargy, irritability, insomnia and difficulty concentrating may develop *(Marginal Vitamin Deficiency)* which, on testing, are associated with objective deficits in cognitive performance; moreover, these deficits can be correlated with electroencephalographic indices of neuropsychological function *(Tucker)*.

Risks

Although, in general, nutrient repletion is quite safe, there is the danger that repletion of one nutrient may worsen a deficiency of another that is not being supplemented. The competitive interaction of copper and zinc is one of the most widely studied. Just a modest increase in dietary zinc can reduce copper absorption *(Forbes)* and, occasionally, even produce a copper-deficiency anemia *(Gordon)*. Zinc also interferes with the intestinal absorption of iron to the extent that zinc supplementation can result in impaired iron nutriture *(Yadrick)*.

So long as nutrient repletion is accomplished by improving the diet, such negative interactions would not be expected to be a problem. A varied diet rich in the nutrients found to be deficient is likely to contain sufficient quantities of micronutrients whose adequacy may be threatened by negative interactions, including those that are marginally deficient but may not have been identified as such.

Sometimes however, a recommendation for improving the diet, even with detailed instructions, is not sufficient to result in adequate nutrient repletion. Patients may fail to follow the recommendation over the long term due to inadequate motivation to make what for them may be a major lifestyle change. Also, a healthy diet, while adequate to *prevent* nutritional deficiencies in most of the general population, may still prove to be inadequate to fully *replete* pre-existing deficiencies. The failure may be due to poor nutrient absorption or to a *nutrient dependency*, that is, a requirement for an unusually large amount of a nutrient to achieve an adequate state of nutriture to satisfy metabolic needs.

For example, some people have an inborn deficiency of the enzyme cystathionine beta-synthase. This enzyme is quite important as it metabolizes homocysteine, a toxic amino acid that contributes to the development of atherosclerosis. For about half of the people with cystathionine beta-synthase deficiency, high supplementary doses of vitamin B_6 will push the reaction forward, markedly reducing or even eliminating the biochemical abnormalities *(Mudd)*. In other words, this sub-group is dependent upon doses of vitamin B_6 well in excess of the RDA in order to prevent their genetic abnormality from promoting the development of atherosclerotic changes.

When dietary recommendations are not adequate to correct nutritional deficiencies, repletion may also require nutrient supplementation. Nutrient repletion using dietary supplements has certain risks which should be considered. Since supplementation consists of a limited list of nutrients, some nutrient deficiencies may not be identified and thus supplemented. Moreover, nutrients that negatively interact with the ones being supplemented may not be provided in adequate dosages to prevent their further depletion. Finally, the active substance may be formulated with other ingredients to facilitate its administration and increase its bioavailability. These preservatives, vehicles and excipients, although considered therapeutically inactive, may occasionally be the cause of adverse reactions *(Napke)*.

These risks can easily be minimized, however, by the addition of carefully chose supplements to a sound diet. Given the obvious benefits of nutrient repletion, they appear to be only a minor consideration.

NUTRIENT PHARMACOTHERAPY

Nutrient pharmacotherapy refers to the use of nutrients, often at dosages well in excess of the recommended dietary allowances, for the purpose of preventing or treating illnesses that are not caused by nutrient deficiencies.

An impressive amount of data suggests that nutrients provided above their RDA level can reduce the risk of illness although, in most cases, the efficacy of preventive nutrient supplementation in greater than RDA dosages has yet to be demonstrated by long-term, randomized, double-blind studies.

As an example of the growing epidemiological evidence, more than 11,000 non-institutionalized adults were followed for a median of 10 years and mortality was related to their total vitamin C intake. The relationship between the standardized mortality ratio for all causes of death and increasing vitamin C intake was found to be strongly inverse for males and weakly inverse for females. The adult RDA for vitamin C is 60 mg daily. When males with a daily vitamin C intake in the 300 to 400 mg range were compared to those who consume less than 50 mg a day, their death rate was 35% lower, while the death rate for females was 10% lower. Even after adjustment for the usual confounding variables, the relationship between vitamin C intake and mortality remained for the males *(Enstrom)*.

In regard to the treatment of established illness, controlled studies demonstrating the efficacy of high-dose nutrient supplementation continue to appear in the literature - although most of the evidence supporting the thousands of applications of nutrient pharmacotherapy is so far only preliminary in nature. Some of the better proven applications include niacin supplementation to reduce elevated cholesterol levels, pyridoxine to reduce infantile seizures and premenstrual symptoms, folic acid in early pregnancy to prevent neural tube defects, and magnesium in acute coronary insufficiency to reduce the risk of myocardial infarction, cardiac arrhythmias and death.

Risks

The risks of nutrient pharmacotherapy can be considerably greater than those of nutrient repletion. Nutrient pharmacotherapy shares with nutrient repletion the risk of negative interactions with other nutrients. However, because of the relatively larger dosages that are provided, the possibility of creating deficiencies is substantially greater.

If a person is taking a medication, nutrient/drug interactions are of concern. Examples are folic acid supplements which decrease the anticonvulsant action of phenytoin, and calcium supplements which practically nullify the efficacy of tetracycline if the two are taken together. (Many of these interactions can be avoided by instructing patients to take their supplements an hour before or at least two hours after taking medication.)

An important risk that is not encountered in nutrient repletion in the risk of nutrient toxicity. Fortunately, the body has a number of mechanisms unique to nutrients for preventing high doses from becoming toxic. For example, as the oral dose of some of the vitamins, major minerals, trace elements and amino acids, as well as the oral dose of glucose, increases beyond a threshold, the percentage of absorption from the gut is reduced. Similarly, the percentage of the dosage excreted tends to increase as the dosage of a nutrient is increased beyond a threshold.

While they add a considerable measure of safety to nutrient pharmacotherapy, these protective biological adjustments can become overwhelmed if the supplemental dosages are too high. Other factors, such as the storage of fat-soluble vitamins in body tissues, also contribute to the danger of toxicity from high dosages of nutrients, particularly when given over a long time period.

The margin of safety between the effective pharmacologic dose of a nutrient and toxicity is highly variable. A number of nutrients, such as vitamin B_{12}, have no known toxicity at any dose. Most, such as calcium, are only therapeutic at doses well below their minimum toxic dose, while a few, such as vitamin A, are sometimes utilized at doses that are at the low end of their toxic range. The chart below summarizes the Recommended Dietary Allowances, Maximal Daily Treatment Dosages and Lowest Observed Adverse Effect Levels (LOAELs) of important vitamins and minerals. (It is important to realize that the lack of an established LOAEL does not mean that a high dosage is necessarily safe.)

NUTRIENT PHARMACOTHERAPY: RISK OF TOXICITY

Nutrient	Adult RDA⁺	Maximum Daily Treatment Dosage#	Lowest Observed Adverse Effect Level*
biotin	30-100 µg**	16 mg	[none established]
calcium	1,000-1,200 mg^	3,000 mg	>2,500 mg
chromium [Cr^{+++}]	50 - 200 mg**	3,000 mg	[none established]
copper	1.5 - 3 mg**	10 mg	[none established]
fluoride	3.8 mg^	80 mg	4 - 20 mg~
folic acid	180 mg (f) 200 µg (m)	75,000 mg	5,000 mg
iodine	150 mg	230 mg	[none established]
iron	15 mg (f) 10 mg (m)	200 mg	100 mg
magnesium	310-320 mg^^ (f)	1,000 mg	[none established]
	400-420 mg^^ (m)	1,000 mg	[none established]
manganese	2 - 5 mg**	190 mg	[none established]
molybdenum	75-250 mg**	2,000 mg	[none established]
niacin	13-15 mg (f) 15-19 mg (m)	4,500 mg	500-1,000 mg++
pantothenic acid	4-7 mg**	1,000 mg	[none established]
phosphorus	700 mg^^	1,500 mg	>2,500 mg
riboflavin	1.2-1.3 (f) 1.4-1.7 mg (m)	400 mg	[none established]
selenium	55 mg (f) 70 µg (m)	1,000 mg	910 mg
thiamin	1-1.1 mg (f) 1.2-1.5 mg (m)	1,500 mg	[none established]
vitamin A	2,670 IU (f) 3,340 IU (m)	150,000 IU	21,600 IU
vitamin B_6	1.6 mg (f) 2.0 mg (m)	1,500 mg	500 mg
vitamin B_{12}	2 mg	2,000 mg	[none established]
vitamin C	60 mg	200,000 mg	[none established]
vitamin D	400-1200 IU^	1,600 IU	2,000 IU
vitamin E	8.8-12 IU (f) 11-15 IU (m)	2,500 IU	[none established]
vitamin K	65 mg (f) 80 mg (m)	100 mg	[none established]
zinc	12 mg (f) 15 mg (m)	150 mg	60 mg

+ = excluding pregnant or lactating women (*except as noted: from the 10th edition, Recommended Dietary Allowances. Washington, DC, National Academy Press, 1989*)

= maximum effective dosage suggested by experimental studies (*see Werbach MR. Nutritional Influences on Illness CD-ROM. Tarzana, CA, Third Line Press Inc., 1998*).

* = *from Hathcock JN. Vitamin and Mineral Safety. Washington, DC, Council for Responsible Nutrition, 1997, and Hathcock JN. Vitamins and minerals: efficacy and safety. Am J Clin Nutr 66:427-37, 1997*

^ = Adequate Intake (*from Dietary Reference Intakes for Calcium, Phosphorus, Magnesium, Vitamin D, and Fluoride. Washington, DC, National Academy Press, 1997*)

^^ = Recommended Dietary Allowance (*from Dietary Reference Intakes for Calcium, Phosphorus, Magnesium, Vitamin D, and Fluoride. Washington, DC, National Academy Press, 1997*)

** = Estimated Safe & Adequate Intake *(from the 10th edition, Recommended Dietary Allowances. Washington, DC, National Academy Press, 1989)*

~ = Hathcock JN. Quantitative evaluation of vitamin safety. Pharmacy Times May, 1985 pp. 104-13

++ = greater than 500 mg for nicotinic acid or 1 g for nicotinamide (1/2 the dosages for sustained release preparations)

NUTRIENTS VERSUS DRUGS (FOREIGN SUBSTANCES) FOR PHARMACOTHERAPY

Nutrients are biological precursors for, or participants in, metabolic processes. Whether they are endogenously synthesized or gain entry to the body as foods, they are normally present, and both their absorption, metabolism and excretion proceed according to physiological mechanisms that are established and in continuous action for that very purpose *(Schneider-Helmert)*. Drugs, by contrast, are foreign substances not normally present in the body; their absorption, metabolism and excretion proceed via detoxification pathways designed for xenobiotics.

In addition to the risks we discussed in regard to nutrient repletion, three other risk factors are shared by drugs and nutritional medicines. First, both seek to alter homeostatic processes; thus adverse effects may develop that can be due to exaggerated responses to their pharmacological effects. (These reactions can often be minimized by reducing the dosage.) Second, there may be unpredictable "allergic" reactions, such as an uncommon reaction to an injection of thiamine at a pharmacological dosage. Lastly, on rare occasions impurities formed during the manufacturing process may cause untoward reactions. Eosinophilia-myalgia syndrome, for example, has been largely traced to a contaminant formed during the manufacture of L-tryptophan *(Belongia)*.

When we compare the risk/benefit ratio of nutrient pharmacotherapy with that of drugs, a general conclusion is more difficult to make. The risks of some nutrients in pharmacological doses are more serious than they are when used at RDA doses, while proof of their efficacy is generally more tenuous than is proof of the efficacy of governmentally-approved drugs.

One generalization we can make is that, for drugs, as compared to nutrients, the therapeutic range generally appears to be much closer to the bottom of the toxic range. This is a powerful argument for evaluating patients for nutritional intervention prior to considering the use of medications.

Adverse reactions to drugs are common and sometimes serious. In the United States alone, the cost of morbidity and mortality from prescription drugs is roughly $76 billion annually *(Johnson)*. A crude estimate is that hospitalizable illness results from one out of every 500 long-term drug treatments per year *(Jick)*. One out of seven hospital days is devoted to the care of drug toxicity *(Melmon)*, one out of three hospital patients suffers from obvious adverse effects of drugs *(Jick)* and an adverse reaction occurs among hospitalized patients once out of every twenty drug exposures *(Jick)*.

Because of the substantial danger of drug toxicity, prescription errors are of concern. Roughly 1% of these errors causes the patient to have notable adverse effects *(Bates)*. Unfortunately, the frequency of dangerous prescription errors appears to be rapidly rising. In one hospital study, for example, the annual number of errors with potential for adverse patient consequences increased more than 400% between 1987 and 1995 *(Lesar)*.

Few statistics comparing the frequency of drug reactions to supplement reactions are available; however notable adverse effects of nutritional supplements, even at pharmacological dosages, appear to be extremely rare. The FDA estimates that 40% of the adult population is taking nutritional supplements *(Stewart)*, so this apparent difference is unlikely to be due to a higher prevalence of medication use than of nutritional supplementation.

One source of data is the annual report complied by the American Association of Poison Control Centers Data Collection System. We have summarized some of the data presented in their 1988 report which includes data for almost one and one-half million poison exposures reported by 64 centers *(Lotovitz)*. The statistics include both intentional and accidental poisonings for all age groups including infants. To make the comparison more meaningful, we excluded street drugs, stimulants and topical preparations from the Drug category.

POISON EXPOSURES: OUTCOME

	VITAMINS	MINERALS	DRUGS
TOTALS	23,870	8416	298,284
No Effect	81%	69%	61%
Minor Effect	18%	27%	32%
Moderate Effect	1.3%	3.2%	6.1%
Major Effect	0.03%	0.25%	1.21%
Death	0.004%	0.05%	0.15%

SOURCE: 1988 Report, Am. Assoc. of Poison Control Centers

These figures support the hypothesis that nutritional supplements are, in general, markedly less toxic than drugs. The major common exception is the serious toxicity of an iron overdose, particularly in infants and small children. Of course, the results of poison exposures may not indicate how the dangers of supplements and medications compare when taken as directed, although there is good reason to suppose that the comparison is similar.

Compare, for example, aspirin (acetylsalicylic acid) with most nutrients that appear to be reasonably safe and effective at pharmacological doses. Because aspirin, for a medication, is relatively free of adverse effects, it does not require a prescription. This does not mean, however, that it is entirely safe. At low doses, it may produce gastric distress, heartburn or nausea. Occult gastrointestinal bleeding, although clinically insignificant, is common.

Epidemiological evidence suggests an association between aspirin given during the prodromal phase of an influenza or varicella infection and the subsequent development of Reye's syndrome. Higher doses can cause hepatotoxicity and hypoprothrombinemia. An acute intolerance occurs in about 0.3% of the population, including people who have taken the drug without incident for many years, which often consists of bronchospasm that may be severe and occasionally is fatal *(Drug Eval)*. Finally, aspirin overdose is one of the most common causes of poisoning from medications.

Few nutrients at appropriate pharmacological doses are so dangerous as this non-prescription drug. Some (such as folacin, pantothenic acid, riboflavin and vitamin B_{12}) fail to show evidence of toxicity even at dosages of 100 times their RDAs and most others have yet to have a Lowest Observed Adverse Effect Level established - although many nutrients may cause adverse effects if the dosage is high enough. So long as the dosage of a nutrient is below the level at which adverse effects have been reported, it is doubtful that it is as dangerous as aspirin. If its therapeutic dosage reaches into the toxic range, however, the risk of toxicity must be weighed against its potential benefits.

For example, vitamin A, the most potentially toxic of the vitamins, is an example of a nutrient with therapeutic applications at dosages that are sometimes above its Lowest Observed Adverse Effect Level of 21,600 IU daily. Its pharmacological benefits can usually be obtained at doses of 100,000 IU daily or less, especially if it is combined with vitamin E with which it has a synergistic effect *(Ayres)*.

Since toxicity is uncommon at doses below 100,000 IU *(Bauernfeind)*, and since adverse effects not due to toxicity are rare, its safety profile at pharmacological doses compares reasonably well with that of many prescription drugs. Iron, by contrast, even though it is an essential trace mineral, should probably not be supplemented other than to prevent or replete a deficiency; otherwise there are no known benefits despite considerable risks.

As is the case for drugs, the level of nutrient supplementation that results in toxicity as well as the length of time that it takes before toxicity develops varies enormously between individuals. Therefore, if the risk/benefit ratio is low enough, it may still be appropriate to utilize a dosage of a nutrient known to be above its Lowest Observed Adverse Effect Level, but only so long as the patient is monitored for the earliest signs of toxicity. Then, if toxicity starts to develop, discontinuing the supplement should be considered although, just as with drug side effects, an adverse effect may not be serious enough to warrant discontinuation.

CLINICAL TRIALS

Whatever the appeal of a specific nutritional supplement, remember that supplements are designed to *supplement* nutrients found in the diet. Whole foods are complex mixtures of numerous chemical substances, many of which have been poorly researched. Our knowledge of the relationship of these substances to health and healing is fragmentary and largely rudimentary. We know even less about the nutritional importance of the ratios that exist between the quantities of these substances within a food, and the importance of the ratios that exist between the quantities of these substances between foods.

In repeated instances, conclusions regarding therapeutic diets have been refuted long after they have become standard clinical practice. Examples are sugar avoidance in diabetic diets (refuted when the actual glycemic responses of individual carbohydrates were measured) and the milk-based diet for the treatment of peptic ulcer (refuted when it was found that milk produces an acid rebound).

We also suffer from limited knowledge about individual differences in nutrient needs, including differences in absorption, metabolism, utilization and excretion. In addition to differences in baseline nutrient intake, these differences are due to numerous factors, including genetics, gender, age, illness, physical exercise, psychological stress, exposure to toxins, and so forth.

The decision to add a specific quantity of a nutrient as a supplement to the diet of a particular person is therefore not an entirely rational one, even when there is an extensive body of scientific literature documenting the efficacy of that nutrient for a proposed clinical application. Therefore, until we better understand the underlying mechanisms by which diet affects health, nutritional supplements should be viewed as adjunctive to the best possible diet.

Nutritional medicines have been claimed to be beneficial for thousands of applications, although often scientific proof of their efficacy has not been well established. We, personally, would not give a patient a trial of a nutrient at a pharmacologic dosage for an unproved application unless the risk of adverse effects is fairly well established. If, however, the risk is known, then we would consider treatment with that nutrient, just as we would consider other treatments, based on what appears to be its relative advantages and disadvantages to our patient when compared to competing treatments.

We take this position because the decision to use a nutritional medicine, just as most other clinical decisions, is based on a number of factors. Science often fails to provide us with enough information to make the decision; then we have to make a subjective judgment when deciding between the treatment alternatives. To be more specific, some of the factors that should be compared before recommending any one treatment over another include:

- risk
- cost
- proof of efficacy
- chances of efficacy
- speed of efficacy
- degree of probable efficacy
- feasibility of combination treatment
- patient beliefs, motivation and ability to follow through

While nutritional science has major limitations, we believe that practitioners should attempt to be as scientific as possible in their practices.

- Give preference to the treatments that have been best validated.
- If you are unsure of which of several treatments, or combinations of treatments, to choose, and there is no time pressure, attempt to proceed with a particular treatment program for a reasonable trial period. Then, if that program fails, try another. (Frequent changes in protocol made before the results of a program become clear make it impossible to determine a program's efficacy.)
- Whenever feasible, perform blinded trials using placebos - but get your patient's consent before using them.

Here are some suggestions that apply specifically to choosing nutritional supplements:

- Start with improving the diet.
- Consider nutrient-nutrient interactions.
- Consider drug-nutrient interactions.
- Investigate the supplement's bioavailability.
- If your patient may be sensitive to foods or food additives, recommend supplements that are not

derived from the inciting foods and minimize the use of excipients.

Most importantly, treat the patient, not the diagnosis. For example, depression may be a manifestation of a somatic illness such as cancer, or an illness that sounds somatic in origin may be simply a physical expression of a depression or of an anxiety state. Always remember these words of Hippocrates:

"Some patients, though their condition is perilous, recover their health simply through their contentment with the goodness of the physician."

REFERENCES

American Dietetic Association. Recommendations concerning supplement usage: ADA statement. J Am Diet Assoc 46:1342-3, 1987

American Medical News, October 5, 1992, p. 32

Anonymous. Interim CDC recommendations for folic acid supplementation for women. JAMA 266:1191, 1991

Ayres S et al. Synergism of vitamins A and E with dermatologic applications. Cutis 23:600-3,689-90, 1979

Bates DW et al. Relationship between medication errors and adverse drug events. J Gen Intern Med 10(4):199-205, 1995

Bauernfeind JC. The Safe Use Of Vitamin A: A Report of the International Vitamin A Consultative Group. Washington, DC, The Nutrition Foundation, 1980

Belongia EA et al. An investigation of the cause of the eosinophilia-myalgia syndrome associated with tryptophan use. N Engl J Med 323(6):357-65, 1990

Beutler E et al. Iron therapy in chronically fatigued non-anemic women: A double-blind study. Ann Intern Med 52:378, 1960

Bowman BB, Rosenberg IH. Assessment of the nutritional status of the elderly. Am J Clin Nutr 35(5 Suppl):1142-51, 1982

Brin M. Erythrocyte as a biopsy tissue in the functional evaluation of thiamin status. JAMA 187:762-6, 1964

Drug Evaluations Subscription. Chicago, American Medical Association, 1990:1:22-6

Enstrom JE et al. Vitamin C intake and mortality among a sample of the United States population. Epidemiology 3(3):194-202, 1992

Folkers K. Renaissance in biomedical and clinical research on vitamins and coenzymes. J Optimal Nutr 1(1):11-15, 1992

Forbes RM, Erdman JW, Jr. Annu Rev Nutr 3:213, 1983

Gordon DJ, in OA Levander, Ed. Nutrition '87. Washington, DC, American Institute of Nutrition, 1987, p. 27

Jick H. Drugs-- remarkably nontoxic. N Engl J Med 291(16):824-8, 1974

Johnson JA, Bootman JL. Drug-related morbidity and mortality. Arch Intern Med 155:1949-56, 1995

Kim TF. Do low levels of iron affect body's ability to regulate temperature, experience cold? News. JAMA 260(5):607, 1988

Lesar TS et al. Medication-prescribing errors in a teaching hospital. A 9-year experience. Arch Intern Med 157(14):1569-76, 1997

Lotovitz TL et al. 1988 annual report of the American Association of Poison Control Centers National Data Collection System. Am J Emerg Med 7(5):495, 1989

Marginal vitamin deficiency: The "gray area" of nutrition. Vitamin Issues Vol II, No. 2, Ca. 1980

Melmon KL. Preventable drug reactions: causes and cures. N Engl J Med 284(24):1361-8, 1971

Mudd SH. Homocystinuria, in JB Wyngaarden & LH Smith Jr, Eds. Cecil: Textbook of Medicine. 18th Edition. Philadelphia, W.B. Saunders, 1988:1160-61.

Napke E, Stevens DG. Excipients and additives: hidden hazards in drug products and in product substitution. Can Med Assoc J 131(12):1449-52, 1984

National Research Council. Nutrient Adequacy: Assessment Using Food Consumption Surveys. Washington, DC, National Academy Press, 1986

Norton L, Wozny MC. Residential location and nutritional adequacy among elderly adults. J Gerontol 39(5):592-5, 1984

Pao EM, Mickle SJ. Problem nutrients in the United States. Food Technol 35:58-62,64,66-9,79, 1981

Recommended Dietary Allowances. Washington, DC, National Academy Press, 1989

Schneider-Helmert D, Spinweber CL. Evaluation of L-tryptophan for treatment of insomnia: a review. Naval Health Res Center, Naval Med Res Develop Com, Rep 84-4, Jan 1984

Stewart ML et al. Vitamin/mineral supplement use: A telephone survey of adults in the United States. J Am Diet Assoc 85:1585-90, 1985

Thurnham DI. Red cell enzyme tests of vitamin status: do marginal deficiencies have any physiological significance? Proc Nutr Soc 40:155-63, 1981

Tucker DM et al. Nutrition status and brain function in aging. Am J Clin Nutr 52:93-102, 1990

Yadrick MK et al. Iron, copper, and zinc status: response to supplementation with zinc or zinc and iron in adult females. Am J Clin Nutr 49:145-50, 1989

HOW TO RULE OUT FOOD SENSITIVITIES

When ingestion of a food is promptly followed by symptoms, the diagnosis is obvious. Often, however, the diagnosis is more elusive, as ingestion of inciting foods fails to elicit immediate symptoms. This occurs most often when inciting foods are eaten frequently, and is thought to be the result of the development of a chronic maladaptive state.

An elimination diet is the direct method for diagnosing food sensitivities; if the eliminated foods contributed to the illness, clinical improvement will occur. Foods must be eliminated for a minimum of 5 days to allow for the removal of their remains from the gastrointestinal tract and to provide time for the effects of their systemic absorption to dissipate. As some of these effects may be protracted, a longer period of food exclusion, ranging from 2 to 6 weeks, is more diagnostically definitive.

The nature of the elimination diet depends upon the history and clinical presentation, as well as upon individual motivation. Foods selected to remain in the diet should be those which are least suspected of causing symptoms. Most definitive, but most severe and potentially unhealthful, is a 5-day <u>water-only fast</u>. An <u>elemental diet</u>, consisting of a liquid mixture in which as few of the ingredients as possible are food-derived, provides basic nourishment but is difficult to tolerate. A <u>two-food diet</u>, such as the lamb and pear diet, consists of one protein- and fat-rich food and one carbohydrate-rich food. People on such limited diets for diagnostic purposes should be in reasonably good health and should be followed medically.

A <u>common food elimination diet</u> is often the most practical. In this diet, only foods which are normally eaten more often than twice a week are eliminated. This diet commonly provides a wide enough variety of foods to ensure nutritional adequacy and minimizes the inconvenience to the patient. To be done correctly, patients must restrict themselves to foods whose exact composition they know. Unless the food sources of all their ingredients are known, medications, nutritional supplements and toothpaste may be sources of eliminated foods which could possibly reduce the diagnostic value of the diet. Of course, medications should not be discontinued without the physician's approval. (Baking soda can be substituted for toothpaste.)

Sometimes only one food, or a few foods, need be eliminated. Occasionally specific foods have been linked to certain illnesses, such as gluten (which is found in wheat, oats, rye and barley) in schizophrenia. While unproven, unusually strong craving for a particular food is believed to suggest sensitivity to that food. Since eliminating only suspicious foods is the easiest elimination diet to follow, it can be tried first, and a more extensive elimination can be tried later if symptoms fail to improve.

Clinicians note that some patients will initially feel worse, usually starting 12 to 24 hours after beginning the diet. Their symptoms may worsen, or they may experience new symptoms, such as headache or a flu-like syndrome. Assuming that symptom production is not a nocebo (negative placebo) effect, this development is a preliminary indication that they are indeed sensitive to one or more of the eliminated foods, and that improvement should be expected with continued adherence to the diet.

If a food elimination diet results in improvement, eliminated foods are systematically reintroduced one at a time in order to identify the specific foods to which the person is sensitive. Nocebo effects can be eliminated if foods and a placebo are dispensed in capsules, each with a coded label.

Ideally, since reactions can be delayed as long as 72 hours, one food should be introduced every 3 days. When many foods have been eliminated, these food challenges may take a month or longer. They can be done more closely together, daily for example, but sometimes identification of inciting foods becomes difficult when delayed reactions overlap, and it may take several days before the patient returns to the baseline state.

During the elimination period, and especially during provocative testing, patients should keep a food diary. One column can be used to record the time each food was ingested, while another column can record changes in signs and symptoms. A particular symptom can be rated on a scale, and ratings at the end of each day can be averaged to provide a comparison over time.

Individualized elimination diets can be based on the results of blood testing. Several types of blood tests for food sensitivities are available. They may evaluate cellular damage when blood cells are exposed to a food (cytotoxic tests) or immune reactions to a food (IgE or IgG RAST; IgG immune complexes). Much of their appeal is due to their convenience, which is counterbalanced by their cost.

Despite improvements in recent years, different types of blood testing done on the same patient will often yield different results; some even yield quite different results when repeated on the same patient. At best, blood tests for food sensitivities only indicate an abnormal response to a food; they are unable to tell whether that food is contributing to the illness, or even whether that food will eventually produce symptoms if it continues to be consumed.

Despite their limitations, elimination diets based on blood testing may be effective in reducing symptoms. When, however, such a diet has proven ineffective, a standard elimination diet should still be considered.

Skin testing is another diagnostic method. Prick and scratch tests, which only test for atopic (IgE-mediated) allergic reactions, are of very limited value for diagnosing food sensitivities. In provocative testing, various dilutions of each food are placed into or under the skin, or under the tongue, and both the patient and the clinician look for changes in signs or symptoms within the next 10 minutes. The attraction of provocative testing is that it is not only diagnostic, but it may also be therapeutic. However, while experienced clinicians report excellent results with this method, its efficacy is highly controversial.

FOR FURTHER INFORMATION

Brostoff J. Complete Guide to Food Allergy and Intolerance. Third Edition. Baillière Tindall, 1998

Lessof MH. Food Intolerance. Chapman & Hall, 1992

Metcalfe DD, Sampson HA, Simon R. Food Allergy. Blackwell, 1997

Trevino RJ, Dixon HS, Eds. Food Allergy. Thieme Medical Publishers, 1997

PART TWO

NUTRITIONAL TREATMENTS FOR SPECIFIC ILLNESSES

EFFICACY RATINGS

In contrast to the standardized testing that governments frequently require before drugs reach the market, nutritional treatments are commonly available without having achieved any consensus of efficacy within the professional community. Proof of efficacy is only one of several criteria in choosing a specific treatment; yet it is of sufficient importance to be addressed.

This has been done with a simple rating system. Each of the following chapters starts with a Nutritional Treatment Guide that lists treatments to be discussed in the text and rates them according to the key that is provided at the bottom of this page.

While a great deal of effort was made to provide accurate ratings, there are undoubtedly classification errors due to the massiveness, and sometimes the inaccessibility, of the nutritional literature. Moreover, no attempt has been made to critique the quality of individual studies.

The ratings are determined, not merely by the scientific quality of the studies, but by the relevance of the outcome measures to clinical efficacy. Thus, a controlled clinical trial that uses an outcome measure other than clinical improvement may be rated as a "[-]" (efficacy suspected from indirect data).

Despite its obvious imperfections, it is hoped that the Guide will prove helpful in providing a quick overview of nutritional treatments in a unique manner that permits a simple comparison of the scientific validation behind each treatment.

EFFICACY *GENERALLY ACCEPTED*

✓ = Generally accepted as effective within the medical and scientific communities.

(Commonly, but not necessarily, acceptance is based on the results of multiple controlled human trials.)

EFFICACY *DEMONSTRATED*

* = Efficacy demonstrated in at least one *controlled* human trial.

EFFICACY *SUSPECTED*

[+] = Efficacy suspected from at least one *uncontrolled* human trial.

[-] = Efficacy suspected from indirect data (animal experiments, epidemiological surveys, *in vitro* studies, outcome measures that are not fundamental to the diagnosis, etc.).

EFFICACY *CHALLENGED*

? = Failure to confirm efficacy in at least one study of similar design (controlled, uncontrolled or indirect).

ACNE ROSACEA

NUTRITIONAL TREATMENT GUIDE

✓ = Efficacy generally accepted.
* = Efficacy *demonstrated* by controlled human trials.
[+] = Efficacy *suspected* from uncontrolled human trials.
[-] = Efficacy *suspected* from indirect data.
? = Efficacy *challenged* in a study of similar design.

VITAMINS

[+] **Vitamin B Complex deficiencies:** repletion (? 800 μg folate, 200 μg vitamin B_{12} and 100 mg of the other B vitamins daily) (6 week trial)
Consider giving intramuscularly and/or giving hydrochloric acid supplements if oral supplementation fails to result in clinical and laboratory evidence of normalization.
[+] **Isotretinoin (13-*cis*-retinoic acid):** 10 mg daily (4 month trial; results begin after 1 week)

OTHER NUTRITIONAL FACTORS

[+] **Betaine or Glutamic Hydrochloride:** 10 to 50 gr as tolerated following meals
(Beware of symptoms of gastric irritation.)
[+] **Pancreatic Enzymes:** potency, and thus dosage, varies with different preparations

TOPICAL AGENT

[+] **Tretinoin (retinoic acid; vitamin A acid):** 0.025% cream (4 month trial)

NUTRITIONAL FACTORS

VITAMINS

Vitamin B Complex Deficiencies

Preliminary data suggests that acne rosacea may be a manifestation of inadequate B vitamin nutriture, either due to dietary inadequacy or to impaired digestion causing poor absorption.

Studies performed in the 1940s found that rosacea patients often have reduced baseline levels of hydrochloric acid which may fail to respond to a gastric stimulus *(Johnson)*. More recently, one study found that, compared to controls, rosacea patients had significantly lower pancreatic lipase concentrations and output. Consistent with the hypothesis that impaired digestion may relate to the dermatologic abnormalities, rosacea patients who complained of digestive symptoms had improvements in both their skin condition and their dyspepsia when supplemented with pancreatic enzymes *(Barba)*.

In open trials, supplementation with niacinamide, riboflavin, vitamin B_6, or with the entire vitamin B complex, was followed by clinical improvement. For example, 89% of 36 patients with rosacea keratitis (including 5 out of 9 with cutaneous rosacea) healed promptly following supplementation with small doses of riboflavin (1-4.5 mg daily). All patients who failed to respond had achlorhydria following histamine stimulation *(Johnson)*.

An open trial of dilute hydrochloric acid given along with vitamin B complex was also followed by clinical improvement. The author of this study noted that the severity of the skin condition seemed to correlate with both the degree of baseline hydrochloric acid deficiency and signs of vitamin B complex deficiency *(Allison)*.

While B vitamins may be beneficial, high supplementary dosages of B complex vitamins can occasionally *cause* a rosacea-like eruption which fades when the supplement is discontinued *(Sheretz)*.

Vitamin A and the Retinoids

The more recent literature has focused on treating rosacea with the retinoids. While supplementation with vitamin A itself appears to be unstudied, isotretinoin (13-*cis*-retinoic acid), a stereoisomer of all-*trans*-retinoic acid that appears to have similar toxicity to that of the vitamin, has been administered in several open trials. Its efficacy may be due to its ability to increase epidermal retinol levels *(Rollman)*.

Papules, pustules and nodules appear to be responsive, while vasomotor lability and telangiectasia fail to respond *(Plewig)*. Also, although too toxic for systemic use, tretinoin (also called vitamin A acid or retinoic acid) is a metabolite that appears effective when applied to the lesions as a cream *(Ertl)*. Its main side effect is skin irritation.

A 39 year-old woman with a long history of rosacea presented with a slightly reddened face with large pimples and dilated capillaries along with bloodshot eyes. She also reported a lifelong history of mild constipation. Physical examination revealed split and cracked fingernails. Gastric analysis by radiotelemetry suggested hypochlorhydria.

She was treated with betaine hydrochloride (45 gr per full meal). In 2 months there was substantial clearing of her lesions, her constipation was gone, and her fingernails were breaking less and starting to regrow. Vitamin B_{12} and folate by injection were added along with oral B complex and other supplements. Two years later, her facial skin was completely free of rosacea, except for traces of dilated capillaries near her nose (Wright).

BIBLIOGRAPHY

Allison JR. The relation of hydrochloric acid and vitamin B complex deficiency in certain skin diseases. South Med J 38:235-41, 1945

Barba A et al. Pancreatic exocrine function in rosacea. Dermatologica 165:601-6, 1982

Ertl GA et al. A comparison of the efficacy of topical tretinoin and low-dose isotretinoin in rosacea. Arch Dermatol 130(3):319-24, 1994

Johnson L, Eckardt R. Rosacea keratitis and conditions with vascularization of the cornea treated with riboflavin. Arch Ophthalmol 23:899, 1940

Plewig G et al. Action of isotretinoin in acne rosacea and gram-negative folliculitis. J Invest Dermatol 86:390-3, 1986

Rollman O, Vahlquist A. Oral isotretinoin (13-cis-retinoic acid) therapy in severe acne: Drug and vitamin A concentrations in sebum and skin. J Invest Dermatol 86(4):384-9, 1986

Sherertz EF. Acneiform eruption due to "megadose" vitamins B6 and B12. Cutis 48(2):119-20, 1991

Wright JV. A case of acne rosacea, in Wright JV. Dr. Wright's Guide to Healing with Nutrition. Emmaus, Penn., Rodale Press, 1984

ACNE VULGARIS

NUTRITIONAL TREATMENT GUIDE

✓ = Efficacy generally accepted.
* = Efficacy *demonstrated* by controlled human trials.
[+] = Efficacy *suspected* from uncontrolled human trials.
[-] = Efficacy *suspected* from indirect data.
? = Efficacy *challenged* in a study of similar design.

DIETARY FACTORS

[+] **High Fiber diet**

- -

[-] **Low Carbohydrate diet**
[-] **Low Fat diet**
[-] ? avoid **Refined Carbohydrates**

NUTRITIONAL FACTORS

✓ **Isotretinoin (13-cis-Retinoic Acid):** 0.5 to 1.0 mg/kg in 2 divided doses daily for 15 to 20 weeks
(Due to side effects, limited to moderate to severe acne unresponsive to other treatments.)

- -

* ? **Vitamin B_6**: pyridoxine 50 mg daily (3 month trial)
(When used to treat premenstrual acne flares: take daily for 1 week prior to and during menses.)
* ? **Zinc deficiency**: *especially for pustular acne:* 135 mg daily *AND* **Copper** 2 mg daily
(preferably effervescent zinc sulfate) (3 month trial)

- -

[+] **Chromium:** high chromium yeast 1 tsp twice daily [400 μg chromium]
[+] **Folic Acid:** 5 to 10 mg daily
[+] **Omega-6 Fatty Acid deficiency:** *example:* evening primrose oil 500 mg capsules [7-10% GLA] 6 to 8 daily
[+] **Pantothenic acid:** 10 g orally daily in divided doses *plus* topical application of pantothenic acid cream (20% by weight) 4 to 6 times daily
[+] **Selenium deficiency**: 200 μg daily
AND **Vitamin E**: 200 IU twice daily (especially for pustular acne) (6 to 12 week trial)
[+] **Vitamin A**: 100,000 IU
AND **Vitamin E:** 800 IU daily (4 month trial) (Do not use with oral isotretinoin.)
(Reduce to maintenance dosage as soon as possible.)

OTHER RELATED FACTORS

[+] ? rule out **Food Sensitivities**

TOPICAL AGENTS

✓ **Isotretinoin (13-*cis*-Retinoic Acid)**: 0.05% gel applied twice daily (8 week trial)
OR
✓ **Tretinoin (Vitamin A Acid)**: cream, gel and liquid available in various strengths

---

* **Niacinamide:** Apply topically as a 4% gel. (8 week trial)

DIETARY FACTORS

Terribly common, but poorly understood, acne vulgaris seems to be a disease of civilization, with far less acne found among Eskimos and African blacks eating native diets than among those eating modern Western diets. The primitive diet was higher in fiber, lower in fat, and devoid of refined carbohydrates. Whether such differences account for the high prevalence of acne in our society has, unfortunately, yet to be fully investigated.

There is evidence that both fat and carbohydrates increase sebum production. In normals, this increase is moderate, but in acne patients, this increase is marked, suggesting that the increased sebum may aggravate the skin lesions *(Lobitz)*.

Eating 'sweets' between meals has been associated with a sharp elevation of blood sugar, and prolonged or repeated hyperglycemia is believed by some to aggravate acne. Consistent with this hypothesis, a survey of over 1000 adults found that refined carbohydrate or sugar intake was significantly correlated with the risk of dermatoses *(Ringsdorf)*. However, when acne patients were placed on a sugar-restricted diet, they showed no differences from controls *(Cornbleet)*. Also, in an early study, 5 out of 10 patients placed on a high carbohydrate diet and given daily infusions of 5% dextrose in water *improved* - and continued to improve for several months after the intravenous infusions were stopped while the diet was continued *(Crawford)*. Further investigations should resolve this controversy.

Dietary fiber, by contrast, may be beneficial. One clinician has reported that several patients showed rapid clearing following supplementation with 1 oz daily of an all-bran cereal *(Kaufman)*. Controlled studies are needed for confirmation of this finding.

Food sensitivities have sometimes appeared to explain acne outbreaks, but careful scientific studies have so far failed to confirm such clinical impressions *(Anderson)*.

A 13 year-old male with severe cystic acne had a history of atopic eczema at age 7 which had failed to respond to topical steroids, but had responded promptly and permanently to a one-week fruit diet. He would regularly have a major exacerbation of the acne the day after the ingestion of chocolate, almonds and possibly other nuts; afterwards it would take about one month for his condition to return to its baseline. The difference was so marked that he was unable to hide his indiscretions from his parents who, by looking at his face the next morning, invariably would recognize that he had eaten one of the foods to which he was sensitive.

NUTRITIONAL FACTORS

VITAMINS

Vitamin A and the Retinoids

Without doubt, the most clinical interest in recent years has been generated by work with vitamin A and its derivatives. Acne patients may have both lower serum and skin vitamin A levels than normals, and Ayres and Mihan have reported success with over 100 patients who received 100,000 IU of vitamin A with 800 IU of vitamin E daily. Most responded within weeks and maintenance control was obtained with lower doses *(Ayres)*. Serious toxicity of vitamin A, even at these dosages, is rare and early signs and symptoms of adverse reactions can be readily noted by the physician. (Because of hepatic storage, long-term use of doses of vitamin A higher than about 10,000 IU should be avoided.)

Isotretinoin (13-cis-retinoic acid), a synthetic derivative of vitamin A which is available by prescription, has been shown to raise epidermal retinol levels *(Vahlquist)* and has been shown in double-blind studies to be effective in the treatment of acne *(Lester;Strauss)*. Because of its toxicity, however, its use is restricted to cases of severe, recalcitrant cystic acne. Fortunately, it has also proved to be effective when applied topically, although benzoyl peroxide gel works more rapidly (*Hughes*).

Unresolved is the question of how large doses of vitamin A combined with vitamin E compare to isotretinoin - which appears to be at least as toxic as vitamin A. In addition to the systemic use of retinoids, topical application of either tretinoin (retinoic acid; vitamin A acid) or isotretinoin, both of which are available by prescription, may be beneficial *(Kligman;Chalker)*.

Vitamin B Complex

Several of the B vitamins may have efficacy in acne treatment. In a small open trial, supplementation with large dosages of folic acid seemed to be helpful *(Callaghan)* and, in a double-blind study, topical application of a topical niacinamide gel has been shown to provide benefit *(Shalita)*. In an open trial of 100 patients, pantothenic acid was given both orally and as a cream for topical application. Within one to two days, serum secretion notably decreased and, within one to two weeks, the frequency of new acne eruptions began to decline and existing lesions started to regress *(Leung)*.

Early work suggests that vitamin B_6, which has been found to be beneficial to women with premenstrual syndrome, may also benefit those with premenstrual acne flares *(Snider)*. Occasionally, however, *stopping* vitamin B_6 - or vitamin B_{12} - supplementation may improve an acneiform exanthema, particularly in women *(Braun-Falco)*. (These supplement-related lesions consist of loosely disseminated small papules or papulopustules on the face and the upper parts of the back and chest spreading to the upper arm.)

A 26 year-old woman with reddened, coarse skin over her forehead, cheeks and nose with slight puffiness, scattered pimples and many cysts and deeply infected pustules. She noted that her acne started one year before menarche, worsened notably following her first menses, and always worsened premenstrually. In addition she complained of marked premenstrual fluid retention and irritability. Oral contraceptives caused depression and anxiety along with headaches, breast tenderness, nausea and increased fluid retention. She also had a history of toxemia of pregnancy twice. Antibiotics, diuretics and tranquilizers were of little help.

She was placed on pyridoxine 100 mg 4 times daily and a topical cream containing vitamin B_6 100 mg/gram. After 3 weeks her fluid retention was gone, energy levels were improved and her acne had greatly improved. After another month, her face was completely free of the rash, but it would break out with fresh lesions if she skipped vitamin B_6 for 48 hours (Wright).

MINERALS

Selenium Deficiency

Selenium may be low both in whole blood and plasma *(Michaëlsson,1990)*. Results of an open trial suggest that selenium supplementation, at least when combined with vitamin E, may be effective, especially for male patients with severe pustular acne and low levels of erythrocyte glutathione peroxidase (a selenium-containing enzyme) *(Michaëlsson,1984)*.

Zinc Deficiency

Acne patients, especially if the acne is severe, may be deficient in zinc. Zinc has an anti-inflammatory effect on cutaneous lesions; this appears to be due to inhibition of polymorphonuclear leukocyte chemotaxis induced by reduced granulocyte zinc levels *(Dreno)*.

While not all studies have shown positive results, the results of several double-blind studies have suggested that zinc supplementation may be effective, especially in regard to treating inflammation and pustules *(Lidën;Verma)*. In one study *(Michaëlsson,1977)*, it was clearly more effective than 300,000 IU of vitamin A.

(Effervescent zinc sulfate was used in some of the most positive studies.)

OTHER NUTRITIONAL FACTORS

Omega-6 Fatty Acid Deficiencies

Also lower than normal are the levels of linoleic acid, an omega-6 fatty acid, in the sebum *(Downing)*. In an open trial *(Hubler)*, patients on a low-fat diet appeared to benefit from supplementation with corn oil (which is rich in linoleic acid).

These results suggest that supplementation with linoleic acid may be beneficial, although controlled trials are needed to confirm this. Theoretically, a source of gamma-linolenic acid (such as borage, blackcurrent or evening primrose oil) may also be beneficial as it may help to normalize impaired omega-6 fatty acid metabolism in the skin.

Linoleic acid is converted to prostaglandins with the first step requiring the enzyme delta-6-desaturase, the synthesis of which is induced by insulin. Skin, but not oral, glucose tolerance appears to be impaired in acne patients *(Abdel)*.

High Chromium Yeast

Since high chromium yeast, which is an excellent source of glucose tolerance factor, has been shown to improve oral glucose tolerance and enhance insulin sensitivity (see Diabetes Mellitus), it is conceivable that it may be of benefit in acne by promoting the normal conversion of linoleic acid within the skin. Indeed, in a preliminary study *(McCarty)*, 10 patients rapidly improved following supplementation with high-chromium yeast.

BIBLIOGRAPHY

Abdel KM et al. Glucose tolerance in blood and skin of patients with acne vulgaris. Int J Dermatol 22:139-49, 1977

Anderson PC. Foods as a cause of acne. Am Fam Physician 3(3):102-3, 1971

Ayres S Jr, Mihan R. Acne vulgaris and lipid peroxidation: New concepts in pathogenesis and treatment. Int J Dermatol 17:305, 1978

Braun-Falco O, Lincke H. The problem of vitamin B6/B12 acne. A contribution on acne medicamentosa. MMW 118(6):155-60, 1976

Callaghan TJ. The effect of folic acid on seborrheic dermatitis. Cutis 3:583-8, 1967

Chalker DK et al. Efficacy of topical isotretinoin 0.05% gel in acne vulgaris. J Am Acad Dermatol 17:251-4, 1987

Cornbleet T, Gigli I. Should we limit sugar in acne? Arch Dermatol 83:968, 1961

Crawford GM, Swatz JH. Acne and the carbohydrates. Arch Dermatol Syphilol 33:1035-41, 1936

Downing DT et al. Essential fatty acids and acne vulgaris. J Am Acad Dermatol 14:221-5, 1986

Dreno B, Trossaert M, Boiteau HL, Litoux P. Zinc salts effects on granulocyte zinc concentration and chemotaxis in acne patients. Acta Derm Venereol 72(4):250-2, 1992

Hubler WR. Unsaturated fatty acids in acne. Arch Dermatol 79:644, 1959

Hughes BR et al. A double-blind evaluation of topical isotretinoin 0.05%, benzoyl peroxide gel 5% and placebo in patients with acne. Clin Exp Dermatol 17(3):165-8, 1992

Kaufman WF. The diet and acne. Letter to the Editor. Arch Dermatol 119(4):276, 1983

Kligman AM et al. Topical vitamin A acid in acne vulgaris. Arch Dermatol 99:469-76, 1969

Lester RS et al. Isotretinoin and tetracycline in the management of severe nodulocystic acne. Int J Dermatol 1985 May;24(4):252-7, 1985

Leung LH. Pantothenic acid deficiency as the pathogenesis of acne vulgaris. Med Hypotheses 44:490-2, 1995

Lidén S et al. Clinical evaluation of acne. Acta Derm Venereol Suppl (Stockh) Suppl 89:49-52, 1980

Lobitz WC. The structure and function of the sebaceous glands. Arch Dermatol 76:162-71, 1957

McCarty M. High chromium yeast for acne? Med Hypotheses 14:307-10, 1984

Michaëlsson G et al. Effects of oral zinc and vitamin A in acne. Arch Dermatol 113(1):31-36, 1977

Michaëlsson G, Edqvist L. Erythrocyte glutathione peroxidase activity in acne vulgaris and the effect of selenium and vitamin E treatment. Acta Derm Venereol (Stockh) 64(1):91-14, 1984

Michaëlsson G. Decreased concentration of selenium in whole blood and plasma in acne vulgaris. Acta Derm Venereol 70(1):92, 1990

Ringsdorf WM Jr, Cheraskin E. Diet and dermatosis. South Med J 69(6):732&734, 1976

Shalita A et al. Topical nicotinamide compared with clindamycin gel in the treatment of inflammatory acne vulgaris. Int J Dermatol 34:434-7, 1995

Snider BL, Dieteman DF. Pyridoxine therapy for premenstrual acne flare. Letter to the Editor. Arch Dermatol 110:130-31, 1974

Strauss JS et al. Isotretinoin therapy for acne: results of a multicenter dose-response study. J Am Acad Dermatol 10(3):490-6, 1984

Vahlquist A. Oral isotretinoin (13-cis-retinoic acid) therapy in severe acne: Drug and vitamin A concentrations in sebum and skin. J Invest Dermatol 86(4):384-9, 1986

Verma KC et al. Oral zinc sulfate therapy in acne vulgaris: a double blind trial. Acta Dermatovener 60:337, 1980

Wright JV. A case of menstrual upset with acne and depression. Dr. Wright's Book of Nutritional Therapy. Emmaus, PA, Rodale Press, 1979

ACQUIRED IMMUNODEFICIENCY SYNDROME (A.I.D.S.)

See Also: IMMUNODEPRESSION
INFECTION

NUTRITIONAL TREATMENT GUIDE

✓ = Efficacy generally accepted.
* = Efficacy *demonstrated* by controlled human trials.
[+] = Efficacy *suspected* from uncontrolled human trials.
[-] = Efficacy *suspected* from indirect data.
? = Efficacy *challenged* in a study of similar design.

DIETARY FACTORS

[+] treat **Malnutrition**

NUTRITIONAL FACTORS

* **L-carnitine:** 6 g daily
* **Cysteine:** N-acetylcysteine 3 to 8 g daily in divided doses
* **Zinc deficiency:** zinc sulfate 220 mg twice daily *AND* **Copper** 2 mg daily
* ? **Beta-carotene:** 30 to 180 mg daily

- -

[+] **alpha-Lipoic acid:** 100 to 300 mg daily
[+] **Coenzyme Q_{10}:** 200 mg daily
[+] **Selenium deficiency:** 200 μg daily
[+] **Vitamin B_6 deficiency:** 50 to 200 mg daily
[+] **Vitamin B_{12} deficiency:** 1,000 μg intramuscularly weekly initially, then monthly
[+] **Vitamin C:** Supplement to bowel tolerance
[+] **Vitamin E deficiency:** D,L alpha-tocopheryl acetate 200 to 2,000 IU or mg daily for 6 weeks; then maintenance levels as needed

- -

[-] **Folic acid deficiency:** 800 μg daily
[-] **Magnesium deficiency:** ≈ 400 mg daily (Consider IM or IV administration, especially in hypomagnesemia.)
[-] **Niacin deficiency:** 50 to 100 mg daily
[-] **Omega-3 fatty acids:** *example:* MaxEPA 1 g capsules [180 mg EPA; 120 mg DHA] 10 to 20 daily
[-] **Omega-6 fatty acids:** *example:* evening primrose oil 500 mg capsules [7-10% GLA] 6 to 8 daily
[-] **Riboflavin deficiency:** 5 to 10 mg daily
[-] **Thiamine deficiency:** 50 mg orally or IM daily

[-] Vitamin A **deficiency:** 50,000 IU daily for 6 weeks (10,000 IU daily during pregnancy); then maintenance levels as needed
[-] Vitamin C **deficiency:** 500 mg twice daily
[-] Vitamin D **deficiency:** 50,000 to 100,000 IU 2 to 3 times during the first week; then, if needed, either 100,000 IU of ergocalciferol or cholecalciferol every 3 to 6 months *OR* 800 to 1600 IU daily

OTHER RELATED FACTORS

[+] rule out **Food Sensitivities**
[+] ? **Egg lipid extract (AL 721):** 10 g daily

- -

[-] **Hydrochloric Acid deficiency:** betaine or glutamic hydrochloride 10 to 50 gr following each meal (Beware of gastric irritation.)

"Nutritional factors play a key role in HIV disease progression and nutritional intervention is a key component of any comprehensive clinical management strategy for HIV infection (Varela)."

In AIDS, not only is the diet often inadequate, but there is also substantial wasting and weight loss due to metabolic disturbances and malabsorption *(Gramlich)*. The danger of malnutrition is serious, and nutritional status represents a major determinant of patient survival *(Chlebowski)*. Besides the more obvious adverse effects of macronutrient deficiencies, developing micronutrient deficiencies may potentiate HIV replication and exacerbate the pathological effects of HIV-induced chronic immune activation/inflammation *(Moseson)*. Yet, due to an inadequate diet, most HIV-positive patients ingest less than 50% of the RDA for at least one nutrient *(Dworkin,1991)*.

NUTRITIONAL FACTORS

VITAMINS

Vitamin A Deficiency

Serum vitamin A concentrations of AIDS patients with low vitamin A intakes are often below the normal range *(Karter)*. Repeated and chronic infections also tend to compromise the vitamin A nutriture of HIV-positive patients *(Ward)*. Vitamin A deficiency tends to be associated with a reduction in CD4 (helper) cell counts as well as with other T-cell subset abnormalities *(Semba)*.

Both HIV-infected children and adults may benefit from vitamin A supplementation *(Coutsoudis; Ward)*. Among other things, normalization is associated with higher T-cell counts *(Baum,1995)*. However, not only low intakes, but also very high intakes, of vitamin A may increase the risk of progression to AIDS in HIV-positive patients *(Tang,1993)*.

Vitamin B Complex Deficiencies

The concentration of reduced homocysteine, a toxic amino acid, may be elevated, suggesting possible deficiencies of vitamins B_6, B_{12}, and folic acid. Increased homocysteine can promote the formation of reactive oxygen species and accelerated immunologic deterioration as well as increased HIV replication *(Müller)*.

Indeed, there is evidence of deficiency for all three of these B vitamins. Folic acid may be reduced *(Downing)*, sometime severely enough to cause neurological degeneration *(Smith)*, although zidovudine (AZT) treatment may increase red cell folate levels *(Baum,1991a)*. Vitamin B_6 may be deficient despite adequate intake which, in turn, is associated with decreased immune function *(Baum,1991b)*.

Supplementation of vitamin B_6 may substantially reduce the risk of progression to AIDS *(Tang,1996)*. It may also help reduce the effects of psychological stress *(Shor-Posner,1994)* and increase T lymphocyte levels in HIV-positive patients *(Folkers,1993)*.

Finally, decreases in vitamin B_{12} status in HIV-infected patients have been associated with peripheral neuropathy and myelopathy *(Kieburtz)*, as well as with increasing immune dysfunction *(Baum,1995)*. Supplementation of vitamin B_{12} in deficient patients has improved memory *(Shor-Posner,1995a)*, reduced dementia *(Herzlich,1993)*, decreased peripheral neuropathy *(Kieburtz)*, and increased depressed T-helper cell counts *(Baum,1995)*.

The hematologic toxicity of zidovudine (AZT) has been a problem. However, there is reason to be believe that adequate folic acid and/or vitamin B_{12} repletion may reduce the risk, although controlled clinical trials remain to be done *(Herzlich,1990)*.

Nutriture of other member of the vitamin B complex may also be reduced. Niacin, riboflavin and thiamine intakes may be inversely related to the risk of AIDS in HIV-positive patients, and the highest quartile of intake of each was independently associated with improved survival over an 8-year follow-up period *(Tang,1996)*. Moreover, neuropathological changes characteristic of Wernicke's encephalopathy (which results from thiamine deficiency) have been described post-mortem in non-alcoholic AIDS patients *(Schwenk)*.

Vitamin C

Plasma levels of vitamin C may be reduced in ARC, AIDS, and asymptomatic HIV-positive patients *(Bogden)*. Furthermore, intake may be inversely related to the risk of AIDS in HIV-positive patients *(Tang,1993)*.

In vitro, ascorbate diminishes HIV viral protein production in infected cells and reverse transcriptase stability in extracellular virion *(Harakeh)*. Ingestion of vitamin C until diarrhea is induced (often referred to as the "ascorbate flush"), at least when performed in informal clinical settings, has been found to improve symptomatology and slow the decline of, or even improve, killer T cell activity and T helper/T suppressor ratios *(Cathcart,1984,1990;Brighthope)*. Also informally, the application of a vitamin C paste up to 4 times daily, while simultaneously prescribing massive oral doses of ascorbate, has been reported to successfully treat early lesions of Kaposi's sarcoma *(Cathcart,1984)*.

A 37-year-old male homosexual with AIDS first noted enlargement of lymph glands in the neck, axilla and groin 2 to 3 years earlier. He then developed a number of infections including herpes simplex, fungal dermatitis, and a number of respiratory tract infections resistant to a variety of antibiotics. General psychological deterioration occurred which resulted in his inability to continue to work. Small reddish/purple flat lesions developed on his arms, legs and soft palate which were diagnosed on biopsy as Kaposi's sarcoma. Bowel intolerance of virtually any food then developed, resulting in severe bowel cramps and diarrhea and the loss of 3 stone in weight over a period of 8 to 10 weeks.

He was told to take hourly doses of sodium ascorbate, even during the night if possible. In this way he consumed 60 to 90 grams of ascorbate daily and increased it when necessary to 200 grams daily (equivalent to roughly a teaspoon every half hour). He was also treated with intravenous sodium ascorbate as required. Ascorbate dosages were determined by his level of well being, especially his energy levels. When his energy levels increased, the ascorbate dosage was reduced. It was found that, when he was placed on antibiotics or had extra stress, his requirements for ascorbate increased. In addition, he was placed on vegetable juices and nutrient supplements, and taught relaxation exercises with mediation and visual imagery.

Over the next 7 months, his general health improved, his appetite increased and he started to gain weight. The bowel symptoms subsided and, as he became able to tolerate more solid foods, he was placed on a vegetarian diet. The Kaposi's lesions faded, some reduced in size, and no new lesions developed during this time period. His T lymphocyte helper/suppressor ratio gradually improved from 0.38 to 0.8. At the gravest point of his illness, the T4 lymphocyte count had dropped to just under 100 x 10^9/L, while during the period of clinical improvement it increased to 350 x 10^9/L (Brighthope).

Vitamin D Deficiency

There is a correlation between serum vitamin D levels and CD+ cell counts. Furthermore, serum vitamin D may be the most important marker of immunodeficiency in HIV-infected patients and can be used to predict survival and progression to AIDS *(Haug)*.

Vitamin E Deficiency

Either plasma or serum levels of vitamin E may be reduced in HIV infected patients *(Periquet;Shor-Posner,1995b;Malvy)*.

Supplementation may enhance immunocompetence *(Odeleye)* and boost plasma glutathione levels *(Hu)*. Moreover, it may increase the therapeutic efficacy of AZT while reducing toxicity *(Gogu,1989,1991)*.

MINERALS

Iron

The question of whether to consider iron supplementation should be dealt with on an individual basis, preferably on the basis of laboratory testing. For HIV-positive patients, results of a prospective study suggest that the risk of progression to AIDS may decrease with higher levels of iron consumption *(Abrams)*. However, since iron stores tend to be excessive in advanced stages of AIDS, limiting its intake and using iron-chelating drugs may be appropriate at this point in the disease *(Boelaert)*.

Magnesium Deficiency

Plasma, serum, and erythrocyte levels of magnesium may be reduced in HIV-positive patients *(Berger;Bogden)*. As magnesium deficiency in erythrocytes may be correlated with fatigue and muscle aches *(Berger)*, it is possible that supplementation would improve these symptoms.

Selenium Deficiency

Deficiency of selenium is common in HIV-positive patients and may be related to the pathogenesis and progression of the disease *(Dworkin,1988; Constans,1995a)*. Serum selenium levels may correlate positively with CD4 counts *(Constans,1995b)*, while glutathione peroxidase, a selenium-dependent enzyme, may be reduced in AIDS and ARC patients *(Dworkin,1994)*.

Supplementation may increase glutathione peroxidase activity and blood glutathione concentration *(Delmas-Beauvieux)*. It may also potentiate the efficacy of AIDS vaccines and other biological or prophylactic therapies as well as reduce the toxicity of drug treatments in AIDS *(Schrauzer,1994)*. According to Gerhard Schrauzer, professor emeritus, University of California, San Diego, "present indications are that selenium supplementation increases energy, reduces gastrointestinal problems and skin infections, prevents weight loss, improves mood and appears to slow down the loss of CD4 cells" *(Schrauzer,1997)*.

Zinc Deficiency

Adequate plasma/serum zinc levels appear to be important to maintain immune function in HIV-infected patients *(Baum,1991a)*, yet these levels are often reduced *(Bogden;Falutz;Periquet)*. While adequate plasma/serum zinc levels may be important for a therapeutic response to AZT *(Baum,1991a)*, AZT treatment may reduce these levels *(Baum,1991a)*.

Supplementation may help increase CD4 levels, either in combination with AZT *(Mocchegiani)* or alone *(Baum,1995)*, and may reduce the development of Kaposi's sarcoma and opportunistic infections *(de Gorden)*.

OTHER NUTRITIONAL FACTORS

Arginine

Arginine supplementation is immunostimulatory; however, in contrast to other immunostimulatory regimens, it does not appear to increase the risk of activating HIV replication *(Wrightham)*. While this makes arginine supplementation theoretically attractive, arginine levels in the plasma/serum rise, rather than fall, during the course of the illness *(Dröge,1988; Ollenschlager)*. Moreover, a recent double-blind study of HIV-infected non-hospitalized patients found that arginine supplementation combined with omega-3 fatty acids failed to show evidence of immunostimulation (when added to a multivitamin/multimineral supplement) after 6 months of treatment *(Pichard)*. Whether other study conditions, such as a larger dosage of arginine, or restricting supplementation to AIDS patients, would be effective remains to be seen.

Carnitine Deficiency

Both serum *(De Simone,1992)* and intracellular *(De Simone,1994)* carnitine levels may be decreased in AIDS patients. Furthermore, AZT-induced myopathy is associated with reduced muscle carnitine levels *(Dalakas)*.

Supplementation with L-carnitine may improve immune function and lipid metabolism in general *(De Simone,1993,1994)*. Moreover, supplementation may prevent and improve both the mitochondrial abnormalities and the lipid accumulation induced by AZT *(Semino-Mora)*.

Carotenoids

The intake of beta-carotene by HIV-infected patients has been shown to be directly related to survival *(Tang,1996)*. Moreover, plasma/serum levels of carotenoids are often reduced in HIV-positive patients *(Branowitz)*.
There is evidence that beta-carotene supplementation may increase CD4 cell levels *(Fryburg;Mckeown)* and activity *(Garewal)*, although a double-blind study failed to find evidence of benefit for a group of HIV-positive patients given a high dosage for 3 months *(Coodley)*. Supplementation may also increase blood glutathione concentration in HIV-positive patients *(Delmas-Beauvieux)* and thereby contribute to cellular defenses against damaging free radicals.

Coenzyme Q_{10} Deficiency

Blood levels of coenzyme Q_{10} may be reduced in both AIDS and ARC patients *(Folkers,1988)*.

Supplementation may increase CD4 lymphocytes and helper/suppressor ratios; it may also raise the level of immunoglobulin G *(Folkers,1993)*.

Cysteine Deficiency

Given that plasma cysteine is often found to be significantly lower in HIV-positive patients than in healthy controls *(deQuay)*, it has been suggested that AIDS may be the consequence of a virus-induced cysteine deficiency *(Dröge,1993)*. Compared to cysteine, *N-acetylcysteine* (NAC), because of the addition of an acetyl group, is more stable and more active biologically.

Glutathione, a tripeptide important to cellular defenses, may be deficient in HIV-positive patients. *(Delmas-Beauvieux)*. While the systemic bioavailability of oral glutathione supplements is uncertain *(Witschi)*, supplementation of HIV-infected patients with NAC has been shown to replenish depleted glutathione levels under double-blind conditions *(Herzenberg)*.

There is also evidence that NAC supplements may enhance antibody-dependent cellular cytotoxicity of neutrophils *(Roberts)*, inhibit HIV replication *(Roederer)*, and inhibit cytokine-mediated cachexia *(Roederer)*. In regard to patient outcome, NAC supplementation may prevent the progression of the HIV-positive patient to AIDS *(Dröge,1992)*, and assist cachectic AIDS patients in overall symptomatic improvement *(James)*. In fact, a recent double-blind study found that patients with very low CD4 cell counts who took NAC survived roughly twice as long as those given placebo *(Herzenberg)*.

Essential Fatty Acids

Due to their important immunomodulating effects, including the ability to destroy enveloped viruses, gamma-linolenic acid (GLA; an *omega-6* fatty acid) and/or eicosapentaenoic acid (EPA; an *omega-3* fatty acid) and their derivatives may be sources of natural endogenous agents against AIDS by preventing the spread of viral infection *(Bĕgin;Marcus;Razzini)*.

The lack of research in this area is disappointing. For a group of non-hospitalized HIV-positive patients, supplementation with omega-3 fatty acids along with arginine, when added to a multivitamin/multimineral supplement, failed to improve immunological parameters under double-blind conditions *(Pichard)*. More studies are needed to clarify the role of essential fatty acid supplement in HIV-related illness.

alpha-Lipoic Acid

In HIV-positive individuals, supplementation with the antioxidant alpha-lipoic acid has been found to increase plasma ascorbate and glutathione levels and to decrease markers of plasma lipid peroxidation. *In vitro*, it increases intracellular glutathione levels and inhibits HIV activation *(Suzuki)*. Furthermore, in many patients the nutrient may increase CD4 counts and improve the helper/suppressor cell ratio *(Packer)*. Controlled trials are needed to establish its efficacy in the clinical setting.

OTHER RELATED FACTORS

Egg Lipid Extract (AL 721) Supplementation

Ingestion of an egg lipid extract (AL 721) has been examined. This substance is a potent membrane fluidizer extracted from egg yolks which operates by extracting cholesterol from the cell membrane. It consists of 70% neutral lipids, 20% phosphatidylcholine, and 10% phosphatidylethanolamine *(Lyte)*.

While reports of the effectiveness of AL 721 have been mixed, one study demonstrated improvements in several signs and symptoms *(Shinitzky)* and two studies have noted reductions in blood HIV levels *(Lippa;Yust)*.

Food Sensitivities

Lactose malabsorption was found in more than one-third of a group of HIV-positive children and could thus be a cause of gastrointestinal complaints *(Halata)*. Furthermore, a clinical report suggests that many patients are sensitive to various foods, exposure to which may aggravate their symptoms *(Cathcart, 1984)*.

Hydrochloric Acid Deficiency

There is evidence that AIDS patients may fail to produce adequate amounts of hydrochloric acid *(Lake-Bakaar, 1988a)*. As this may be a cause of nutrient malabsorption *(Lake-Bakaar, 1988b)*, repletion should be considered.

COMBINED TREATMENT REGIMEN

A 45-year-old Caucasian male with a history of ulcerative colitis and ankylosing spondylitis had been HIV positive for 5 years. He presented with emaciation, pallor, flattened soft nails with many transverse lines, anal fissures, coated tongue, monilia, frequent bowel movements, dry skin, leg and foot cramps, painful stiff shoulders and hips, muscle pains in the arms, lassitude, poor memory and concentration, insomnia, anxiety and a purple skin lesion on his right leg. He was taking AZT 100 mg 3 times daily, Salazopyrin 0.5 g 4 times daily (for his ulcerative colitis) and, at times, diclofenac sodium (for his ankylosing spondylitis). He was mildly anemic. Nutriture for riboflavin (EBRA), thiamine (TPP effect; ETKA), vitamin B_6 (EGOT; P5P effect), phosphate and selenium was below the normal ranges. Evaluation for food sensitivities revealed reactions to several foods.

He was told to discontinue eating the foods to which he reacted adversely, and supplemented with riboflavin, thiamine, vitamin B_6, phosphate and selenium. Energy, strength and mentation dramatically improved. He gained several kilograms in weight and the girth of his arm muscles doubled. While before treatment he had been barely able to swim one length of a pool, he now was able to swim 40 lengths (Reading).

BIBLIOGRAPHY

Abrams B, Duncan D, Hertz-Picciotto I. A prospective study of dietary intake and acquired immune deficiency syndrome in HIV-seropositive homosexual men. J Acquir Immune Defic Syndr 6(8):949-58, 1993

Baum MK et al. Zidovudine-associated adverse reactions in a longitudinal study of asymptomatic HIV-1 infected homosexual males. J Acquir Immune Defic Syndr 4(12):1218-26, 1991a

Baum MK et al. Association of vitamin B_6 status with parameters of immune function in early HIV-1 infection. J Acquir Immune Defic Syndr 4:1122-32, 1991b

Baum MK et al. Micronutrients and HIV-1 disease progression. AIDS 9:1051-6, 1995

Bĕgin ME, Das UN. A deficiency in dietary gamma-linolenic and/or eicosapentaenoic acids may determine individual susceptibility to AIDS. Med Hypotheses 20(1):1-8, 1986

Berger DS et al. Prevalence of red blood cell magnesium deficiency in HIV-1 infected patients and its association with fatigue and myalgia. Abstract. J Am Coll Nutr 13(5):522, 1994

Bodgen JD et al. Micronutrient status and human immunodeficiency virus (HIV) infection. Ann NY Acad Sci 587:189-95, 1990

Boelaert JR et al. Altered iron metabolism in HIV infections: mechanisms, possible consequences, and proposals for management. Infect Agents Dis 5:36-46, 1996

Branowitz SA et al. Carotene deficiency in HIV patients. AIDS 10(1):115, 1996

Brighthope I. AIDS - Remissions using nutrient therapies and megadose intravenous ascorbate. Int Clin Nutr Rev 7(2):53-75, 1987

Cathcart RF 3rd. Vitamin C in the treatment of acquired immune deficiency syndrome (AIDS). Med Hypotheses 14(4):423-33, 1984

Cathcart RF 3rd. Glutathione and HIV infection. Letter. Lancet i:235, 1990

Chlebowski RT et al. Nutritional status, gastrointestinal dysfunction, and survival in patients with AIDS. Am J Gastroenterol 84(10):1288-93, 1989

Constans J et al. Fatty acids and plasma antioxidants in HIV-positive patients: correlation with nutritional and immunologic status. Clin Biochem 28:421-6, 1995a

Constans J et al. Serum selenium predicts outcome in HIV infection. J Acquir Immune Defic Syndr 10(3):392, 1995b

Coodley GO et al. Beta-carotene in HIV infection: An extended evaluation. AIDS 10(9):967-73, 1996

Coutsoudis A et al. The effects of vitamin-A supplementation on the morbidity of children born to HIV-infected women. Am J Public Health 85(8):1076-81, 1995

Dalakas MC et al. Zidovudine-induced mitochondrial myopathy is associated with muscle carnitine deficiency and lipid storage. Ann Neurol 35:482-7, 1994

de Gordon AM. Effects of adjuvant therapy with zinc in human immunodeficiency infection. Abstract. J Am Coll Nutr 11(5):601, 1992

Delmas-Beauvieux M-C et al. The enzymatic antioxidant system in blood and glutathione status in human immunodeficiency virus (HIV)-infected patients: effects of supplementation with selenium or β-carotene. Am J Clin Nutr 64:101-7, 1996

de Quay B et al. Glutathione depletion in HIV-infected patients: role of cysteine deficiency and effect of oral N-acetylcysteine. AIDS 6(8):815-9, 1992

DeSimone C et al. AIDS 6:203-5, 1992

DeSimone C et al. High dose L-carnitine improves immunologic and metabolic parameters in AIDS patients. Immunopharmacol Immunotoxicol 15(1):1-12, 1993

DeSimone C et al. Carnitine depletion in peripheral blood mononuclear cells from patients with AIDS: effect of oral L-carnitine. AIDS 8(5):655-60, 1994

Dowling S et al. Vitamin B12 and folate status in human immunodeficiency virus infection. Eur J Clin Nutr 47:803-7, 1993

Dröge W et al. Abnormal amino-acid concentrations in the blood of patients with acquired immunodeficiency syndrome (AIDS) may contribute to the immunological defect. Biol Chem Hoppe-Seyler 369:143-8, 1988

Dröge W et al. HIV-induced cysteine deficiency and T-cell dysfunction - a rationale for treatment with N-acetylcysteine. Immunology Today 13(6):211-14, 1992

Dröge W. Cysteine and glutathione deficiency in AID patients: a rationale for the treatment with N-acetyl-cysteine. Pharmacology 46(2):61-5, 1993

Dworkin BM et al. Abnormalities of blood selenium and glutathione peroxidase activity in patients with acquired immunodeficiency syndrome and AIDS-related complex. Biol Trace Elem Res 15:167-77, 1988

Dworkin BM et al. Dietary intake in patients with acquired immunodeficiency syndrome (AIDS), patients with AIDS-related complex, and serologically positive human immunodeficiency virus patients: correlations with nutritional status. J Parenter Enteral Nutr 14(6): 605-9, 1991

Dworkin BM Selenium deficiency and HIV infection and the acquired immunodeficiency syndrome (AIDS). Chem Biol Interact 91:181-6, 1994

Falutz J et al. Zinc as a cofactor in human immunodeficiency virus-induced immunosuppression. Letter. JAMA 259(19):2850-1, 1988

Folkers K et al. Biochemical deficiencies of coenzyme Q_{10} in HIV-infection and exploratory treatment. Biochem Biophys Res Commun 153:888-96, 1988

Folkers K et al. The activities of coenzyme Q_{10} and vitamin B_6 for immune response. Biochem Biophys Res Commun 193:88-92, 1993

Fryburg DA et al. The effect of supplemental beta-carotene on immunologic indices in patients with AIDS: a pilot study. Yale J Biol Med 1995 Jan;68(1-2):19-23, 1995

Garewal H et al. A preliminary trial of beta-carotene in subjects infected with the human immunodeficiency virus. J Nutr 122:728-32, 1992

Gogu SR et al. Increased therapeutic efficacy of zidovudine in combination with vitamin E. Biochem Biophys Res Commun 165(1): 401-7, 1989

Gogu SR et al. Protection of zidovudine-induced toxicity against murine erythroid progenitor cells by vitamin E. Exp Hematol 19(7):649-52, 1991

Gramich LM et al. Nutrition and HIV infection. J Nutr Biochem 6:2-11, 1995

Halata MS et al. Lactose malabsorption in children with human immunodeficiency virus (HIV) infection. Abstract. J Am Coll Nutr 12:593, 1993

Harakeh S et al. Suppression of human immunodeficiency virus replication by ascorbate in chronically and acutely infected cells. Proc Natl Acad Sci U S A 87(18):7245-9, 1990

Haug S et al. Subnormal serum concentrations of 1,25-vitamin D in human immunodeficiency virus infection: Correlation with degree of immune deficiency and survival. J Infect Dis 169:889-92, 1994

Herzenberg LA, De Rosa SC, Dubs JG, et al. Glutathione deficiency is associated with impaired survival in HIV disease. Proc Natl Acad Sci U S A 94:1967-72, 1997

Herzlich BC et al. Synergy of inhibition of DNA synthesis in human bone marrow by azidothymidine plus deficiency of folate and /or vitamin B_{12}? Am J Hematology 33:177-83, 1990

Herzlich B, SchianaT. Case report: Reversal of apparent AIDS dementia complex following treatment with vitamin B_{12}. J Intern Med 233:495-7, 1993

Hu JJ et al. Effects of dietary supplementation of alpha-tocopherol on plasma glutathione and DNA repair activities. Canc Epidemiol Biomark Preven 5(4):263-70, 1996

James JS. AIDS Treatment News, Issue #88, October 6, 1989

Karter DL et al. Vitamin A deficiency in non-vitamin-supplemented patients with AIDS: a cross-sectional study. J Acquir Immune Defic Syndr Hum Retrovirol 8:199-203, 1995

Kieburtz K et al. Abnormal vitamin B_{12} metabolism in human immunodeficiency virus infection. Arch Neurol 48:312-14, 1991

Lake-Bakaar G et al. Gastric secretory failure in patients with the acquired immunodeficiency syndrome (AIDS). Ann Intern Med 109(6):502-4, 1988a

Lake-Bakaar G et al. Gastropathy and ketoconazole malabsorption in the acquired immunodeficiency syndrome (AIDS). Ann Intern Med 109(6) 471-3, 1988b

Lippa AS et al. Presentation at the International Symposium on AIDS, Washington, D.C., June, 1987

Lyte M, Shinitzky M. A special lipid mixture for membrane fluidization. Biochem Biophys Acta 812:133-8, 1985

Malvy DJM et al. Relationship of plasma malondialdehyde, vitamin E and antioxidant micronutrients to human immunodeficiency virus. 1. Seropositivity. Clin Chim Acta 224:89-94, 1994

Marcus SH. Breakdown of PGE_1 synthesis is responsible for the acquired immunodeficiency syndrome. Med Hypotheses 15:39-46, 1984

McKeown LA. Beta carotene lifts CD4 counts. Study reported in Medical Tribune Feb. 25, 1993, p. 1

Mocchegiani E et al. Benefit of oral zinc supplementation as an adjunct to zidovudine (AZT) therapy against opportunistic infections in AIDS. Int J Immunopharmacol 17(9):719-27, 1995

Moseson M et al. The potential role of nutritional factors in the induction of immunologic abnormalities in HIV-positive homosexual men. J Acquir Immune Defic Syndr 2(3):235-47, 1989

Müller F et al. Elevated plasma concentration of reduced homocysteine in patients with human immunodeficiency virus infection. Am J Clin Nutr 63:242-8, 1996

Odeleye OE, Watson RR. The potential role of vitamin E in the treatment of immunologic abnormalities during acquired immune deficiency syndrome. Prog Food Nutr Sci 15(1-2):1-19, 1991

Ollenschlager G et al. Plasma amino acid pattern of patients with HIV infection. Clin Chem 34(9):1787-9, 1998

Packer L et al. Antioxidant properties and clinical implications of α-lipoic acid, in L Packer, E. Cadenas, Eds. Biothiols in Health and Disease. New York, Marcel Dekker, 1995, pp. 479-516

Periquet BA et al. Micronutrient levels in HIV-1-infected children. AIDS 9:887-93, 1995

Pichard C et al. A randomized double-blind controlled study of 6 months of oral nutritional supplementation with arginine and omega-3 fatty acids in HIV-infected patients. Swiss HIV Cohort Study. AIDS 12(1):53-63, 1998

Razzini E, Baronzio GF. Omega-3 fatty acids as coadjuvant treatment in AIDS. Med Hypotheses 41(4):300-5, 1993

Reading CM. Case Report: Nutritional intervention for AIDS patients. J Nutr Med 3:145-8, 1992

Roberts, RL et al. N-acetylcysteine enhances antibody-dependent cellular cytotoxicity in neutrophils and mononuclear cells from healthy adults in human immunodeficiency virus-infected patients. J Infect Dis 172:1492-502, 1995

Roederer M et al. N-acetylcysteine: a new approach to anti-HIV therapy. AIDS Res Hum Retroviruses 8(2):209-17, 1992

Schrauzer GN, Sacher J. Selenium in the maintenance and therapy of HIV-infected patients. Chem Biol Interact 91:199-205, 1994

Schrauzer GN interviewed by Kirk Hamilton in Clinical Pearls News 7(4), April, 1997

Schwenk J et al. Wernicke's encephalopathy in two patients with acquired immunodeficiency syndrome. J Neurol 7:445-7, 1990

Semba RD, Park S, Royal W, Griffin DE. Vitamin A deficiency and T-cell subpopulation in HIV-infected adults. Nutr Res 16:915-23, 1996

Semino-Mora C et al. Lab Invest 71:102-12, 1994

Shinitzky M et al. Lipid regimens for the treatment of AIDS, in RR Watson, Ed. Cofactors in HIV-1 Infection and AIDS. Boca Raton, FL, CRC Press, 1990

Shor-Posner G et al. Impact of vitamin B_6 status on psychological distress in a longitudinal study of HIV-1 infection. Int J Psychol Med 24(3):209-22, 1994

Shor-Posner G et al. Plasma cobalamin levels affect information processing speed in a longitudinal study of HIV-1 disease. Arch Neurol 52(2):195-201, 1995a

Shor-Posner G et al. Elevated IgE levels in relationship to nutritional status and immune parameters in early human immunodeficiency virus type I disease. J Allergy Clin Immunol 95:886-92, 1995b

Smith I et al. Folate deficiency and demethylation in AIDS. Lancet ii:215, 1987

Suzuki YJ et al. Alpha-lipoic acid is a potent inhibitor of NF-kappa B activation in human T cells. Biochem Biophys Res Commun 189(3):1709-15, 1992

Tang AM et al. Dietary micronutrient intake and the risk of progression to Acquired Immunodeficiency Syndrome (AIDS) in Human Immunodeficiency Virus Type 1 (HIV-1) infected homosexual men. Am J Epidemiol 138:937-51, 1993

Tang AM et al. Effects of micronutrient intake on survival in human immunodeficiency virus type 1 infection. Am J Epidemiol 143(12):1244-56, 1996

Varela P et al. Effects of human immunodeficiency virus infection and detoxification time on anthropometric measurements and dietary intake of male drug addicts. Am J Clin Nutr 66:509S-14S, 1997

Ward BJ et al. Vitamin A status in HIV infection. Nutr Res 13:157-66, 1993

Witschi A et al. The systemic availability of oral glutathione. Eur J Clin Pharmacol 43(6):667-9, 1992

Wrightham MN et al. L-arginine: a therapeutic option for AIDS/HIV infection? Med Hypotheses 38(3):236-9, 1992

Yust I et al. Reduction of circulating HIV antigens in seropositive patients after treatment with AL-721. Isr J Med Sci 26(1):20-6, 1990

AGGRESSIVE BEHAVIOR

See Also: **ATTENTION-DEFICIT HYPERACTIVITY DISORDER**
'HYPOGLYCEMIA' (FUNCTIONAL)
LEARNING DISORDERS

NUTRITIONAL TREATMENT GUIDE

✓ = Efficacy generally accepted.
* = Efficacy *demonstrated* by controlled human trials.
[+] = Efficacy *suspected* from uncontrolled human trials.
[-] = Efficacy *suspected* from indirect data.
? = Efficacy *challenged* in a study of similar design.

DIETARY FACTORS

✓ avoid **Alcohol**

- -

* ? avoid **refined Sugar**

NUTRITIONAL FACTORS

* **Lithium (high dose):** 900,000 to 1,500,00 μg daily (available by prescription)
* **Lithium (low-dose):** ? 200 to 400 μg daily (available as a vegetable concentrate) (4 week trial)
* **Tryptophan**: 6 to 10 g daily in divided doses (available by prescription)
(Warning: Do not consider using 5-hydroxytryptophan as a substitute.)

- -

[+] **Iron deficiency:** 30 mg twice daily until repletion; then minimal possible dosage
[+] **Niacin deficiency:** 50 to 100 mg daily
[+] **Omega-3 fatty acids:** *example:* MaxEPA 1 g caps [180 mg EPA; 120 mg DHA] 10 to 20 daily
[+] **Pantothenic acid deficiency:** 100 to 200 mg daily
[+] **Thiamine deficiency:** 50 mg orally or IM daily
[+] **Vitamin B_6 deficiency:** 50 to 100 mg daily
[+] **Vitamin C deficiency:** 500 mg twice daily
[+] **Zinc deficiency:** zinc sulfate 220 mg twice daily *AND* **Copper** 2 mg daily

- -

[-] **Magnesium deficiency:** ≈ 400 mg daily (Consider IM or IV administration, especially in hypomagnesemia.)
[-] rule out **Manganese toxicity**

OTHER RELATED FACTORS

✓ rule out **Food Sensitivities**

The aggressive behavioral syndrome is marked by restlessness, irritability, impulsivity and a proneness to violence. Diagnostically, it overlaps the DSM-IV *(American Psychiatric Association)* diagnoses of Attention-deficit/Hyperactivity Disorder, Conduct Disorder, Oppositional Defiant Disorder and Antisocial Personality Disorder.

DIETARY FACTORS

See *alcohol* under Tryptophan, and *refined sugar* under Sugar Intake and Reactive Hypoglycemia, below.

NUTRITIONAL FACTORS

VITAMIN DEFICIENCIES

Deficiencies of several vitamins are known to be associated with irritability. These include niacin *(Gelenberg)*, pantothenic acid *(Hodges)*, thiamine *(Lonsdale)*, vitamin B_6 *(McLaren)* and vitamin C *(Wilmot)*. In industrialized societies, the classic vitamin deficiency diseases are rare, although marginal vitamin nutriture due either to inadequate intake or to vitamin dependency appears to be fairly common. Moreover, under laboratory conditions, adverse behavioral changes precede specific clinical findings in a number of vitamin deficiencies *(Brin)*.

It is not known how frequently overaggressive behaviors are a manifestation of marginal vitamin nutriture. While little has been published to prove a relationship between the aggressive behavioral syndrome in humans and marginal vitamin nutriture, Lonsdale and Shamberger, writing in *The American Journal of Clinical Nutrition*, reported on 20 people eating "junk food" diets who were found to have biochemical evidence of marginal thiamine deficiency. Their subjects, and particularly the adolescents, were impulsive, highly irritable, aggressive and sensitive to criticism.

Following thiamine supplementation, their behavior improved concurrent with laboratory evidence of improved thiamine nutriture, suggesting that marginal thiamine deficiency may have contributed to their aggressive behavioral syndrome *(Lonsdale)*. Hopefully, well-controlled studies will eventually provide a clearer picture of the importance of marginal vitamin deficiencies in promoting overaggressive behaviors.

MINERALS

Iron Deficiency

The most common nutritional deficiency in industrialized societies, 10% of American males and 3% of American females are overtly iron-deficient (ferritin less than 10 ng/mL) *(Bailey)*. A deficiency of iron is known to interfere with proper brain function. Dopamine is a major neurotransmitter in the brain, iron is highly concentrated in the dopamine pathways, and animal studies have shown that iron deficiency may cause learning deficits and consequent behavioral impairment by diminishing dopamine neurotransmission *(Youdim)*. Iron is also needed as a co-factor for the enzymes which metabolize not only dopamine, but also serotonin and norepinephrine, other major neurotransmitters which have a potent influence on behavior.

Evidence is now emerging that iron deficiency may be an important contributor to the aggressive behavioral syndrome. Among adolescent males, iron deficiency has been shown to be directly associated with aggressive behavior (Conduct Disorder) *(Tu; Webb)* and, in a population of incarcerated adolescents, the prevalence of iron deficiency was nearly twice that found in their non-incarcerated peers *(Rosen)*.

While there has been little research on the effects of iron repletion, a report suggests that iron supplementation may have helped normalize impulsive, overaggressive behaviors in two iron-deficient adolescents *(Tu)*.

Lithium

There is considerable evidence that pharmacologic doses of lithium, which has no known essential function, can reduce abnormal aggressive behaviors including self-mutilation *(Wickham)*. Lithium has been used successfully with treatment-resistant hospitalized children with diagnoses of Conduct disorder, Aggressive Type

(Campbell), as well as with brain-injured *(Glenn)* and mentally retarded *(Spreat)* patients with aggressive, combative or self-destructive behavior.
While often effective, lithium at pharmacologic doses (generally 900,000 µg or more daily) has serious limitations. It suffers from many potential side effects, some of which are common. Because it becomes toxic at a serum level that is not much higher than the therapeutic range, serum lithium levels must be tested periodically. For these reasons, patients must be under medical supervision so long as they are taking the drug.

It is possible that lithium may exert a powerful effect on overaggressive behaviors at far lower levels of intake. Using data from 27 Texas counties, Schrauzer and Shrestha found that the incidences of suicide, homicide and rape were significantly higher in counties whose drinking water supplies contained little or no lithium than in counties with higher water lithium levels, even after correcting for population density. Corresponding associations with the incidences of robbery, burglary and theft were also significant, as were associations with the incidences of arrests for possession of opium, cocaine and their derivatives *(Schrauzer, 1990)*. Moreover, there is evidence suggesting that hair lithium levels of violent imprisoned offenders may be significantly reduced *(Schrauzer, 1992)*.

Low-dose lithium supplementation (400 µg daily) was compared to placebo in a 4-week study of 24 young men and women, all of whom were former drug users; some were violent offenders or had a history of domestic violence. Subjects completed weekly questionnaires measuring mental and physical activity, ability to think and work, mood and emotionality. Based on the questionnaires as well as the comments of the subjects, low-dose lithium supplementation appeared to have both a mood-improving and mood stabilizing effect *(Schrauzer, 1994)*.

If we assume that a person consumes about one liter of water daily from municipal supplies, it is striking that the level of lithium provided from the vegetable concentrates approximates that consumed by residents of the Texas counties with higher lithium levels:

"Natural" lithium dosage: 150 µg daily

Lithium level of drinking water in the Texas counties with higher levels: 70 -170 µg per liter

Source: Schrauzer, 1994

Magnesium Deficiency

Rodent studies suggest that magnesium has a complex relationship with aggressive behaviors. Magnesium deficiency reduces offensive aggressive behavior but increases defensive aggressive behavior *(Kantak)*. Lower levels of magnesium supplementation increase the number of attacks on intruders, while higher levels have the opposite effect *(Izenwasser)*.

In humans, magnesium deficiency, which enhances catecholamine secretion and sensitivity to stress, may promote aggressive behavior. Increased catecholamines, in turn, induce intracellular magnesium losses and, eventually, increase urinary losses of magnesium *(Henrotte)*.

It has been suggested that the Type A behavior pattern - which is associated with chronic stress and aggressive behavior - may both cause and be caused by magnesium deficiency *(Henrotte)*. Also, suicide attempts, which are violently aggressive acts against the self, have been correlated with lowered magnesium levels in the cerebrospinal fluid *(Banki)*. In one group of 155 psychiatric patients, more disturbed, excitable behavior was strongly associated with low plasma magnesium levels. Interestingly, there was also a similar association with *elevated* plasma magnesium levels *(Kirow)*.

Manganese Toxicity

Manganese is an essential trace mineral. Massive overexposure produces "manganese madness" which may initially be marked by violence, criminal acts and a state of mental excitement; later, neurological impairment slowly develops, with signs and symptoms which resemble Parkinson's disease.

A study of 285 counties in the states of New York, California, and Florida found that, in examining counties *without* manganese toxicity, violent crime rates in those counties with the greatest share of the population at risk were 3 times higher than in those counties with the lowest share. In contrast, for counties in which manganese toxicity was present, this difference jumped to 11 times the base rate *(Masters)*.

The behavioral effects of marginal levels of manganese toxicity have not been described. Gottschalk and his associates consistently found elevated hair manganese in a population of violent male offenders, suggesting that marginal manganese toxicity may be associated with violent criminal behavior. Compared to the hair manganese levels which they found, people exposed to levels of manganese pollution which are known to be toxic possess hair values that are 2 to 6 times higher *(Gottschalk)*. Similar findings were noted in a group of violence-prone boys *(Marlowe)*.

Elevated hair manganese levels have also been reported in hyperkinetic children *(Barlow;Collipp)*, and men with a history of childhood hyperactivity have an increased rate of antisocial and drug use disorders *(Mannuzza)*. In rats, chronic manganese exposure initially produces hyperactivity with an increased tendency to fight *(Chandra)*. While any hypothesis concerning the behavioral effects of marginal manganese toxicity in humans is highly speculative, these findings suggest that marginal manganese toxicity may promote overaggressive behaviors in adults.

Zinc Deficiency and the Zinc to Copper Ratio

A deficiency of zinc increases brain norepinephrine *(Walwork)* and may be associated with emotional disorders including irritability and impulsivity. In an informal clinical report of more than 4,000 behavior disordered patients, Walsh noted that zinc depletion was common as manifested by symptoms of deficiency along with depressed plasma zinc levels *(Walsh,1995)*. He suggests that these patients may suffer from a failure to properly utilize dietary zinc, resulting in high urinary zinc excretion *(Walsh,1995)*. This lowers the zinc to copper ratio, one of the most important mineral ratios in human biological chemistry.

For example, in a study of assaultive young men, the median serum zinc to copper ratio was significantly depressed *(Walsh,1997)*. Moreover, a study of chronic juvenile offenders found that their diets were richer in zinc, and poorer in copper, than those of normals *(Schauss,1979b)*; thus the *dietary* zinc to copper ratio may actually be elevated, suggesting an unconscious attempt to rectify the mineral imbalance through diet.

Several studies have investigated the relationship between hair copper and proneness to violence. The results have been inconsistent. Hair copper has been found to be elevated *(Marlowe)*, depressed *(Cromwell)*, and normal *(Gottschalk)*, suggesting that there may be biologically different sub-populations.

Walsh notes that his patients eventually responded to zinc supplementation augmented by L-cysteine (to mobilize and excrete copper while enhancing zinc absorption) along with vitamin B_6, vitamin C and vitamin E, although lifelong zinc supplementation appeared to be necessary to maintain benefits *(Walsh,1995)*. Controlled clinical trials remain to be done to confirm his observations.

A 9 year-old boy who lived near a smelter was charged with attempted murder and had been on 8 different medications including Ritalin. His hair copper levels were markedly elevated at 15 ppm. Hair zinc levels were quite low and his zinc/copper ratio was 1:1 (ideally 8-12:1). His hair manganese levels were also elevated to the 90th percentile.

After 4 months of nutritional treatment, his hair zinc levels had increased, although his hair copper was still elevated. One year later, his hair analysis was normal. Subsequently he graduated from a junior college with an almost straight A average and, when last contacted, was in his senior year of a four-year college on scholarship (Schauss,1993).

OTHER NUTRITIONAL FACTORS

Omega-3 Essential Fatty Acids

Concern has been expressed in the literature about a frequent finding that very low cholesterol levels appear to be associated with higher incidences of accidents and violent acts. While lower serum cholesterol was found to be associated with higher mortality due to accidents and violence in western Finland, which is by the coast, this was not true in eastern Finland, which is inland *(Pekkanen)*, suggesting that fish consumption may have protected the coastal inhabitants *(Hibbeln)*.

Similarly, when 355 men and women were switched to a cholesterol-lowering diet in which fish consumption was increased, aggressive hostility as well as depression decreased *(Weidner)*. Since fish are a major source of omega-3 fatty acids, this finding suggests that a higher intake of omega-3 fatty acids may decrease violent acts - at least if, as in the usual Western diet, the ratio of omega-6 to omega-3 fatty acids is relatively high.

This hypothesis was confirmed in a study of non-human primates that were given a diet that substantially increases the ratio of omega-6 to omega-3 fatty acids above their baseline of about a 6:1 ratio. The result was an increase in aggressive behavior *(Kaplan)*.

Tryptophan

Serotonin, a major neurotransmitter, has been found to play an important role in modulating aggressive behavior. Impulsive, violent and suicidal behaviors have repeatedly been shown to be associated with a reduction in serotonergic activity in the central nervous system *(Roy)*.

Alcohol ingestion, which is well known to magnify the potential for aggression *(Lau)*, appears to transiently increase brain serotonin turnover *(Goodwin)*. This effect would initially improve mood, but result in further serotonin depletion and thus promote aggressive behavior.

The combination of excessive alcohol intake and a low tryptophan diet (tryptophan is the dietary precursor of serotonin) has been found to be associated with decreased brain serotonin and increased aggression *(Pihl,1995)*. In a study of alcoholic impulsive offenders with antisocial personality disorder, aggressive behavior was found to be related to depressed cerebrospinal fluid (CSF) serotonin levels. Depressed CSF levels of 5-HIAA (a serotonin metabolite) were associated with elevated CSF testosterone levels. While 5-HIAA levels were related to impulsivity, testosterone levels were related to aggressiveness and interpersonal violence *(Virkkunen,1994)*.

In addition to alcoholics, depressed CSF 5-HIAA levels have also been found in suicidal/aggressive patients and violent offenders who were not alcoholic *(Linnoila;van Praag)*.

Several lines of evidence suggest that the amount of tryptophan in the diet relates closely to aggressive behavior. For example, rats given a diet almost lacking in tryptophan develop aggressive behavior towards mice *(Giammanco)*. In humans, tryptophan intake is inversely correlated with aggressive traits *(Cleare,1994,1995)*. Moreover, bimodal seasonal patterns (emotional changes related to the seasons) are related to plasma L-tryptophan availability, and this data matches known seasonal patterns in the prevalence of violent suicide and depression *(Maes)*.

Tryptophan must compete with other large neutral amino acids to cross the blood-brain barrier; therefore the ratio of the amount of tryptophan to the amount of competing amino acids (the tryptophan ratio) may provide a rough indication of the availability of tryptophan in the brain for conversion into serotonin. Kitahara has calculated the dietary tryptophan ratio for 18 European countries to attempt to relate it to homicide rates. While initially no correlation was found between low tryptophan ratios and homicide, once social and cultural differences were controlled for, low tryptophan ratios were found to be associated with high homicide rates *(Kitahara)*.

A more direct method of examining the relationship between the tryptophan ratio and aggression is by measuring the actual ratio in the blood plasma. When a group of depressed alcoholics was evaluated in this manner, those with a history of aggression, including suicide attempts, also had the lowest tryptophan ratios *(Branchey)*.

If a low ratio of tryptophan to competing amino acids is associated with aggressive behavior, will tryptophan supplementation reduce that behavior? Dietary tryptophan was manipulated in social groups of vervet monkeys by providing them with amino acid mixtures that were tryptophan-free, nutritionally balanced, or excessively high in tryptophan. These mixtures were shown to have a marked effect on plasma tryptophan levels.

During spontaneous activity, the only effect of the different mixtures was increased aggression in the males on the tryptophan-free mixture. During competition for food, however, while the tryptophan-free mixture continued to increase male aggression, the high-tryptophan mixture reduced aggression in both males and females *(Chamberlain)*. These data suggest that tryptophan supplementation may be most effective in reducing aggression during times of stress.

When hospitalized male schizophrenics were given tryptophan, only those patients with high levels of hostility and a high lifetime frequency of aggressive incidents benefited; these patients showed a lessening of hostility and depression, a reduction in ward incidents and improvement on a standardized psychiatric rating scale *(Morand)*. In another study of 20 aggressive patients, 6 grams of tryptophan daily for one month failed to reduce the number of violent incidents, although it significantly reduced the need for potent medications to control violent or agitated behavior *(Volavka)*.

The rate of firing of serotonergic neurons in the brain increases as the level of behavioral arousal increases; thus increased serotonin levels would be more likely to influence brain function at higher levels of arousal. Indeed, this fact probably explains why the vervet monkeys only responded to tryptophan supplementation when they were put under competitive stress. It also may explain why altered tryptophan levels failed to affect aggression in a study of normal human males, while overaroused, hostile and aggressive psychiatric patients responded well.

In the conversion of tryptophan to serotonin, the intermediate step is its conversion to 5-hydroxy-tryptophan. Surprisingly, supplementation with 5-hydroxytryptophan may *increase* aggressive behavior, apparently because, while tryptophan appears to enhance the serotonergic system exclusively, 5-hydroxytryptophan also appears to enhance the catecholaminergic system *(Raleigh)*.

COMBINED NUTRIENT SUPPLEMENTATION

Several studies have investigated the effect of supplementing violence-prone subjects with a combination of nutrients. Perhaps the best study to date concerned 62 confined delinquents aged 13 to 17 years. They randomly received either a vitamin/mineral supplement or a placebo. After 3 months, both violence and non-violence rule infractions decreased only in the supplemented group.

Twenty-six of the subjects donated pre- and post-intervention blood samples. While, for the 10 subjects who maintained their normal or low blood vitamin levels throughout the trial, there was little change in violence (29 acts during baseline vs. 37 during intervention), the 16 subjects whose initially low blood vitamin levels were corrected produced 131 violent acts during baseline and 11 during interventions *(Schoenthaler,1997)*.

OTHER RELATED FACTORS

Sugar Intake and Reactive Hypoglycemia

There is early evidence that hypoglycemia during glucose tolerance testing is related to hostile, aggressive behavior such as that seen in habitually violent and impulsive criminals *(Roy)*. Virkkunin, for example, found that a group of habitually violent adult criminals had lower basal glucose levels during glucose tolerance testing than controls *(Virkkunen,1982)*. Even in the normal population, there is evidence of a relationship between hypoglycemic tendencies and both frustration and hostility *(Benton)*.

Assuming that there is an association between hypoglycemia and the aggressive behavioral syndrome, the question of whether hypoglycemia causes the syndrome remains. One method of investigating the issue of causality is by changing the amount of sugar in the diet and examining the behavioral effects. Since dietary sugar provokes insulin production which may cause a reactive hypoglycemia, a change in behavior following a change in sugar intake would be consistent with the hypothesis that dietary sugar influences that behavior.

In a series of increasingly sophisticated double-blind studies, Schoenthaler addressed this question by reducing the sugar intake of thousands of incarcerated juvenile offenders in different locations around the United States. Compared to offenders on a placebo diet, he found a significant reduction in various forms of antisocial behavior (such as assaultiveness, fighting, self-injury and suicide attempts) in offenders restricted to a minimal amount of sugar in their diet - but only for the males *(Schoenthaler,1982-6)*.

While Schoenthaler's work suggests that dietary sugar may influence behavior, he did not examine blood sugar levels; it thus fails to address the role of reactive hypoglycemia in the aggressive behavioral syndrome. The finding that only males responded may either be because males are more likely to engage in aggressive behaviors, or because males are more sensitive to nutritional influences on aggression. (Remember that the lack of tryptophan in the diet only increased aggression during spontaneous play in the male monkeys.)

However, *JAMA* has published a meta-analysis of 16 placebo-controlled studies that failed to support Schoenthaler's work *(Wolraich)*, and Schoenthaler's work has been criticized on the basis of serious methodological flaws *(White)*. Moreover, much of the work in this area has been criticized for failing to control for the possibility that subjects may be hypersensitive to sugar, and thus even a modest amount of sugar in the control diets could theoretically mask any behavioral differences between the experimental and control groups *(Miller)*. Further studies are clearly needed to bring clarity to this contentious issue.

Even if a high sugar diet does not provoke hypoglycemia, it may foster aggressive behavior due to its low content of micronutrients. In fact, Schoenthaler reached this conclusion after finding that a group of incarcerated juvenile offenders responded to a low sugar diet with a significant reduction in conduct problems, but failed to show improvement until after the first month, and then showed a linear improvement over 18 weeks *(Schoenthaler,1986)*.

Food Sensitivities

It appears that overaggressive behaviors can be provoked by a reaction to common foods. Reactions range from irritability to a psychotic aggressive reaction. Children who improved after food eliminations had previously been irritable, fretful, quarrelsome and could not get along with others. Often they had to be taken out of school as they upset the classes and were considered incorrigible. After food eliminations, however, their personalities dramatically changed, and they became happy and social *(Clarke)*.

A study reported in the *Lancet* suggests that food sensitivities may be quite common among behaviorally-disturbed children. 81 out of a group of 140 children with behavior disorders (almost two-thirds) experienced significant improvement following the elimination of certain foods along with food additives. When they were challenged with the specific foods which had been eliminated, their behavior problems returned. Moreover, 75% of these children reacted to a double-blind challenge with salicylates but not to placebo *(Swain)*.

When he was five years and one month old, G.L. was seen because of uncontrollable temper tantrums. He was believed aphasic because of poor speech development, and was too uncomfortable to do initial IQ testing. The EEG showed 14-per-second spikes, large amounts of sharp activity in the motor leads, temporal single, polyphasic sharp waves, and a long run of sharp waves in the right temporal area. Allergy tests revealed strong reactions to milk, chocolate and yeast.

He was placed on a diet free of milk, chocolate, and cola drinks. Seven and one half months later, his EEG was normal. Six months after the repeat EEG, he was learning better and his behavior was much improved. He was challenged again with the suspected foods for one week, during which time his behavior again became uncontrollable.

The EEG now showed two-and-one-half to six-per-second activity on the right, greater in the mid-temporal and parietal leads, accentuated by drowsiness. Light cerebral dysfunction was diagnosed (Moyer).

Adults may also display overaggressive behaviors due to food sensitivities. For example, MacKarness has written of a woman who had been hospitalized 13 times for violent behavior and depression; after common foods were eliminated from her diet, she no longer became violent or depressed. Instead she felt fine and obtained a regular job *(MacKarness)*.

While the research literature suggests that any commonly ingested food or food additive may be responsible for provoking pathological psychological and behavioral reactions, milk may be a special case. Schauss and Simonsen found that chronic juvenile delinquents consumed much more milk than matched controls without a history of delinquency. The male offenders consumed an average of a gallon of milk daily compared to a little less than a quart a day for the controls, and the females showed similar differences *(Schauss, 1979a)*.

Schauss believes that overconsumption of milk causes antisocial behavior. He has reported that, when several Michigan detention centers reduced their inmates' milk consumption, the incidence of antisocial behavior declined; when they permitted milk consumption to increase again, antisocial behavior also increased *(Schauss, 1984)*.

Schauss has also suggested that the link between cow's milk and delinquency may only apply to homogenized milk. *(Schauss, 1993)*. His hypothesis is strengthened by a mouse study which found increased antigenicity with homogenized bovine milk compared to raw or pasteurized milk. Furthermore, as the fat content of the homogenized milk increased, so did the antigenicity. The researchers theorize that homogenization alters the relationship between proteins and fats, thus increasing the risk of allergic manifestations *(Poulsen, 1987)*.

Serum Triglycerides

In a study of 1592 men and women aged 55 to 74 years, a relationship was found between serum triglyceride levels and both hostile acts and a domineering attitude. This relationship, which was especially prevalent in men, was independent of age, total and HDL cholesterol, cigarette smoking, and alcohol consumption *(Fowkes)*. Since nutritional intervention can lower serum triglyceride levels (see Atherosclerosis), these findings suggest yet another interrelationship between nutrition and aggressive behavior.

Heavy Metal Toxicity

Aluminum

Exposure to aluminum may contribute to overaggressive behaviors. Hair aluminum levels of a group of 22 juvenile offenders *(Schmidt)*, as well as of another group of 10 severely delinquent, psychotic or prepsychotic adolescent boys *(Rees)*, were elevated. However, both studies compared aluminum levels to laboratory norms rather than to matched controls; thus other differences between the groups could account for the findings.

Cadmium

Studies comparing hair cadmium levels of violent male offenders to matched controls have had conflicting results. One study looked at hair cadmium levels of 40 apparently normal young men entering US Navy recruit training and found a highly significant relationship between hair cadmium levels and the number of demerits each recruit had received. Moreover, the 3 recruits who had the highest cadmium levels all displayed serious behavior difficulties during training *(Struempler)*. Similar findings were noted in a study of emotionally disturbed boys which compared 23 violence-prone boys to 31 boys who were not prone to violence: a significant association was found between increased hair cadmium levels and violence-prone behavior *(Marlowe)*.

Lead

Brain damage due to toxic metal exposure may promote aggressive, antisocial and violent behaviors. Lead exposure is known to cause learning and behavioral problems, problems which are found in a substantial portion of juvenile delinquents.

The strongest evidence to date that lead exposure increases the frequency of aggressive behaviors comes from the Edinburgh Lead Study which included over 500 children between the ages of 6 and 9. After taking 30 possible confounding variables into account, the investigators still found a significant relationship between the log of blood lead levels and teachers' ratings of the children's behavior on an "aggressive/antisocial" scale and on a "hyperactive" scale, but not on a "neurotic" scale. As in other studies on the relationship between lead exposure and brain damage, a dose-response relationship was found between blood lead and behavior ratings, with no evidence of a threshold *(Thomson)*.

Other measures of body lead levels have shown similar associations. Hair lead levels have been found to be directly associated with violence-prone behavior in a group of violence-prone boys *(Marlowe)*. The relationship between bone lead levels and delinquent behavior was explored in a retrospective cohort study published in *JAMA*. From a group of 850 seven-year-old boys, all who scored in the upper 30th percentile of the distribution on a self-reported antisocial behavior scale were matched with an equal number randomly drawn from the lower 70% of the distribution. Bone lead levels which were obtained when they were 12 years old were compared to earlier behavior assessments using the Child Behavior Checklist (CBCL), teachers' and parents' reports, and their own self-report of antisocial behavior and delinquency.

At 7 years of age, borderline associations were found between bone lead levels and teachers' aggression, delinquency, and externalizing scores. Four years later, bone lead levels were significantly associated with teachers' ratings of somatic complaints and delinquent, aggressive, internalizing, and externalizing behavior. Moreover, a significant association had developed between bone lead levels and several parent-rated CBCL cluster scores.

High bone lead children reported higher scores in their self-reports of delinquency at 11 years of age, and were more likely to obtain worse scores on all items of the CBCL during the 4-year period of observation. High bone lead levels were also associated with an increased risk of exceeding the threshold score of the CBCL which indicated a clinical problem in regard to attention, aggression, and delinquency *(Needleman)*.

Pihl and associates have addressed the relationship of lead exposure and violent behavior in adults. Hair lead levels from 19 violent criminals were found to be elevated as compared with those of 10 nonviolent criminals *(Pihl,1982)*. This study was repeated 8 years later by the same research team with essentially the same results. However, their results were contradicted by those of the Gottschalk study on hair manganese levels; in that study, no significant differences were found between hair lead levels of 104 violent criminals, prison guards and local townspeople *(Gottschalk)*.

BIBLIOGRAPHY

American Psychiatric Association: Diagnostic and Statistical Manual of Mental Disorders, Fourth Edition. Washington, DC, American Psychiatric Association, 1994

Bailey L et al. Serum ferritin as a measure of iron stores in adolescents. J Pediatr 101:774-6, 1982

Banki CM et al. Cerebrospinal fluid magnesium and calcium related to amine metabolites, diagnosis, and suicide attempts. Biol Psychiatry 20(2):163-71, 1985

Barlow PJ. A pilot study on the metal levels in the hair of hyperactive children. Med Hypotheses 11(3):309-18, 1983

Benton D et al. Mild hypoglycaemia and questionnaire measures of aggression. Biol Psychol 14(1-2):129-35, 1982

Branchey L et al. Depression, suicide and aggression in alcoholics and their relationship to plasma amino acids. Psychiatry Res 12(3):219-26, 1984

Brin M. Examples of behavioral changes in marginal vitamin deficiency in the rat and man, in J Brozek, Ed. Behavioral Effects of Energy and Protein Deficits. United States Department of Health, Education and Welfare Publ. no. (National Institutes of Health) 79-1906, 1979

Campbell M et al. Behavioral efficacy of haloperidol and lithium carbonate. A comparison in hospitalized aggressive children with conduct disorder. Arch Gen Psychiatry 41(7):650-6, 1984

Chamberlain B et al. The effect of raising or lowering tryptophan levels on aggression in vervet monkeys. Pharmacol Biochem Behav 28(4):503-10, 1987

Chandra SV. Psychiatric illness due to manganese poisoning. Acta Psychiatr Scand Suppl 303:49-54, 1983

Clarke TW. The relation of allergy to character problems in children: A survey. Ann Allergy March-April, 1950, pp. 175-87

Cleare AJ, Bond AJ. Effects of alterations in plasma tryptophan levels on aggressive feelings. Arch Gen Psychiatry 51:1004-5, 1994

Cleare AJ, Bond AJ. The effect of tryptophan depletion and enhancement on subjective and behavioral aggression in normal male subjects. Psychopharmacology 118: 72-81, 1995

Collipp PJ. Manganese in infant formulas and learning disability. Ann Nutr Metab 27:488-94, 1983

Cromwell PF, Abadie BP, Stephens JT, Kyler M. Hair mineral analysis: biochemical imbalances and violent criminal behavior. Psychol Rep 64(1):259-66, 1989

Fowkes FGR et al. Serum cholesterol, triglycerides, and aggression in the general population. Lancet 340:995-8, 1992

Gelenberg AJ. Psychiatric Disorders, in DM Paige, Ed. Clinical Nutrition, Second Edition. St. Louis, The C.V. Mosby Company, 1988

Giammanco S et al. Short term diet of precooked corn meal almost lacking in tryptophan and interspecific rat-mouse aggressive behavior. Arch Int Physiol Biochim 98(1):23-6, 1990

Glenn MB et al. Lithium carbonate for aggressive behavior or affective instability in ten brain-injured patients. Am J Phys Med Rehabil 68(5):221-6, 1989

Goodwin FK. Alcoholism research: delivering on the promise. Public Health Rep 103(6):569-74, 1988

Gottschalk LA et al. Abnormalities in hair trace-elements as indicators of aberrant behavior. Compr Psychiatry 32:229-37, 1991

Henrotte JG. Type A behavior and magnesium metabolism. Magnesium 5:201-10, 1986

Hibbeln JR, Salem N Jr. Dietary polyunsaturated fatty acids and depression: when cholesterol does not satisfy. Am J Clin Nutr 62:1-9, 1995

Hodges RE et al. J Clin Invest 38:1421, 1959

Izenwasser SE et al. Stimulant-like effects of magnesium on aggression in mice. Pharmacol Biochem Behav 25(6):1195-9, 1986

Kantak KM. Magnesium deficiency alters aggressive behavior and catecholamine function. Behav Neurosci 102(2):304-11, 1988

Kaplan JR et al. The effects of fat and cholesterol on social behavior in monkeys. Psychosom Med 53(6):634-42, 1991

Kirow GK et al. Plasma magnesium levels in a population of psychiatric patients: correlation with symptoms. Neuropsychobiology 30(2-3): 72-8, 1994

Kitahara M. Dietary tryptophan ratio and homicide in Western and Southern Europe. J Orthomol Med 1(1):13-6, 1986

Lau MA, Pihl RO. Alcohol and the Taylor aggression paradigm: a repeated measures study. J Stud Alcohol 55(6):701-6, 1994

Linnoila VMI et al. Aggression, suicidality, and serotonin. J Clin Psychiatry 53:10 (suppl) 46-51, 1992

Lonsdale D, Shamberger R. Red cell transketolase as an indicator of nutritional deficiency. Am J Clin Nutr 33(2):205-11, 1980

MacKarness R. Eating Dangerously. New York, Harcourt, Brace, Jovanovich, 1976

Maes M et al. Seasonal variation in plasma L-tryptophan availability in healthy volunteers: relationships in violent suicide occurrence. Arch Gen Psychiatry 52: 937:45, 1995

Mannuzza S et al. Hyperactive boys almost grown up. V. Replication of psychiatric status. Arch Gen Psychiatry 48:77-83, 1991

Marlowe M et al. Hair trace element content of violence prone male children. J Advancement Med 7(1):5-18, 1994

Masters RD, Nelson A. Rockefeller Professor of Government, Dartmouth College, Hanover, New Hampshire. Unpublished data, June, 1995

McLaren DS. Clinical manifestations of nutritional disorders, in ME Shils & VR Young. Modern Nutrition in Health and Disease, Seventh Edition. Philadelphia, Lea & Febiger, 1988

Miller JB. Sweets are a cause of hyperactivity! The Environmental Physician, Spring, 1995

Morand C et al. Clinical response of aggressive schizophrenics to oral tryptophan. Biol Psychiatry 18(5):575-8, 1983

Moyer KE. Allergy & aggression: The physiology of violence. Psychol Today July, 1975, pp. 77-9

Needleman HL et al. Bone lead levels and delinquent behavior. JAMA, 275(5):363-9, 1996

Pekkanen J et al. Serum cholesterol and risk of accidental or violent death in a 25-year follow-up. The Finnish cohorts of the Seven Countries Study. Arch Intern Med 149(7):1589-91, 1989

Pihl RO et al. Hair element content of violent criminals. Can J Psychiatry 27:533, 1982

Pihl RO et al. Acute effect of altered tryptophan levels and alcohol on aggression in normal human males. Psychopharmacology 119:353-60, 1995

Poulsen OM et al. Effect of homogenization and pasteurization on the allergenicity of bovine milk analysed by a murine anaphylactic shock model, Clin Allergy 17(5):449-58, 1987

Raleigh MJ. Differential behavioral effects of tryptophan and 5-hydroxytryptophan on vervet monkeys: influence of catecholaminergic systems. Psychopharmacology (Berlin) 93(1):44-50, 1987

Rees EL. Aluminum toxicity as indicated by hair analysis. J Orthomol Psychiatry 8:37, 1979

Rosen GM, Deinard AS, Schwartz S et al. Iron deficiency among incarcerated juvenile delinquents. J Adolesc Health Care 6:419-23, 1985

Roy A et al. Monamines, glucose metabolism, aggression towards self and others. Int J Neurosci 41(3-4):261-4, 1988

Schauss AG. Nutrition and antisocial behaviour. Int Clin Nutr Rev 4(4):172-7, 1984

Schauss AG. Nutrition and crime: update - presentation at the Well Mind Symposium 1992 - reported in Townsend Letter for Doctors, June, 1993

Schauss AG et al. Critical analysis of the diets of chronic juvenile offenders: Part II. J Orthomol Psychiatry 8(3):222-6, 1979b

Schauss AG, Simonsen CE. Critical analysis of the diets of chronic juvenile offenders: Part I. J Orthomol Psychiatry 8(3):149-57, 1979a

Schmidt K et al. Clinical ecology treatment approach for juvenile offenders. J Behav Ecology: Biosocial 2(1), 1981

Schoenthaler SJ. Int J Biosoc Res Vol. 3-7, 1982-6

Schoenthaler SJ. Diet and delinquency: empirical testing of seven theories. Int J Biosoc Res 7(2):108-31, 1986

Schoenthaler S, Amos S, Doraz W, et al. The effect of randomized vitamin-mineral supplementation on violent and non-violent antisocial behavior among incarcerated juveniles. J Nutr Environ Med 7:343-52, 1997

Schrauzer GN et al. Effects of nutritional lithium supplementation on mood: A placebo-controlled study with former drug users. Biol Trace Elem Res 40(1):89-101, 1994

Schrauzer GN et al. Lithium in scalp hair of adults, students, and violent criminals. Biol Trace Elem Res 34(2):161-76, 1992

Schrauzer GN, Shrestha KP. Lithium in drinking water and the incidences of crimes, suicides, and arrests related to drug addictions. Biol Trace Elem Res 25(2):105-13, 1990

Spreat S et al. Lithium carbonate for aggression in mentally retarded persons. Comp Psychiatry 30(6):505-11, 1989

Struempler RE et al. Hair mineral analysis and disruptive behavior in clinically normal young men. J Learn Disabil 18(10):609-12, 1985

Swain A et al. Salicylates, oligoantigenic diets, and behaviour. Letter. Lancet ii:41-2, 1985

Thomson GO et al. Blood-lead levels and children's behaviour: results from the Edinburgh Lead Study. J Child Psychol Psychiatry 30(4):515-28, 1989

Tu JB et al. Iron deficiency in two adolescents with conduct, dysthymic and movement disorders. Can J Psychiatry 39(6):371-5, 1994

van Praag HM. Affective disorders and aggression disorders: evidence for a common biological mechanism. Suicide Life Threat Behav 16(2): 103:32, 1986

Virkkunen M. Reactive hypoglycemic tendency among habitually violent offenders. A further study by means of the oral glucose tolerance test. Neuropsychobiology 8:35-40, 1982

Virkkunen M et al. CSF biochemistries, glucose metabolism, and diurnal activity rhythms in alcoholic, violent offenders, fire setters, and healthy volunteers. Arch Gen Psychiatry 51(1):20-7, 1994

Volavka J et al. Tryptophan treatment of aggressive psychiatric patients. Biol Psychiatry 28(8):728-32, 1990

Walsh WJ. Zinc deficiency, metal metabolism, and behavior disorders. Unpublished monograph. Health Research Institute, 1804 Centre Point Dr., Suite 106, Naperville, IL 60503, March, 1995

Walsh WJ et al. Elevated blood copper/zinc ratios in assaultive young males. Physiol Behav 62(2):327-9, 1997

Walwork JC et al. Distribution of minerals and catecholamines in rat brain: effects of zinc deficiency, in CJ Frederickson et al, Eds. The Neurobiology of Zinc, Part B: Deficiency, Toxicity and Pathology (Neurology and Neurobiology V. 11B). New York, Alan R. Liss, 1984:49-64

Webb TE, Oski FA. Behavioral status of young adolescents with iron deficiency anemia. J Special Ed 8(2):153-6, 1974

Weidner G et al. Improvements in hostility and depression in relation to dietary change and cholesterol lowering. Ann Intern Med 117(10):820-3, 1992

White JW, Wolraich M. Effect of sugar on behavior and mental performance. Am J Clin Nutr 62 (suppl): 242S-9S, 1995

Wickham EA, Reed JV. Lithium for the control of aggressive and self-mutilating behaviour. Int Clin Psychopharmacol 2(3):181-90, 1987

Wilmot CA et al. Ascorbic acid inhibits isolation-induced fighting in mice. Fed Proc 42:1160, 1983

Wolraich ML et al. The effect of sugar on behavior or cognition in children. JAMA, 274:1617-21, 1995

Youdim MB et al. Putative biological mechanisms of the effect of iron deficiency on brain biochemistry and behavior. Am J Clin Nutr 50(3 Suppl.):607-15, 1990

ALCOHOLISM

See Also: ANXIETY
DEPRESSION
'HYPOGLYCEMIA'
NEURALGIA & NEUROPATHY
ORGANIC MENTAL DISORDERS

NUTRITIONAL TREATMENT GUIDE

✓ = Efficacy generally accepted.
* = Efficacy *demonstrated* by controlled human trials.
[+] = Efficacy *suspected* from uncontrolled human trials.
[-] = Efficacy *suspected* from indirect data.
? = Efficacy *challenged* in a study of similar design.

I. TO REDUCE ALCOHOL TOXICITY AND PROMOTE HEALING

✓ **Well-balanced, nutritionally adequate diet** (including at least 1 g protein/kg/d) with repletion of deficient nutrients [see table below]

- -

* **L-Carnitine:** acetylcarnitine 2 g daily (3 month trial)
* **Glutathione deficiency:** S-adenosylmethionine 1.2 g daily (6 month trial)
* **Vitamin C:** ? 2 g daily

- -

[+] **Magnesium deficiency:** ≈ 400 mg daily (Consider parenteral administration.)
[+] **Niacin** or **Niacinamide:** ? 250 mg twice daily
[+] **Pantethine:** ? 300 mg 2 to 3 times daily
[+] **Thiamine deficiency:** 50 mg daily
(Alkyl disulfide derivatives are preferable, if available.)
(Consider intramuscular administration, especially during alcohol withdrawal.)
[+] **Tryptophan:** 1 g 3 times daily
[+] **Vitamin A deficiency:** 50,000 IU daily (only if the patient is not drinking)
[+] **Vitamin E deficiency:** D,L-alpha-tocopheryl acetate 200-2000 mg or IU daily for 6 weeks

- -

[-] rule out **Food Sensitivities**
[-] rule out elevated **Homocysteine** levels
[-] **L-Carnitine:** ? 750 mg twice daily
[-] **Omega-3 Fatty Acids:** *example:* MaxEPA 1 g caps [180 mg EPA; 120 mg DHA] 10 to 20 daily
[-] **Omega-6 Fatty Acids:** *example:* evening primrose oil 500 mg caps [7-10% GLA] 6 to 8 daily
[-] **Phosphatidylcholine:** ? 900 mg 3 times daily
[-] **Selenium deficiency:** 200 μg daily
[-] **Taurine:** ? 1 g 3 times daily
[-] **Zinc deficiency:** zinc sulfate 220 mg twice daily *AND* **Copper** 2 mg daily

II. TO REDUCE ALCOHOL WITHDRAWAL SYMPTOMS

* **Evening Primrose oil**: 500 mg caps [7-10% GLA] 6 to 8 daily
* **gamma-Hydroxybutyric Acid**: 50 mg/kg body weight daily
* **Taurine**: 1 g 3 times daily

- -

[+] **Phosphorus**: Correct hypophosphatemia.

III. TO REDUCE CRAVING FOR ALCOHOL

* **Well-balanced, nutritionally adequate diet** with nutritional supplementation and nutrition education (to reduce recidivism)
* **L-Glutamine**: 2 g (1/2 tsp) daily in divided doses

- -

[+] Increase consumption of **Raw Foods**
[+] **Niacin:** 500 to 1000 mg in time-release form daily (3 to 4 week trial)

- -

[-] avoid **Coffee** (including decaffeinated coffee)
[-] rule out **Food Sensitivities**
[-] rule out **Reactive Hypoglycemia**
[-] **Thiamine**: ? 100 mg daily
[-] **Tryptophan**: ? 1 g 3 times daily
[-] **Zinc deficiency:** zinc sulfate 220 mg twice daily *AND* **Copper** 2 mg daily

DIET AND THE ALCOHOLIC

While alcohol itself has been shown to cause liver disease, myopathy and cardiomyopathy, some of the adverse effects of alcoholism (such as polyneuropathy and Wernicke's encephalopathy) which were formerly ascribed to the direct toxic effects of alcohol are now recognized as resulting primarily from nutritional deficiencies.

These deficiencies have several causes. Since alcoholic beverages tend to be calorie-rich while nutrient-poor, alcoholics commonly fail to ingest a nutritionally-adequate diet. Alcohol has been shown to cause maldigestion and malabsorption. It does so by inflaming the lining of the esophagus, stomach and duodenum, and by causing changes in the wall of the small intestines which interfere with the enzymatic digestion of foodstuffs.

The blocking action of alcohol may prevent the normal interaction among nutrients, and its toxic effects on the liver may interfere with that organ's ability to utilize nutrients. Finally, alcohol causes mineral depletion through hyperexcretion in the urine and stool.

Nutritional treatment of alcoholism must therefore be built on the foundation of a well-balanced, nutritionally adequate diet with additional supplementation designed to provide nutrient repletion. No matter how good the nutritional intake, however, the alcohol-induced changes in the gastrointestinal system may continue to impair the alcoholic's ability to utilize nutrients even long after drinking has ceased. While the esophagitis and gastritis heal quickly, it can take up to 2 years for the small bowel to repair the damage, and the liver may never fully recover.

SOME COMMON NUTRITIONAL DEFICIENCIES AMONG ALCOHOLICS

Macronutrients
- Protein

Vitamins
- Vitamin A
- Vitamin B Complex, including:
  - Folic Acid
  - Niacin
  - Riboflavin
  - Thiamine
  - Vitamin B_6
  - Vitamin B_{12}*
- Vitamin C
- Vitamin D
- Vitamin E

Minerals
- Magnesium
- Phosphorus
- Selenium
- Zinc

Other Nutritional Factors
- Choline
- Gamma-linolenic acid
- Glutathione

* *In the presence of alcoholic liver disease, serum B_{12} levels correlate with the severity of the hepatitis, and thus should not be used as a measure of B_{12} nutriture. This is due to the failure of the diseased liver to remove cobalamin and its analogues from the serum; thus liver B_{12} levels may be low despite normal or elevated serum B_{12}.*

A 35 year-old longshoreman was a typical "spree" drinker who consumed large quantities of alcohol and ingested very little food during a period of several weeks prior to hospitalization. He was severely jaundiced, and had an enlarged and tender liver.

Upon hospitalization he voluntarily consumed 4,000 to 6,500 kcal/d including 200 to 250 g of protein. A liver biopsy done several days after admittance showed a moderate fatty change and cellular infiltration. He gained 15 kg body weight. The serum bilirubin concentration returned to normal, liver size decreased and tenderness promptly subsided. After 3 weeks, no clinical or laboratory stigmata of liver disease remained. The histologic appearance of a second biopsy obtained after about 3 and one-half weeks of hospitalization was essentially normal (Chalmers).

Coffee

Most research suggests that heavy coffee intake may have an adverse impact on health. However, epidemiological studies have found coffee consumption to be inversely related to serum levels of gamma-glutamyltransferase, a marker for alcoholic liver disease as well as other hepatobiliary diseases. Since green tea, despite its caffeine content, does not show the same effect, factors other than caffeine appeared to explain the relationship *(Kono;Poikolainen)*. Still lacking, however, is direct evidence that coffee consumption protects from hepatobiliary diseases.

I. REDUCING ALCOHOL TOXICITY AND PROMOTING HEALING

ACETALDEHYDE

The primary metabolite of ethanol, acetaldehyde may promote the development of liver disease, cardiomyopathy and atherosclerosis. Chronic alcoholics are believed to develop elevated acetaldehyde levels due to accelerated degradation of ethanol to acetaldehyde coupled with slowing of the degradation of acetaldehyde *(Davis)*.

Niacin, Pantethine and Taurine

Niacin, by oxidizing ethanol, may be beneficial by reducing acetaldehyde levels *(Cleary,1986)*. *Niacinamide* appears to be equally effective *(Eriksson)*.

The effects of acetaldehyde may also be reduced by supplementation with *pantethine (Watanabe,1985a)*, a derivative of pantothenic acid, or *taurine (Watanabe,1985b)*, an amino acid. Both increase the activity of alcohol dehydrogenase, the enzyme that metabolizes acetaldehyde. Pantethine is ineffective, however, for patients who flush after alcohol ingestion, as flushing appears to be correlated with a deficient hepatic capacity to produce the enzyme. It is likely that taurine has the same limitation.

ANTIOXIDANTS

Alcohol toxicity can also be reduced by employing antioxidants. Vitamin C, vitamin E and selenium, three antioxidants that are commonly depressed in the serum of alcoholics *(Lecomte)*, appear to reduce the toxic effects of alcohol, especially the development of alcoholic liver disease.

Vitamin C

Pretreatment with vitamin C appears to protect against fatty infiltration of the liver *(DeLuzio)*. For normals, 5 grams given daily for 2 weeks prior to alcohol ingestion enhanced blood ethanol clearance and reduced the detrimental effects of ethanol on motor coordination and color discrimination (but not on intellectual function) in half of the subjects *(Susick)*. A shorter period of pretreatment (1 hour) with a lower dosage (2 grams) has also been shown to enhance blood alcohol clearance *(Chen)*.

Vitamin E Deficiency

Animal work suggests that chronic alcohol ingestion may reduce vitamin E in liver parenchymal cells *(Bjorneboe,1987)*. Several human studies have shown that plasma/serum levels of the vitamin are depressed in alcoholics *(Clot)*. Furthermore, alcoholics with reduced plasma/serum and hepatic vitamin E levels have shown evidence of increased oxidative stress *(Bjorneboe,1993)*.

There is preliminary evidence from animal studies that vitamin E, like vitamin C, when taken before or during alcohol ingestion, may prevent fatty infiltration of the liver *(Kawase)* although, in alcoholics, it seems ineffective against advanced cirrhosis *(Pía de la Maza)*. Other animal work suggests that vitamin E may also reduce alcohol's cardiotoxic effects *(Redetzki)*.

Selenium Deficiency

The lower the level of liver selenium, the worse the liver disease *(Korpela)*, and alcoholics who are deficient in both selenium and vitamin E suffer from more active liver disease than those who are deficient in only one of these two antioxidant nutrients; they also show evidence of increased lipid peroxidation *(Tanner)*. Moreover, alcoholic cirrhotics with reduced selenium levels have been found to show improved liver function following selenium supplementation *(Van Gossum)*.

Glutathione and S-adenosylmethionine Deficiencies

Erythrocyte levels of glutathione may be low in alcoholics, whether or not they have cirrhosis. Similarly, chronic ethanol ingestion decreases hepatic levels of S-adenosylmethionine (SAMe), a glutathione precursor *(Duce)*.

Parenteral administration of *reduced glutathione* may decrease the extent of ethanol-induced macroscopic injury to the mucosa of the gastric body and antrum *(Loguercio,1993)*. Also, a controlled study found that low hepatic glutathione levels could be normalized with the administration of SAMe *(Loguercio,1994; Vendemiale)*.

The value of SAMe supplementation was demonstrated in a study of ethanol-fed baboons. It was found that dietary SAMe offset the ethanol-mediated reduction in hepatic levels of both SAMe and glutathione. Moreover, it moderated the ethanol-induced increases in plasma glutamate dehydrogenase and aspartate aminotransferase, and normalized the morphology of hepatic mitochondria, thus attenuating alcohol-induced liver injury *(Lieber,1990)*.

HOMOCYSTEINE

Plasma levels of homocysteine, a toxic amino acid, are often elevated in chronic alcohol consumers *(Cravo;Hultberg)*.

Folic Acid, Vitamin B_6 and/or Vitamin B_{12}

Elevated homocysteine not only indicates an interference with one-carbon metabolism, but suggests a need for additional *folic acid, vitamin B_6*, and/or *vitamin B_{12}*, vitamins that lower homocysteine levels by serving as coenzymes in its metabolism *(Cravo)*. (See Atherosclerosis.)

OTHER NUTRIENTS

L-Carnitine

L-carnitine, according to the results of animal work, may inhibit the development of alcohol-induced fatty liver, apparently by facilitating the oxidation of the increased fatty acid load due to alcohol ingestion *(Sachan)*.

The efficacy of supplemental carnitine in preventing the development of alcoholic liver disease is not yet clear *(McCarty)*. However, *acetylcarnitine*, a patented derivative, has been shown under double-blind conditions to reverse the cognitive defects found in chronic alcoholics *(Tempesta)*.

Choline Deficiency

Choline appears to be hepatoprotective. This is relevant since chronic alcohol ingestion results in a decrease of liver phospholipids, especially phosphatidylcholine, and this decrease is correctable with phosphatidylcholine supplementation *(Lieber, 1992)*.

Animal studies (including monkeys) suggest that a deficiency of choline is particularly important if liver damage is to occur *(Rogers AE; Takada)*, and a small pilot study found that some fatty livers respond nicely to a purified diet of just a vitamin/mineral-enhanced glucose solution so long as choline is added *(Phillips)*.

Omega-3 Fatty Acid Deficiencies

Chronic alcohol intoxication causes depletion of these essential polyunsaturates from neuronal membranes *(Salem)*. This can foster the development of depressive symptoms *(Hibbeln)*.

Omega-6 Fatty Acids

In animal studies, both prostaglandin E_1 and its omega-6 fatty acid precursor, gamma-linolenic acid, have been shown to retard or prevent the development of fatty liver during ethanol administration *(Segarnick)*. Evening primrose oil, the best-studied of the natural substances that have a high content of gamma-linolenic acid (other than mother's milk), may be of value in preventing liver damage in patients who are continuing to drink *(Horrobin)*. More speculative is the possibility that it may promote hepatic regeneration.

Magnesium Deficiency

Magnesium deficiency is yet another development that may contribute to tissue damage. Hypomagnesemia, which is common in hospitalized alcoholics, results from deficient intake, malabsorption, excessive renal losses, and reduced cellular uptake *(Rivlin)*. Magnesium deficiency may cause cardiomyopathy *(Burch)* as well as a myopathy *(Pall)* that responds rapidly to magnesium administration. Magnesium deficiency may also contribute to osteoporosis *(Abbott)*.

Finally, the N-methyl-D-aspartate (NMDA) receptor is an important part of the brain's neuroexcitatory pathway. Magnesium inhibits this receptor; thus deficiency may cause or contribute to a variety of neuromuscular and psychiatric symptoms.

While hypocalcemia is primarily due to hypoalbuminemia, magnesium deficiency is another possible cause, in which case it is rapidly responsive to magnesium supplementation *(Pall)*. Serum magnesium levels may be low before and during the early stages of delirium tremens (although low magnesium does not appear to provoke the syndrome), and serum levels may later return to normal on their own *(Jermain)*.

Magnesium supplementation can reverse many of the changes due to deficiency. It has been shown to improve hepatic function *(Gullestad)* to successfully treat alcoholic myopathy *(Pall)*, and to dramatically reverse hypomagnesemic encephalopathy *(Glick)*.

Thiamine Deficiency

Thiamine deficiency is a frequent finding *(Darnton-Hill)*, especially when there is evidence of alcoholic liver disease. Causes include inadequate intake, interference of ethanol with absorption and utilization of the vitamin for the synthesis of coenzyme and thiamine-dependent haloenzymes, and reduced hepatic storage.

The neuropsychiatric complications of alcoholism, such as Wernicke's syndrome and Korsakoff's psychosis, are commonly believed to be due to deficiency of this vitamin *(Cook)*, while polyneuropathy may be specifically due to a defect in thiamine utilization *(Paladin)*. Alcoholic cirrhosis is also associated with inadequate thiamine nutriture *(Tallaksen)*.

There is general agreement that thiamine supplementation is required for the chronic alcoholic, especially during withdrawal. Oral supplementation will often restore tissue levels *(Baines)*; however, because of problems with absorption, intramuscular administration, or the use of derivatives that are more readily absorbed, may be preferable. The latter include *benfotiamine*, a lipophilic derivative, and *thiamine tetrahydrofurfuryl disulfide*, a synthetic derivative of allithiamine - a substance that is naturally formed in garlic bulbs and other plants of the allium species by the conjugation of allicin with thiamine.

L-Tryptophan

Chronic alcoholism leads to a deficiency in brain serotonin due to a decreased ratio of tryptophan, its essential amino acid precursor, to the other amino acids competing with tryptophan for brain transport *(Branchey)*. Depression (especially when associated with aggression and suicidal acts), blackouts, memory impairment and epilepsy are all associated with a deficiency in brain serotonin *(Virkkunen)*. While the diet of the alcoholic is likely to be tryptophan-deficient, tryptophan deficiency may also be due to enhanced tryptophan catabolism associated with increased glucocorticoid activity *(Buydens-Branchey)*.

It would seem that tryptophan supplementation should therefore be advisable. Unfortunately the benefits of supplementation have not been carefully explored. A pilot study found that tryptophan pretreatment prevented ethanol-induced impairment of one aspect of memory (facial recognition), although it failed to prevent impairment of verbal recall *(Westrick)*.

Vitamin A Deficiency

Vitamin A is frequently markedly deficient in the liver *(Lieber, 1983)* and serum *(McCauley)* of alcoholics, although serum levels usually remain normal until liver stores are exhausted *(Majumdar)*. Supplementation is especially indicated for alcoholics suffering from liver or sexual dysfunction as well as from night blindness *(Lieber, 1988)*, and it may also improve the sense of taste and olfaction *(Garett-Laster)*.

The one caveat is that, if the alcoholic continues to drink heavily, vitamin A supplementation may actually *promote* the development of liver disease *(Lieber, 1988)*. For this reason, it has been suggested that, for this population, beta-carotene supplementation be given to enhance vitamin A levels *(McCauley)*; however, alcohol-fed baboons fed supplemental beta-carotene still developed histological changes in the liver *(Leo)*. Thus, even beta-carotene supplementation needs to be coupled with control of drinking to avoid all danger of hepatic damage *(Ahmed)*.

Zinc Deficiency

Zinc deficiency, common in alcoholics, may cause liver damage through impairment of ethanol clearance from the blood *(Milne)*. Because vitamin A is necessary for zinc absorption while zinc, in turn, is crucial to vitamin A metabolism, zinc and vitamin A deficiencies are commonly associated *(Scholmerich)*; in fact, vitamin A supplementation alone may improve taste and olfaction (sensations which are impaired by zinc deficiency), possibly by improving zinc absorption.

Low brain zinc levels are often found in chronic alcoholics. As with magnesium deficiency, zinc deficiency increases NMDA receptor excitotoxicity; among other things this increases an alcoholic's susceptibility to withdrawal seizures. Zinc deficiency can also produce neuronal damage through increased free radical formation; thus zinc replacement is part of a rational approach to treating alcohol-related withdrawal seizures and brain dysfunction *(Menzano)*.

II. REDUCING SYMPTOMS OF ALCOHOL WITHDRAWAL

gamma-Hydroxybutyric Acid

Gamma-hydroxybutyric acid is an endogenous substance that appears promising when given in pharmacologic doses. A constituent of the mammalian brain that is concentrated in the hypothalamus and basal ganglia, it suppresses the ethanol withdrawal syndrome in ethanol-dependent rats, and has been shown to be dramatically effective in minimizing the withdrawal syndrome in humans *(Biggio; Gessa)*. Its use, however, must be carefully regulated as it can cause seizures and coma *(Dyer)* and physical dependence may develop with chronic use *(Galloway)*.

Omega-6 Fatty Acids

Evening primrose oil, discussed earlier as an hepatoprotectant, appears to have some value as a source of omega-6 fatty acids in reducing both alcohol craving and the alcohol withdrawal syndrome. The results of animal studies with both PGE_1 and primrose oil have been confirmed in a human double-blind study. Among the patients who received the oil for 3 weeks, there was a significant reduction in the amount of diazepam needed to ease symptoms and a modest but consistent lowering of the score for measures of withdrawal severity *(Glen)*.

A Norwegian fisherman with severe depressions would binge drink for 2 weeks at a time, consuming a bottle of whiskey a day; then, because he became sick and run down, he would sober up for one or two weeks. He was given evening primrose oil or placebo in a double-blind manner and logged each day's alcohol consumption, degree of alcohol craving and depression on a rating scale.

Primrose oil resulted in an 80% reduction in depression and alcohol craving within a week, and he had no alcohol consumption for 6 weeks for the first time in years. Shortly after being switched to placebo, however, he went on a binge and dropped out of the study (Bates).

Phosphorus

Among hospitalized alcoholics, blood phosphorus levels are commonly below normal *(Stein)*, particularly 2 to 4 days after hospitalization. When it is severe, hypophosphatemia produces visual hallucinations as well as neurological features that may be confused with delirium tremens *(Knochel)*. Furthermore, it has been suggested that delirium tremens could be fostered by hypophosphatemia *(Larner)*.

Taurine

Another nutrient that holds promise in alcohol withdrawal is the amino acid taurine. An inhibitory neurotransmitter, taurine significantly ameliorated symptoms of alcohol withdrawal in a controlled study *(Ikeda)*.

In addition, data from open trials suggest that taurine supplementation is effective in relieving muscle cramps in patients with liver cirrhosis *(Matsuzaki;Yamamoto)*.

III. REDUCING ALCOHOL CRAVING

DIETARY FACTORS

It is possible that nutritional interventions may reduce the alcoholic's compulsive need to drink. For example, rats fed a typical teenage "junk food" diet continuously increased their alcohol consumption, while rats fed a healthy, well-balanced diet maintained a low level of alcohol intake *(Register)*. When caffeine or coffee was added to the diet of either group, alcohol intake significantly increased *(Register)*.

While, unfortunately, few studies have investigated the effects of nutritional interventions on alcohol craving in humans, one such study suggests that increasing the percentage of raw foods in the diet can be strikingly effective (at least for those patients who are motivated to make such a major dietary change.) When a group of hypertensives ate an average of 2/3 of their calories as uncooked food for several months, 80% of those who smoked or drank alcohol abstained spontaneously *(Douglass)*.

ACETALDEHYDE

Acetaldehyde has been blamed for promoting alcohol addiction by its ability to combine with monamine metabolites to form addicting morphine-like alkaloids *(Davis)*. Thus, nutritional treatments aimed at reducing acetaldehyde (*see above*) may also benefit the alcoholic by reducing alcohol craving.

NUTRITIONAL FACTORS

L-Glutamine

Not only did the administration of L-glutamine to rats diminish their urge to drink alcohol *(Rogers LL,1956)* but, in a crossover study, 9 out of 10 patients stated that glutamine diminished their desire to drink as well as decreased their anxiety and improved their sleep. Relatives and friends observing them agreed. When placebo was substituted, only 2 or 3 of the 10 continued to do well, and none who failed to respond to glutamine responded to placebo *(Rogers LL,1957)*.

A secretary in her early thirties had been drinking heavily for several years and was extremely despondent. She showed no response to one week on placebo. During the following 2 weeks she received L-glutamine 1 g daily. She stopped drinking completely and her outlook improved tremendously. She was shifted to placebos and, by the end of the sixth week, she had started to drink occasionally. By the end of the tenth week, she was drinking as heavily as before taking glutamine and had stopped taking the placebo capsules.

She agreed to resume the trial and was switched back to glutamine. Her drinking stopped again almost immediately. Over the next 3 months, she was followed while continuing on glutamine. She reported drinking a little beer occasionally but claimed not to have had hard liquor or to have overindulged at any time. She also commented frequently on her ability to sleep better and on her decreased nervousness (Rogers LL,1957).

Lithium

Administration of lithium has been examined as a possible agent to reduce alcohol intake. Unfortunately, human studies have shown that this approach has limited or no efficacy *(Backlage;Jefferson;Lejoyeux).*

L-Tryptophan

Supplementation with the essential amino acid tryptophan which, as noted above, is frequently deficient in alcoholics, may be beneficial. So far the only evidence of the efficacy of tryptophan supplementation comes from a study of cats that ate nutritionally adequate diets and had been permitted for at least several months to choose freely between water and alcohol. When they received intraperitoneal tryptophan injections, they reduced their alcohol intake *(Baskina).*

Vitamin B Complex

When rats were given diets deficient in the B complex vitamins, they were more likely to choose alcohol over water. After they were supplemented with vitamin B complex, however, they preferred water over alcohol *(Norton).*

Subsequent studies have sought to identify components of the vitamin B complex that reduce drinking behavior. *Niacin*, by reducing acetaldehyde levels, is believed to contribute to the effect *(Cleary,1986)*, and niacin supplementation was followed by a reduction in alcohol craving in an open trial *(Cleary,1990)*. Animal studies also suggest that *thiamine* deficiency contributes to the relationship between the vitamin B complex deficiency and increased alcohol intake *(Eriksson).*

Zinc

Rat studies have also linked zinc nutriture to alcohol craving. When rats are made zinc-deficient, their alcohol intake increases *(Collipp)*. When they are then supplemented with zinc, their alcohol intake declines *(Skal'nyi).*

FOOD SENSITIVITIES

Food sensitivities have been blamed for contributing to alcohol addiction. Alcoholics have been found to have "leaky guts" making them more vulnerable than normals to absorb food antigens and toxic compounds *(Bjarnason)*. However, evidence that food reactions actually provoke ethanol craving is lacking.

REACTIVE HYPOGLYCEMIA

An interesting theory suggests that craving for alcoholic beverages may be related to their high sugar content which attracts people experiencing reactive hypoglycemia. Alcohol ingestion is known to increase gastric acidity; this could lead to excessive insulin release due to augmented beta-cell responsiveness in response to the increased release of gut secretagogues *(Freinkel)*. Also, results of an animal study suggest that insulin production may be directly correlated with alcohol intake *(Forander).*

Although it is conceivable that an alcoholic experiencing reactive hypoglycemia would reach for the bottle, studies demonstrating that hyperinsulinism causes alcoholism are lacking.

BIBLIOGRAPHY

Abbott L et al. Magnesium deficiency in alcoholism: possible contribution to osteoporosis and cardiovascular disease in alcoholics. Alcohol Clin Exp Res 18(5):1076-82, 1994

Ahmed S et al. Interactions between alcohol and beta-carotene in patients with alcoholic liver disease. Am J Clin Nutr 60:430-6, 1994

Backlage NE, Jefferson JW. Alternative uses of lithium in psychiatry. Psychosomatics 28(5): 239-56, 1987

Baines M et al. Tissue thiamin levels of hospitalized alcoholics before and after oral or parenteral vitamins. Alcohol Alcohol 23(1):49-52, 1988

Baskina NF, Lapin IP. [Changes in alcohol choice by chronically alcoholized cats affected by tryptophan, its metabolites and preparations affecting its metabolism.] Farmacol Toksikol 45(1):70-76, 1982

Bates C. Essential Fatty Acids and Immunity in Mental Health. Tacoma, WA, Life Sciences Press, 1987, p. 71

Biggio, G et al. Suppression of voluntary alcohol intake in rats and alcoholics by gamma-hydroxybutyric acid: a non-GABAergic mechanism. Adv Biochem Psychopharmacol 47:281-8, 1992

Bjarnason I et al. The leaky gut of alcoholism: Possible route of entry for toxic compounds. Lancet i:179-82, 1984

Bjorneboe GE et al. Reduced hepatic alpha tocopherol content after long-term administration of ethanol to rats. Biochim Biophys Acta 918:236-41, 1987

Bjorneboe A, Bjorneboe GE. Antioxidant status and alcohol-related diseases. Alcohol Alcohol 28(1):111-16, 1993

Branchey L et al. Ethanol impairs tryptophan transport into the brain and depresses serotonin. Life Sci 29(26):2751-5, 1981

Burch GE, Giles TD. The importance of magnesium deficiency in cardiovascular disease. Am Heart J 94:649-57, 1977

Buydens-Branchey L et al. Increase in tryptophan oxygenase activity in alcoholic patients. Alcoholism (NY) 12(1):163-7, 1988

Chalmers TC, Davidson CS. Survey of recent therapeutic measures in cirrhosis of the liver. N Engl J Med 240:449, 1949

Chen MF et al. Effect of ascorbic acid on plasma alcohol clearance. J Am Coll Nutr 9(3):185-9, 1990

Cleary JP. The NAD deficiency diseases. J Orthomol Med 1(3):149-57, 1986

Cleary JP. Niacinamide and addictions. Letter. J Nutr Med 1:83-4, 1990

Clot P et al. Monitoring oxidating damage in patients with liver cirrhosis and different daily alcohol intake. Gut 35:1637-43, 1994

Collipp PJ et al. The effects of dietary zinc deficiency on voluntary alcohol drinking in rats. Alcoholism (NY) 8(6):556-9, 1984

Cook CCH, Thomson AD. B-complex vitamins in the prophylaxis and treatment of Wernicke-Korsakoff syndrome. Br J Clin Pract 57(9):461-5, 1997

Cravo ML et al. Hyperhomocysteinemia in chronic alcoholism: correlation with folate, vitamin B-12, and vitamin B-6 status. Am J Clin Nutr 63:220-4, 1996

Darnton-Hill I, Truswell AS. Thiamin status of a sample of homeless clinic attenders in Sydney. Med J Aust 152(1):5-9, 1990

Davis BE, Walsh MJ. Alcohol, amines and alkaloids: A possible biochemical basis for alcohol addiction. Science 167:1005-7, 1970

DeLuzio NR. A mechanism of the acute ethanol-induced fatty liver and the modification of liver injury by antioxidants. Lab Invest 15:50-61, 1966

Douglass J et al. Effects of a raw food diet on hypertension and obesity. South Med J 78(7):841, 1985

Duce AM et al. S-adenosyl-L-methionine synthetase and phospholipid methyltransferase are inhibited in human cirrhosis. Hepatology 8:65-8, 1988

Dyer JE. gamma-Hydroxybutyrate: a health-food product producing coma and seizurelike activity. Am J Emerg Med 9(4):321-4, 1991

Eriksson K et al. The effects of dietary thiamin on voluntary ethanol drinking and ethanol metabolism in the rat. Br J Nutr 43(1):1-13, 1980

Forander et al. Q J Stud Alcohol. 19:379, 1958

Freinkel N, Getzger BE. Oral glucose tolerance curve and hypoglycemias in the fed state. N Engl J Med 280:820-8, 1969

Galloway GP et al. Physical dependence on sodium oxybate. Letter. Lancet 343:57, 1994

Garrett-Laster M et al. Impairment of taste and olfaction in patients with cirrhosis: The role of vitamin A. Hum Nutr Clin Nutr 38C:203-14, 1984

Gessa GL. Gallimberti L. Gamma-hydroxybutyric acid in the treatment of alcohol dependence. Clin Neuropharmacol 15 Suppl 1 Pt A:303A-304A, 1992

Glen I et al. Possible pharmacological approaches to the prevention and treatment of alcohol-related CNS impairment: Results of a double blind trial of essential fatty acids, in G Edwards, J Littleton, Eds. Pharmacological Treatments for Alcoholism. London, Croom, Helm, 1984:331-50

Glick JL. Use of magnesium in the management of dementias. Med Sci Res 18:831-3, 1990

Gullestad L, et al. Oral magnesium supplementation improves metabolic variables and muscle strength in alcoholics. Alcohol Clin Exp Res 16(5):986-90, 1992

Hibbeln JR and Salem N Jr. Dietary polyunsaturated fatty acids and depression: when cholesterol does not satisfy. Am J Clin Nutr 62:1-9, 1995

Horrobin DF. A biochemical basis for alcoholism and alcohol-induced damage including the fetal alcohol syndrome and cirrhosis: Interference with essential fatty acid and prostaglandin metabolism. Med Hypotheses 6:929-42, 1980

Hultberg B et al. Elevated plasma homocysteine in alcoholics. Alcohol Clin Exp Res 17(3):687-9, 1993

Ikeda H. Effects of taurine on alcohol withdrawal. Letter to the Editor. Lancet ii:509, 1977

Jefferson JW. Lithium: The present and the future. J Clin Psychiatry 51:8(Suppl):4-8, 1990

Jermain DM et al. Controversies over the use of magnesium sulfate in delirium tremens. Ann Pharmacother 26(5):650-2, 1992

Kawase T et al. Lipid peroxidation and antioxidant defenses in rat liver after chronic ethanol feeding. Hepatology 10:815-21, 1989

Knochel JP. The pathophysiology and clinical characteristics of severe hypophosphatemia. Arch Intern Med 137:203-20, 1977

Kono S et al. Coffee and serum gamma-glutamyltransferase; a study of self-defense officials in Japan. Am J Epidemiol 139:723-7, 1994

Korpela H et al. Decreased serum selenium in alcoholics as related to liver structure and function. Am J Clin Nutr 42:147-51, 1985

Larner AJ. Hypophosphataemia, hallucinations, and delirium tremens. Letter. Lancet 338:1467, 1991

Lecomte E et al. Effect of alcohol consumption on blood antioxidant nutrients and oxidative stress indicators. Am J Clin Nutr 60(2):255-61, 1994

Lejoyeux M et al. Evaluation of lithium treatment in alcoholism. Alcohol Alcohol 28(3):273-9, 1993

Leo MA et al. Interaction of ethanol with beta carotene: delayed blood clearance and enhanced hepatotoxicity. Hepatology 15:883-91, 1992

Lieber CS. Alcohol-nutrition interaction: 1983. Contemp Nutr December 1983

Lieber CS. Biochemical and molecular basis of alcohol-induced injury to liver and other tissues. N Engl J Med 391(25):1639-50, 1988

Lieber CS et al. S-adenosyl-L-methionine attenuates alcohol-induced liver injury in the baboon. Hepatology 11:165-72, 1990

Lieber CS et al. Dietary dilinoleoylphosphatidylcholine (CLPC) is incorporated into liver phospholipids, protects against alcoholic cirrhosis, enhances collagenase activity and prevents acetaldehyde-induced collagen accumulation in cultured lipocytes. Abstract. Hepatology 16:87A, 1992

Loguercio C et al. Glutathione prevents ethanol induced gastric mucosal damage and depletion of sulphhydryl compounds in humans. Gut 34:161-5, 1993

Loguercio C et al. Effect of S-adenosyl-L-methionine administration on red blood cell cysteine and glutathione levels in alcoholic patients with and without liver disease. Alcohol Alcohol 29(5):597-604, 1994

Majumdar SK et al. Vitamin A utilization status in chronic alcoholic patients. Int J Vitam Nutr Res 53(3):273-9, 1983

Matsuzaki Y et al. Is taurine effective for treatment of painful muscle cramps in liver cirrhosis? Am J Gastroenterol 88:1466-7, 1993

McCarty MF. Nutritional prevention of alcoholic liver disease - present and future prospects. Letter. J Optimal Nutr 3(2):102-7, 1994

McCauley, CK et al. Vitamin status of alcoholics upon admission and after two weeks of hospitalization. J Am Coll Nutr 12(1):77-83, 1993

Menzano E and Carlen PL. Zinc deficiency and corticosteroids in the pathogenesis of alcoholic brain dysfunction - a review. Alcohol Clin Exp Res 18(4): 894-901, 1994

Milne DB et al. Effect of short-term dietary zinc intake on ethanol metabolism in adult men. Clin Res 39:A652, 1991

Norton VP. Interrelationships of nutrition and voluntary alcohol consumption in experimental animals. Br J Addition 72(3):205-12, 1977

Paladin F, Russo Perez G. The haematic thiamine level in the course of alcoholic polyneuropathy. Eur Neurol 26(3):129-33, 1987

Pall HS et al. Hypomagnesaemia causing myopathy and hypocalcaemia in an alcoholic. Postgrad Med J 63:665-7, 1987

Pía de la Maza M et al. Effects of long-term vitamin E supplementation in alcoholic cirrhotics. J Am Coll Nutr 14(2):192-6, 1995

Phillips GB, Davidson CS. Nutritional aspects of cirrhosis in alcoholism - Effect of a purified diet supplemented with choline. Ann N Y Acad Sci 57:812, 1954

Poikolainen K, Vartiainen E. Determinants of gamma-glutamyltransferase: positive interaction with alcohol and body mass index, negative association with coffee. Am J Epidemiol 15;146(12):1019-24, 1997

Register UD et al. Influence of nutrients on intake of alcohol. J Am Diet Assoc 61(2):159-62, 1972

Redetzki JE et al. Amelioration of cardiotoxic effects of alcohol by vitamin E. J Toxicol Clin Toxicol 20(4):319-31, 1983

Rivlin RS. Magnesium deficiency and alcohol intake: mechanisms, clinical significance and possible relation to cancer (a review). J. Am Coll Nutr 13(5): 416-23, 1994

Rogers AE et al. Acute and chronic effects of ethanol in non human primates, in KC Hayes, Ed. Primates in Nutritional Research. New York, Academic Press, 1979:249-89

Rogers LL et al. Voluntary alcohol consumption by rats following administration of glutamine. J Biol Chem 220(1):321-23, 1956

Rogers LL, Pelton RB. Glutamine in the treatment of alcoholism: A preliminary report. Quart J Stud Alcohol 18(4):581-87, 1957

Sachan DS et al. Ameliorating effects of carnitine and its precursors on alcohol-induced fatty liver. Am J Clin Nutr 39:738-44, 1984

Salem, N Jr, Ward G. The effects of ethanol on polyunsaturated fatty composition, in C Alling, I Diamond, SW Leslie et al., Eds. Alcohol, Cell Membranes and Signal Transduction in Brain. New York, Plenum Press, 1993:33-46

Scholmerich J et al. Zinc and vitamin A deficiency in liver cirrhosis. Hepatogastroenterology 30:1333-8, 1982

Segarnick DJ et al. Gamma-linolenic acid inhibits the development of the ethanol-induced fatty liver. Prostaglandins Leukotrienes Med 17:277-82, 1985

Skal'nyi AV et al. [Reduction of voluntary alcohol consumption under the effects of prolonged-action zinc.] Biull Eksp Biol Med 113(4):383-5, 1992

Stein JH et al. Hypophosphatemia in acute alcoholism. Am J Med Sci 252:78-83, 1966

Susick RL, JR, Zannoni VG. Effect of ascorbic acid on the consequences of acute alcohol consumption in humans. Clin Pharmacol Ther 41(5):502-09, 1987

Takada A et al. Regression of a dietary cirrhosis in rats fed alcohol and a "super diet." Evidence for the non-hepatotoxic nature of ethanol. Am J Clin Nutr 20:213-15, 1967

Tallaksen CM et al. The concentration of thiamin and thiamin phosphate esters in patients with alcoholic liver cirrhosis. Alcohol Alcohol 27(5):523-30, 1992

Tanner AR et al. Depressed selenium and vitamin E levels in an alcoholic population: Possible relationship to hepatic injury through increased lipid peroxidation. Dig Dis Sci 31:1307-12, 1986

Tempesta E et al. Role of acetyl-L-carnitine in the treatment of cognitive deficit in chronic alcoholism. Int J Clin Pharmacol Res 10:101-7, 1990

Van Gossum A, Neve J. Low selenium status in alcoholic cirrhosis is correlated with aminopyrine breath test. Biol Trace Elem Res 47:201-7, 1995

Vendemiale G et al. Effects of oral S-adenyl-L-methionine on hepatic glutathione in patients with liver disease. Scand J Gastroenterol 24(4):407-15, 1989

Virkkunen M, Linnoila M. Brain serotonin, type II alcoholism and impulsive violence. J Stud Alcohol Suppl 11:163-9, 1993

Watanabe A et al. Lowering of blood acetaldehyde but not ethanol concentrations by pantethine following alcohol ingestion: Different effects in flushing and non-flushing subjects. Alcohol Clin Exp Res 9:272, 1985a

Watanabe A et al. Lowering of liver acetaldehyde but not ethanol concentrations by pretreatment with taurine in ethanol-loaded rats. Experientia 41(11):1421-2, 1985b

Westrick ER et al. Dietary tryptophan reverses alcohol-induced impairment of facial recognition but not verbal recall. Alcoholism (NY) 12(4):531-3, 1988

Yamamoto S et al. [Painful muscle cramps in liver cirrhosis and effects of oral taurine administration]. Nippon Shokakibyo Gakkai Zasshi 91(7):1205-9, 1994) (in Japanese)

ALLERGY
(ALTERED REACTIVITY)

See Also: BRONCHIAL ASTHMA

NUTRITIONAL TREATMENT GUIDE

✓ = Efficacy generally accepted.
* = Efficacy *demonstrated* by controlled human trials.
[+] = Efficacy *suspected* from uncontrolled human trials.
[-] = Efficacy *suspected* from indirect data.
? = Efficacy *challenged* in a study of similar design.

NUTRITIONAL FACTORS

I. *GENERAL*

* **Calcium:** 1 g daily

- -

[+] **Essential Fatty Acid deficiencies**: individualized program based on laboratory testing
[+] **Magnesium deficiency:** ≈ 400 mg daily
[+] **Niacin:** ? 50 mg 3 times daily
[+] **Pantothenic Acid:** 100 to 500 mg daily
[+] **Vitamin B_{12}:** 1000 μg weekly (Consider intramuscular administration.)
[+] **Vitamin C:** 1,000 to 2,250 mg daily
[+] **Vitamin E:** 400 IU daily

- -

[-] **Quercetin:** 1 to 2 g daily divided into 3 to 6 doses
[-] **Zinc deficiency:** zinc sulfate 220 mg twice daily *AND* **Copper** 2 mg daily

II. *FORMALDEHYDE SENSITIVITY*

[+] **Pantethine:** 300 mg twice daily

III. *MONOSODIUM GLUTAMATE SENSITIVITY*

* **Vitamin B_6:** 50 mg daily for prophylaxis

- -

[-] **Vitamin C** ? 500 mg daily for prophylaxis

IV. *SULFITE SENSITIVITY*

* **Vitamin B_{12}:** 2,000 to 4,000 μg sublingually daily for prophylaxis

[+] **Molybdenum** ? 20 to 250 μg daily

OTHER RELATED FACTORS

* rule out **Food Sensitivities**

NUTRIENTS

There is some evidence that several nutrients may play a role in both atopic and non-atopic reactions.

VITAMINS

Niacin

Both niacin and niacinamide inhibit mast cell degranulation and histamine release *(Bekier; Moussatche)*. An early report noted rapid improvement in patients with bronchial asthma or hay fever following intramuscular or intravenous administration of niacinamide *(Dainow)*.

Although controlled human intervention trials in the treatment of allergy are lacking, it is known that pruritus, a common side effect of chloroquine treatment for malaria, is prevented about half of the time by the use of a concurrent antihistamine *(Okor)*. Fifty milligrams of niacin has been shown under double-blind conditions to be effective in reducing pruritus in these patients *(Ajayi)*, suggesting that a similar oral dosage may have some efficacy in reducing allergic reactions.

Pantothenic Acid

Anecdotal reports suggest that pantothenic acid supplementation may reduce allergic rhinitis and possibly other allergic conditions *(Martin; Williams)*. Controlled trials are needed for confirmation.

Vitamin B_6

The results of a double-blind study suggest that supplementation with the vitamin may prevent reactions to monosodium glutamate (MSG) even though, at baseline, reactive patients had similar levels of red cell glutamic-oxaloacetic transaminase activity (a measure of B_6 nutriture) as non-reactive controls *(Folkers)*.

Vitamin B_{12}

In an open trial, 18 out of 20 patients with intractable asthma, 9 out of 10 patients with chronic urticaria, and all 6 patients with chronic contact dermatitis improved following weekly vitamin B_{12} injections *(Simon)*. Also, vitamin B_{12} (delivered sublingually) has been shown in a double-blind study to protect against reactions to sulfite-containing foods *(Bhat)*.

Vitamin C

Low plasma ascorbate levels are correlated with elevated blood histamine *(Johnston)*, and supplementation with vitamin C reduces blood histamine in subjects with either low plasma ascorbate or elevated blood histamine *(Clemetson)*. There are anecdotal reports of patients with allergic rhinitis responding to ascorbate supplementation, with a greater percentage of patients responding to higher doses *(Brown)*. However, it appears that, in doses up to 4 grams daily, ascorbic acid fails to suppress both the histamine skin response and the nasal response to allergens *(Fortner)*; thus its efficacy at that dosage for allergic responses remains questionable.

Results of animal studies suggest that vitamin C may be able to prevent reactions to MSG *(Ahmad)*. Controlled human trials are needed to ascertain if it can prevent similar reactions in humans.

Vitamin E

While the research is preliminary, it appears that vitamin E may have antihistaminic properties. In one study, volunteers were injected intra-cutaneously with histamine. When they were given vitamin E for 5 to 7 days prior to the injection, there was far less swelling around the injection site *(Kamimura)*.

A physician with allergies took pantothenic acid 100 mg at bedtime and found that his nasal stuffiness cleared in less than 15 minutes and that he stopped awakening at 4 or 5 A.M. with cough and mucous secretion. He subsequently found that many of his patients also noted significant relief of nasal congestion following pantothenic acid supplementation (Crook).

MINERALS

Calcium

For several decades, calcium administration has been used to treat allergic disorders of the skin and respiratory tract *(Bachert)* although, until recently, controlled studies were lacking. In a double-blind crossover study published in the *Journal of Allergy and Clinical Immunology*, oral supplementation with 1 gram of calcium significantly inhibited allergen-induced swelling of the nasal mucosa (but not sneezing or nasal secretions) *(Bachert)*. In a similar type of study, oral calcium supplements in combination with calciferol (vitamin D_2) were effective in reducing airway resistance and intrathoracic gas volume, as well as increasing forced expiratory and expiratory one-second volumes in patients with bronchial asthma and airway obstruction *(Utz)*.

Magnesium Deficiency

Intracellularly, magnesium inhibits the action of calcium in releasing chemical mediators of allergic reactions from basophils and mast cells *(Fantidis)*. Chronic magnesium deficiency may provoke atopic allergic reactions *(Durlach)*, and animal work has demonstrated a synergism of antigen challenge and severe (but not moderate) magnesium deficiency on blood and urinary histamine levels *(Wei)*.

While marginal magnesium deficiency is common, magnesium supplementation in the absence of deficiency has not been demonstrated to be beneficial.

Molybdenum

Sulfite, which is known to provoke bronchospasm and other allergic reactions, is detoxified by the enzyme sulfite oxidase (sulfoxidation) to sulfate, a harmless, inert substance which is excreted in the urine. Sulfite is not normally present in urine, but it has been reported to be present in the urine of allergic and hypersensitive individuals. While poor sulfoxidizers constitute the minority (34%) of normals, they constitute the majority (78%) of both atopic and non-atopic food-sensitive patients *(Scadding)*.

Since molybdenum is required for the activation of sulfite oxidase, a molybdenum deficiency would contribute to a sulfite overload *(Abumrad)* and consequently may theoretically provoke symptoms. Indeed, blood molybdenum was reduced or absent in the majority of a group of people with sulfite sensitivity *(Papaioannou)*. Moreover, in a case report, intravenous molybdenum appeared to alleviate asthmatic symptoms while reducing urinary sulfite *(Wright)*. Whether molybdenum supplementation is an effective treatment for food sensitivities remains to be determined.

Zinc Deficiency

Physiologic concentrations of zinc have been shown to inhibit the release of histamine from human basophils and tissue mast cells *(Marone)*. Whether zinc supplementation has antihistaminic effects is unknown, although reduced red cell zinc has been reported to be associated with chemical sensitivities *(Rogers)*.

OTHER NUTRITIONAL FACTORS

Essential Fatty Acids

Individuals with atopic allergies may demonstrate abnormalities in the omega-6 series of essential fatty acids with elevated levels of *cis*-linoleic acid, and depressed levels of the products of linoleic acid metabolism - suggesting a defect in the functioning of delta-6-desaturase which converts linoleic acid to gamma-linolenic acid *(Manku)*. The metabolites of alpha-linolenic acid, members of the omega-3 family of essential fatty acids, may also be depressed *(Galland)*.

Since the essential fatty acids are the precursors to the prostaglandins, these abnormalities may result in prostaglandin deficiencies and imbalances which could affect the allergic response *(Galland)*. In fact, there is evidence from anecdotal reports that supplementation with essential fatty acids may reduce allergic symptoms in certain individuals for whom these symptoms are part of a larger picture of essential fatty acid deficiency.

Supplementation with either or both families of essential fatty acids should be individualized based on laboratory findings and clinical response.

A 6-year-old boy suffered from chronic nasal congestion with occasional cough and wheezing, developed hives if licked by a dog, and had episodes of irritability and crying after eating sweets. Since infancy he had a history of excessive thirst. On examination, he had dry skin, lackluster hair, numerous follicular keratoses, puffiness, a pale, boggy nasal lining, and white spots on his fingernails. Basic laboratory testing showed hypereosinophilia and low serum ferritin. Essential fatty acid analysis showed an elevation of linoleic acid in serum phospholipids with depressed levels of its prostaglandin precursors, and low concentrations of all the omega-3 fatty acids.

He was treated with evening primrose oil (EPO). After 1 month, he no longer developed hives when licked by his neighbor's dog, he had less nasal congestion, his skin and hair were less dry, and he appeared calmer. Salmon oil extract and an iron supplement were added, and a program of immunotherapy (allergy shots) was started.

Over the next 9 months, his hair and skin became lustrous, the eye puffiness disappeared, and he had no congestion or behavioral problems. Two weeks after EPO was stopped, he became more thirsty, sniffles, cough and wheezing developed, irritability reappeared, and he again developed hives upon contact with dogs. EPO was restarted and the symptoms disappeared within the next two weeks (Galland).

Pantethine

A derivative of pantothenic acid and precursor of coenzyme A, pantethine supplementation may increase the activity of aldehyde dehydrogenase *(Watanabe)*. Since this enzyme metabolizes formaldehyde, it has been postulated that supplementation with pantethine may reduce hypersensitivity to formaldehyde. Unfortunately, except for an unpublished case report *(Anonymous)*, this hypothesis has not been tested.

Quercetin

Like disodium chromoglycate, quercetin possesses a benzopyrone nucleus. It is believed to reduce allergic responses by at least 3 mechanisms: It stabilizes mast cells and basophils, thereby inhibiting degranulation and the subsequent release of histamine and other inflammatory mediators *(Ogasawara)*. It interacts with calmodulin to dampen the inflammatory response by inhibiting the action of several enzymes involved in that response *(Nishino)*, and it decreases leukotriene formation by inhibiting various steps in eicosanoid metabolism *(Yoshimoto)*. Controlled clinical trials are lacking, however.

FOOD SENSITIVITIES

Several reports have noted improvements in perennial allergic rhinitis, chronic urticaria and angioedema, and bronchial asthma following the elimination of foods and/or food additives. In a study published in the *Lancet*, for example, 24 of 43 children suffering from urticaria and/or angioedema who had responded to an additive-free diet reacted to double-blind challenges of food additives; the others remained well when a normal diet was reintroduced *(Supramaniam)*.

BIBLIOGRAPHY

Abumrad NN et al. Amino acid intolerance during prolonged parenteral nutrition reversed by molybdate therapy. Am J Clin Nutr 34:2551-9, 1981

Ahmad K, Jahan K. Studies on the preventive and curative action of ascorbic acid on the neurological toxicity of monosodium glutamate. Food Nutr Bull 7(4):51-3, 1985

Ajayi AA, Akinleye AO, Udoh SJ, et al. The effects of prednisone and niacin on chloroquine-induced pruritus in malaria. Eur J Clin Pharmacol 41(4):383-5, 1991

Anonymous. Pantethine: possible treatment for formaldehyde sensitivity. Ecological Formulas, 1061-B Shary Circle, Concord, CA 94518, 1986

Bachert C, Drechsler S, Hauser U, et al. Influence on oral calcium medication on nasal resistance in the nasal allergen provocation test. J Allergy Clin Immunol 91(2):599-604, 1993

Bekier E, Maslinski CZ. Antihistaminic action of nicotinamide. Agents Actions 4(3):196, 1974

Bhat NK. Presentation at the 43rd Annual Meeting, American Academy of Allergy and Immunology, 1987

Brown EA, Ruskin S. The use of cervitaminic acid in the symptomatic and coseasonal treatment of pollinosis. Ann Allergy 7:65-70, 1949

Clemetson CA. Histamine and ascorbic acid in human blood. J Nutr 110(4):662-8, 1980

Crook WG. Letter to the Editor. Ann Allergy 49:45-46, 1987

Dainow I. Recherches cliniques sur certaines proprietes anti-allergiques de la nicotinamide. Z Vitamin-forsch 15:245-50, 1944

Durlach J. Repports experimentaux et cliniques entre magnesium et hypersensibilite. Rev Fr Allergo 15:133-46, 1975

Fantidis P, Ruiz Cacho J, Marin M, et al. Intracellular (polymorphonuclear) magnesium content in patients with bronchial asthma between attacks. J R Soc Med 88(8):441-5, 1995

Folkers K et al. Biochemical evidence for a deficiency of vitamin B6 in subjects reacting to monosodium-L-glutamate by the Chinese restaurant syndrome. Biochem Biophys Res Commun 100:972-77, 1981

Fortner BR Jr et al. The effect of ascorbic acid on cutaneous and nasal response to histamine and allergen. J Allergy Clin Immunol 69(6):484-88, 1982

Galland L. Increased requirements for essential fatty acids in atopic individuals: A review with clinical descriptions. Am J Clin Nutr 5:213-28, 1986

Johnston CS, Solomon RE, Corte C. Vitamin C depletion is associated with alterations in blood histamine and plasma free carnitine in adults. J Am Coll Nutr 15(6):586-91, 1996

Kamimura M. Antiinflammatory activity of vitamin E. J Vitaminol 18(4):204-09, 1972

Manku MS et al. Reduced levels of prostaglandin precursors in the blood of atopic patients: Defective delta-6-desaturase function as a biochemical basis for atopy. Prostaglandins Leukotrienes Med 9(6):615-28, 1982

Marone G et al. Physiological concentrations of zinc inhibit the release of histamine from human basophils and lung mast cells. Agents Actions 18(1-2):103-106, 1986

Martin W. On treating allergic disorders. Letter to the Editor. Townsend Letter for Doctors Aug/Sept, 1991:670-1

Moussatche H, Prouvost-Danon A. Inhibition by nicotinamide and nicotinic acid of histamine release in the anaphylactic reaction in vitro. Influence of some metabolites. An Acad Brasileira de Ciencias 33:173-8, 1961

Nishino H et al. Quercetin interacts with calmodulin, a calcium regulatory protein. Experientia 40(2):184-5, 1984

Ogasawara H, Middleton E Jr. Effect of selected flavonoids on histamine release (HR) and hydrogen peroxide (H_2O_2) generation by human leukocytes. J Allergy Clin Immunol 75:184, 1985

Okor RS. Responsiveness of chloroquine-induced pruritus to antihistamine therapy - a clinical survey. J Clin Pharm Ther 15(2):147-50, 1990

Papaioannou R, Pfeiffer CC. Sulfite sensitivity - unrecognized threat. Is molybdenum the cause? J Orthomol Psychiatry 13(2):105-10, 1984

Rogers SA. Zinc deficiency as model for developing chemical sensitivity. Int Clin Nutr Rev 10(1):253-9, 1990

Scadding GK et al. Poor sulphoxidation ability in patients with food sensitivity. Br Med J 297:105-07, 1988

Simon SW. Vitamin B12 therapy in allergy and chronic dermatoses. J Allergy 2:183-85, 1951

Supramaniam G, Warner JO. Artificial food additive intolerance in patients with angio-oedema and urticaria. Lancet 2:907-09, 1986

Utz G, Hauck AM. [Oral application of calcium and vitamin D2 in allergic bronchial asthma.] MMW 118(43):1395-8, 1976

Watanabe A et al. Lowering of blood acetaldehyde but not ethanol concentrations by pantethine following alcohol ingestion: Different effects in flushing and non-flushing subjects. Alcohol Clin Exp Res 9:272, 1985

Wei W, Kranz KB. A synergism of antigen challenge and severe magnesium deficiency on blood and urinary histamine levels in rats. J Am Coll Nutr 9(6):616-22, 1990

Williams RJ. The expanding horizon in nutrition. Texas Rep Biol Med 19(2):245-58, 1961

Wright J, Littleton K. Defects in sulphur metabolism. Int Clin Nutr Rev 9(3):118-19, 1989

Yoshimoto T et al. Flavonoids: Potent inhibitors of arachidonate 5-lipoxygenase. Biochem Biophys Res Commun 116:612-18, 1983

ANEMIA

See Also: CELIAC DISEASE
INFERTILITY

NUTRITIONAL TREATMENT GUIDE

✓ = Efficacy generally accepted.
* = Efficacy *demonstrated* by controlled human trials.
[+] = Efficacy *suspected* from uncontrolled human trials.
[-] = Efficacy *suspected* from indirect data.
? = Efficacy *challenged* in a study of similar design.

NUTRITIONAL FACTORS

✓ **Folic acid deficiency:** 800 μg daily
✓ **Iron deficiency:** 30 mg twice daily; then minimal possible dosage
✓ **Vitamin B_{12} deficiency:** 1000 μg intramuscularly weekly initially and monthly afterwards

\- -

* **Vitamin A deficiency:** 50,000 IU daily for 6 weeks (10,000 IU daily during pregnancy)
* **Zinc deficiency:** zinc sulfate 220 mg twice daily *AND* **Copper** 2 mg daily

\- -

[+] **Pantothenic acid deficiency:** 100 to 200 mg daily
[+] **Riboflavin deficiency:** 5 to 10 mg daily
[+] **Thiamine deficiency:** 50 mg daily orally or intramuscularly
[+] **Vitamin B_6 deficiency:** 50 to 100 mg daily
[+] **Vitamin C deficiency:** 500 mg twice daily
[+] **Vitamin E deficiency:** D,L-alpha-tocopheryl acetate 200 to 2,000 mg or IU daily for 6 weeks
[+] **Copper deficiency:** 2 mg twice daily for up to 6 weeks along with 50 mg zinc daily
[+] **Magnesium deficiency:** usual oral dosage ≈ 400 mg daily (Consider IM or IV administration.)

OTHER FACTORS

* **Hydrochloric Acid deficiency:** betaine or glutamic hydrochloride 10 to 50 gr following meals (Beware of gastric irritation.)

\- -

[+] rule out **Gluten Sensitivity**
[+] rule out **Milk Sensitivity** (infants with iron-deficiency anemia)

OVERVIEW

The microcytic anemia of iron deficiency, and the megaloblastic anemia of folate or vitamin B_{12} deficiency, are widely known. While nutritional pharmacotherapy does not appear to be indicated in the treatment of anemia, many anemias are fostered by deficiencies of any of a variety of vitamins and minerals, repletion of which will often cause a reticulocytosis.

Hydrochloric acid deficiency should be considered as a cause of iron-deficiency and sickle cell anemias. Gluten sensitivity may present as anemia, while milk sensitivity may cause an iron deficiency by provoking intestinal bleeding.

NUTRIENT DEFICIENCIES IN ANEMIAS

	Anemia (general)	Beta-Thalassemia	Sickle Cell	Sideroblastic
Copper	X		X	
Folic Acid	X		X	
Iron	X		X	
Magnesium	X	X	X	
Riboflavin	X		X	
Thiamine	X			
Vitamin A	X		X	
Vitamin B_6	X		X	X
Vitamin B_{12}	X		X	
Vitamin C	X	X		
Vitamin E	X	X	X	
Zinc		X	X	

VITAMIN DEFICIENCIES

Vitamin A Deficiency

Anemia gradually develops several months after starting a diet deficient in vitamin A. Serum hemoglobin begins to decline well before the loss of night vision or the development of 'deficient' serum levels of the vitamin *(Hodges)*. The anemia, which is due to impaired hemoglobin synthesis, is reversible with supplementation *(West)*. Vitamin A may also be deficient in sickle cell anemia *(Sindel)*.

Vitamin B Complex Deficiencies

Folic acid deficiency is a well-known cause of megaloblastic anemia. Deficiency can also be related to sickle cell anemia *(Pierce)* which, in turn, is responsive to supplementation *(Reed)*. When deficient, folate supplementation may also be beneficial in treating aplastic anemia *(Branda)* or red cell aplasia *(Gothoni)*.

When deficient, pantothenic acid supplementation can be helpful in alleviating anemia *(McCurdy)*.

A 53 year-old black female was admitted with anorexia, weight loss, lethargy, incontinence and hypochromic anemia with increased iron storage in the bone marrow. After an unsuccessful trial of pyridoxine, all symptoms and signs improved dramatically following the administration of pantothenic acid (pantothenyl alcohol 50 to 200 mg IM daily).

Several years later, a similar clinical picture developed and there was a clinical, but probably not a hematologic, response to a multivitamin preparation containing large amounts of pantothenic acid (McCurdy).

Riboflavin deficiency can cause a normochromic, normocytic anemia and reticulocytopenia that responds to supplementation *(Lane)*. Riboflavin deficiency also may be associated with sickle cell anemia, usually in conjunction with other deficiencies *(Sindel)*.

Thiamine deficiency may be associated with a megaloblastic anemia *(Mangel)* which, in turn, may respond to supplementation.

A child with megaloblastic anemia failed to respond to vitamin B_{12} or folic acid but responded to supplementation with oral thiamine 20 mg daily. When, on two occasions, the thiamine supplement was stopped, anemia recurred (Rogers).

Vitamin B_6 deficiency may be associated with both a microcytic anemia *(Bernat,1983a)* and a megaloblastic anemia *(Hines,1964)*; both respond to supplementation. When the vitamin is deficient, sickle cell anemia may also show a response to vitamin supplements *(Natta,1984)*. Furthermore, if a sideroblastic anemia is unresponsive to pyridoxine, supplementation with pyridoxal-5'-phosphate may be effective, as the anemia may be due to defective phosphorylation of pyridoxine to its active form *(Hines,1975)*.

A patient with primary acquired sideroblastic anemia was unresponsive to pyridoxine 100 mg daily, but showed a prompt reticulocytosis when given pyridoxal-5-phosphate 20 mg daily (Hines,1970).

Of course, vitamin B_{12} deficiency is a well known cause of pernicious anemia, a megaloblastic anemia, and supplementation may be able to reverse the neurologic damage *(Berk)*. Moreover, a B_{12} deficiency may be associated with sickle cell anemia which can respond to intramuscular supplementation *(al-Momen)*.

Vitamin C Deficiency

Vitamin C deficiency is occasionally associated with a normochromic, normocytic, or macrocytic anemia *(Sauberlich)*. Furthermore, the nutrient may be reduced in beta-thalassemia *(Ginberti)*. Vitamin C enhances non-heme iron absorption, which can aid in the prevention and treatment of iron-deficiency anemia *(Monsen)* and may stimulate hematopoiesis *(Ajayi)*.

Vitamin E Deficiency

When a non-specific anemia is found to be associated with vitamin E deficiency, it may respond to supplementation *(Drake)*. In addition, there are a number of specific forms of anemia that are associated with deficiency, all of which may also respond to repletion. These include sickle cell anemia *(Sindel;Natta,1980)*, beta-thalassemia *(Giuberti;Osoylu)*, and the anemias associated with cystic fibrosis *(Farrell)* and Mediterranean G_6PD deficiency *(Corash)*..

MINERAL DEFICIENCIES

Copper Deficiency

Copper deficiency, which can be due instigated by a high level of zinc supplementation, is associated with a hypochromic, microcytic anemia *(Williams)*. In addition, due to its effects on ceruloplasmin, copper deficiency may cause an *iron* deficiency anemia due to impaired iron absorption and reduced heme synthesis while iron accumulates in storage tissues. When induced by a copper deficiency, iron deficiency anemia can only be corrected with copper supplementation *(Watts)*. Serum copper levels may also be reduced in sickle cell anemia *(Ishir)*.

A 35-year-old Caucasian woman ingested 110 to 165 mg elemental zinc as zinc sulfate for 10 months. She developed a slowly worsening microcytic, hypochromic anemia found to be due to copper deficiency. Zinc supplementation was eliminated and she was supplemented with 2 mg copper daily. After 2 months, her anemia was unchanged. She received 10 mg copper chloride intravenously over a period of 5 days, and responded (Hoffman).

Iron Deficiency and Overload

Iron deficiency is likely to be the most frequent cause of anemia. It responds well to iron supplementation *(Bernat,1983b)*. In addition, iron is often deficient in pernicious anemia *(Carmel)* as well as in sickle cell anemia *(Reed)*. (See Hydrochloric Acid Deficiency and Food Sensitivities below, and Copper Deficiency above.)

By contrast, beta-thalassemia major (Cooley's anemia), an inherited microcytic anemia, may be associated with iron overload, and levels of ferritin, an iron storage protein, may be positively correlated with lipid peroxidation product concentrations in this disorder *(Livrea)*. Iron supplementation is therefore contraindicated in the treatment of a microcytic anemia unless there is evidence of iron deficiency.

Magnesium Deficiency

Magnesium nutriture may be reduced in a number of anemias, including sickle cell anemia *(Ishir)*, beta-thalassemia *(Hyman)* and sideropenic anemia *(Abbasciano)*. In sickle cell anemia, magnesium depletion appears to be at least partly due to excessive urinary excretion *(Olukoga)*. Supplementation may increase the absolute reticulocyte count and the number of immature reticulocytes, while reducing the number of dense sickle erythrocytes *(De Franceschi,1997a)*.

In regard to beta-thalassemia, results of a study in mice suggest that dietary magnesium supplementation may improve the anemia *(De Franceschi,1997b)*; the results of human trials have yet to be reported.

Zinc Deficiency

Plasma levels of zinc may be low in sickle cell anemia *(Ishir)* which may be corrected by supplementation *(Sindel)*. Pharmacologic doses of zinc (100-300 mg daily) for several months can, however, produce a severe *copper* deficiency causing a sideroblastic anemia with hypocupremia, anemia, leukopenia, and neutropenia *(Broun)*.

In beta-thalassemia, chronic hemolysis causing hyperzincuria appears to be the cause of zinc deficiency *(Vatanavicharn)*.

COMBINED NUTRIENT DEFICIENCIES

A handicapped child initially presented with iron-deficiency anemia. Despite treatment with iron supplements, after 5 weeks the anemia had worsened and symptoms of bruising and joint pain appeared.

When biochemical tests indicated deficiencies of vitamin C and folic acid, the child was then given vitamin C and folic acid supplementation to which he responded. The initial lack of response to iron suggests that vitamin C deficiency may have been the primary cause for the decreased utilization of iron. Alternatively, iron supplementation could have precipitated scurvy by increasing the oxidation of ascorbic acid. Because of a lack of bone marrow response, it is unlikely that iron supplementation precipitated folic acid deficiency, but ascorbic acid deficiency may have further depleted the patient's low folate stores (Clark).

OTHER RELATED FACTORS

Hydrochloric Acid deficiency

A deficiency of hydrochloric acid may impair iron absorption, leading to an iron-deficiency anemia *(Jacobs,1966)*. Conversely, hydrochloric acid output may improve following iron supplementation *(Shearman)*, although atrophic gastritis does not appear to be causally related to the anemia *(Cater)*. Adequate supplementation with glutamic or betaine hydrochloride should normalize iron nutriture and correct the anemia *(Jacobs,1964)*.

Also, patients with sickle cell anemia may have intestinal bacterial overgrowth which can be associated with nutritional deficiencies *(Heyman)*. This overgrowth, in turn, could be secondary to hydrochloric acid deficiency causing increased survival of ingested bacteria *(Giannella)*.

Food Sensitivities

In infants, milk sensitivity may cause intestinal bleeding. This can lead to the development of iron deficiency anemia *(Oski)*. Also, anemia is a characteristic sign of celiac disease due to gluten sensitivity, although it is rarely the only sign *(Kaiser)*.

For about 2 years, a 23-year-old asymptomatic, normal-weight woman had been known to have an iron-deficiency anemia. Radiography of the small intestine revealed a coarse rugal pattern of the duodenum. Endoscopically-obtained duodenal biopsy demonstrated villous atrophy. Elevated anti-gliadin antibody titers, as well as her response to a gluten-free diet, confirmed the diagnoses of celiac disease (Kaiser).

BIBLIOGRAPHY

Abbasciano V et al. Serum and erythrocyte levels of magnesium in microcytosis: comparison between heterozygous beta-thalassemia and sideropenic anemia. Haematologica 76(4):339-41, 1991

Ajayi OA, Nnaji UR. Effect of ascorbic acid supplementation on haematological response and ascorbic acid status of young female adults. Ann Nutr Metab 34:32-6, 1990

al-Momen AK. Diminished vitamin B_{12} levels in patients with severe sickle cell disease. J Intern Med 23796:551-5, 1995

Berk L et al. Effectiveness of vitamin B12 in combined system disease. N Engl J Med 239:328, 1948

Bernat I. Pyridoxine responsive anemias, in Iron Metabolism. New York, Plenum Press, 1983a:313-14

Bernat I. Iron deficiency, in Iron Metabolism. New York, Plenum Press, 1983b:215-74

Branda RF et al. Folate-induced remission in aplastic anemia with familial defect of cellular folate uptake. N Engl J Med 298(9):469-75, 1978

Broun RE et al. Excessive zinc ingestion: a reversible cause of sideroblastic anemia and bone marrow depression. JAMA 264:1441-3, 1990

Carmel R et al. Iron deficiency occurs frequently in patients with pernicious anemia. JAMA 257(8):1081-83, 1987

Cater RE II. The clinical importance of hypochlorhydria. (A consequence of chronic Helicobacter infection): Its possible etiological role in mineral and amino acid malabsorption, depression, and other syndromes. Med Hypotheses 39:375-83, 1992

Clark NG et al. Treatment of iron-deficient anemia complicated by scurvy and folic acid deficiency. Nutr Rev 50(5):134-7, 1992

Corash L et al. Reduced chronic hemolysis during high-dose vitamin E administration in Mediterranean type glucose-6-phosphate dehydrogenase deficiency. N Engl J Med 303:416-20, 1980

De Franceschi L et al. Oral magnesium supplements reduce erythrocyte dehydration in patients with sickle cell disease. J Clin Invest 100(7):1847-52, 1997a

De Franceschi L et al. Dietary magnesium supplementation ameliorates anemia in a mouse model of beta-thalassemia. Blood 90(3):1283-90, 1997b

Drake JR, Fitch CD. Status of vitamin E as an erythropoietic factor. Am J Clin Nutr 33:2386-93, 1980.

Farrell PM et al. The occurrence and effects of human vitamin E deficiency. A study in patients with cystic fibrosis. J Clin Invest 60:233-41, 1977

Giannella RA et al. Influence of gastric acidity on bacterial and parasitic enteric infections. Ann Intern Med 78:271-6, 1973

Giuberti M et al. Plasma vitamin E, platelet vitamin C and plasma ferritin levels in heterozygous beta-thalassemia. Nutr Rep Int 35(6):1141-50, 1987

Gothoni G et al. High-dose folic acid treatment for red-cell aplasia. Letter. Lancet 345:1645-6, 1995

Heyman MB et al. Elevated fasting breath hydrogen and abnormal hydrogen breath tests in children with sickle cell disease: a preliminary report. Am J Clin Nutr 49:654-7, 1989

Hines JD, Harris JW. Pyridoxine-responsive anemia: Description of three patients with megaloblastic erythropoiesis. Am J Clin Nutr 14:137-46, 1964

Hines JD, Grasso JA. The sideroblastic anemias. Semin Hematol 7(1):86-106, 1970

Hines JD, Love D. Abnormal vitamin B_6 metabolism in sideroblastic anemia: Effect of pyridoxal phosphate therapy. Clin Res 23:403A, 1975

Hodges RE et al. Hematopoietic studies in vitamin A deficiency. Am J Clin Nutr 31:876-85, 1978

Hoffman HN et al. Zinc-induced copper deficiency. Gastroenterology 94:508-12, 1988

Hyman CB et al. The clinical significance of magnesium depletion in thalassemia. Ann N Y Acad Sci 344:436-43, 1980

Ishir T et al. Zinc, copper, magnesium and sickle cell anemia. Trace Elem Electrolytes 12(3):161, 1995

Jacobs A et al. Role of hydrochloric acid in iron absorption. J Appl Physiol 19(2):187-8, 1964

Jacobs A et al. Gastric acidity and iron absorption. Br J Haematol 12:728-36, 1966

Kaiser U. [Monosymptomatic endemic sprue as a cause of iron-deficiency anemia. Dtsch Med Wochenschr 116(42):1588-90, 1991

Lane M, Alfrey CP Jr. The anemia of human riboflavin deficiency. Blood 25(4):432-42, 1965

Livrea MA et al. Oxidative stress and antioxidant status in b-thalassemia major: iron overload and depletion of lipid-soluble antioxidants. Blood 88(9):3608-14, 1996

Mangel H et al. Thiamine-dependent beriberi in the "thiamine-responsive anemia syndrome." N Engl J Med 311:836-8, 1984

McCurdy PR. Is there an anemia responsive to pantothenic acid? J Am Geriatr Soc 21(2):88-91, 1973

Monsen ER. Ascorbic acid: An enhancing factor in iron absorption, in Nutritional Bioavailability of Iron. American Chemical Society, 1982, pp. 85-95

Natta CL et al. A decrease in irreversibly sickled erythrocytes in sickle cell anemia patients given vitamin E. Am J Clin Nutr 33:968-71, 1980

Natta CL, Reynolds RD. Apparent vitamin B_6 deficiency in sickle cell anemia. Am J Clin Nutr 40:235-9, 1984

Olukoga AO et al. Urinary magnesium excretion in steady-state sickle cell anaemia. Acta Haematol 90(3):136-8, 1993

Oski FA. Don't Drink Your Milk! Syracuse, Mollica Press, 1983

Osoylu S, Gurgey A. Vitamin E treatment in triplicated alpha-globin gene-heterozygous beta-thalassemia. Am J Hematol 38:335-6, 1991

Pierce LE, Rath, CE. Evidence for folic acid deficiency in the genesis of anemic sickle cell crisis. Blood 20:19, 1962

Reed JD et al. Nutrition in sickle cell disease. Am J Hematol 24(4):441-45, 1987

Rogers LE et al. Thiamine-responsive megaloblastic anemia. J Pediatr 74(4):494-504, 1969

Sauberlich HE. Ascorbic acid, in Nutrition Reviews' Present Knowledge in Nutrition, Fifth Edition. Washington, D.C., The Nutrition Foundation, Inc., 1984

Shearman DJC et al. Gastric function and structure in iron deficiency. Lancet i:845-8, 1966

Sindel LJ et al. Nutritional deficiencies associated with vitamin E deficiency in sickle cell patients: the effect of vitamin supplementation. Nutr Res 10:267-73, 1990

Vatanavicharn S et al. Zinc and copper status in hemoglobin H disease and beta-thalassemia/hemoglobin E disease. Acta Haematol 68(4):317-20, 1982

Watts DL. The nutritional relationships of copper. J Orthomol Med 4(2):99-108, 1989

West CE, Roodenburg AJC. Role of vitamin A in iron metabolism. Voeding 53:201-5, 1992

Williams DM. Copper deficiency in humans. Semin Hematol 20(2):118-28, 1983

ANXIETY

See Also: MITRAL VALVE PROLAPSE

NUTRITIONAL TREATMENT GUIDE

✓ = Efficacy generally accepted.
* = Efficacy *demonstrated* by controlled human trials.
[+] = Efficacy *suspected* from uncontrolled human trials.
[-] = Efficacy *suspected* from indirect data.
? = Efficacy *challenged* in a study of similar design.

DIETARY FACTORS

* avoid **Alcohol**
* avoid **Caffeine**

- -

[+] avoid **Sugar**

NUTRITIONAL FACTORS

* **L-5-Hydroxytryptophan:** 200 to 900 mg daily in divided doses (2 month trial)
* **Inositol:** 500 mg to 12 g daily in divided doses
* **Selenium deficiency:** 200 μg daily

- -

[+] **Calcium:** ? 1,000 mg daily for the treatment of hypocalcemia (along with treatment of the underlying metabolic disorder). Administer IM if necessary.
[+] **Magnesium deficiency:** ≈ 400 mg daily (Consider IM or IV administration, especially in hypomagnesemia.)
[+] **Niacinamide:** ? 500 mg twice daily
[+] **Omega-3 Fatty Acid deficiency:** *example:* MaxEPA 1 g caps [180 mg EPA; 120 mg DHA] 10 to 20 daily
[+] **Thiamine deficiency:** 50 mg daily orally or intramuscularly
[+] **Vitamin B_6 deficiency:** 50 to 100 mg daily
[+] **Vitamin B_{12} deficiency:** 1,000 μg intramuscularly weekly initially and monthly afterwards
[+] **Vitamin C deficiency:** 500 mg twice daily
[+] **Vitamin E deficiency:** D,L-alpha-tocopheryl acetate 200 to 2,000 mg or IU daily for 6 weeks

OTHER RELATED FACTORS

* rule out **Food Sensitivities**

- -

[+] rule out **'Reactive Hypoglycemia'**

Pathologically anxious patients often report that physical exertion can elicit or increase their anxiety and its somatic manifestations, and it has been known for about half a century that patients with panic attacks demonstrate excessive blood lactic acid production during exercise. Proof that excessive blood lactate could cause an attack of intense anxiety in patients came in 1967, when Pitts and McClure found that a lactate infusion yielding concentrations equivalent to those produced during strenuous exercise would elicit anxiety symptoms in patients but not in normals *(Pitts,1967)*.

In glycolysis, glucose is converted into pyruvate. Under aerobic conditions, pyruvate is then converted into acetyl-co A and then, through the Krebs cycle, into energy. However, during strenuous exercise or other situations creating anaerobic conditions, pyruvate is converted into lactate instead of going through the Krebs cycle. The resulting elevation of the lactate/pyruvate ratio suggests a basic intracellular chemical disturbance in energy formation and utilization which, when energy needs to be rapidly mobilized, may produce the experience of anxiety *(Wendel)*.

DIETARY FACTORS

Sugar

Sugar (sucrose) consumption may be followed by heightened anxiety or panic in some patients. By stimulating insulin release, the elevation in blood sugar following sucrose ingestion may cause a reactive decrease in blood glucose which, in susceptible people, may be associated with anxiety *(Wendel)*. In addition, glucose infusion has been shown to increase lactate production and elevate the lactate/pyruvate ratio *(Wendel)*. Fructose, under anaerobic conditions, is metabolized more rapidly than glucose to lactate and therefore, theoretically, should also be avoided, as should sorbitol and xylitol for which fructose is a metabolite *(Cook)*.

Caffeine

Results of controlled studies have shown that patients with anxiety, especially if they are prone to panic attacks, are unusually sensitive to the anxiogenic effects of caffeine, another substance which increases the lactate/pyruvate ratio *(Alberti)*, although even normal schoolchildren tend to feel more anxious after caffeine ingestion *(Bernstein)*. Moreover, withdrawal from regular caffeine intake may temporarily exacerbate anxiety *(Silverman)*. Both the anxiogenic effects of caffeine and withdrawal anxiety in chronic caffeine-containing beverage users have also been demonstrated in rats *(Bhattacharya)*.

Alcohol

Alcohol causes a sharp rise in the hepatic ratio of NAD to NADH. This inhibits gluconeogenesis from lactate, raising the lactate/pyruvate ratio *(Alberti)*. While alcohol is often taken to relieve anxiety, under double-blind conditions its ingestion may actually *increase* anxiety *(Monteiro)*. Also, anxiety along with hyperventilation and alcohol craving occur together both acute and subacute alcohol withdrawal syndromes *(Roelofs)*.

NUTRITIONAL FACTORS

VITAMINS

Vitamin B Complex

Deficiencies of members of the vitamin B complex appear to be common in agoraphobia (fear of open spaces) *(Abbey)*. The same is likely to be true for other anxiety-related conditions.

Inositol

Inositol is a key intermediate of the phosphatidyl-inositol cycle, a second-messenger system use by several noradrenergic, serotonergic and cholinergic receptors *(Benjamin,1995a)*. Since ingestion has been shown to raise inositol levels in the cerebrospinal fluid *(Levine)*, this nutrient could potentially serve as an anti-anxiety agent.

Indeed, when a group of 21 patients with panic disorder either with or without agoraphobia received 12 grams daily of inositol or placebo in random order for 4 weeks each, the inositol supplement was associated with a significantly greater reduction in the frequency and severity of panic attacks and of agoraphobia than the placebo. Moreover, while the efficacy of the nutrient was judged to be comparable to that of imipramine, in contrast to imipramine, the side effects were minimal *(Benjamin,1995b)*.

Niacinamide

Niacinamide, but not niacin, passes readily from the plasma to the cerebrospinal fluid where it is taken up into brain cells by a high-affinity accumulation system

(Hankes), suggesting it is the preferred form of the vitamin for the treatment of anxiety. It was found in an animal study to have benzodiazepine-like actions including anti-conflict, anti-aggressive, muscle relaxant and hypnotic effects *(Mohler)*.

Lactate reacts with niacinamide-adenine dinucleotide (NAD^+) to form pyruvic acid and reduced NAD (NADH + H^+). The equilibrium of this reaction favors lactate and NAD^+, but it can be driven by adding excess NAD^+. It may be that supplementation with niacinamide helps to drive the reaction, thus reducing lactate concentrations *(Wendel)*.

Gaby and Wright have reported that, in the clinical setting, niacinamide supplementation sometimes appears to be effective, especially for patients whose anxiety is secondary to reactive hypoglycemia. They typically prescribe doses of 500 mg twice daily and 1,000 mg 3 times daily *(Gaby)*.

Thiamine Deficiency

Elevated lactate may also be caused by inadequate pyruvate dehydrogenase activity resulting from a thiamine deficiency or dependency. In that case, the conversion of pyruvate to acetyl CoA is inhibited, fostering its conversion to lactic acid *(Wick)*. Symptoms of a prolonged moderate thiamine deficiency may include fearfulness progressing to agitation as well as emotional instability and psychosomatic complaints *(Williams)*.

In a study of more than 1,000 healthy young men, those who were chronically borderline thiamine-deficient (based on measurements of erythrocyte transketolase activity) were significantly more anxious on a measure of current mental state. They were not, however, significantly more nervous on a test that measures personality factors (long-term patterns) *(Heseker)*.

Vitamin B_6 Deficiency

Gamma aminobutyric acid (GABA), an inhibitory neurotransmitter which is involved in the regulation of anxiety, requires vitamin B_6 for its synthesis; thus a deficiency of this vitamin may theoretically result in heightened anxiety. Vitamin B_6 is also required for the conversion of tryptophan to serotonin, a neurotransmitter which is suspected of being involved in anxiety - although the data are so far inconclusive *(Johnston)*. When over 1,000 healthy young men were studied, those found to be chronically deficient in vitamin B_6 based on repeated measures of erythrocyte enzyme activity (alpha-EAST) were significantly more nervous on a measure of personality, although they were not significantly more anxiety on a measure of current mental state *(Heseker)*. In an open trial, patients with hyperventilation syndrome who were found to have abnormal xanthurenic acid excretion (an indicator of vitamin B_6 deficiency) improved following the administration of pyridoxine and tryptophan, suggesting that a marginal B_6 deficiency may have produced the syndrome by causing serotonin depletion *(Hoes)*.

Vitamin B_{12} Deficiency

When cobalamin levels of more than 1,000 healthy young men were studied, those who were chronically borderline vitamin B_{12}-deficient were significantly more anxious on a measure of current mental state, although not significantly more nervous on a test based on personality factors *(Heseker)*.

Where there are no large, controlled clinical trials investigating the efficacy of B_{12} supplementation in lowering anxiety levels, there is a report of two women in their sixties who, despite normal vitamin B_{12} absorption, believed that weekly injections of the vitamin relieved their nervousness and fatigue. They randomly received either the vitamin or placebo by injection once weekly for 25 weeks. Just prior to each injection, they were asked questions concerning the effects of their previous injection. No difference was found between vitamin B_{12} and placebo, suggesting that the placebo effect may account for clinical impressions of its efficacy for treating anxiety in patients with normal vitamin B_{12} nutriture *(Schilling)*.

Whether B_{12} supplementation reduces anxiety when the vitamin is borderline deficient remains to be investigated, although it is known that anxiety may be part of the neuropsychiatric syndrome seen in advanced cases of pernicious anemia *(Ambrosino)*.

Vitamin C Deficiency

There is early evidence that a chronic borderline deficiency of vitamin C may contribute to anxiety. While healthy young men found to have chronic borderline deficiencies of vitamin C (based on plasma ascorbic acid levels) were significantly more anxious than normals on a measure of current mental state, their rating of nervousness as a personality factor was similar *(Heseker)*.

Vitamin E Deficiency

The literature on anxiety in borderline vitamin E deficiency is as skimpy as that concerning vitamin C.

When the same population of more than 1,000 healthy young men as described previously was tested for chronic borderline plasma alpha-tocopherol levels, those who had borderline deficiencies were not significantly more anxious in regard to current mental state; however, they were significantly more nervous in regard to their personality *(Heseker)*.

MINERALS

Calcium: hypocalcemia

Hypocalcemia may be associated with an organic anxiety syndrome which is relieved by calcium supplementation *(Lawlor)*. It has been theorized that, since lactate infusions can lower the ionized calcium level, anxiety resulting from elevated blood lactate may be due to hypocalcemia. However, the blood lactate level at the onset of anxiety symptoms can only complex less than 3% of ionized calcium, while ionized calcium levels would have to be reduced at least 30% to produce symptoms of hypocalcemia *(Grosz)*.

Also, infusions of other agents which chelate ionized calcium produce profound hypocalcemic symptoms but fail to produce panic attacks in patients with a history of such attacks *(Pitts,1979)*. These data suggest that anxiety as part of the presentation of hypocalcemia has a different origin than anxiety due to excess blood lactate.

1. A 49-year-old postmenopausal vegetarian female with a 30-year history of generalized anxiety with inability to relax, trembling, sweating, apprehensiveness, worry, insomnia, and occasional depression with worsening of symptoms associated with stress. After 1 ½ years of psychotherapy, her symptoms suddenly increased despite a lack of precipitating stresses, and were unrelieved by oxazepam. Five weeks later, she developed severe chest pain which was found to be due to two spontaneous rib fractures. Evaluation revealed marked osteoporosis and a serum calcium of 7.2 mg/dL (normal = 8.5-10.5 mg/dL). Her anxiety was reduced to its former level following correction of the hypocalcemia and the addition of estrogens (Carlson).

2. A 58 year-old insulin-dependent diabetic female had a 35-year history of generalized anxiety disorder with worry, fear, sweating, shaking, insomnia, and mild depression. One day she reported increasing severity of all symptoms, with frequent panic attacks and a "completely different feeling." She proceeded to develop muscle spasms, stuttering, and tetany with a positive Chvostek's sign. Her serum calcium was 6.1 mg/dL. Further evaluation revealed idiopathic hypoparathyroidism. Following medical treatment her anxiety decreased to its previous level (Carlson).

Magnesium Deficiency

A chronic marginal magnesium deficiency, which is common in countries consuming the Western diet, is associated with anxiety along with neuromuscular irritability. Roughly half of all patients with panic attacks have mitral valve prolapse, and there is evidence that the symptoms of mitral valve prolapse may be related to marginal magnesium status (see Mitral Valve Prolapse). In addition, since magnesium is the most important activator of the enzymes of glycolysis, magnesium deficiency is yet another cause of an increased lactate/pyruvate ratio *(Buist)*.

An anxious 34 year-old man had a lifetime history of being easily startled, especially when he was relaxed or very tired. Even a slight noise would make him jump or cringe. In addition, he experienced constant calf tension which sometimes became painful. His diet was restricted due to multiple food intolerances; lactose, oils, coarse grains and most fresh fruits and vegetables would cause stomach cramps, gas and diarrhea.

Serum calcium and magnesium were normal; however both leukocyte and lymphocyte magnesium levels were reduced. He was placed on a multivitamin/multimineral along with an additional 300 mg of magnesium. Six weeks later, he noted that he was slightly calmer, less tense, and his exaggerated startle response had disappeared. However, he continued to have calf tightness and hypersensitivity to noise.

Five months after starting magnesium, there were no further changes, and lymphocyte and leukocyte magnesium levels were unimproved from baseline. Lymphocyte calcium was normal, while leukocyte calcium was reduced. He was started on calcium 750 mg daily without further improvement.
He was then given 15 cc intravenously of 20% magnesium chloride. Within one hour, he noted a general feeling of relaxation, and his calf tenseness entirely disappeared for the next two to three weeks. He subsequently had additional injections whenever the calf tightness returned. Each time the effects lasted longer until the injections were no longer needed.

Selenium Deficiency

In a double-blind crossover study, 50 unselected subjects received either selenium or placebo for 5 weeks. Selenium supplementation was associated with improvement in mood and, in particular, a decrease in anxiety. Moreover, the lower the level of selenium in the diet, the more the reports of anxiety, depression, and tiredness decreased following selenium therapy *(Benton)*.

OTHER NUTRITIONAL FACTORS

Omega-3 Essential Fatty Acid Deficiency

Rudin has argued that agoraphobia may be a manifestation of a deficiency of the series 3 prostaglandins caused by a deficiency of omega-3 essential fatty acids - since the omega-3 fatty acids provide the substrate upon which niacin and the other B vitamin co-enzymes act to form these prostaglandins. If agoraphobia were due to an omega-3 fatty acid deficiency, it would be associated with other features of the deficiency syndrome, such as signs and symptoms of drying dermatoses, autonomic neuropathies, tinnitus and/or fatigue.

Rudin reports improvement in appropriately selected patients following administration of a titrated dosage of linseed oil, 50% of which is alpha-linolenic acid, an omega-3 fatty acid *(Rudin)*. His clinical experience has yet to be confirmed by controlled studies.

A 58 year-old man was able to travel in public but, for 40 years, could not cross an open square or field by himself without having a severe panic attack. He had slight osteoarthritis, marked tinnitus, slight food allergies, mild autonomic and somatic neuropathy, mild dermatosis, mild fatigue and alcohol intolerance.

He was placed on linseed oil supplementation. Starting about 2 to 3 months later, he reported consistent and definite reduction of agoraphobia associated with an increased sense of calm (Rudin).

5-Hydroxytryptophan

Dietary tryptophan is converted in the body into the neurotransmitter serotonin and may have a mild sedating effect. Its efficacy in anxiety states is largely untested, although it appears to be effective in certain patients *(Hoyse)*. (See Vitamin B_6 above.) After contamination in the manufacturing procedure used by one company resulted in the development of a serious illness (eosinophilia-myalgia syndrome), tryptophan has been unavailable except by prescription in many countries.

5-Hydroxytryptophan is the metabolite of tryptophan and the immediate precursor of serotonin. Under double-blind conditions, it has been shown to cause a moderate reduction in anxiety for patients suffering from anxiety disorders *(Kahn)*.

OTHER RELATED FACTORS

Food Sensitivities

Anecdotal reports have suggested that food sensitivities may provoke anxiety; the experimental evidence, however, is meager. In a double-blind study, 30 patients complaining of anxiety or another psychological symptom reported significantly greater cognitive-emotional symptoms after exposure to sub-lingual antigens (foods, chemicals or mold) than after exposure to placebos - for which symptoms were equal to their base rate *(King)*. Further controlled studies are needed for confirmation.

'Reactive Hypoglycemia'

In an informal study of 300 patients who were found to exhibit a drop in blood glucose of at least 20% below their fasting level during a 6-hour glucose tolerance test, half complained of anxiety. Physical symptoms, especially neurologic symptoms, were common. Previous treatments with tranquilizers, sedatives and/or electroconvulsive therapy, had been ineffective. About 85% responded to a high protein, low carbohydrate, caffeine-free diet *(Salzer)*.

BIBLIOGRAPHY

Abbey LC. Agoraphobia. J Orthomol Psychiatry 11:243-59, 1982

Alberti KG, Nattrass M. Lactic Acidosis. Lancet ii:25-9, 1977

Ambrosino SV. Neuropsychiatric aspects of pernicious anemia: report of a case. Psychosomatics 7(1):24-8, 1966

Benjamin J et al. Inositol treatment in psychiatry. Psychopharmacol Bull 31(1):167-75, 1995a

Benjamin J et al. Double-blind, placebo-controlled, crossover trial of inositol treatment for panic disorder. Am J Psychiatry 152(7):1084-6, 1995b

Benton D, Cook R. The impact of selenium supplementation on mood. Biol Psychiatry 29(11):1092-8, 1991

Bernstein GA et al. Caffeine effects on learning, performance, and anxiety in normal school-age children. J Am Acad Child Adolesc Psychiatry 33(3):407-15, 1994

Bhattacharya SK et al. Anxiogenic action of caffeine: an experimental study in rats. J Psychopharmacol (Oxf) 11(3):219-24, 1997

Buist RA. Anxiety neurosis: The lactate connection. Int Clin Nutr Rev 5:1-4, 1985

Carlson RJ. Longitudinal observations of two cases of organic anxiety syndrome. Psychosomatics 27(7):529-31, 1986

Cook GC, Jacobson J. Individual variation in fructose metabolism in man. Br J Nutr 26(2):187-95, 1971

Gaby AR. Vitamin B3 (Part 2): Powerful tool in nutritional medicine. Nutrition & Healing December, 1995

Grosz HJ, Farmer BB. Blood lactate in the development of anxiety symptoms. Arch Gen Psychiatry 21(5):611-19, 1969

Hankes LV. Nicotinic acid and nicotinamide, in LJ Machlin, Ed. Handbook of Vitamins. New York, Marcel Dekker, 1984:329-77

Heseker H et al. Psychological disorders as early symptoms of mild-moderate vitamin deficiency. Ann NY Acad Sci 669:352-7, 1992

Hoes M et al. Hyperventilation syndrome, treatment with L-tryptophan and pyridoxine; predictive values of xanthurenic acid excretion. J Orthomol Psychiatry 10(1):7-15, 1981

Hoyse SE. Experiences with L-tryptophan in a child and family psychiatric department. J Int Med Res 10(3):157-9, 1982

Johnston AL, File SE. 5-HT and anxiety: promises and pitfalls. Pharmacol Biochem Behav 24(5):1467-70, 1986

Kahn RS et al. Effect of a serotonin precursor and uptake inhibitor in anxiety disorders; a double-blind comparison of 5-hydroxytryptophan, clomipramine and placebo. Int Clin Psychopharmacol 2(1):33-45, 1987

King DS. Can allergic exposure provoke psychological symptoms? A double-blind test. Biol Psychiatry 16(1):3-19, 1981

Lawlor BA. Hypocalcemia, hypoparathyroidism, and organic anxiety syndrome. J Clin Psychiatry 49(8):317-18, 1988

Levine J et al. Inositol treatment raises CSF inositol levels. Brain Res 627(1):168-70, 1993

Mohler H et al. Nicotinamide is a brain constituent with benzodiazepine-like actions. Nature 278:563-65, 1979

Monteiro MG et al. Subjective feelings of anxiety in young men after ethanol and diazepam infusions. J Clin Psychiatry 51(1):12-16, 1990

Pitts FN Jr, McClure JN Jr. Lactate metabolism in anxiety neurosis. N Engl J Med 277(25):1329-36, 1967

Pitts FN, Allen RE. Biochemical induction of anxiety, in WE Fann, I Karacan, AD Pokorny et al, Eds. Phenomenology and the Treatment of Anxiety. New York, Spectrum Publications, 1979

Roelofs SM. Hyperventilation, anxiety, craving for alcohol: a subacute alcohol withdrawal syndrome. Alcohol 2(3):501-5, 1985

Rudin DO. The major psychoses and neuroses as omega-3 essential fatty acid deficiency syndrome: Substrate pellagra. Biol Psychiatry 16(9):837-50, 1981

Salzer HM. Relative hypoglycemia as a cause of neuropsychiatric illness. J Natl Med Assoc 58(1):12-17, 1966

Schilling RF, Morris FK. Is vitamin B12 a tonic? Wis Med J 70(5):143-4, 1971

Silverman K et al. Withdrawal syndrome after the double-blind cessation of caffeine consumption. N Engl J Med 327:1109-14, 1992

Wendel OW, Beebe WE. Glycolytic activity in schizophrenia, in D Hawkins & L Pauling, Eds. Orthomolecular Psychiatry: Treatment of Schizophrenia. San Francisco, W. H. Freeman, 1973

Wick H et al. Thiamine dependency in a patient with congenital lactiacidaemia. Agents Actions 7(3):405-10, 1977

Williams RD et al. Induced thiamine (Vitamin B1) deficiency in man; relation of depletion of thiamine to development of biochemical defect and of polyneuropathy. Arch Intern Med 71:38-53, 1943

APHTHOUS STOMATITIS

NUTRITIONAL TREATMENT GUIDE

✓ = Efficacy generally accepted.
* = Efficacy *demonstrated* by controlled human trials.
[+] = Efficacy *suspected* from uncontrolled human trials.
[-] = Efficacy *suspected* from indirect data.
? = Efficacy *challenged* in a study of similar design.

NUTRITIONAL FACTORS

[+] **Folic Acid deficiency:** 800 μg daily
[+] **Iron deficiency:** 30 mg twice daily until repletion; then minimal possible dosage
[+] **Lysine:** 500 mg daily; 1000 mg 4 times daily during recurrence
[+] **Niacin deficiency:** 50 to 100 mg daily
[+] **Riboflavin deficiency:** 5 to 10 mg daily
[+] **Thiamine deficiency:** 50 mg daily orally or intramuscularly
[+] **Vitamin B_6 deficiency:** 50 mg to 100 mg daily
[+] **Vitamin B_{12} deficiency:** 1,000 μg IM weekly initially and monthly afterwards
[+] **Zinc deficiency:** zinc sulfate 220 mg twice daily *AND* **Copper** 2 mg daily

OTHER RELATED FACTORS

* rule out **Food Sensitivities**

- -

[+] ***Lactobacillus acidophilus*:** local application and oral administration

NUTRITIONAL FACTORS

VITAMINS

Vitamin B Complex Deficiencies

Occasional patients are deficient in certain members of the vitamin B complex. Repletion of a deficiency of folic acid *(Nally)*, niacin *(Barthelemy)*, riboflavin *(Nolan)*, thiamine *(Nolan)*, vitamin B_6 *(Nolan)* or vitamin B_{12} *(Nally)*, whether based on low serum or erythrocyte levels, is sometimes followed by remission. However, controlled trials to prove the relationship have yet to be undertaken.

A woman with repeated episodes of aphthous stomatitis also had glossitis. She was found to be anemic and to have a serum vitamin B_{12} level of 50 pg/ml (normal: 200-1000). She was absorbing less than one percent of her dietary intake of the vitamin, and had no intrinsic factor activity.

Intramuscular injections of vitamin B_{12} produced immediate improvements, with complete and lasting remission of all oral ulcerations as well as of the glossitis and the anemia (Palopoli).

MINERALS

Iron Deficiency

Similar to deficiencies of the B complex vitamins, the results of open trials suggest that repletion of a deficiency of iron may be beneficial. For example, of a group of 100 affected children, 5 had iron deficiency anemia while another 13 had iron deficiency without anemia. Four of the anemic children received iron supplements. Six months later, 2 of them had a dramatic improvement in the lesions while one other had a slight improvement. All 3 now had normal serum iron levels. Lesions in the fourth child had worsened. However, she had a combination of low iron and low folate levels and both had failed to normalize *(Field)*.

In another study, 23 of a group of 330 patients were found to be deficient in iron, 6 in vitamin B_{12}, 7 in folic acid, and 11 in two or more of these nutrients, for a total of 47 patients (14%). After 33 of the patients with demonstrated deficiencies received 6 months of supplementation, 70% of them had a complete remission and 33% improved, while the rest showed no changes *(Wray, 1978)*.

Zinc Deficiency

In open trials, zinc administration, both as an oral supplement and as a local application, has been reported to be effective *(Wang)*. As with the above nutrients, the efficacy of zinc may depend upon the level of zinc nutriture. When, for example, zinc supplementation was provided to a group of 17 patients, all 9 patients with lower serum zinc levels (<110 μg/dL) improved, compared to only 3 of the 8 patients with higher zinc levels *(Merchant)*.

A 15 year-old boy with a 6-year history of recurrent aphthous ulceration on a monthly basis despite local treatment as well as systemic treatment with steroids, Isoprinosine, interferon, and lysozyme. He was found to have zinc deficiency (serum zinc level 65 μg/dl) and a cellular immune deficiency (confirmed by lymphoblastic transformation assay).

He was placed on 50 mg zinc sulfate 3 times daily. After 3 months, the aphthae disappeared and did not reappear for 1 year. Moreover, serum zinc levels and the lymphoblastic transformation assay normalized (Entre).

There is a double-blind crossover study of zinc supplementation in the literature. It found zinc to have a small, but statistically insignificant, effect *(Wray, 1982b)*. However, the study only lasted 3 months; a longer trial, perhaps restricted to zinc-deficient patients, may have more positive findings.

OTHER NUTRITIONAL FACTORS

Lysine

In an open trial, 28 patients received lysine 500 mg daily for prophylaxis which was increased to 1000 mg 4 times daily at the earliest sign of an outbreak. Nearly everyone reported that lysine reduced the number of recurrences, although a few required 1000 mg daily for effective prophylaxis. When an episode occurred, the high dosage of lysine reduced their duration by 25% to 50% *(Wright)*.

If a trial of lysine is successful, there is some concern about continuing it over the long term, since excessive dietary lysine may contribute to the risk of atherosclerosis *(Kritchevsky)*. On a theoretical basis, supplementation with a smaller dosage of arginine (with which lysine competes) may possibly reduce the risk; however, whether arginine will interfere with the therapeutic effect of lysine is unknown. The alternative is to monitor serum cholesterol levels, as the increase in risk may be due to enhanced hepatic cholesterol production *(Schmeisser)*.

OTHER RELATED FACTORS

Lactobacillus Acidophilus

The results of anecdotal reports suggest that *L. acidophilus*, with or without *L. bulgaricus*, may be of benefit if applied locally by swishing a liquefied product in the mouth, sometimes followed by swallowing the product *(James)*.

A double-blind study failed to confirm its efficacy in reducing the duration of healing. However, since the patients in that study were severely mentally retarded, its effect on pain could not be assessed *(Gertenrich)*.

A 39 year-old woman developed almost continuous canker sores following treatment with an antibiotic 2 years earlier. The sores failed to respond to any medication that her husband, a physician, was able to obtain. She was treated with tablets containing viable Lactobacillus acidophilus and Lactobacillus bulgaricus which she dissolved in her mouth with milk 4 times a day with prompt disappearance of her symptoms (Weekes).

Food Sensitivities

There are many anecdotal reports relating specific food sensitivities to recurrent aphthae, although scientific documentation is meager, and it appears that the majority of patients are not atopic. In a double-blind study, 60 patients' leukocytes were first tested to discover which food antigens caused them to release histamine. When the test-positive foods were eliminated, 30% of patients had a decreased ulcer incidence and, following re-challenge with foods which had been eliminated, 30% of those foods were associated with an increased incidence of oral lesions *(Wray, 1982a)*. More controlled studies are needed before the relative importance of food sensitivities will be known.

BIBLIOGRAPHY

Barthelemy H et al. Skin and mucosal manifestations in vitamin deficiency. J Am Acad Dermatol 15(4-6):1263-74, 1986

Entre L. Recurrent aphthous ulceration with zinc deficiency and cellular immune deficiency. Oral Surg Oral Med Oral Pathol 72(5):559-61, 1991

Field EA et al. Clinical and haematological assessment of children with recurrent aphthous ulceration. Br Dent J 163:19-22, 1987

Gertenrich RL, Hart RW. Treatment of oral ulcerations with Bacid (Lactobacillus acidophilus). Oral Surg 30(2):196-200, 1970

James APR. Common dermatologic disorders. CIBA Clinical Symposia 19(2):38-64, 1967

Kritchevsky D, Dietary protein and experimental atherosclerosis. Ann N Y Acad Sci 676:180-7, 1993

Merchant HW et al. Zinc sulfate supplementation for treatment of recurring oral ulcers. South Med J 70(5):559-61, 1977

Nally FF, Blake GC. Recurrent aphthae: treatment with vitamin B12, folic acid, and iron. Letter. Br Med J 3:308, 1975

Nolan A et al. Recurrent aphthous ulceration: vitamin B1, B2, and B6 status and response to replacement therapy. J Oral Pathol Med 20:389-91, 1991

Palopoli J, Waxman J. Recurrent aphthous stomatitis and vitamin B12 deficiency. South Med J 83:475-7, 1990

Schmeisser DD et al. Effect of excess dietary lysine on plasma lipids of the chick. J Nutr 113(9):1777-83, 1983

Wang SW et al. [The trace element zinc and aphthosis.] Rev Stomatol Chir Maxillofac 87(5):339-43, 1986

Weekes DJ. N Y State J Med 58(16), August 15, 1958

Wray D et al. Food allergens and basophil histamine release in recurrent aphthous stomatitis. Oral Surg oral Med Oral Pathol 54(4):388-95, 1982a

Wray D. A double blind trial of systemic zinc sulfate in recurrent aphthous stomatitis. Oral Surg 53(5):469-72, 1982b

Wray D et al. Nutritional deficiencies in recurrent aphthae. J Oral Pathol 7(6):418-23, 1978

Wright EF. Clinical effectiveness of lysine in treating recurrent aphthous ulcers and herpes labialis. Gen Dent Jan/Feb 1994:40-2

ATHEROSCLEROSIS

including CORONARY THROMBOSIS

See Also: CARDIAC ARRHYTHMIAS
CEREBROVASCULAR DISEASE
HYPERTENSION
PERIPHERAL VASCULAR DISEASE

NUTRITIONAL TREATMENT GUIDE

✓ = Efficacy generally accepted.
* = Efficacy *demonstrated* by controlled human trials.
[+] = Efficacy *suspected* from uncontrolled human trials.
[-] = Efficacy *suspected* from indirect data.
? = Efficacy *challenged* in a study of similar design.

I. DIETARY FACTORS

✓ restrict dietary **Cholesterol** (especially if cholesterol-sensitive) to below 300 to 400 mg daily
✓ restrict **Fat**, generally to 30% of calories
✓ restrict **Saturated Fat** to below 10% of calories
✓ emphasize **Vegetables**, especially sources of **Soluble Fibers**
Examples: oats, carrots, peas, potatoes, apples
✓ moderate **Alcohol** consumption (up to 2 drinks daily)

- -

[-] avoid **Sucrose** and **Fructose**
[-] avoid **Unfiltered Coffee**
[-] ? avoid **Hydrogenated Oils**
[-] ? consume **Fish** regularly
[-] ? minimize **Caffeine** intake

II. NUTRITIONAL FACTORS

A. To Generally Combat Atherogenesis and Coronary Thrombosis

* **L-Arginine:** *to improve impaired endothelium-dependent dilation:* ? 7 g 3 times daily
* **Glycosaminoglycans:** Mesoglycan 200 mg daily
* **N-Acetylcysteine:** *to reduce oxidative damage during an acute MI:* ? 15 g
* **Vitamin E:** 800 IU daily

- -

[+] **Folic Acid:** 1 to 2 mg daily

- -

[-] rule out **Cadmium** toxicity
[-] **Calcium deficiency:** 1 to 2 g daily
[-] **Carotenoids**
[-] **Chromium:** ? 200 μg daily
[-] **Copper deficiency:** 2 mg twice daily for up to 6 weeks along with **zinc** 50 mg daily
[-] rule out **Copper** toxicity
[-] **Iron deficiency:** 30 mg twice daily until repletion; then minimal dosage possible
[-] rule out **Iron** toxicity
[-] **Magnesium deficiency:** ≈ 400 mg daily (Consider IM or IV administration, especially in hypomagnesemia.)
[-] **Omega-3 fatty acids**: *example:* MaxEPA 1 g caps [180 mg EPA; 120 mg DHA] 10 to 20 daily
[-] **Omega-9 fatty acids** (oleic acid)
[-] **Potassium deficiency:** ? 80 to 100 meq daily total intake, preferably from potassium-rich foods
[-] **Selenium deficiency:** 200 μg daily
[-] **Taurine**
[-] **Vitamin B_6 deficiency:** 50 to 100 mg daily
[-] **Vitamin C deficiency:** 500 mg twice daily
[-] **Vitamin D deficiency:** 50,000 to 100,000 IU 2 or 3 times daily during the first week; then, if needed, either 100,000 IU of ergo- or cholecalciferol every 3 to months *OR* 800 to 1600 IU daily
[-] rule out **Vitamin D** toxicity
[-] **Vitamin E:** ? 400 to 800 IU daily
[-] **Zinc deficiency:** zinc sulfate 220 mg twice daily *AND* **Copper** 2 mg daily

B. To *Specifically* Reduce the Risk of, or Death from, Myocardial Infarction

* **L-Carnitine:** 1 to 3 g twice daily
* **Glycosaminoglycans:** chondroitin polysulfate ? 1 g 3 times daily
* **Niacin:** Start with 100 mg 3 times daily with meals. Increase by 100 mg 3 times daily each week to a maximum of 1 g 3 times daily if needed to achieve adequate results.
* **Potassium deficiency:** ? 80 to 100 meq daily total intake, preferably from potassium-rich foods
* **Vitamin E:** 800 IU daily
* ? **Magnesium:** ? 400 mg daily orally *or* IV infusion following acute MI

- -

[-] rule out **Arsenic** toxicity
[-] rule out **Cadmium** toxicity
[-] **Calcium:** ? 800 to 1,500 mg daily
[-] **Carotenoids**
[-] **Flavonoids**
[-] **Iron deficiency:** 30 mg twice daily until repletion; then minimal dosage possible
[-] rule out **Mercury** toxicity
[-] **Omega-3 Fatty Acids:** *example:* MaxEPA 1 g caps [180 mg EPA; 120 mg DHA] 10 to 20 daily
[-] **Vitamin B_6:** ? 50 mg daily
[-] **Vitamin C deficiency:** 500 mg twice daily
[-] ? **Omega-6 Fatty Acids:** *example:* evening primrose oil 500 mg caps [7-10% GLA] 6 to 8 daily

C. To *Specifically* Reduce the Risk of Arterial Thrombosis

* **L-Arginine:** *to normalize increased platelet aggregability:* ? 8.4 g daily
* **Glycosaminoglycans:** Mesoglycan ? 100 to 200 mg daily

* **Vitamin C**: ? 1 g twice daily
* **Vitamin E**: ? 400 to 800 IU daily

- -

[+] **Coenzyme Q_{10}**: *to reduce blood viscosity and inhibit platelets:* 100 to 200 mg daily
[+] **Magnesium**: ? 400 mg daily
[+] **Pantethine**: *to inhibit platelet aggregation:* 300 mg 4 times daily with food (1 month trial)
[+] **Taurine**: *to inhibit platelet aggregation:* 1.5 g daily
[+] **Vitamin B_6**: ? 50 mg daily

- -

[-] **Calcium**: ? 800 to 1,500 mg daily
[-] **Copper deficiency**: 2 mg twice daily for up to 6 weeks along with **zinc** 50 mg daily
[-] rule out **Mercury** toxicity
[-] **Omega-3 Fatty Acids**: *example:* MaxEPA 1 g caps [180 mg EPA; 120 mg DHA] 10 to 20 daily
[-] **Omega-6 Fatty Acids**: *example:* evening primrose oil 500 mg caps [7-10% GLA] 6 to 8 daily
[-] **Selenium**: 200 μg daily

D. To Improve Poor Myocardial Oxygenation (resulting in improved cardiac function)

* **L-Carnitine**: 1 to 2 g twice daily *OR*
L-Propionylcarnitine: 500 mg 3 times daily (1 month trial)
* **Coenzyme Q_{10}**: 30 to 150 mg daily in divided doses (1 month trial)
* **Omega-3 Fatty Acids**: *example:* MaxEPA 1 g caps [180 mg EPA; 120 mg DHA] 10 to 20 daily
* **Vitamin C**: 500 mg daily

E. To Reduce the Risk of Restenosis in Coronary Artery Bypass Grafts

* **Vitamin C**: 500 mg daily
* ? **Omega-3 Fatty Acids**: *example:* MaxEPA 1 g caps [180 mg EPA; 120 mg DHA] 10 to 20 daily

F. To Improve Abnormal Lipid Metabolism

✓ **Niacin**: Start with 100 mg 3 times daily with meals. Increase by 100 mg 3 times daily each week to a maximum of 1 g 3 times daily if needed to achieve adequate results.

- -

* **Calcium**: ? 1,500 mg daily
* **L-Carnitine**: 2 g twice daily (2 month trial)
* **Chromium**: ? 200 μg daily (3 month trial)
* **Glycosaminoglycans**: mesoglycan ? 70 mg daily
* **Omega-3 Fatty Acids**: *for hypertriglyceridemia: example:* MaxEPA 1 g caps [180 mg EPA; 120 mg DHA] 10 to 20 daily
* **Omega-6 Fatty Acids**: *example:* evening primrose oil 500 mg caps [7-10% GLA] 6 to 8 daily
* **Phytosterols**: sitostanol ester 3 g daily *OR* beta-sitosterol 6 g daily (2 month trial)
* **Vitamin C**: 500 mg twice daily
* ? **Pantethine**: 300 mg 3 times daily with food (Does *not* increase HDL cholesterol.) (Results start in 1 to 2 months; maximal benefits take at least 4 months.)
* ? **Vitamin E**: *to increase HDL cholesterol:* 400 to 800 IU daily (3 month trial)

- -

[+] **Coenzyme Q_{10}**: 50 mg twice daily (10 week trial)
[+] **Copper deficiency**: 2 mg twice daily for up to 6 weeks *AND* **Zinc** 50 mg daily
[+] **Magnesium**: ≈ 400 mg daily

[+] **N-Acetylcysteine:** 1,200 to 3,600 mg daily
[+] **Vitamin B_6 deficiency:** 50 to 100 mg daily

- -

[-] rule out **Copper** toxicity
[-] rule out **Lead** toxicity
[-] rule out **Vitamin D** toxicity

G. To Reduce Elevated Homocysteine Levels

* **N-Acetylcysteine:** ? 3,600 mg daily

- -

[+] **Betaine:** *for vitamin B_6-unresponsive homocystinuria:* 3 g twice daily (up to 20 g daily may be required)
[+] **Folic Acid:** 800 μg daily (6 week trial)
[+] **Vitamin B_6:** 50 to 100 mg daily (6 week trial)
[+] **Vitamin B_{12}:** 200 to 400 μg daily (6 week trial) (Consider intramuscular administration.)

Perhaps because it is the most common cause of death among adults in our society, there has been more clinical research into nutritional factors contributing to atherosclerosis and coronary heart disease than into any other illness. Factors relating to the general topic of atherogenesis as well as to atherogenic coronary heart disease will be discussed in this chapter; cardiac arrhythmias, cerebrovascular disease and peripheral vascular disease, even when atherogenesis is the underlying cause, are discussed in their own chapters.

Nutritional factors are now known to play a major role in the development of atherosclerosis and we are gradually learning how to manipulate these factors to affect the course of the disease. In fact, the results of early studies suggest that it may even be possible to slowly *reverse* the process through nutritional means.

There are several different types of outcome measures which have been used in clinical studies. Morbidity and mortality as related to progression of the disease process is perhaps the ultimate measure of clinical significance, but is frequently impossible to assess due to practical limitations of study designs. The size of atherosclerotic lesions give us important information on the pathology of the disease, while measures of platelet aggregation, platelet adhesiveness and fibrinolysis provide us with clues as to the tendency for acute ischemic events to occur in plaque-laden vessels. Angina pectoris provides us with a functional measure of coronary vascularization, and certain blood lipid and apolipoprotein levels have been repeatedly correlated with the risk of atherogenesis and subsequent morbidity and mortality from the disease.

DIETARY FACTORS

OBESITY

Obesity, and especially fat storage in the area of the abdominal viscera, is associated with increased cardiovascular morbidity and mortality. These individuals frequently present with an atherogenic lipid profile and are more frequently characterized by hemostatic, metabolic and anatomical abnormalities compatible with insulin resistance and increased atherothrombotic risk. By improving tissue sensitivity to insulin, weight loss improves many of the cardiovascular risk factors in these patients *(Nielsen)*.

LIPIDS AND THEIR METABOLISM

Dietary fat is directly correlated with mortality from coronary heart disease and total serum cholesterol levels *(Dietschy)*. High fat diets raise glucose and total cholesterol levels. They reduce the postprandial increase in plasminogen activator inhibitor, suggesting that they impair the fibrinolytic response *(Ho)*. They also decrease the ability of blood vessels to dilate *(Tomaino)*.

Generally, about 30% of caloric intake from fat is recommended, although there are reasons to believe that diets that are high in monounsaturates can safely contain up to 40% of calories from fat *(Jeppesen)*. Diets containing less than 30% of calories from fat carry a number of risks including increased plasma triglyceride levels *(Schaefer)*, inadequate intake of essential fatty acids *(Siguel)*, and reduction of HDL cholesterol levels

(Schaefer) - although there are no data showing that the reduction of HDL cholesterol levels by consumption of a low fat diet is harmful *(Brinton;Connor WE)*.

There may also be symptoms such as fatigue, impaired concentration, lack of stamina, and personality change *(Gould)*. Furthermore, low fat, low cholesterol diets are contraindicated for children under 2 years of age since the diets may retard proper development *(Lifshitz)*.

The manner in which fats and oils are processed, stored and used has important implications for their metabolism and consequently for their nutritional value. Oils high in essential fatty acids are more prone to rancidity (which has prompted manufacturers to reduce or avoid them in many products). Light, oxygen and heat are detrimental *(Erasmus)*, while adding a small amount of vitamin E, an antioxidant, to the oil reduces peroxidation *(Chow)*. Similarly, high blood levels of polyunsaturates make LDL more susceptible to oxidation. As oxidized LDL increases its atherogenicity *(Steinberg)*, adequate antioxidant protection is particularly important *(Reaven,1991)*.

In this section, we will review the literature concerning the relationship between the general categories of fats and atherosclerosis. Later, in the discussion of individual nutritional factors, we will review the literature concerning specific fatty acids.

Saturates

Not all dietary fats have the same effects, and the picture has become increasingly complicated as the effects of individual fatty acids have been ascertained. Saturated fatty acids appear to be bear much of the responsibility for the adverse effects of fats. Their intake has been found to be positively related to total *(Caggiula)* and LDL *(Millen)* cholesterol levels, and negatively related to HDL cholesterol levels *(Cobb)*, and is believed to be closely related, not only to atherosclerosis, but also to arterial and venous thromboses *(Renaud,1985)*.

Polyunsaturates

Generally, polyunsaturated fats are half as powerful in lowering total serum cholesterol levels as saturated fats are in raising them *(Keys)*. Compared to saturated fats, they lower LDL and VLDL cholesterol levels, while HDL cholesterol levels are relatively unaffected *(Iacono)*. Polyunsaturated fat intake has been inversely related to carotid artery wall thickness *(Tell)*, while decreased concentrations of polyunsaturates in skeletal muscle phospholipids are associated with insulin resistance, a primary risk factor for coronary heart disease *(Borkman)*.

Monounsaturates

The predominant dietary monounsaturate is oleic acid, which is abundant in olive oil, certain other oils such as canola oil, and nuts such as almonds and walnuts. When monounsaturates are substituted for carbohydrates in an isocaloric diet, they have a neutral effect on serum total cholesterol levels. At realistic levels of intake, they have comparable effects to those of polyunsaturates on serum lipoprotein levels *(Mensink)*. At high levels of intake (greater than 15% of calories), they continue to have a neutral effect on HDL cholesterol - while polyunsaturates have been shown to *lower* HDL cholesterol *(Knapper)*.

On the other hand, polyunsaturates appear to be superior to monounsaturates in regard to possible effects on arterial thickening. While, as stated above, polyunsaturate intake has been inversely related to carotid artery wall thickness, there is evidence of a *direct* correlation between monounsaturate intake and carotid artery wall thickness *(Tell)*. Moreover, the monounsaturated fatty acid content of plasma phospholipids and cholesterol esters has been positively correlated with intima-media thickness of the carotid arterial wall *(Ma,1997)*. For patients experiencing progressive carotid artery intima-media thickening, however, increased monounsaturated fat intake relative to saturated fat intake predicts a *reduction* in the annual progression rate *(Markus)*, suggesting that replacing saturates with monounsaturates retards the process.

Hydrogenation and Trans Fats

Saturating an unsaturated vegetable oil by hydrogenation to make it harder, or to increase its shelf life, is a popular process that may create atherogenic products. The dietary intake of hydrogenated vegetable oils is associated epidemiologically with atherosclerosis *(Martin)*. Hydrogenation may increase the content of artificial *trans* fats which interfere with essential fatty acid metabolism *(Hill)* and may well be atherogenic *(Booyens)*.

In regard to serum cholesterol levels, their effect appears to be between that of saturated fats and unhydrogenated oils *(Longnecker)*. As the effects of some of these *trans* fats are still unexplored, a better appreciation of the extent of their contribution to atherogenesis awaits further research. In the meantime, it is considered prudent to minimize their intake *(Lichtenstein)*. (They are widely found in "fast foods," commercial bakery products and commercially prepared foods.)

Dietary Cholesterol

In patients with atherosclerosis, dietary cholesterol predicts the rate of progression of intima-media thickness *(Markus)*. Animal studies have repeatedly shown that cholesterol feeding causes atherosclerosis *(Stamler)*. Even when monkeys were fed amounts of cholesterol that were too small to cause high blood cholesterol levels, they developed atherosclerosis *(Armstrong)*.

Although dietary cholesterol contributes to serum cholesterol levels, these levels are considerably more sensitive to saturated fat intake than to dietary cholesterol *(Hegsted)*. About one-third of the population lacks precise cholesterol regulatory mechanisms and should minimize dietary cholesterol, while others probably have little to gain by limiting cholesterol to less than average levels of intake *(McNamara)*. Moreover, hyper-response to dietary cholesterol does not appear to occur in individuals following a low-fat, high-fiber diet. For such people, reduction in dietary cholesterol below 400 mg a day produces no further substantial cholesterol lowering *(Edington)*.

The heating of animal fat oxidizes cholesterol to 25-hydroxy cholesterol which may accelerate degeneration of smooth muscle cells in arterial tissue and initiate atherosclerotic plaques. Oxysterols are commonly found in dried egg products, powdered milk, cheeses and in a variety of high-temperature dried animal products *(Hubbard)*.

Thus, based upon current knowledge, it is advisable to minimize fats in the diet. Fat should come primarily from monounsaturates (e.g. olive oil) and the essential polyunsaturated fatty acids. Cholesterol intake may be moderate so long as the diet is also high in soluble fiber and serum cholesterol level is not elevated. For example, a recent meta-analysis of metabolic ward studies determined that replacing 60% of saturated fats with polyunsaturates and avoiding 60% of dietary cholesterol reduced total blood cholesterol levels by 10 to 15% (about 0.8 mmol/L), with 80% of this reduction coming from LDL cholesterol *(Clarke)*.

A 36-year-old white male presented with a total cholesterol of 264 mg/dl, HDL cholesterol of 38, LDL cholesterol of 192, and triglycerides of 171. He ate most meals out, kept high-fat snacks at home, and ate high-fat foods at mealtimes.

He was counseled about his diet and began eating breakfast at home (usually oatmeal), carrying his lunch to work and cooking at home using low-fat cookbooks for recipes. When he had to have meals out, he learned to choose lower fat foods. After 3 months, his total cholesterol had dropped to 212 mg/dl (20% decrease), HDL cholesterol had increased to 49 (23% increase), LDL cholesterol had dropped to 128 (34% decrease), while triglycerides were 212 (Greene).

EGGS

Because egg yolks are particularly rich in cholesterol, there has been substantial concern about their ingestion. Human trials, however, have had mixed results. For example, here are summaries of two crossover studies that examined the addition of eggs to the diet of healthy subjects. In the first, lactovegetarians who usually consumed 3 eggs a week received, under double-blind conditions, either 1 egg a day or an egg-free diet. Compared to the control diet, the egg diet raised LDL cholesterol levels but failed to affect HDL cholesterol levels *(Sacks,1984)*. In the other crossover study, subjects added 2 boiled eggs to their usual daily diet. While total cholesterol levels increased by 4%, HDL cholesterol increased by 10% and LDL cholesterol was unchanged *(Schnohr)*.

Until the picture clarifies, moderation is probably the best course for healthy people, while those who are predisposed to coronary heart disease are probably best served by avoiding egg yolks. As previously discussed, egg yolks should not be cooked under high temperatures to avoid oxidizing the cholesterol; thus scrambled and dried eggs should be avoided.

DAIRY PRODUCTS

The effect of milk upon cholesterol depends upon its butterfat content. Whole milk (4% fat by weight; 48% of energy from fat) appears to raise LDL cholesterol about 3 times as much as it raises HDL cholesterol *(Sacks,1985)*; it also raises apolipoprotein B *(Steinmetz)*. Reduced fat milk (2% fat by weight; 31% of energy from fat) may have a slight total cholesterol-lowering effect *(Hepner)*, while skim milk appears to effectively lower total cholesterol, apolipoprotein B, and triglyceride levels *(Buonopane;Steinmetz)*.

The results of early studies suggest that cheese consumption may have little effect on serum fatty acid levels. This is presumably because the palmitic and stearic acids found in cheese are poorly absorbed because they form insoluble calcium soaps in the gastrointestinal tract *(Renaud,1992)*.

Yogurt, even without reduction of its fat content, may reduce total cholesterol *(Hepner)*. Lowering the fat content most likely increases its efficacy in lowering cholesterol, but studies are lacking.

FISH

Fish consumption is generally believed to have a positive effect on lipid metabolism and thus may help to protect against atherosclerosis. The benefit is commonly ascribed to the high levels of the essential omega-3 fatty acids in fatty fish.

While findings of some epidemiological studies question this belief *(Pietinen)*, results of controlled clinical studies are generally consistent with this hypothesis. Particularly impressive in regard to its clinical implication was a study of more than 2,000 men who had recovered from a myocardial infarction. Some received advice to increase fatty fish intake to 2 to 3 portions a week, others were told to reduce fat intake and increase the ratio of polyunsaturated to saturated fat, and still others were told to increase their intake of cereal fiber. Of the 3 groups, only those advised to increase fish intake showed a significant change in subsequent mortality, with a 29% reduction in all-cause mortality over the next 2 years - although the incidence of reinfarction plus death from coronary heart disease was unaffected *(Burr)*.

One of the confounding factors is the *mercury* content of non-fatty freshwater fish. In a prospective study of almost 2,000 Finnish men who were initially free of cardiovascular disease and cancer, those who consumed local non-fatty fish species had elevated hair mercury contents, and dietary fish intake, like mercury, was associated with significantly increased risks acute myocardial infarction and death from coronary heart disease, cardiovascular disease and all causes *(Salonen,1995a)*.

Evidence for the superiority of fish over meat comes from a study of 20 patients who had suffered an acute myocardial infarction and were placed for 8 weeks on a diet that followed the standard "healthy heart" guidelines. Fish was then substituted for meat and the men continued the diet for another 4 weeks. Compared to their plasma fatty acid composition on the meat diet, there were definite improvements on the fish diet, including a decline in arachidonic acid levels and increases in the levels of the essential omega-3 fatty acids EPA and DHA *(Santos)*.

VEGETABLES

Any diet designed to combat atherosclerosis should emphasize the consumption of vegetables. Low in saturated fatty acids and cholesterol-free, vegetables are high in complex carbohydrates and dietary fiber.

Water-soluble fibers appear moderately effective in improving lipid metabolism by binding dietary and biliary cholesterol to prevent its absorption from the gut *(Spiller)*. Soluble fibers reduce total and LDL cholesterol levels in both hypercholesterolemic and normocholesterolemic subjects, although LDL cholesterol reductions are greater with the hypercholesterolemics. HDL cholesterol and triglyceride levels are usually unaffected. While they have a greater lipid-lowering effect than insoluble fibers, this effect varies. A 2 to 3 week trial of any of the following fibers would be adequate *(Glore)*:

pectin 6-40 g
guar gum 8-36 g
dried legumes 100-150 g (0.5-.75 cups)
dry oat bran 25-100 g (0.3-1.2 cups)
dry oatmeal 57-140 g (0.7-1.7 cups)
dried psyllium 10-30 g (3-9 tbsp)

Other components of vegetables also improve cholesterol metabolism. *Saponins* decrease cholesterol absorption and inhibit the resorption of bile acids *(Oakenfull)*. *Phytosterols* are cholesterol analogs which decrease cholesterol absorption by displacing cholesterol from bile salt micelles *(Ikeda)*.

Several vegetables have been investigated for their specific benefits. Common <u>beans</u>, such as pinto, navy and kidney beans, and <u>alfalfa</u> seeds have been shown to lower total serum cholesterol levels *(Anderson,1990)*. <u>Buckwheat</u> intake is associated with lower serum total and LDL cholesterol and a higher ratio of HDL to total cholesterol *(He)*. <u>Eggplant</u> inhibited the development of atheromatous plaques in rabbits *(Mitschek)*. <u>Garlic</u> and <u>onion</u>, both members of the genus Allium, may normalize plasma lipids, enhance fibrinolytic activity and inhibit platelet aggregation *(Ernst)*. <u>Ginger</u>, a potent inhibitor of thromboxane synthetase, is as potent an inhibitor of platelet aggregation as is aspirin *(Backon)*, and one study found it to be more effective than onion or garlic *in vivo* *(Srivastava)*. Konjac glucomannan has been found to be effective in lowering total and LDL cholesterol and triglycerides *(Arvill)*.

Not surprisingly, when cholesterol levels were compared, vegans (who avoid all animal products) have the lowest total and LDL cholesterol levels and meat eaters have the highest; vegetarians and fish eaters who avoid meat have similar intermediate values. HDL cholesterol was highest in the fish eaters (whose diets are rich in EPA and DHA), and did not differ between the other groups *(Thorogood)*. Furthermore, vegans have lower triglycerides, glucose, and uric acid and higher apolipoprotein A-1 and antithrombin III than nonvegetarians *(Melby;Pan)*.

SUGARS

Long-term consumption of excessive sucrose and fructose has repeatedly been shown to enhance risk factors associated with coronary heart disease *(Reiser,1985)*. Associations have been found with increased total and LDL cholesterol and triglycerides *(Reiser,1979;Frayn)*, as well as with decreased HDL cholesterol *(Frayn;Yudkin)*.

There is some evidence that the portion of the population which responds to sucrose with hyperinsulinism is most prone to its atherogenic effects *(Szanto)*. In addition, urinary chromium loss is increased *(Kozlovsky)*, and chromium deficiency is a risk factor for coronary heart disease (see below). Restricting sugars to below 10% of calories appears reasonable.

ALCOHOL

Although heavy alcohol consumption is clearly detrimental *(Criqui)*, there is a strong argument that moderate alcohol consumption (up to 2 drinks per day) may be beneficial. The results of most epidemiological studies have suggested an inverse association between moderate drinking and both the incidence of and death from coronary heart disease *(Kannel;Pearson)*.

There has been considerable research attempting to determine whether specific alcoholic beverages are preferable. A recent literature review suggests that all alcoholic drinks are linked with lower risk and that a substantial portion of the benefit is from alcohol itself rather than from the components of each type *(Rimm,1996)*.

However, there is also evidence that *red* wine, which is rich in polyphenols, is more beneficial that *white* wine, which has a lower polyphenol concentration, and that the alcohol content of wine is not necessary for it to enhance plasma antioxidant capacity *(Serafini)*. In fact, the antioxidant effects of red wine may be similar to those of red grape juice *(Day)*, probably due to the flavonoid content *(Miyagi)*. Results of an animal study suggest that 6 glasses of grape juice or 2 glasses of red wine have equivalent effects in inhibiting platelet activity in thrombosis in stenosed coronary arteries *(Demrow)*.

There have also been many studies investigating changes in markers of coronary heart disease risk with moderate alcohol consumption. Moderate drinking has been found to be associated, for example, with an increased ratio of apolipoprotein A-1 to LDL-B *(Moore)*. It has also been found to be associated with an increase in total, HDL2 and HDL3 cholesterol levels *(Gaziano,1993)*, while results of other studies have suggested that alcohol exerts salutary effects through its action on fibrinolytic factors *(Ridker)*.

Moderate alcohol consumption may also exert positive effects concerning postmenopausal coronary heart disease by increasing serum estradiol levels *(Gavaler)*. This effect may be due to the phytoestrogen content of some alcohol-containing beverages such as beer *(Rosenblum)* which can aromatize androgens, converting them into estrogens *(Gavaler)*.

Despite growing evidence of the benefit of moderate drinking in reducing the risk of coronary heart disease, moderate alcohol consumption increases the risk of stroke, breast cancer and other diseases *(Eichner)*. It therefore cannot be routinely recommended as a healthy component of the diet.

COFFEE

For several years, the results of studies exploring whether coffee consumption promotes coronary heart disease have been confusing due to their contradictory findings *(Kawachi)*. The picture has gradually become clearer, however, as confounding variables affecting the relationship have become identified.

For example, coffee, as opposed to tea, is directly associated with behavioral factors, such as smoking and animal fat consumption, that promote coronary heart disease, and negatively associated with factors, such as the intake of fresh fruits and physical activity, that are preventative *(Schwarz)*. Other confounding factors include alcohol use, serum cotinine, lipid and selenium levels, body mass index, blood pressure, Lewis blood group, hypertension, type II diabetes mellitus and social class *(Gyntelberg)*.

Similarly, confounding variables have also obscured the relationship of caffeine intake to coronary heart disease. In one study, men who drank decaffeinated coffee exclusively had lower body mass indices, a diet lower in fat, and consumed more cruciferous vegetables. Women who consumed decaffeinated coffee exclusively also exercised, consumed cruciferous vegetables and took vitamin supplements more regularly *(Leviton)*.

A major breakthrough in clarifying these relationships was the discovery that *boiled* coffee had a greater effect on serum lipids than *filtered* coffee *(Bønaa)*. The reason for this difference was traced to the presence of lipid-soluble substances present in boiled preparations but removed during filtering *(Kawachi)*. These have been identified as cafestol and kahweol, diterpenes that are present in coffee in oil droplets and floating fines *(Urgert,1995)*.

Even in regard to unfiltered coffee, the exposure to cafestol and kahweol differs. Turkish or Scandinavian boiled coffee contains 2 to 5 gram of floating fines per liter, while French press (cafetiere) coffee contains 1.5 grams of fines per liter *(Urgert,1995)*. Cafestol and kahweol may raise serum cholesterol levels due to the adverse effect on the integrity of liver cells *(Urgert,1996)*.

Caffeine may also make a contribution to the adverse effects of coffee. There is evidence that it alters coronary vasomotor tone at rest, which might lower the threshold for ischemic events in patients with coronary artery disease *(Bottcher)*. Consumption of 3 cups per daily of caffeinated filtered coffee increased plasma levels of total, LDL and HDL cholesterol in one study *(Fried)*, although failed to do so in another *(Bak)*. Also, ingestion of 100 milligrams of caffeine caused a 4-fold rise in plasma beta-thromboglobulin, a measure of platelet reactivity *(Ammaturo)*.

Thus, it now appears that the major danger of coffee drinking in regard to promoting coronary heart disease may be due to the drinker's failure to use a coffee filter, although caffeine may also make a contribution.

TOWARDS THE IDEAL CARDIOVASOPROTECTIVE DIET

Patients seeking to reduce their fat intake often substitute carbohydrates for fats. High carbohydrate, high fiber diets that are low in fat lower total and LDL serum cholesterol and triglyceride levels by about 20% *(Anderson,1987)*. They also lower HDL cholesterol levels, however *(Mensink)*.

Diets that are markedly high in carbohydrate do have a risk. Insulin production increases which could lead to insulin resistance *(Heller)*, a key component of "syndrome X." Other components of this syndrome include obesity, elevated LDL cholesterol and triglycerides, decreased HDL cholesterol, diabetes mellitus and hypertension *(Reaven,1995)*. While the substitution of carbohydrate for fat increases insulin and triglycerides *(Jeppesen)*, when low-fat sources of protein are exchanged for carbohydrate, LDL cholesterol and triglyceride levels decrease and HDL cholesterol levels rise *(Wolfe)*.

Further complicating the issue is evidence that reducing fat intake may not be as important as changing the ratio of dietary fatty acids. A diet high in monounsaturates appears preferable, not only to a high saturated fat diet, but also to a low fat, high carbohydrate diet. For example, a high monounsaturate diet can lower total plasma and LDL cholesterol levels below those resulting from a low fat, high carbohydrate diet while also reducing the proneness of LDL to oxidation *(Berry)*. Also, while a low fat, high carbohydrate diet may lower HDL cholesterol levels, the high monounsaturate diet does not *(Grundy,1988)*.

Until the picture clarifies further, it seems that moderation is the best approach to macronutrient balance. Diets that are too low in fat, or too high in carbohydrate, are probably best avoided. Rather than attempting to define an exact ratio between macronutrient categories, the emphasis on diet composition seems better placed on the choice of foods within each category. Positive attributes of a cardiovasoprotective diet are likely to include carbohydrates with a high content of soluble fiber, proteins that are high in quality, and fats that are low in saturates and adequate in essential fatty acids.

HOMOCYSTEINE ACCUMULATION

See *Homocysteine Accumulation* in Nutrition and Integrative Medicine, one of the introductory chapters, for a general discussion of homocysteine, its adverse effects, and its metabolism.

Homocysteine is a toxic amino acid which is an independent risk factor for atherosclerosis. Normalizing homocysteine metabolism is usually easily accomplished with nutritional supplementation and appears to be protective. In a study of 750 patients with atherosclerotic vascular disease who were younger than 60 years old, when compared to nonusers of vitamin supplements, the

58 subjects taking vitamin supplements containing folate, vitamin B_6 and cobalamin appeared to have only 38% of the risk of vascular disease, a proportion of which was attributable to lower plasma homocysteine levels (although they may have been more health conscious in other ways) *(Graham)*.

Currently in process are the long-term prospective randomized double-blind studies needed to provide definitive scientific verification that lowering elevated plasma homocysteine levels will retard the progression of atherosclerosis.

Folic Acid

Folic acid is coenzyme for the conversion of homocysteine to methionine. Current thinking is that inadequate folate intake is the main determinant of the destructive effects of homocysteine (*Stampfer*). In fact, one study found that supplementation with the combination of the 3 relevant B-vitamins did not lower plasma homocysteine any further than supplementation with folic acid alone (*Ubbink, 1994*). Supplementation with 1 to 2 mg of folate daily is usually adequate to normalize homocysteine levels even if the problem is *not* due to folate insufficiency (*Stampfer*).

Vitamin B_6

Vitamin B_6 is coenzyme for the conversion of homocysteine to cystathionine. In contrast to a folate or a vitamin B_{12} deficiency, a vitamin B_6 deficiency does not usually raise basal serum homocysteine concentrations, although failure to detoxify homocysteine can be brought out by first giving the patient a methionine load (100 mg/kg body weight) *(Brattström, 1996)*.

Patients with homocysteine accumulation because of heterozygous homocystinuria due to a deficiency of the enzyme cystathionine beta-synthase often respond well to high supplemental dosages of the vitamin *(Boers)*. (This is a classic example of a vitamin dependency syndrome.)

Vitamin B_{12}

As vitamin B_{12} is utilized in the remethylation of homocysteine to methionine, a deficiency, even in healthy people without other evidence of B_{12} deficiency, is frequently associated with increased homocysteine levels *(Lussier-Cacan)*. These levels, which can sometimes be higher than those seen in heterozygous homocystinuria, return to normal with supplementation *(Brattström, 1988)*.

Trimethylglycine (Betaine)

Trimethylglycine is the oxidative product of choline and cofactor for the enzyme betaine homocysteine methyltransferase. When added to the other nutrients, trimethylglycine may normalize amino acid metabolism in patients with pyridoxine-unresponsive homocystinuria, a genetically determined cause of abnormal homocysteine metabolism *(Dudman)*.

NUTRITIONAL FACTORS

VITAMINS

Folic Acid

(Also see the discussion under HOMOCYSTEINE ACCUMULATION above.)

Folate intake has been inversely related to the risk of myocardial infarction *(Verhoef)*. In fact, in a prospective study of more than 80,000 nurses recently published in the *Journal of the American Medical Association*, nurses with a median daily folate intake of about 700 micrograms had only 69% of the risk of coronary heart disease of nurses whose median daily intake was about 150 micrograms *(Rimm, 1998)*. (The 1989 RDA for adult females is 180 micrograms.) Similarly, plasma folate levels are inversely correlated with the risk of myocardial infarction *(Schwartz)*.

Besides its efficacy in lowering raised homocysteine levels, high levels of folate supplementation have been found in open trials to prevent the progression of atherosclerosis in patients with angina *(Oster)* and to increase capillary blood flow in patients with diffuse, chronic arteriosclerosis *(Kopjas)*.

Niacin

Niacin is well established as being effective in the treatment of hyperlipidemia. It has been shown to reduce coronary death and non-fatal myocardial infarction. It reduces total cholesterol, LDL cholesterol and triglycerides and increases HDL cholesterol. Sustained-release niacin may be associated with more dramatic changes in LDL cholesterol and triglyceride, whereas the short-acting preparation causes greater increases in HDL cholesterol. Niacin also favorably influences other lipid parameters including lipoprotein(a), alimentary lipemia, familial defective apolipoprotein B-100 and small dense LDL *(Crouse)*.

Doses of 2.5 grams daily have raised HDL cholesterol by 27% in patients with normal triglycerides and by 41% in patients with hypertriglyceridemia *(Brown)*. The increase of HDL cholesterol occurs at a lower dose (1,500 mg/day) than the reduction of LDL cholesterol (>1500 mg/day). Niacin can be effectively combined with a bile acid sequestrant or a reductase inhibitor as the combination has a synergistic effect in reducing LDL cholesterol *(Crouse)*.

Unfortunately, at recommended doses, niacin may have significant side effects. Common is a histamine flush due to the release of histamine from mast cells which starts in 20 minutes and can last for one and one-half hours. The flush usually is reduced after 3 days and may later disappear. It can be minimized by taking niacin with meals, raising the dosage gradually and, if necessary, by taking temporarily aspirin 300 mg 15 to 30 minutes before ingestion. It may also be helpful to take niacin with a fiber supplement and to avoid alcohol and spicy foods for one hour before and after its ingestion *(Jancin)*. Since niacin competes with uric acid for excretion, hyperuricemia may occur and hepatic toxicity is possible. Pruritus, hyperpigmentation and glucose intolerance have also been reported.

Vitamin B_6

(Also see the discussion under HOMOCYSTEINE ACCUMULATION above.)

The intake of vitamin B_6 appears to be inversely related to the risk of myocardial infarction *(Verhoef;Zoler)*; in fact, at least in women, it now appears that an intake of vitamin B_6 above the RDA may be important for the primary prevention of coronary heart disease *(Rimm,1998)*. Similarly plasma levels of the vitamin have been inversely related to the risk of both coronary artery disease *(Robinson)* and myocardial infarction *(Verhoef)*.

Animal studies have repeatedly found that a vitamin B_6-deficient diet results in the development of widespread atherosclerotic lesions *(Kuzuya)*. The reasons for this finding are only gradually becoming understood. We have already referred to two important roles for vitamin B_6 in atherogenesis: it is a coenzyme for both a key step in essential fatty acid metabolism (the action of delta-6-desaturase) and for the conversion of the toxic amino acid homocysteine to cystathionine.

There is also evidence vitamin B_6 supplementation may inhibit platelet aggregation and prolong clotting time *(Subbarao)*, and animal work suggests that vitamin B_6 may have a role to play in regulating blood cholesterol levels *(Rinehart)*. Vitamin B_6 may inhibit the glycosylation of LDL cholesterol, and glycosylated LDL cholesterol is believed to promote the development of atherosclerosis *(Kuzuya)*. Moreover, especially if the vitamin is marginally deficient, supplementation may reduce total and LDL cholesterol levels *(Brattström,1990)*.

Vitamin B_{12}

(See the discussion under HOMOCYSTEINE ACCUMULATION above.)

Vitamin C

While some of the larger epidemiological studies have found an inverse relationship between vitamin C intake and coronary heart disease *(Knekt,1994;Manson,1992a)*, this finding has not been confirmed by other large studies *(Kushi;Rimm,1993)*.

The evidence that a known ascorbate deficiency is associated with coronary heart disease is more consistent. In an animal model, ascorbate deficiency causes abnormalities of the arterial intima that is typical of atherosclerosis *(Willis,1957)*. Similarly, in human observational studies, low plasma ascorbate levels have been related to a increased risk of myocardial infarction *(Nyyssonen)*.

There are several reasons why a marginal vitamin C deficiency may contribute to atherogenesis:

1. *Cholesterol metabolism:* It is coenzyme for cholesterol-7-alpha hydroxylase, an enzyme required for synthesizing bile acids from cholesterol.
2. *Triglyceride metabolism:* It stimulates plasma lipoprotein lipase, an enzyme required for triglyceride catabolism.
3. *Arterial wall integrity:* It is required for the hydroxylation of proline for collagen formation *(Ginter;Turley)*.
4. *Antioxidant:* Vitamin C plays an important role as an antioxidant against the oxidative modification of LDL by scavenging active free radicals, and by reducing the alpha-tocopheroxyl radical *(Niki)*.

Plasma ascorbic acid correlates directly with HDL cholesterol and inversely with total cholesterol, systolic and diastolic blood pressure, and indicators of lipid peroxidation *(Toohey)*.

Supplementation

Even without evidence of a marginal deficiency, supplementation may raise HDL cholesterol *(Jacques)*, lower LDL cholesterol levels *(Gatto,1995)*, and diminish the tendency towards thrombosis by reducing platelet adhesiveness and aggregation *(Bordia,1985)*, and fibrinogen concentrations *(Khaw)*, while increasing fibrinolytic activity *(Bordia,1980)*.

Under double-blind conditions, supplementation with ascorbic acid reverses endothelial vasomotor dysfunction in patients with coronary artery disease *(Levine)*. There is also evidence from controlled studies that supplementation may improve the outcome of cardiopulmonary bypass surgery *(Dingchao)* and reduce the incidence of coronary restenosis after angioplasty *(Tomoda)*.

There is very early evidence that vitamin C supplementation may retard, and possibly even reverse, plaque formation. In a controlled study, 10 patients with intermittent claudication received ascorbate supplements while 6 served as controls. After 2 to 6 months, atherosclerotic plaques showed enlargement in only 3 of the 10 treated patients compared to 3 of the 6 controls. In addition, repeat femoral arteriograms revealed definite improvement in some of the involved arteries for 6 of these patients but for none of the controls *(Willis, 1954)*; however, this could be due to the ability of ascorbate to improve endothelium-dependent vasodilation *(Solzbach)*.

Vitamin D

A marginal vitamin D deficiency may promote coronary heart disease as serum levels of 1,25-vitamin D (the active form of the vitamin) have been found to be inversely related to the extent of coronary calcification *(Watson)*.

Vitamin D Toxicity: A Warning

Excessive exposure to vitamin D is also detrimental. The results of studies on swine suggest that an excess intake may accelerate the frequency of degenerated smooth muscle cell death in the intima of arterial tissue *(Kummerow)*, and there is epidemiologic evidence that elevated cholesterol levels may be associated with a high daily intake of vitamin D *(Dalderup)*.

Proof that excess vitamin D enhances human atherogenesis is lacking; it seems prudent, however, to guard against excessive vitamin D intake. With so many foods fortified with vitamin D, multivitamins which include vitamin D, and livestock which have been fed high levels of vitamin D prior to slaughter, the possibility of vitamin D toxicity should not be neglected.

Vitamin E

Vitamin E is a potent antioxidant which prevents lipid peroxidative tissue damage. It appears to regulate endothelial cell proliferation and repair while protecting them against oxidative injury *(Hennig,1988)*.

In a large study involving 24 countries, the intake of vitamin E was strongly inversely correlated with the risk of death from coronary heart disease. Sunflower seed oil was the major source of alpha-tocopherol. This oil has 7 times the vitamin E content of soybean oil, the main oil consumed in most countries studied with higher rates of coronary artery disease *(Bellizzi)*. Moreover, vitamin E intake has been found to be inversely related to carotid arterial wall thickness *(Kritchevsky)*.

Plasma vitamin E levels have shown similar inverse correlations. For example, in a study of middle-aged men from 16 European countries, there was a high inversely correlation between age-specific mortality from ischemic heart disease and lipid-standardized vitamin E levels *(Gey)*.

Once standardized for cholesterol levels, vitamin E levels within atherosclerotic plaques are significantly lower than in normal arterial wall, while the products of lipid oxidation are significantly higher *(Carpenter)*; in fact, the severity of coronary atherosclerotic lesions have been found to be inversely related to vitamin E levels in arterial tissue *(Mezzetti)*.

Supplementation

Numerous studies have examined the effects of vitamin E supplementation on coronary heart disease and acute myocardial infarction. Vitamin E supplementation of at least 100 IU daily appeared to slow the progression of coronary artery atherosclerosis in men with previous coronary bypass surgery. *(Hodis)*. In a double-blind study published in the *Lancet*, supplementation of 800 IU per day significantly reduced the risk of cardiovascular death and non-fatal MI for over 2000 patients with coronary atherosclerosis when reassessed after a mean of 510 days *(Stephens)*. Moreover, for patients with variant angina, 300 mg of vitamin E acetate daily reduced the frequency of attacks *(Miwa)*.

When the use of vitamin supplements was related to the incidence of ischemic heart disease, supplement use was consistently associated with a decreased incidence, and vitamin E was more consistently and strongly associated with a lower incidence of the disease than any other vitamin *(Meyer)*. Also, in a 4-year prospective study of almost 40,000 male health professionals who were free of diagnosed coronary heart disease, diabetes and hypercholesterolemia at the start, men who took at least 100 IU of vitamin E daily for at least 2 years have a multivariate relative risk of coronary disease of only two-thirds of those who did not take vitamin E supplements *(Rimm,1993)*.

Under controlled conditions, high-dosage vitamin E supplementation prior to cardiac bypass surgery has improved the outcome *(Yau)* and prevented the usual increase in free radicals during surgery *(Cavarocchi)*. Furthermore, high-dosage alpha tocopherol supplementation may reduce the risk of restenosis following percutaneous transluminal coronary angioplasty *(DeMaio)* as well as the risk of thrombosis following heart transplantation *(DeLorgeril)*.

While vitamin E (alpha-tocopherol) has not been noted for lowering elevated LDL cholesterol levels, supplementation has raised HDL cholesterol levels in some studies *(Cloarec)*, but not in others *(Kalbfleisch)*. It has been suggested that this may be because only certain people are responders *(Muckle)*.

Vitamin E is also the nutrient that has been shown most consistently to prevent LDL oxidation *(Jialal)*. This effect appears to be dose-related with a threshold of about 400 IU daily *(Cockcroft)*, although 1,200 IU daily is significantly more effective *(Fuller)*. There is also evidence from double-blind studies that Vitamin E may reduce platelet adhesiveness *(Steiner)* and aggregation *(Calzada)*.

MINERALS

Calcium balance

Intracellular calcium regulates many of the physiological, biochemical and molecular processes known to function abnormally in atherosclerosis. Moreover, increased intracellular calcium levels appear to be causally related to atherogenesis *(Phair)*.

While human studies are few, both inadequate *(Fujita)* and excessive *(Seely)* calcium intake have been blamed for promoting the development of atherosclerosis. The evidence appears stronger for a relationship between inadequate calcium intake and atherosclerosis since, in the elderly, low calcium and vitamin D intake, short solar exposure, decreased intestinal absorption, and falling renal function all contribute to calcium deficiency, secondary hyperparathyroidism, bone loss and possibly calcium shift from the bone to soft tissue, and from the extracellular to the intracellular compartment. Calcium deposition in the vascular wall then promotes the development of atherosclerosis and hypertension *(Fujita)*.

Consistent with this hypothesis are the findings of a study which found elevated plasma parathyroid hormone levels in almost half of a group of 56 patients with coronary heart disease. Moreover, parathyroid hormone levels were highest in those patients whose disease affected 3 coronary vessels and in patients who had had a myocardial infarction *(Herrmann G)*.

Supplementation

Based on results derived from an animal model of atherosclerosis, calcium supplementation may protect against atherogenesis. Beneficial effects included a prolongation of clotting time, decreased platelet aggregation and decreased total plasma cholesterol and slightly decreased plasma triglycerides with a greatly increased fecal excretion of fecal lipids and saturated fatty acids *(Renaud,1983;Yacowitz)*.

In a controlled human trials, calcium supplementation decreased total and LDL cholesterol in hyperlipidemic patients. While bile acid excretion was unaffected, the excretion of saturated fat more than doubled, perhaps because supplemental calcium facilitates the incorporation of free saturated fatty acids into micelles with bile acids for excretion, thus reducing the absorption of saturated fats *(Denke)*.

Chromium Deficiency

Research suggests that inadequate chromium nutriture, because of its involvement in lipid and glucose metabolism, increases the risk of atherosclerosis *(Simonoff,1984a)*. Aortic tissue of victims of coronary heart disease has decreased chromium levels *(Vlad)*. Even though plasma chromium levels are not in equilibrium with tissue stores, low plasma chromium levels suggest the presence of coronary atherosclerosis *(Simonoff,1984b)*. However, the lack of an adequate measure of marginal chromium status has hampered research on the hypolipidemic effects of chromium *(Lefavi)*.

Supplementation

In controlled human studies, chromium supplementation is often effective in lowering serum triglycerides *(Abraham,1992)*, and both total and LDL cholesterol *(Hermann)*, while it raises HDL cholesterol *(Abraham,1992)*. Both inorganic and organic (Brewer's yeast; "GTF chromium") forms of chromium were used successfully in these studies. As the efficacy of chromium supplementation in normalizing blood lipids has varied between studies, Mertz has suggested that only certain cases of abnormal lipid metabolism, possibly those specifically related to impaired glucose tolerance, are related to chromium deficiency *(Mertz)*.

Copper Balance

Copper deficiency is theorized to be "of prime importance" in the etiology of coronary artery disease. Copper-deficient animals are hypercholesterolemic, hyperuricemic, have glucose intolerance and display EKG abnormalities. Their hearts and arteries have abnormal connective tissue, lipid deposits, and inflammatory changes *(Klevey,1983)*.

Moreover, copper-deficient female mice develop alterations in blood clotting mechanisms that could increase the risk of coronary heart disease *(Lynch)*. Low copper diets are common in the industrialized nations, and some have ratios of zinc to copper greater than those that have produced hypercholesterolemia in animals *(Klevay,1983)*.

When healthy men were fed low-copper diets, LDL cholesterol increased and HDL cholesterol declined. These changes reversed after they received copper supplements *(Reiser,1987)*. Furthermore, atherosclerotic lesions have low copper concentrations *(Vijaya,1995; Vlad)*. It has been suggested that, in coronary artery disease, copper is released from arterial tissue into the blood *(Vlad)*.

The diet of a healthy 29-year-old male was designed to reduce his dietary copper intake to 0.83 mg daily. After 3.5 months, his total serum cholesterol concentration had risen by 15% (Klevay,1984).

In contrast to many other important nutrients, an *elevated* serum copper concentration is a common finding in patients with this disease *(Vijaya,1996)*, and elevated plasma or serum copper levels may be directly correlated with the risk of atherosclerosis and myocardial infarction *(McMaster;Salonen,1991)*. This may be because plasma or serum copper may fail to reflect either copper intake or organ copper. In fact, animal experiments reveal that high serum copper may reflect low copper nutritional status *(Klevey,1992)*.

Copper Toxicity: A Warning

In addition, excessive dietary copper, like copper deficiency, is associated with hyperlipidemia and hypertension *(Vijaya,1996)*, both important risk factors for atherosclerosis. It now appears that an optimum level of copper is required to maintain antioxidant defenses; thus both copper excess and copper deficiency increases antioxidant stress *(Strain)*.

Iron Balance

As with copper, if iron nutriture is either inadequate or excessive, atherosclerosis may be promoted. When available in moderate quantities and attached to protein, it is essential to cell growth and metabolism, but it becomes toxic when freed. It is both a strong biological oxidant and reductant because of its ability to switch back and forth between ferrous and ferric oxidation states *(Herbert)*.

Probably due to the two-sided effects of iron, the results of much of the research have been inconsistent. Most epidemiological studies have failed to support the hypothesis that high body iron increases the risk of coronary heart disease *(Sempos)*, while the larger studies have found lower iron to be a risk factor, especially in older populations *(Corti,1997a)*.

Elevated serum ferritin levels appear to be harmful. For example, high serum ferritin has been related to elevated total cholesterol, triglycerides, fibrinogen, and blood pressure, and decreased HDL cholesterol *(Oshaug)*. Moreover, in a prospective study, elevated serum ferritin more than doubled the risk of acute myocardial infarction *(Salonen,1992)*. There is also evidence from a controlled crossover study that decreasing elevated ferritin levels by blood letting may promote increased oxidation resistance of serum VLDL and LDL cholesterol *(Salonen,1995b)*.

While it is too early to draw firm conclusions, both high and low serum iron levels may promote coronary artery disease. In a large 17-year prospective study, men with elevated serum iron levels (>175 mg/dL) had over twice the relative risk of a fatal myocardial infarction, while women had more than 5 times the relative risk *(Morrison HI)*. By contrast, in another prospective study, this one lasting an average of 4 ½ years, men in the highest iron quartile were one-fifth as likely to die of coronary artery disease as men in the lowest quartile, while women in the highest quartile had one-half the risk of those in the lowest quartile *(Corti, 1997b)*.

While certainly not definitive, research linking elevated iron levels to the risk of coronary heart disease seems convincing enough to recommend that supplemental iron be avoided unless a need can be documented through laboratory testing.

Magnesium

Deficiency

Magnesium deficiency is associated with an increased risk of coronary artery disease, myocardial infarction, ventricular tachyarrhythmias and sudden cardiac death *(Lauler)*. In a study of more than 15,000 subjects, those with cardiovascular disease had significantly lower serum magnesium levels than those free from disease *(Ma, 1995)*. Moreover, magnesium loading tests have demonstrated that tissue magnesium is not only depressed, but actually deficient in many patients with acute myocardial infarction *(Rasmussen, 1988)*.

Although direct proof of a causal relationship is lacking *(Weiss)*, animal studies suggest that magnesium deficiency promotes the disorder. For example, magnesium deficiency markedly augments atherogenesis in the rabbit model *(Altura)*, and reduces rat myocardial tolerance to transitory ischemia *(Borcyhgrevink)*.

Several studies have found angina pectoris to be inversely related to magnesium status. For example, when men with variant angina were divided into those who had more than 4 attacks per week and those who had less attacks, magnesium status (as determined by 24-hour magnesium loading tests as well as by serum, mononuclear cell, erythrocyte and urine magnesium levels) was poorer in the group with the more frequent attacks *(Satake)*.

Even in the absence of significant organic stenosis, vasospastic angina appears to be promoted by magnesium deficiency *(Igawa)*. However, following at acute myocardial infarction, serum magnesium levels decrease while urinary magnesium excretion remains stable, suggesting that there is a shift of the mineral from the extracellular to the intracellular space *(Rasmussen, 1986)*; thus a reduced serum magnesium level in these patients does not necessarily mean that magnesium nutriture is compromised.

Supplementation

While it is clear that magnesium deficiency should be corrected, magnesium has also been used extensively for its pharmacologic effects at higher dosages. High calcium to magnesium ratios favor excessive release or formation of vasoconstrictive and platelet aggregating factors and directly enhance intravascular blood coagulation, both in the microcirculation and in large blood vessels *(Seelig, 1994)*. Conversely, pharmacologic dosages of magnesium inhibit of calcium influx which may alter the electrophysiological properties of heart cells, decrease catecholamine secretion, influence the synthesis of prostacyclin and/or alter platelet function *(Weiss)*.

When administered by intravenous infusion following acute myocardial infarction, magnesium has been shown to decrease myocardial damage and reduce mortality, and appears to be especially valuable for the elderly and patients who are ineligible for thrombolysis *(Shechter)*. Not all studies have found magnesium administration to be effective in this situation, however, so its use remains controversial *(Visser)*. Several suggestions have been made to increase its efficacy *(Seelig, 1996)*.

Also, extracellular magnesium has an antithrombotic action due mainly to its anti-platelet effect, which suggests that magnesium supplementation may help to prevent coronary thrombosis *(Gawaz)*. However, a controlled study found no changes in hemostatic variables in patients who had a non-thrombolytic-treated acute myocardial infarction after they received intravenous magnesium *(Torgersen)*.

When HDL cholesterol levels are abnormally low, even despite elevated LDL cholesterol, results of an open trial suggest that oral magnesium supplementation may help to raise HDL cholesterol while lowering total cholesterol levels *(Davis WH)*. Whether only magnesium-deficient patients will benefit is unclear *(Nozue)*. Moreover, among people without cardiovascular disease, one survey found an *inverse* relationship between dietary magnesium and serum HDL cholesterol levels *(Ma, 1995)*.

Since the myocardium cannot retain potassium when myocardial magnesium is deficient *(Dychner)*, concurrent potassium supplementation is recommended whenever magnesium deficiency is discovered.

Potassium Deficiency

A high potassium intake is associated with protection from cardiovascular disease. Theoretically, high dietary potassium could increase plasma potassium concentration, thereby inhibiting free radical formation, smooth muscle proliferation, and thrombus formation. In addition, the increase in glomerular filtration rate will probably cause a shift in the relationship between arterial pressure and sodium excretion that will lead to a reduction in arterial blood pressure *(Young)*.

Following an acute myocardial infarction, potassium supplementation may be as effective as magnesium in reducing the risk of subsequent coronary events; in fact, administration of either increases the serum level of both *(Singh,1996a)*.

Selenium Deficiency

Epidemiological and clinical studies have provided evidence of an inverse relationship between selenium status and ischemic heart disease. Prospective studies have produced conflicting results, although the cumulative data tend to show an inverse association between very low serum selenium concentrations and the risk of ischemic heart disease *(Bunker)*, although much of the increase in risk appears to be explained by smoking *(Kardinaal,1997)*.

In open trials, selenium supplementation has reduced platelet aggregation *(Stead)* and resulted in a substantial increase in bleeding time *(Schiavon)*.

Zinc Deficiency

In vitro studies suggest that zinc is vital to endothelial integrity and may play an important role in vascular endothelial barrier function *(Hennig,1992)*. Moreover, the susceptibility of the endothelium to damage by unsaturated fatty acids may be greatly increased by low levels of zinc *(Hennig,1990)*.

Probably due to its antioxidant activity, zinc protects the structural integrity of myocardial cells against catecholamine-induced myocardial damage *(Singal)*. While zinc supplementation decreases lipid peroxides *(Fortes)*, it does not appear to protect against LDL oxidation *(Gatto,1996)*.

A Warning

Despite the importance of adequate zinc nutriture, excessive zinc levels appear to be detrimental. For example, high serum zinc levels are directly associated with increased concentrations of total serum cholesterol, LDL cholesterol, and triglycerides *(Hiller)*. Moreover, zinc supplementation has been shown to *decrease* HDL cholesterol without changing total cholesterol, LDL cholesterol or triglycerides *(Black)* and, even at a minimal dosage of more than 15 mg daily, to prevent the enhancement of HDL cholesterol from exercise *(Goodwin)*. These adverse changes may well be due, not to zinc directly, but to low copper levels due to the depression of copper by zinc *(Bremner)*.

OTHER NUTRITIONAL FACTORS

L-Arginine

Arginine has gained a new prominence over the last several years as the precursor for nitric oxide *(Palmer,1988)*, and accumulating evidence indicates that supplemental administration of L-arginine restores endothelium-derived nitric oxide production in many disorders in which it is altered *(Maxwell)*. While it plays many roles throughout the body, nitric oxide is especially important in cardiovascular health because it has been identified as the endothelium-derived relaxing factor, an important regulator of vascular tone *(Vallance)*. It also inhibits platelet adhesion and aggregation as well as monocyte adherence and chemotaxis *(Flavahan)*.

Both plasma L-arginine *(Jeserich)* and arterial nitric oxide *(Beswick)* have been found to be reduced in patients with hypercholesterolemia. Moreover, in hypercholesterolemic rabbits, supplemental arginine at levels commonly found in the diet normalized low levels of nitric oxide *(Cooke)*.

Supplementation

Supplemental L-arginine can restore endothelium-dependent dilatation of the coronary circulation that has been impaired by hypercholesterolemia *(Drexler)* and inhibit platelet aggregation *(Adams)*. In one study, 27 young hypercholesterolemic patients with endothelial dysfunction and elevated LDL cholesterol received L-arginine and placebo for 4 weeks each in random order with a 4-week wash-out period. Supplemented patients showed significant improvement in endothelium-dependent dilation, a change which may slow or inhibit the atherosclerosis process *(Clarkson)*.

Supplementation appears to have other benefits which are just starting to be recognized. In a double-blind study, oral supplementation with L-arginine normalized the increased platelet aggregability of hypercholesterolemic patients *(Wolf)*, thus reducing the risk of thrombosis. Furthermore, in the rabbit model of atherosclerosis, L-arginine added to the drinking water reduced intimal hyperplasia and enhanced vascular healing following balloon angioplasty *(Tarry)*.

L-Carnitine

A naturally occurring amino acid found in all living tissue, carnitine is ingested preformed in foods, with animal foods its primary dietary source, or synthesized in the liver from lysine and methionine. As it is the co-factor required for the transport of long chain fatty acids across the inner mitochondrial membrane, depletion is believed to cause intracellular lipid accumulation.

Supplementation

Supplementation with carnitine allows the ischemic heart increased energy expenditure before coronary insufficiency develops *(Cherchi)*, probably by increasing its ability to oxidize fatty acids. It has been found effective for the treatment of angina pectoris in several controlled trials *(Davini)*. Moreover, controlled studies have demonstrated taht oral or intravenous supplementation reduces the immediate adverse effects of acute myocardial infarction, including reduction in the infarct size, reduced QRS score, reduced serum aspartate transaminase, lactate dehydrogenase and lipid peroxides. Clinical improvements include reductions in angina pectoris, heart failure with left ventricular enlargement, arrhythmias and total cardiac events *(Singh,1996b)*.

Following an acute myocardial infarction *(Rebuzzi)*, intravenous L-carnitine administration has been found to decrease cardiac necrosis and to improve the survival rate after cardiogenic shock *(Corbucci)*.

In addition to its striking effects on cardiac function, L-carnitine supplementation has beneficial effects on blood lipids. One year after 160 patients discharged after an acute myocardial infarction randomly received L-carnitine or just standard treatment, the carnitine-supplemented group had highly significant improvements in their lipid patterns *(Davini)*. Supplementation may reduce total cholesterol and triglyceride levels and increase HDL cholesterol *(Pola)*.

L-Propionylcarnitine

L-propionylcarnitine is a naturally-occurring derivative of L-carnitine which appears to be used by the myocardium to stimulate the tricarboxylic (energy) cycle via succinate synthesis *(Siliprandi)*. In a double-blind crossover study of 46 patients with stable exercise-induced angina, L-propionylcarnitine was compared to diltiazem, a calcium-channel blocker. The effects of the two substances were generally comparable. However, during diltiazem treatment, 8 patients complained of palpitations compared to 3 patients during L-propionylcarnitine treatment, a significant difference *(Bartels)*.

Carotenoids

Numerous epidemiological studies have found an inverse relationship between carotenoid intake and the risk of coronary artery disease and/or myocardial infarction. This finding has been noted for all carotenoids *(Gaziano,1995)* as well as specific carotenoids such as beta-carotene *(Manson,1992b)*, lutein and zeaxanthin *(Iribarren)*.

Adipose tissue beta-carotene concentrations were found to be strongly inversely correlated to the incidence of myocardial infarction - although this finding was dependent upon polyunsaturated fatty acid levels *(Kardinaal,1995)*. Levels of plasma or serum carotenoids *(Morris)* and beta-carotene *(Singh,1995)* have also been found to be inversely related to the risk of coronary heart disease and/or myocardial infarction.

Supplementation

Supplementation of synthetic *trans*-beta-carotene (STBC), the form used in most clinical trials, is controversial since, in large, double-blind studies, STBC supplementation failed to reduce the risk of coronary heart disease both in smokers and non-smokers *(Hennekens)*, and actually *increased* the risk of angina pectoris and deaths from coronary heart disease in smokers *(Rapola,1996,1997)*. Furthermore, in smokers, former smokers, and workers exposed to asbestos, supplementation of STBC plus vitamin A increased the risk of death from coronary heart disease *(Omenn)*.

This result had been unexpected - although the results of an epidemiological study had already suggested that the protective effect of beta-carotene among smokers may be reduced *(Rimm,1993)*. Numerous explanations have been offered in an attempt to explain this worrisome finding. One is that supplementation with beta-carotene may promote deficiencies of other carotenoids *(White)*. This would be particularly relevant for heavy smokers, who may already have a marginal carotenoid status *(Sulsky)*. Others have suggested that STBC performs differently than the beta-carotene found in food as it is only one out of the 272 configurational beta-carotene isomers *(von Eggers Doering)*. Also, beta-carotene from food may only be a marker for other dietary behaviors conducive to lower risk of coronary heart disease *(Kohlmeier)*.

While STBC supplementation has been found in some studies to increase HDL cholesterol levels *(Ringer)*, other studies have found no effect *(Ribaya-Mercado)*, leaving the issue unresolved. Similarly, the ability of STBC supplementation to protect LDL from oxidation is questionable *(Nenseter)*.

Therefore, at this time, we advise against the use of synthetic *trans*-beta-carotene supplements for atherosclerosis, either preventively or therapeutically.

One alternative to the problem is to supplement with a *natural* form of beta-carotene instead of STBC. The 9-*cis*-beta-carotene isomer, which is about half the beta-carotene content of *Dunaliella bardawil*, an algae which is a source of natural beta-carotene, appears to act *in vivo* more efficiently than STBC as a lipophilic antioxidant *(Ben-Amotz)* and supplementation with this algae as a source of beta-carotene is just starting to be explored. When, for example, 5 healthy volunteers received natural beta-carotene, plasma lipid peroxidation decreased by 22% and LDL susceptibility to oxidation decreased by 40% *(Levy)*. Further studies should clarify whether natural beta-carotene is an effective supplement, or whether beta-carotene in foods is only a marker for other beneficial nutrients or other confounding factors.

Coenzyme Q_{10} (ubiquinone)

This is a lipoidal, vitamin-like substance found primarily in the myocardium which facilitates the bioenergetic reactions of cellular respiration. It also appears to be an important lipid-soluble antioxidant whose presence in the reduced form (ubiquinol-10) in low-density lipoprotein suppresses the pro-oxidant, or complements the antioxidant, activity of alpha-tocopherol *(Thomas)*. In fact, it may well be the most effective lipid antioxidant present in LDL *(Mohr)*.

Patients with atherosclerosis may have reduced blood levels of CoQ_{10} *(Hanaki;Judy)*. Ubiquinol-10, its reduced form, may also be lower, and the percentage of ubiquinol-10 to CoQ_{10} may be reduced as a result of oxidative stress *(Kontush)*.

Supplementation

Coenzyme Q_{10} supplements have been shown in double-blind studies to reduce the frequency of anginal episodes and, as documented by reduced S-T segment depression during exercise, to increase exercise tolerance *(Kamikawa)*. Supplementation appears to reduce the risk of coronary thrombosis by inhibiting platelets *(Serebruzny)* and by reducing blood viscosity *(Kato)*.

CoQ_{10} supplementation may be of considerable value in protecting the myocardium during coronary artery bypass surgery and promoting healing *(Chello)*. For example, when, under double-blind conditions, high-risk cardiac surgery patients received CoQ_{10} starting 14 days before surgery and continuing for 30 days afterwards, their recovery period was only 3 to 5 days versus 15 to 30 days for the controls *(Judy)*.

Coenzyme Q_{10} supplementation has also been found to decrease total serum cholesterol and raise HDL cholesterol, at least in hypertensives *(Digiesi)*. In regard to its antioxidant effects, supplementation with CoQ_{10} increases the level of ubiquinol-10, its reduced form, in all classes of lipoproteins, and increases the resistance of LDL to free radical oxidation *(Aejmelaeus;Mohr)*.

Fatty Acids, Essential

While earlier studies examined the effects of polyunsaturated fatty acids as a group, more recent research has focused on those polyunsaturates that are also essential fatty acids and separating them into their two families, the omega-3 and omega-6 fatty acids. Their importance lies in their role as precursors to the prostaglandins, prostacyclins, thromboxanes and leukotrienes. These are families of hormone-like substances that have important influences on immune function, smooth muscle function, platelet aggregation and inflammation.

Omega-3 Fatty Acids

alpha-linolenic acid → EPA → 3 series prostaglandins
↳ DHA

Dietary alpha-linolenic acid (18:3 n3) is parent to the omega-3 fatty acids. It is transformed into the 3 series prostaglandins first by desaturation (through the action of delta-6-desaturase) to stearidonic acid (18:4 n3), then by elongation to eicosatetraenoic acid (20:4 n3). Next, by desaturation, eicosapentaenoic acid (EPA) (20:5 n3), the immediate precursor to the 3 series of prostaglandins, is formed. Further elongation and desaturation results in the formation of docosahexaenoic acid (DHA) (22:6 n3)

Adequate dietary alpha-linolenic acid does not insure adequate supplies of the 3 series prostaglandins. Both series of essential fatty acids require the enzyme delta-6-desaturase; specifically for the conversion of alpha-linolenic acid to stearidonic acid. The activity of this enzyme may be reduced by, for example, alcohol, saturated and *trans* fats, deficiencies of vitamin B_6 and zinc, ageing, viral infections, chemical carcinogens and radiation. In addition, alpha-linolenic acid, which is abundant in flaxseed oil, is found in greatest quantities in oils from northern plants, while oils from southern plants are currently more widely available in most Western countries.

Certain plant oils, such as flaxseed oil, are rich in alpha-linolenic acid. However, because they are structurally closer to their key biological metabolites, and do not require the limiting enzyme delta-6-desaturase, EPA and DHA are preferable as metabolic precursors of the 3 series prostaglandins. Fish oils are excellent sources of both of these fatty acids and thus have been utilized in most of the experimental studies.

The relationship of EPA and DHA to cardiovascular disease appears to be an intimate one. Their beneficial effects are numerous. They prevent cardiac arrhythmias, are antithrombotic, retard the growth of atherosclerotic plaque, promote the synthesis of the beneficial nitric oxide in the endothelium, are profoundly hypolipidemic (especially lowering plasma triglycerides), inhibit both VLDL production and apolipoprotein B synthesis, have a mild blood pressure lowering effect *(Connor SL)*, and reduce the susceptibility of LDL to oxidation *(Wander)*.

Cardiovascular mortality has been shown to be inversely related to omega-3 fatty acid intake in some, but not all, observational studies *(Pritchard)*. Moreover, adipose tissue *(Seidelin)*, platelet *(Hodgson)*, erythrocyte membrane *(Shamberger)* and serum *(Simon)* levels have been shown to be inversely related to the risk of coronary heart disease.

Supplementation

Supplementation with omega-3 fatty acids has been shown to improve cardiac function in patients with coronary artery disease *(Salachas)* and inhibit occlusion of coronary artery bypass grafts *(Eritsland)*. There is also evidence from 4 randomized trials omega-3 fatty acids may inhibit restenosis after percutaneous transluminal angioplasty *(Gapinski)*, although later studies *(Cairns; Leaf)* have failed to confirm this.

Based on a review of placebo-controlled studies providing less than 7 grams of omega-3 fatty acids daily for at least 2 weeks:

1. serum triglyceride concentrations decrease by 25 to 30%
2. LDL cholesterol concentrations tend to rise by 5 to 10%
3. HDL cholesterol concentrations tend to rise by 1 to 3%
4. total cholesterol concentrations are not materially affected *(Harris, 1997a)*.

Omega-3 fatty acids are unique among the polyunsaturates in their ability to lower triglycerides. In patients with elevated triglycerides, this may cause LDL cholesterol to rise - since elevated triglycerides are associated with abnormally low LDL levels which, with all treatments, normalize when triglycerides come down *(Davidson)*.

The one caution in taking supplements of omega-3 fatty acids is to ensure that they are taken with adequate vitamin E to prevent increased membrane peroxidation and cellular damage *(Wander)*.

For the reasons already stated, relatively little research has been done on alpha-linolenic acid, the precursor to both EPA and DHA. Flaxseed, with over 50% alpha-linolenic acid in its oil, when provided either as a supplement or in baked bread, reduced both total and LDL cholesterol *(Cunnanae)* and has a powerful inhibitory effect on hypercholesterolemic atherosclerosis induced in rabbits *(Prasad, 1997)*. However, flaxseed oil with almost no alpha-linolenic acid has a similar anti-atherosclerosis effect on rabbits, suggesting that its therapeutic effects cannot simply be explained by its alpha-linolenic acid content *(Prasad, 1998)*.

There are similar problems in accepting the simple explanation that the beneficial cardiovascular effects of fish oils on coronary artery disease are due to EPA and DHA. For example, not all omega-3-rich fish oils have the same effect, possibly due to differences in their ratios of EPA to DHA *(Grimsgaard; Harris, 1997b)*:

Oil	EPA:DHA
Pollack	3.8
MaxEPA (North Sea fish)	1.6
Salmon	0.8
Tuna	0.35

In fact, recent findings suggest that EPA is not elongated to DHA, while some DHA is retroconverted to EPA *(Grimsgaard)*. Future studies will likely focus on the specific effects of each of these important fatty acids.

Omega-6 Fatty Acids

linoleic acid → GLA → DGLA → 1 series prostaglandins

Dietary *cis*-linoleic acid (18:2 n6), the parent compound of the omega-6 fatty acids, is found in abundance in safflower and a number of other commonly-used vegetable oils. It is transformed into the 1 series prostaglandins first by desaturation to form gamma-linolenic acid (GLA) (18:3 n6) and then by elongation to form dihomogamma-linolenic acid (DGLA) (20:3 n6), the immediate precursor of prostaglandin E_1 (PGE_1).

While omega-3 fatty acids primarily decrease triglyceride concentrations, omega-6 fatty acids mainly reduce LDL cholesterol *(Klor)*. There is some evidence that the risk of coronary heart disease is inversely correlated with a low dietary intake of linoleic acid *(Gartside)*. However, while adipose tissue linoleic acid has been inversely correlated with the risk of coronary heart disease *(Rapley)* and with the risk of sudden cardiac death *(Roberts)*, a positive correlation between tissue linoleic acid levels and the risk of coronary artery disease has also been found *(Hodgson)*. The relationship of plasma linoleic acid levels to coronary artery disease is also uncertain *(Bang,1987)*.

A low intake of linoleic acid, however, is only one of the reasons for inhibition of PGE_1 synthesis:

1. A high intake of refined carbohydrate will block mobilization of linoleic acid stores.
2. The activity of delta-6-desaturase. Earlier we discussed how delta-6-desaturase is required for the conversion of alpha-linolenic acid to stearidonic acid. The same enzyme is also required to convert linoleic acid to GLA. As noted above, its activity is reduced by many factors, including alcohol, saturated and *trans* fats, deficiencies of vitamin B_6 and zinc, ageing, viral infections, chemical carcinogens and radiation.
3. Free DGLA may either be converted to PGE_1 or stored in membrane phospholipids. Zinc enhances the mobilization of DGLA for transformation to PGE_1; the conversion of free DGLA to PGE1 is enhanced by alcohol, ascorbic acid and probably niacin.

Thus, in certain people, PGE_1 may be deficient despite an adequate dietary intake of linoleic acid. Reducing the intake of saturated and *trans* fats while insuring adequate supplies of vitamin B_6 and zinc appears prudent. In addition, the administration of a plant oil which has a relatively high content of gamma-linolenic acid (such as evening primrose and borage oil) may be indicated when delta-6-desaturase activity may be inadequate in order to bypass the metabolic block *(Horrobin)*.

As with omega-3 fatty acid supplementation, supplementation with omega-6 fatty acids in the presence of low antioxidant status carries a risk for atherosclerosis promotion due to their susceptibility to oxidation *(Louheranta)*. Therefore, vitamin E should always be given along with omega-6 fatty acid supplements.

Omega-3 vs. Omega-6 Fatty Acids

Several studies have examined the relative benefits of omega-3 versus omega-6 ingestion. In most cases, omega-3 fatty acids have been found to be more hypolipidemic *(Kinsella)* and yield better risk lowering for coronary heart disease *(Bang,1980)*. In addition, omega-3 fatty acids are superior in reducing triglyceride and lipoprotein (a) levels *(Herrmann W)* as well as in increasing HDL cholesterol *(Herrmann W)* and lipoprotein lipase levels *(Zampelas)*. However, omega-3 and omega-6 fatty acids may be equally effective in reducing fibrinogen levels *(Radack)*.

Human beings evolved on a diet in which the omega-3 and omega-6 fatty acids were balanced, a situation that appears to be more physiologic in terms of prostaglandin and leukotriene metabolism and interleukin-1 production *(Simopoulos)*. Both require the limiting enzyme delta-6-desaturase for their metabolism and, if either linoleic acid (omega-6) or alpha-linolenic acid (omega-3) is administered in high levels, it inhibits the metabolism of the other (*Holman*).

Available evidence suggests that a balance between the omega-3 and omega-6 fatty acids in the diet may help to prevent degenerative diseases. The modern Western diet is usually relatively deficient in omega-3 fatty acids, with a ratio of omega-6 to omega-3 of between 10 and 14 to 1 instead of 1 to 1 as in the case of the diets of wild animals.

Populations with a low ratio of dietary omega-3 to omega-6 fatty acids have an increased risk for cardiovascular diseases. In Israel, for example, the consumption of omega-6 fatty acids is unusually high for a Western country (8% higher than in the United States and 10 to 12% higher than in most European countries). There is also a high prevalence of cardiovascular disease and related syndromes (hypertension and non-insulin-dependent diabetes mellitus), suggesting that the high consumption of omega-6 fatty acids may aggravate hyperinsulinemia and insulin resistance; it may also serve as a substrate for lipid peroxidation and free radical formation *(Yam)*. Similar results were found when the Danish diet (polyunsaturates mainly from the omega-6 family) was compared to that of the Greenland Eskimo (polyunsaturates mainly from the omega-3 family) *(Bang,1980)*.

More of a balance could be achieved if cold-water fish replaced meat and eggs as a major protein source, and if linseed oil, which is high in alpha-linolenic acid, became a common dietary oil. When there is reason to believe that delta-6-desaturase activity is impaired, supplementation with both fish oils that are high in eicosapentaenoic acid and plant oils that are high in gamma linolenic acid may be indicated.

Fatty Acids, Omega-9

(Also see Monounsaturates above under Lipids and Their Metabolism.)

Oleic acid, an omega-9 fatty acid, is the major fatty acid in olive oil and other oils that are rich in this family of fatty acids. It is considered to be their primary ingredient for cardiovascular protection, although other constituents of high-monounsaturated oils may be involved *(Muriana)*.

The incidence of coronary heart disease has been found to be inversely correlated with the concentration of oleic acid in red blood cells *(Fan)*. A high-oleic acid diet is believed to inhibit arachidonic acid incorporation into platelet phospholipids which would inhibit production of thromboxane A2, a promotor of platelet aggregation and arterial wall spasm *(Barradas)*. In fact, compared to linoleic acid (omega-6), it raises the threshold for platelet aggregation *(Burri)*. Oleic acid also may be superior to both the omega-3 and omega-6 fatty acids in reducing the susceptibility of LDL to peroxidative damage *(Mata)*, and has even been shown to reduce the susceptibility of HDL to oxidative modification *(Sola)*.

Although oleic acid appears to be relatively neutral in terms of its effects on cholesterol levels *(Heyden)*, it may tend to slightly lower LDL cholesterol while raising HDL cholesterol *(Katan,1994)*.

Fatty Acids, Saturated

The effect of a dietary saturated fat upon blood fats depends upon the effects of its constituent fatty acids. Only some of the longer-chain saturated fatty acids appear to be atherogenic. Based on serial quantitative angiography, progression of coronary heart disease was found to be directly, strongly and independently associated with the intake of saturated fatty acids with a chain length 14 to 18 carbon atoms *(Watts)*. However, the association between *stearic acid* (18 carbon atoms) and coronary heart disease is unsettled *(Markus)* - possibly because it is rapidly unsaturated to the monounsaturate *oleic acid (Grundy,1990)* which has been shown in rabbits to slow the progression of atherosclerosis *(Parthasarathy)*.

saturated fatty acid	# of carbon atoms
lauric	12
myristic	14
palmitic	16
stearic	18

The results of studies investigating the effect of saturated fatty acids are difficult to evaluate as they are strongly influenced by confounding dietary and metabolic factors. For example, while the 12-carbon *lauric* acid seems able to raise LDL cholesterol levels *(Derr)*, the 18-carbon *stearic acid* does not appear to do so *(Yu)*. Moreover, even though serum levels of the 16-carbon *palmitic acid* have been found to be directly associated with the risk of coronary heart disease *(Simon)*, it appears to have no effect on blood lipids so long as dietary lipids are reasonably sound (low cholesterol, adequate linoleic acid, and not too high a percentage of calories from fat) *(Hayes,1992;Temme)*.

Saturated Fatty Acid Composition Of Some Popular Fats And Oils

Fat or Oil	Lauric	Myristic	Palmitic	Stearic	Total Saturates
beef tallow		3%	24%	19%	46%
butterfat			38%	9%	63%
coconut oil	47%	18%	9%	3%	92%
corn oil			11%	2%	13%
cottonseed oil		1%	22%	3%	26%
lard		2%	26%	14%	42%
palm oil		1%	45%	4%	50%
palm kernel oil	48%	16%	8%	3%	82%

Flavonoids

Several studies have found an inverse correlation between flavonoid intake and risk of myocardial infarction. Major sources of flavonoids in the studies were fruit and vegetables, tea and red wine; onions and apples were the riches source of flavonoids *(Knekt,1996)*.

Flavonoids could function by any of a number of mechanisms such as free-radical scavenging, chain-breaking antioxidant activity or metal chelation. In addition, this diverse group of compounds can inhibit LDL oxidation, or reduce platelet aggregation or damage from ischemia *(Muldoon)*.

Randomized clinical trials are needed to determine whether flavonoids are actually protective against atherosclerosis *(Katan,1997)*.

Glutathione

Glutathione is a tripeptide composed of the amino acids cysteine, glycine, and glutamic acid. It functions as a major intracellular antioxidant and as a primary component of detoxication pathways.

Compared to normals, erythrocyte glutathione levels have been found to be lower in patients with unstable angina pectoris *(Dubois-Rende)*, suggesting that increasing cellular glutathione levels may be beneficial. However, due to its hydrolysis by intestinal and hepatic gamma-glutamyltransferase, the bioavailability of dietary glutathione has been questioned *(Witschi)*. Therefore, studies have examined supplementation with *N-acetylcysteine*, which is converted in the body into metabolites capable of stimulating glutathione synthesis *(Kelly)*, to increase intracellular glutathione levels. (See N-acetylcysteine below).

Glycosaminoglycans

Heparin is a specific glycosaminoglycan which is the drug of choice in most situations that require an anticoagulant. However, it has many side effects, including hemorrhage, thrombocytopenia, eosinophilia and osteoporosis *(Walenga)*; close medical supervision is therefore required.

Extracts rich in a mixture of the glycosaminoglycans found in the aorta are well absorbed orally *(Zanolo)*. *Mesoglycan*, which has been employed in many of the studies, is a natural heparin-like extract obtained from the bovine intestinal mucosa whose components include chondroitin, dermatan and heparan sulfates, hyaluronic acid, and related hexosaminoglycans.

Glycosaminoglycans appear to protect the vascular endothelium *(Tanganelli)* and reduce the progression of atherosclerosis *(Laurora)* and the danger of thrombosis *(Vecchio)*. They may decrease triglyceride and total, VLDL and LDL cholesterol levels *(Postiglione;Saba; Vecchio)* and increase HDL cholesterol *(Saba;Vecchio)*.

Chondroitin sulfate is a glycosaminoglycan composed of repeating units of N-acetylchondrosine with one sulfate group per disaccharide unit. In a controlled study of chondroitin sulfate A, after 6 years only 6 out of 120 patients with coronary heart disease who were randomly treated with chondroitin sulfate A in addition to conventional treatment experienced coronary incidents compared to 42 controls. Moreover, only 4 of the treated patients died of myocardial infarction verses 14 of the controls *(Morrison LM)*.

N-Acetylcysteine

N-acetylcysteine (NAC) supplementation has been increasingly utilized as a means of increasing intracellular glutathione levels (see Glutathione above). Specifically, an animal study found that oral NAC supplementation increased myocardial glutathione content in a dose-dependent manner *(Ferrari)*.

NAC has been shown to have several beneficial effects for patients with coronary artery disease. It increased HDL cholesterol levels in hyperlipidemic patients in a dose-dependent manner *(Franseshini)*. In a controlled study, a high dosage of oral NAC reduced the oxidative stress seen during an acute myocardial infarction due to myocardial ischemia and reperfusion, with a trend towards more rapid reperfusion and better preservation of left ventricular function *(Arstall)*. Also of interest, high-dosage NAC supplementation, in a double-blind crossover study, reduced plasma homocysteine levels by 45% *(Wiklund)*.

A Warning

Despite its apparent benefits to patients, results of a controlled study suggest that NAC may have a *pro-oxidant* effect on *healthy* subjects. When 6 healthy volunteers took NAC supplements for 6 weeks, the glutathione concentration in treated subjects as compared to controls was reduced by 48% and oxidized glutathione was 80% higher. The percent of glutathione to reduced glutathione, a marker of oxidative stress, was 83% lower in treated subjects. Also, there was no effect on oxidized LDL, suggesting that NAC was not acting as an antioxidant *(Kleinveld)*. These findings suggest that NAC may be contraindicated in the primary prevention of atherosclerosis.

Pantethine

Pantethine, the active form of pantothenic acid, is the fundamental moiety of coenzyme A.

Supplementation with pantethine has been shown to decrease total and LDL cholesterol and triglyceride levels in several studies, 2 of which were double-blind and crossed-over *(Angelico;Gaddi)*, although a third double-blind study found it ineffective for patients who had failed to respond to a combination of drug and dietary therapy *(Da Col)*. HDL cholesterol levels appear to be unaffected *(Gaddi)*. In addition, pantethine supplementation may inhibit platelet aggregation and production of thromboxane A2 *(Prisco)*.

When compared in a randomized study to fenofibrate, a cholesterol-lowering drug (fenofibrate), it was just as effective in lowering total and LDL cholesterol levels, but without the side effects of the drug *(Cattin)*.

Phytosterols

These are cholesterol analogs found in vegetables. Their administration may decrease cholesterol absorption by displacing cholesterol from bile salt (taurocholate) micelles *(Ikeda)*. Both *sitostanol* and *beta-sitosterol* have been utilized in a number of studies.

Phytosterols reduce plasma total and LDL cholesterol levels. They generally appear to not affect HDL cholesterol or triglyceride levels *(Miettinen)*, although there is some evidence for an HDL cholesterol-raising effect of sitostanol *(Jones)*.

In a double-blind crossover study, sitostanol has been shown to reduce total serum cholesterol LDL cholesterol levels *(Gylling)*. Reduction in campesterol resorption, which reflects intestinal absorption of cholesterol, has been used as an indicator of its efficacy *(Richter)*.

The administration of beta-sitosterol also appears promising. When given along with a meal containing 500 mg of cholesterol, beta-sitosterol decreased cholesterol absorption by 42% *(Mattson)*. Beta-sitosterol also improved the reduction of LDL cholesterol achieved with lovastatin by an additional 13 to 15% *(Richter)*.

Taurine

During myocardial ischemia, and particular during an acute myocardial infarction, blood taurine levels rise and peak 12 to 24 hours later *(Bhatnagar)*.

In the rabbit model, supplementation with taurine reduces the development of atherosclerotic plaques without affecting serum lipids *(Petty)*. The failure of taurine to affect serum lipid concentrations in rabbits has been confirmed in humans, at least in healthy males *(Tanno)*. Taurine may, however, reduce the tendency of platelets to aggregate by 30 to 70% *(Hayes,1989)*.

COMBINED NUTRITIONAL INTERVENTIONS

Although controlled clinical trials rarely investigate the additive, or even synergistic, benefits of using supplements in combination, clinicians often observe improved results by using cardioprotective nutrients in combination:

A 50 year-old man began to note mild chest pain with exercise at age 47. His father had died of a MI at age 61 and his father's father had died of a MI at age 71. His cholesterol and triglycerides were elevated and there were EKG abnormalities on the treadmill. He was told by his cardiologist to enroll in a medically supervised exercise program and prescribed nitroglycerin for pain. His angina worsened and he was switched to long-acting nitroglycerin and begun on propanolol. Later, an anti-thrombotic agent and ASA were added.

He failed to improve until 3 years prior to evaluation when he began his own nutritional program. This consisted of avoiding red meat, reducing animal protein, avoiding sugar and refined carbohydrates, avoiding caffeine, restricting alcohol and supplementing with vitamin C 3 gm daily, vitamin E 800 IU daily, lecithin 2 tbsp daily, dolomite (a source of calcium and other minerals) 3 tabs daily, selenium 100 mcg daily, garlic oil 6 caps daily, sunflower or safflower oil 1 tbsp daily, brewer's yeast 2 tbsp daily and zinc 30 mg daily along with a multi-vitamin.

Over the next 2 years, his total cholesterol dropped from 388 to 255, triglycerides dropped from 417 to 165, and angina improved "80%" (although he continued to show exercise-related EKG changes) so his cardiologist slowly discontinued his medications. At the time of evaluation he required nitroglycerin only occasionally but had made no further progress in the past year. Total cholesterol was 260, HDL cholesterol was 38 and triglycerides were 163.

He was started on D,L-carnitine 750 mg twice daily. Six months later his angina was gone, even with maximal exertion and EKG changes on the treadmill were nearly gone. Triglycerides were 114, total cholesterol 195 and HDL cholesterol 46 (Wright).

OTHER RELATED FACTORS

TOXIC MINERALS

High levels of several toxic minerals are associated with increased risk of coronary heart disease and/or myocardial infarction. For example, the risk of mortality for ischemic heart disease rises with increasing arsenic levels *(Chen;Engel)*. Deaths from cardiovascular diseases appear to be strongly correlated with high concentrations of cadmium contamination *(Carroll)* and even long-low-level chromic cadmium exposure is associated with a higher frequency of atherosclerosis *(Houtman)*.

Lead toxicity among workers engaged in lead production is associated with elevations of total, LDL and VLDL cholesterol and triglycerides as well as decreases in HDL cholesterol *(Gatagonova)*. Mercury toxicity is related to LDL cholesterol oxidation *(Salonen,1995b)* and increased platelet activity *(Kostka)*.

CAN NUTRITIONAL SUPPLEMENTATION CAUSE PLAQUE REGRESSION?

The possibility for atherosclerotic plaque to regress is no longer controversial. Magnetic resonance imaging of the aorta and of the carotid and iliac arteries of humans receiving fat-free total parenteral nutrition have shown plaque regression in as little as 2 to 3 weeks *(Dudrick)* and, in experimental animals, including primates, cholesterol-free diets have resulted in regression of atherosclerosis *(Malinow)*.

Despite the promise, almost all the work concerning the use of nutritional supplements to promote plaque regression has been done in animals. There is, for example, very early evidence suggesting that vitamin C supplementation may promote regression of atherosclerotic plaques. When guinea pigs developed atherosclerosis due to scurvy (vitamin C deficiency), the early lesions resorbed rapidly following ascorbate supplementation. Advanced lesions, however, were considerably more resistant to reversal, apparently because the only contact of the islands of lipid with the resorbing process is at the surface *(Willis,1957)*.

When rabbits were fed a high-cholesterol diet, those fed chromium supplements had only 50% as much plaque formation as the rest of the group *(Abraham,1982)*. Moreover, when rabbits who already had established atherosclerotic plaques were supplemented with chromium, there was significant plaque regression *(Abraham,1980)*. Rabbits with established atherosclerotic plaques due to cholesterol feeding showed significant plaque regression when supplemented with 3% soya lecithin *(Hunt)*.

The results of studies on animal models suggest that magnesium supplementation may prevent calcification of the blood vessels and the development of atherosclerosis, apparently by modulating cholesterol accumulation in the aortic wall *(Ouchi)*. Moreover, lesions in animals that were induced by atherogenic diets and magnesium deficiency regressed upon supplementation with 4 to 6 times the normal magnesium requirements *(Vitale)*.

Since there are so few human studies in this area, the results of a controlled study of 50 patients with coronary artery disease and hyperlipidemia are particularly intriguing. Half of the group received a 300 mg capsule daily of Palmvitee, a vitamin E supplement which contains alpha-tocopherol 16 mg, gamma and alpha-tocotrienols 40 mg as well as palm superolein 240 mg. Subsequent bilateral duplex ultrasonography revealed apparent carotid atherosclerotic regression in 7 of the supplemented patients compared to none of the 25 controls, and there was progression of the lesion in 2 of the supplemented patients compared to 10 of the controls *(Tomeo)*.

BIBLIOGRAPHY

Abraham AS et al. The effect of chromium on established atherosclerotic plaques in rabbits. Am J Clin Nutr 33:2294-8, 1980

Abraham AS et al. The effect of chromium on cholesterol-induced atherosclerosis in rabbits. Atherosclerosis 41:371-9, 1982

Abraham A et al. The effects of chromium supplementation on serum glucose and lipids in patients with and without non-insulin-dependent diabetes. Metabolism 41:768-71, 1992

Adams MR et al. Oral L-arginine inhibits platelet aggregation but does not enhance endothelium-dependent dilation in healthy young men. J Am Coll Cardiol 26(4):1054-61, 1995

Aejmelaeus R et al. Ubiquinol-10 and total peroxyl radical trapping capacity of LDL lipoproteins during aging: the effects of Q-10 supplementation. Mol Aspects Med 18 Suppl:S113-S120, 1997

Altura BT et al. Magnesium dietary intake modulates blood lipid levels and atherogenesis. Proc Natl Acad Sci U S A 87(5):1840-4, 1990

Ammaturo V et al. Caffeine stimulates in vivo platelet reactivity. Acta Med Scand 224:245-47, 1988

Anderson JW, Gustafson NJ. High-carbohydrate, high-fiber diet: Is it practical and effective in treating hyperlipidemia? Postgrad Med 82(4):40-55, 1987

Anderson JW et al. Serum lipid response of hypercholesterolemic men to single and divided doses of canned beans. Am J Clin Nutr 51:1013-19, 1990

Angelico M et al. Improvement in serum lipid profile in hyper-lipoproteinaemic patients after treatment with pantethine: a crossover, double-blind trial versus placebo. Curr Ther Res 33:1091, 1983

Armstrong ML et al. Intimal thickening in normocholesterolemic rhesus monkeys fed low supplements of dietary cholesterol. Circ Res 34(4):447-54, 1974

Arstall MA et al. N-acetylcysteine in combination with nitroglycerin and streptokinase for the treatment of evolving acute myocardial infarction: safety and biochemical effects. Circulation 92(10):2855-62, 1995

Arvill A, Bodin L. Effect of short-term ingestion of konjac glucomannan on serum cholesterol in healthy men. Am J Clin Nutr 61:585-9, 1995

Backon J. Ginger: Inhibition of thromboxane synthetase and stimulation of prostacyclin: Relevance for medicine and psychiatry. Med Hypotheses 20:271, 1986

Bak AA, Grobbee DE. Caffeine, blood pressure, and serum lipids. Am J Clin Nutr 53:971-5, 1991

Bang HO et al. The composition of the Eskimo food in north western Greenland. Am J Clin Nutr 33:2657-61, 1980

Bang HO, Dyerberg J. Fatty acid pattern and ischaemic heart disease. Lancet i:663, 1987

Barradas M et al. The effect of olive oil supplementation on human platelet function, serum cholesterol-related variables and plasma fibrinogen concentrations: A pilot study. Nutr Res 10:403-11, 1990

Bartels GL et al. Effects of L-propionylcarnitine on ischemia-induced myocardial dysfunction in men with angina pectoris. Am J Cardiol 74:125-30, 1994

Bellizzi MC et al. Vitamin E and coronary heart disease: the European paradox. Eur J Clin Nutr 48:822-31, 1994

Ben-Amotz A, Levy Y. Bioavailability of a natural isomer mixture compared with synthetic all-trans β-carotene in human serum. Am J Clin Nutr 63:729-34, 1996

Berry EM et al. Effects of diets rich in monounsaturated fatty acids on plasma lipoproteins - the Jerusalem Nutrition Study. II Monounsaturated fatty acids vs carbohydrates. Am J Clin Nutr 56:394-403, 1992

Beswick AD et al. Long-term diet modification and platelet activity. J Intern Med 229:511-5, 1991

Bhatnagar SK et al. Significance of blood taurine levels in patients with first time acute ischaemic cardiac pain. Int J Cardiol 27(3):361-6, 1990

Black MR et al. Zinc supplements and serum lipids in young adult white males. Am J Clin Nutr 47:970-5, 1988

Bønaa K et al. Coffee and cholesterol: Is it all in the brewing? The Tromso study. Br Med J 297:1103-04, 1988

Booyens J et al. The role of unnatural dietary trans and cis unsaturated fatty acids in the epidemiology of coronary heart disease. Med Hypotheses 25(3):175-82, 1988

Borcyhgrevink P, Jynge P. Acquired magnesium deficiency and myocardial tolerance to ischemia. J Am Coll Nutr 6:355-63, 1987

Bordia AK. The effect of vitamin C on blood lipids, fibrinolytic activity and platelet adhesiveness in patients with coronary artery disease. Atherosclerosis 35:181-7, 1980

Bordia A et al. Effect of vitamin C on platelet adhesiveness and platelet aggregation in coronary artery disease patients. Clin Cardiol 8(10):552-4, 1985

Borkman M et al. The relation between insulin sensitivity and the fatty-acid composition of skeletal-muscle phospholipids. N Engl J Med 328(4)8:238-44, 1993

Bottcher M et al. Effect of caffeine on myocardial blood flow at rest and during pharmacological vasodilation. J Nucl Med 36(11):2016-21, 1995

Boushey CJ et al. A quantitative assessment of plasma homocysteine as a risk factor for vascular disease: Probable benefits of increasing folic acid intakes. JAMA 274(13):1049-57, 1995

Brattström LE et al. Higher total plasma homocysteine in vitamin B12 deficiency than in heterozygosity for homocystinuria due to cystathionine beta-synthase deficiency. Metabolism 37(2):175-8, 1988

Brattström L et al. Pyridoxine reduces cholesterol and low-density-lipoprotein and increases antithrombin III activity in 80-year-old men with low plasma pyridoxal 5-phosphate. Scand J Clin Lab Invest 50(8):873-7, 1990

Brattström L. Vitamins as homocysteine-lowering agents. J Nutr 126:1276S-1280S, 1996

Bremner I, Beattie JH. Copper and zinc metabolism in health and disease: speciation and interactions. Proc Nutr Soc 54:489-99, 1995

Brinton EA. A low-fat diet decreases high density lipoprotein (HDL) cholesterol levels by decreasing HDL apolipoprotein transport rates. J Clin Invest 85(1):144-51, 1990

Brown WV. Niacin for lipid disorders: indications, effectiveness and safety. Postgrad Med 98(2):185-93, 1995

Bunker VW, Clayton BE. Selenium status in disease: the role of selenium as a therapeutic agent. BJCP 44(8):401-3, 1990

Buonopane GJ et al. Effect of skim milk supplementation on blood cholesterol concentration, blood pressure, and triglycerides in a free-living human population. J Am Coll Nutr 11(1):56-57, 1992

Burr ML et al. Effects of changes in fat, fish, and fibre intakes on death and myocardial reinfarction: diet and reinfarction trial (DART). Lancet ii:757-61, 1989

Burri BJ et al. Platelet aggregation in humans is affected by replacement of dietary linoleic acid with oleic acid. Am J Clin Nutr 54:359-62, 1991

Caggiula AW, Mustad VA. Effects of dietary fat and fatty acids on coronary artery disease risk and total and lipoprotein concentrations: epidemiologic studies. Am J Clin Nutr 65(suppl):1597S-610S, 1997

Cairns JA et al. Fish oils and low-molecular weight heparin for the reduction of restenosis after percutaneous transluminal coronary angioplasty: the EMPAR study. Circulation 94(7):1553-60, 1996

Calzada C et al. The influence of antioxidant nutrients on platelet function in healthy volunteers. Atherosclerosis 128(1):97-105, 1997

Carpenter KLH et al. Depletion of alpha-tocopherol in human atherosclerotic lesions. Free Rad Res 23:549-58, 1995

Carroll RE. The relationship of cadmium in the air to cardiovascular disease death rates. JAMA 198(3):267-9, 1966

Cattin L et al. Treatment of hypercholesterolemia with pantethine and fenofibrate: An open randomized study on 43 subjects. Curr Ther Res 38(3):386-95, 1985

Cavarocchi NC et al. Superoxide generation during cardiopulmonary bypass: is there a role for vitamin E? J Surg Res 40:519-27, 1986

Chello M et al. Protection by coenzyme Q10 from myocardial reperfusion injury during coronary artery bypass grafting. Ann Thorac Surg 58(5):1427-32, 1994

Chen C-J et al. Dose-response relationship between ischemic heart disease mortality and long-term arsenic exposure. Arterioscler Thromb Vasc Biol 16(4):504-10, 1996

Cherchi A et al. Effects of L-carnitine on exercise tolerance in chronic, stable angina: A multicenter, double-blind, randomized, placebo controlled crossover study. Int J Clin Pharmacol Ther Toxicol 23(10569-72, 1985

Chow CK. Nutritional influences on cellular antioxidant defenses systems. Am J Clin Nutr 32:1066-81, 1979

Clarke R et al. Dietary lipids and blood cholesterol: quantitative meta-analysis of metabolic ward studies. BMJ 314:112-17, 1997

Clarkson P et al. Oral L-Arginine improves endothelium-dependent dilation in hypercholesterolemic young adults. J Clin Invest 97(8):1989-94, 1996

Cloarec MJ et al. Alpha-tocopherol: effect on plasma lipoproteins in hypercholesterolemic patients. Isr J Med Sci 23(8):869-72, 1987

Cobb MM et al. Determinants of plasma cholesterol responsiveness to diet. Br J Nutr 71(2):271-82, 1994

Cockcroft J, Chowienczyk P. Beyond cholesterol reduction in coronary heart disease: Is vitamin E the answer? Heart 76:293-4, 1996

Connor SL, Connor WE. Are fish oils beneficial in the prevention and treatment of coronary artery disease? Am J Clin Nutr 66(4 Suppl):1020S-1031S, 1997

Connor WE, Connor SL. Clinical Debate: Should a low-fat, high-carbohydrate be recommended for everyone? Rebuttal. N Engl J Med 337(8):566, 1997

Cooke JP et al. Antiatherogenic effects of L-arginine in the hypercholesterolemic rabbit. J Clin Invest 90:1168-72, 1992

Corbucci GG, Loche F. L-carnitine in cardiogenic shock therapy: pharmacodynamic aspects and clinical data. Int J Clin Pharmacol Res 13:87-91, 1993

Corti M et al. Iron status and risk of cardiovascular disease. Ann Epidemiol 7(1):62-8, 1997a

Corti M-C et al. Serum iron level, coronary artery disease, and all-cause mortality in older men and women. Am J Cardiol 79:120-7, 1997b

Criqui MH, Ringel BL. Does diet or alcohol explain the French paradox? Lancet 344:1719-23, 1994

Crouse JR 3rd. New developments in the use of niacin for treatment of hyperlipidemia: new considerations in the use of an old drug. Coron Artery Dis 7:321-6, 1996

Cunnanae SC et al. High alpha-linolenic acid flaxseed (Linum usitatissimum): some nutritional properties in humans. Br J Nutr 69:443-53, 1993

Da Col PG et al. Pantethine in the treatment of hyper-cholesterolemia: A randomized double-blind trial versus tiadenol. Curr Ther Res 36:314, 1984

Dalderup LM. Vitamin D, cholesterol, and calcium. Lancet i:645-6, 1968

Davidson MH. Fish oil vs. total lipid profile. Letter. Medical World News February 22, 1988, p. 10

Davini P et al. Controlled study on L-carnitine therapeutic efficacy in post-infarction. Drugs Exp Clin Res 18(8):355-65, 1992

Davis WH et al. Monotherapy with magnesium increases abnormally low high density lipoprotein cholesterol: A clinical essay. Curr Ther Res 36:341, 1984

Day AP et al. Effect of concentrated red grape juice consumption on serum antioxidant capacity and low-density lipoprotein oxidation. Ann Nutr Metab 41(6):353-7, 1997

De Lorgeril M et al. The beneficial effect of dietary antioxidant supplementation on platelet aggregation and cyclosporine treatment in heart transplant recipients. Transplantation 58:193-4, 1994

DeMaio SJ et al. Vitamin E supplementation, plasma lipids and incidence of restenosis after percutaneous transluminal coronary angioplasty (PTCA). J Am Coll Nutr 11(1):68-73, 1992

Demrow HS et al. Administration of wine and grape juice inhibits in vivo platelet activity and thrombosis in stenosed canine coronary arteries. Circulation 91(4):1182-8, 1995

Denke M et al. Short-term dietary calcium fortification increases fecal saturated fat content and reduces serum lipids in men. J Nutr 123:1047-53, 1993

Derr J et al. The role of fatty acid saturation on plasma lipids, lipoproteins, and apolipoproteins: II. The plasma total and low-density lipoprotein cholesterol response of individual fatty acids. Metabolism 42(1):130-4, 1993

Dietschy JM. Dietary fatty acids and the regulation of plasma low density lipoprotein cholesterol concentrations. J Nutr 128(2 Suppl):444S-448S, 1998

Digiese V et al. Coenzyme Q_{10} in essential hypertension. Molec Aspects Med 15(Suppl):S257-263, 1994

Dingchao H et al. The protective effects of high-dose ascorbic acid on myocardium against reperfusion injury during and after cardiopulmonary bypass. Thorac Cardiovasc Surg 42(5):276-8, 1994

Drexler H et al. Correction of endothelial dysfunction in coronary microcirculation of hypercholesterolaemic patients by L-arginine. Lancet 338:1546-50, 1991

Dubois-Rende JL et al. Oxidative stress in patients with unstable angina. Eur Heart J 15:179-83, 1994

Dudman NP et al. Disordered methionine/homocysteine metabolism in premature vascular disease. Its occurrence, cofactor therapy, and enzymology. Arterioscler Throm 13(9):1253-60, 1993

Dudrick SJ et al. Experimental and clinical atherosclerosis: Their experimental reversal. Trans Stud Coll Physicians Phila 10(1-4):35-61, 1988

Dychner T, Wester PO. Magnesium and potassium in serum and muscle in relation to disturbances of cardiac rhythm, in Magnesium in Health and Disease. Spectrum Publishing Company, 1980:551-7

Edington JD et al. Serum lipid response to dietary cholesterol n subjects fed a low-fat, high-fiber diet. Am J Clin Nutr 50:58-62, 1989

Eichner ER. Alcohol versus exercise for coronary protection. Am J Med 79(2):231-40, 1985

Engel RR, Smith AH. Arsenic in drinking water and mortality from vascular disease: an ecological analysis in 30 counties in the United States. Arch Environ Health 49(5):418-27, 1994

Erasmus U. Fats and Oils. Vancouver, Alive Books, 1986

Eritsland J et al. Effect of dietary supplementation with n-3 fatty-acids on coronary-artery bypass graft patency. Am J Cardiol 77(1):31-6, 1996

Ernst E. Cardiovascular effects of garlic (Allium sativum): A review. Pharmatherapeutica 5(2):83-9, 1987

Fan WX et al. Erythrocyte fatty acids, plasma lipids, and cardiovascular disease in rural China. Am J Clin Nutr 52:1027-36, 1990

Ferrari R et al. Oxygen free radicals and myocardial damage: protective role of thiol-containing agents. Am J Med 91(3C):95S-105S, 1991

Flavahan NA. Atherosclerosis or lipoprotein-induced endothelial dysfunction. Circulation 85:1927-38, 1992

Fortes C et al. Zinc supplementation and plasma lipid peroxides in an elderly population. Eur J Clin Nutr 51(2):97-101, 1997

Franseshini G et al. Dose-related increase of HDL-cholesterol levels after N-acetylcysteine in man. Pharmacol Res 28(3):213-18, 1993

Frayn KN, Kingman SM. Dietary sugars and lipid metabolism in humans. Am J Clin Nutr 62(suppl):250S-63S, 1995

Fried RE et al. The effect of filtered-coffee consumption on plasma lipid levels. JAMA 267(6):811-15, 1992

Fujita T. Aging and calcium as an environmental factor. J Nutr Sci Vitaminol (Tokyo) 31 Suppl S15-9, 1985

Fuller CJ et al. Effects of increasing doses of alpha-tocopherol in providing protection of low-density lipoprotein from oxidation. Am J Cardiol 81(2):231-3, 1998

Gaddi A et al. Controlled evaluation of pantethine, a natural hypolipidemic compound, in patients with different forms of hypolipoproteinemia. Atherosclerosis 50(1):73-83, 1984

Gapinski JP et al. Preventing restenosis with fish oils following coronary angioplasty. Arch Intern Med 153(13):1595-601, 1993

Gartside PS, Glueck CJ. Relationship of dietary intake to hospital admission for coronary heart and vascular disease: The NHANES II National Probability Study. J Am Coll Nutr 12(6):5676-84, 1993

Gatagonova TM. [Characteristics of the serum lipids in lead industry workers.] Med Tr Prom Ekol (12):17-21, 1994

Gatto LM, Samman S. The effect of zinc supplementation on plasma lipids and low-density lipoprotein oxidation in males. Free Rad Biol Med 19(4):517-21, 1995

Gatto LM et al. Ascorbic acid induces a favorable lipoprotein profile in women. J Am Coll Nutr 15(2):154-8, 1996

Gavaler JS, Van Thiel DH. The association between moderate alcoholic beverage consumption and serum estradiol and testosterone levels in normal postmenopausal women: relationship to the literature. Alcohol Clin Exp Res 16(1):87-92, 1992

Gawaz M. [Antithrombocytic effectiveness of magnesium.] Fortschr Med 114:329-32, 1996

Gaziano JM et al. Moderate alcohol intake, increased levels of high-density lipoprotein and its subfractions, and decreased risk of myocardial infarction. N Engl J Med 329:1829-34, 1993

Gaziano JM et al. A prospective study of consumption of carotenoids in fruits and vegetables and decreased cardiovascular mortality in the elderly. Ann Epidemiol 5:255-60, 1995

Gey KF et al. Inverse correlation between plasma vitamin E and mortality from ischemic heart disease in cross-cultural epidemiology. Am J Clin Nutr 53:326S-34S, 1991

Ginter E et al. Vitamin C in the control of hypercholesterolemia in man. Int J Vitam Nutr Res Suppl 23:137-52, 1982

Glore SR et al. Soluble fiber and serum lipids: a literature review. J Am Diet Assoc 94:425-36, 1994

Goodwin JS et al. Relationship between zinc intake, physical activity and blood levels of high density lipoprotein cholesterol in a healthy elderly population. Metabolism 34(6):519-23, 1985

Gould KL. Very low-fat diets for coronary heart disease: perhaps, but which one? Letter. JAMA 275(18):1402-3, 1996

Graham IM et al. Plasma homocysteine as a risk factor for vascular disease. JAMA 277(22):1775-81, 1997

Greene JM, Feldman EB. Physician's office guide to a lipid-lowering diet. J Am Coll Nutr 5:443-52, 1991

Grimsgaard S et al. Highly purified eicosapentaenoic acid and docosahexaenoic acid in humans have similar triacylglycerol-lowering effects but divergent effects on serum fatty acids. Am J Clin Nutr 66:649-59, 1997

Grundy SM et al. Comparison of monounsaturated fatty acids and carbohydrates for reducing raised levels of plasma cholesterol in man. Am J Clin Nutr 47(6):965-9, 1988

Grundy SM, Denke MA. Dietary influences on serum lipids and lipoproteins. J Lipid Res 31:1149-72, 1990

Gylling H et al. Reduction of serum cholesterol in postmenopausal women with previous myocardial infarction and cholesterol malabsorption induced by dietary sitostanol ester margarine: women and dietary sitostanol. Circulation 96(12):4226-31, 1997

Gyntelberg F et al. Coffee consumption and risk of ischaemic heart disease--a settled issue? J Intern Med 237(1):55-61, 1995

Hanaki Y et al. Coenzyme Q10 and coronary artery disease. Clin Investig 71(8 Suppl):S112-S115, 1993

Harris WS. n-3 Fatty acids and serum lipoproteins: human studies. Am J Clin Nutr 65(suppl):1645S-54S, 1997a

Harris WS et al. n-3 Fatty acids and urinary excretion of nitric oxide metabolites in humans. Am J Clin Nutr 65:459-64, 1997b

Hayes KC et al. Taurine modulates platelet aggregation in cats and humans. Am J Clin Nutr 49:1211-16, 1989

Hayes KC, Khosla P. Dietary fatty acid thresholds and cholesterolemia. FASEB 6:2600-7, 1992

He J et al. Oats and buckwheat intakes and cardiovascular disease risk factors in an ethnic minority of China. Am J Clin Nutr 61:366-72, 1995

Hegsted DM et al. Dietary fat and serum lipids: an evaluation of the experimental data. Am J Clin Nutr 57:875-83, 1993

Heller RF, Heller RF. Hyperinsulinemic obesity and carbohydrate addiction: the missing link is the carbohydrate frequency factor. Med Hypotheses 42(5):307-12, 1994

Hennekens CH et al. Lack of effect of long-term supplementation with beta carotene on the incidence of malignant neoplasms and cardiovascular disease. N Engl J Med 334(18):1145-9, 1996

Hennig B, Boissonneault GA. The roles of vitamin E and oxidized lipids in atherosclerosis. Int Clin Nutr Rev 8(3):134-9, 1988

Hennig B et al. Zinc protects against linoleic acid-induced disruption of endothelial barrier function in culture. J Am Coll Nutr 9:535, 1990

Hennig B et al. Zinc deficiency alters barrier function of cultured porcine endothelial cells. J Nutr 122:1242-7, 1992

Hepner G et al. Hypocholesterolemic effect of yogurt and milk. Am J Clin Nutr 32(1):19-24, 1979

Herbert V et al. Most free-radical injury is iron-related: it is promoted by iron, hemin, holoferritin and vitamin C, and inhibited by desferoxamine and apoferritin. Stem Cells (Dayt) 12(3):289-303, 1994

Hermann J et al. Effects of chromium supplementation on plasma lipids, apolipoproteins, and glucose in elderly subjects. Nutr Res 14(5):671-4, 1994

Herrmann G et al. Parathyroid hormone in coronary artery disease--results of a prospective study. J Endocrinol Invest 9(4):265-71, 1986

Herrmann W et al. Comparison of effects of N-3 and N-6 fatty acids on serum level of lipoprotein(a) in patients with coronary artery disease. Am J Cardiol 76(7):459-62, 1995

Heyden S. Polyunsaturated and monounsaturated fatty acids in the diet to prevent coronary heart disease via cholesterol reduction. Ann Nutr Metab 38(3):117-22, 1994

Hill EG et al. Intensification of essential fatty acid deficiency in the rat by dietary trans-fatty acids. J Nutr 109:1759-67, 1979

Hiller R et al. Serum zinc and serum lipid profiles in 778 adults. Ann Epidemiol 5:490-6, 1995

Ho C-H et al. The influence of the high fat diet on fibrinolytic activity. Thromb Res 77(3):201-8, 1995

Hodgson JM et al. Can linoleic acid contribute to coronary artery disease? Am J Clin Nutr 58:228-34, 1993

Hodis HN et al. Serial coronary angiographic evidence that antioxidant vitamin intake reduces progression of coronary artery atherosclerosis. JAMA 273(23):1849-54, 1995

Holman RT. Nutritional and metabolic interrelationships between fatty acids. Fed Proc 23:1062-7, 1964

Horrobin DF. The importance of gamma-linolenic acid and prostaglandin E1 in human nutrition and medicine. J Holistic Med 3:118-39, 1981

Houtman JP. Prolonged low-level cadmium intake and atherosclerosis. Sci Total Environ 138(1-3):31-6, 1993

Hubbard RW et al. Atherogenic effect of oxidized products of cholesterol. Prog Food Nutr Sci 13(1):17-44, 1989

Hunt C et al. Hyperlipoproteinaemia and atherosclerosis in rabbits fed low-level cholesterol and lecithin. Br J Exp Pathol 139(12):1633-4, 1982

Iacono JM, Dougherty RM. Lack of effect of linoleic acid on the high-density-lipoprotein cholesterol fraction of plasma proteins. Am J Clin Nutr 53:660-4, 1991

Igawa A et al. Comparison of frequency of magnesium deficiency in patients with vasospastic and fixed coronary artery disease. Am J Cardiol 75:728-31, 1995

Ikeda I et al. Inhibition of cholesterol absorption in rats by plant sterols. J Lipid Res 29(12):1573-82, 1988

Iribarren C et al. Association of serum vitamin levels, LDL susceptibility to oxidation, and autoantibodies against MDA-LDL with carotid atherosclerosis. Arteriol Thromb Vasc Biol 17:1171-7, 1997

Jacques PF et al. Effect of vitamin C supplementation on lipoprotein cholesterol, apolipoprotein, and triglyceride concentrations. Ann Epidemiol 5(1):52-9, 1995

Jancin B. Try niacin yourself and improve patient rapport. Family Practice News November 1, 1995:18

Jeppesen J et al. Effects of low-fat, high-carbohydrate diets on risk factors for ischemic heart disease in postmenopausal women. Am J Clin Nutr 65:1027-33, 1997

Jeserich M et al. Reduced plasma L-arginine in hypercholesterolaemia. Letter. Lancet 339:561, 1992

Jialal I, Fuller CJ. Effect of vitamin E, vitamin C and beta-carotene on LDL oxidation and atherosclerosis. Can J Cardiol 11(Suppl G):97G-103G, 1995

Jones PJH et al. Dietary phytosterol as cholesterol-lowering agents in humans. Can J Physiol Pharmacol 75:217-27, 1997

Judy WV et al. Myocardial preservation by therapy with coenzyme Q10 during heart surgery. Clin Investig 71:S155-S161, 1993

Kalbfleisch JH et al. Alpha-tocopherol supplements and high-density-lipoprotein-cholesterol levels. Br J Nutr 55(1):71-8, 1986

Kamikawa T et al. Effects of coenzyme Q10 on exercise tolerance in chronic stable angina pectoris. Am J Cardiol 56:247, 1985

Kannel WB, Ellison RC. Alcohol and coronary heart disease: the evidence for a protective effect. Clin Chim Acta 246(1-2):59-76, 1996

Kardinaal A et al. Association between beta-carotene and acute myocardial infarction depends on polyunsaturated fatty acid status - The Euramic Study. Arterioscler Thromb Vasc Biol 15(6):726-32, 1995

Kardinaal AF et al. Association between toenail selenium and risk of acute MI in European men. The EURAMIC study. European antioxidant MI and breast cancer. Am J Epidemiol 145(4):373-9, 1997

Katan MB et al. Effects of fats and fatty acids on blood lipids in humans: an overview. Am J Clin Nutr 60(6 Suppl):1017S-1022S, 1994

Katan MB. Flavonoids and heart disease. Editorial. Am J Clin Nutr 65:1542-3, 1997

Kato T et al. Reduction of blood viscosity by treatment with coenzyme Q10 in patients with ischemic heart disease. Int J Clin Pharmacol Ther Toxicol 28(3):123-6, 1990

Kawachi K et al. Does coffee drinking increase the risk of coronary heart disease? Results from a meta-analysis. Br Heart J 72:269-75, 1994

Kelly GS. Clinical applications of N-acetylcysteine. Altern Med Rev 3(2):114-27, 1998

Keys A, Parlin RW. Serum cholesterol response to changes in dietary lipids. Am J Clin Nutr 19:175, 1966

Khaw K-T, Woodhouse P. Interrelation of vitamin C, infection, hemostatic factors and cardiovascular disease. BMJ 310:1559-63, 1995

Kinsella JE et al. Dietary n-3 polyunsaturated fatty acids and amelioration of cardiovascular disease: possible mechanisms. Am J Clin Nutr 52:1-28, 1990

Kleinveld HA et al. Failure of N-acetylcysteine to reduce low-density lipoprotein oxidizability in healthy subjects. Eur J Clin Pharmacol 43:639-42, 1992

Klevay L. Copper and ischemic heart disease.. Biol Trace Element Res 5:245-55, 1983

Klevay LM, Inman L, Johnson LK, et al. Increased cholesterol in plasma in a young man during experimental copper depletion. Metabolism 33:1112-18, 1984

Klevay LM. Re: serum copper and the risk of acute myocardial infarction: a prospective population study in men in eastern Finland. Letter. Am J Epidemiol 135(7):832-4, 1992

Klor HU et al. Nutrition and cardiovascular disease. Eur J Med Res 2(6):243-57,1997

Knapper JME et al. Substitution of dietary monounsaturated fatty acids for saturated fatty acids in a free-living population: a feasibility study. J Hum Nutr Diet 9:273-82, 1996

Knekt P et al. Antioxidant vitamin intake and coronary mortality in an longitudinal population study. Am J Epidemiol 139:1180-9, 1994

Knekt P et al. Flavonoid intake and coronary mortality in Finland: a cohort study. BMJ 312:478-81, 1996

Kohlmeier L, Hastings SB. Epidemiologic evidence of a role of carotenoids in cardiovascular disease prevention. Am J Clin Nutr 62(suppl):1370S-6S, 1995

Kontush A et al. Plasma ubiquinol-10 is decreased in patients with hyperlipidaemia. Atherosclerosis 129(1):119-26, 1997

Kopjas TL. Effect of folic acid on collateral circulation in diffuse chronic arteriosclerosis. J Am Geriatr Soc 14(11):1187-92, 1966

Kostka B. Toxicity of mercury compounds as a possible risk factor for cardiovascular disease. Br J Indust Med 48:845-6, 1991

Kozlovsky AS et al. Effects of diets high in simple sugars on urinary chromium losses. Metabolism 35:515, 1986

Kritchevsky SB et al. Dietary antioxidants and carotid artery wall thickness: the ARIC study. Circulation 92(8):2142-50, 1995

Kummerow FA. Nutrition imbalance and angiotoxins as dietary risk factors in coronary heart disease. Am J Clin Nutr 32:58-83, 1979

Kushi KH et al. Dietary antioxidant vitamins and death from coronary heart disease in postmenopausal women. N Engl J Med 334:1156-62, 1996

Kuzuya F. Vitamin B6 and arteriosclerosis. Nagoya J Med Sci 55(1-4):1-9, 1993

Lauler DP, Ed. A symposium: magnesium deficiency - pathogenesis, prevalence, and strategies for repletion. Am J Cardiol 16(14):G1G-46G, 1989

Laurora G et al. Delayed arteriosclerosis progression in high risk subjects treated with mesoglycan. Evaluation of intima-media thickness. J Cardiovasc Surg (Torino) 34(4):313-8, 1993

Leaf A et al. Do fish oils prevent restenosis after coronary angioplasty? Circulation 90(5):2248-57, 1994

Lefavi RG. Has chromium been overlooked as a hypolipidemic agent? Nutr Rep 9(9), Sept. 1991

Levine GN. Ascorbic acid reverses endothelial vasomotor dysfunction in patients with coronary artery disease. Circulation 93(6):1107-13, 1996

Leviton A, Allred EN. Correlates of decaffeinated coffee choice. Epidemiol 5:537-40, 1994

Levy Y et al. Effect of dietary supplementation of β-carotene on human monocyte-macrophage-mediated oxidation of low density lipoprotein. Isr J Med Sci 32(6):473-8, 1996

Lichtenstein AH. Trans fatty acids, plasma lipid levels, and risk of developing cardiovascular disease: a statement for healthcare professionals from the American heart association. Circulation 95(11):2588-90, 1997

Lifshitz F. Children on adult diet: is it harmful? J Am Coll Nutr 11(suppl): 84S-90S, 1992

Longnecker MP. Food labels, trans fatty acids, and coronary heart disease. Editorial. Epidemiology 8(2):122-3, 1997

Louheranta AM et al. Linoleic acid intake and susceptibility of very-low-density and low-density lipoproteins to oxidation in men. Am J Clin Nutr 63:698-703, 1996

Lussier-Cacan S et al. Plasma total homocysteine in healthy subjects: sex-specific relation with biological traits. Am J Clin Nutr 64:587-93, 1996

Lynch S, Klevay L. Effects of a dietary copper deficiency on plasma coagulation factor activities in male and female mice. J Nutr Biochem 3:387, 1992

Ma J et al. Associations of serum and dietary magnesium with cardiovascular disease, hypertension, diabetes, insulin and carotid artery wall thickness: the ARIC study. J Clin Epidemiol 48(7):927-40, 1995

Ma J et al. Relation of plasma phospholipid and cholesterol ester fatty acid composition to carotid artery intima-media thickness: the Atherosclerosis Risk in Communities (ARIC) Study. Am J Clin Nutr 65:551-9, 1997

Malinow MR. Experimental models of atherosclerosis regression. Atherosclerosis 48:105, 1983

Manson J et al. A prospective study of vitamin C and incidence of coronary heart disease in women. Circulation 85:865, 1992a

Manson JE et al. A prospective study of antioxidant vitamins and incidence of coronary heart disease in women. Abstract. J Am Coll Nutr 11(5):633, 1992b

Markus RA et al. Influence of lifestyle modification on atherosclerotic progression determined by ultrasonographic change in the common carotid intima-media thickness. Am J Clin Nutr 65:1000-4, 1997

Martin W. Margarine (not butter) the culprit? Letter. Lancet ii:407, 1983

Mata P et al. Monounsaturated and polyunsaturated n-6 fatty acid-enriched diets modify LDL oxidation and decrease human coronary smooth muscle cell DNA synthesis. Arterioscler Thromb Vasc Biol 17(10):2088-95, 1997

Mattson FH et al. Optimizing the effect of plant sterols on cholesterol absorption in man. Am J Clin Nutr 35(4):697-700, 1982

Maxwell AJ, Cooke JP. Cardiovascular effects of L-arginine. Curr Opin Nephrol Hypertens 7(1):63-70, 1998

McMaster D, et al. Serum copper and zinc in random samples of the population in Northern Ireland. Am J Clin Nutr 56:440-6, 1992

McNamara DJ. Dietary cholesterol and the optimal diet for reducing risk of atherosclerosis. Can J Cardiol 11(Suppl G):113G-126G, 1995

Melby CL et al. Blood pressure and blood lipids among vegetarian, semivegetarian, and nonvegetarian African Americans. Am J Clin Nutr 59:103-9, 1994

Mensink RP, Katan MB. Effect of dietary fatty acids on serum lipids and lipoproteins: a meta-analysis of 27 trials. Arterioscler Thromb 12:911-19, 1992

Mertz W. Chromium in human nutrition: A review. J Nutr 123:626-33, 1993

Meyer F et al. Lower ischemic heart disease incidence and mortality among vitamin supplement users. Can J Cardiol 12:930-4, 1996

Mezzetti A et al. Vitamins E, C and lipid peroxidation in plasma and arterial tissue of smokers and nonsmokers. Atherosclerosis 112:91-9, 1995

Miettinen TA et al. Reduction of serum cholesterol with sitostanol-ester margarine in a mildly hypercholesterolemic population. N Engl J Med 333(20):1308-12, 1995

Millen BE et al. Diet and plasma lipids in women. I. Macronutrients and plasma total and low-density lipoprotein cholesterol in women: The Framingham Nutrition Studies. J Clin Epidemiol 49(6):657-63, 1996

Mitschek GH. [Histological studies on cholesterol-induced atheromatosis in rabbits in mean- and long-term tests.] Exp Pathol (Jena) 10 (3-4): 156-66, 1975

Miwa K et al. Vitamin E deficiency in variant angina. Circulation 94(1):14-18, 1996

Miyagi Y et al. Inhibition of human low-density lipoprotein oxidation by flavonoids in red wine and grape juice. Am J Cardiol 80(12):1627-31, 1997

Mohr D et al. Dietary supplementation with coenzyme Q_{10} results in increased levels of ubiquinol-10 within circulating lipoproteins and increased resistance of human low-density-lipoprotein to the initiation of lipid peroxidation. Biochim Biophys Acta 1126(3):247-54, 1992

Moore RD et al. Effect of low-dose alcohol versus abstention on apolipoproteins A-I and B. Am J Med 84(5):884-90, 1988

Morris DL et al. Serum carotenoids and coronary heart disease. The Lipid Research Clinics Coronary Primary Prevention Trial and Follow-up Study. JAMA 272(18):1439-41, 1994

Morrison HI et al. Serum iron and risk of fatal acute myocardial infarction. Epidemiology 5(2):243-6, 1994

Morrison LM, Enrick L. Coronary heart disease: reduction of death rate by chondroitin sulfate A. Angiology 24:269-8766, 1973

Muckle T, Hazir D. Variation in human blood high-density lipoprotein response to oral vitamin E megadosage. Am J Clin Pathol 91:165-71, 1989

Muldoon MF, Kritchevsky SB. Flavonoids and heart disease. Evidence of benefit still fragmentary. BMJ 312:458-9, 1996

Muriana FJG et al. Intake of olive oil can modulate the transbilayer movement of human erythrocyte membrane cholesterol. Cell Molec Life Sci 53:496-500, 1997

Nenseter M et al. No effect of beta-carotene supplementation on the susceptibility of low-density-lipoprotein to in-vitro oxidation among hypercholesterolemic, postmenopausal women. Scand J Clin Invest 55(6):477-85, 1995

Nielsen S, Jensen MD. Obesity and cardiovascular disease: is body structure a factor? Curr Opin Lipidol 8(4):200-4, 1997

Niki E, Noguchi N. Protection of human low-density lipoprotein from oxidative modification by vitamin C, in Lester Packer & Jurgen Fuchs, Eds. Vitamin C in Health and Disease. Chapter 10:183-192, 1997

Nozue T et al. Magnesium status, serum HDL cholesterol, and apolipoprotein A-1 levels. J Pediatr Gastroenterol Nutr 20:316-18, 1995

Nyyssonen K et al. Vitamin C deficiency and risk of myocardial infarction: prospective population study of men from Eastern Finland. BMJ 314:634-8, 1997

Oakenfull D, Sidhu GS. Could saponins be a useful treatment for hypercholesterolaemia? Europ J Clin Nutr 44:79-88, 1990

Omenn GS et al. Effects of a combination of beta carotene and vitamin A on lung cancer and cardiovascular disease. N Engl J Med 334:1150-5, 1996

Oshaug A et al. Associations between serum ferritin and cardiovascular risk-factors in healthy-young-men. A cross-sectional study. Eur J Clin Nutr 49:430-8, 1995

Oster KA. The treatment of bovine xanthine oxidase initiated atherosclerosis by folic acid. Clin Res 24:512A, 1976

Ouchi Y et al. Effect of dietary magnesium on development of atherosclerosis in cholesterol-fed rabbits. Atherosclerosis 10:732-7, 1990

Palmer RMJ et al. Vascular endothelial cells synthesise nitric oxide from L-arginine. Nature 333:664-6, 1988

Pan W-H et al. Hemostatic factors and blood lipids in young Buddhist vegetarians and omnivores. Am J Clin Nutr 58:354-9, 1993

Parthasarathy S et al. Low density lipoprotein rich in oleic acid is protected against oxidative modification: implications for dietary prevention of atherosclerosis. Proc Natl Acad Sci U S A 87:3494-8, 1990

Pearson TA. Alcohol and heart disease. Circulation 94(11):3023-5, 1996

Petty MA et al. The effects of taurine on atherosclerosis development in cholesterol-fed rabbits. Eur J Pharmacol 180(1):119-27, 1990

Phair RD. Cellular calcium and atherosclerosis: A brief review. Cell Calcium 9(5-6):275-84, 1988

Pietinen P et al. Intake of fatty acids and risk of coronary heart disease in a cohort of Finnish men: the alpha-tocopherol, beta-carotene cancer prevention study. Am J Epidemiol 145(10):876-87, 1997

Pola P et al. Statistical evaluation of long-term L-carnitine therapy in hyperlipoproteinaemias. Drugs Exp Clin Res 9:925034, 1983

Postiglione A et al. Effect of oral mesoglycan on plasma lipoprotein concentration and on lipoprotein lipase activity in primary hyperlipidemia. Pharmacol Res Commun 16(1):1-8, 1984

Prasad K. Dietary flax seed in prevention of hypercholesterolemic atherosclerosis. Atherosclerosis 132(1):69-76, 1997

Prasad K. Reduction of hypercholesterolemic atherosclerosis by CDC-flaxseed with very low alpha-linolenic acid. Atherosclerosis 136(2):367-75, 1998

Prichard BN et al. Fish oils and cardiovascular disease. BMJ 310:819-20, 1995

Prisco D et al. Effect of pantethine treatment on platelet aggregation and thromboxane A2 production. Curr Ther Res 35:700, 1984

Radack K et al. The comparative effects of n-3 and n-6 polyunsaturated fatty acids on plasma fibrinogen levels: A controlled clinical trial in hypertriglyeridemic subjects. J Am Coll Nutr 9(4):352-7, 1990

Rapley CH et al. Fatty acid pattern and ischaemic heart disease. Lancet i:1202, 1987

Rapola JM et al. Effect of vitamin E and beta carotene on the incidence of angina pectoris. JAMA 275(9):693-8, 1996

Rapola JM et al. Randomised trial of α-tocopherol and β-carotene supplements on incidence of major coronary events in men with previous myocardial infarction. Lancet 349:1715-20, 1997

Rasmussen HS. Magnesium and acute myocardial infarction. Arch Intern Med 146:872, 1986

Rasmussen HS et al. Magnesium deficiency in patients with ischemic heart disease with and without acute myocardial infarction uncovered by intravenous loading test. Arch Intern Med 148:329-32, 1988

Reaven GM. Pathophysiology of insulin resistance in human disease. Physiol Rev 75(3):473-86, 1995

Reaven P et al. Feasibility of using an oleate-rich diet to reduce the susceptibility to low-density lipoprotein to oxidative modification in humans. Am J Clin Nutr 54:701-6, 1991

Rebuzzi A et al. Beneficial effects of L-carnitine in the reduction of the necrotic area in acute myocardial infarction. Drugs Exp Clin Res 10:219-23, 1984

Reiser S et al. Isocaloric exchange of dietary starch and sucrose in humans. I. Effects on levels of fasting blood lipids. Am J Clin Nutr 32(8):1659-69, 1979

Reiser S. Effect of dietary sugars on metabolic risk factors associated with heart disease. Nutr Health 3:203-16, 1985

Reiser S et al. Effect of copper intake on blood cholesterol and its lipoprotein distribution in men. Nutr Rep Int 36(3):641-50, 1987

Renaud S et al. Protective effects of dietary calcium and magnesium on platelet function and atherosclerosis in rabbits fed saturated fat. Atherosclerosis 47:187-98, 1983

Renaud S. Dietary fats and platelet function. Proc Nutr Soc Aust 10:1-13, 1985

Renaud SC. What is the epidemiologic evidence for the thrombogenic potential of dietary long-chain fatty acids? Am J Clin Nutr 56:823S, 1992

Ribaya-Mercado JD et al. Effect of β-carotene supplementation on the concentrations of distribution of carotenoids, vitamin E, vitamin A, and cholesterol in plasma lipoprotein and non-lipoprotein fractions in healthy older women. J Am Coll Nutr 14(6):614-20, 1995

Richter WO et al. Treatment of severe hypercholesterolemia with a combination of beta-sitosterol and lovastatin. Curr Ther Res 57(7):497-505, 1996

Ridker PM et al. Association of moderate alcohol consumption and plasma concentration of endogenous tissue-type plasminogen activator. JAMA 272(12):929-33, 1994

Rimm EB et al. Vitamin E consumption and the risk of coronary heart disease in men. N Engl J Med 328(20):1450-6, 1993

Rimm EB et al. Review of moderate alcohol consumption and reduced risk of coronary heart disease: is the effect due to beer, wine, or spirits. BMJ 312(7033):731-6, 1996

Rimm EB et al. Folate and vitamin B6 from diet and supplements in relation to risk of coronary heart disease among women. JAMA 279(5):359-64, 1998

Rinehart JF, Greenberg LD. Vitamin B6 deficiency in the Rhesus monkey. Am J Clin Nutr 4:318-25, 1956

Ringer TV et al. Beta-carotene's effects on serum lipoproteins and immunologic indices in humans. Am J Clin Nutr 53(3):688-94, 1991

Roberts TL et al. Linoleic acid and the risk of sudden cardiac death. Br Heart J 70(6):524-9, 1993

Robinson K et al. Hyperhomocysteinemia and low pyridoxal phosphate: common and independent reversible risk factors for coronary artery disease. Circulation 92(10):2825-30, 1995

Rosenblum ER et al. Isolation and identification of phytoestrogens from beer. Alcohol Clin Exp Res 16(5):843-5, 1992

Saba P et al. Hypolipidemic effect of mesoglycan in hyperlipidemic patients. Curr Ther Res 40:761-8, 1986

Sacks E et al. Ingestion of egg raises plasma low-density lipoproteins in free-living subjects. Lancet ii:647-9, 1984

Sacks FM et al. Plasma lipoprotein levels in vegetarians. The effect of ingestion of fats from dairy products. JAMA 254(10):1337-41, 1985

Salachas A et al. Effects of low-dose fish oil concentrate on angina, exercise tolerance time, serum triglycerides, and platelet function. Angiology 45(12):1023-31, 1994

Salonen J et al. Serum copper and the risk of acute myocardial infarction: A prospective population study in men in eastern Finland. Am J Epidemiol 134:268-76, 1991

Salonen JT et al. High stored iron levels are associated with excess risk of myocardial infarction in eastern Finnish men. Circulation 86(3):803-11, 1992

Salonen JT et al. Intake of mercury from fish, lipid peroxidation, and the risk of myocardial infarction and coronary, cardiovascular and any death in Eastern Finnish men. Circulation 91:645-55, 1995a

Salonen JT et al. Lowering of body iron stores by blood letting and oxidation resistance of serum lipoproteins: a randomized, cross-over trial in male smokers. J Intern Med 237:161-8, 1995b

Santos MJ et al. Influence of dietary supplementation with fish on plasma fatty acid composition in coronary heart disease patients. Ann Nutr Metab 39(1):52-62, 1995

Satake K et al. Relation between severity of magnesium deficiency and frequency of anginal attacks in men with variant angina. J Am Coll Cardiol 28:897-902, 1996

Schaefer EJ et al. Body weight and low-density lipoprotein cholesterol changes after consumption of a low-fat libitum diet. JAMA 274(18):1450-5, 1995

Schiavon R et al. Selenium enhances prostacyclin production by cultured epithelial cells: Possible explanation for increased bleeding times in volunteers taking selenium as a dietary supplement. Thrombosis Res 34:389, 1984

Schnohr P et al. Egg consumption and high-density-lipoprotein cholesterol. J Intern Med 235(3):249-51, 1994

Schwartz SM. Myocardial infarction in young women in relation to plasma total homocysteine, folate, and a common variant in the methylenetetrahydrofolate reductase gene. Circulation 96(2):412-7, 1997

Schwarz B et al. Coffee, tea and lifestyle. Prev Med 23:377-84, 1994

Seelig MS. Consequences of magnesium deficiency on the enhancement of stress reactions; preventive and therapeutic implications (a review). J Am Coll Nutr 13(5):429-46, 1994

Seelig MS et al. Is there a place for magnesium in the treatment of acute MI? Am Heart J 132(2):471-7, 1996

Seely S. Is calcium excess in western diet a major cause of arterial disease? Int J Cardiol 33(2):191-8, 1991

Seidelin KN et al. n-3 fatty acids in adipose tissue and coronary artery disease are inversely related. Am J Clin Nutr 55:1117-9, 1992

Sempos CT et al. Body iron stores and the risk of coronary artery disease. N Engl J Med 330:1119-24, 1994

Serafini M et al. Alcohol-free red wine enhances plasma antioxidant capacity in humans. J Nutr 128:1003-7, 1998

Serebruzny VL et al. Dietary coenzyme Q10 supplementation alters platelet size and inhibits human vitronectin (CD5/CD61) receptor expression. J Cardiovasc Pharmacol 29(1):16-22, 1997

Shamberger RJ. Erythrocyte fatty acid studies in patients. J Advancement Med 10(3):195-205, 1997

Shechter M et al. Is there a role for supplemental magnesium in acute myocardial infarction in high-risk populations (patients ineligible for thrombolysis and the elderly)? Coronary Artery Disease 7:352-8, 1996

Siguel E et al. Very low-fat diets for coronary heart disease. Perhaps, but which one? Letter. JAMA 275(18):1402, 1996

Siliprandi N et al. Propionyl-L-carnitine: biochemical significance and possible role in cardiac metabolism. Cardiovasc Drugs Ther 5 Suppl 1:11-15, 1991

Simon JA et al. Serum fatty acids and risk of coronary heart disease. Am J Epidemiol 142(5):469-76, 1995

Simonoff M. Chromium deficiency and cardiovascular risk. Cardiovasc Res 18(10):591-6, 1984a

Simonoff M et al. Low plasma chromium in patients with coronary artery and heart diseases. Biol Trace Element Res 6:431, 1984b

Simopoulos AP. Omega-3 fatty acids in health and disease and in growth and development. Am J Clin Nutr 54:438-63, 1991

Singal PK et al. Protective action of zinc against catecholamine-induced myocardial changes. Electrocardiographic and ultrastructural studies. Lab Invest 44:426, 1981

Singh RB et al. Dietary intake and plasma levels of antioxidant vitamins in health and disease: a hospital-based case-control study. J Nutr Environ Med 5:235-42, 1995

Singh RB et al. Effect of treatment with magnesium and potassium on mortality and reinfarction rate of patients with suspected acute myocardial infarction. Int J Clin Pharmacol Ther 34:219-25, 1996a

Singh RB et al. A randomized, double-blind placebo-controlled trial of L-carnitine in suspected acute myocardial infarction. Postgrad Med J 72:45-50, 1996b

Sola R et al. Oleic acid rich diet protects against the oxidative modification of high density lipoprotein. Free Radical Biol Med 22(6):1037-45, 1997

Solzbach U et al. Vitamin C improves endothelial dysfunction of epicardial coronary arteries in hypertensive patients. Circulation 96(5):1513-9, 1997

Spiller RC. Cholesterol, fibre, and bile acids. Editorial. Lancet 347:415-15, 1996

Srivastava KC. Effects of aqueous extracts of onion, garlic and ginger on platelet aggregation and metabolism of arachidonic acid in the blood vascular system: In vitro study. Prostagl Med 13:227, 1984

Stamler J, Shekelle R. Dietary cholesterol and human coronary heart disease. The epidemiologic evidence. Arch Pathol Lab Med 112(10):1032-40, 1988

Stampfer MJ, Malinow MR. Can lowering homocysteine reduce cardiovascular risk? Editorial. N Engl J Med 332(5):328-9, 1995

Stead NW et al. Selenium (Se) balance in the dependent elderly. Am J Clin Nutr 39:677, 1984

Steinberg D et al. Beyond cholesterol: modifications of low-density lipoprotein that increase its atherogenicity. N Engl J Med 320:915-24, 1989

Steiner M et al. Vitamin E plus aspirin compared with aspirin alone in patients with transient ischemic attacks. Am J Clin Nutr 62(suppl):1381S-4S, 1995

Steinmetz KA et al. Effect of consumption of whole milk and skim milk on blood lipid profiles in healthy men. Am J Clin Nutr 59:612-18, 1994

Stephens NG et al. Randomised controlled trial of vitamin E in patients with coronary disease: Cambridge Heart Antioxidant Study (CHAOS). Lancet 347:781-6, 1996

Strain JJ. Newer aspects of micronutrients in chronic disease: copper. Proc Nutr Soc 53(3):583-98, 1994

Subbarao K et al. Pyridoxal 5'-phosphate - a new physiological inhibitor of blood coagulation and platelet function. Biochem Pharmacol 28:531-4, 1979

Sulsky SI et al. Nutritional status of elderly smokers and non-smokers. J Nutr Med 1:187-94, 1990

Szanto S, Yudkin J. Dietary sucrose and the behaviour of blood platelets. Proc Nutr Soc 29(1):Suppl 3A, 1970

Tanganelli P et al. Updating on in-vivo and in-vitro effects of heparin and other glycosaminoglycans (mesoglycan) on arterial endothelium: a morphometrical study. Int J Tissue React 14(3):149-53, 1992

Tanno N et al. Effect of taurine administration on serum lipid and biliary lipid composition in man. Tohoku J Exp Med 159(2):91-100, 1989

Tarry WC, Makhoul RB. L-Arginine improves endothelium-dependent vasorelaxation and reduces intimal hyperplasia after balloon angioplasty. Arteriosclerosis Thrombosis 14:938-43, 1994

Tell GS et al. Dietary fat intake and carotid artery wall thickness: The atherosclerosis risk in communities (ARIC)study. Am J Epidemiol 139: 979-89, 1994

Temme EHM et al. Comparison of the effects of diets enriched in lauric, palmitic, or oleic acids on serum lipids and lipoproteins in healthy women and men. Am J Clin Nutr 63:897-903, 1996

Thomas SR. Inhibition of LDL oxidation by ubiquinol-10. A protective mechanism for coenzyme Q in atherogenesis? Mol Aspects Med 18 Suppl:S85-S103, 1997

Thorogood M et al. Plasma lipids and lipoprotein cholesterol concentration in people with different diets in Britain. Br Med J 295:351-53, 1987

Tomaino RM, Decker EA. High-fat meals and endothelial function. Nutr Rev 56(6):182-5, 1998

Tomeo AC et al. Antioxidant effects of tocotrienols in patients with hyperlipidemia and carotid stenosis. Lipids 30(12):1179-83, 1995

Tomoda H et al. Possible prevention of postangioplasty restenosis by ascorbic acid. Am J Cardiology 78(11):1284-6, 1996

Toohey L et al. Plasma ascorbic acid concentrations are related to cardiovascular risk factors in African-Americans. J Nutr 126:121-8, 1996

Torgersen AM et al. Magnesium therapy, fibrinolytic parameters and von Willebrand Factor in acute myocardial infarction. Int J Cardiol 56:53-9, 1996

Turley S et al. Role of ascorbic acid in the regulation of cholesterol metabolism and the pathogenesis of atherosclerosis. Atherosclerosis 24:1-18, 1976

Ubbink J et al. Vitamin requirements for the treatment of hyperhomocysteinemia in humans. J Nutr 124:1927-33, 1994

Urgert R et al. Effects of cafestol and kahweol from coffee grounds on serum lipids and serum liver enzymes in humans. Am J Clin Nutr 61:149-54, 1995

Urgert R et al. Comparison of effect of cafetiere and filtered coffee on serum concentrations of liver aminotransferases and lipids: six month randomised controlled trial. BMJ 313:1362-6, 1996

Vallance P et al. Effects of endothelium-derived nitric oxide on peripheral arteriolar tone in man. Lancet ii:997-1000, 1989

Vecchio F et al. Mesoglycan in treatment of patients with cerebral ischemia: effects on hemorrheologic and hematochemical parameters. Acta Neurol (Napoli) 15(6):449-56, 1993

Verhoef P et al. Homocysteine metabolism and risk of myocardial infarction: relation with vitamin B6, B12, and folate. Am J Epidemiol 143(9):845-59, 1996

Vijaya J et al. Trace metal analysis in the aorta with and without atherosclerotic lesions. Trace Elem Electrolytes 12(4):200-2, 1995

Vijaya J et al. Serum copper levels and lipid profile of ischemic heart disease patients and hypertensives. Trace Elem Electrol 13(3):147-50, 1996

Visser PJ et al. Magnesium therapy in acute myocardial infarction. Neth J Med 46(3):156-65, 1995

Vitale JJ. Magnesium deficiency and cardiovascular disease. Letter. Lancet 340:1224-5, 1992

Vlad M et al. Concentration of copper, zinc, chromium, iron and nickel in the abdominal aorta of patients deceased with coronary heart disease. J Trace Elem Electrolytes Health Dis 8(2):111-14, 1994

von Eggers Doering W. Antioxidant vitamins, cancer, and cardiovascular disease. Letter. N Engl J Med 335(14):1065, 1996

Walenga JM, Bick RL. Heparin-induced thrombocytopenia, paradoxical thromboembolism, and other side effects of heparin therapy. Med Clin North Am 82(3):635-58, 1998

Wander RC et al. Effects of interaction of RRR-α-tocopheryl acetate and fish oil on low-density-lipoprotein oxidation in postmenopausal women with and without hormone-replacement therapy. Am J Clin Nutr 63:184-93, 1996

Watson KE et al. Active serum vitamin D levels are inversely correlated with coronary calcification. Circulation 96:1755-60, 1997

Watts GF et al. Relationships between nutrient intake and progression/regression of coronary atherosclerosis as assessed by serial quantitative angiography. Can J Cardiol 11(Suppl G):110G-114G, 1995

Weiss M, Lasserre B. Should magnesium therapy be considered for the treatment of coronary heart disease? I. A critical appraisal of current facts and hypotheses. Magnes Res 7(2):135-44, 1994

White WS et al. Pharmacokinetics of beta-carotene and canthaxanthin after individual and combined doses by human subjects. J Am Coll Nutr 13:665-71, 1994

Wiklund O et al. N-acetylcysteine treatment lowers plasma homocysteine but not serum lipoprotein(a) levels. Atherosclerosis 119:99-106, 1996

Willis GC et al. Serial arteriography in atherosclerosis. Can Med Assoc J 71:562-8, 1954

Willis GS. The reversibility of atherosclerosis. Can Med Assoc J 77:106-10, 1957

Witschi A et al. The systemic availability of oral glutathione. Eur J Clin Pharmacol 43(6):667-9, 1992

Wolf A et al. Dietary L-arginine supplementation normalizes platelet aggregation in hypercholesterolemic humans. J Am Coll Cardiol 29(3):479-85, 1997

Wolfe BM et al. Potential role of raising dietary protein intake for reducing risk of atherosclerosis. Can J Cardiol 11(Suppl G):127G-130G, 1995

Wright JV. Dr. Wright's Guide to Healing with Nutrition. Emmaus, Penn., Rodale Press, 1984

Yacowitz H et al. Calcium and lipid metabolism: Effects of increased dietary calcium on atherosclerosis in rabbits. Trans N Y Acad Sci 33(3):344-50, 1971

Yam D et al. Diet and disease - the Israeli paradox: possible dangers of a high omega-6 polyunsaturated fatty acid diet. Isr J Med Sci 32:1134-43, 1996

Yau TM et al. Vitamin E for coronary bypass operations. A prospective, double-blind, randomized trial. J Thorac Cardiovasc Surg 108(2):302-10, 1994

Young DB et al. Potassium's cardiovascular protective mechanisms. Am J Physiol 268(4 Pt 2):R825-R837, 1995

Yu S et al. Plasma cholesterol-predictive equations demonstrate that stearic acid is neutral and monounsaturated fatty acids are hypocholesterolemic. Am J Clin Nutr 61:1129-39, 1995

Yudkin J. Effects of high dietary sugar. Br Med J 281:1396, 1980

Zampelas A et al. Postprandial lipoprotein lipase, insulin and gastric inhibitory polypeptide responses to test meals of different fatty acid composition: comparison of saturated,n-6 and n-3 polyunsaturated fatty acids. Eur J Clin Nutr 48:849-58, 1994

Zanolo G et al. Pharmacokinetic aspect of tritium-labeled glycosaminoglycans (mesoglycan), their absorption in rat and monkey and tissue distribution in rat. Boll Chim Farm 123:223-35, 1984

Zoler ML. High folic acid intake lowers heart attack risk: every additional 100 μg cuts MI risk 6%. Family Practice News August 1, 1997;1

ATTENTION-DEFICIT HYPERACTIVITY DISORDER

See Also: LEARNING DISORDERS

NUTRITIONAL TREATMENT GUIDE

✓ = Efficacy generally accepted.
* = Efficacy *demonstrated* by controlled human trials.
[+] = Efficacy *suspected* from uncontrolled human trials.
[-] = Efficacy *suspected* from indirect data.
? = Efficacy *challenged* in a study of similar design.

DIETARY FACTORS

* **Caffeine:** 100 to 200 mg 3 times daily
* ? avoid **Sugar**

- -

[+] **high Protein, low Carbohydrate diet**

NUTRITIONAL FACTORS

* **Magnesium deficiency:** ≈ 400 mg daily. (Consider IM or IV administration, especially in hypomagnesemia.)
* **Niacin:** 500 to 2,000 mg 3 times daily
* **Thiamine:** 100 mg 4 times daily
* **Vitamin B_6:** 20 to 30 mg/kg/d (only if blood serotonin is low)

- -

[+] **Calcium deficiency:** ≈ 1 g daily
[+] **Choline:** 500 to 3,000 mg daily *OR* **Deanol** (See dosage schedule below in the text.)
[+] rule out **Copper toxicity**
[+] **Iron deficiency:** 30 mg twice daily until repletion; then minimal possible dosage
[+] **Omega-6 Fatty Acids:** evening primrose oil 0.5 to 1 g 3 times daily

- -

[-] **Copper deficiency:** 2 mg twice daily *AND* **Zinc** 50 mg daily
[-] rule out **Manganese toxicity**
[-] **Zinc deficiency:** zinc sulfate 220 mg twice daily *AND* **Copper** 2 mg daily

OTHER FACTORS

* ? rule out **Food Sensitivities**

- -

[-] rule out **Aluminum toxicity**

[-] rule out **Cadmium toxicity**
[-] rule out **Lead toxicity**

DIETARY FACTORS

Hyperkinetic children and adults may respond to a high protein, low carbohydrate, sugar-free diet. In addition to being calmer, they may be better able to discriminate between different stimuli and thus better able to learn *(Conners,1987;Kershner;Prinz)*. The finding that hyperkinetic boys excrete more nitrogen than normals following meals of equal protein content is consistent with a need for increased dietary protein *(Stein)*. Also, hyperinsulinism has been suggested as one of the causes of the disorder.

An 8-year-old boy presented with a history of temper tantrums and overly aggressive behavior. He was also irritable and difficult to reach, particularly in the morning and around meal times. An uncle and some cousins had diabetes mellitus. His serum glucose level was found to be abnormally low, while his serum insulin level was elevated, which suggested a prediabetic condition.

After being placed on a high protein, low carbohydrate diet, his hyperactivity soon abated, his aggressive tantrums stopped, and he began to perform well in school (Walker).

Sugar

Studies investigating the hypothesis that refined sugar worsens symptoms have had contradictory results, suggesting that any adverse effects of acute sugar ingestion are limited to a small minority of patients *(Benton;White;Wolraich)*. The inconsistencies found in many of the findings relating sugar ingestion to behavior and cognitive function may be due to methodological shortcomings. These include:

- a failure to control for energy intake.
- possible drowsiness causing a drop in cognitive performance due to an increase in the carbohydrate to protein ratio.
- Only acute effects were assessed.
- Only sugar (sucrose), which is the minority of all added sugars, was assessed; not the variety of sugars (e.g. corn syrup, high fructose corn syrup, glucose, and fructose) commonly used.
- Foods that parents think of as containing sugar may also contain other ingredients that are the true cause of behavioral reactions.
- Some children may be sensitive to many food components; reactions may result from a combination of other ingredients and sugar *(Jacobson;White)*.

Another hypothesis which may explain these inconsistencies is that the combination of sugar with a meal consisting almost entirely of starch (such as sugar-sweetened breakfast cereals) or even of protein may have a more powerful effect on behavior than sugar alone *(Conners,1985;Wells)*. While this theory is interesting, it needs further testing.

Caffeine

Since stimulants may be an effective treatment, and caffeine is a stimulant, several studies have investigated the behavioral effects of caffeine. While perhaps less effective than methylphenidate, caffeine calms at least some children with the disorder. Improvements in both general behavior and impulsivity have been reported *(Firestone)*; however, some children will experience nausea, abdominal pain or insomnia *(Schecter)*.

NUTRITIONAL FACTORS

VITAMIN B COMPLEX

It appears that megadose supplementation with members of the vitamin B complex may be beneficial to occasional patients, perhaps because their symptoms are a manifestation of a specific vitamin dependency. Supplementation with niacin as niacinamide has been found effective under placebo-controlled conditions for some severely disturbed hyperkinetic children, especially those with psychotic features and family histories consistent with niacin dependency disorders *(Hoffer)*.

One author found thiamine supplementation to be effective under double-blind conditions. He studied a group of 100 children aged 4 to 15 years, the majority of whom had minimal cerebral dysfunction syndrome with hyperkinesis. Parents were given coded envelopes containing a 3-day supply. The first of these contained thiamine 100 mg to be given 4 times daily; the second contained a lactose placebo. About one-quarter of these children seemed to respond to thiamine. Twenty-one of them received a one-week trial of the vitamin followed by one week of placebo. About half of these children responded dramatically to thiamine and relapsed on placebo *(Brenner)*.

Finally, vitamin B_6, which is required for the conversion of tryptophan to serotonin, appears to be effective for some children under double-blind conditions - particularly those whose blood serotonin levels are low *(Coleman,1979;Haslam)*. Both more information on baseline nutriture B complex vitamins and controlled clinical trials are needed to clarify the picture.

At age ten, a boy who had demonstrated auditory memory and discrimination difficulties on testing 2 years earlier developed hyperkinesis and became unable to concentrate, overly aggressive, easily frustrated and agitated, intolerant of noises, fearful of crossing the street, and confused while playing basketball. At night he suffered from nightmares and complained that his blankets felt like stones and that familiar objects in his bedroom appeared far away.

Physical examination was normal, as was the EEG, glucose tolerance test and CBC. The Feingold diet was ineffective. He began a series of single nutrient trials. Although placebo had no effect, pyridoxine 100 mg 3 times daily precipitated hallucinations, and both calcium pantothenate and riboflavin also appeared to have deleterious effects.

Following supplementation with thiamine 100 mg 4 times daily, his behavioral symptoms and nightmares disappeared. School performance, emotional lability, and memory improved dramatically and his letter reversals disappeared.

He did well until 2 months after discontinuation of thiamine, when the hyperactivity, poor memory, letter reversals and behavioral disturbances returned. On testing, levels of thiamine, lactic acid and pyruvic acid were all normal. Another 3-month course of thiamine was associated again with dramatic improvement. In all, each of 3 trials of thiamine withdrawal and one placebo substitution were associated with relapse. However, thiamine could be reduced to 100 mg daily without adverse effects once ascorbic acid 100 mg twice daily was added. On maintenance thiamine, he has continued to do well over 3 years of follow-up (Brenner).

MINERALS

While hyperkinesis associated with abnormal blood levels of several nutrient minerals is known to respond to effective nutritional interventions, the clinical significance of mineral levels in the lower (or, in the case of copper, upper) end of the normal range has, in general, not been scientifically investigated. However, anecdotal reports do suggest that nutritional interventions to move those levels closer to the mean may be worth trying.

Calcium Deficiency

Although we have yet to determine how frequently a marginal calcium deficiency contributes to hyperkinesis, a study of 50 hyperactive children aged 4 to 13 years found that, compared to normals, their average plasma, erythrocyte, urine and hair calcium levels were lower, with hair showing the greatest deficit *(Kozielec,1994)*.

Hyperactivity caused by hypocalcemia without hypercalciuria may respond to calcium supplementation:

A 9 year-old boy diagnosed as hyperactive at age 4 had been treated with methylphenidate for 2 ½ years. An EEG revealed unusual electrical discharges in the right temporal region. On laboratory testing, he had a very low blood calcium level with normal urinary calcium excretion.

Within 2 months after his milk intake was increased, his behavior markedly improved and he was able to stop medication. On retesting, his blood calcium level had returned to normal (Walker).

Copper

Toxicity

Copper excess may be associated with irritability, and directly influences neurotransmitter systems, although its role in hyperkinesis is poorly understood. *In vitro*, it inhibits the enzyme 5-hydroxytryptophane decarboxylase, which is necessary for the production of serotonin; both increased *(Irwin)* and decreased *(Coleman,1971)* blood serotonin levels have been reported in hyperkinesis.

Copper is part of the metalloenzyme dopamine B hydroxylase, which is necessary for the production of noradrenaline, and increased dopamine B hydroxylase levels have been reported in hyperkinesis *(Rapoport)*. Copper elevations are also tied to dopamine activity, and reducing elevated copper levels has been shown to sometimes reduce schizophrenic symptoms *(Bowman)*.

A hyperactive 8 year-old Caucasian boy with Attention Deficit Disorder showed evidence of paranoid ideation and depression. He had tantrums and complained of constant tinnitus at bedtime. His serum copper was 144 mg%

He was supplemented with vitamin C, manganese, molybdenum and zinc and prescribed deanol (an acetylcholine precursor) 10 drops daily. Three months later his parents reported that, although compliance had been a problem, his hyperactivity had improved slightly. Serum copper had fallen to 132 mg%

The following year his parents reported a significant decrease in hyperactivity and cessation of tinnitus. Serum copper had fallen further to 124 mg% (Pfeiffer).

Deficiency

Results of an epidemiological study of 50 hyperactive children suggest that insufficient copper nutriture may also contribute to hyperkinesis *(Kozielec,1994)*. Further studies are needed for confirmation.

Iron Deficiency

Iron deficiency is common in our society, and there is evidence that iron nutriture in hyperkinetic children may be reduced *(Kozielec,1994; Ward)*. Moreover, when 14 nonanemic boys aged 7 to 11 years old with attention deficit-hyperactivity disorder received an iron supplement (Ferrocal 5 mg/kg/day for 30 days), there was a significant decrease on the parents' Conners Hyperactivity Rating Scale scores, although the teachers' scores were unchanged *(Sever)*.

A 13 year-old male adolescent had a 2-year history of being aggressive, irritable, destructive, and dysphoric. He had previously been diagnosed as having attention-deficit hyperactivity disorder and treated with stimulants without success. He was considered to be a sexual offender against young children and, during the previous year, had been charged with assault for violent outbursts and for threatening people with a knife. He laughed and cried inappropriately, complained of visual hallucinations and had run away from home in his pajamas.

Despite treatment with psychotropic drugs for one month, he remained restless, irritable and unable to sit still. After several attempts to adjust his medication had failed to control his disruptive behavior, he was eventually hospitalized on an emergency basis in a psychotic state.

On admission, he appeared undernourished, tremulous, restless and extremely disruptive. He moved constantly and complained of visual hallucinations. There was no evidence of thought disorganization. A marginally low mean corpuscular volume lead to the discovery of iron deficiency; all psychotropic medication was then gradually replaced by ferrous sulfate 300 mg twice daily. Concurrently, he was placed in a conjoint behavior modification program. Although the circulating iron deficit was corrected within 3 weeks, it took 2 months before steady behavioral improvement and diminution of akathisia became noticeable, and he became less impulsive and more manageable. A trial of withdrawing ferrous sulfate for 4 weeks during the fifth month of hospitalization was followed by a drop in the serum iron level to 9 mmol/L coincident with a slight increase in irritability and restlessness. Ferrous sulfate supplementation was resumed and, 9 months later, he has remained stable in a community group home without recurrence of akathisia or any major management problem (Tu).

Magnesium Deficiency

Children with magnesium deficits may present with a hyperkinetic syndrome. They are characterized by excessive fidgeting, anxious restlessness, psychomotor instability, and learning difficulties *(Durlach).*

Among children with Attention Deficit-Hyperactivity Disorder (DSM-IV), magnesium deficiency appears to be quite common. In one group of 94 boys and 20 girls aged 9 to 12 years old, 95% had evidence of deficiency based on levels in the hair (78%), red blood cells (59%) or blood serum (34%) *(Kozielec,1997).*

Repletion of a chronic borderline magnesium deficiency, while not well studied, appears to be an effective treatment. In one study, 50 children aged 7 to 12 years with Attention Deficit-Hyperactivity Disorder (DSM-IV) and magnesium deficiency received 200 mg magnesium daily for 6 months. Compared to both untreated, matched controls and their own clinical state before supplementation, treated children demonstrated a significant decrease in hyperactivity on standard psychometric scales *(Starobrat-Hermelin).*

Manganese Toxicity

Elevated manganese levels could theoretically cause increased locomotor activity by decreasing dopamine turnover *(Collipp).* Consistent with this hypothesis, two studies of hair manganese levels in hyperactive children found them to be elevated *(Barlow;Collipp).*

Zinc Deficiency

Zinc deficiency may be associated with irritability, and hyperactive children may have lower zinc levels in serum, urine, hair and fingernails than normals *(Bekaroglu; Kozielec,1994).* Tartrazine, sunset yellow, and perhaps other food additives, may increase both abnormal behavior and urinary zinc excretion *(Ward)*; this suggests that reactions to food additives may be mediated by a further lowering of already low zinc levels. Moreover, zinc and copper each reduces the other's absorption; thus zinc supplementation would help to counteract the adverse effects of elevated copper.

The following case report suggests that zinc deficiency may contribute to the adverse behavioral effects sometimes reported following sugar consumption:

A girl diagnosed as having minimal brain dysfunction had learning problems and displayed antagonism, uncooperativeness, and unprovoked raging temper tantrums. At 13 she was placed on a high-protein, sugar-free diet with vitamin C, nicotinamide and pyridoxine. Tantrums ceased after a few days but recurred after candy.

Because she was unusually alert and cooperative after eating oysters (which have a high zinc content), a trial of zinc supplementation was begun. After chelated zinc 80 mg in the morning and 200 mg in the afternoon was added, there was dramatic behavioral improvement within 24 hours. Discontinuation of zinc supplements was followed by tantrums (Kronick).

OTHER NUTRITIONAL FACTORS

Choline

The efficacy of nutritional precursors to the neurotransmitter acetylcholine has been explored. In a study of 70 children and adolescents with Attention Deficit-Hyperactivity Disorder (DSM III-R), choline or lecithin supplementation, either alone or in combination, was employed along with psychotropic medication. Choline was started with a 500 mg dose and then titrated upwards as tolerated to 3000 mg daily. All demonstrated some degree of positive response, some more dramatic than others *(Woodbury)*.

Deanol

Deanol is a salt of dimethylaminoethanol (DMAE), a substance native to the body. It has been theorized to be superior to choline salts as an acetylcholine precursor because:

- in contrast to choline, it is not metabolized by gut bacteria and crosses the blood-brain barrier easily.
- it uniquely inhibits the enzyme choline oxidase which diverts choline from acetylcholine production into the production of betaine.

Five hundred milligrams daily, and sometimes as much as 1,000 mg daily, is often needed, although occasionally only 10 mg to 20 mg is adequate. Side effects from acetylcholine excess may occur (headache, muscle tension, irritability and/or depression restlessness, insomnia); they can be minimized by starting at 10 mg to 100 mg and then waiting a week before raising the dosage. If symptoms appear, the supplement should be discontinued for 1 or 2 days and restarted at a lower dosage *(South)*.

Under double-blind conditions, deanol was been found superior to placebo in the treatment of childhood hyperkinesis and related problems in multiple studies *(Coleman,1976;Geller;Lewis)*.

Essential Amino Acids

Theoretically, supplemental phenylalanine or tyrosine, both nutritional precursors to norepinephrine, would appear to be beneficial. Neither, however, has shown evidence of efficacy *(Eisenberg;Zametkin)*. Moreover, low platelet serotonin and blood tryptophan levels are evidence of defective serotonin metabolism *(Comings)*, yet an open trial of tryptophan, the nutritional precursor to serotonin, resulted in only minimal improvement after one week *(Nemzer)*.

In summary, then, nutritional precursor therapy for hyperkinesis seems to be ineffective.

Essential Fatty Acid Deficiency

Children with attention deficit-hyperactivity disorder may be deficient in essential fatty acids (EFAs) *(Stevens)*, and supplementation with *evening primrose oil*, a source of omega-6 essential fatty acids, was effective in a small open trial *(Colquhoun)*. However, as supplementation was unsuccessful in the only controlled study - a double-blind crossover study involving 90 children *(Gibson)* - omega-6 fatty acid deficiency appears to be a relatively rare cause of hyperkinesis. Repletion of a possible deficiency of omega-3 fatty acids (the other family of essential fatty acids) has not been studied.

The best candidates for supplementation appear to be males (whose EFA requirements are much higher than females) complaining of excessive thirst (a cardinal sign of EFA deficiency) with dry hair and skin and an allergic history. Since zinc is required for the conversion of EFAs to prostaglandins, concurrent supplementation with zinc may be helpful.

A 6 year-old boy had been diagnosed as having Attention Deficit Disorder with visual motor incoordination and developmental immaturity at the child study center of a major university. He had episodes of irritability and crying which his mother attributed to eating sweets. In addition, he had a history of excessive thirst since infancy, as well as a history of chronic nasal congestion with occasional cough and wheezing, and developed hives if licked by a dog.

On physical examination, he was cooperative and pleasant. He had dry skin, lackluster hair, numerous follicular keratoses, puffy eyes, a pale boggy nasal mucosa, and white spots on his fingernails. Laboratory testing revealed eosinophilia and low serum ferritin. Linoleic acid was elevated in serum phospholipids, the other omega-6 prostaglandin precursors were depressed, and all omega-3 essential fatty acid concentrations were depressed.

He was treated with evening primrose oil 2 grams daily with a prompt reduction in thirst. One week later, his teacher noted increased irritability while his mother noted a loss of appetite. The dosage of EPO was reduced to 500 milligrams. After 1 month, his mother reported that he no longer developed hives when licked by a dog, he had less nocturnal congestion, his skin and hair were less dry, and he was calmer. An iron supplement and MaxEPA (fish oil extract) were added and he was started on immunotherapy.

When, after 9 months of treatment, EPO was stopped, his parents noted increased thirst after 2 weeks, along with sniffles, cough and wheezing, irritability, and hives following contact with dogs. EPO was restarted, and all symptoms remitted in 10 to 14 days. He continued to do well during 19 months of follow-up (Galland).

OTHER RELATED FACTORS

Food Sensitivities

Food sensitivities will sometimes provoke hyperkinesis *(Boris)*, and elimination of offending foods and food additives has been repeatedly shown to sometimes improve behavior under double-blind conditions *(Schmidt)*. There is also recent evidence suggesting that children with Pervasive Developmental Disorders marked by loss of acquired skills and intestinal symptoms may exhibit ileal-lymphoid-nodular hyperplasia *(Wakefield)*. This finding suggests that a reactive inflammatory response in the adjacent lymphoid tissue of Peyer's patches may result in the entry of antigens across the inflamed mucosa of the bowel resulting in adverse effects on central nervous system function *(Sabra)*.

However, the prevalence of food sensitivities in hyperkinesis remains an issue for debate.

A 4 ½-year-old boy had been diagnosed as mentally retarded at the child development center of a leading medical school. He was hyperactive, drooled, and could not sit still or pay attention.

He was placed on an elimination diet and made a dramatic improvement. Food offenders were identified, including milk, chocolate, egg, wheat, and chicken. By following his diet, his symptoms were controlled. At the age of 23, he had graduated from college and was pursuing a masters degree (Crook).

The Finegold (salicylate and food additive-free) diet has been particularly popular *(Finegold)*; in double-blind studies, reactions to both salicylates *(Swain)* and food additives *(Egger)* were found to be common in this population.

When, for example, 23 hyperactive children given doses of tartrazine (yellow dye #5) after a ingesting a diet free of synthetic colorings, there was a significant increase in irritability, restlessness, and sleep disturbances *(Rowe)*.

A 7-year-old boy had a history of severe hyperkinesis for several years. When at home, he stomped around, slamming doors, kicking walls and charging oncoming cars with his bicycle. At school he was disruptive and unable to learn. Numerous pediatricians, neurologists, psychiatrists and psychologists were consulted, and he had a complete medical and neurological work-up at a teaching medical center. All attempts at treatment failed.

He was then placed on a salicylate-free diet. Within a few weeks, he became well adjusted both at home and at school. However, every infraction of the dietary program led almost immediately to a recurrence of the hyperkinetic behavior patterns (Finegold).

THE FINEGOLD DIET

I. Avoid foods that contain artificial colors and flavors.

II. Avoid foods containing natural salicylates:

Almonds	Mint flavors
Apples (cider & cider vinegars)	Nectarines
Apricots	Oranges
Blackberries	Peaches
Cherries	Plums or prunes
Cloves	Raspberries
Cucumbers and pickles	Strawberries
Currents	All tea
Gooseberries	Tomatoes
Grapes or raisins (wine & wine vinegars)	Oil of wintergreen

III. Miscellaneous items to avoid:

All aspirin-containing compounds
All medications with artificial colors and flavors
Toothpaste and toothpowder (substitute salt and soda)
All perfumes

Heavy Metal Toxicity

Aluminum

Hyperkinetic children may suffer from aluminum toxicity. In a study of 28 children with hyperactivity or learning disorders, their mean serum aluminum levels were found to be elevated (17 ± 6.9 μg; normal: <10 μg) *(Howard)*, while among a group of 486 hyperactive children, there were many cases in which aluminum levels in the urine and scalp hair showed highly significant elevations *(Ward)*.

Cadmium

In some cases of childhood hyperactivity, urine and scalp hair cadmium levels are significantly elevated when compared to normals *(Ward)*. A study of children treated with methylphenidate found that, especially for those with socially inappropriate behavior, hair phosphorus and zinc, both markers of cadmium toxicity, were low, while hair cadmium was high compared to the hair lead level *(Stewart-Pinkham)*.

Lead

Young rats exposed to lead become hyperactive *(Tang)*. Recent studies have found lead levels of hyperactive children as measured in bone, hair, blood and urine tend to be higher than in normals *(Needleman;Tuthill)*, although other studies suggest that such elevated levels are not common *(David;Gittleman)*.

When moderate lead poisoning is found, treatment of affected children with chelation therapy has been found to improve cognitive performance *(Ruff)*.

BIBLIOGRAPHY

Barlow PJ. A pilot study on the metal levels in the hair of hyperactive children. Med Hypotheses 11(3):309-18, 1983

Benton D. Dietary sugar, hyperactivity and cognitive functioning: a methodological review. J Appl Nutr 41(1):13-22, 1989

Bekaroglu M et al. Relationships between serum free fatty acids and zinc, and attention deficit hyperactivity disorder: a research note. J Child Psychol Psychiatry 37(2):225-7, 1996

Boris M, Mandel FS. Food and additives are common causes of the attention deficit hyperactive disorder in children. Ann Allergy 72:462-7, 1994

Bowman MB, Lewis MS. The copper hypothesis of schizophrenia: A review. Neurosci Biobehav Rev 5(6):321-8, 1982

Brenner A. The effects of megadoses of selected B complex vitamins on children with hyperkinesis: Controlled studies with long-term follow-up. J Learn Disabil 15(5):258-64, 1982

Coleman M. Serotonin concentrations in whole blood in hyperactive children. J Pediatr 78(6):985-90, 1971

Coleman N et al. Deanol in the treatment of hyperkinetic children. Psychosomatics 17(2):68-72, 1976

Coleman M et al. A preliminary study of the effect of pyridoxine administration in a subgroup of hyperkinetic children: A double-blind crossover comparison with methylphenidate. J Biol Psych 14(5):741-51, 1979

Collipp PJ et al. Manganese in infant formulas and learning disability. Ann Nutr Metab 27:488-94, 1983

Comings DE. Serotonin and the biochemical genetics of alcoholism: lessons from studies of attention deficit hyperactivity disorder (ADHD) and Tourette syndrome. Alcohol Alcohol Suppl 2:237-41, 1993

Conners CK, George Washington U. School of Medicine - reported in Med Tribune January 8, 1985

Conners CK, George Washington U. School of Medicine - reported in New Medical Science. December, 1987

Colquhoun I, Bunday S. A lack of essential fatty acids as a possible cause of hyperactivity in children. Med Hypotheses 7:673-79, 1981

Crook WG. Nutrition, food allergies, and environmental toxins. Letter. J Learn Disabil 20(5):260-61, 1987

David O et al. Lead and hyperactivity. Lancet ii:900-03, 1972

Durlach J. Clinical aspects of chronic magnesium deficiency, in MS Seelig, Ed. Magnesium in Health and Disease. New York, Spectrum Publications, 1980

Egger J, Carter CM, Graham PJ, Gumley D, Soothill JF. Controlled trial of oligoantigenic treatment in the hyperkinetic syndrome. Lancet i:540-5, 1985

Eisenberg J et al. Effect of tyrosine on attention deficit disorder with hyperactivity. J Clin Psychiatry 49(5):193-95, 1988

Finegold BF. Hyperkinesis and learning disabilities linked to the ingestion of artificial food colors and flavors. J Learn Disabil 9(9):551-9, 1976

Firestone P et al. The effects of caffeine on hyperactive children. J Learn Disabil 11(3):133-41, 1978

Galland L. Increased requirements for essential fatty acids in atopic individuals: A review with clinical descriptions. J Am Coll Nutr 5:213-28, 1986

Geller SJ. Comparison of a tranquilizer and a psychic energizer. JAMA 174:89-92, 1960

Gibson RA. The effect of dietary supplementation with evening primrose oil on hyperkinetic children. Proc Nutr Soc Aust 10:196, 1985

Gittelman R, Eskenazi B. Lead and hyperactivity revisited. An investigation of nondisadvantaged children. Arch Gen Psychiatry 40:827-33, 1983

Haslam RH, Dalby JT. Blood serotonin levels in the attention-deficit disorder. Letter. N Engl J Med 309(21):1328-9, 1983

Hoffer A. Vitamin B3 dependent child. Schizophrenia 3:107-13, 1971

Howard JMH. Clinical import of small increases in serum aluminum. Clin Chem 30(10):1722-3, 1984

Irwin M et al. Tryptophan metabolism in children with attentional deficit disorder. Am J Psychiatry 138(8):1082-5, 1981

Jacobson MF. Effects of sugar on behavior in children. Letter. JAMA 275(10):756-7, 1996

Kershner J, Hawke W. Megavitamins and learning disorders: A controlled double-blind experiment. J Nutr 109(5):819-26, 1979

Kozielec T et al. [Deficiency of certain trace elements in children with hyperactivity.] Psychiatr Pol 28(3):345-53, 1994 (in Polish)

Kozielec T, Starobrat-Hermelin B. Assessment of magnesium levels in children with attention deficit hyperactivity disorder (ADHD). Magnes Res 10(2):143-8, 1997

Kronick D. A case history: Sugar, fried oysters, and zinc. Acad Therap 11:119, 1975

Lewis JA, Young R Deanol and methylphenidate in minimal brain dysfunction. Clin Pharmacol Ther 17(5):534-40, 1975

Needleman HL et al. Bone lead levels and delinquent behavior. JAMA 275(5):363-9, 1996

Nemzer ED et al. Amino acid supplementation as therapy for attention deficit disorder. J Am Acad Child Psychiatry 25:509-13, 1986

Pfeiffer CC, Mailloux R. Excess copper as a factor in human diseases. J Orthomol Med 2(3):171-82, 1987

Prinz RJ et al. Dietary correlates of hyperactive behavior in children. J Consult Clin Psychol 48:760-9, 1980

Rapoport J et al. Minor physical anomalies and plasma dopamine beta hydroxylase activity in hyperactive boys. Am J Psychiatry 131:386, 1974

Rowe KS, Rowe KJ. Synthetic food coloring and behavior: A dose response effect in a double-blind, placebo-controlled, repeated-measures study. J Pediatrics, November, 1994:691-8

Ruff HA et al. Declining blood lead levels and cognitive changes in moderately lead-poisoned children. JAMA 269(13):1679-81, 1993

Sabra A et al. Ileal-lymphoid-nodular hyperplasia, non-specific colitis, and pervasive developmental disorder in children. Letter. Lancet 352:234-5, 1998

Schecter MD, Timmons GD. Objectively measured hyperactivity. II. Caffeine and amphetamine effects. J Clin Pharmacol 25:276-80, 1985

Schmidt MH et al. Does oligoantigenic diet influence hyperactive/conduct-disordered children—a controlled trial. Eur Child Adolesc Psychiatry 6(2):88-95, 1997

Sever Y et al. Iron treatment in children with attention deficit hyperactivity disorder. Neuropsychobiology 35:178-80, 1997

South J. Natural remedies for ADD. Nutritional News 11(9), September 1997

Starobrat-Hermelin B, Kozielec T. The effects of magnesium physiological supplementation on hyperactivity in children with attention deficit hyperactivity disorder (ADHD). Positive response to magnesium oral loading test. Magnes Res 10(2):149-56, 1997

Stein TP, Sammaritano AM. Nitrogen metabolism in normal and hyperkinetic boys. Am J Clin Nutr 39(4):520-4, 1984

Stevens LJ et al. Essential fatty acid metabolism in boys with attention-deficit hyperactivity disorder. AM J Clin Nutr 62:761-8, 1995

Stewart-Pinkham SM. Attention deficit disorder: a toxic response to ambient cadmium air pollution. Int J Biosoc Med Res 11(2):134-43, 1989

Swain A et al. Salicylates, oligoantigenic diets, and behavior. Letter. Lancet July 6, 1985, pp. 41-2

Tang HW et al. Effects of low level lead exposure on behavior of young rats. Chung Kuo Yao Li Hsueh Pao 15(4):316-19, 1994

Tu J-B et al. Iron deficiency in two adolescents with conduct, dysthymic and movement disorders. Can J Psychiatry 39:371-7, 1994

Tuthill RW. Hair lead levels relation to children's classroom attention-deficit behavior. Arch Environ Health 51(3):214-20, 1996

Wakefield AJ et al. Ileal-lymphoid-nodular hyperplasia, non-specific colitis, and pervasive developmental disorder in children. Lancet 351:637-41, 1988

Walker S III. Drugging the American child: We're too cavalier about hyperactivity. J Learn Disabil 8:354, 1975

Ward NI. Assessment of chemical factors in relation to child hyperactivity. J Nutr Environ Med 7:333-42, 1997

Wells KC. Laboratory of Behavioral Medicine, Children's Hospital, Washington, D.C., 1985

White JW, Wolraich M. Effect of sugar on behavior and mental performance. Am J Clin Nutr 62(suppl):242S-9S, 1995

Wolraich ML et al. The effect of sugar on behavior or cognition in children. JAMA 274:1617-21, 1995

Woodbury MM, Woodbury MA. Neuropsychiatric development: two case reports about the use of dietary fish oils and/or choline supplementation in children. J Am Coll Nutr 12(3):239-45, 1993

Zametkin AJ et al. Treatment of hyperactive children with D-phenylalanine. Am J Psychiatry 144(6):792-4, 1987

AUTISM

NUTRITIONAL TREATMENT GUIDE

✓ = Efficacy generally accepted.
* = Efficacy *demonstrated* by controlled human trials.
[+] = Efficacy *suspected* from uncontrolled human trials.
[-] = Efficacy *suspected* from indirect data.
? = Efficacy *challenged* in a study of similar design.

NUTRITIONAL FACTORS

* **Vitamin B_6:** ? 10 to 15 mg/kg body weight daily
* ? **Folic acid:** 10 mg daily (autistic males with fragile X syndrome)
* ? **Magnesium:** ? 30 mg/kg body weight daily (up to 1 g) *AND*
Vitamin B_6: ? 10 to 15 mg/kg body weight daily

- -

[-] **Vitamin B_{12} deficiency:** 1,000 μg intramuscularly weekly initially and monthly afterwards

OTHER RELATED FACTORS

[+] rule out **Food Sensitivities**

NUTRITIONAL FACTORS

VITAMINS

Folic Acid

The fragile X syndrome, which frequently manifests as behaviors from the autistic spectrum, is the most common familial form of mental retardation. Folate supplementation has been found to be beneficial in occasional patients under double-blind conditions *(Gillberg;Hagerman)*. The most likely responders are prepubertal males; the most likely symptoms to respond are those of attention deficit-hyperactivity disorder *(Bregman)* (see Attention-deficit Hyperactivity Disorder).

An 8-year-old white male with fragile X syndrome had an IQ in the high-moderate to mild range of mental retardation and met the DSM-III-R criteria for Pervasive Developmental Disorder, Not Otherwise Specified. His behavioral problems included restlessness, overactivity, excitability, impulsivity, fidgetiness and inattentiveness, meeting criteria for Attention-deficit Hyperactivity Disorder.

After the patient was drug-free for 3½ weeks, he was started on 10 mg folic acid daily (0.3 mg/kg body weight) for 14 weeks. Folate was then discontinued for 8½ weeks while he continued to be monitored. The teacher, but not the mother, was completely blind as to the child's treatment status.

Initially, both teacher and parent reported stable baseline behaviors on the Conners Behavior Checklist with mean baseline scores of 15.3 (teacher-unstructured time), 14.7 (teacher-structured time), and 10.7 (parent). While on folic acid, the scores, which were calculated weekly, decreased to 6.7 (teacher-unstructured), 5.8 (teacher-structured) and 6.9 (parent).

Following discontinuation of folic acid, subsequent scores did not revert to pre-trial levels immediately; however the trend was toward increased distractibility and overactivity. Scores were 7.2 (teacher-unstructured), 6.3 (teacher-structured) and 8.4 (parent) (Greenblatt).

Vitamin B_6

Vitamin B_6 may be deficient in autistic patients *(Raiten)*. Several studies, including a double-blind crossover study *(Rimland)*, have found that supplementation with high dosages may result in improved behavior as well as in objective improvements in biochemical and electrophysiological values *(Lelord,1979)*. Whether the vitamin is exerting a pharmacologic effect, or whether the supplement is merely repleting a deficiency, is unclear.

Vitamin B_{12} Deficiency

Of a group of 12 children aged 3 to 10 years, 9 of whom were autistic, who had a history of normal development followed by a loss of language and other acquired skills, and who presented with diarrhea and abdominal pain, 8 were tested for urinary methylmalonic acid excretion. All had elevated levels, suggesting a functional vitamin B_{12} deficiency.

As these children were also found to have intestinal abnormalities, and as vitamin B_{12} is essential for myelinogenesis in the developing central nervous system, the investigators theorized that the intestinal lesions may have interfered with cobalamin resorption from bile and thus contributed to their developmental regression *(Wakefield)*.

MINERALS

Magnesium

Magnesium levels in hair may be reduced in autistic children *(Marlow)*. When combined with vitamin B_6, magnesium supplementation has lead to behavioral improvements in several double-blind studies *(Lelord,1982)*, and there is evidence that the combination of the 2 nutrients is more effective than either nutrient alone *(Martineau,1985)*. Objective changes include improvement in conditioned evoked potentials *(Martineau,1988)* and decreases in the excretion of urinary homovanillic acid, the principal metabolite of dopamine *(Martineau,1985)*.

The two nutrients have a close biological relationship. Both magnesium and vitamin B_6 deficiencies produce comparable clinical disorders *(Seelig)*, and vitamin B_6 has a powerful influence on magnesium nutriture *(Durlach;Majumdar;Turnlund)*.

A 4-year old autistic child was treated with vitamin B_6 30 mg/kg body weight daily and magnesium 15 mg/kg body weight daily for 8 months. There was clear improvement in behavior, urinary levels of homovanillic acid (the principal metabolite of dopamine), and EEG evoked potentials.

Six weeks after supplementation was discontinued, deterioration necessitated reinstitution of nutritional treatment (Martineau,1986).

OTHER NUTRITIONAL FACTORS

L-Tryptophan

Serotonin, whose nutritional precursor is L-tryptophan, is the neurotransmitter that is most consistently implicated in the pathophysiology of autism and related disorders *(Potenza)*. Plasma/serum and whole blood levels of serotonin and tryptophan, its nutritional precursor, are often elevated *(Anderson;Hoshino)*. Moreover, plasma free tryptophan levels are positively correlated with the severity of autistic symptoms and hyperactivity, and negatively with the Developmental Quotient *(Hoshino)*.

A low-tryptophan diet, however, will only worsen autistic behaviors *(McDougle)*.

OTHER RELATED FACTORS

Food Sensitivities

Food sensitivities may be relevant in that elimination of allergenic foods from the diet has been demonstrated in open trials to improve behavior, especially social contact, stereotypy, self-mutilation like head banging, and 'dreamy state' periods. Furthermore, alimentary problems may be improved dramatically as well as sleep disturbances and seizure activity *(Torisky;Reichelt)*.

The "opioid excess" theory of autism proposes that autistic disorders result from the incomplete breakdown and excessive absorption of gut-derived peptides from foods, including barley, rye, oats, and casein from milk and dairy products. These peptides may exert central opioid effects, disrupting neuroregulation and brain development *(Panksepp;Reichelt;Shattock)*.

While this theory remains to be validated, there is recent evidence suggesting that those children with Pervasive Developmental Disorder who exhibit loss of acquired skills complain of intestinal symptoms may exhibit ileal-lymphoid-nodular hyperplasia *(Wakefield)*. This finding suggests that a reactive inflammatory response in the adjacent lymphoid tissue of Peyer's patches may result in the entry of antigens across the inflamed mucosa of the bowel *(Sabra)*.

BIBLIOGRAPHY

Anderson GM. Monamines in autism: an update of neurochemical research on a pervasive developmental disorder. Med Biol 65:67-74, 1987

Bregman JD et al. Fragile X syndrome: variability of phenotypic expression. J Am Acad Child Adolesc Psychiatry 26:463-71, 1987

Durlach J. Donnees Actuelles Sur les mecanismes de Synergie entre Vitamin B6 et Magnesium. J Medicine de Besancon 5:349, 1969

Gillberg C et al. Folic acid as an adjunct in the treatment of children with the autism fragile-X syndrome (AFRAX). Dev Med Child Neurol 28(5):624-7, 1986

Greenblatt JM et al. Folic acid in neurodevelopment and child psychiatry. Prog Neuropsychopharmacol Biol Psychiatry 18:647-60, 1994

Hageman RJ et al. Oral folic acid versus placebo in the treatment of males with the Fragile X Syndrome. Am J Med Genet 23:241-62, 1986

Hoshino Y et al. Blood serotonin and free tryptophan concentration in autistic children. Neuropsychobiology 11:22-7, 1984

Lelord G et al. Electrophysiological and biochemical studies in autistic children treated with vitamin B6, in D Lehmann, E Callaway, Eds. Human Evoked Potentials: Applications and Problems. New York, Plenum Press, 1979

Lelord G et al. Clinical and biological effects of high doses of vitamin B6 and magnesium on autistic children. Acta Vitaminol Enzymol 4(1-2):27-44, 1982

Marlow M et al. Decreased magnesium in the hair of autistic children. J Orthomol Psychiatry 13(2):117-22, 1984

Martineau J et al. Vitamin B_6, magnesium, and combined B_6-Mg: Therapeutic effects in childhood autism. Biol Psychiatry 20:467-78, 1985

Martineau J et al. Long-term effects of combined vitamin B6-magnesium administration in an autistic child. Biol Psychiatry 21:511-18, 1986

Martineau J et al. The effects of combined pyridoxine plus magnesium administration on the conditioned evoked potentials in children with autistic behavior. Curr Top Nutr Dis 19:357-62, 1988

Majumdar P, Boylan M. Alteration of tissue magnesium levels in rats by dietary vitamin B6 supplementation. Int J Vitam Nutr Res 59:300-3, 1989

McDougle CJ et al. Effects of tryptophan depletion in drug-free adults with autistic disorder. Arch Gen Psychiatry 53:993-1000, 1996

Panksepp J. A neurochemical theory of autism. Trends Neurosci 2:174-7, 1979

Potenza MN, McDougle CJ. The role of serotonin in autism-spectrum disorders. CNS Spectrums 2(5):25-42, 1997

Raiten DJ et al. Vitamin and trace element assessment of autistic and learning disabled children. Nutr Behav 2:9-17, 1984

Reichelt KL et al. Biologically active peptide-containing fractions in schizophrenia and childhood autism. Adv Biochem Psychopharmacol 28:627-43, 1993

Rimland B et al. The effect of high doses of vitamin B_6 on autistic children: A double-blind crossover study. Am J Psychiatry 135:472-5, 1978

Sabra A et al. Ileal-lymphoid-nodular hyperplasia, non-specific colitis, and pervasive developmental disorder in children. Letter. Lancet 352:234-5, 1998

Seelig MS. Magnesium requirements in human nutrition. Magnes Bull 3(Suppl 1a):26-47, 1981

Shattock P et al. Role of neuropeptides in autism and their relationships with classical neurotransmitters. Brain Dysfunction 3:328-45, 1991

Torisky DM et al. The NAC pilot project: a model for nutrition screening and intervention for developmentally disabled children with behavior disorders. J Orthomol Med 8(1):25-42, 1993

Turnlund JR et al. Vitamin B-6 depletion followed by repletion with animal- or plant-source diets and calcium and magnesium metabolism in young women. Am J Clin Nutr 56:905-10, 1992

Wakefield AJ et al. Ileal-lymphoid-nodular hyperplasia, non-specific colitis, and pervasive developmental disorder in children. Lancet 351:637-41, 1988

BENIGN BREAST DISEASE

See Also: CANCER
PREMENSTRUAL SYNDROME

NUTRITIONAL TREATMENT GUIDE

✓ = Efficacy generally accepted.
* = Efficacy *demonstrated* by controlled human trials.
[+] = Efficacy *suspected* from uncontrolled human trials.
[-] = Efficacy *suspected* from indirect data.
? = Efficacy *challenged* in a study of similar design.

DIETARY FACTORS

* **low Fat diet**
* avoid **Methylxanthines**

NUTRITIONAL FACTORS

* **Iodine:** *example:* Lugol's iodine or SSKI 2-10 drops daily depending upon body weight and severity of the disorder. *(If available, aqueous iodine 0.07 to 0.09 mg/kg daily.)*
* ? **Omega-6 Fatty Acids:** *example:* evening primrose oil 500 mg caps [7-10% GLA] 6 to 8 daily (3 month trial)
* ? **Vitamin E:** 600 IU daily (3 month trial)

- -

[+] **Vitamin A:** 150,000 IU daily (only under medical supervision)

DIETARY FACTORS

Low Fat Diet

There appears to be a correlation between the percentage of calories derived from fat and the risk of benign breast disease. When the dietary patterns of 854 biopsied cases were compared to those of matched controls, women with atypical lesions had a greater intake of high-fat foods, with the odds ratio in the highest quartile of fat consumption close to 3.0. Also, there was a trend for increasing ductal atypica with increasing saturated fat consumption *(Lubin)*.

The risk of atypical lesions may not be the only effect of dietary fat. When, in a controlled study, women with severe persistent cyclical mastopathy were taught how to reduce dietary fat to 15% of calories, there was a significant reduction in the severity of premenstrual breast tenderness and swelling in the intervention group. On examination, 6 out of 10 patients in the intervention group showed reduced breast swelling, tenderness and nodularity. In the control group, which had simply been given general dietary advice, only 2 out of 9 patients improved *(Boyd)*. These findings have since been replicated in a different country *(Mishra)*.

Total dietary fat intake may not be as important as the percentage of fatty acids that are saturated and/or essential. When the plasma fatty acid profiles of women with either mastalgia or breast cysts were examined, the results were abnormal, with increased proportions of saturated fatty acids and reduced proportions of essential fatty acids *(Gately)*.

Methylxanthines

Benign breast disease as diagnosed by x-rays has been found to be positively correlated with both caffeine and total methylxanthine ingestion *(Bullough)*.

Avoidance of methylxanthines (found in coffee, chocolate and some teas and cola beverages) may be beneficial, although some study results suggest that total abstention may be necessary *(Minton)*. For example, 4 months after 158 patients randomly received a methylxanthine-free diet or no dietary advice, there was a statistically significant reduction in clinically palpable breast findings in the abstaining group compared to the controls *(Ernster)*. Some of the open trials and observational studies, however, have failed to find a relationship *(Lecos)*.

NUTRITIONAL FACTORS

VITAMINS

Vitamin A

Three months after 12 women with moderate to severe breast pain which had failed to respond to mild painkillers or caffeine withdrawal were supplemented with vitamin A 150,000 IU daily, 9 of them had marked pain reduction and, in 5, breast masses decreased at least 50%. Three of the patients had to have therapy stopped or interrupted because of side effects, all of which were fully reversible. At follow-up 8 months later, the responding patients showed continued benefit *(Band)*.

There is early data suggesting that the efficacy of vitamin A supplementation may be primarily confined to women with *proliferative* benign breast disease, as the risk of this diagnosis among women taking vitamin A supplements is only half that of unsupplemented women, while the risk of developing other histologic types of benign breast disease appears to be unaffected *(Hislop)*. Results of this latter study (which found an even lower risk for women who frequently consumed green vegetables) suggest that a much lower dosage of vitamin A may be adequate, although this hypothesis has yet to be tested prospectively.

Because of the potential toxicity of high dosages of vitamin A, they should only be given under close medical supervision after other treatments have proven to be ineffective. If effective, an attempt should be made to reduce or eliminate supplementation as soon as possible, as hepatic storage increases over time.

Vitamin E

Studies investigating supplementation with vitamin E have had mixed results. Earlier studies, some of which were controlled, found that most women responded *(London 1981,1982)*. More recent controlled studies, however, have had negative results *(London,1985;Meyer)*. The reason for the difference in results is unknown. Thus, the efficacy of vitamin E is, at best, uncertain - even though a recent report from a university hospital noted that 40% of a group of 234 women with benign breast disorders, 70% of whom had breast pain and nodularity, seemed to benefit from taking the supplement *(Khanna)*.

> *A woman had a 25-year history of breast tenderness. Once she began taking vitamin E 400 IU daily, she had complete relief of her symptom. Eliminating the supplement, or even reducing the dosage, resulted in return of the tenderness, however (Bricklin).*

MINERALS

Iodine

When rats, especially older rats, are made iodine-deficient, they develop breast lesions which histologically resemble human fibrocystic breast disease. In humans, supplementation with *inorganic iodides* or *iodine caseinate* has been found effective in treating the symptoms of fibrocystic breast disease, with remissions in roughly 90% of patients.

The usual dose of *Lugol's iodine* (95% sodium iodide; 5% iodine) is between 2 and 10 drops daily depending upon body weight and the severity of the disorder *(Gaby;Ghent,1993)*. Side effects include occasional changes in thyroid indices, acne and iodism *(Ghent,1993)*. Moreover, while symptoms may remit, the fibrosis remains which, when substantial, may have precancerous potential *(Ghent,1986,1993)*.

More recently, experimentation with *diatomic (elemental) iodine* suggests that it may be superior as it not only relieves pain, typically in 2 to 8 weeks, but it also gradually resolves the fibrosis *(Eskin;Ghent,1986)*.

Once iodine supplementation is found to be effective, it should not be stopped, or there is a 90% chance of recurrence within 9 months *(Eskin)*.

OTHER NUTRITIONAL FACTORS

Omega-6 Fatty Acids

Supplementation with omega-6 fatty acids by the oral administration of evening primrose oil has been found to be effective in treating patients with mastalgia, especially when the pain and tenderness is cyclical *(Pashby;Pye)*. Treatment is accompanied by an increase in the percentage of essential fatty acids in the plasma towards normal, although this finding is not necessarily associated with a clinical response *(Gateley)*. Women with proven breast cysts may not be responsive, however *(Mansel)*.

COMBINED NUTRITIONAL INTERVENTIONS

A 48 year-old woman gave a history of premenstrual breast tenderness since adolescence. In her early 30's, she began to note breast lumps which were diagnosed as fibrocystic disease. Around age 40, the premenstrual breast tenderness worsened and she began to develop benign breast cysts which were drained or surgically removed. Her mother, who had had a similar history, eventually developed breast cancer.

Physical examination revealed painful, tender breasts with numerous lumps.

She was given dietary counseling (no refined sugar or refined flour, emphasize fresh, raw foods, eliminate artificial flavors, colors and preservatives), and iodine was applied intravaginally (to increase its absorption) immediately after which she was given intravenous magnesium. In addition, she was started on supplementation with pyridoxine 100 mg 3 times daily (to modulate prolactin production and to counteract the effects of elevated levels of undetoxified estrogen), vitamin B complex "50" 3 times daily, iodine 1 drop daily (to reduce the overproduction of estrogen and for its effect on breast tissue), chelated magnesium 135 mg twice daily, essential fatty acid capsules 400 mg 3 daily (to make iodine more available) and vitamin E 600 IU daily (to protect against toxicity from the essential fatty acids).

One week later her breasts were softer and less tender, and many of the cystic lumps were slightly smaller. The intravaginal iodine and IV magnesium treatments were repeated. Eight months later her breasts were soft and pain-free, and there were only some small residual lumpy areas remaining. Her supplementation was continued to prevent recurrence, but was reduced in quantity (Wright).

BIBLIOGRAPHY

Band PR et al. Treatment of benign breast disease with vitamin A. Prev Med 13:549-54, 1984

Boyd NF et al. Effect of a low-fat high-carbohydrate diet on symptoms of cyclical mastopathy. Lancet ii:128-32, 1988

Bricklin M, Ed. Rodale's Encyclopedia of Natural Home Remedies. Emmaus, Pa, Rodale Press, 1982

Bullough B et al. Methylxanthines and fibrocystic breast disease: a study of correlations. Nurse Pract 15(3):36-8, 43-4, 1990

Ernster VL et al. Effects of a caffeine-free diet on benign breast disease: a randomized trial. Surgery 91(3):263-7, 1982

Eskin B and Ghent W - reported in Medical World News January 11, 1988, p. 25

Gaby AR. Fibrocystic breasts: Commentary. Health & Healing 2(7), July, 1995

Gateley CA et al. Plasma fatty acid profiles in benign breast disorders. Br J Surg 79(5):407-9, 1992

Ghent WR, Eskin BA. Elemental iodine supplementation in clinical breast dysplasia. Abstract. Proc Annu Meet Am Assoc Cancer Res 27:189, 1986

Ghent WR et al. Iodine replacement in fibrocystic disease of the breast. Can J Surg 36(5):453-60, 1993

Hislop TG et al. Diet and histologic types of benign breast disease defined by subsequent risk of breast cancer. Am J Epidemiol 131(2):263-70, 1990

Khanna AK et al. Spectrum of benign breast disorders in a university hospital. J Indian Med Assoc 95(1):5-8, 1997

Lecos CW. Caffeine jitters: Some safety questions remain. FDA Consumer 12/87-1/88

London RS et al. Endocrine parameters and alpha-tocopherol therapy of patients with mammary dysplasia. Cancer Res 41 (9 Pt2):3811-13, 1981

London RS et al. Mammary dysplasia: Endocrine parameters and tocopherol therapy. Nutr Res 2:243-47, 1982

London RS et al. The effect of vitamin E on mammary dysplasia: A double-blind study. Obstet Gynecol 65:104-6, 1985

Lubin F et al. Nutritional factors associated with benign breast disease etiology: a case-control study. Am J Clin Nutr 50:5516, 1989

Mansel RE et al. A randomized trial of dietary intervention with essential fatty acids in patients with categorized cysts. Ann N Y Acad Sci 586:288-94, 1990

Meyer EC et al. Vitamin E and benign breast disease. Surgery 107(5):549-51, 1990

Minton JP, Aboud-Issa H. Nonendocrine theories of the etiology of benign breast disease. World J Surg 13(6):680-4, 1989

Mishra SK et al. Efficacy of low fat diet in the treatment of benign breast disease. Natl Med J India 7(2):60-2, 1994

Pashby NL et al. Br J Surg 68:801, 1981

Pye JK et al. Clinical experience of drug treatments for mastalgia. Lancet ii:373-7, 1985

Wright JV. Dr. Wright's Guide to Healing with Nutrition. Emmaus, PA, Rodale Press, 1984

BENIGN PROSTATIC HYPERPLASIA

NUTRITIONAL TREATMENT GUIDE

✓ = Efficacy generally accepted.
* = Efficacy *demonstrated* by controlled human trials.
[+] = Efficacy *suspected* from uncontrolled human trials.
[-] = Efficacy *suspected* from indirect data.
? = Efficacy *challenged* in a study of similar design.

NUTRITIONAL FACTORS

✓ **L-Alanine:** 200 mg,
L-Glutamic Acid: 530 mg *AND*
Glycine: 90 mg (PPC, Nikken-Kagagu, Japan) 3 times daily (3 month trial)

---

* ? **Beta-sitosterol:** free beta-sitosterol 130 mg (6 month trial)

[+] **Zinc:** zinc sulfate 220 mg twice daily *AND* **Copper** 2 mg daily

---

[-] **Selenium:** 200 μg daily

NUTRITIONAL FACTORS

MINERALS

Selenium

See Cadmium Toxicity below.

Zinc

The prostate contains a higher concentration of zinc than any other organ in the body *(Zaichick)*. Zinc exerts an important influence on prostatic androgens. Prolactin is a hormone that increases testosterone uptake by the prostate. While zinc increases prolactin uptake into the prostate, it inhibits prolactin secretion by the pituitary gland *(Judd)* and reduces the specific binding of the hormone to the receptor *(Leake, 1984a)*. It also inhibits the activity of 5-alpha-reductase, the enzyme that irreversibly converts testosterone to dihydrotestosterone *(Leake, 1984b)*, and inhibits the specific binding of androgens to the prostatic cytosol and nuclear androgen receptors *(Leake, 1984c)*.

In BPH, plasma zinc levels may increase *(Bandlish)* suggesting that zinc is interacting with the enlarged gland on a systemic basis. Prostatic zinc levels may also rise, although the increase is in the prostatic fluid rather than within cells *(Schrodt)* as tissue binding is reduced *(Györkey)*.

Since benign prostatic hyperplasia is an androgen-dependent metabolic disorder marked by increased intraprostatic concentration of dihydrotestosterone, zinc supplementation could theoretically be beneficial. Back in 1974, the chairman of the Department of Urology of the Chicago Medical school and his colleagues revealed the positive results of an open trial of zinc supplementation at the American Urological Association's annual meeting, reporting that supplementation successfully reduced both symptoms and prostatic size in the majority of a group of 19 patients *(Bush)*. Unfortunately, the results of these early findings have yet to be confirmed by other investigators.

A 67 year-old man with urinary urgency and frequency, dysuria and reduced size of urinary stream who could only pass a small amount of urine at a time. The bladder always seemed full and there was a continual dull ache across his lower abdomen. Sleep was disturbed due to the need to urinate 5 to 6 times nightly.

Dietary analysis showed an extremely low zinc intake and he was placed on 30 mg zinc daily. Within a month, his condition began to improve and, after 6 months, he was asymptomatic (Van Fleet).

OTHER NUTRITIONAL FACTORS

Amino Acids

A number of double-blind studies have found the combination of L-glutamic acid, L-alanine and glycine to have some efficacy. Subjective improvement, reduction in residual urine and shrinkage of the prostate have been reported *(Dumrau)*. In fact, the efficacy of this combination has become so well accepted that it is being used as the control drug against which to test the efficacy of other agents such as prazosin (a selective alpha 1-adrenoceptor blocker) *(Yamaguchi)* and Cernilton (a flower pollen extract) *(Maekawa)*.

Essential Fatty Acids

When testosterone enters the prostate cell, it both converts to dihydrotestosterone (which stimulates growth) and stimulates the synthesis and release of prostaglandins. Released prostaglandins, in turn, inhibit further testosterone binding to the prostate. It has been suggested that, with aging, testosterone binding may increase due to declining prostaglandin synthesis, causing unrestrained cell growth leading to prostatic hypertrophy *(Klein)*.

In an uncontrolled, unpublished study whose results were reported in 1941, 19 patients received a combination of linoleic, linolenic and arachidonic acids. After several weeks, all showed a reduction in the size of the prostate, an increase in the force of the urinary stream and a diminution of residual urine. Twelve no longer had any residual urine and 13 no longer had nocturia *(Hart)*. Controlled studies with specific essential fatty acids are needed to ascertain the efficacy of the essential fatty acids.

Beta-Sitosterol

Phytosterols are cholesterol analogs found in vegetables which decrease cholesterol absorption by displacing cholesterol from bile salt (taurocholate) micelles *(Ikeda)*. Various extracts of one phytosterol, beta-sitosterol, have been studied for the treatment of BPH under double-blind conditions, and in most studies have shown efficacy *(Klippel)*. While this phytosterol is known to have a potent effect on cholesterol metabolism in the prostate *(Kadow)*, its specific mechanism of action is unknown *(Lowe)*.

OTHER RELATED FACTORS

Cadmium Toxicity

A research team has found prostatic cadmium concentrations in BPH to be considerably higher than in normal tissue, with the dihydrotestosterone level directly proportional to cadmium concentrations *(Habib)*. Although another investigator failed to confirm these findings *(Lahtonen)*, prostatic hyperplasia has been produced in animals by injecting cadmium into the prostate *(Hoffman)*. Furthermore, *in vitro*, cadmium stimulates the growth of human prostatic epithelium.

Selenium

Also *in vitro*, the proper concentration of selenium inhibited cadmium-stimulated prostatic growth *(Webber)*. Animal work has also demonstrated that selenium supplementation, at least when given concurrent with cadmium exposure, protects against cadmium toxicity *(Wahba)*. As selenium intake is frequently inadequate in Western-type diets, insurance against inadequate selenium nutriture may therefore be protective, at least in theory.

BIBLIOGRAPHY

Bandlish U et al. Plasma zinc level estimation in enlarged prostate. Indian J Pathol Microbiol 31(3):231-4, 1988

Bush IM. Zinc and the prostate. Presented at the annual meeting of the American Medical Association. Chicago, 1974

Dumrau F. Benign prostatic hyperplasia: Amino acid therapy for symptomatic relief. Am J Geriatr 10:426-30, 1962

Györkey F, Sato CS. In vitro 65-Zinc-binding capacities of normal, hyperplastic and carcinomatous human prostate gland. Exp Mol Pathol 8:216-24, 1968

Habib FK et al. Metal-androgen interrelationships in carcinoma and hyperplasia of the human prostate. J Endocrinol 71(1):133-41, 1976

Hart JP, Cooper WL. Vitamin F in the treatment of prostatic hyperplasia. Report Number 1, Lee Foundation for Nutritional Research, Milwaukee, WI, 1941

Hoffman L et al. Carcinogenic effects of cadmium on the prostate of the rat. J Cancer Res Clin Oncol 109(3):193-9, 1985

Ikeda I et al. Inhibition of cholesterol absorption in rats by plant sterols. J Lipid Res 29(12):1573-82, 1988

Judd AM et al. Zinc acutely, selectively and reversibly inhibits pituitary prolactin secretion. Brain Res 294:190-2, 1984

Kadow C, Abrams PH. A double-blind trial of the effect of beta-sitosteryl glucoside (WA184) in the treatment of benign prostatic hyperplasia. Eur Urol 12(3):187-9, 1986

Klein LA, Stoff JS. Prostaglandins and the prostate: An hypothesis on the etiology of benign prostatic hyperplasia. Prostate 4(3):247-51, 1983

Klippel KF et al. A multicentric, placebo-controlled, double-blind clinical trial of sitosterol (phytosterol) for the treatment of benign prostatic hyperplasia. Br J Urol 80(3):427-32, 1997

Lahtonen R. Zinc and cadmium concentrations in whole tissue and in separated epithelium and stroma from human benign prostatic hypertrophic glands. Prostate 6(2):177-83, 1985

Leake A et al. Interaction between prolactin and zinc in the human prostate gland. J Endocrinol 102(1):73-6, 1984a

Leake A et al. The effect of zinc on the 5-alpha-reduction of testosterone by the human prostate gland. J Steroid Biochem 20:651-5, 1984b

Leake A et al. Subcellular distribution of zinc in the benign and malignant human prostate: Evidence for a direct zinc androgen interaction. Acta Endocrinol 105:281-8, 1984c

Lowe FC, Ku JC. Phytotherapy in treatment of benign prostatic hyperplasia: a critical review. Urology 48(1):12-20, 1996

Maekawa M et al [Clinical evaluation of Cernilton on benign prostatic hypertrophy--a multiple center double-blind study with Paraprost]. Hinyokika Kiyo 36(4):495-516, 1990

Schrodt GR et al. The concentration of zinc in diseased human prostate glands. Cancer 17:1555-66, 1964

Van Fleet JK. A Doctor's Private Healing Secrets. Parker Publishing Company, 1977

Wahba ZZ et al. Protective effects of selenium on cadmium toxicity in rats: role of altered toxicokinetics and metallothionein. J Toxicol Environ Health 38:171-82, 1993

Webber MM. Selenium prevents the growth stimulatory effects of cadmium on human prostatic epithelium. Biochem Biophys Res Commun 127(3):871-7, 1985

Yamaguchi O et al. Clinical evaluation of effects of prazosin in patients with benign prostatic obstruction. A double-blind, multi-institutional, Paraprost-controlled study. Urol Int 45 Suppl 1:40-6, 1990

Zaichick VY et al. Zinc in the human prostate gland: normal, hyperplastic and cancerous. Int Urol Nephrol 29(5):565-74, 1997

BIPOLAR DISORDER

See Also: DEPRESSION

NUTRITIONAL TREATMENT GUIDE

✓ = Efficacy generally accepted.
* = Efficacy *demonstrated* by controlled human trials.
[+] = Efficacy *suspected* from uncontrolled human trials.
[-] = Efficacy *suspected* from indirect data.
? = Efficacy *challenged* in a study of similar design.

NUTRITIONAL FACTORS

✓ **Lithium ('pharmacologic'):** 900 mg to 1,500 mg daily (only under medical supervision)

- -

* **Folic Acid:** *to enhance lithium pharmacotherapy:* 200 μg daily
* **Phosphatidylcholine:** *to treat manic symptoms:* 5 to 10 g 3 times daily (if 90% pure)
* **L-Tryptophan** 6 to 12 g daily
with **vitamin B_6** 50 mg daily: *to potentiate the effect of lithium*
* **L-Tryptophan:** 6 to 12 g daily
with **vitamin B_6** 50 mg daily: *to treat bipolar depression*
* **Vitamin C deficiency:** 500 mg twice daily
* **Vitamin C:** 3 g daily
* ? **L-Tryptophan:** 6 to 12 g daily
with **vitamin B_6** 50 mg daily: *to treat manic symptoms*

- -

[+] avoid **L-Glutamine** supplementation at dosages of 2 or more grams daily
[+] avoid **Inositol** supplementation
[+] **Lithium ('nutritional'):** *to treat bipolar depression:* 50 μg daily (2 week trial)
[+] **L-Phenylalanine:** *to treat bipolar depression:* 500 mg twice daily *WITH* **vitamin B_6:** 100 mg twice daily
[+] **Potassium:** *to reduce lithium toxicity:* high dietary intake *OR* potassium chloride 20 meq twice daily
[+] **S-Adenosyl-L-Methionine:** *to treat bipolar depression:* 800 mg daily (beware of switch to mania)
[+] **Safflower Oil:** *to reverse lithium neurotoxicity:* 3-5000 ml twice daily (*not* during a manic episode)
[+] **Vitamin B_{12} deficiency:** 1,000 μg intramuscularly weekly initially and monthly afterwards

- -

[-] **Folic Acid deficiency:** 800 μg daily
[-] avoid **Vanadium** (low vanadium diet)

OTHER RELATED FACTORS

[+] rule out **Food Sensitivities**

NUTRITIONAL FACTORS

VITAMIN DEFICIENCIES

Folic Acid Deficiency

Folic acid deficiency is the most common nutrient deficiency and may be found in over one-quarter of hospitalized psychiatric patients *(Lipton)*. Folate deficiency appears to affect mood by impairing the synthesis of tetrahydrobiopterin (BH_4), a cofactor essential for the synthesis of serotonin and other monoamines involved in the pathogenesis of affective disorders *(Coppen,1989)*. One study has reported an inverse association between plasma folate levels and affective morbidity *(Coppen,1982)*; however, later studies have failed to confirm this relationship *(McKeon;Stern)*.

Vitamin B_{12} Deficiency

Vitamin B_{12} may be deficient in hospitalized psychiatric patients. In fact, one study noted that the percentage of hospitalized mental patients with below normal levels of vitamin B_{12} was 30 times higher than in the general population *(Edwin)*.

Deficiency of this nutrient may cause a secondary mania, even in the absence of clinical features of pernicious anemia. Neurological signs are usually present, although they may be subtle. Supplementation appears to be effective in resolving the manic symptoms *(Dommisse; Holmes)*.

An 81-year-old man presented with a full manic syndrome and low serum B_{12} in the absence of clinical features of pernicious anemia, but with a positive Schilling test and antibodies to parietal cells and intrinsic factor. Mental status normalized rapidly with B_{12} replacement and, during the initial week of treatment, haloperidol (Goggans).

Vitamin C

Certain bipolar patients may be in a state of 'subscurvy' *(Schorah)*, and excitement has been found to increase the breakdown of ascorbic acid *(Maas)*.

If vitamin C is deficient, results of a small double-blind study suggest that supplementation may reduce both manic and depressive symptoms *(Milner)*.

There is also evidence that vitamin C supplementation may be of value even when ascorbic acid nutriture is unknown - and thus could be adequate. In a double-blind study, 23 hospitalized patients (11 manic; 12 depressed) were rated as to symptoms, given 3 grams of ascorbic acid or placebo, and then rated hourly for the next 6 hours. The same procedure was repeated the following day except that the ascorbic acid and placebo were switched. On both days, illness severity fell slowly during the day in the placebo group but much more rapidly in the treated group. These differences were significant at 3, 4 and 5 hours post-ingestion *(Naylor,1981a)*.

Another double-blind study investigated the combined effects of ascorbic acid with EDTA in bipolar disorder. The experimental regime was as effective as amitriptyline (an antidepressant drug) for depressed patients, while manic patients responded better to lithium *(Kay)*.

It has been theorized that vitamin C may reduce symptoms of bipolar disorder by decreasing the detrimental effects of vanadium on erythrocyte Na^+-K^+-ATPase activity. It is believed to do so by reducing vanadate (+5) to the vanadyl ion (+4), the latter being a much less effective inhibitor of Na^+-K^+-ATPase activity *(Anonymous)*. (See Vanadium below.)

MINERALS

Lithium

Given that pharmacologic doses of lithium are a major form of therapy in bipolar disorder, much has been written on the subject. However, a small amount of data also exists concerning the nutritional aspects of lithium. Specifically, low nutritional levels of lithium intake may be inversely related to the risk of serious mental illness *(Dawson)*.
Furthermore, the results of a small pilot study suggest that supplementation with low-dose natural lithium supplementation may be effective in alleviating bipolar depression *(Fierro)*. The possibility that nutritional lithium supplementation may be effective is intriguing because of the common problem of side effects from pharmacologic administration of lithium.

Lithium pharmacotherapy has multiple effects upon nutrient distribution and metabolism. For example, lithium reduces calcium absorption from the gut *(Carman)* while it decreases urinary calcium excretion *(Crammer)*, and blood calcium levels may rise *(Smigan)*. The efficacy of lithium treatment is directly correlated with serum folate levels *(Lee)*, and folate supplementation has been shown under double-blind conditions to enhance the efficacy of lithium treatment *(Coppen,1986)*.

Potassium

Evidence from an animal model suggests that dietary potassium protects against lithium toxicity, particularly in regard to renal function *(Everts)*, and it is clear that hypokalemia should be avoided or corrected by patients taking lithium *(Jefferson)*. Moreover, there is early evidence suggesting that potassium supplements may reduce the side effects of pharmacological levels of lithium administration *(Bhaskara)*.

Vanadium

Bipolar patients may have increased plasma vanadium levels, even after recovery *(Dick,1982)*. While plasma, but not hair, vanadium may be increased during depression, vanadium levels in both plasma and hair have been found to be elevated during mania *(Naylor,1984)*. In addition, vanadium toxicity is known to be associated with depression and melancholia *(Witkowska)*.

Vanadium is a powerful inhibitor of Na^+-K^+-ATPase activity *(Cantley)*. It has been suggested that a reduction in the activity of the Na^+-K^+-ATPase pump may be responsible for both the manic and depressive phases of the disorder *(el-Mallakh)*. In bipolar disorder, but not in normals, increased plasma vanadium is negatively correlated with Na^+-K^+-ATPase activity *(Dick,1981)*. Moreover, lymphocytes from manic-depressives are impaired in their ability to produce new Na^+-K^+-ATPase pump sites in response to challenges *(Naylor,1981b)*.

Medications utilized in the treatment of bipolar disorder antagonize the effects of vanadium, suggesting that this may be an important explanation for their effects. Lithium administration, which increases Na^+-K^+-ATPase activity *(Naylor,1981b)*, appears to lower vanadium levels *(Campbell)*. Phenothiazines, much like vitamin C, catalyze the reduction of vanadate to the less active vanadyl ion *(Naylor,1981c)*, while carbamazepine has been shown *in vitro* to largely reverse the inhibition by vanadate of the Na^+-K^+-ATPase of erythrocytes *(Naylor,1985)*.

Therapies based on decreasing vanadate levels in the body (e.g. ascorbic acid, EDTA, methylene blue) have been reported to be effective in both depression and mania (*Naylor,1981b*). In fact, decreasing dietary vanadium intake along with the administration of the mineral chelator EDTA has been shown to reduce both mania and depression under double-blind conditions *(Naylor,1981a)*.

An 82 year-old female had a severe bipolar disorder unresponsive to lithium and other treatments. Within 2 weeks after starting the low vanadium, high EDTA, high ascorbate regime, she settled into a mild hypomanic state and showed no depressive phases for 8 weeks. Five days after withdrawal of the supplements, she became severely depressed, but returned to the hypomanic condition upon their resumption (Naylor,1981a).

OTHER NUTRITIONAL FACTORS

Choline

Supplementation with an exogenous source of choline that enhances biosynthesis of the neurotransmitter acetylcholine was found to be effective in the treatment of mania in a small double-blind study *(Cohen)*. Moreover, in open trials it appears to be effective for rapidly cycling bipolar patients who are refractory to lithium *(Stoll)*.

Phosphatidylcholine is the preferred substance for this purpose; *choline salts* and *lecithin* have also been used as acetylcholine precursors.

A 13-year-old girl with stress-related, early-onset bipolar illness who was in a manic state responded poorly to neuroleptics and not at all to lithium. However, she responded well to lecithin (15 to 23 grams daily of 90% pure phosphatidyl choline) over several weeks (Schreier).

L-Glutamine: A Warning

While low dosages of supplemental L-glutamine appear to be safe, supplementation with 2 grams or more daily can precipitate a manic episode in susceptible people. High-dosage glutamine supplementation is therefore contraindicated in bipolar disorder *(Mebane)*.

A man with no prior psychiatric history was hospitalized with a one-week history of increasing motor and verbal activity culminating in grandiose delusions, hypersexuality, and insomnia. Two weeks earlier, he had begun to ingest up to 4 grams of L-glutamine daily. Symptoms ceased within one week of stopping the supplement (Mebane).

Inositol: A Warning

Lithium may treat mania by reducing inositol, which is a key intermediate of the phosphatidyl-inositol (PI) cycle, a second messenger system used by several noradrenergic, serotonergic and cholinergic receptors *(Benjamin)*. Moreover, there is evidence that inositol supplementation may precipitate a manic episode *(Levine)*.

Essential Fatty Acids

Results of a small open trial suggest that supplementation with safflower oil may reverse tremor and other neurotoxic side effects of lithium treatment *(Lieb)*. While these results were attributed to the high linoleic acid content of the oil, a similar trial using evening primrose oil was unsuccessful *(Schou)*. Controlled trials are needed to clarify the issue.

A Warning

Omega-6 essential fatty acid supplements are contraindicated during manic episodes *(Horrobin)*. They are believed capable of causing an exacerbation as the manic phase of the disorder is associated with elevated levels of prostaglandin E_1 *(Abdulla)*, for which these fatty acids serve as precursors.

L-Phenylalanine

The results of open trials suggest that supplementation with L-phenylalanine may be effective for treating the depressive phase of the illness *(Sabelli;Simonson)*. Vitamin B_6 supplements were also provided in order to enhance the amino acid's metabolism.

Stimulant-type side effects may occur, such as transient headaches, constipation, transient nausea, insomnia, irritability, increased blood pressure and increased anxiety. Also, as L-phenylalanine is a dopamine agonist, it should not be combined with a monoamine oxidase inhibitor. Because of the lack of long-term studies, it has been suggested that supplementation only be given for a short period of time *(Simonson)*.

S-adenosyl-L-methionine

S-adenosyl-L-methionine (SAMe) is produced from L-methionine and ATP through the action of methionine-adenosyltransferase (MAT). Normalization of MAT activity has been associated with clinical improvement in depressives *(Tolbert)*.

Despite its impressive results in treating unipolar depression (see Depression), its use in bipolar disorder appears to be limited. In an open trial, supplementation of SAMe seemed to elevate mood in 9 out of 11 depressed bipolar patients *(Carney)*. However, all patients who responded switched to an elevated mood state (mania, hypomania or euphoria). These results suggest the SAMe should only be used for unresponsive patients and when other agents are planned to be used to control the resulting mood elevation. Controlled studies would help to clarify its treatment role.

L-Tryptophan

L-Tryptophan is the dietary precursor of serotonin, a neurotransmitter with powerful effects on mood; thus is not surprising that supplementation with this nutrient has several applications to the treatment of bipolar disorder. L-tryptophan supplements have been found effective in double-blind studies in the treatment of mania *(Chouinard)* and in the treatment of bipolar depression *(Murphy)*. Moreover, again in a double-blind study, L-tryptophan has been shown to potentiate the effects of lithium in bipolar patients *(Brewerton)*.

Giving vitamin B_6 concomitantly is believed to boost the effective tryptophan dosage by reducing the competition between tryptophan and kynurenine, a tryptophan metabolite, for passage across the blood-brain barrier *(Green;Möller)*.

L-tryptophan supplements have become much less available in recent years after a faulty manufacturing procedure led to the production of a highly toxic contaminant which caused eosinophilia-myalgia syndrome.

L-5-Hydroxytryptophan: A Warning

Because *L-5-hydroxytryptophan*, its immediate metabolite, is more readily available and is also an effective anti-depressant, it is tempting to utilize it to substitute for supplementation with tryptophan. In contrast to tryptophan, however, L-5-hydroxytryptophan also stimulates noradrenergic neurons and thus is more likely to precipitate mania in bipolar patients *(van Hiele)*.

FOOD SENSITIVITIES

The contribution of food sensitivities to symptoms of bipolar disorder is not well defined. One study has found an association between a possible secondary mania and the presence of IgE antibodies to wheat or rye *(Rix)*.

A 32-year-old art teacher had a 10-year history of severe mood swings which were diagnosed as bipolar disorder. Lithium controlled her severe mood swings; however she felt very depressed and lethargic. Nutritional evaluation revealed mild magnesium and zinc deficiencies, but supplementation with these nutrients made little difference in her mental state.

She was then started on a diet restricted to fruit, vegetables, rice, meat and fish. After a month she felt distinctly less depressed and had few mood swings. After 2 months she had increased her work from 2 days a week to 4, and her friends and colleagues had noticed a remarkable improvement in her mood and in her previously glum appearance. Three days after eating bread, however, she became severely depressed and had to stop work for 6 weeks. She returned to her strict diet, and her depression cleared in 6 to 8 weeks (Davies).

BIBLIOGRAPHY

Abdulla YH, Hamadah K. Effect of ADP on prostaglandin E1 formation in blood platelets from patients with depression, mania and schizophrenia. Br J Psychiatry 127:591-5, 1975

Anonymous. Vanadium, vitamin C and depression. Nutr Rev 40(10):293-5, 1981

Benjamin J et al. Inositol treatment in psychiatry. Psychopharmacol Bull 31(1):167-75, 1995

Bhaskara Rao Tripuraneni, fellow in child psychiatry, Harbor-UCLA Medical Center, Torrance, California - reported in Clin Psychiatry News 18(10):3, October, 1990 an presented to the 143rd Annual Mtg. of the Am. Psychiatric Assoc., May 12-17, 1990, Abstracts NR 100 and NR 210

Brewerton TD, Reus VI. Lithium carbonate and L-tryptophan in the treatment of bipolar and schizoaffective disorders. Am J Psychiatry 140:757-60, 1983

Campbell CA et al. Vanadium and other trace elements in patients taking lithium. Biol Psychiatry 24(7):775-81, 1988

Cantley LC et al. Vanadate is a potent (Na,K)-ATPase inhibitor found in ATP derived from muscle. J Biol Chem 252:7421-3, 1977

Carman JS, Wyatt RJ. Calcium: bivalent cation in the bivalent psychoses. Biol Psychiatry 14(2):295-336, 1979

Carney MWP et al. The switch mechanism and the bipolar/unipolar dichotomy. Br J Psychiatry 154:48-51, 1989

Chouinard G et al. A controlled clinical trial of L-Tryptophan in acute mania. Biol Psychiatry 20:546-57, 1985

Cohen BM et al. Lecithin in the treatment of mania: Double-blind, placebo-controlled trials. Am J Psychiatry 139:1162-4, 1982

Coppen A, Abou-Saleh MT. Plasma folate and affective morbidity during long-term lithium therapy. Br J Psychiatry 141:87-89, 1982

Coppen A et al. Folic acid enhances lithium prophylaxis. J Affect Disord 10(1):9-13, 1986

Coppen A et al. Depression and tetrahydrobiopterin: The folate connection. J Affect Disord 16(2-3):103-7, 1989

Crammer J. Lithium, calcium, and mental illness. Letter. Lancet i:215-16, 1975

Davies S, Stewart A. Nutritional Medicine. London, Pan Books, 1987:403

Dawson EB. The relationship of tap water and physiological levels of lithium to mental hospital admission and homicide in Texas, In Schrauzer & Klippel, Eds Lithium in Biology and Medicine. Cambridge, VCH, 1991:169-88

Dick DA et al. Plasma vanadium concentrations in manic-depressive illness. J Physiol 310:27, 1981

Dick DA et al. Plasma vanadium concentration in manic-depressive illness. Psychol Med 12(3):533-7, 1982

Dommisse J. Subtle vitamin-B12 deficiency and psychiatry: a largely unnoticed but devastating relationship? Med Hypotheses 34:131-40, 1991

Edwin E et al. Vitamin B_{12} hypovitaminosis in mental diseases. Acta Med Scand 177:68;9-99, 1965

el-Mallakh RS. The Na,K-ATPase hypothesis for manic-depression. I. General considerations. Med Hypotheses 12(3):253-68, 1983

Everts HB et al. A compartmental model predicts that dietary potassium affects lithium dynamics in rats. J Nutr 126(5):1445-54, 1996

Fierro AA. Natural low dose lithium supplementation in manic-depressive disease. Nutr Perspectives January, 1988, pp. 10-11

Goggans FC. A case of mania secondary to vitamin B12 deficiency. Am J Psychiatry 141(2):300-1, 1984

Green AR, Aronson JK. The pharmacokinetics of oral L-tryptophan: Effects of dose and concomitant pyridoxine, allopurinol or nicotinamide administration. Adv Biol Psychiatry 10:67-81, 1983

Holmes JM. Cerebral manifestations of vitamin B_{12} deficiency. Br Med J 2:1394-8, 1956

Horrobin DF. The regulation of prostaglandin biosynthesis by the manipulation of essential fatty acid metabolism. Rev Pure Appl Pharmacol Sci 4:339-83, 1983

Jefferson JW. Potassium supplementation in lithium patients: a timely intervention or premature speculation? J Clin Psychiatry 53:10, 1992

Kay DS et al. The therapeutic effect of ascorbic acid and EDTA in manic-depressive psychosis: Double-blind comparisons with standard treatments. Psychol Med 14(3):533-8, 1984

Lee S et al. Folate concentration in Chinese psychiatric outpatients on long-term lithium treatment. J Affect Disord 24(4):265-70, 1992

Levine J et al. Inositol-induced mania? Am J Psychiatry 153(6):839, 1996

Lieb J. Linoleic acid in the treatment of lithium toxicity and familial tremor. Prostaglandins Med 4:275-9, 1980

Lipton M et al. Vitamins, megavitamin therapy and the nervous system, in R Wurtman, J Wurtman, Eds. Nutrition and the Brain Vol. 33. New York, Raven Press, 1979:183-264

Maas JW. Arch Gen Psychiatry 4:109, 1961

McKeon P et al. Serum and red cell folate and affective morbidity in lithium prophylaxis. Acta Psychiatr Scand 83(3):199-201, 1991

Mebane AH. L-Glutamine and mania. Letter. Am J Psychiatry 141(10), October, 1984

Milner G. Ascorbic acid in chronic psychiatric patients: A controlled trial. Br J Psychiatry 109:294-9, 1963

Möller SE et al. Tryptophan availability in endogenous depression - relation to efficacy of L-tryptophan treatment. Adv Biol Psychiatry 10:30-46, 1983

Murphy DL et al. L-tryptophan in affective disorders: indoleamine changes and differential clinical effects. Psychopharmacologia 34(1):11-20, 1974

Naylor GJ, Smith AHW. Vanadium: A possible aetiological factor in manic-depressive illness. Psychol Med 11:249-56, 1981a

Naylor GJ, Smith AHW. Defective genetic control of sodium-pump density in manic-depressive psychosis. Psychol Med 11:257-63, 1981b

Naylor GJ et al. Possible explanation for therapeutic action of lithium, and a possible substitute (methylene-blue). Letter. Lancet ii:1175-6, 1981c

Naylor GJ. Vanadium and manic depressive psychosis. Nutr Health 3(1-2):79-85, 1984

Naylor GJ. Reversal of vanadate-induced inhibition of Na-K ATPase. A possible explanation of the therapeutic effect of carbamazepine in affective illness. J Affect Disord 8(1):91-3, 1985

Rix KJ et al. Food antibodies in acute psychoses. Psychol Med 15(2):347-54, 1985

Sabelli HC et al. Clinical studies on the phenylethylamine hypothesis of affective disorder: Urine and blood phenylacetic acid and phenylalanine dietary supplements. J Clin Psychiatry 47(2):66-70, 1986

Schorah CJ et al. Plasma vitamin C concentrations in patients in a psychiatric hospital. Hum Nutr Clin Nutr 37C:447-52, 1983

Schou M. Linoleic acid in the treatment of lithium-induced tremor: A pilot study with negative outcome. Prostaglandins Med 5:343-4, 1980

Schreier HA. Mania responsive to lecithin in a 13-year old girl. Am J Psychiatry 139:108-10, 1982

Simonson M. L-Phenylalanine. Letter. J Clin Psychiatry 46(8):355, 1985

Smigan L. Long -term lithium treatment. Some clinical, psychological and biological aspects. Acta Psychiatr Scand 71(2):160-70, 1985

Stern SL et al. Serum and red cell folate concentrations in outpatients receiving lithium carbonate. Int Clin Psychopharmacol 3(1):49-52, 1988

Stoll AL et al. Choline in the treatment of rapid-cycling bipolar disorder: clinical and neurochemical findings in lithium-treated patients. Biol Psychiatry 40:382-8, 1996

Tolbert LC et al. Clinical correlations of one-carbon metabolism abnormalities. Prog Neuropsychopharmacol Biol Psychiatry 12(4):491-502, 1988

van Hiele LJ. L-5-Hydroxytryptophan in depression: the first substitution therapy in psychiatry? Neuropsychobiology 6(4):230-40, 1980

Witkowska D, Brzezinski, J. Alteration of brain noradrenaline, dopamine and 5-hydroxy-tryptamine levels during vanadium poisoning. Pol J Pharmacol Pharm 31:393-8, 1979

BRONCHIAL ASTHMA

See Also: ALLERGY

NUTRITIONAL TREATMENT GUIDE

✓ = Efficacy generally accepted.
* = Efficacy *demonstrated* by controlled human trials.
[+] = Efficacy *suspected* from uncontrolled human trials.
[-] = Efficacy *suspected* from indirect data.
? = Efficacy *challenged* in a study of similar design.

DIETARY FACTORS

* minimize **Salt** intake
* **Caffeine:** 350 mg or more (coffee, cola or caffeine tablets) (in emergencies only)

- -

[+] **low Tryptophan diet**

- -

[-] increase **Fresh Fruit** and **Vegetable** intake

NUTRITIONAL FACTORS

✓ **N-acetylcysteine:** deliver by inhalation. (Efficacy of oral preparation is uncertain.)

- -

* **Magnesium:** *symptomatic relief:* 400 mg daily (3 week trial)
* **Selenium:** 100 μg daily
* avoid **Tryptophan** supplementation
* **Vitamin B_6:** *to reduce theophylline side effects:* pyridoxal hydrochloride at least 15 mg daily
* ? **Magnesium:** *to treat an acute episode:* IV magnesium sulfate 25 mg/kg body weight over 20 minutes; maximum 2 g in 100 ml normal saline
* ? **Omega-3 fatty acids:** *example:* MaxEPA 1 g caps [180 mg EPA; 180 mg DHA] 10 to 20 daily (4 week trial) (See discussion in the text under Essential Fatty Acids.)
* ? **Vitamin B_6:** ? 50 to 100 mg daily (Prescribe pyridoxal-5'-phosphate if the patient is receiving theophylline.)
* ? **Vitamin C:** 2 g daily; in an acute episode: 8 to 10 g

- -

[+] **Betaine or glutamic hydrochloride:** 10 to 50 gr as tolerated at the start of meals. (Watch for signs of gastric irritation.)
[+] **Molybdenum:** 250 μg IV twice weekly for 2 weeks, then 500 μg twice weekly for 8 weeks, then 750 μg weekly for 4 weeks (Monitor copper levels and supplement if needed.)
[+] **Vitamin B_{12}:** 1 to 3 cc hydroxycobalamin IM daily for 30 days, then 3 times weekly for 2 weeks, then once weekly as needed

- -

[-] **Magnesium deficiency:** ≈ 400 mg daily (Consider IM or IV administration, especially in hypomagnesemia.)
[-] **Niacin deficiency:** 50 to 100 mg daily
[-] **Riboflavin deficiency:** 5 to 10 mg daily

OTHER RELATED FACTORS

* rule out **Food Sensitivities**

DIETARY FACTORS

Fruit And Vegetable Consumption

A recent study of 2,650 children aged 8 to 11 years found that one-second forced expiratory volume (FEV1) was positively associated with the frequency of fresh fruit consumption. While most of these children were not asthmatic, the association was strongest for the wheezers. There was a similar, although weaker, association with the consumption of salads and green vegetables *(Cook)*.

Sodium Chloride

Double-blind crossover studies have shown that increasing salt intake worsens the severity of the asthmatic condition *(Burney,1989;Carey)*. These results are consistent with epidemiological observations. For example, sales of table salt in the different regions of England and Wales were found to be independently correlated with mortality from asthma for both adult men and for children of both sexes *(Burney,1986)* while, in an Italian study, table salt use was strongly related to wheezing, especially in boys *(Pistelli)*.

Caffeine

Caffeine has been shown to relieve asthmatic airway constriction under double-blind conditions *(Becker)*; in fact, theophylline is actually a metabolic product of caffeine, and caffeine is 40% as effective as theophylline *(Gong)*. In fact, while the protective effect is small, coffee ingestion may contribute to the reduced prevalence of asthma in adults as compared to children *(Schwartz,1992)*.

Caffeine and theophylline together, however, can be toxic. Because of its adverse effects on health, caffeine on a regular basis for the purpose of reducing asthmatic symptoms is not recommended. However, since even a single cup of coffee produces as much as a 15% increase in FEV1 *(Gong)*, it can be quite useful for treating acute symptoms when other treatment is unavailable.

NUTRITIONAL FACTORS

VITAMINS

Vitamin B Complex

Niacin

Niacin appears to inhibit mast cell degranulation and histamine release *(Bekier)*. Both niacin intake and serum levels are inversely correlated with the incidence of wheezing *(Schwartz,1990)* and, in a Russian study, 83% of a group of asthmatics were niacin-deficient *(Rozanov)*.

Only very early work has investigated whether niacin supplementation reduces asthmatic symptoms, and whether any efficacy is limited to repletion of a pre-existing deficiency. In a placebo-controlled study, intramuscular niacin administration was effective for 16 out of a group of 19 patients with acute asthma, although 2 of the 19 had marked exacerbations and side effects were common - which suggests that it should not be used routinely until it is better studied. The efficacy of oral supplementation with niacin remains to be shown.

A 35 year-old Puerto Rican woman developed asthma 8 years earlier following an upper respiratory infection. She presented with a severe episode of acute asthma.

Treatment consisted of intravenous administration of niacin 100 mg. Within a few minutes the wheezing diminished, and her breathing became less labored. Although she felt better, there were still scattered rhonchi present. She was told to take 100 mg of niacin orally every 2 hours.

Two months later, she returned due to recurrent attacks. She was told to increase niacin to 200 mg before meals and before retiring. The severity of her attacks abated, and epinephrine, which was formerly used every few hours, was now needed only on rare occasions.

However, she awoke one morning a month later with a very severe attack which was not relieved by epinephrine but was partially controlled by Aminophyllin IV. She then received 100 mg of niacin IV which reduced the severity of the paroxysm for 3 hours. Subsequently, oral niacin completely controlled the asthma again (Maisel).

Riboflavin Deficiency

Asthmatic inflammation results in increased oxygen free radical generation. As flavin adenine dinucleotide, riboflavin is a cofactor for the antioxidant enzyme, glutathione reductase, and it is believed that the activity of this enzyme protects against asthmatic pathophysiology *(Misso)*. Thus, by reducing glutathione generation, a riboflavin deficiency may increase the risk of bronchial asthma *(Greene)*.

Vitamin B_6

In asthmatics, both plasma and red cell levels of pyridoxal-5'-phosphate, the activated form of the vitamin, have been found to be reduced *(Delport;Reynolds)*. This may be due, at least in part, to the effect of theophylline, which is a pyridoxal kinase antagonist.

There have been a few controlled studies investigating whether vitamin B_6 supplementation reduces asthmatic symptoms. In one study, 76 children with moderate or severe asthma received 200 mg pyridoxine daily or placebo. After 5 months, the children in the pyridoxine group had significantly less symptoms; moreover, the dosage of bronchodilators and corticosteroids had been reduced *(Collipp)*. However, a 9-week study, this one of adults with steroid-dependent asthma, failed to find differences between patients supplemented with 300 mg pyridoxine and those given placebo *(Sur)*.

Vitamin B_6 supplementation may have another application for patients receiving theophylline. A dosage of 15 mg daily of pyridoxal hydrochloride was found, in a double-blind crossover study, to markedly reduce theophylline-related tremor. There was also a tendency for it to reduce many other adverse effects of theophylline on the nervous system *(Bartel)*.

Vitamin B_{12}

In open trials, vitamin B_{12}, when given intramuscularly in massive doses, seems to reduce asthmatic symptoms, with children having the best results *(Crocket)*. Of roughly 50 children who were under age 10 (only a few of whom had taken intermittent steroids), about 60% quit wheezing entirely, 20 to 30% had substantial relief and only 10% had fair to poor results. Side effects were minimal *(Wright, 1989a)*. Double-blind studies are needed for confirmation.

Vitamin B_{12} may be especially indicated for the many asthmatics (perhaps as many as 1 in 500) who are *sulfite-sensitive*. When 1,500 micrograms was given orally to sulfite-sensitive asthmatics before they were exposed to sulfites, the vitamin supplement was more effective than drugs in blocking asthmatic reactions - and its effects lasted longer *(Anibarro;Simon)*.

When first seen at age 3, a boy was receiving maximum doses of bronchodilators and inhalers, yet his asthma was getting worse. Prednisone controlled his wheezing, but he developed edema.

He was started on daily injections of vitamin B_{12} (hydroxycobalamin). After 2 injections, the boy was breathing more easily. By 2 weeks, his wheezing was so much less that his parents stopped his inhaler. By 3 weeks, they stopped his bronchodilator. When he was seen after one month, he was doing "just fine" and therefore the frequency of the injections began to be tapered. Based on the results of previous testing, he also began treatment for food sensitivities and supplemental hydrochloric acid was added.

In the ensuing 9 years, he only wheezed one other time. That was at age 5 when his vitamin B_{12} injections were tapered too far and his foods were not being adequately restricted. He was placed back on bronchodilators for a short time, but recovered quickly with the resumption of daily B_{12} shots and strict dietary control. Stomach acid levels were normal when tested at age 9, and the infrequent B_{12} injections were stopped. On follow-up at age 12, he was fine (Wright, 1986).

Vitamin C

The intake and serum level of vitamin C are inversely correlated with the incidence of wheezing *(Schwartz, 1990)* and pulmonary function deficits *(Schwartz, 1994)*. A Russian study found 96.8% of 124 patients to be deficient in vitamin C *(Rozanov)*. Likewise, in India, Singh found that asthmatics have a significantly lower intake and plasma level of vitamin C than controls *(Singh)*, while a study in Scotland of patients with seasonal symptoms of bronchial reactivity found more than a 5-fold risk of bronchial reactivity in patients with the lowest intakes of vitamin C *(Soutar)*.

In a double-blind experiment, asthmatics receiving 1 gram of vitamin C daily had fewer than one-fourth as many asthmatic attacks as those receiving placebo *(Anah)*. In some studies *(Cohen; Mohsenin, 1987)*, but not in others *(Kordansky; Malo)*, vitamin C protected asthmatics from bronchoconstriction and other asthma-related symptoms. Moreover, vitamin C has been shown under double-blind conditions to reduce the tendency of exercise to cause bronchospasm *(Schachter)*.

Vitamin C may be effective in bronchial asthma due to its ability to lower blood histamine levels. Among people with low levels of vitamin C, the lower the level of their vitamin C, the higher their histamine levels; when they take vitamin C, their histamine levels fall. In fact, even when vitamin C is not low, but histamine levels are high, vitamin C supplementation will cause histamine levels to fall *(Clemetson)*. There is also evidence that vitamin C may favorably alter arachidonic acid metabolism *(Mohsenin, 1983)*.

Vitamin E

Vitamin E intake appears to be reduced in asthmatics *(Singh)* and its intake has been inversely related to the risk of bronchial asthma *(Troisi)*.

While supplementation with this vitamin has been poorly investigated, vitamin E supplements have been shown to help normalize immune function in asthmatic patients *(Pletsktyi)*. Moreover, results of a pilot study suggest that vitamin E can dramatically decrease asthmatic symptoms *(Ahrot-Westerlund)*, although controlled trials are needed to reliably ascertain its clinical efficacy.

MINERALS

Magnesium

How often magnesium deficiency plays a role in provoking asthmatic symptoms is uncertain, although some clinicians believe it to be a common finding *(Gaby, 1995)*. Studies relating asthma to blood magnesium levels have so far produced a confusing picture. In one study, reduced serum magnesium levels were found in one-quarter of a group of asthmatics; this finding extended to half of the group during acute attacks *(Haury)*. Other studies, however, found serum magnesium to be normal *(Falkner)* or even elevated *(Petrov)*.

Yet another study found normal levels of serum and erythrocyte magnesium, but reduced magnesium levels in polymorphonuclear leukocytes *(Fantidis)*. Durlach suggests that these latter findings reflect dysregulation of the control mechanisms of magnesium metabolism (what he calls magnesium *depletion*) rather than a magnesium deficiency *(Durlach)*.

Others studies have lent weight to the hypothesis that magnesium nutriture is closely related to asthmatic episodes in susceptible people. Magnesium intake has been found to be inversely related to the risk of airway hyper-reactivity and wheezing *(Britton)*. Moreover, abnormally high intracellular calcium levels may exist during an asthmatic attack *(Landon)*, and magnesium blocks calcium's entry into smooth muscle cells and may inhibit the action of calcium in releasing chemical mediators from basophils and mast cells *(Fantidis)*.

Finally, prostanoids, which stimulate mucus secretion and bronchial smooth muscle contraction, are magnesium-dependent, and rats made magnesium-deficient have been found to have increased tissue prostanoid levels *(Fantidis)*.

Several double-blind studies have demonstrated the value of magnesium therapy in the treatment of an acute episode when administered either by intravenous injection *(Clarallo)* or by intranasal inhalation *(Nannini)*, although not all studies have found intravenous magnesium to be effective *(Bernstein;Green)*. Recently, a double-blind crossover study explored the efficacy of magnesium supplementation following 3 weeks of a low magnesium diet. Magnesium supplements were associated with a significant reduction in asthma symptom scores, although no objective improvements could be demonstrated *(Hill)*.

The efficacy of long-term magnesium supplementation in preventing asthma attacks, especially as to how it relates to borderline magnesium deficiency, remains to be elucidated.

A 62-year-old man with acute respiratory failure secondary to a severe asthma attack had clinically deteriorated despite aggressive standard treatment and evidenced acidosis and hypercarbia by arterial blood gas determination.

An intravenous dose of one gram magnesium sulfate produced rapid clinical and arterial blood gas improvement and enabled management of the patient without endotracheal intubation and mechanical ventilation (McNamara).

Molybdenum

Sulfites, with their tendency to provoke bronchospasm, are derived exogenously from foods and endogenously from amino acid metabolism. The enzyme sulfite oxidase oxidizes sulfite to the inert and harmless sulfate. Molybdenum, the trace element contained in the enzyme, has been found to be deficient in the blood of the majority of a group of people with sulfite sensitivity *(Papaioannou)*. Urinary sulfite has been suggested as a measure of sulfoxidation *(Wright,1989b)*. If so, reduced molybdenum may be reflected by increased urinary sulfite.

In a case report, a female asthmatic with increased urinary sulfite was treated with intravenous molybdenum. Urinary sulfite decreased, wheezing considerably decreased, and she was able to greatly reduce her medications *(Wright,1989b)*. Controlled studies are needed to confirm this early report. Wright, the co-author of the report, has treated a number of similar patients and reports that oral molybdenum is far less effective *(Wright,1991)*.

It is interesting that the proportion of a group of patients with food sensitivities who were poor sulfoxidizers was significantly higher than that of normal controls *(Scadding)*. This finding suggest that food-sensitive asthmatics may be more likely to respond to intravenous molybdenum. (See Food Sensitivities below.)

Selenium

Plasma and erythrocyte selenium levels as well as glutathione peroxidase activity (which is selenium-dependent) are often decreased *(Kadrabova)*. These levels appear to be even lower in aspirin-intolerant asthmatics *(Malmgren;Pearson)*, suggesting that there may be a genetic syndrome-specific factor related to aspirin intolerance *(Pearson)*.

One double-blind study has examined the effects of sodium selenite supplementation with asthmatics. After 14 weeks, the selenium group showed significant increases in serum selenium levels and glutathione peroxidase activity, while the placebo group showed no changes. Six of the 24 patients in the selenium group demonstrated clinical improvements in a variety of asthmatic symptoms compared to improvement in only one patient in the placebo group. However, the improvement could not be validated by parameters of lung function or airway hyperresponsiveness. The investigators hypothesize that selenium and glutathione peroxidase may alter the activities of prostaglandins and the lipoxygenase metabolites that are implicated as mediators of asthma *(Hasselmark,1993)*.

OTHER NUTRITIONAL FACTORS

N-acetylcysteine

N-acetylcysteine has been found to be an effective mucolytic agent when given by inhalation *(Millman)*. However, a possible side effect may be inhibition of the usual decreasing bronchial reactivity to allergens after repeated allergen inhalation challenges *(Dorsch)*.

N-acetylcysteine is also available for oral administration. Open trials have found it to be equally effective as when it is given by inhalation, and it lacks the side effects (such as bronchospasm) that sometimes force the drug to be discontinued *(Fischer;Volkl)*. However, a double-blind crossover study failed to find effects of orally-administered preparation on any spirometric, lung mechanic or gas exchange variable, nor on the frequency of pulmonary symptoms in chronic asthma *(Bylin)*. Further controlled studies are thus needed to ascertain its efficacy.

Essential Fatty Acids

Omega-3 Fatty Acids

Analyses of dietary questionnaires have revealed that increased dietary fish oil intake may be associated with reduced rates of active bronchitis and wheezing *(Schwartz,1990)*. Furthermore, among asthmatic children, those who ate oily fish had a significantly reduced risk of current asthma *(Hodge,1996)*.

Several controlled experiments have examined the effects of providing asthmatics with omega-3 fatty acid supplements derived from fish oil. Unfortunately, the results have been highly conflicting, with some studies finding both subjective and objective improvement along with a decline of the late allergic response and other evidence of improved immunoregulation *(Masuev)*, while others failing to find evidence of benefit *(Stenius-Aarniala,1989)* or even, in aspirin-intolerant asthmatics, suppression of neutrophil function *(Arm)*.

Omega-6 Fatty Acids

linoleic acid → GLA → DGLA → 1 series prostaglandins

Evening primrose oil is a rich source of gamma linolenic acid (GLA) which is a precursor to the synthesis of the series 1 prostaglandins. Double-blind studies have failed to find evidence that supplementation with this oil is beneficial *(Hederos;Stenius-Aarniala,1989)*.

Omega-6 to Omega-3 Ratio

The prevalence of bronchial asthma has grown simultaneously with an increase in dietary omega-6-containing vegetable oils coupled with a decrease in consumption of omega-3-containing oily fish. Omega-6 fatty acids are precursors to arachidonic acid which can be converted to pro-inflammatory prostaglandin E2 (PGE2) which promotes allergic sensitization. By contrast, eicosapentaenoic acid, an omega-3 fatty acid found in fatty fish, inhibits PGE2 production. Several authors have attributed the increasing prevalence of bronchial asthma to the increased ratio of omega-6 to omega-3 fatty acids in the diet *(Black;Chang;Hodge)*. If they are correct, then either dietary changes in the ratio, or supplementation with fish oils, may be effective in reducing the asthmatic diathesis.

Results of a recent study that took the dietary ratio between the two families of essential fatty acids into consideration may finally explain the contradictory findings of prior studies of omega-3 fatty acid supplementation (see Omega-3 Fatty Acids above). Asthmatics first received low-dosage fish oil supplementation designed to result in a dietary ratio of omega-3 to omega-6 fatty acids of 0.1 to 10 for 4 weeks followed by high-dosage supplementation with a ratio of 0.5 to 1 for another 4 weeks. With low omega-3 ingestion, methacholine-induced respiratory distress increased; with high omega-3 ingestion, more than 40% of patients improvement in methacholine-induced bronchoprovocation, while the rest of the group lost further respiratory capacity.

Responders could be separated from non-responders on the basis of urinary 5-series leukotriene excretion, leading the investigators to suggest that the patients who are likely to respond to fish oils are those for whom a trial of omega-3 fatty acids results in a urinary ratio of 4-series to 5-series leukotrienes of less than one *(Broughton)*. In the absence of such testing, it appears that a 4 week trial of fish oil supplementation may be appropriate. Unless there is clear benefit, the supplement should not be continued.

Tryptophan: A Warning

Tryptophan should not be used as a nutritional supplement in this patient population as it is the precursor of serotonin, a neurotransmitter known to cause bronchoconstriction in asthmatics. In one double-blind study, when tryptophan was removed from a standard diet, asthmatics actually improved *(Urge)*. This suggests that a low-tryptophan diet may be beneficial.

OTHER RELATED FACTORS

Increased Gut Permeability

New findings are revealing that asthma is more than simply a disorder of the respiratory system; a mucosal defect in distant locations may be an etiology. For example, in a study of 37 men and women, 21 with allergic and 16 with nonallergic asthma, intestinal permeability was significantly increased compared to controls. Furthermore, this increase was unrelated to serum IgE level, eosinophilia, disease severity, steroid or NSAID treatment, alcoholism, smoking, or food allergy. The investigators suggest that asthmatics suffer from "a primary general mucosal defect simultaneously in several organs and clinically expressed in a single organ [the lungs] after an exogenous stimulation, such as antigenic or environmental factors *(Benard)*."

We know that that a wide variety of influences can provoke an asthma attack in susceptible people by penetrating the protective barrier of the intestinal lining. These include foods *(Gardner)* as well as translocated intestinal bacteria or the endotoxins they produce *(Matuschak)*. The gut barrier could even be compromised by diversion of splanchnic blood flow caused by sustained sympathoadrenal activation *(Matuschak)*.

Food Sensitivities

The literature suggesting that a wide variety of foods may provoke asthma, often despite the lack of immediate reactions, is continuing to grow. In one study, for example, 107 patients with perennial allergic bronchial asthma underwent food ingestion challenges. Seventy-one percent of patients with a history of food reactions developed symptoms following challenges as did 56% of the 45 patients without a known history of such reactions. Some reactions were within 2 hours; however, others were delayed as long as 56 hours after challenge. A few days later, 22 of the patients were tested with the same foods under double-blind conditions; there were no statistically significant differences in their bronchial responses *(Pelikan)*.

In another double-blind study, 21 hospitalized severe asthmatics with symptoms all year long kept to a liquid diet which was almost entirely free of food antigens, while 17 similar patients drank a liquid consisting of the regular hospital diet blended to have a similar taste and texture as the experimental diet. Both groups also received their doctors' usual medical treatment during the study.

After only 2 weeks, there were major differences between the two groups. Nine of the 21 asthmatics on the antigen-free diet improved, 3 of them dramatically, and none of them got worse. In the other group, only 1 of the 17 asthmatics improved, while 5 got worse. The researchers were so impressed by their findings that they suggested that similar patients should all try an antigen-free diet, even if they have little or no evidence of allergies *(Hoj)*. A longer period on the diet may well have resulted in still better results.

One reason why so many asthmatics are food sensitive was discovered over half a century ago. In 1931, Dr. George Bray studied the secretion of hydrochloric acid by the stomach in 200 asthmatic children and compared it to that of children without asthma. Four out of 5 asthmatic children had reduced levels of gastric acid, while only 1 out of 10 of the non-asthmatic children was found to be deficient. When the children with gastric hypoacidity were given hydrochloric acid before or during meals, and they continued to avoid foods to which they were sensitive, they had immediate improvements in appetite, weight, sleep and asthmatic attacks, and the attacks became less severe and shorter in duration *(Bray)*.

It would be a mistake to conclude from such studies that food reactions are responsible for most asthma attacks. Not surprisingly, other studies have found a smaller percentage of asthmatics to be food-sensitive and there is evidence that both parents and physicians sometimes overdiagnose food reactions in asthmatics *(May)*.

COMBINED NUTRITIONAL TREATMENT

Gaby has noted that acute asthma attacks may resolve within a few minutes following an intravenous injection of nutrients (vitamin C 3-12 g, pyridoxine 1-300 mg, pantothenic acid 250-500 mg, hydroxycobalamin 1-2,000 µg, magnesium chloride 400-1000 mg, calcium glycerophosphate 2-5 ml., and niacinamide 1-200 mg) *(Gaby, 1987)*. He has also reported excellent long-term results from combined nutritional treatment:

In the year prior to nutritional treatment, a 5 year-old asthmatic boy had visited an emergency room 20 times and had been hospitalized several times for asthma and twice for bronchial pneumonia.

He was placed on a food elimination diet and given daily supplements of pyridoxine 50 mg, pantothenic acid 100 mg, vitamin C 500 mg, calcium 300 mg and magnesium 150 mg. He quickly became symptom-free but would develop symptoms within hours after ingesting milk or wheat.

After one year, an upper respiratory infection produced moderately severe wheezing and coughing which was treated with vitamin C 1 g, pyridoxine 50 mg., niacinamide 50 mg., hydroxycobalamin 1000 µg, magnesium chloride 300 mg. and calcium glycerophosphate 1.5 ml. His wheezing and coughing subsided within 3 minutes (Gaby, 1987).

BIBLIOGRAPHY

Ahrot-Westerland B. Letter. Acta Ophthalmol (Copenh) 66:237-8, 1988

Anah, CO et al. High dose ascorbic acid in Nigerian asthmatics. Tropical Geograph. Med. 32:132-37, 1980

Anibarro B et al. Asthma with sulfite intolerance in children: a blocking study with cyanocobalamin. J Allergy Clin Immunol 90(1):103-9, 1992

Arm JP et al. Effect of dietary supplementation with fish oil lipids on mild asthma. Thorax 43(2):84-92, 1988

Bartel PR et al. Vitamin B-6 supplementation and theophylline-related effects in humans. Am J Clin Nutr 60:93-9, 1994

Becker AJ et al. The bronchodilator effects and pharmacokinetics of caffeine in asthma. N Engl J Med 310(12):743-6, 1984

Bekier E, Maslinski CZ. Antihistaminic action of nicotinamide. Agents Actions 4(3):196, 1974

Benard A et al. Increased intestinal permeability in bronchial asthma. J Allergy Clin Immunol 97(6):1173-78, June, 1996

Bernstein WK et al. Lack of effectiveness of magnesium in chronic stable asthma. Arch Intern Med 155:271-6, 1995

Black PN, Sharpe S. Dietary fat and asthma: is there a connection? Eur Res J 10:6-12, 1997

Bray GW. The hypochlorhydria of asthma of childhood. Quart J Med 24:181-97, 1931

Britton J et al. Dietary magnesium, lung function, wheezing, and airway hyper-reactivity in a random adult population sample. Lancet 344:357-62, 1994

Broughton KS et al. Reduced asthma symptoms with n-3 fatty acid ingestion are related to 5-series leukotriene production. Am J Clin Nutr 65:1011-7, 1997

Burney PG et al. Response to inhaled histamine and 24 hour sodium excretion. Br Med J 292:1483-6, 1986

Burney PG et al. The effect of changing dietary sodium on the bronchial response to histamine. Thorax 44(1):36-41, 1989

Bylin G et al. No influence of acetylcysteine on gas exchange and spirometry in chronic asthma. Eur J Respir Dis 71(2):102-7, 1987

Carey OJ et al. Effect of alterations of dietary sodium on the severity of asthma in men. Thorax 48:714-18, 1993

Chang CC et al. Asthma mortality: another opinion - is it a matter of life and . . . bread? J Asthma 30(2):93-103, 1993

Clarallo L et al. Intravenous magnesium therapy for moderate to severe pediatric asthma: results of a randomized, placebo-controlled trial. J Pediatr 129:809-14, 1996

Clemetson CA. Histamine and ascorbic acid in human blood. J Nutr 110(4):662-8, 1980

Cohen HA et al. Blocking effect of vitamin C in exercise-induced asthma. Arch Pediatr Adolesc Med 151(4):367-70, 1997

Collipp PJ et al. Pyridoxine treatment of childhood bronchial asthma. Ann Allergy 35:93-97, 1975

Cook DG et al. Effect of fresh fruit consumption on lung function and wheeze in children. Thorax 52:628-33, 1997

Crocket JA. Cyanocobalamin in asthma. Acta Allergologica 11:261-8, 1957

Delport R et al. Vitamin B6 nutritional status in asthma: The effect of theophylline therapy on plasma pyridoxal-5'-phosphate and pyridoxal levels. Int J Vitam Nutr Res 58(1):67-72, 1988

Dorsch W et al. Adverse effects of acetylcysteine on human and guinea pig bronchial asthma in vivo and on human fibroblasts and leukocytes in vitro. Int Arch Allergy Appl Immunol 82(1):33-9, 1987

Durlach J. Commentary on recent clinical advances: Magnesium depletion, magnesium deficiency and asthma. Magnes Res 8(4):403-5, 1995

Falkner D et al. Serum magnesium levels in asthmatic patients during acute exacerbations of asthma. Am J Emerg Med 10(1):1-3, 1992

Fantidis P et al. Intracellular (polymorphonuclear) magnesium content in patients with bronchial asthma between attacks. J R Soc Med 88(8):441-5, 1995

Fischer JF, Scheuler D. [Comparative studies on the mucolytic effectiveness of Mucosolvin oral and Mucosolvin inhalant]. Z Erkr Atmungsorgane 167(1-2):96-102, 1986

Gaby AR. Editorial: Asthma. The Townsend Letter for Doctors, April, 1987, p.73

Gaby AR. Literature review and commentary. Townsend Letter for Doctors & Patients December 1995

Gardner G. Gastrointestinal absorption of intact proteins. Ann Rev Nutr 8:329-50, 1988

Gong H Jr et al. Bronchodilator effects of caffeine in coffee. A dose-response study of asthmatic subjects. Chest 89(3):335-42, 1986

Green SM, Rothrock SG. Intravenous magnesium for acute asthma: failure to decrease emergency treatment duration or need for hospitalization. Ann Emerg Med 21(3):260-5, 1992

Greene LS. Asthma and oxidant stress: nutritional, environmental, and genetic factors. J Am Coll Nutr 14(4):317-24, 1995

Hasselmark L et al. Selenium supplementation in intrinsic asthma. Allergy 48:30-6, 1993

Haury VG. Blood serum magnesium in bronchial asthma and its treatment by the administration of magnesium sulfate. J Lab Clin Med 26:340-4, 1940

Hederos C-H, Berg A. Epogam evening primrose oil treatment in atopic dermatitis and asthma. Arch Dis Child 75:494-7, 1996

Hill J et al. Investigation of the effect of short-term change in dietary magnesium intake in asthma. Eur Respir J 10(10):2225-9, 1997

Hodge L et al. Increased consumption of polyunsaturated oils may be a cause of increased prevalence of childhood asthma. Aust N Z J Med 24:727, 1994

Hodge L. Consumption of oily fish and childhood asthma risk. Med J Australia 164:137-40, 1996

Hoj L et al. A double-blind controlled trial of elemental diet in severe, perennial asthma. Allergy 36:257-62, 1981

Kadrabova J et al. Selenium status is decreased in patients with intrinsic asthma. Biol Trace Elem Res 52:241-8, 1996

Kordansky DW et al. Effect of vitamin C on antigen induced bronchospasm. J Allergy Clin Immunol 63(1):61-4, 1979

Landon RA, Young, EA. Role of magnesium in regulation of lung function. J Am Diet Assoc 93(6):674-7, 1993

Maisel FE, Somkin E. Treatment of asthmatic paroxysm with nicotinic acid. J Allergy 13:397-403, 1942

Malmgren R et al. Lowered glutathione-peroxidase activity in asthmatic patients with aspirin intolerance. Allergy 41:43-5, 1986

Malo J-L et al. Lack of acute effects of ascorbic acid on spirometry and airway responsiveness to histamine in subjects with asthma. J Allergy Clin Immunol 78(6):1153-58, 1986

Masuev KA. [The effect of polyunsaturated fatty acids on the biochemical indices of bronchial asthma patients]. Ter Arkh 69(3):33-5, 1997

Matuschak GM. Liver-lung interactions in critical illness. New Horizons: The Science and Practice of Acute Medicine 2(4):488-504, November, 1994

May C. Objective clinical and laboratory studies of immediate hypersensitivity reactions to foods in asthmatic children. J. Allergy Clin. Immunol. 58:500-512, 1978

McNamara RM et al. Intravenous magnesium sulfate in the management of acute respiratory failure complicating asthma. Ann Emerg Med 18(2):197-9, 1989

Millman M et al. Use of acetylcysteine in bronchial asthma - another look. Ann Allergy 54(4):294-6, 1985

Misso NL et al. Reduced platelet glutathione peroxidase activity and serum selenium concentration in atopic asthmatic patients. Clin Exp Allergy 26(7):838-47, 1996

Mohsenin V et al. Effect of ascorbic acid on response to methacholine challenge in asthmatic subjects. Am Rev Resp Dis 127:143-7, 1983

Mohsenin V et al. Effect of vitamin C on NO2-induced airway hyporesponsiveness in normal subjects. Am Rev Respir Dis 136:1408-11, 1987

Nannini LJ Jr, Hofer, D. Effect of inhaled magnesium sulfate on sodium metabisulfite-induced bronchoconstriction in asthma. Chest 111(4):858-61, 1997

Papaioannou R, Pfeiffer CC. Sulfite sensitivity - unrecognized threat. Is molybdenum the cause? J Orthomol Psychiatry 13(2):105-10, 1984

Pearson D et al. Selenium status in relation to reduced glutathione peroxidase activity in aspirin-sensitive asthma. Clin Exp Allergy 21:203-8, 1991

Pelikan Z, Pelikan-Filipek M. Bronchial response to the food ingestion challenge. Ann Allergy 58(3):164-72, 1987

Petrov D, Stoeva N. [Sodium, potassium, calcium and magnesium metabolism in patients with allergic-infectious bronchial asthma.] Vutr Boles 23(1):85-90, 1984

Pistelli R et al. Respiratory symptoms and bronchial responsiveness are related to dietary salt intake and urinary potassium excretion in male children. Eur Respir J 6(4):517-22, 1993

Pletsityi KD et al. [Vitamin E: immunocorrecting effect in bronchial asthma patients]. Vopr Med Khim 41(4):33-36, 1995

Reynolds RD, Natta CL. Depressed plasma pyridoxal phosphate concentrations in adult asthmatics. Am. J. Clin. Nutr. 41:684-88, 1985

Rozanov EM et al. [Vitamin PP and C allowances and their correction in the treatment of bronchial asthma patients.] Vopr Pitan (6):21-24, 1987

Scadding GK et al. Poor sulphoxidation ability in patients with food sensitivity. Br Med J 297:105-7, 1988

Schachter EN, Schlesinger A. The attenuation of exercise-induced bronchospasm by ascorbic acid. Ann Allergy 49:146-50, 1982

Schwartz J, Weiss ST. Dietary factors and their relation to respiratory symptoms. The Second National Health and Nutrition Examination Survey. Am J Epidemiol 132(1):67-76, 1990

Schwartz J, Weiss ST. Caffeine intake and asthma symptoms. Ann Epidemiol 2:672-35, 1992

Schwartz J, Weiss ST. Relationship between dietary vitamin C intake and pulmonary function in the First National Health and Nutrition Examination Survey (NHANES I). Am J Clin Nutr 59:110-14, 1994

Simon RA et al. Sulfite-sensitive asthma. Res. Instit. of Scripps Clinic Scientific Report 39:57-58, 1982-83

Singh RB et al. Dietary intake and plasma levels of antioxidant vitamins in health and disease: a hospital-based case-control study. J Nutr Environ Med 5:235-42, 1995

Soutar A et al. Bronchial reactivity and dietary antioxidant. Thorax 52(2):166-70, 1997

Stenius-Aarniala B et al. Evening primrose oil and fish oil are ineffective as supplementary treatment of bronchial asthma. Ann Allergy 62(6):534-47, 1989

Sur S et al. Double-blind trial of pyridoxine (vitamin B6) in the treatment of steroid-dependent asthma. Ann Allergy 70:147-52, 1993

Troisi RJ et al. A prospective study of diet and adult-onset asthma. Am J Respir Crit Care Med 151:1401-8, 1995

Urge G et al. Effect of dietary tryptophan restrictions on clinical symptoms in patients with endogenous asthma. Allergy 38:211-12, 1983

Volkl KP, Schneider B. [Therapy of respiratory tract diseases with N-acetylcysteine. An open therapeutic observation study of 2,512 patients]. Fortschr Med 110(18):346-50, 1992

Wright JV. Vitamin B-12 and asthma. Let's Live, June, 1986, pp. 16 & 18

Wright J. Vitamin B12: Powerful protection against asthma. Int Clin Nutr Rev 9(4):185-8, 1989a

Wright J, Littleton K. Defects in sulphur metabolism. Int Clin Nutr Rev 9(3):118-19, 1989b

Wright JV. Asthma and molybdenum Part I. Let's Live, May, 1991

CANCER

See Also: BENIGN BREAST DISEASE
CERVICAL DYSPLASIA
IMMUNODEPRESSION

NUTRITIONAL TREATMENT GUIDE

✓ = Efficacy generally accepted.
* = Efficacy *demonstrated* by controlled human trials.
[+] = Efficacy *suspected* from uncontrolled human trials.
[-] = Efficacy *suspected* from indirect data.
? = Efficacy *challenged* in a study of similar design.

I. PREVENTION

A. Dietary Factors that may Reduce Cancer Risk:

* high **Dietary Fiber** intake *(in familial adenomatous polyposis, to reduce risk of colon cancer)*

- -

[-] **high Dietary Fiber diet** *(in general)*
[-] high **Fish** intake
[-] high **Fruit and Vegetable** intake
[-] **low Cholesterol diet**
[-] **low Fat diet**
[-] **low Protein, high Carbohydrate diet**
[-] avoid **Alcohol**
[-] avoid **Fried** foods
[-] avoid **Cured, Smoked, Browned or Charred Meats**
[-] drink **Hard, Unchlorinated Water**
[-] minimize **Salt**
[-] avoid **Sugar**

B. Nutrients that may Reduce Cancer Risk:

* **Gamma Linolenic Acid:** *to reduce rectal mucosal cell proliferation:* 2.5-7.7 g omega-3 fatty acids from fish oil
* **Lactulose:** *to reduce risk of colorectal cancer:* 20 g daily
* **Selenium:** 200 μg daily
* **Vitamin A:** *in oral leukoplakia, to reverse lesions:* 60 mg per week
* **Vitamin E:** *to reduce risk of prostate cancer:* 50 mg daily
* ? **Beta-Carotene** (Warning: may possibly increase cancer risk.)
* ? **Folic Acid:** *in cervical dysplasia, to reduce risk of cervical carcinoma:* 10 mg daily
* ? **Vitamin E:** *to reduce risk of colorectal cancer:* ? 50-400 IU daily
to reduce risk of stomach cancer: ? 50-400 IU daily

- -

[+] **Folic Acid**: *in ulcerative colitis, to reduce risk of colon cancer:* 10 mg daily
in bronchial squamous metaplasia, to reduce risk of lung cancer: 10 mg daily
[+] **Vitamin A**: *to reduce risk of squamous cell carcinoma:* 25,000 IU daily
[+] **Vitamin E**: (in general) ? 50 to 400 IU daily

- -

[-] **Butyric Acid**: (colon cancer)
[-] **Calcium deficiency:** ≈ 1 g daily
[-] **Carotenoids** (mixed)
[-] **Flavonoids**
[-] **Folic Acid deficiency:** 800 μg daily
[-] **Glutathione**
[-] **Inositol Hexaphosphate** (phytic acid)
[-] **Iodine deficiency:** repletion
[-] **Magnesium deficiency:** ≈ 400 mg daily
[-] **N-acetylcysteine**
[-] **Niacin deficiency:** 50 to 100 mg daily
[-] **Omega-3 Fatty Acids**: *example:* MaxEPA 1 g caps [180 mg EPA; 120 mg DHA] 10 to 20 daily
[-] **Omega-6 Fatty Acids**: *example:* evening primrose oil 500 mg caps [7-10% GLA] 6 to 8 daily
[-] **Omega-9 Fatty Acids**: olive oil
[-] **Phytosterols**: (colon cancer)
[-] **Riboflavin deficiency:** 5 to 10 mg daily
[-] **Selenium deficiency:** 200 μg daily
[-] **Vitamin A deficiency:** 50,000 IU daily for 6 weeks (10,000 IU daily during pregnancy)
[-] **Vitamin B_6 deficiency:** 50 to 100 mg daily
[-] **Vitamin C**: ? 500 mg twice daily
[-] **Zinc**: zinc sulfate 220 mg twice daily *AND* **Copper** 2 mg daily

C. Other Nutritional Factors that may Reduce Cancer Risk:

[-] ***Lactobacillus acidophilus*** (colon cancer)

D. Toxic Exposures that may Increase Cancer Risk:

[-] **Arsenic**
[-] **Cadmium**
[-] **Nickel**

II. TREATMENT

A. Administration may Treat Cancer:

* **Alkylglycerols** (A.B. Astra, Sweden): 200 mg 3 times daily
* ***Lactobacillus casei***: *in bladder cancer, to reduce relapses:* 1 g 3 times daily
* **Niacin**: *in bladder cancer, to reduce relapses following surgery and radiation when combined with aspirin*
* **Proteolytic enzymes** (example: Wobe-Mucos® 4 tablets 3 times daily)
* **Vitamin A and the Retinoids**

- -

* ? **Vitamin C**: 10 g to 50 g daily in divided doses as tolerated, starting with IV administration

- -

[+] **Cartilage Extract**: *example:* Catrix 3 g every 8 hours (4 month trial)

[+] **Coenzyme Q_{10}**: 90 mg to 390 mg daily
[+] **reduced Glutathione**: (hepatocellular carcinoma) 5 g daily dissolved in juice
[+] **Omega-3 Fatty Acids**: 18 g fish oil daily
[+] **Shark Cartilage Extract**: ? 30 g daily orally, or delivered vaginally or rectally as a suspension
[+] **Vitamin D** and **Calcium**: (parathyroid cancer)

- -

[-] **Butyric Acid**
[-] **L-Glutamine**
[-] **Magnesium**: (hemolymphoreticular malignancies)
[-] **Vitamin D** (in general)
[-] **Zinc deficiency:** *to restore failing immune function:* zinc sulfate 220 mg twice daily *AND* **Copper** 2 mg daily

B. Administration may Enhance the Therapeutic Effect of Radiation and/or Chemotherapy:

* **Vitamin C**: 5 g daily in divided doses (radiation)

- -

[+] **Vitamin A**: 200,000 IU daily for 10 days (radiation & chemotherapy)

- -

[-] **L-Glutamine**: (radiation & chemotherapy)
[-] **Vitamin E**: (chemotherapy)

C. Administration may Reduce the Adverse Effects of Chemotherapy:

* **Glutamine**: *to reduce GI side effects (diarrhea and the need for parenteral nutrition and antifungal treatment):* 6 g 3 times daily dissolved in water starting 3 days prior to chemotherapy
* **Glutathione (reduced)**: *cisplatin:* 1.5 g/m^2 in 100 mg normal saline over 15 minutes
* **Vitamin E**: *to prevent and treat oral mucositis:* topical application

- -

[+] **Coenzyme Q_{10}**: *adriamycin:* 30 mg daily
[+] **L-Glutamine:** *to reduce oral mucositis:* 4 g twice daily given as a suspension (swish & swallow)
[+] **Proteolytic enzymes**: *example:* Wobe-Mucos®
[+] **Selenium**: *cisplatin and others:* 200 μg or more daily
[+] **Vitamin E**: *adriamycin:* 1600 IU dl-α-tocopherol acetate starting 5-7 days prior to chemotherapy

- -

[-] **Niacin**: *adriamycin*
[-] ? **N-Acetylcysteine**: *cyclophosphamide, ifosfamide, adriamycin:* ? 2 to 3 g every 6 hours

D. Administration may Reduce Radiation Injuries:

* **Alkylglycerols (A.B. Astra, Sweden):** 200 mg 3 times daily
* **Glutathione (reduced)**: 1200 mg IV
* ***Lactobacillus acidophilus***: *to protect against damage to the GI tract:* product containing 2 x 10^9 viable organisms in a 6.5% lactulose-containing yogurt starting 5 days before radiotherapy
* **Niacin**: 0.5 to 1 g 3 times daily *with* aspirin 500 mg daily

- -

[+] **Hydrolyzed Protein**: *to protect against damage to the GI tract*
[+] **N-Acetyl-Cysteine**: *to protect against skin damage* (topical ointment)
[+] **Proteolytic enzymes**: *example:* Wobe-Mucos®

- -

[-] **Glutamine**: *to protect against enteritis*

There are vast numbers of epidemiologic, animal and *in vitro* studies whose results suggest that dietary factors exert a powerful influence upon cancer risk. Once a precancerous lesion has developed, results of small human intervention trials suggest that nutritional factors may help to determine whether certain lesions will either recede or progress to cancer.

One estimate is that 35% of cancer deaths are attributable to diet, with a range of 10 to 70%; another is that 40% of cancer deaths in men and 60% in women are attributable to diet. Surprisingly, considering the vastness of the research literature, the experimental evidence that nutritional interventions will affect an established cancer in humans is quite meager.

DIETARY FACTORS

Malnutrition

Malnutrition may be of the *marasmus* type when food intake in general is inadequate, or of the *kwashiorkor* type when there is specifically inadequate protein intake. It is a common finding in cancer patients, and one that adversely affects both survival and the quality of life *(Rivadeneira)*. For example, although acute weight loss is, by itself, an inadequate measure of nutritional status *(Delmore)*, a study of over 3,000 patients enrolled in 12 chemotherapy protocols found that median survival was significantly shorter for patients enrolled in 9 of the protocols who had experienced weight loss prior to chemotherapy *(Dewys)*.

In addition to its overall salutary effects upon survival and the quality of life, nutritional repletion is specifically associated with the return of immunocompetence, a reduction in sepsis, normalization of wound healing, and an apparent increase in tumor response to chemotherapy *(Copeland)*.

Low Fat Diets

Fat intake, more often than any other dietary factor, has been repeatedly found to be directly correlated with the risk of cancer in a number of locations. While many cancers have been implicated, these especially include cancers of the colon, breast and prostate *(Bueno-de-Mesquita;Hursting)*.

Whether this association indicates a causal relationship is unclear. Indirect evidence suggesting a causal relationship does exist. For example, animals fed high-fat diets do develop cancers at these same sites more readily *(Carroll,1991)*, and decreasing dietary fat has been shown to increase natural-killer-cell activity in healthy humans *(Barone,1989)*. However, since fat is calorie-dense, it may simply be an indicator of a high total energy intake *(Klurfeld)*, and a high energy intake is suspected of increasing the risk of these same three cancers *(Bueno-de-Mesquita)*. Other criticisms include the crudeness of the dietary assessments, the lack of supporting human intervention trials, and the failure to detail the type of fat *(Mann)*.

For example, the importance of detailing the type of fat has been shown in studies concerning the risk of colon cancer. While the intake of animal fat is positively associated with colon cancer risk, the intake of vegetable fat is negatively associated and thus may actually be protective *(Galli)*; thus grouping animal and vegetable fats together could result in misleading conclusions.

The prevailing theory to explain the relationship between a high fat diet and colon cancer postulates that fat promotes this disease by increasing the levels of fatty and bile acids within the colon. These acids irritate and damage the epithelial cells of the colon. As a result of this cellular destruction, an increase in the rate of cellular proliferation occurs *(Cats)*.

Fried foods

The intake of fried foods has been found to be directly associated with the risk of several cancers. This includes malignant glioma *(Böing,1993)*, ovarian cancer *(Snowdon)*, and urothelial cancer *(Bruemmer)*. In regard to colorectal cancer, while cancer risk for the frequent intake of meat fried until it developed a medium or lightly browned surface was actually lower than that for frequent intake of boiled meat, the *highest* risk was clearly associated with the frequent intake of meat fried with a heavily browned surface *(Gerhardsson de Verdier)*.

Moreover, fats tend to oxidize during deep frying, and women with mammary dysplasia (which indicates a high risk for developing breast cancer) have been shown to excrete about twice as much urinary malonaldehyde, a marker of lipid peroxidation, as normals *(Boyd)*.

Hydrogenated Oils and Trans Fats

Avoidance of partially hydrogenated oils containing *trans* fats has also been advocated as helpful in preventing cancer as a positive relationship between *trans* fat intake and cancer incidence has been noted *(Enig;Kinsella)*. Others, however, believe that reliable data have yet to support concerns about the intake of *trans* fats so long as people consume a balanced diet containing adequate linoleic acid (an omega-6 essential fatty acid) *(Hunter)*. Indeed, other studies have found no relationship between the intake of *trans* fats and cancer risk *(Petrek)*. Further studies should help to clarify the issue.

Low Cholesterol Diets

Cancer risk has been positively correlated with dietary cholesterol in several epidemiological studies of specific cancers, including glioma (a form of brain cancer) *(Kaplan)*, laryngeal cancer *(Kolonel)*, lung cancer *(Hinds)* and ovarian cancer *(Risch)*.

In a study of the diets of over 16,000 Seventh-Day Adventist women, consumption of fried eggs showed the strongest association between specific dietary components and fatal ovarian cancer. The authors hypothesized that the production of cytotoxic oxidation products of cholesterol by frying eggs may interfere with cholesterol biosynthesis and consequently the manufacture of ovarian hormones *(Snowdon)*.

The relationship of cancer risk to *serum* cholesterol concentrations is more complex - possibly because a lowering of serum cholesterol is a very early sign of established cancer *(Sherwin)*. Both elevated *(Holtzman)* and very low *(Sherwin)* serum cholesterol levels have been found to be associated with an increased risk of colon cancer. However, evidence has yet to appear that demonstrates a causal relationship between low serum cholesterol and an increased risk of developing cancer *(Kritz)*.

Low Protein Diets

In addition to keeping the percent of energy from fat low (see the discussion above), the evidence suggests that protein intake should be kept relatively low, especially in relation to carbohydrates. For example, milk, liver, butter and oil (primarily unsaturated) intake (foods high in protein and/or fat) was found to be associated with a high risk of non-Hodgkin's lymphoma, while the intake of whole-grain bread and pasta (high carbohydrate foods) was associated with a low risk of the disease *(Franceschi,1989)*. Similarly, compared to normals, women with endometrial cancer were found to consume a greater percentage of their calories from fat and a lower percentage of their calories from carbohydrates *(Goodman,1997a)*.

Other malignancies whose incidence have shown a positive association with protein intake and/or a negative association with carbohydrate intake, include breast cancer *(Kolonel)*, brain cancer *(Kaplan)*, colorectal cancer *(Sandler)*, pancreatic cancer *(Böing,1985)*, prostate cancer *(Vlajinac)* and stomach cancer *(Harrison)*, although the data are not entirely consistent.

The results of animal experiments agree with the observations of human dietary habits. Even though they consume more calories, protein-restricted animals have been shown to develop fewer pre-neoplastic lesions and tumors than those fed a high protein diet *(Youngman)*.

Hydrolyzed Protein

Protein that has been partly broken down into its components by hydrolysis may have a special application in cancer treatment. When provided prior to radiation therapy, the ingestion of hydrolyzed protein has been found to minimize the damage to the gastrointestinal tract caused by the treatment. While the mechanism is not known, the protective effect may be because of reduced damage to the gut due to protein hydrolysis *(Chlebowski)*.

Red Meat

Red meat, an important source of dietary protein, has certain cancer risks associated with its consumption, one of which - its fat content - has already been discussed. For example, a strong correlation has been found between red meat consumption and colon cancer, possibly due to the formation of N-nitroso compounds in the gut *(Bingham)*. In one study, subjects were fed either beef, lamb or pork 60 g or 600 g daily which was fried in butter to maximize mutagen content. Higher red meat intakes led to much higher levels of N-nitroso compounds in the feces *(Bingham)*.

Higher levels of N-nitroso compounds are also formed when the meat has been cured with nitrate or nitrite (which turns it red). These substances are not only carcinogenic in animals, but are also linked epidemiologically with, for example, stomach cancer *(van Loon)*, glioma *(Böing,1993)*, laryngeal cancer *(Esteve)*, leukemia *(Peters)* and urinary tract cancer *(Wilkens)*.

Moreover, browning and charring of meat results in the formation of carcinogenic heterocyclic amines from the pyrolysis of proteins and amino acids. The longer the meat is cooked, and the higher the temperature, the more carcinogens are created *(Anonymous,1996)*.

Both curing and broiling were investigated in a study of 234 children with cancer. Maternal hot-dog consumption of one or more times per week was associated with twice the risk of childhood brain tumors. Among children, eating hamburgers one or more times a week was also associated with twice the risk of brain tumors, and the combination of no supplemental vitamins and eating meats was associated more strongly with both acute lymphocytic leukemia and brain tumors *(Sarasua)*.

Fish

Fish consumption has a very different relationship to cancer risk and mortality than that of red meat consumption. For example, data from 66 countries showed that the consumption of animal products was most strongly associated with breast cancer mortality, while fish products appeared to exert protective effects *(Hebert)*. Similar protective effects have been noted in regard to the risk of colorectal cancer *(Franceschi,1997)* and of laryngeal cancer *(Esteve)*.

However, one study found the intakes of both fish protein and fish fat (but not the intake of animal fat) to be *positively* associated with the risk of stomach cancer *(Kolonel)*. While this finding is unexplained, one possible explanation is that the population examined (people living in Hawaii) fried much of their fish, but not much of their meat.

Dietary Fiber

Numerous epidemiological studies have found an inverse relationship between the intake of dietary fiber and cancer risk. However, a recent large cohort study, reported in *The New England Journal of Medicine*, found no association between dietary fiber intake and the risks of colorectal cancer and colorectal adenoma *(Fuch)*.

Food fibers are complex carbohydrates which are subdivided into soluble and insoluble fibers. *Soluble fibers* are present in fruits, vegetables, and certain grains like oats. They are metabolized in the small intestine and especially in the large intestine through bacterial enzymes. The resulting products increase stool size only moderately, but have appreciable effects in modifying the metabolism of colon carcinogens.

In contrast, *insoluble fibers*, present in sizable amounts in bran cereals, like wheat or rice, are not significantly metabolized by enzymes in the intestinal flora. They increase stool size substantially through water retention and other mechanisms. The larger bulk dilutes carcinogens, especially tumor promoters such as secondary bile acids, resulting in lower risk of colon cancer in animals and in humans *(Weisburger,1993)*.

The data from epidemiological studies, however, often fail to clarify whether the associations are due to dietary fiber (and specifically which fibers), or due to other factors linked to a high fiber diet. For example, phytic acid (inositol hexaphosphate) (found, for example, in cereal grains, nuts, and seeds) could be as important as fiber in suppressing colon cancer *(Graf)*, and the same may apply to other nutrients found in fiber-rich food such as beta-carotene and vitamin C *(Ausman)*. There is even reason to question whether dietary fiber is truly protective against colon cancer, as fermentable (soluble) fiber substrates can stimulate the proliferation of colonic epithelial cells *(Wasan)*.

In addition to its possible value in preventing colon cancer, evidence from animal models and human studies also suggests that dietary fiber - or perhaps a high fiber diet - may lower the risk of breast cancer *(Weisburger,1993)*.

Several hypotheses have been advanced to explain its efficacy which center around the salutary effects of a high fiber diet on estrogen metabolism. A high fiber diet reduces circulating estrogens by reducing their enterohepatic circulation, and it usually has a high content of isoflavones and lignans, substances that compete with estrogen for binding sites. Diets high in fiber are usually rich in complex carbohydrates, and a high fiber, high complex carbohydrate diet reduces circulating estrogen levels by improving insulin sensitivity. They are also low in fat and, as noted above, dietary fat appears to increase breast cancer risk. Finally, obesity, which is relatively rare in people whose fiber intake is high, is associated with the biologically active, pro-carcinogenic, 16-alpha estrone metabolites *(Stoll,1996)*.

There are also inverse associations between dietary fiber intake and other cancers. Endometrial cancer risk is inversely related to dietary fiber from cereals, vegetables and fruit *(Goodman,1997a)*. In one study, women who consumed several servings daily of vegetables, fresh fruits, and whole grain breads and cereals had a 40 to 60% lower risk of endometrial cancer *(Levi)*. Gastric cancer risk is inversely related to fruit and vegetable intake *(Zheng)* as well as whole grain intake *(Jacobs)*. Ovarian cancer risk is inversely related to the consumption of vegetable, but not fruit or cereal fiber *(Risch)*, while pancreatic cancer risk is inversely related to the consumption of fiber from vegetable, fruit and cereals *(Howe)*.

In regard to prostate cancer, plasma levels of both testosterone and estradiol-17 beta (both of which are directly related to cancer risk) have a significant inverse relationship with dietary fiber intake *(Howie)*. Moreover, the more fiber consumed (especially lignin and insoluble fibers), the greater was the binding of estrogen and testosterone, suggesting that the free levels of these hormones in the circulation was lowered *(Ross)*. In one recent study, however, men in the highest quartile for fiber intake had 4 times the risk of developing prostate cancer *(Vlajinac)*.

Fruits and Vegetables

Consumption of fruits and vegetables has been suggested to be protective against a wide range of cancers, although the data regarding hormone-related cancers are weak *(Bueno-de-Mesquita)*. In fact, for most cancer sites, even after controlling for potentially confounding factors, persons with low fruit and vegetable intakes (the lower quartile) experience about twice the risk of cancer of those with a high intake *(Block)*. A review of 206 human epidemiologic studies and 22 animal studies found that the evidence suggested a protective effect against cancers of the stomach, esophagus, lung, oral cavity and pharynx, endometrium, pancreas and colon.

Raw vegetables appeared to have the most protective effect against cancers, followed by allium vegetables (garlic and onions), carrots, green vegetables, cruciferous vegetables and tomatoes *(Steinmetz)*. Yellow-orange vegetables were also protective, as were tomatoes and strawberries *(Colditz)*.

Soy products lower the risk of cancer over and above their low-fat, high-fiber content. They contain several anti-cancer compounds, including phytoestrogens such as isoflavones, protease inhibitors, phytosterols and saponins. Moreover, in addition to human epidemiologic studies, there are numerous animals studies that found soy or soy isoflavones to be protective against experimental carcinogenesis *(Messina)*.

Vegetarian diets

Low in fat while high in protective nutrients such as fiber, phytoestrogens and carotenoids, it is not surprising that a vegetarian diet is associated with a reduced incidence of several cancers. In one study, cancer mortality was decreased by more than one-half in people who followed a vegetarian lifestyle for at least 20 years *(Frentzel-Beyme)*.

The differences in vegetarians responsible for their reduced cancer risk are not clear; however, there is evidence, for example, that the cytotoxicity of their peripheral blood lymphocytes are twice as high as in omnivores *(Malter)*. Also, many neoplastic cells have lost activity of the enzyme delta-6-saturase, and most vegetables lack this enzyme. Thus a vegetarian diet would deprive these cells of higher-chain fatty acids which would result in alterations that would make them easier prey for immune defenses *(Siguel)*.

Vegetarians have reduced risks of several specific cancers. Breast cancer risk is reduced *(Hebert)*, possibly because of lowering of estrogen levels *(Goldin, 1982)*. Colon cancer risk is reduced *(Galli)*, possibly by reducing the levels of enzymes in the fecal microflora that may result in the formation of proximal carcinogens *(Goldin, 1980)*, the formation of N-nitroso compounds, the action of heterocyclic amines produced during cooking of meat protein, or the pro-oxidative effect of its iron content *(Hill)*.

The risks of esophageal cancer *(Srivastava)* and non-Hodgkin lymphoma *(Chiu)* are both lower. Inhibition of nitrosamine formation is believed to explain the reduced risk of stomach cancer *(Barale)*. As to the risk of pancreatic cancer, animal sources of calories, protein and fat all appear to contribute *(Ghadirian, 1991)*.

Milk Products

Conflicting results have been seen in studies relating the consumption of products derived from cow's milk and cancer incidence, undoubtedly because these are highly complex substances containing numerous factors with opposing actions in various proportions. The results of both epidemiologic and experimental studies suggest that dietary milk products may exert an inhibitory effect on the development of several types of tumors. For example, various types of cheeses and yogurt suppress the growth of several experimental tumors in mice. Recent studies have also shown improvement in cases of cancer of the oral cavity, stomach, rectum, lung and cervix with increased milk consumption.

It appears that the protective effect of dairy products may be largely explained by their whey protein content. Very rich in substrate for glutathione synthesis, whey protein diets result in increased glutathione concentration in certain tissues, and glutathione is an immune enhancer *(Bounous)* (See Glutathione below.)

Milk fat, on the other hand, could be the major explanation for the tumor-promoting effects. In a study of over 3,000 cancer patients, and 1,300 matched controls, cancer patients more often reported frequent *whole* (i.e. high animal fat) milk consumption, while control subjects were more likely to report never drinking whole milk. Moreover, although the overall pattern of effects were not fully explained by variations in milk fat content, some associations with cancer risk were found for a computerized index of milk fat intake *(Mettlin)*. These findings complement those from another study that found an inverse association between the intake of *low fat* dairy products and cancer risk at 5 sites in people from 20 countries *(Hursting)*.

Sugar

In addition to the possibility of procarcinogenic effects of dietary sugar itself, a high sugar intake is associated with the ingestion of low-fiber processed foods. Therefore, an association between sugar and cancer could be due to these other aspects of the diet that are commonly associated with a high sugar intake.

Chronic consumption of high amounts of sugar has been positively associated with the risk of biliary tract cancer. Experimental studies have shown that the chronically high sugar consumption may enhance biliary cholesterol saturation by elevating triglyceride levels and reducing HDL-lipoprotein levels, thereby increasing the risk of gallstone formation. The presence of gallstones may give rise to carcinogenesis through damage of the wall of the biliary system and subsequent increased cell division *(Moerman)*.

Sugar consumption has been consistently associated with the risk of colorectal cancer in a dose-response fashion *(WCRF Panel)*. This may be because a high sucrose diet increases mouth-to-anus transit time, despite decreasing the mouth-to-cecum time, and increases the fecal concentration of both total and secondary bile acids *(Bostick,1994)*.

Breast cancer mortality shows a positive correlation with dietary sugar, and a negative correlation with complex carbohydrates in the diet *(Carroll,1977)*. In fact, an epidemiologic survey of 21 countries has suggested that high sucrose intake is a major risk factor for the development of breast cancer in women over 45 years of age *(Seely)*. An adverse influence of sugar in promoting the development of breast cancer *(Hoehn)* as well as the mortality rate from breast cancer *(Santisteban)* has been shown in animal studies.

There is also epidemiological evidence relating sugar consumption to endometrial *(Levi)* and stomach *(Böing,1985;Cornee)* cancers.

Salt

Epidemiological studies have linked a high intake of dietary salt (sodium chloride) with a number of cancers. These include cancers of the bladder *(Vena)*, colorectal area *(Kune.1989)*, esophagus *(Gao)*, and Stomach *(Joossens)*. However, when 139 cases of confirmed brain tumors were compared to matched controls, the intake of sodium was *inversely* related to the risks of both types of tumors *(Kaplan)*.

Alcohol

Ethanol intake has been repeatedly associated with an increased cancer risk *(Mufti)*. Cancers whose risks are positively associated with alcohol intake include breast cancer *(Longnecker)*, colorectal cancer *(Giovannucci,1995)*, endometrial cancer *(Parazzini)*, esophageal cancer *(Cheng)*, laryngeal cancer *(Freudenheim)*, lung cancer *(Potter)*, malignant melanoma *(Bain)*, stomach cancer *(D'Avanzo)*, and upper aerodigestive tract (larynx, pharynx, mouth, esophagus) cancer *(Kune,1992)*.

Despite these frequent associations, ethanol is neither tumorigenic nor genotoxic in animals *(Anderson)*. One theory that is supported by animal research is that ethanol potentiates the carcinogenic risk associated with other environmental factors *(Anderson)*. Other experimental evidence suggests that ethanol promotes tumors under conditions in which it produces free radicals during its metabolism *(Mufti)*. The fact that ethanol is immunosuppressive may also be relevant *(Mufti)*. Finally, alcoholism, independent of the amount of alcohol ingested, may itself be a risk factor for as yet undetermined reasons *(Hedberg)*.

Coffee

Due to conflicting results, the relationship between coffee consumption and cancer risk remains unclear despite numerous studies. In animal studies, caffeine can either increase or decrease malignant cell development depending upon the carcinogen it is used with, the type of host cell, and the stage of the cell cycle in which it is introduced *(Pozniak)*. One animal study found that caffeine in a dosage roughly equivalent to that consumed in a typical Western diet had little or no effect unless the animals were folate-deficient. In that case, they developed increased chromosomal damage (micronuclei) in nucleated erythrocyte precursors *(MacGregor)*.

Other variables may also confound and thus obscure the relationship. A study of close to 3,000 people found that men who drank decaffeinated coffee exclusively had lower body mass indices, a diet lower in fat, and consumed more cruciferous vegetables. Women who consumed decaffeinated coffee exclusively also exercised, consumed cruciferous vegetables and took vitamin supplements more regularly *(Leviton)*.

A recent literature review concludes that, in the usual doses, coffee consumption appears to be safe in that it produces no potential genotoxic, mutagenic or carcinogenic effect. The authors warn, however, that coffee's effects with regard to the risk of cancers of the pancreas, colon, and urinary tract remain debatable *(Nehlig)*.

NUTRITIONAL FACTORS

VITAMINS

Folic Acid Deficiency

Cervical Cancer

Because folate may play a role in the carcinogenic process by affecting DNA synthesis and the speed of cell division *(González)*, numerous studies have examined the relationship between this nutrient and various cancers.

Women with untreated cervical cancer may have reduced levels of plasma folate *(Orr),* although this finding was not confirmed in another study *(Potischman)*. More important in regard to carcinogenesis is the presence of a *localized* deficiency of the vitamin, as deficiency of folic acid within the cervical tissues has been repeatedly shown to be positively associated with the development of cervical dysplasia - which may then progress to cervical cancer. Apparently, a folate deficiency in the cervical tissues facilitates the incorporation of human papilloma virus genomes at a fragile chromosomal site; then multiple nutritional, hormonal, and immunologic factors interact in a synergistic manner to determine whether the cell line becomes immortalized and invasive *(Butterworth,1992)*.

Oral folate supplementation is sometimes effective in reversing cervical dysplastic changes associated with a localized cervical folate deficiency *(Butterworth,1982)*. However, once the lesion is no longer early and preneoplastic, folate supplementation has not been shown to be effective *(Pottischman)*.

Colon Cancer

Colon cancer risk varies inversely with folate intake *(Ferraroni)* as well as with plasma and erythrocyte folate levels *(Porcelli)*. Theories to explain why folate deficiency may predispose to colon cancer include:

- Global and/or gene-specific DNA hypomethylation
- Increased DNA damage and abnormal DNA repair,
- Increased chromosomal fragility
- Impairment of immune function
- Secondary choline deficiency and activation of secondary transcellular signals *(Kim Y-I)*.

DNA methylation is an intermediate biomarker in the development of colorectal cancer and is significantly lower in carcinomas than adenomas *(Cravo)*. Evidence of the role of folate comes from a study in which folic acid 10 mg daily was found to increase the degree of DNA methylation of the rectal mucosa from patients with either adenomas or carcinomas whose neoplasms had been removed *(Cravo)*.

Patients with ulcerative colitis have both an increased risk of colon cancer and decreased folate levels, the latter due in part to treatment with sulfasalazine, a competitive inhibitor of folate absorption. They are thus an excellent sub-group to test the efficacy of folate supplementation in preventing colon cancer. Indeed, one research team has conducted retrospective studies to examine the issue and found that folate supplementation appeared to reduce the risk of colon dysplasia and cancer in this group of patients *(Lashner)*.

Lung Cancer

Localized folate deficiency may promote the development of lung cancer. Smokers have lower circulating folate levels than nonsmokers, but smokers with bronchial metaplasia (a precursor to lung cancer) have still lower folate levels.

When these smokers are supplemented with folate as well as with vitamin B_{12} under double-blind conditions, there is histological improvement of their lesions *(Heimberger,1988;Saito)*. Similarly, folate supplementation has been shown to suppress epithelial hyperplasia and metaplasia of the bronchial epithelium in a rat model *(Kamei)*.

Other Cancers

Early studies suggest that folate deficiency may increase the risk of other aerodigestive tract cancers *(Heimberger,1992)*. These include esophageal cancer *(van Helden)* and gastric cancer *(González)*.

Niacin

Neither deficiencies or excess of niacin have been shown to produce a consistent effect on carcinogenesis in animals *(Bryan)*. However, limiting niacin intake in humans results in a decrease of up to 70% of intracellular NAD, and evidence is accumulating that maintenance of intracellular NAD is a critical factor in responses to DNA damage *(Jacobson,1993a,b)*.

In a study of the cardiotoxicity of adriamycin in mice, niacin supplementation reduced the drug's cardiotoxicity without interfering with its antitumor effect *(Schmitt-Gräff)*. Also, when combined with aspirin and given during conventional treatment, niacin supplementation reduced relapses and increased 5-year survival in patients with advanced bladder carcinomas treated with surgery along with both pre- and post-operative gamma radiation, possibly due to the efficacy of the antithrombogenic effect of the two substances in reducing late complications of radiation therapy *(Popov)*.

Riboflavin Deficiency

The intake of riboflavin has been found to be inversely correlated with the risk of colorectal cancer *(La Vecchia)* and prostate cancer *(Kaul)*. Moreover, low blood riboflavin levels may be inversely correlated with the risk of esophageal cancer *(Guo)*.

It has been theorized that the protective effect of riboflavin may be due to its ability to induce DNA-repair enzymes *(La Vecchia)*.

Thiamine: A Warning

Not only is there little evidence that thiamine intake reduces cancer risk, but there is concern over whether thiamine supplementation should be contraindicated for cancer patients.

In a recent review, the authors noted that clinical and experimental data demonstrate increased thiamine utilization of human tumors and its interference with experimental chemotherapy. Moreover, anti-thiamine compounds significantly inhibit nucleic acid synthesis and tumor cell proliferation in *in vitro* and *in vivo* in several tumor models. They suggest that excessive thiamine supplementation may thwart cancer therapies, and recommend limiting thiamine supplementation while providing concomitant treatment with transketolase inhibitors *(Boros)*.

Not all authors agree, however. Based on human and animal studies, earlier investigators found that tumor formation was accompanied by the development of thiamine deficiency. They also found that, when cancer patients received thiamine supplements, not only was cancer growth not stimulated, but the impairment of vitamin metabolism seen in cancer was partially restored. Because of these findings, they have recommended that thiamine be included as part of the treatment program *(Trebukhina)*.

Until the picture clarifies, it appears rational to avoid massive thiamine supplementation in the treatment of cancer.

Vitamin A

Retinol (vitamin A alcohol) and its metabolites play a crucial role in regulating the differentiation and proliferation of epithelial cells, and are potent induces of apoptosis (cellular death). The effects of retinoids are thought to be mediated through the metabolite retinoic acid, which binds to nuclear retinoic acid receptors that then interact with specific retinoic acid response elements *(Sankaranarayanan)*.

Vitamin A intake has been shown to be inversely correlated to risk of several cancers. These include cancers of the bladder *(Bruemmer)*, colon *(Ghadirian,1997)*, endometrium *(Goodman,1997b)*, larynx *(Graham)*, liver *(Pan)*, lung *(Bond)*, and stomach *(Zheng)*. Multiple inverse correlations have been found between serum or plasma concentrations of vitamin A and both the risk of cancer in general *(Eichholzer)* and the risk of many specific cancers. In addition, low serum retinol levels have been found to be associated with a diminished response to chemotherapy *(Brown,1981)*.

Supplementation

Under double-blind conditions, supplementation with vitamin A reverses leukoplakia *(Stich)*. Moreover, in an open trial, supplementation with vitamin A for 5 years reduced the incidence of squamous cell carcinomas, but not of basal cell carcinomas, in a group of patients who were at moderate risk for skin cancer *(Moon)*. In another open trial, short-term, massive doses of vitamin A enhanced the therapeutic response of solid tumors to radiation and cyclophosphamide, although it increased leukopenia in response to the drug and delayed the recovery of the white blood count *(Hoefer-Janker)*.

Since, at clinically tolerable doses, vitamin A has shown only limited activity against neoplastic processes, synthetic derivatives are being developed to have an improved benefit-to-risk ratio. Retinoids have shown anti-cancer activity in regard to certain premalignancies such as actinic keratoses *(Alirezai)* as well as for several malignancies *(Muindi)*. Their efficacy appears to be limited because they primarily inhibit the promotion of carcinogenesis, but not the later phases of conversion and progression *(Muto)*.

Vitamin B_6 Deficiency

Since pyridoxine is a coenzyme in the biosynthesis of thymidine, a deficiency of which can increase mutagenesis, a vitamin B_6 deficiency could theoretically increase the vulnerability to cancer *(Prior)*. Indeed, mice exposed to experimental viral-induced cancer who are B_6-deficient demonstrate enhanced tumor susceptibility, increased tumor size and a lengthened regression time *(Ha)*. Moreover, occasional surveys have found that cancer patients were more likely than controls to have a reduced intake of vitamin B_6 *(Harrison)*.

Patients with both solid tumors *(Chrisley)* or leukemias *(Pais)* may be low in pyridoxal phosphate, the activated form of the vitamin, although both this finding and the finding of reduced intake in cancer patients fail to suggest whether the deficiency may have fostered carcinogenesis.

Vitamin B_{12}

There is some interesting, although fragmentary, literature relating vitamin B_{12} nutriture to hematopoietic malignancies. Vitamin B_{12} deficiency may present a blood picture and bone marrow appearance which can be mistaken for leukemia *(Dokal)*; thus the evaluation of vitamin B_{12} status is advisable when leukemia is suspected.

Marked elevation of serum concentrations of the both vitamin B_{12} and its binding proteins appears to be characteristic of acute promyelocytic leukemia *(Groopman)*. Moreover, in the case of hematopoietic malignancies, excessive replacement of vitamin B_{12} may have the potential of accelerating the progress of the malignancy *(Ahmann)*. Supplementation with the vitamin is therefore not advisable unless there is evidence of deficiency.

Vitamin C

Intake and Nutriture

There is strong evidence from numerous epidemiologic studies that the intake of vitamin C is inversely correlated with cancer risk *(Bendich)*. Moreover, there is an inverse correlation between cancer risk and plasma/serum levels of the vitamin *(Gey)*, as well as with other measures such as urinary levels in bladder cancer *(Schlegal)*, intragastric levels in intestinal metaplasia (a premalignant condition) *(Zhang)*, and leukocyte levels in familial adenomatous polyposis (another premalignant condition) *(Spigelman)*.

Specific effects of vitamin C have been identified in regard to its protective effect against the development of gastric cancer. These effects appear to be at an early stage of development, perhaps before gastric pH has increased as a result of extensive atrophy *(O'Toole)*. The results of both observational *(Rood)* and experimental *(Correa)* studies suggest that the presence of *Helicobacter pylori*, an established risk factor for gastric cancer, may be associated with reduced availability of ascorbic acid.

Supplementation

A comprehensive review of the published literature suggests that supplementation with pharmacologic dosages of vitamin C may reduce the risk of cancer at several sites *(Bendich)*. Not only may supplemental vitamin C kill tumor cells, but it may stimulate the host's immune system against the residual tumor cells *(Prasad,1980a)*. Unresolved, however, is disagreement over whether vitamin C supplementation can increase the survival time of terminal cancer patients *(Cameron,1978; Moertel;Riordan)*. A protocol for the use of vitamin C in cancer treatment has been published *(Cameron,1991)*.

Both *in vitro* and *in vivo*, the vitamin substantially inhibits the endogenous formation of carcinogenic nitrosamines and nitrosamides from dietary nitrites and nitrates, perhaps due to the reduction of nitrites into nitric oxide *(Singh VN)*. In addition, supplementation with vitamin C has been shown to reduce the mutagenicity of gastric juice *(O'Connor)* and to reduce gastric mucosal DNA damage *(Dyke)*.

The results of *in vitro* studies suggest that high, but not toxic, levels of vitamin C may enhance the effect of such chemotherapeutic agents as doxorubicin, cisplatin, paclitaxel *(Kurbacher)*, 5-flurouracil and bleomycin *(Prasad,1979)*. There is also early evidence that vitamin C supplementation may enhance the effect of radiation therapy. In an intriguing study which has only been published in summary form, 50 previously untreated cancer patients randomly received radiation therapy either with or without vitamin C 5 grams daily in divided doses. After 1 month, 87% of the study group compared to 55% of the controls showed a complete response to treatment (disappearance of all known disease). After 4 months, 63% of the study group compared to 45% of the controls continued to show a complete response.

After 1 month, progressive disease was seen in 3% of the study group and 5% of the controls; after 4 months, progressive disease was seen in 20% of the study group compared to 7% of the controls. In the control group, the 6-month survival rate was 45% in patients without disease and 55% in those with disease; in the study group it was 67% in those without disease and 33% in those with disease. Moreover, subjective responses, including ratings of pain and anorexia, favored vitamin C, and a comparison of other objective parameters such as weight loss and anemia also favored the vitamin *(Gupta)*.

A 42-year-old man with histologically proven, widely disseminated, reticulum cell sarcoma had a complete regression of his fatal illness exactly after receiving intravenous high-dose ascorbate administration. Some months later, a reduction in dosage coincided with reactivation of the disease process. The dosage was increased and the cancer quickly went back into remission. Seventeen years later, he was still alive (Cameron,1975;Campbell).

Vitamin D

The intake of vitamin D has been inversely related to the risk of colorectal cancer *(Martinez)*. An inverse relationship between serum levels of 25-hydroxy vitamin D and colorectal cancer risk has also been noted *(Garland,1989)*. Moreover, when sigmoidoscopic biopsies were taken from patients with familial adenomatous polyposis and exposed to the vitamin *in vitro*, cell production rates were reduced *(Thomas)*.

Exposure to sunlight is a measure of vitamin D nutriture, and breast cancer rates in the northeastern United States are almost twice as high as in the south and southwest where sunlight exposure is higher *(Garland,1990)*. A similar relationship has been found for the risk of death from both ovarian *(Lefkowitz)* and prostate *(Schwartz)* cancers.

Women with breast carcinomas whose tumors have vitamin D receptors have a significantly longer disease-free survival than those whose tumors are receptor-negative, thus suggesting a possible role for the vitamin in controlling breast cancer cell proliferation *(Colston)*. Similarly, men with a particular variant of the vitamin D receptor gene appear to have a reduced risk of requiring surgery for prostate cancer *(Taylor JA)*.

Supplementation

The results of *in vitro* studies suggest that supplementation with calcitriol (1,25-dihydroxyvitamin D) may inhibit cell proliferation of several types of cancer cells, including melanoma, breast, bone, leukemia *(Anonymous,1987)*, prostate and osteosarcoma *(Fife)*. Calcitriol is known to decrease the proliferation of parathyroid cells *(Silver)*. While little is known about the efficacy of vitamin D or calcitriol in treating cancer of the parathyroid, a young woman with parathyroid cancer whose parathyroid hormone levels rose 3 months following cancer surgery had normalization of parathyroid levels so long as she received either vitamin D or calcitriol daily along with calcium *(Palmierei-Sevier)*.

Many questions concerning its efficacy and toxicity in treating cancer patients remain to be answered before vitamin D, or a synthetic analogue, becomes an acceptable cancer treatment *(Reichel)*.

Vitamin E

Vitamin E intake has been inversely correlated with the risk of several cancers, including those of the breast *(Negri)*, cervix *(Verreault)*, skin *(Kirkpatrick)*, and the aerodigestive tract: mouth, pharynx and larynx *(Nomura)*, lung *(Albanes)*, esophagus *(Gao)*, stomach *(Zheng)*, colon and rectum *(Ghadirian,1997)*. Similarly blood levels of vitamin E have been negatively correlated with cancer risk *(Malvy;Singh RB)*.

Supplementation

In a prospective study of over 11,000 elderly people, the use of separate vitamin E supplements at baseline reduced the risk of cancer mortality by 29%. Even more striking was the finding that, if vitamin E supplements were used both in the past and at baseline, the relative risk was reduced by 59% *(Losonczy)*. These findings are consistent with the results of many animal and *in vitro* experiments which have shown that the supplementation of the diet with vitamin E within a certain dose range reduced the risk of chemical- and radiation-induced cancers *(Prasad,1992)*.

Like vitamin C, vitamin E blocks the formation of carcinogenic nitrosamines in the stomach *(Lathia)*. Supplementation also dramatically reduces the level of mutagens in the stool *(Bruce)*.

Although, *in vitro*, vitamin E induces apoptosis in colorectal cancer cells *(Chinery)*, whether vitamin E supplementation reduces the risk of colorectal cancer remains uncertain. Under double-blind conditions, older male smokers who took a relatively small-dosage vitamin E supplement (50 mg daily) had fewer incident cases (68 versus 81) *(Albanes)*. However, assuming this reduction is confirmed, it does not appear to be due to decreased formation of colorectal adenomas since, in another double-blind study, 4 years after a group of patients colorectal adenomas took either vitamin E 400 mg daily or placebo, the relative risk of new adenomas for both groups was virtually identical *(Greenberg)*.

Moreover, two other double-blind studies investigated the combination of vitamins C and E for patients with colorectal polyps. One found a reduction in risk that could have been due to chance *(DeCosse)*, while the other found no effect *(McKeown-Eyssen)*.

The results of other vitamin E supplementation trials are also mixed. In a double-blind Finnish study of male older male smokers, after 5 to 8 years, supplementation with 50 mg daily had no apparent effect on the incidence of lung cancer *(Anonymous,1994)*. In regard to stomach cancer, a small study of patients with atrophic gastritis, roughly half of whom would be expected to have precancerous changes, 55 mg daily of vitamin E caused a moderate decrease in the activity of ornithine decarboxylase, an enzyme that may have a role in gastric carcinogenesis *(Bukin)*. However, in the same double-blind Finnish study of older male smokers alluded to earlier, 50 mg of alpha tocopherol given for 5 to 8 years was associated with an increase in cases of stomach cases (70 cases) versus placebo controls (56 cases) *(Albanes)*.

In an open trial, 43 patients with oral leukoplakia, a precancerous condition, received 400 IU daily of alpha tocopherol. For 20 of them, the lesions decreased by at least 50%, while 9 had improvement in the stage of dysplasia *(Benner)*. This finding is consistent with the results of 2 retrospective studies which found vitamin E supplementation to be associated with a lower risk of oral cancer *(Barone,1992;Gridley)*.

As to prostate cancer, the double-blind Finnish study of older male smokers also examined subsequent cases of prostate cancer 5 to 8 years following supplementation with 50 mg of alpha-tocopherol. The supplemented group had only 99 cases of prostate cancer compared to 151 cases in the control group, a 32% decrease. Also, mortality from prostate cancer was 40% lower in men receiving vitamin E *(Heinonen)*.

Vitamin E supplementation may also be useful as an adjuvant to chemotherapy. Results of *in vitro* studies suggest that it may enhance the effect of adriamycin (doxorubicin), 5-flurouracil *(Chinery)* and vincristine *(Prasad,1980b)*, thus permitting reductions in dosage. Vitamin E supplementation has had mixed results in preventing alopecia from developing in patients receiving adriamycin *(Martin-Jimenez;Wood)*. While research is still preliminary, other adverse effects of adriamycin that may possibly be reduced by vitamin E are cardiac and skin toxicity *(Faber)* and hepatic injury *(Pascoe)*. Topical vitamin E supplementation may also reduce chemotherapy-induced oral mucositis *(Wadleigh)*.

MINERALS

Minerals in Drinking Water

Water hardness, which is usually due to dissolved calcium and magnesium, is inversely correlated with the risk of cancers of the digestive tract *(Norie)*, including gastric *(Yang,1998)* and colon *(Yang,1997)* cancers. Since water is free of chelating agents, the minerals it contains are usually absorbed twice as well as the minerals in foods, although their concentrations are usually small in relation to their concentrations in foods. Because of the low pH, toxic elements such as lead and cadmium may be leached from pipes in soft water areas while, in hard water areas, intestinal absorption of these elements may be reduced due to competition from calcium and magnesium ions *(Borgman)*.

Calcium

While *in vitro* and animal studies support a protective effect of calcium intake on colorectal cancer, the overall results from case-control and cohort studies suggest that calcium intake is *not* associated with a substantially lower risk *(Martinez)*.

There is evidence, however, that calcium supplementation modulates the proliferative behavior of the colonic mucosa in humans at increased risk for colon cancer *(Wargovich)*. For example, in a study from Memorial Sloan-Kettering Cancer Center in New York, 10 patients with rectal mucosal biopsies that showed patterns of proliferation of the epithelial cells lining colonic crypts which were characteristic of familial colon cancer were given 1.25 gm calcium daily. After two to three months, the number of rapidly proliferating cells in the colonic epithelium had significantly decreased and was almost the same as in people at low risk for colon cancer *(Lipkin)*.

Also, human feces contain substantial amounts of calcium long-chain fatty acid soaps which increase during calcium supplementation *(Owen,1995)*, and it has been suggested that calcium may reduce the mutagenic effects of bile acids and free ionized fatty acids in aqueous phase feces within the colon by forming these soaps *(Newmark)*.

It may be that the epidemiological evidence suggesting the efficacy of calcium supplementation for preventing colon cancer is due to the confounding effect of vitamin D nutriture. In a case-control study, when the combined effect of intakes of calcium, vitamin D and selected antioxidants was evaluated, the odds ratio reached 0.46 in the high-intake subjects *(La Vecchia)*. Similarly, a prospective study of men found that those who had the lowest combined index of dietary calcium and vitamin D were 2 ½ times more likely to develop colorectal cancer as men who had the highest index *(Garland,1985)*. Another prospective study, however, this time of women, found that, after adjustment for risk factors, the reduction in risk lost significance *(Bostick,1993)*.

Chlorine Toxicity

Several studies over the past few years have examined the relationship between exposure to chlorine found in chlorinated tap water and risk of certain cancers. In addition to ingestion, exposure can be via skin absorption and inhalation of the aerosol from baths and showers *(Brown,1984;Weisel)*.

Cancers most frequently related to chlorine exposure in epidemiologic studies are colorectal cancers *(Flaten)* and lower urinary tract cancers *(Wilkens)*.

Fluorine Toxicity

Fluoridated water has been suggested to be carcinogenic, and fluoride exposure as low as 1 ppm (roughly the level in fluoridated drinking water) has been shown to cause genetic damage *(Yiomouyiannis)*. It has also been suggested that the high levels of sodium fluoride found in certain toothpastes and mouthwashs may be carcinogenic *(Sutton)*.

Based on data from animal and/or epidemiological studies, cancers whose risks may be increased due to fluorine exposure include osteosarcoma, thyroid follicular cell adenomas, oral and nasal squamous dysplasia, and hepatocholangiocarcinoma *(Lee JR)*.

Iodine

The dietary intake of iodine appear to be negatively correlated with cancers of the female reproductive system *(Stadel)*. This finding suggests that a low iodine intake may produce increased gonadotrophin stimulation leading to a hyperestrogenic state characterized by relatively high production of estrone and estradiol and a relatively low estriol to estrone plus estradiol ratio *(Stadel)*.

Moreover, women with low iodine levels often have severe hyperplasia and fibrocystic breast disease, precancerous conditions which respond to iodine supplementation *(Eskin)*.

Iron

Numerous laboratory and clinical studies have observed that iron can favor neoplastic cell growth. In both animals and humans, primary neoplasms develop at body sites of excessive iron deposits. The invaded host attempts to withhold iron from the cancer cells by sequestering the metal in newly formed ferritin *(Weinberg)*. Since iron can catalyze the production of free oxygen radicals *(Halliwell)*, it may be a limiting nutrient for the growth and development of cancer cells.

While many epidemiologic studies have been conducted, the findings have been inconsistent. Dietary iron intake in the usual range appears to be unrelated to cancer risk *(Stevens,1986)* - or may even be protective for some cancers such as stomach *(Harrison)* and prostate *(Vlajinac)* cancers which appear to be promoted by low body iron stores *(Akiba;Picurelli)*. By contrast, high body iron stores may increase the risk of certain cancers, such as colorectal and pulmonary cancers *(Knekt,1994)*.

Until the picture clarifies, iron supplementation should be avoided unless there is evidence of an iron deficiency.

Magnesium

The results of epidemiologic studies suggest that magnesium intake is inversely correlated with cancer mortality *(Blondell;Seelig)*. Magnesium appears to protect against precancerous cellular changes, so a deficiency could predispose to neoplastic cell division *(Seelig)*. In studies of experimental cancer in animals, magnesium-deficient diets increased cancer development, while excess dietary magnesium reduced it *(Blondell)*.

Hemolymphoreticular malignancies are stimulated by magnesium deficiency and therefore magnesium supplementation appears to be beneficial *(Durlach)*. Solid cancers, however, have high metabolic requirements that require magnesium, so magnesium supplementation when there is no deficiency may stimulate their growth *(Seelig)*.

Selenium

Selenium status has been found to be inversely related to cancer risk in numerous *in vitro*, animal and epidemiologic studies. Serum selenium is an excellent predictor of the subsequent development of cancer *(Willett)*, and it appears that lower serum selenium levels are probably antecedent to the development of the tumor rather than caused by it *(Ujiie)*. The results of prospective studies have been mixed, however, with some suggesting an inverse relationship between selenium levels and cancer and others failing to confirm this finding *(Garland,1995;Watrach)*.

An interesting example of both the success and failure of selenium supplementation is a recent randomized, double-blind study of over 1,300 patients with histories of basal or squamous cell carcinomas of the skin that was reported in the *Journal of the American Medical Association*. Patients were treated for a mean of 2.8 years (standard deviation of 2.8 years) and had a total follow-up of 6.4 years with a standard deviation of 2 years. Selenium supplementation failed to affect the incidences of the cancers under study. However, it was associated with reductions in total cancer mortality, total cancer incidence, and incidences of lung, colorectal, and prostate cancers. These latter findings were so impressive that the blinded phase of the study was stopped early *(Clark)*.

In addition to reducing cancer risk, selenium supplementation may reduce tissue damage from chemotherapy while it is extremely well tolerated *(Hu;Sundstrom)*.

Zinc

In animal models, both zinc deficiency and zinc excess may inhibit tumor growth *(Song,1984)*. Experimental tumors lower intestinal zinc absorption capacity while raising the rate of zinc uptake. As a result, other tissues become zinc-deficient. In tumor bearing mice, for example, a zinc-excess diet is beneficial as they are generally zinc-deficient; the diet normalizes zinc organ concentrations resulting in increased survival time *(Song,1989)*.

Of all the trace elements, both epidemiological and experimental studies have found dietary zinc deficiency to be the one most strongly linked to the risk of developing esophageal carcinoma *(Barch)*. While plasma zinc concentrations are lower in patients with the disease, the concentration of zinc in diseased esophageal tissue is no different from that of adjacent normal tissue *(Lipman)*. Findings from prospective studies, however, have so far suggested that zinc supplementation is ineffective in preventing esophageal cancer *(Muñoz)*.

Since zinc concentration in the prostate is much higher than in other tissues, the relationship of zinc nutriture to prostate cancer has been explored. Prostatic zinc levels are lower in patients with prostatic cancer than either those of normals or of patients with prostatic hyperplasia *(Zaichick)*. Similarly, serum zinc levels are lower in prostate cancer patients than in patients with benign prostatic hyperplasia *(Whelen)*.

A possible role for zinc in preventing prostate cancer is also suggested by the antagonism between zinc and the toxic metal cadmium. Cadmium, a known cause of prostatic cancer *(Elinder)*, has been shown to stimulate the growth of human prostatic epithelium at low concentrations, suggesting that it may promote prostate cancer by replacing zinc *(Webber)*.

There is some evidence for this hypothesis. Compared to biopsies from both normals and patients with benign prostatic hyperplasia, one study found the highest levels of cadmium, and the lowest levels of zinc, in patients with poorly-differentiated carcinomas *(Feustel)*. Not only are the cadmium levels markedly increased in prostatic carcinomas, but dihydrotestosterone levels are proportional to the cadmium concentrations *(Habib)*, suggesting that hormonal stimulation may be involved. As in regard to esophageal cancer, however, there is no direct evidence that zinc supplementation reduces the risk of prostatic cancer.

Although the data concerning the reduction of cancer risk is disappointing, there is evidence that zinc supplementation may restore failing immune function in cancer patients by repleting a zinc deficiency *(Weide;Allen)*. Improved immune status will hopefully translate into a better quality of life and improved survival.

OTHER NUTRITIONAL FACTORS

Alkylglycerols

Outside of human bone marrow and mother's milk, these natural substances are highest in shark liver oil. In an early controlled trial, they were shown to enhance the regression of uterine cancer when administered prior to radiation therapy *(Brohult,1986)*. Furthermore, administration prior to, during and after radiation therapy for the treatment of uterine cancer reduced radiation injuries by as much as two-thirds *(Brohult,1979)*.

Amino Acids

L-Arginine

Arginine serves as dietary precursor to nitric oxide, an intracellular secondary messenger affecting cellular regulation, interaction and defense. Nitric oxide may either promote tumor growth or inhibit it *(Chinje)*; it appears that arginine may also have either effect.

In mice, supplementation with L-arginine retards tumor growth through immunomodulation. *(Reynolds)*. *In vitro*, it inhibits tumor target cells in leukemia *(Hibbs)*. In human breast cancer, it enhances host defenses *(Brittenden)*, although it also increases tumor protein synthesis *(Park)*; thus its effect on the clinical course is uncertain.

Because of its opposing effects, L-arginine cannot be recommended for cancer patients until further research is completed.

Cysteine

N-acetylcysteine, which is closely related to the amino acid cysteine and a precursor to intracellular glutathione (see Glutathione below), may protect against some of the adverse effects of chemotherapy. Animal studies suggest that it may prevent the hemorrhagic cystitis commonly caused by treatment with cyclophosphamide *(Levy)* or ifosfamide *(Watson)*. However, a randomized controlled human trial found it to be ineffective in blocking the cardiotoxicity of doxorubicin *(Myers)*.

When applied topically as an ointment, N-acetylcysteine protects against skin reactions, alopecia and damage to the mucus membranes of the eyes from radiation therapy *(Kim JA)*.

As a source of intracellular glutathione, N-acetylcysteine may eventually prove to be an effective agent to prevent cancer by detoxifying carcinogenic xenobiotics *(De Flora;Van Zandwijk)*. Controlled clinical trials are currently in process.

Glutamine

Glutamine is the most abundant amino acid in the blood and tissues. As it is important to the synthesis of glutathione in the liver and kidney, supplementation may be another means of modulating glutathione levels. Animal studies suggest that glutamine may suppress the growth of cancers *(Klimberg,1996a)*. Moreover, it may render tumor cells more sensitive to radiation and chemotherapy by decreasing their intracellular glutathione levels, while it also restores depressed glutathione levels in normal tissues *(Rouse)*. This latter effect suggests that glutamine supplementation may be superior in cancer therapy to treatment with other antioxidants as, unlike glutamine, they enhance glutathione nutriture in both normal *and* tumor cells *(Klimberg,1996b)*.

Glutamine supplementation may also reduce the adverse effects of chemotherapy. In a controlled study, the diarrhea that developed in patients with acute myelogenous leukemia who received glutamine starting 3 days prior to multi-drug chemotherapy was less severe and lasted a shorter period of time. Moreover, both the use of parenteral nutrition and systemic antifungal therapy was reduced *(Muscaritoli)*. Similar benefits were noted in an open trial in regard to chemotherapy-induced oral mucositis *(Skubitz)*.

Patients undergoing radiation therapy may also achieve some protection from radiation damage since, in an animal study, glutamine supplementation improved healing of radiation enteritis *(Klimberg,1991)*.

While intriguing, these possible benefits of glutamine supplementation need confirmation by controlled clinical trials.

Carotenoids

Carotenoids exhibit biological activities as antioxidants, affect cell growth regulation, and modulate gene expression and immune response *(Rock)*. The relationship between their intake and cancer has been extensively examined in the literature. Carotenoids have been shown to be antineoplastic in animal models of cancer. *In vitro*, they are anti-mutagenic *(Santamaria)* and may protect human lymphocytes from x-ray-induced genetic damage *(Umegaki)*.

Carotenoid intake and both blood and tissue concentrations have been repeatedly found to be inversely associated with the risk of numerous cancers *(Rock)*. Moreover, tissue carotenoid levels may be lower in cancerous tissues than in adjacent normal tissues *(Palan)*.

Of course, inverse associations do not indicate causal relationships. For example, there is evidence that the lower carotenoid blood levels found in cancer patients may be due to malnutrition rather than to the presence of cancer *(Meguid)*. Since fruits and vegetables are major sources of dietary carotenoids, and there is considerable evidence that their intake is protective against cancer, it is possible that carotenoids serve as markers of fruit and vegetable intake, and that other substances contained in fruits and vegetables explain their benefits.

Unfortunately, little human research has been performed relating supplementation with carotenoids other than beta-carotene to cancer prevention.

Beta-Carotene

An efficient quencher of singlet oxygen, beta-carotene prevents tissue damage by trapping organic free radicals. Results of a large number of studies suggest that people with the highest dietary intakes or blood levels of beta-carotene have a 20 to 40 percent lower risk of cancer than those with the lowest intakes or blood levels *(Hennekens)*, and controlled studies have reported its efficacy in reversing precancerous lesions such as oral leukoplakia *(Garewal)* and intestinal metaplasia *(Bukin)*.

However, despite promising findings from small clinical trials, the results of 4 large-scale randomized trials suggest that, in well-nourished populations, beta-carotene supplementation has no overall anticancer effect *(Hennekens)*. In fact, there is even early evidence that beta-carotene supplementation may increase the risk of lung cancer in certain susceptible populations, namely smokers *(Albanes)* and workers exposed to asbestos *(Omenn)*.

Many theories have been advanced to explain this disappointing finding. These include, for example, suggestions that the dosages were too low and that the supplement needs to be used for a longer period of time to prevent cancer. Experimental evidence suggests that natural beta-carotene may be more effective than the synthetic form *(Yeum)*, and the suggestion that the provision of a more natural formulation of mixed carotenoids may be more effective than beta-carotene alone is particularly intriguing *(White)*. Further clarification awaits the outcome of controlled clinical trials.

Coenzyme Q_{10} (ubiquinone)

In patients with cancer, blood levels of coenzyme Q_{10} may be reduced *(Folkers,1997)*.

Thiry-five cases of advanced breast cancer have been reported who received coenzyme Q_{10} in addition to other nutritional supplements and conventional treatment. While it is, of course, impossible to separate out the efficacy of the various components of the treatment program, patients appeared to do unusually well. For example, 6 of the initial 32 patients showed tumor regression and none died during 18 months of treatment whereas 4 deaths had been expected. None of the initial 32 patients developed further distant metastases during the 18 months, and 2 of the 3 additional cases had evidence of disappearance of metastases *(Lockwood,1994a,1994b,1995)*.

In addition, 10 other case histories have been published of patients with cancers of the lung, pancreas, larynx, breast and prostate, many of whom were considered terminal, who survived at least 5 to 15 years after starting treatment with coenzyme Q_{10} *(Folkers,1993)*.

Clinical studies have also shown that the administration of coenzyme Q_{10} reduces the adverse side-effects of chemotherapy with adriamycin. In controlled studies, coenzyme Q_{10} prevented the expected depression in cardiac output, and reduced the frequency of EKG abnormalities, cardiac arrhythmias, hypotension and anginal symptoms. Hair loss was also reduced *(Yamawaki)*. Moreover, it is believed to double the anti-tumor activity of the drug *(Yamanaka)*.

A 48-year-old man with inoperable lung cancer was treated with coenzyme Q_{10}. His cancer went into remission and, in 17 years of follow-up, he has had no signs of recurrence of cancer or of congestive heart failure (Folkers,1993).

Fatty Acids

Trans Fatty Acids

Partially-hydrogenated oils contain a relatively high percent of the unnatural *trans* form of fatty acids. It has been suggested that they may be a major contributor to the carcinogenic effect of fats since there are positive correlations of cancer mortality with the intake of both total and vegetable fat, but not with animal fat or with total or individual unsaturated fatty acids *(Enig)*.

Only some of the large number of unnatural fatty acids produced by hydrogenation have been investigated. So far, however, studies using animal models have failed to find evidence of their carcinogenicity at levels likely to be found in the human diet, and they do not appear to pose a significant risk of fostering carcinogenesis so long as they are ingested as part of a balanced diet containing adequate linoleic acid *(Hunter)*.

Polyunsaturates

Concern has also been voiced about the possible carcinogenicity of polyunsaturated fatty acids. By increasing the synthesis of series-2 (pro-inflammatory) prostaglandins, they could depress the activity of natural killer cells, the first line of defense against tumor cells *(Barone,1989)*. Moreover, animal studies have found that polyunsaturates are required for the growth of cancers in a quantity that is greater than that needed by the host *(Dupont)*. Epidemiological studies have been of little help in clarifying the issue, as some studies have found a direct relationship between the intake of polyunsaturates and cancer risk *(Pearce)* while others have found an inverse relationship *(Witte)*.

Recent evidence, however, has shown that the tumorigenicity of foods varies inversely with their content of polyunsaturates, and *in vitro* studies have found that polyunsaturates killed human cancer cells at concentrations which had no adverse effects on normal cells. While the sensitivity of cancer cells to specific polyunsaturates varied, all cancer cell lines could be killed by one or more combinations *(Bëgin,1985,1990)*.

Carcinogenicity could possibly result from the susceptibility of these fatty acids (especially the omega-3 fatty acids) to lipid peroxidation *(Giovannucci,1993; Oldeleye)*. For this reason, additional vitamin E should be ingested when polyunsaturated acid intake is high *(Laganiere)*.

Since the biological effects of the various polyunsaturates differ greatly, it is more heuristic to explore their effects by families or even separately. Investigations of the separate effects of the two families of essential fatty acids (the omega-3 and the omega-6 fatty acids) have been particularly revealing.

Omega-3 Essential Fatty Acids

Results of studies using experimental animal models *(Pritchard)* as well as *in vitro* studies *(Reich)* suggest that fish oils that are high in the omega-3 fatty acid eicosapentaenoic acid may inhibit carcinogenesis.

Human trials have also suggested that fish oils are beneficial. In a placebo-controlled study, 40 days after patients with generalized solid tumors began daily doses of fish oils, there was a significant increase in the T-helper/T-suppressor cell ratio among the malnourished patients (who had a lower ratio at baseline). Moreover, mean survival was significantly prolonged in the supplemented patients *(Gogos)*.

Repeated double-blind studies have found fish oil supplementation to be effective in reducing colonic epithelial cell proliferation, especially in patients at high risk for colon cancer *(Anti;Huang)*. Also, based on the results from experimental animal models, omega-3 fatty acids may be beneficial in cancer cachexia by protecting against the development of cancer-induced tumors, the growth of solid tumors, and metastatic disease *(Karmali)*.

Omega-6 Essential Fatty Acids

The effects of the omega-6 fatty acids are more mixed. The results of *in vitro* studies and animal experimental models suggest promotional *(Carroll,1986)* as well as inhibitory *(Norman)* effects. This lack of clarity has also been reflected in human studies. In regard to breast cancer, for example, there is evidence that linoleic acid intake may reduce cancer risk *(Witte)*, while there is also evidence suggesting that it enhances the metastatic process *(Rose)*. There is also evidence that both linoleic acid and total omega-6 fatty acid nutriture are inversely related to natural killer cell activity, a first-line defense against cancer *(Rasmussen)*.

The results of similar types of studies do suggest that gamma-linolenic acid (GLA), the metabolite of linoleic acid, may inhibit carcinogenesis *(Dippenaar)*. It is generally accepted that production of GLA is sometimes blocked because of inadequate activity of the enzyme delta-6-desaturase. It has been theorized that this blockage could promote carcinogenesis. If so, supplementation with a source of GLA may inhibit carcinogenesis by restoring normal prostaglandin E series metabolism *(Booyens,1983)*. Indeed, transformed and malignant cell lines frequently show loss or greatly reduced activity of delta-6-desaturase *(Hrelia,1994)*.

The evidence to date for the efficacy of GLA is promising, and it is now considered to be the most effective differential cytotoxic agent among the different polyunsaturates tested *(Hrelia,1996)*. When human breast, lung and prostate cancer cells and normal human fibroblasts were co-cultured in the absence of polyunsaturates, the malignant cells outgrew the normal ones. When, however, GLA was added to the co-cultures, the normal cells outgrew the malignant ones at concentrations which had no adverse effects on human fibroblasts or on normal animal cell lines *(Bëgin,1986)*.

GLA has been found to kill about 40 different human cancer cell lines *in vitro* without harming normal cells *(Fearon)*. Other *in vitro* evidence suggests that the toxicity of GLA to tumor cells is not dependent upon metabolites but is due to GLA itself *(Hrelia,1996)*. In accord with the results of the *in vitro* studies, animal models of breast cancer have also responded well to high dietary levels of evening primrose oil *(Prichard)*.

The results of early human studies are also encouraging. In an open trial, the administration of evening primrose oil, a rich source of GLA, to 21 patients with untreatable malignancies produced marked subjective improvement and, in some patients, objective improvement *(van Der Merwe,1987)*, and the combined administration of evening primrose oil and vitamin C doubled the mean survival time for 11 patients with primary hepatic carcinoma *(van der Merwe,1984)*. Even 48 patients with inoperable pancreatic cancer appeared to benefit, with the highest dose of the lithium salt of GLA being associated with a longer survival time than the lowest dose *(Fearon)*. However, in a controlled trial, 54 patients with colorectal cancer failed to benefit *(McIllmurray)*. More and better studies are needed before the therapeutic value of GLA supplementation in cancer treatment can be well evaluated.

Omega-3 to Omega-6 Fatty Acid Ratio

A great deal of evidence has accumulating showing that the modern diet in the industrialized countries has suffered from a relative lack of omega-3 saturated fatty acids, especially as compared to the intake of omega-6 fatty acids *(Labadarios)*. This imbalance may be contributing to the prevalence of cancer, If so, increasing the ratio of omega-3 to omega-6 essential fatty acids may reduce cancer risk *(Bueno-de-Mesquita; Weisburger,1997)*.

Omega-9 Fatty Acids

Oleic acid is a monounsaturated, nonessential omega-9 fatty acid found primarily in olive oil. When compared to omega-3 and omega-6 essential fatty acids, it may enhance or more weakly inhibit tumor growth *(Booyens,1985;Pritchard)*. In epidemiological studies, there is increasing evidence that it may help to protect against breast cancer. Evidence for a protective effect in regard to other cancers is promising but very limited *(Lipworth)*.

Butyric Acid

Butyric acid is a 4-carbon fatty acid produced by the anaerobic bacteria of the human colon which serves as a major energy source for colorectal epithelium. It is also the major metabolite when dietary fiber is exposed to colonic flora.

Several actions of butyrate protect against colon cancer *(Velazquez)*. The results of *in vitro* studies suggest that it promotes the differentiation of malignant cells and apoptosis (cell death) in premalignant and malignant colonic epithelial cells *(Hague)*. In an animal model of colon cancer, its direct application significantly reduced the number of tumors and the incidence of malignancies and carcinoma in the rat colon *(Medina)*; thus it may be a major colon cancer-inhibiting metabolite *(Hague)*.

Flavonoids

These are a family of plant-derived polyphenol compounds found in common foods. In animal studies, dietary flavonoids inhibit both the initiation and promotion phases of cancer *(Fujiki;Kuhnau)*. Epidemiological studies also suggest that flavonoid intake may be protective.

In one study, there was an inverse association between their intake and the incidence of cancer at all sites combined *(Knekt,1997)*. Another study failed to find decreased risk to be associated with total flavonoid intake, although a high flavonoid intake from fruits and vegetables was protective against cancers of the alimentary and respiratory tracts *(Hertog)*.

Phytoestrogens

Diphenolic plant substances such as isoflavonoids (isoflavones and coumestrans), lignans, and resorcyclic acid lactones are converted in the bowel to compounds with weak estrogenic properties. Since they bind to estrogen receptor sites, they also compete with endogenous estrogen and thus reduce its effects in states of estrogen excess. These attributes make them attractive as potential inhibitors of estrogen-related carcinogenesis *(Adlercreutz)*.

Soy isoflavones such as genistein show cytostatic activity against human mammary cancer cell lines *in vitro* and can suppress carcinogen-induced mammary cancer in rats *(Stoll,1997)*. Urinary excretion of the phytoestrogens enterolactone and equol have been inversely related to the risk of breast cancer *(Ingram)*. Similarly, higher concentrations of the phytoestrogens daidzein and equol (probably due to the consumption of soy) may be inversely related to the risk of prostate cancer *(Morton)*.

Quercetin

Although found to be mutagenic *in vitro*, quercetin has been shown to be anticarcinogenic *in vivo (Stavric)*. *In vitro*, it limits the growth of human acute leukemias in a dose-dependent manner and enhances the anti-proliferative activity of anti-leukemia agents *(Hoffman;Larocca)*. Also *in vitro*, it synergistically enhances the anti-proliferative effect of cisplatin, a widely used treatment for ovarian, testicular, and head and neck cancer *(Cross)*.

Glutathione

A tripeptide found in a variety of foods, glutathione may function as an anticarcinogen by acting as an antioxidant and by binding with cellular mutagens *(Flagg)*. Its dietary intake may be inversely associated with, for example, oral and pharyngeal cancer risk *(Flagg)*, and total plasma levels are markedly decreased in many types of cancer *(Beutler)*.

In animal models, oral or enteral supplementation with reduced glutathione inhibits carcinogenesis *(Novi;Trickler)*. While controlled human trials of glutathione as the sole treatment for cancer are lacking, there is an interesting report of an open trial involving 8 patients with hepatocellular carcinoma (a neoplasm with an extremely poor prognosis) who were not candidates for surgery. Two patients were unable to tolerate the supplement due to gastrointestinal irritation and the sulfur odor. Five of the 6 patients died within one year.

At follow-up the patient who survived remained in good condition without progression of the tumor, and his alpha-1-feroprotein (the reference diagnostic test for this carcinoma) was normal. Two women with moderately advanced tumors survived almost one year, tumor growth stopped or regressed and, in one of them, an initially abnormal alpha-1-fetoprotein returned to normal, while alpha-1-fetoprotein remained normal in the other patients *(Dalhoff)*.

In double-blind studies, glutathione supplementation reduced the neurotoxicity of cisplatin without reducing its efficacy *(Cascinu;Smyth)*. Also, in a controlled study of women with endometrial cancer, intravenous glutathione given just prior to adjuvant radiotherapy reduced the occurrence of diarrhea to nearly half, suggesting that it reduced the oxidative damage of radiation to the intestinal mucosa *(De Maria)*.

Inositol Hexaphosphate (phytic acid)

Ubiquitous in plants and animals, inositol hexaphosphate is not only a natural antioxidant, but may also be the precursor of intracellular inositol phosphates, important for various cellular functions including cell proliferation and differentiation *(Yang)*. Both *in vitro* and *in vivo*, it has a striking anti-cancer action, and may even cause differentiation of malignant cells resulting in reversion to a normal phenotype *(Shamsuddin)*.

Because inositol hexaphosphate is present in high quantities in high fiber diets, it may help to explain the inverse relationship between high fiber intake and cancer risk. For example, in an animal model of breast cancer, inositol hexaphosphate was clearly more effective as a cancer preventive agent than the addition of 20% bran to the diet *(Vucenik)*.

While the results of human trials are yet to be reported, results of animal and *in vitro* studies have already suggested that inositol hexaphosphate may reduce both the risk and the early expression of breast and colorectal cancers *(Graf)*.

Lactulose

A non-digestible dietary fiber and prebiotic, lactulose is believed to inhibit the promotion stages of colon carcinogenesis. For example, it has been shown to reduce dehydroxylation of chenodeoxycholic acid to the potentially toxic secondary bile acid lithocholic by over 90% *(Owen, 1997).*

In a randomized study, 209 patients who had undergone polypectomy for colonic adenomas randomly received either lactulose, antioxidant vitamins (vitamin A 30,000 IU, vitamin C 1 g and D,L-alpha-tocopherol acetate 70 mg daily), or no treatment. After an average follow-up of 18 months, the recurrence rates of adenomas were 5.7%, 14.7% and 35.9% in the vitamin, lactulose and untreated groups, suggesting that lactulose, while less effective than a combination of antioxidant vitamins, may have some efficacy in preventing the formation of colonic adenomas *(Roncucci).*

Phytosterols

Phytosterols are cholesterol analogs found in plant oils, seeds, nuts, cereals, and legumes. Poorly absorbed by the intestinal lumen, they appear to interfere with cholesterol and bile acid metabolism and absorption, thus reducing serum cholesterol levels and altering cholesterol's effect on colon carcinogenesis *(Rao).*

In one study, for example, 3-day composite diets of 18 pure vegetarians, 50 lacto-ovo-vegetarians and 100 nonvegetarians were analyzed for their sterol composition and the plant sterol/cholesterol ratios. The findings suggested that the absolute amounts of cholesterol consumed may not be as significant in colon carcinogenesis as its relationship to total plant sterols in the diet *(Nair).*

COMBINED NUTRIENT SUPPLEMENTATION

Many clinical trials of nutritional treatments for cancer have used nutrients in combination in an attempt to maximize their benefits. Most have reported good results. Hoffer and Pauling have reported their findings from an ongoing informal clinical trial of a combined diet and supplement regimen. Generally, their program consists of dietary instructions to reduce red meats, increase green vegetables, and avoid sugar, coffee, cocoa and milk products. Nutritional supplements consist of:

- Vitamin C (mixture of ascorbic acid, sodium ascorbate and calcium ascorbate): 12 g or to bowel tolerance
- Vitamin B_3 (niacin, niacinamide): 1.5-3 g
- Vitamin B_6 (pyridoxine): 250 mg
- Folic acid: 5-10 mg
- other B vitamins: 25 or 50 times the RDAs
- Vitamin E: 800 IU
- Beta carotene: 25,000-50,000 IU
- Selenium: 0.2-0.5 mg
- Zinc sulfate: 220 mg
- Calcium, magnesium or a multimineral tablet (sometimes)
- Coenzyme Q_{10} 300 mg (later modification)

A progress report published in 1993 noted that 101 out of a group of 134 patients who entered the study followed the program. For analysis, survival of study patients who failed to follow the program (controls) was compared to survival of those who followed it. Forty percent of those who followed the program were judged to be excellent responders, with survival times after study entry of at least 5 years, while 60 percent were good responders, with mean survival times about 4 times that of the controls. Similar results were noted for about 170 subsequent patients *(Hoffer, 1993).*

The contribution of vitamin C supplementation to survival appeared to be especially important. Unless patients ingested the high dosages of the vitamin for at least 2 months, their prognosis was very poor *(Hoffer, 1989).* However, the efficacy of the program was not attributable to vitamin C alone, as only about 10% of patients who *only* ingested supplemental ascorbate were judged to be excellent responders versus the 60% of patients on the full regimen who were excellent responders *(Hoffer, 1993).*

Numerous formal studies, most of them double-blind, have reported efficacy using various combinations of supplemental nutrients. These include studies of cancers of the bladder *(Lamm)*, breast *(Pagnanelli)*, colon *(Roncucci)*, esophagus and stomach *(Taylor PR; Wang)*, and lung *(Jaakkola).* In addition to responses seen in solid tumors, a case of pre-leukemia may have responded to a nutritional supplementation program:

A 25-year-old male complained of a 2 to 3 year period of progressive malaise, fatigue and headache. Pre-leukemia was diagnosed on the basis of blood and bone marrow studies.

He was placed on a regime which included large daily doses of antioxidants consisting of a multivitamin along with folic acid 1 mg, vitamin A 25 mg, vitamin C 1 gm, vitamin E 800 IU, selenium 400 µg, zinc 30 mg, beta-carotene 50 mg, cysteine 2 gm and N-acetyl cysteine 3 gm. He was also given phenylalanine 3 gm and tyrosine 3 gm for the treatment of depression.

After 3 months, his full blood count was entirely normal. Six months after his bone marrow biopsy, a repeat biopsy was entirely normal (Braverman).

OTHER RELATED FACTORS

Hydrochloric Acid Deficiency

Intestinal metaplasia, a premalignant condition, occurs in chronic atrophic gastritis and is associated with reduced output of hydrochloric acid *(Sobala)*. Also, cancer of the gastric remnant after partial gastrectomy for peptic ulcer disease could be due to alkaline bile reflux *(Domellof)*. However, there is no evidence that providing hydrochloric acid supplementation will reduce the risk of gastric cancer.

Cartilage-derived Anti-angiogenesis Factor

Angiogenesis has been shown to be necessary for tumor growth and the establishment of metastases; thus a substance that inhibits tumor angiogenesis may be anti-neoplastic. It has been shown in animal studies that such a factor is present in both shark *(Lee A)* and bovine *(Langer)* cartilage.

Catrix, an acidic glycosaminoglycan complex derived from bovine tracheal cartilage rings, was found effective *in vitro* against a human myeloma cell line as well as against colon, ovarian, pancreatic, sarcoma and testicular cancer biopsy specimens at concentrations which appeared achievable *in vivo (Durie)*. When tested in an open trial, the results suggested that administration of the complex may safely treat a variety of cancers with a high rate of positive responses. Following years of therapy with this substance, 90% of a group of 31 malignancies improved, and 61% of them went into complete remission. Apparent responders included patients with glioblastoma multiforme and cancers of the cervix, lungs, ovary, pancreas, prostate, rectum and thyroid, as well as an inoperable squamous cancer of the nose. No toxic effects were observed *(Prudden)*.

As in regard to bovine cartilage, the results of early trials with extracts of shark cartilage have been reported. For example, after 7 weeks, 7 of 8 advanced cancers treated daily rectally and intravaginally with suspensions of shark cartilagenous material demonstrated a reduction in tumor size *(Lane)*.

Since the angiogenesis-inhibiting factor is 1000 times more concentrated in shark cartilage than in calf cartilage *(Lee A)*, shark cartilage would, in theory, be a better source. Folkman *(Kirchhof)* and Langer *(Matthews)* have stated, however, that the stomach inactivates the specific peptide that inhibits angiogenesis, and thus any anti-neoplastic effect following oral administration must be due to other mechanisms.

Hopefully, controlled clinical trials will eventually determine the efficacy of cartilage extracts in cancer treatment and clarify any differences in efficacy between shark- and bovine-derived substances.

A 69-year-old jaundiced woman was found to have a carcinoma of the head of the pancreas with nodal involvement. A Whipple procedure was done, but microscopic sections showed a transection of the cancer on the common duct. She refused chemotherapy and was started on a bovine cartilage preparation (Catrix) 3 gm daily orally which was raised over the next year to 9 gm daily and reduced over the following year back to 3 gm daily. There was no concomitant therapy.

Four to eight months after starting treatment, her alkaline phosphatase level increased sharply to 10 times normal. It then declined and reached normal by 26 months. Her weight increased steadily from 106 lbs to 136 lbs 2 years after starting treatment and subsequently has remained steady.

Eight years after starting treatment, physical exam and blood chemistries are normal and she feels well (Prudden).

Lactobacilli

Lactobacillus acidophilus

Colon cancer is believed to be due, at least in part, to the alterations in fecal bacterial enzyme activity induced by the high fat, low fiber Western diet *(Gorbach, 1982)*. *L. acidophilus* reduces the fecal concentrations of bacterial enzymes that catalyze the conversion of procarcinogens to proximal carcinogens *(Goldin, 1984)*. Moreover, total concentrations of some Lactobacillus species have the closest associations with a low risk of colon cancer *(Moore)*. Controlled clinical trials are needed to ascertain the efficacy of this important bacterium in the prevention and treatment of colon cancer.

The evidence for the efficacy of *L. acidophilus* in preventing radiotherapy-associated diarrhea is far stronger. In controlled trials, women undergoing pelvic radiotherapy for cancer treatment had a significant reduction in diarrhea by ingesting acidophilus starting several days prior to radiotherapy *(Salminen, 1988, 1995)*.

Lactobacillus casei

Under double-blind conditions, 138 patients with transitional cell carcinoma of the bladder that had been surgically removed randomly received *L. casei* or placebo. On average, it took 30% longer for the lactobacillus-treated patients to have a recurrence of their bladder cancer compared to placebo controls, and the cancer returned significantly less often in patients receiving *L. casei* than in those receiving placebo *(Aso)*.

Proteolytic Enzymes

Circulating immune complexes suppress cellular immunity *(Hellstrom)* and their concentration may be related to cancer prognosis *(Nydegger)*. The administration of hydrolytic enzymes may by beneficial by reducing the concentration of immune complexes, resulting in symptomatic improvement and weight gain *(Wrba, 1993)*. Moreover, cellular immunity may improve *(Kim J-P)*, the production of tumor necrosis factor-alpha is stimulated *(Desser)*, and there are both fibrinolytic and thrombolytic effects on tumor cells *(Ransberger)*.

In animal experiments, tumor incidence is reduced and survival is increased *(Ransberger)*. A number of human trials have been conducted, some of which were controlled. For example, 90% of a group of 50 patients with breast cancer stages I to III who received pre- and post-operative treatment with Wobe-Mucos®, a standardized mixture of proteolytic enzymes, survived 10 years and showed no signs of relapses or metastases compared to 70% of patients who did not receive the enzyme mixture *(Rokitansky)*.

Proteolytic enzymes have also shown efficacy in inoperable bronchial *(Wrba, 1978)* and gastric *(Kim J-P)* carcinomas by providing a better quality of life. Dramatic improvements in survival have been reported in pancreatic carcinoma when administered along with megadoses of vitamin A, with many of the patients surviving at least several years *(Anonymous, 1985)*, and pleural exudation appears to respond well to local application in the pleural cavity in pleural carcinoma *(Kokron)*.

Their administration as an adjunct to radiation or chemotherapy appears to reduce adverse effects *(Glenk)*. In one clinic, for example, the percentage of patients requiring corticosteroids to counteract the side effects of radiation therapy was reduced from 60% to 3.3%, and the need for opiates and other analgesics was decreased, when proteolytic enzymes were provided *(Ransberger)*.

Toxic Minerals

Arsenic

Arsenic toxicity is associated with a greater risk of fatal internal organ cancers *(Chen)* such as urinary tract cancers *(Guo)* and lung cancer *(Lee-Feldstein)* as well as with non-lethal skin cancers *(Chen)*.

Cadmium

In addition to increasing the risk of prostatic cancer (*see discussion under Zinc above*) *(Feustel;Habib)*, cadmium toxicity is associated with an increased risk of lung cancer *(Elinder)*.

Nickel

Nickel toxicity increases the risk of nasopharyngeal *(Ling-Wei)* and lung carcinomas *(Doll)*.

BIBLIOGRAPHY

Adlercreutz H, Mazur W. Phyto-oestrogens and Western diseases. Ann Med 29:95-120, 1997

Ahmann FR, Durie BG. Acute myelogenous leukaemia modulated by B12 deficiency: a case with bone marrow blast cell assay corroboration. Br J Haematol 58(1):91-4, 1984

Akiba S et al. Serum ferritin and stomach cancer risk among a Japanese population. Cancer 67:1707-12, 1991

Albanes D et al. Effects of alpha-tocopherol and beta-carotene supplements on cancer incidence in the Alpha-Tocopherol Beta-Carotene Cancer Prevention Study. Am J Clin Nutr 62(suppl):1427S-30S, 1995

Alirezai M et al. Clinical evaluation of topical isotretinoin in the treatment of actinic keratoses. J Am Acad Dermatol 30(3):447-51, 1994

Allen JI et al. Association between urinary zinc excretion and lymphocyte dysfunction in patients with lung cancer. Am J Med 79(2):209-15, 1985

Anderson LM et al. Alcohol-related cancer risk: a toxicokinetic hypothesis. Alcohol 12(2):97-104, 1995

Anonymous. WOBE-MUGOS® in Therapy of Tumour-and Virus Diseases. Unpublished monograph. MUCOS Pharma GmbH & Co., Alpenstraße 29, 8192 Geretsried 1, Germany, Ca. 1985

Anonymous. Editorial. Vitamin D: New perspectives. Lancet i:1122-3, 1987

Anonymous. Alpha-tocopherol, Beta-carotene Cancer Prevention Study Group. The effect of vitamin E and beta-carotene on the incidence of lung cancer and other cancers in male smokers. N Engl J Med 330:1029-35, 1994

Anonymous. Diet said to be major contributor to development of breast cancer. Primary Care and Cancer 1996:13

Anti M et al. Effects of different doses of fish oil on rectal cell proliferation in patients with sporadic colonic adenomas. Gastroenterology 107:1709-18, 1994

Aso Y et al. Preventive effect of a lactobacillus casei preparation on the recurrence of superficial bladder cancer in a double-blind trial. Eur Urol 27:104-9, 1995

Ausman LM. Fiber and colon cancer: does the current evidence justify a preventive policy? Nutr Rev 51(2):57-63, 1993

Bain C et al. Diet and melanoma. An exploratory case-control study. Ann Epidemiol 3(3):235-8, 1993

Barale R et al. Vegetables inhibit, in vivo, the mutagenicity of nitrite combined with nitrosable compounds. Mutation Res 120:145, 1983

Barch DH. Esophageal cancer and microelements. J Am Coll Nutr 8(2):99-107, 1989

Barone J et al. Dietary fat and natural-killer-cell activity. Am J Clin Nutr 50:861-7, 1989

Barone J et al. Vitamin supplement use and risk for oral and esophageal cancer. Nutr Cancer 18:31-41, 1992

Bĕgin ME et al. Selective killing of human cancer cells by polyunsaturated fatty acids. Prostaglandins Leukotrienes Med 19(2):177-86, 1985

Bĕgin ME et al. Differential killing of human carcinoma cells supplemented with n-3 and n-6 polyunsaturated fatty acids. J Natl Cancer Inst 77:1053-62, 1986

B3gin ME. Fatty acids, lipid peroxidation and diseases. Proc Nutr Soc 49:261-7, 1990

Bendich A, Langseth L. The health effects of vitamin C supplementation: a review. J Am Coll Nutr 14(2):124-36, 1995

Benner SE et al. Regression of oral leukoplakia with alpha-tocopherol: a community clinical oncology program chemoprevention study. J Natl Cancer Inst 85:44-7, 1993

Beutler E, Gelbart T. Plasma glutathione in health and in patients with malignant disease. J Lab Clin Med 105:581-4, 1985

Bingham SA et al. Does increased endogenous formation of N-nitroso compounds in the human colon explain the association between red meat and colon cancer? Carcinogenesis 17:515-23, 1996

Block G et al. Fruit, vegetables, and cancer prevention: a review of the epidemiological evidence. Nutr Cancer 18:1-20, 1992

Blondell JM. The anticarcinogenic effect of magnesium. Med Hypotheses 6:863-71, 1980

Böing H et al. Regional nutritional pattern and cancer mortality in the Federal Republic of Germany. Nutr Cancer 7(3):121-30, 1985

Böing H et al. Dietary carcinogens and the risk for glioma and meningioma in Germany. Int J Cancer 53:561-5, 1993

Bond GG et al. Dietary vitamin A and lung cancer: Results of a case-control study among chemical workers. Nutr Cancer 9:109-21, 1987

Booyens J, Katzeff IE. Cancer: A simple metabolic disease? Med Hypotheses 12(3):195-201, 1983

Booyens J et al. Dietary fats and cancer. Med Hypotheses 17:351-62, 1985

Borgman RF. Dietary factors in essential hypertension. Prog Food Nutr Sci 9:109-47, 1985

Boros LG et al. Thiamine supplementation to cancer patients: a double edged sword. Anticancer Res 18(1B):595-602, 1998

Bostick R et al. Relation of calcium, vitamin D, and dairy food intake to incidence of colon cancer among older women. Am J Epidemiol 137:1302-17, 1993

Bostick RM et al. Sugar, meat, and fat intake, and non-dietary risk factors for colon cancer incidence in Iowa women (United States). Cancer Causes Control 5:38-52, 1994

Bounous G et al. Whey proteins in cancer prevention. Cancer Lett 57:91-4, 1991

Boyd NF, McGuire V. The possible role of lipid peroxidation in breast cancer risk. Free Rad Biol Med 10(3-4):185-90, 1991

Braverman ER. Reversal of pre-leukemia with antioxidants: a case report. J Nutr Med 2:313-15, 1991

Britteden J et al. L-arginine stimulates host defenses in patients with breast cancer. Surgery 115(2):205-12, 1994

Brohult A et al. Reduced mortality in cancer patients after administration of alkoxylglycerols. Acta Obstet Gynecol Scand 65(7):779-85, 1986

Brohult A et al. Effect of alkoxylglycerols on the frequency of fistulas following radiation therapy for carcinoma of the uterine cervix. Acta Obstet Gynecol Scand 58(2):203-07, 1979

Brown HS et al. The role of skin absorption as a route of exposure for volatile organic compounds (VOCs) in drinking water. Am J Public Health 74(5):479-84, 1984

Brown RR et al. Correlation of serum retinol levels with response to chemotherapy in breast cancer. Meeting abstract. Proc Am Assoc Cancer Res 22:184, 1981

Bruce WR, Dion PW. Studies relation to a fecal mutagen. Am J Clin Nutr 33:2511-12, 1980

Bruemmer B et al. Nutrient intake in relation to bladder cancer among middle-aged men and women. Am J Epidemiol 144(5):485-95, 1996

Bryan BT. The influence of niacin and niacinamide on in vivo carcinogenesis. Adv Exp Med Biol 206:331-8, 1986

Bueno-de-Mesquita HB, Gonzalez CA. Main hypotheses on diet and cancer investigated in the EPIC study. Eur J Canc Prev 6:107-17, 1997

Bukin YV et al. Effect of prolonged beta-carotene or DL-alpha-tocopheryl acetate supplementation on ornithine decarboxylase activity in human atrophic stomach mucosa. Cancer Epidemiol Biomark Prevent 4:865-70, 1995

Butterworth CE Jr et al. Improvement in cervical dysplasia associated with folic acid therapy in users of oral contraceptives. Am J Clin Nutr 35:73-82, 1982

Butterworth CE Jr. Effect of folate on cervical cancer. Synergism among risk factors. Ann N Y Acad Sci 669:293-9, 1992

Cameron E et al. The orthomolecular treatment of cancer. III. Reticulum cell sarcoma: double complete regression induced by high-dose ascorbic acid therapy. Chem Biol Interact 11(5):387-93, 1975

Cameron E, Pauling L. Supplemental ascorbate in the supportive treatment of cancer: Reevaluation of prolongation of survival times in terminal human cancer. Proc Nat Acad Sci USA 75:4538-42, 1978

Cameron E. Protocol for the use of vitamin C in the treatment of cancer. Med Hypotheses 36(3):190-4, 1991

Campbell A et al. Reticulum cell sarcoma: two complete 'spontaneous' regressions, in response to high-dose ascorbic acid: a report on subsequent progress. Oncology 48(6):495-7, 1991

Carroll KK. Dietary factors in hormone-dependent cancers, in M Winick, Ed. Current Concepts in Nutrition, Volume 6: Nutrition and Cancer. New York, John Wiley & Sons, 1977:25-40

Carroll KK. Lipid oxidation and carcinogenesis. Prog Clin Biol Res 206:237-44, 1986

Carroll KK. Dietary fats and cancer. Am J Clin Nutr 53:1064S-7S, 1991

Cascinu S et al. Neuroprotective effect of reduced glutathione on cisplatin-based chemotherapy in advanced gastric cancer: a randomized double-blind placebo-controlled trial. J Clin Oncol 13:26-32, 1995

Cats A et al. Randomized, double-blinded, placebo-controlled intervention study with supplemental calcium in families with hereditary nonpolyposis colorectal cancer. J Natl Cancer Inst 87(8):598-603, 1995

Chen C-J et al. Arsenic and cancer. Letter. Lancet i:414-15, 1988

Cheng KK et al. Stopping drinking and risk of oesophageal cancer. Br Med J 310:1094-7, 1995

Chinery R et al. Antioxidants enhance the cytotoxicity of chemotherapeutic agents in colorectal cancer: A p53-independent induction of p21WAF1/CIP1 via C/EBPb. Nature Med 3(11):1233-41, 1997

Chinje EC, Stratford IJ. Role of nitric oxide in growth of solid tumours: a balancing act. Essays Biochem 32:61-72, 1997

Chiu B C-H et al. Diet and risk of non-Hodgkin lymphoma in older women. JAMA 275(17):1315-31, 1996

Chlebowski RT et al. New directions in the nutritional management of the cancer patient. Nutr Res 13:3-21, 1993

Chrisley BM et al. Vitamin B6 status of a group of cancer patients. Nutr Res 6(9):1023-30, 1986

Clark LC et al. Effects of selenium supplementation for cancer prevention in patients with carcinoma of the skin. JAMA 276(24):1957-63, 1996

Colditz GA et al. Increased green and yellow vegetable intake and lowered cancer deaths in an elderly population. Am J Clin Nutr 41(1):32-6, 1985

Colston KW et al. Possible role for vitamin D in controlling breast cancer proliferation. Lancet i:188-91, 1989

Cornee J et al. A Case-control study of gastric cancer and nutritional factors in Marseille, France. Eur J Epidemiol 11: 55-65, 1995

Copeland EM 3rd et al. Nutrition and cancer. Int Adv Surg Oncol 4:1-13, 1981

Correa P et al. Gastric juice ascorbic acid after intravenous injection: effect of ethnicity, pH and Helicobacter pylori infection. J Natl Cancer Inst 87:52-3, 1995

Cravo M et al. DNA methylation as an intermediate biomarker in colorectal cancer: modulation by folic acid supplementation. Eur J Cancer Prev 3(6):473-9, 1994

Cross JH et al. Effect of quercetin on the genotoxic potential of cisplatin. Int J Cancer 66:404-9, 1996

Dalhoff K et al. Glutathione treatment of hepatocellular carcinoma. Liver 12:341-3, 1992

D'Avanzo B et al. Alcohol consumption and the risk of gastric cancer. Nutr Cancer 22:57-64, 1994

DeCosse JJ et al. Effect of wheat fiber and vitamins C and E on rectal polyps in patients with familial adenomatous polyposis. J Natl Cancer Inst 81(17):1290-7, 1989

De Flora S et al. In vivo effects of N-acetylcysteine on glutathione metabolism and on the biotransformation of carcinogenic and/or mutagenic compounds. Carcinogenesis 6:1735-45, 1985

Delmore G. Assessment of nutritional status in cancer patients: widely neglected? Support Care Cancer 5(5):376-80, 1997

De Maria D et al. Adjuvant radiotherapy of the pelvis with or without reduced glutathione: a randomized trial in patients operated on for endometrial cancer. Tumori 78:374-6, 1992

Desser L, Rehberger A. Induction of tumor necrosis factor in human peripheral-blood mononuclear cells by proteolytic enzymes. Oncology 47(6):475-7, 1990

Dewys WD et al. Prognostic effect of weight loss prior to chemotherapy in cancer patients. Am J Med 69:491-7, 1980

Dippenaar N et al. The reversibility of cancer: Evidence that malignancy in melanoma cells is gamma-linolenic acid deficiency-dependent. S Afr Med J 62:505-9, 1982

Dokal IS et al. Vitamin B-12 and folate deficiency presenting as leukeamia. Br Med J 300:1263-4, 1990

Doll R et al. Cancers of the lung and nasal sinuses in nickel workers. Br J Cancer 24:623-32, 1970

Domellof L. Gastric carcinoma promoted by alkaline reflux gastritis -- with special reference to bile and other surfactants as promoters of postoperative gastric cancer. Med Hypotheses 5(4):463-76, 1979

Dupont J et al. Food uses and health effects of corn oil. Am J Clin Nutr 9(5):438-70, 1990

Durie BG et al. Antitumor activity of bovine cartilage (Catrix-S) in the human tumor stem cell assay. J Biol Response Mod 4(6):590-95, 1985

Durlach J, Bara M. Magnesium and its relationship to oncology, in H. Sigel, A. Sigel, Eds. Metal Ions in Biological Systems, Vol. 26: Compendium on magnesium and its role in biology. New York-Basel, Marcel Dekker, 1990

Dyke GW et al. Effect of vitamin C supplementation on gastric mucosal damage. Carcinogenesis 15(2):291-5, 1994

Eichholzer M et al. Prediction of male cancer mortality by plasma levels of interacting vitamins: 17 year follow-up of the prospective Basal study. Int J Cancer 66:145-50, 1996

Elinder CG et al. Cancer mortality of cadmium workers. Br J Ind Med 42(10):651-5, 1985

Enig MG et al. Dietary fat and cancer trends - A critique. Fed Proc 37:2215-20, 1978

Eskin BA. Iodine and breast cancer. A 1982 update. Biol Trace Elem Res 5:399-412, 1983

Esteve J et al. Diet and cancers of the larynx and hypopharynx: the IARC multi-center study in southwestern Europe. Cancer Causes Control 7:240-52, 1996

Faber M et al. Lipid peroxidation products, and vitamin and trace element status in patients with cancer before and after chemotherapy, including adriamycin: a preliminary study. Biol Trace Elem Res 47:117;24, 1995

Fearon KC et al. An open-label phase I/II dose escalation study of the treatment of pancreatic cancer using lithium gammalinolenate. Anticancer Res 16(2):867-74, 1996

Ferraroni M et al. Selected micronutrient intake and the risk of colorectal cancer. Br J Cancer 70(6):1150-5, 1994

Feustel A, Wennrich R. Zinc and cadmium in cell fractions of prostatic cancer tissues of different histological grading in comparison to BPH and normal prostate. Urol Res 12(2):147-50, 1984

Fife RS et al. Effects of vitamin D3 on proliferation of cancer cells in vitro. Cancer Lett 120(1):65-9, 1997

Flagg EW et al. Dietary glutathione intake and the risk of oral and pharyngeal cancer. Am J Epidemiol 139:453-65, 1994

Flaten TP. Chlorination of drinking water and cancer incidence in Norway. Int J Epidemiol 21(1):6-15, 1992

Folkers K et al. Survival of cancer patients on therapy with coenzyme Q10. Biochem Biophys Res Commun 192(1):241-5, 1993

Folkers K et al. Activities of vitamin Q10 in animal models and a serious deficiency in patients with cancer. Biochem Biophys Res Commun 234(2):296-9, 1997

Franceschi S et al. Dietary factors and non-Hodgkin's lymphoma: a case-control study in the north-eastern part of Italy. Nutr Cancer 12:333-41, 1989

Franceschi SI et al. Food groups and risk of colorectal cancer in Italy. Int J Cancer 72:56-61, 1997

Frentzel-Beyme R, Chang-Claude J. Vegetarian diets and colon cancer: the German experience. Am J Clin Nutr 59(suppl):1143S-52S, 1994

Freudenheim JL et al. Diet, smoking, and alcohol in cancer of the larynx: a case-control study. Nutr Cancer 17:33-45, 1992

Fuch CS et al. Dietary fiber and the risk of colorectal cancer and adenoma in women. N Engl J Med 230(3):169-76, 1999

Fujiki H et al. Inhibition of tumor promotion by flavonoids, in Plant Flavonoids in Biology and Medicine, vol. 1. New York, Alan R. Liss, 1986:429-40

Galli C, Butrum R. Dietary omega-3 fatty acids and cancer: an overview, in AP Simopoulos et al, Eds. Health Effects of omega-3 polyunsaturated Fatty Acids in Seafoods. World Rev Nutr Diet 66:3446-61, 1991

Gao YT et al. Risk factors for esophageal cancer in Shanghai, China. II. Role of diet and nutrients. Int J Cancer 58(2):197-202, 1994

Garewal HS. Potential role of β-carotene in prevention of oral cancer. Am J Clin Nutr 53:294S-7S, 1991

Garland C et al. Dietary vitamin D and calcium and risk of colorectal cancer: A 19-year prospective study in men. Lancet i:307-9, 1985

Garland CF et al. Serum 25-hydroxyvitamin D and colon cancer. Eight-year prospective study. Lancet i:176-8, 1989

Garland FC et al. Geographic variation in breast cancer mortality in the United States: A hypothesis involving exposure to solar radiation. Prev Med 19:614-22, 1990

Garland M et al. Prospective study of toenail selenium levels and cancer among women. J Natl Cancer Inst 87(7):497-505, 1995

Gerhardsson de Verdier M. Epidemiologic studies on fried foods and cancer in Sweden. Princess Takamatsu Symp 23:292-8, 1995

Gey KF et al. Plasma levels of antioxidant vitamins in relation to ischemic heart disease and cancer. Am J Clin Nutr 45(5 Suppl):1368-77, 1987

Ghadirian P et al. International comparisons of nutrition and mortality from pancreatic cancer. Cancer Detect Prev 15(5):357-62, 1991

Ghadirian P et al. Nutritional factors and colon carcinoma: a case-control study involving French Canadians in Montreal, Quebec, Canada. Cancer 80:858-64, 1997

Giovannucci E et al. A prospective study of dietary fat and risk of prostate cancer. J Natl Cancer Inst 85(19):1571-9, 1993

Giovannucci E et al. Alcohol, low-methionine-low-folate diets, and risk of colon cancer in men. J Natl Cancer Inst 87(4):265-73, 1995

Glenk W, Neu S. Enzyme Die Bausteine des Lebens Wie sie wirken, helfen und heilen. Munich, Wilhelm Heyne Verlag, 1990:118 (in German)

Gogos CA et al. Dietary omega-3 polyunsaturated fatty acids plus vitamin E restore immunodeficiency and prolong survival for severely ill patients with generalized malignancy: a randomized control trial. Cancer 82(2):395-402, 1998

Goldin BR et al. Effect of diet and Lactobacillus acidophilus supplements on human fecal bacterial enzymes. J Natl Cancer Inst 64(2):255-61, 1980

Goldin BR et al. Estrogen excretion patterns and plasma levels in vegetarian and omnivorous women. N Engl J Med 307:1542-7, 1982

Goldin BR, Gorbach SL. The effect of milk and lactobacillus feeding on human intestinal bacterial enzyme activity. Am J Clin Nutr 39(5):756-61, 1984

González CA et al. Nutritional factors and gastric cancer in Spain. Am J Epidemiol 139:466-73, 1994

Goodman MT et al. Diet, body size, physical activity, and the risk of endometrial cancer. Cancer Res 57:5077-85, 1997a

Goodman MT et al. Association of soy and fiber consumption with the risk of endometrial cancer. Am J Epidemiol 146(4):294-306, 1997b

Gorbach SL. The intestinal microflora and its colon cancer connection. Infection 10(6):379-84, 1982

Graf E, Eaton J. Suppression of colon cancer by dietary phytic acid. Nutr Cancer 19(1):11-19, 1993

Graham S et al. Dietary factors in the epidemiology of cancer of the larynx. Am J Epidemiol 113(6):675-80, 1981

Greenberg ER et al. A clinical trial of antioxidant vitamins to prevent colorectal adenoma. N Engl J Med 331:141-7, 1994

Gridley G et al. Vitamin supplement use and reduced risk of oral and pharyngeal cancer. Am J Epidemiol 135(10):1083-92, 1992

Groopman J, Ellman L Acute promyelocytic leukemia. Am J Hematol 7(4):395-408, 1979

Guo How-Ran et al. Arsenic in drinking water and incidence of urinary cancers. Epidemiology 8(5):545-50, 1997

Gupta S. Effect of radiotherapy on plasma ascorbic acid concentration in cancer patients. Unpublished thesis - summarized in Hanck AB. Vitamin C and cancer. Prog Clin Biol Res 259:307-20, 1988

Ha C et al. The effect of B-6 on host susceptibility to Moloney Sarcoma Virus-induced tumor growth in mice. J Nutr 114:938-45, 1984

Habib FK et al. Metal-androgen interrelationships in carcinoma and hyperplasia of the human prostate. J Endocrinol 71(1):133-41, 1976

Hague A et al. The role of butyrate in human colonic epithelial cells: an energy source or inducer of differentiation and apoptosis? Proc Nutr Soc 55:937-43, 1996

Hallivell B, Gutteridge JM. Oxygen free radicals and iron in relation to biology and medicine: Some problems and concepts. Arch Biochem Biophys 246:501-14, 1986

Harrison LE et al. The role of dietary factors in the intestinal and diffuse histologic subtypes of gastric adenocarcinoma: a case-control study in the U.S.. Cancer 80(6):1021-8, 1997

Hebert J, Rosen A. Nutritional, Socioeconomic, and reproductive factors in relation to female breast cancer mortality: findings from a cross-national study. Cancer Detect Preven 20(3):234-44, 1996

Hedberg K et al. Alcoholism and cancer of the larynx: a case-control study in western Washington (United States). Cancer Causes and Control 5:3-8, 1994

Heimburger DC et al. Improvement in bronchial squamous metaplasia in smokers treated with folate and vitamin B12: Report of a preliminary randomized, double-blind intervention trial. JAMA 259(10):1525-30, 1988

Heimberger DC. Localized deficiencies of folic acid in aerodigestive tissues. Ann NY Acad Sci 669:87-96, 1992

Heinonen OP et al. Prostate cancer and supplementation with alpha-tocopherol and beta-carotene: incidence and mortality in a controlled trial. J Natl Cancer Inst 90(6):440-6, 1998

Hellstrom & Hellstrom, in Salinas and Hanna, Eds. Immune Complexes and Cancer. Vol. 15, 1985

Hennekens CH et al. Lack of effect of long-term supplementation with beta carotene on the incidence of malignant neoplasms and cardiovascular disease. N Engl J Med 334(18):1145-9, 1996

Hertog MGL et al. Dietary flavonoids and cancer risk in the Zutphen Elderly Study. Nutr Cancer 22:175-84, 1994

Hibbs JB et al. L-arginine is required for the expression of he activated macrophage effector mechanism causing selective metabolic inhibition in target cells. J Immunol 138:550-65, 1987

Hill M. Epidemiology of meat and colorectal cancer - historical aspects. Eur Cancer Prevent News 31:8-10, 1997

Hinds MW et al. Dietary cholesterol and lung cancer among men in Hawaii. Am J Clin Nutr 37:192-3, 1983

Hoefer-Janker H et al. [Initial clinical experiences with subtoxic doses of vitamin A during radiotherapy and cytostatic treatment of tumors.] Krebsarzt 24(4):203-7, 1969 (in German)

Hoehn SK, Carroll KK. Effects of dietary carbohydrate on the incidence of mammary tumors induced in rats by 7,12-dimethylbenz(a)-anthracene. Nutr Cancer 1(3):27-30, Spring, 1979

Hoffer A. Orthomolecular Medicine for Physicians. New Canaan, CT, Keats Publishing, 1989

Hoffer A, Pauling L. Hardin Jones biostatistical analysis of mortality data for a second set of cohorts of cancer patients with a large fraction surviving at the termination of the study and a comparison of survival times of cancer patients receiving large regular doses of vitamin C and other nutrients with similar patients not receiving these doses. J Orthomol Med 8(3):157-67, 1993

Hoffman R et al. Enhanced anti-proliferative action of busulphan by quercetin on the human leukaemia cell line K562. Br J Cancer 59:347-8, 1989

Holtzman EJ et al. Serum cholesterol and the risk of colorectal cancer. N Engl J Med July 9, 1987, p. 114

Howe G et al. Dietary factors and risk of pancreatic cancer: Results of a Canadian population-based case-control study. Int J Cancer 45:604-8, 1990

Howie BJ, Shultz TD. Dietary and hormonal interrelationships among vegetarian Seventh-Day Adventists and nonvegetarian men. Am J Clin Nutr 42(1):127-34, 1985

Hrelia S et al. The role of delta-6- and delta-9-desaturase in the fatty acid metabolism of hepatomas with different growth rate. Biochem Mol Biol Int 34(3):449-55, 1994

Hrelia S et al. gamma-Linolenic acid supplementation can affect cancer cell proliferation via modification of fatty acid composition. Biochem Biophys Res Commun 225(2):441-7, 1996

Hu Y-J et al. The protective role of selenium on the toxicity of cisplatin-contained chemotherapy regimen in cancer patients. Biol Trace Elem Res 56:331-41, 1997

Huang Y-C et al. N-3 fatty acids decrease colonic epithelial cell proliferation in the high-risk bowel mucosa. Lipids 31(suppl):S313-S317, 1996

Hunter JE, Applewhite TH. Isomeric fatty acids in the US diet: Levels and health perspectives. Am J Clin Nutr 44(6):707-17, 1986

Hursting S et al. Types of dietary fat and the incidence of cancer at five sites. Prev Med 19:242-53, 1990

Ingram D et al. Case-control study of phyto-oestrogens and breast cancer. Lancet 350:990-4, 1997

Jaakkola K et al. Treatment with antioxidant and other nutrients in combination with chemotherapy and irradiation in patients with small-cell lung cancer. Anticancer Res 12:599-606, 1992

Jacobs DR Jr et al. Whole grain intake and cancer: a review of the literature. Nutr Cancer 24(3):221-9, 1995

Jacobson EL, Jacobson MK. A biomarker for the assessment of niacin nutriture as a potential preventive factor in carcinogenesis. J Intern Med 233:59-62, 1993a

Jacobson EL. Niacin deficiency and cancer in women. J Am Coll Nutr 12(4):412-16, 1993b

Joossens JV et al. Dietary salt, nitrate and stomach cancer mortality in 24 countries. Int J Epidemiol 25(3):494-502, 1996

Kamei T et al. Experimental study of the therapeutic effects of folate, vitamin A, and vitamin B_{12} on squamous metaplasia of the bronchial epithelium. Cancer 71(8):2477-83, 1993

Kaplan S et al. Nutritional factors in the etiology of brain tumors. Am J Epidemiol 146(10):832-41, 1997

Karmali RA. Historical perspective and potential use of omega-3 fatty acids in therapy of cancer cachexia. Nutrition 12(1) suppl:S2-S4, 1996

Kaul L et al. The role of diet in prostate cancer. Nutr Cancer 9:123-8, 1987

Kim JA et al. Topical use of N-acetylcysteine for reduction of skin reaction to radiation therapy. Semin Oncol 10(1 Suppl 1):86-88, 1983

Kim J-P et al. Effect on rosette forming T-lymphocyte level in immunochemotherapy using Picibanil and Wobe-Mugos in gastric cancer patients. J Korean Surg Soc 23, 1981

Kim Y-I et al. Folate, epithelial dysplasia and colon cancer. Proc Assoc Am Physicians 107:218-27, 1995

Kinsella JE et al. Metabolism of trans fatty acids with emphasis on the effects of trans, trans-octadecadienoate on lipid composition, essential fatty acid, and prostaglandins: An overview. AM J Clin Nutr 34:2307, 1981

Kirchhof D, Kirchhof E. The Successful Use of Bovine Tracheal Cartilage in the Treatment of Cancer. Belgrade, Montana, Kriegel & Assoc., 1995

Kirkpatrick CS et al. Case-control study of malignant melanoma in Washington State. II. Diet, alcohol, and obesity. Am J Epidemiol 139:869-80, 1994

Klimberg VS. Prevention of radiogenic side effects using glutamine-enriched elemental diets. Recent Results Cancer Res 121:283-5, 1991

Klimberg VS et al. Glutamine suppresses PGE2 synthesis and breast cancer growth. J Surg Res 63(1):293-7, 1996a

Klimberg VS, McClellan JL. Glutamine, cancer and its therapy. Am J Surg 172(5):418-24, 1996b

Klurfeld DM, Kritchevsky D. Wistar Institute, Philadelphia - quoted in Med World News, April 25, 1988

Knekt P et al. Body iron stores and risk of cancer. Int J Cancer 56(3):379-82, 1994

Knekt P et al. Dietary flavonoids and the risk of lung cancer and other malignant neoplasms. Am J Epidemiol 146(3):223-30, 1997

Kokron O. Österr Zschr Onkol 4:82-5, 1977 (in German)

Kolonel LN et al. Nutrient intakes in relation to cancer incidence in Hawaii. Br J Cancer 44(3):332-9, 1981

Kritz H et al. Low cholesterol and cancer. J Clin Oncol 14(11):3043-8, 1996

Kuhnau J. The flavonoids. A class of semi-essential food components: their role in human nutrition. World Rev Nutr Diet 24:117-91, 1976

Kune G et al. Dietary sodium and potassium intake and colorectal cancer risk. Nutr Cancer 12:351-9, 1989

Kune GA, Vitetta L. Alcohol consumption and the aetiology of colorectal cancer: a review of the scientific evidence from 1957 to 1991. Nutr Cancer 18:97-111, 1992

Kurbacher CM et al. Ascorbic acid (vitamin C) improves the antineoplastic activity of doxorubicin, cisplatin, and paclitaxel in human breast carcinoma cells in vitro. Cancer Lett 103:183-9, 1996

Labadarios D, Walker ARP. Dietary avoidance of coronary heart disease - How practicable is the Mediterranean Diet? Cardiovasc J So Afr Cardiovascular Suppl. 1:C30-C36, 1996

Laganiere S, Fernandes G. High peroxidizability of subcellular membrane induced by high fish oil diet is reversed by vitamin E. Clin Res 35:A565, 1987

Lamm DL et al. Megadose vitamins in bladder cancer: a double-blind clinical trial. J Urol 151(1):21-6, 1994

Lane IW, Contreras E Jr. High rate of bioactivity (reduction in gross tumor size) observed in advanced cancer patients treated with shark cartilage material. J Naturopath Med 3(1):86-8, 1992

Langer R, Murray J. Angiogenesis inhibitors and their delivery systems. Appl Biochem Biotechnol 8(1):9-24, 1983

Larocca LM et al. Quercetin and the growth of leukemic progenitors. Leuk Lymphoma 23(1-2):49-53, 1996

Lashner BA et al. The effect of folic acid supplementation on the risk for cancer or dysplasia in ulcerative colitis. Gastroenterology 112(1):29-32, 1997

Lathia D, Blum A. Role of vitamin E as nitrite scavenger and N-nitrosamine inhibitor: a review. Int J Vitam Nutr Res 59(4):430-8, 1989

La Vecchia C et al. Intake of selected micronutrients and risk of colorectal cancer. Int J Cancer 73:525-30, 1997

Lee A, Langer R. Shark cartilage contains inhibitors of tumor angiogenesis. Science 221:1185-7, 1983

Lee JR. Fluoridation and bone cancer. Editorial. Fluoride 26(2):79-82, 1993

Lee-Feldstein A. A comparison of several measures of exposure to arsenic. Matched case-control study of copper smelter employees. Am J Epidemiol 129(1):112-24, 1989

Lefkowitz ES, Garland CF. Sunlight, vitamin D and ovarian cancer mortality rates in US women. Epidemiol 23(6):1133-6, 1994

Levi F et al. Dietary factors and the risk of endometrial cancer. Cancer 71:3575-81, 1993

Leviton A, Allred EN. Correlates of decaffeinated coffee choice. Epidemiology 5:537-40, 1994

Levy L, Vredevoe DL. The effect of N-acetyl cysteine on cyclophosphamide immunoregulation and antitumor activity. Semin Oncol 10(1 Suppl 1):7-16, 1983

Ling-Wei X et al. Trace element content of drinking water of nasopharyngeal carcinoma patients. Trace Elements in Medicine 5(3):93-6, 1988

Lipkin M, Newmark H. Effect of added dietary calcium on colonic epithelial-cell proliferation in subjects at high risk for familial colonic cancer. N Engl J Med 313:1381-4, 1985

Lipman T et al. Esophageal zinc content in human squamous esophageal cancer. J Am Coll Nutr 6:41-6, 1987

Lipworth L et al. Olive oil and human cancer: an assessment of the evidence. Prev Med 26:181-90, 1997

Lockwood K et al. Partial and complete regression of breast cancer in patients in relation to dosage of coenzyme Q10. Biochem Biophys Res Commun 199(3):1504-8, 1994a.

Lockwood K et al. Apparent partial remission of breast cancer in 'high risk' patients supplemented with nutritional antioxidants, essential fatty acids and coenzyme Q10. Molec Aspects Med 15(suppl):S231-S240, 1994b

Lockwood K et al. Progress on therapy of breast cancer with vitamin Q10 and the regression of metastases. Biochem Biophys Res Commun 212(1):172-7, 1995

Longnecker MP. Alcoholic beverage consumption in relation to risk of breast cancer: meta-analysis and review. Cancer Causes Control 5(1):73-82, 1994

Losonczy KG et al. Vitamin E and vitamin C supplement use and risk of all-cause and coronary heart disease mortality in older persons: the Established Populations for Epidemiologic Studies of the Elderly. Am J Clin Nutr 64:190-6, 1996

MacGregor JT et al. Cytogenetic damage induced by folate deficiency in mice is enhanced by caffeine. Proc Natl Acad Sci U S A 87(24):9962-5, 1990

Malter M et al. Natural killer cells, vitamins and other blood components of vegetarian and omnivorous men. Nutr Cancer 12(3):271-8, 1989

Malvy DJM et al. Assessment of serum antioxidant micronutrients and biochemical indicators of nutritional status in children with cancer in search of prognostic factors. Int J Vitam Nutr Res 67:267-71, 1997

Mann, J. Position statement: nutrition options when reducing saturated fat intake. J Am Coll Nutr 11(S):82S-83S, 1992

Martinez ME, Willett WC. Calcium, vitamin D, and colorectal cancer: a review of the epidemiologic evidence. Cancer Epidemiol Biomarkers Prev 7(2):163-8, 1998

Martin-Jimenez M et al. Failure of high-dose tocopherol to prevent alopecia induced by doxorubicin. Letter. N Engl J Med 315(14):894-5, 1986

Matthews J. Sharks still intrigue cancer researchers. J Natl Cancer Inst 84(13):1000-2, 1992

McKeown-Eyssen G et al. A randomized trial of vitamins C and E in the prevention of recurrence of colorectal polyps. Cancer Res 48(16):4701-5, 1988

McIllmurray MB, Turkie W. Controlled trial of gamma linolenic acid in Dukes's C colorectal cancer. Br Med J 294:1260, 1987

Medina V et al. Sodium butyrate inhibits carcinoma development in a 1,2-dimethylhydrazine-induced rat colon cancer. JPEN J Parenter Enteral Nutr 22(1):14-17, 1998

Meguid M et al. Plasma carotenoid profiles in normals and patients with cancer. J Parenter Enteral Nutr 12(2):147-51, 1988

Messina, MJ et al. Soy intake and cancer risks: a review of the in vitro and in vivo data. Nutr Cancer 21:113-31, 1994

Mettlin CJ et al. Patterns of milk consumption and risk of cancer. Nutr Cancer 13:89-99, 1990

Moerman CJ et al. Consumption of foods and micronutrients and the risk of cancer of the biliary-tract. Prev Med 24(6):591-602, 1995

Moertel CG et al. High-dose vitamin C versus placebo in the treatment of patients with advanced cancer who have had no prior chemotherapy: A randomized double-blind comparison. N Engl J Med 312:137-41, 1985

Moon TE et al. Retinoids in prevention of skin cancer. Cancer Lett 114:203-5, 1997

Moore WE, Moore LH. Intestinal floras of populations that have a high risk of colon cancer. Appl Environ Microbiol 61(9):3202-7, 1995

Morton MS et al. Lignans and isoflavonoids in plasma and prostatic fluid in men: samples from Portugal, Hong Kong, and the United Kingdom. Prostate 32:122-8, 1997

Mufti SI. Alcohol acts to promote incidence of tumors. Cancer Detect Prev 16(3):157-62, 1992

Muindi JR. Retinoids in clinical cancer therapy. Cancer Treat Res 87:305-42, 1996

Muñoz N et al. No effect of riboflavine, retinol, and zinc on prevalence of precancerous lesions of oesophagus. Randomised double-blind intervention study in high-risk population of China. Lancet ii:111-14, 1985

Muscaritoli M et al. Oral glutamine in the prevention of chemotherapy-induced gastrointestinal toxicity. Eur J Cancer 33:319-20, 1997

Muto Y et al. Prevention of second primary tumors by an acyclic retinoid, polyprenoic acid, in patients with hepatocellular carcinoma. N Engl J Med 334:1561-7, 1996

Myers C et al. A randomized controlled trial assessing the prevention of doxorubicin cardiomyopathy by N-acetylcysteine. Semin Oncol 10(1 Suppl 1):53-5, 1983

Nair PP et al. Diet, nutrition intake, and metabolism in populations at high and low risk for colon cancer: Dietary cholesterol, beta-sitosterol, and stigmasterol. Am J Clin Nutr 40(4 suppl):927-30, 1984

Negri E et al. Intake of selected micronutrients and the risk of breast cancer. Int J Cancer 65:140-4, 1996

Nehlig A, Debry G. Coffee and cancer: a review of human and animal data. World Rev Nutr Diet 79:185-221, 1997

Newmark HL et al. Colon cancer and dietary fat, phosphate, and calcium: A hypothesis. J Natl Cancer Inst 72(6):1323-5, 1984

Nomura AM et al. Serum micronutrients and upper aerodigestive tract cancer. Cancer Epidemiol Biomark Prevent 6:407-12, 1997

Norie IH, Foster HD. Water quality and cancer of the digestive tract: The Canadian experience. J Orthomol Med 4(2):59-69, 1989

Norman A et al. Antitumor activity of sodium linoleate. Nutr Cancer 11(2):107-15, 1988

Novi AM. Regression of aflatoxin B1-induced hepatocellular carcinomas by reduced glutathione. Science 212:541-2, 1981

Nydegger UE, Davis JS. Soluble immune complexes in human disease. Crit Rev Clin Lab Sci 12:123, 1980

O'Conner HJ et al. Effect of increased intake of vitamin C on the mutagenic activity of gastric juice and intragastric concentrations of ascorbic acid. Carcinogenesis 6(11):1675-6, 1985

Odeleye OE, Watson RR. Health implications of the n-3 fatty acids. Letter. Am J Clin Nutr 53:177-81, 1991

Omenn GS et al. Effects of a combination of beta carotene and vitamin A on lung cancer and cardiovascular disease. N Engl J Med 334:1150-5, 1996

Orr JW Jr et al. Nutritional status of patients with untreated cervical cancer. II. Vitamin assessment. Am J Obstet Gynecol 151(5):632-5, 1985

O'Toole P, Lombard M. Vitamin C and gastric cancer: Supplements for some or fruit for all? Gut 39:345-7, 1996

Owen RW et al. Analysis of calcium-lipid complexes in faeces. Eur J Cancer Prev 43(3):247-55, 1995

Owen RW. Faecal steroids and colorectal carcinogenesis. Scand J Gastroenterol Suppl 222:76-82, 1997

Pagnanelli GM et al. Effect of vitamin A, C and E supplementation on rectal cell proliferation in patients with colorectal adenomas. J Natl Cancer Inst 84:47-51, 1992

Pais RC et al. Abnormal vitamin B6 status in childhood leukemia. Cancer 66(11):2421-8, 1990

Palan P et al. Decreased b-carotene tissue levels in uterine leiomyomas and cancers of reproductive and nonreproductive organs. Am J Obstet Gynecol 161:1649-52, 1989

Palmierei-Sevier A et al. Case report: long-term remission of parathyroid cancer: possible relation to vitamin D and calcitriol therapy. Am J Med Sci 306(5):309-12, 1993

Pan WH et al. Vitamin A, vitamin E, or beta-carotene status and hepatitis B-related hepatocellular carcinoma. Ann Epidemiol 3:217-24, 1993

Parazzini F et al. Alcohol and endometrial cancer risk: findings from an Italian case-controlled study. Nutr Cancer 23(1):55-61, 1995

Park K et al. Stimulation of human breast cancers by dietary L-arginine. Clin Sci 82:413-17, 1992

Pascoe GA, Reed DJ. Vitamin E protection against chemical-induced cell injury. II. Evidence for a threshold effect of cellular alpha-tocopherol in prevention of adriamycin toxicity. Arch Biochem Biophys 256:159-66, 1987

Petrek JA et al. Fatty acid composition of adipose tissue, an indication of dietary fatty acids, and breast cancer prognosis. J Clin Oncol 15(4):1377-84, 1997

Peters JM, Preston-Martin S, London SJ, et al. Processed meats and risk of childhood leukemia. Cancer Causes Control 5(2):195-202, 1994

Picurelli L et al. [Determination of serum Fe in prostatic pathology.] Actas Urol Esp 14(4):262-3, 1990 (in Spanish)

Pearce ML, Dayton S. Incidence of cancer in men on a diet high in polyunsaturated fats. Lancet i:464-7, 1971

Popov AI. [Effect of the nonspecific prevention of thrombogenic complications on late results in the combined treatment of bladder cancer.] Med Radiol (Mosk) 32(2):42-45, 1987

Porcelli B et al. Levels of folic acid in plasma and red blood cells of colorectal cancer patients. Biomed Pharmacother 50(6-7):303-5, 1996

Potter JD, McMichael AJ. Alcohol, beer, and lung cancer: A meaningful relationship? Int J Epidemiol 13(2):240-2, 1984

Potischman N et al. A case-control study of serum folate levels and invasive cervical cancer. Cancer Res 51(18):4785-9, 1991

Pozniak PC. The carcinogenicity of caffeine and cancer: A review. J Am Diet Assoc 85(9):1127-33, 1985

Prasad KN et al. Sodium ascorbate potentiates the growth inhibitory effect of certain agents on neuroblastoma cells in culture. Proc Natl Acad Sci U S A 76(2):829-32, 1979

Prasad KN. Modulation of the effects of tumor therapeutic agents by vitamin C. Life Sci 27(4):275-80, 1980a

Prasad KN et al. Vitamin E increases the growth inhibitory and differentiating effects of tumor therapeutic agents on neuroblastoma and glioma cells in culture. Proc Soc Exp Biol Med 164(2):158-63, 1980b

Prasad KN, Edwards-Prasad J. Vitamin E and cancer prevention: recent advances and future potentials. J Am Coll Nutr 11(5):487-500, 1992

Prior F. Theoretical involvement of vitamin B6 in tumor initiation. Med Hypotheses 16:421-8, 1985

Pritchard GA et al. Lipids in breast carcinogenesis. Br J Surg 76(10):1069-73, 1989

Prudden JF. The treatment of human cancer with agents prepared from bovine cartilage. J Biol Response Mod 4(6):551-84, 1985

Ransberger K, Maehder K. [The significance of proteolytic enzyme therapy as a component of cancer treatment.] Osterr Z Erforsch Bekampf Krebskr 28(5-6):187-93, 1973 (in German)

Rao AV et al. Effect of fiber-rich foods on the composition of intestinal flora. Nutr Res 14(4):523-35, 1994

Rasmussen LB et al. Effect of diet and plasma fatty acid composition on immune status in elderly men. Am J Clin Nutr 59:572-7, 1994

Reich R et al. Eicosapentaenoic acid reduces the invasive and metastatic activities of malignant tumor cells. Biochem Biophys Res Commun 160:559-64, 1989

Reichel H et al. The role of the vitamin D endocrine system in health and disease. N Engl J Med 320(15):980-91, 1989

Reynolds J et al. Arginine as an immunomodulator. Abstract. Surg Forum 38:415-18, 1987

Riordan NH et al. Intravenous ascorbate as a tumor cytotoxic chemotherapeutic agent. Med Hypotheses 44:207-13, 1995

Risch HA et al. Dietary fat intake and risk of epithelial ovarian cancer. J Natl Cancer Inst 86(18):1409-15, 1994

Rivadeneira DE et al. Nutritional support of the cancer patient. CA Cancer J Clin 48(2):69-80, 1998

Rock CL. Carotenoids: biology and treatment. Pharmacol Ther 75(3):185-97, 1997

Rokitansky O. Präoperative tumortherapie zur Verbessrung der Heilungsergebnisse beim Mammakarzinom. Krebegeschehan 12:127-30,1980 (in German)

Roncucci L et al. Antioxidant vitamins or lactulose for the prevention of the recurrence of colorectal adenomas. Dis Colon Rectum 36:227-34, 1993

Rood JC et al. Helicobacter pylori-associated gastritis and the ascorbic acid concentration in gastric juice. Nutr Cancer 22:65-72, 1994

Rose DP, Hatala MA. Dietary fatty acids and breast cancer invasion and metastasis. Nutr Cancer 21:103-11, 1994

Ross J et al. Dietary and hormonal evaluation of men at different risks for prostate cancer: Fiber intake, excretion, and composition, with in vitro evidence for an association between steroid hormones and specific fiber components. Am J Clin Nutr 51:365-70, 1990

Rouse K et al. Glutamine enhances selectivity of chemotherapy through changes in glutathione metabolism. Ann Surg 221(4):420-6, 1995

Santisteban GA et al. Glycemic modulation of tumor tolerance in a mouse model of breast cancer. Biochem Biophys Res Commun 132(3):1174-9, 1985

Saito M, Kato H, Tsuchida T, et al. Chemoprevention effects on bronchial squamous metaplasia by folate and vitamin B12 in heavy smokers. Chest 102(2):496-9, 1994

Salminen E et al. Preservation of intestinal integrity during radiotherapy using live Lactobacillus acidophilus cultures. Clin Radiol 39:435-7, 1988

Salminen E et al. Adverse effect of pelvic radiotherapy. Fifth Int. Mtg. Progress in Radio-Oncology May, 1995; 10-14:501-4

Sandler RS et al. Diet and risk of colorectal adenomas: macronutrients, cholesterol, and fiber. J Natl Cancer Inst 85(11):846-8, 1993

Sankaranarayanan R, Mathew B. Retinoids as cancer-preventive agents. IARC Sci Publ 139:47-5, 1996

Santamaria L, Bianchi-Santamaria A. Carotenoids in cancer chemoprevention and therapeutic interventions. J Nutr Sci Vitaminol (Tokyo) Spec No: 321-6, 1992

Sarasua S, Savitz DA. Cured and broiled meat consumption in relation to childhood cancer: Denver, Colorado (United States). Cancer Causes Control 5(2):141-8, 1994

Schlegel JU et al. The role of ascorbic acid in the prevention of bladder tumor formation. J Urol 103(2):155-9, 1970

Schmitt-Gräff A, Scheulen ME. Prevention of adriamycin cardiotoxicity by niacin, isocitrate or N-acetyl-cysteine in mice. A morphological study. Pathol Res Pract 181(2):168-74, 1986

Schwartz GG, Hulka BS. Is vitamin D deficiency a risk factor for prostate cancer? Anticancer Res 10(5A):1307-11, 1990

Seely S, Horrobin DF. Diet and breast cancer: The possible connection with sugar consumption. Med Hypotheses 11(3):319-27, 1983

Seelig MS. Magnesium and other nutritional clinical deficiencies in immunologic abnormalities including allergies and neoplasms. Abstract. J Am Coll Nutr 12:579, 1993

Shamsuddin AM et al. IP6: a novel anti-cancer agent. Life Sci 61(4):343-54, 1997

Sherwin RW et al. Serum cholesterol levels and cancer mortality in 361,662 men screened for the multiple risk factor intervention trial. JAMA 257(7):943-8, 1987

Siguel EN. Cancerostatic effect of vegetarian diets. Nutr Cancer 4(4):285-91, 1983

Silver J et al. Regulation of parathyroid cell proliferation. Curr Opin Nephrol Hypertens 6(4):321-6, 1997

Singh RB et al. Dietary intake and plasma levels of antioxidant vitamins in health and disease: a hospital-based case-control study. J Nutr Environ Med 5:235-42, 1995

Singh VN, Gaby SK. Premalignant lesion: role of antioxidant vitamins and beta-carotene in risk reduction and prevention of malignant transformation. Am J Clin Nutr 53:386S-90S, 1991

Skubitz KM et al. Oral glutamine to prevent chemotherapy-induced stomatitis: a pilot study. J Lab Clin Med 127:223-8, 1996

Smyth JF et al. Glutathione reduces the toxicity and improves quality of life of women diagnosed with ovarian cancer treated with cisplatin: results of a double-blind, randomised trial. Ann Oncol 8(6):569-73, 1997

Snowdon DA. Diet and ovarian cancer. Letter to the Editor. JAMA 254(3):356-57, 1985

Sobala GM et al. Levels of nitrite, nitrate, N-nitroso compounds, ascorbic and total bile acids in gastric juice of patients with and without precancerous conditions of the stomach. Carcinogenesis 12(2):193-8, 1991

Song MK et al. Effect of different levels of dietary zinc on longevity of Balb/c mice inoculated with plasmacytoma MOPC 104E. J Natl Cancer Inst 72:647-52, 1984

Song MK et al. Zinc, calcium, and magnesium metabolism: effects on plasmacytomas in Balb/c mice. Am J Clin Nutr 49:701-7, 1989

Spigelman AD et al. Vitamin C levels in patients with familial adenomatous polyposis. Br J Surg 77(5):508-9, 1990

Srivastava M et al. Nutritional risk factors in carcinoma of the esophagus. Nutr Res 15(2):177-85, 1995

Stadel VV. Dietary iodine and the risk of breast, endometrial and ovarian cancer. Lancet i:890-1, 1976

Stavric B. Quercetin in our diet: from potent mutagen to probable anticarcinogen. Clin Biochem 27(4):245-8, 1994

Steinmetz KA, Potter JD. Vegetables, fruit and cancer prevention: a review. J Am Diet Assoc 96:1027-9, 1996

Stevens RG et al. Iron-binding proteins and risk of cancer in Taiwan. J Natl Cancer Inst 76:605-10, 1986

Stich HF et al. Remission of precancerous lesions in the oral cavity of tobacco chewers and maintenance of the protective effect of β-carotene or vitamin A. Am J Clin Nutr 53:298S-304S, 1991

Stoll BA. Can supplementary dietary fiber suppress breast cancer growth? Br J Cancer 73:557-9, 1996

Stoll BA. Eating to beat breast cancer: potential role for soy supplements. Ann Oncol 8:223-5, 1997

Sundstrom H et al. Supplementation with selenium, vitamin E and their combination in gynaecological cancer during cytotoxic chemotherapy. Carcinogenesis 10:273-8, 1989

Sutton PR. Sodium fluoride as an oral carcinogen. Letter. N Z Med J 98(775):207, 1985

Taylor JA et al. Association of prostate cancer with vitamin D receptor gene polymorphism. Cancer Res 56(18):4108-10, 1996

Taylor PR et al. Effect of nutrition intervention on intermediate endpoints in esophageal and gastric carcinogenesis. Am J Clin Nutr 62(suppl):1420S-3S, 1995

Thomas MG et al. Vitamin D and its metabolites inhibit cell proliferation in human rectal mucosa and colon cancer cell line. Gut 33(12):1660-3, 1992

Trebukhina RV et al. [Metabolism of vitamins B1 and PP and their use in oncological practice]. Vopr Med Khim 38(5):33-6, 1992) (in Russian)

Trickler D et al. Inhibition of oral carcinogenesis by glutathione. Nutr Cancer 20:139-44, 1993

Ujiie S et al.. Serum selenium contents in cancer patients. Gan To Kagaku Ryoho 24(4):401-5, 1997

Umegaki K et al. Beta-carotene prevents x-ray induction of micronuclei in human lymphocytes. Am J Clin Nutr 53:238S-46S, 1991

van der Merwe CF et al. Oral gamma-linoleic acid in 21 patients with untreatable malignancy. An ongoing pilot open clinical trial. Br J Clin Pract 41(9):907-15, 1987

van der Merwe CF. The reversibility of cancer. S Afr Med J 65:712, 1984

van Helden PD et al. Esophageal cancer: vitamin and lipotrope deficiencies in an at-risk South African population. Nutr Cancer 10(4):247-55, 1987

van Loon AJ et al. Nitrate intake and gastric cancer risk: results from the Netherlands cohort study. Cancer Lett 114:259-61, 1997

Van Zandwijk N. N-acetylcysteine for lung cancer prevention. Chest 107(5):1437-41, 1995

Velazquez MC et al. Butyrate and the colonocyte: implications for neoplasia. Dig Dis Sci 41(4):727-39, 1996

Verreault R et al. A case-control study of diet and invasive cervical cancer. Int J Cancer 43:1050-4, 1989

Vlajinac HD et al. Diet and prostate cancer: a case-control study. Eur J Cancer 33(1):101-7, 1997

Vucenik I et al. Comparison of pure inositol hexaphosphate and high-bran diet in the prevention of DMBA-induced rat mammary carcinogenesis. Nutr Cancer 28(1):7-13, 1997

Wadleigh RG et al. Vitamin E in the treatment of chemotherapy-induced mucositis. Am J Med 92(5):481-4, 1992

Wang GQ et al. Effects of vitamin/mineral supplementation on the prevalence of histological dysplasia and early cancer of the esophagus and stomach: results from the General Population Trial in Linxian, China. Cancer Epidemiol Biomarkers Prev 3(2):161-6, 1994

Wargovich MJ. Calcium and colon cancer. J Am Coll Nutr 7(4):295-300, 1988

Wasan HS, Goodlad RA. Fibre-supplemented foods may damage your health. Viewpoint. Lancet 348:319-20, 1996

Watrach AM et al. Inhibition of human breast cancer cells by selenium. Cancer Lett 25:41-7, 1984

Watson RA. Ifosfamide: Chemotherapy with new promise and new problems for the urologist. Urology 24(5):465-8, 1984

WCRF Panel. Diet, Nutrition, and the Prevention of Cancer: A Global Perspective. Washington, DC, World Cancer Research Fund/American Institute for Cancer Research, 1997

Webber MM. Effects of zinc and cadmium on the growth of human prostatic epithelium in vitro. Nutr Res 6:35-40, 1986

Weide M et al. Study of immune function of cancer patients influenced by supplemental zinc or selenium-zinc combination. Biol Trace Elem Res 28:11-20, 1991

Weinberg ED. The role of iron in cancer. Eur J Cancer Prev 5(1):19-36, 1996

Weisburger JH et al. Protective mechanisms of dietary fibers in nutritional carcinogenesis. Basic Life Sci 61:45-63, 1993

Weisburger JH. Dietary fat and risk of chronic disease: mechanistic insights from experimental studies. J Am Diet Assn 97(Suppl):S16-S23, 1997

Weisel CP, Chen WJ. Exposure to chlorination by-products from hot water uses. Risk Anal 14(1):101-6, 1994

Whelen P et al. Zinc, vitamin A and prostatic cancer. Br J Urol 55(5):525-8, 1983

White WS et al. Pharmacokinetics of beta-carotene and canthaxanthin after individual and combined doses by human subjects. J Am Coll Nutr 13:665-71, 1994

Wilkens LR et al. Risk factors for lower urinary tract cancer: the role of total fluid consumption, nitrites and nitrosamines, and selected foods. Cancer Epidemiol Biomark Prevent 5:161-6, 1996

Willett WC, MacMahon B. Diet and cancer: An overview. N Engl J Med 310(11):697-703, 1984

Witte JS et al. Diet and premenopausal bilateral breast cancer: a case-control study. Breast Cancer Res Treat 42:243-51, 1997

Wood L. Possible prevention of adriamycin-induced alopecia by tocopherol. N Engl J Med 312:1060, 1985

Wrba H, Kodras B. Unterstüzung der Chemotherapie inoperabler bronchopulmonaler Karzinome durch proteolytische Ferment. Wien Med Wschr 128:153-8, 1978 (in German)

Wrba H, Pecher O. Enzyme - Wirkstoffe der Zukunft Mit der Enzymtherapie das Immunsystem stärken. Vienna, Verlag Orac, 1993 (in German)

Yamanaka N et al, in Y Yamamura, K Folkers, Y Ito, Eds. Biochemical and Clinical Aspects of Coenzyme Q, Volume 2. Amsterdam, Elsevier/North Holland Biomedical Press, 1980:213-24

Yamawaki S et al. Jpn J Cancer Clin 25:1081-6, 1979 (in Japanese)

Yang CY et al. Calcium and magnesium in drinking water and risk of death from colon cancer. Jpn J Cancer Res 88(10):928-33, 1997

Yang CY et al. Calcium, magnesium, and nitrate in drinking water and gastric cancer mortality. Jpn J Cancer Res 89(2):124-130, 1998

Yang GY, Shamsuddin AM. IP6-induced growth inhibition and differentiation of HT-29 human colon cancer cells: involvement of intracellular inositol phosphates. Anticancer Res 15(6B):2479-87, 1995

Yeum K-J et al. β-carotene intervention trial in premalignant gastric lesions. Abstract. J Am Coll Nutr 14(5):536, 1995

Yiomouyiannis JA. Fluoridation and cancer - the biology and epidemiology of bone and oral cancer related to fluoridation. Fluoride 26(2):83-96, 1993

Youngman LD. Protein restriction (PR) and caloric restriction (CR) compared: effects on DNA damage, carcinogenesis, and oxidative damage. Mutat Res 295(4-6):165-79, 1993

Zaichick Vye at al. Zinc in the human prostate gland: normal, hyperplastic and cancerous. Int Urol Nephrol 29(5):565-74, 1997

Zhang L et al. Serum micronutrients in relation to pre-cancerous gastric lesions. Int J Cancer 56(5):650-4, 1994

Zheng W et al. Retinol, antioxidant vitamins, and cancer of the upper digestive tract in a prospective cohort study of postmenopausal women. Am J Epidemiol 142:955-60, 1995

CANDIDIASIS

(OVERGROWTH OF, OR HYPERSENSITIVITY TO, *Candida albicans*)

See Also: IMMUNODEPRESSION
INFECTION

NUTRITIONAL TREATMENT GUIDE

✓ = Efficacy generally accepted.
* = Efficacy *demonstrated* by controlled human trials.
[+] = Efficacy *suspected* from uncontrolled human trials.
[-] = Efficacy *suspected* from indirect data.
? = Efficacy *challenged* in a study of similar design.

DIETARY FACTORS

[+] avoid **Sugar** (to minimize candida growth)
[+] **Yeast and mold-free diet** (to minimize cross-reactivity)

NUTRITIONAL FACTORS

[+] **Caprylic acid:** *to kill candida:* 1,800 mg daily (2 week trial)
[+] **Iron deficiency:** 30 mg twice daily until repletion; then minimal possible dosage
[+] **Magnesium deficiency:** ≈ 400 mg daily (Consider IM or IV administration.)
[+] **Magnesium dependency:** individualized dosage

- -

[-] **Beta-carotene deficiency:** 30 to 120 mg daily
[-] **Copper deficiency:** 2 mg twice daily for up to 6 weeks along with 50 mg **Zinc** daily
[-] avoid **Cysteine** or **Cystine** supplementation
[-] **Folic acid deficiency:** 800 µg daily
[-] **Omega-3 fatty acid deficiency:** *example:* MaxEPA 1 g caps [180 mg EPA; 120 mg DHA] 10 to 20 daily
[-] **Riboflavin deficiency:** 5 to 10 mg daily
[-] **Selenium deficiency:** 200 µg daily
[-] **Vitamin A deficiency:** 50,000 IU daily for 6 weeks (10,000 IU daily during pregnancy)
[-] **Vitamin B_6 deficiency:** 50 to 100 mg daily
[-] **Vitamin C:** 500 mg twice daily
[-] **Zinc deficiency:** zinc sulfate 220 mg twice daily *AND* **Copper** 2 mg daily

OTHER RELATED FACTORS

* ***Lactobacillus acidophilus:*** 8 ounces daily of yogurt containing live cultures (6 month trial)

- -

[+] **Hydrochloric Acid deficiency:** betaine or glutamic hydrochloride 10 to 50 gr following meals. (Beware of gastric irritation.)

Overgrowth of *Candida albicans* in mucous membranes, or hypersensitivity to the organism, is claimed by some authors to cause a poly-symptomatic syndrome (which may include mental symptoms, irritable bowel syndrome, premenstrual syndrome, etc.) even in the absence of infection.

At the present time, however, the American Academy of Allergy and Immunology considers the concept of a 'candidiasis hypersensitivity syndrome' to be unsubstantiated. According to the Academy, "the diagnosis, the special laboratory tests, and the special aspects of treatment should be considered experimental and reserved for use with informed consent in appropriate controlled trials" (*American Academy of Allergy and Immunology*).

DIETARY FACTORS

Sugar

Candida albicans multiplies in a medium that contains sugar, and animal work has shown that dietary glucose intake is a key determinant of candida growth in the gastrointestinal tract *(Vargas)*. When women with a history of candida vulvovaginitis were compared to controls, carbohydrate intake was associated with a history of candida vulvovaginitis *(Reed)*.

In fact, when women with this diagnosis were placed on a sugar-free diet, the incidence and severity of their episodes were reduced *(Horowitz)*. The women in this study demonstrated elevated urinary sugar patterns that correlated well with excessive oral ingestion of dairy products, artificial sweeteners, and sucrose.

Moreover, *Candida albicans* appears to be unable to grow in human saliva unless it is supplemented with glucose *(Samaranayake LP)*. This appears to be due to the ability of dietary sugars to enhance candida's resistance to salivary lysozyme *(Samaranayake YH)*.

At least initially, a sugar-free diet should avoid all sources of sugar, including lactose (milk sugar) and fructose (fruit sugar). Then, if the patient improves, dairy products and fruits can be reintroduced on a trial basis.

A 31-year-old woman with recurrent candida vaginitis complained of fatigue, 'spaciness', mood swings, and sugar cravings. Physical examination revealed allergic 'shiners' below her eyes and a heavy, whitish coating on her tongue.

She was treated with oral nystatin, vitamins and minerals, and an elimination diet followed by individual food testing. After 6 weeks her symptoms had improved considerably and food provocation testing was performed. While other foods were well tolerated, refined sugar in various forms provoked her symptoms. A month later, thinking she was cured, she went on a two-day sugar binge during a holiday. The white coating on her tongue along with her symptoms rapidly returned. She was once again started on nystatin and an elimination diet and responded well.

She did well over the next month, but then was hospitalized for elective surgery. She informed the doctor and dietitian of her sensitivity to sugar and was given a sugar-free diet. However, by the next morning, her tongue had a heavy, whitish coating and she was seriously depressed and very anxious. At that time, she noticed that the label on her IV bottle, which had been dripping into her veins for the past 24 hours, indicated that the contents contained 5% dextrose. After she informed the doctor and the IV was removed, her symptoms gradually resolved over a 7 day period (Gaby).

Yeast- and Mold-free Diet

Some clinicians have advocated a yeast- and mold-free diet because there is considerable cross-reactivity between several genera of fungi *(Hoffman)*. Crook finds that about half of his patients with "candida-related complex" are hypersensitive to yeast *(Crook)*. In patients with chronic urticaria, for example, there may be reactivity both to candida and to other types of yeasts and fungi *(James)*.

The clinical relevance of this finding was demonstrated in a study of 49 chronic urticaria patients who reacted to *Candida albicans* antigens (19% of patients who were tested). Fifty-five percent of these 49 patients also reacted to brewer's yeast. After treatment with a low-yeast diet and anti-fungal therapy, 55% of them experienced a clinical cure. Similar results were obtained employing a yeast-free diet in the treatment of mucous colitis *(Holti)*. Also, Galland has reported that, in the clinical setting, even women whose chief complaint is chronic vaginal candidiasis often experience improvement in vaginal itching and discharge on a yeast/mold elimination diet as well as symptom exacerbation following exposure to yeast- or mold-containing foods *(Galland,1986)*.

NUTRITIONAL FACTORS

VITAMINS

Folic Acid Deficiency

Folate deficiency alone does not appear to promote the growth of candida on mucous membranes; in fact, folate antagonists can inhibit candida growth *(Bush)*. However, in susceptible individuals, folate deficiency may facilitate epithelial invasion of candida hyphae *(Jenkins)*. This finding is probably of clinical relevance as one study found that 15% of patients with candida hypersensitivity or toxicity presented with deficient serum folate levels *(Galland,1985a)*.

The effect of repletion of a folate deficiency has not been investigated by controlled studies. However, because of the numerous adverse effects of such a deficiency, repletion is probably justified.

Riboflavin Deficiency

The only study to report on riboflavin nutriture for patients with candida hypersensitivity or toxicity reported differing results depending upon which test was performed. Twenty-nine percent of 17 patients had deficiency based on the erythrocyte glutathione reductase activity coefficient, although not a single one of 59 patients was riboflavin-deficient based on microbiological assays *(Galland,1985a)*.

Dietary riboflavin must be activated by conversion to riboflavin-5-phosphate, the cofactor of pyridoxine oxidase. As this conversion is magnesium-dependent, it is possible that magnesium deficiency causes abnormal riboflavin metabolism resulting in a functional deficiency of the vitamin. Research is needed to better determine the role of riboflavin in this infection.

Vitamin A Deficiency

Two studies, one of patients with mucocutaneous candidiasis and one of patients with candida hypersensitivity or toxicity, found evidence that, based on serum levels, vitamin A deficiency was common despite normal serum carotene levels *(Galland,1985a;Montes)*. The latter study found deficient levels in 13% of patients.

While controlled human trials are lacking, vitamin A supplementation has been shown to enhance the resistance of mice to candida infections *(Cohen)*. More generally, supplementation causing vitamin A excess enhances lymphocytic response to antigens and antibody responses, and may diminish host susceptibility to infection *(Beisel)*.

Vitamin B_6 Deficiency

Two-thirds of a group of 39 patients with candida hypersensitivity or toxicity were found to be deficient in plasma pyridoxal-5-phosphate, the activated form of the vitamin, while only 5 out of a group of 59 were deficient in pyridoxine. These findings suggest impaired phosphorylation of vitamin B_6 may be more common than dietary insufficiency *(Galland,1985a)*.

Riboflavin is required for the oxidation of pyridoxine phosphate to pyridoxal-5-phosphate. Moreover, Galland has found an association between elevated glutathione reductase activity (suggesting riboflavin deficiency) and low pyridoxal-5-phosphate levels *(Galland,1986)*, thus suggesting that a riboflavin deficiency may cause abnormal vitamin B_6 metabolism. Further studies are needed to clarify the picture.

Vitamin C

Animal work suggests that vitamin C deficiency increases susceptibility to the early stages of candidiasis. However, supplemental levels of the vitamin greater than that needed to replete a deficiency may fail to increase resistance to this microorganism *(Rogers)*.
Vitamin C supplements may have another benefit beside repleting a deficiency. When added to amphotericin B, ascorbic acid enhanced the drug's lethality in regard to *Candida albicans* cells, augmenting the oxygen-dependent killing of the cells induced by the drug *(Brajtburg)*.

MINERALS

Copper Deficiency

Neutrophils from copper-deficient animals have a reduced ability to kill ingested *Candida albicans (Babu;Boyne)*, suggesting that copper deficiency could promote the infection. However, supplementary copper should be limited to the dosage needed to replete a deficiency as, when copper was injected into mice, the filamentous phase of the organism, normally the less virulent phase, became as virulent as the yeast phase *(Vaughn)*.

Iron

The relationship between iron nutriture and candida infection is complex. Reduced serum ferritin levels were found in 10 of a group of 101 patients with candida hypersensitivity or toxicity. However, iron repletion failed to affect the infection in all but those with sideropenic anemia *(Galland,1985a)*.

Iron deficiency is no more common in oral candidosis than in normals, suggesting that the deficiency itself does not promote candida growth on mucous membranes; it may, however, facilitate epithelial invasion by candida hyphae in susceptible people *(Jenkins)*. This may include those with reduced cellular immunity, as mucocutaneous lesions in such patients rapidly improve following iron supplementation *(Higgs)*. Also, *C. albicans* was isolated more often and in greater number from patients with oral candida lesions who had a hypochromic anemia and low serum iron levels, and these patients responded to iron therapy with a rapid clearing of mouth lesions *(Fletcher)*.

Yet another group consists of patients with familial chronic mucocutaneous candidiasis. In one study, 23 out of 31 (74%) had overt or latent iron deficiency based on serum iron and iron-binding capacity and bone marrow biopsies. Eleven of these patients were treated with oral iron, parenteral iron, or a combination of both for several months; nine (82%) showed clinical improvement *(Wells)*.

A Warning

Iron supplementation is contraindicated unless there is evidence of iron deficiency. Animal studies have found that excessive iron encourages candida infection *(Mencacci)*. Endothelial cell injury caused by candida appears to be iron-dependent *(Fratti)*; thus, iron overload may increase the pathogenicity of the organism.

Magnesium Deficiency or Dependency

Magnesium deficiency may be the most common biochemical abnormality in chronic candidiasis patients and could explain functional deficiencies in riboflavin and vitamin B_6 *(Galland,1986)*. Of 41 patients with candida hypersensitivity or toxicity who underwent a magnesium loading test, none had a normal result *(Galland,1985a)*. Conversely, among 50 patients with normocalcemic latent tetany (primarily due to magnesium deficiency), one-third suffered from recurrent or chronic candida infection by history, one-quarter showed evidence of active infection, and one-half demonstrated type I hypersensitivity to an extract of the organism on intradermal testing *(Galland,1985b)*.

Based on his clinical experience, Galland suggests that organic magnesium salts are more likely to be effective than magnesium oxide, even when mixed with amino acids. He recommends that magnesium supplements be combined with pyridoxine 50 to 1,000 mg daily (to improve cellular magnesium uptake) and vitamin D 400 to 1000 IU daily (to increase magnesium absorption). He also suggests that patients with normocalcemic latent tetany, a history of prolonged antibiotic exposure or recurrent candida infection who have refractory symptoms should be considered for oral antifungal therapy and candida desensitization *(Galland,1986)*.

A 43-year-old female with refractory hypomagnesemia had been well until age 30 when she was treated with multiple courses of antibiotics because of urinary tract infections. She developed recurrent candida vaginitis which persisted for 2 years. After starting a stressful job she began to experience symptoms of vertigo, muscle spasms, palpitations, fatigue and depression and became sensitive to many foods, molds and chemicals. Her serum magnesium was measured, and found to be only 1.3 mEq/l.

She was started on oral magnesium supplements with improvement in a number of symptoms, especially muscle pain and spasm. She found, however, that she needed to take over 1,500 mg magnesium daily, enough to produce diarrhea, to relieve her muscle spasms. When re-evaluated, her serum magnesium had increased to 1.94 mEq/l and she was in neutral magnesium balance. She still had a number of symptoms, notably depression and fatigue. Moreover, if she stopped magnesium supplementation, serum magnesium fell to 1.4 mEq/l within 3 days despite a urine magnesium excretion of only 64 mg a day and the absence of diarrhea.

When evaluated later while on magnesium supplementation, Chvostek's sign was positive and electromyography confirmed the presence of latent tetany. She had no visible evidence of candidiasis; however, she was so sensitive to C. albicans extract that immunotherapy was impossible.

She was treated with oral nystatin 8 million units daily, but developed asthma that persisted until the drug was stopped. She was then switched to ketoconazole 200 mg daily for 6 weeks. During this period her diarrhea improved and her depression lifted; however, the drug was stopped because of a skin rash.

Subsequently she was able to decrease her oral magnesium intake by 20% and felt well enough for regular employment. She was also receiving a longer course of an antifungal drug in the hope of reducing her magnesium requirement (Galland,1985b).

Selenium Deficiency

In animals, a deficiency of selenium may reduce the ability of neutrophils to kill candida *(Kukreja)*. Moreover, when selenium-deficient animals receive intravenous injections of *Candida albicans*, the organism multiplies faster and death occurs sooner *(Boyne)*.

However, the effect of selenium supplementation remains to be studied.

Zinc Deficiency

There is some evidence suggesting that zinc deficiency may contribute to candidiasis. When rhesus monkey infants are made zinc-deficient, there is impairment in the ability of their polymorphonuclear leukocytes to phagocytose *Candida albicans (Haynes)*, while zinc-deficient mice have been shown to become more susceptible to candida infection *(Salvin)*.

In humans, candida hypersensitivity or toxicity may be associated with reduced plasma zinc levels - while erythrocyte zinc levels may be elevated *(Galland)*. While one human study found reduced plasma zinc levels in women with recurrent vaginal candidiasis *(Edman)*, another failed to confirm this finding in a similar population *(Bohler)*. Moreover, not only may zinc deficiency encourage candidiasis, but candida infection may cause a zinc deficiency *(Parratt)*.

Results of a study in mice suggest that zinc supplementation may combat infection with *C. albicans*. When mice which are normally susceptible to these infections were fed a high-zinc diet, they became more resistant *(Salvin)*.

OTHER NUTRITIONAL FACTORS

Beta-Carotene Deficiency

Vaginal cell beta-carotene has been found to be significantly reduced in women with vaginal candidiasis *(Mikhail)*. This finding suggests that inadequate beta-carotene may alter the local immune response, resulting in disturbances in the vaginal flora, overgrowth of candida, and the development of vaginal candidiasis.

Caprylic Acid

Caprylic acid is an aliphatic straight-chain fatty acid which occurs naturally in coconut oil. When complexed with a resin, it has been found to be effective in reducing intestinal candidiasis as determined by stool culture *(Crinnion;Neuhauser)*. Administration has also been found to be helpful for treating thrush *(Keeney)*. Formulations from different manufacturers appear to vary greatly in clinical efficacy.

Cysteine or Cystine: A Warning

Like glucose, cysteine and cystine are readily utilized carbon sources for *C. albicans* growth in the yeast form *(Griffin)*. Supplementation with these sulfur amino acids should thus be avoided by patients.

Omega-3 Fatty Acid Deficiency

Members of the omega-3 family of essential fatty acids are often reduced in patients with candida hypersensitivity or toxicity *(Galland,1985;Truss)*. By contrast, levels of certain members of the omega-6 family of essential fatty acids may be elevated, and elevation of pro-inflammatory arachidonic acid, which is derived from the omega-6 family, is a common finding *(Galland, 1985)*.

Findings suggesting of essential fatty acid deficiency are common. In one study, two-thirds of a group of over 100 patients with candida hypersensitivity or overgrowth had two or more findings suggestive of deficiency, including dry skin, flaky paint dermatitis, follicular keratoses, brittle nails and dry, straw-like hair *(Galland, 1985)*.

For these reasons, supplementation with omega-3 fatty acids may theoretically be beneficial *(Galland, 1985)*.

OTHER RELATED FACTORS

Hydrochloric Acid Deficiency

As *Candida albicans* requires a pH of 7.4 for optimal growth, while it becomes completely inhibited at pH 4.5, a deficiency of hydrochloric acid will encourage overgrowth of candida in gastric juice *(Bolivar)*. In fact, H_2-receptor antagonists, by decreasing gastric acidity, frequently encourage such overgrowth, especially in women *(Boero)*.

Lactobacillus acidophilus

Lactobacillus acidophilus has a beneficial effect on the distribution of intestinal and vaginal microflora and on the metabolic activities of fecal enzymes in addition to having a direct anti-candida effect *(Anonymous)*.

This effect has been demonstrated with vaginal candidiasis with both oral *(Hilton)* and vaginal *(Collins; Will)* administration. For example, 13 women with recurrent candidal vaginitis consumed 8 ounces of yogurt containing *L. acidophilus* daily and a yogurt-free diet for 6 months each. After 6 months on the yogurt-containing diet, there was a 3-fold decrease in infections and a decrease in candidal colonization *(Hilton)*.

BIBLIOGRAPHY

American Academy of Allergy and Immunology. Position statement: Candidiasis hypersensitivity syndrome. J Allergy Clin Immunol 78(2):271-3, 1986

Anonymous. Lactobacillus feeding alters human colonic bacterial enzyme activities. Nutr Rev 42(11):374-6, 1984

Babu U, Failla ML. Copper status and function of neutrophils are reversibly depressed in marginally and severely copper-deficient rats. J Nutr 120(12):1700-9, 1990

Beisel WR. Single nutrients and immunity. Am J Clin Nutr 35:417-68 (suppl), 1982

Boero M et al. Candida overgrowth in gastric juice of peptic ulcer subjects on short- and long-term treatment with H_2-receptor antagonists. Digestion 28(3):158-63, 1983

Bohler K et al. Zinc levels of serum and cervicovaginal secretion in recurrent vulvovaginal candidiasis. Genitourin Med 70(5):308-10, 1994

Bolivar R, Bodey GP. Candidiasis of the gastrointestinal tract, in GP Bodey, V Fainstein, Eds. Candidiasis. New York, Raven Press, 1985

Boyne R, Arthur R. The response of selenium-deficient mice to candida albicans infection. J Nutr 116(5):816-22, 1986

Brajtburg J. Effects of ascorbic acid on the antifungal action of amphotericin B. J Antimicrob Chemother 24(3):333-7, 1989

Bush K et al. Activity of sulfa drugs and dihydrofolate reductase inhibitors against Candida albicans. Experientia 38(4):436-7, 1982

Cohen BE, Elin RJ. Enhanced resistance to certain infections in vitamin A-treated mice. Plast Reconstr Surg 54(2):192-4, 1974

Collins EB, Hardt P. Inhibition of candida albicans by lactobacillus acidophilus. J Dairy Sci 63:830-2, 1980

Crinnion WJ. Clinical trial results on Neesby's Capricin. Unpublished manuscript. Probiologic, Inc., 1803 132nd Ave., NE, Bellvue, WA 98005, USA, September 10, 1985

Crook William G interviewed in the Townsend Letter for Doctors, November, 1989, p. 592

Edman J et al. Zinc status in women with vulvovaginal candidiasis. Am J Obstet Gynecol 155(5):1082-5, 1986

Fletcher J et al. Mouth lesions in iron-deficient anemia: Relationship to candida albicans, saliva and to impairment of lymphocyte transformation. J Infect Dis 131:44-50, 1975

Fratti RA et al. Endothelial injury caused by Candida albicans is dependent on iron. Infect Immunol 66(1):191-6, 1998

Gaby AR. Literature review and commentary. Townsend Letter for Doctors, Feb/March 1988

Galland L. Nutrition and candidiasis. J Orthomol Psychiatry 14:50-60, 1985a

Galland L. Normocalcemic tetany and candidiasis. Magnesium 4(5-6):339-44, 1985b

Galland LD. Nutrition and Candida albicans, in J Bland, Ed. 1986: A Year in Nutritional Medicine. New Canaan, Connecticut, Keats Publishing, 1986

Griffin D. Fungal Physiology. Wiley-Interscience, 1981:124-5

Haynes DC et al. Studies of marginal zinc deprivation in rhesus monkeys: VI. Influence on the immunohematology of infants in the first year. Am J Clin Nutr 42(2):252-62, 1985

Higgs JM, Wells RS. Mucocutaneous candidiasis. Br J Dermatol (Suppl) 86:88-102, 1972

Hilton E et al. Ingestion of yogurt containing Lactobacillus acidophilus as prophylaxis for candidal vaginitis. Ann Intern Med 116(5):353-7, 1992

Hoffman DR, Kozak PP. Shared and specific allergens in mold extracts. J Allergy Clin Immunol 63:213, 1979

Holti G. Candida allergy, in Winner & Hurley, Eds. Symposium on Candida Infections. Edinburgh, Livingstone Publishers, 1966

Horowitz BJ et al. Sugar chromatography studies in recurrent Candida vulvovaginitis. J Reprod Med 29(7):441-3, 1984

James J, Warren RP. An assessment of the role of candida albicans and food yeast in chronic urticaria. Br J Dermatol 84:227-37, 1971

Jenkins WM et al. Nutritional deficiency in oral candidosis. Int J Oral Surg 6(4):204-10, 1977

Keeney E. Bull Johns Hopkins Hosp 78:333-9, 1946

Kukreja R, Khan A. Effect of experimental selenium deficiency and its supplementation on the candidacidal activity of neutrophils in albino rats. Indian J Biochem Biophys 31(5):427-9, 1994

Mencacci A et al. Iron overload alters innate and T helper cell responses to Candida albicans in mice. J Infect Dis 175(6):1467-76, 1997

Mikhail MS et al. Decreased beta-carotene levels in exfoliated vaginal epithelial cells in women with vaginal candidiasis. Am J Reprod Immunol 32:221-5, 1994

Montes LF et al. Hypovitaminosis A in patients with mucocutaneous candidiasis. J Infect Dis 128(2):227-30, 1973

Neuhauser I, Gustus E. Successful treatment of intestinal moniliasis with fatty acid-resin complex. Arch Intern Med 93:53-60, 1954

Parratt D. Nutrition and immunity. Proc Nutr Soc 39(2):133-40, 1980

Reed BD et al. The association between dietary intake and reported history of Candida vulvovaginitis. J Fam Pract 29(5):509-15, 1989

Rogers TJ et al. Dietary ascorbic acid and resistance to experimental renal candidiasis. J Nutr 113(1):178-83, 1983

Salvin SB, Rabin BS. Resistance and susceptibility to infection in inbred murine strains. IV. Effects of dietary zinc. Cell Immunol 87(2):546-52, 1984

Samaranayake LP et al. The proteolytic potential of candida albicans in human saliva supplemented with glucose. J Med Microbiol 17(1):13-22, 1984

Samaranayake YH et al. The in vitro lysozyme susceptibility of Candida albicans cultured in carbohydrate-supplemented media. Oral Microbiol Immunol 8(3):177-81, 1993

Truss CO. Metabolic abnormalities in patients with chronic candidiasis: The acetaldehyde hypothesis. J Orthomol Psychiatry 13:66-93, 1984

Vargas SL et al. Modulating effect of dietary carbohydrate supplementation on Candida albicans colonization and invasion in a neutropenic mouse model. Infect Immunol 61(2):619-26, 1993

Vaughn VJ, Weinberg ED. Candida albicans dimorphism and virulence: Role of copper. Mycopathologia 64(1):39-42, 1978

Wells RS et al. Familial chronic muco-cutaneous candidiasis. J Med Genet 9:302, 1972

Will TE. Lactobacillus overgrowth for treatment of moniliary vulvovaginitis. Letter. Lancet ii:482, 1979

CAPILLARY FRAGILITY

See Also: DIABETES MELLITUS

NUTRITIONAL TREATMENT GUIDE

✓ = Efficacy generally accepted.
* = Efficacy *demonstrated* by controlled human trials.
[+] = Efficacy *suspected* from uncontrolled human trials.
[-] = Efficacy *suspected* from indirect data.
? = Efficacy *challenged* in a study of similar design.

NUTRITIONAL FACTORS

* **Hesperidin:** 25 to 200 mg 4 times daily *with* **Vitamin C** 25 to 200 mg 4 times daily
* **Vitamin C:** 500 mg twice daily (2 to 4 month trial)

- -

[+] **Anthocyanosides:** Bilberry extract (standardized for an anthocyanidin content of 25%) 160 to 480 mg daily
[+] **Rutin:** 200 to 500 mg daily
[+] **Vitamin E:** 200 to 600 IU daily (3 week trial)

- -

[-] **Zinc deficiency:** zinc sulfate 220 mg twice daily *AND* **Copper** 2 mg daily

NUTRITIONAL FACTORS

VITAMINS

Vitamin C

Increased capillary fragility is a sign of scurvy, the disease caused by marked vitamin C deficiency. In fact, capillary fragility has been proposed as a functional measure of vitamin C status *(Johnston)*.

The results of controlled studies suggest that ascorbate supplementation may increase the strength of fragile capillaries. Its efficacy is best established for patients who are ascorbate-deficient *(Schorah)*; whether supplementation benefits people with fragile capillaries whose ascorbate nutriture is normal is uncertain.

Vitamin E

Open trials have reported resolution of purpura following supplementation with alpha-tocopherol. Purpura due to various causes seems to respond, including purpura secondary to infection or drugs *(Fujii)*. As with vitamin C, whether benefits are limited to patients who are deficient in the vitamin is unknown.

MINERALS

Zinc Deficiency

Compared to age-matched controls, a group of 20 elderly patients with senile purpura had lower fasting serum zinc levels, while mean serum levels of albumin, the main binder of zinc, were similar, and no other clinical or laboratory findings differentiated the 2 groups *(Haboubi)*. These as yet unconfirmed findings suggest that zinc deficiency may foster the development of senile purpura;

however, no clinical trials of zinc supplementation have been published

OTHER NUTRITIONAL FACTORS

Flavonoids

Anthocyanosides

When patients with varicose veins and ulcerative dermatitis received an oral extract of anthocyanosides, there was a substantial drop in capillary leakage. Anthocyanosides were found to protect altered capillary walls by increasing the endothelium barrier-effect through stabilization of membrane phospholipids, and by increasing the biosynthetic processes of the acid mucopolysaccharides of the connective ground substance through restoration of the altered mucopolysaccharidotic pericapillary sheath *(Mian)*.

Bilberry *(Vaccinium myrtillus)* is a rich source of these flavonoids.

Hesperidin

The combination of hesperidin and vitamin C has been investigated in number of studies. When patients with rheumatoid arthritis and increased capillary fragility received either hesperidin, vitamin C or the combination, the greatest improvement occurred in those taking the combination *(Warter, 1946)*, suggesting that the two substances had at least an additive, if not a synergistic, effect *(Beiler)*. In another study of similar patients, capillary fragility was restored to normal in 90% of patients *(Warter, 1948)*.

In an open trial, menopausal women with easy bruising or spontaneous nosebleeds that worsened at the time of the month in which their menses formerly occurred also responded. Of 15 women with easy bruising, 11 improved after 8 weeks, while the rest responded by 16 weeks. Nosebleeds were stopped in 6 to 11 weeks in 8 cases which were moderate. Of the 3 patients with severe nosebleeds, 1 was successfully treated in 3 months. The other 2 patients improved but their nosebleeds were never completely eliminated until they eventually stopped spontaneously in the fourth year *(Horoschak)*.

Rutin

The frequency of abnormal forearm petechiae counts among diabetics following inflation of a blood pressure cuff ranges from 50 to 100% *(Kornerup)*. Rutin supplementation has been found to improve capillary fragility in this group of patients. In three-quarters of cases, petechiae counts return to normal *(Donegan; Rodriguez)*.

BIBLIOGRAPHY

Beiler JM. Biochemistry of the synergists. Ascorbic acid and hesperidin. Exp Med Surg 12:563-9, 1955

Donegan JM, Thomas WA. Capillary fragility and cutaneous lymphatic flow in relation to systemic and retinal vascular manifestations: rutin therapy. Am J Ophthalmol 31:671-8, 1948

Fujii T. The clinical effects of vitamin E on purpuras due to vascular defects. J Vitaminology 18:125-30, 1972

Haboubi NY et al. Zinc deficiency in senile purpura. J Clin Pathol 38:1189-91, 1985

Horoschak A. Nocturnal leg cramps, easy bruisability and epistaxis in menopausal patients: Treated with hesperidin and ascorbic acid. Del State Med J January, 1959, pp. 19-22

Johnston CS, Collison R. Capillary fragility as a functional measure of vitamin C status. Abstract. J Am Coll Nutr 15(5):536, 1996

Kornerup T. Capillary fragility and diabetic retinopathy. Acta Ophthalmol 33:583-97, 1955

Mian E et al. [Anthocyanosides and the walls of microvessels: further aspects of the mechanism of action of their protective effect in syndromes due to abnormal capillary fragility.] Minerva Med 68(52):3565-81, 1977 (in Italian)

Rodriguez R, Root HG. Capillary fragility and diabetic retinitis. N Engl J Med 238:391-7, 1948

Schorah CJ et al. The effect of vitamin C supplements on body weight, serum proteins, and general health of an elderly population. Am J Clin Nutr 34(5):871-6, 1981

Warter PJ et al. Effect of hesperidin and ascorbic acid on capillary fragility in rheumatic arthritis. J Med Soc N J 43:228-30, 1946

Warter PJ et al. Influence of hesperidin-C on abnormal capillary fragility in rheumatic arthritis patients. Del State Med J 20(3):41-5, 1948

CARDIAC ARRHYTHMIAS

See Also: ATHEROSCLEROSIS

NUTRITIONAL TREATMENT GUIDE

✓ = Efficacy generally accepted.
* = Efficacy *demonstrated* by controlled human trials.
[+] = Efficacy *suspected* from uncontrolled human trials.
[-] = Efficacy *suspected* from indirect data.
? = Efficacy *challenged* in a study of similar design.

DIETARY FACTORS

[+] ? avoid **Caffeine**

- -

[-] avoid heavy **Alcohol** intake
[-] minimize **Saturated Fat**

NUTRITIONAL FACTORS

✓ **Magnesium:** IV infusion (acutely) followed by a trial of oral supplementation (≈ 400 mg daily)

- -

* **L-Carnitine:** 6 to 10 g daily in divided doses

- -

* **Beta-carotene deficiency:** 30 to 120 mg daily
* **Coenzyme Q_{10}:** 30 to 150 mg daily
* **Omega-3 fatty acids:** MaxEPA 1 g caps [180 mg EPA; 120 mg DHA] 10 to 20 daily
* **Potassium deficiency:** ? 80 to 100 mEq daily total intake, preferably from potassium-rich foods
* **Vitamin A deficiency:** 50,000 IU daily for 6 weeks (10,000 IU daily during pregnancy)
* **Vitamin C deficiency:** 500 mg twice daily
* **Vitamin E deficiency:** D,L-alpha-tocopheryl acetate 200 to 2,000 mg or IU daily for 6 weeks; then maintenance levels as needed

- -

[+] **Copper deficiency:** 2 mg twice daily for up to 6 weeks *AND* **Zinc** 50 mg daily
[+] **Folic acid:** 15 to 40 mg daily *AND* **Niacin** 1.5 to 4.5 g daily
[+] **Selenium deficiency:** 200 µg daily
[+] **Vitamin D:** *for sick sinus syndrome:* ? 800 IU daily

- -

[-] **Selenium:** 200 µg daily
[-] **Taurine:** ? 500 mg to 5 g daily
[-] **Vitamin E:** *for ventricular fibrillation:* ? 800 IU daily

OTHER RELATED FACTORS

* rule out **Food Sensitivities**

DIETARY FACTORS

Saturated Fat

The results of several epidemiological surveys have suggested that altering the habitual intake of the *type* of dietary fat, rather than altering the *quantity* of fat, may offer a nutritional means of reducing mortality from severe cardiac arrhythmias better than that achieved by the post hoc administration of anti-arrhythmic agents *(Charnock,1994a)*. Specifically, the intake of saturated fat appears to increase myocardial vulnerability, while the intake of polyunsaturates appears to decrease that risk.

A series of studies using the marmoset monkey have confirmed that this relationship is a causal one. When the heart was subjected to pharmacological or ischemic stress, diets rich in saturated fatty acids promoted arrhythmias, while diets enriched with either omega-3 or omega-6 polyunsaturates reduced arrhythmia vulnerability *(Charnock,1994b)*.

Furthermore, in a retrospective study of patients who experienced an acute myocardial infarction, those with ventricular fibrillation or tachycardia had a higher concentration of long-chain saturated fatty acids than those without *(Abraham)*.

Alcohol

Atrial fibrillation might be the first sign of heart damage due to alcohol abuse, while it usually takes over 10 years of chronic abuse before symptoms become overt *(Moushmoush)*. Also, acute ventricular fibrillation following an alcoholic binge, during which the QTc interval is often prolonged *(Otero-Anton)*, is so well recognized that it is called the "holiday heart syndrome" *(Fuenmayor,1997)*.

Caffeine

Caffeine increases the serum concentrations of epinephrine and norepinephrine *(Robertson)*, so it is not surprising that it has a pro-arrhythmic effect. This effect was recently documented in a canine model. Small doses mostly generated benign arrhythmias due to vagal stimulation, while more severe arrhythmias like ventricular tachycardia, multifocal ventricular premature contractions, atrial flutter and atrial fibrillation were generated with higher doses of caffeine *(Mehta)*.

Despite the arrhythmogenicity of caffeine, even cardiac patients can usually consume it in moderate doses of perhaps 300 mg (equivalent to 3 cups of coffee) without experiencing changes in cardiac rhythm *(Myers)*. However, in an open trial, only 200 mg increased the effective refractory period of the left atrium and caused arrhythmias in a group of cardiac patients who normally consumed 3 to 5 cups of coffee daily but abstained for 48 hours prior to testing *(Dobmeyer)*.

NUTRITIONAL FACTORS

VITAMINS

The literature on the efficacy of vitamin supplements in preventing and treating cardiac arrhythmias is very limited. Patients with acute myocardial infarction may have reduced plasma levels of vitamin A, vitamin C, vitamin E and beta carotene, and those who also have cardiac arrhythmias have even lower levels *(Singh,1994a)*. Moreover, when, in a double-blind study, patients suspected of an acute myocardial infarction were supplemented with these vitamins starting within a few hours of their symptoms, there was a reduction in the frequency of arrhythmias *(Singh,1996)*.

While little work has been done to investigate the individual actions of these nutrients, when rats developed myocardial ischemia due to coronary artery occlusion, there was a significant decrease in the ventricular fibrillation threshold in the placebo group, while no decrease in threshold occurred in the vitamin E-treated rats *(Fuenmayor,1989)*. This suggests that vitamin E supplementation may help protect against this serious arrhythmia.

Supplementation with other vitamins also may be helpful. Three elderly patients have been described whose atrial fibrillation ceased so long as their nutritional supplement program included adequate folic acid and niacin, and another 3 patients are said to have responded similarly *(Hoffer)*.

A single case report of an elderly woman suggests that vitamin D supplementation may cure the sick sinus syndrome. The vitamin appears to have a role in the impulse formation of the sinus node by facilitating transport of calcium during the action potential *(Kessel)*.

MINERALS

Magnesium

Magnesium is a cofactor in myocardial sodium-potassium ATPase which regulates the electrical activity of the heart. There is considerable research suggesting that magnesium deficiency increases the danger of cardiac arrhythmias. When, for example, dogs were made acutely magnesium-deficient, their coronary arteries became more likely to go into spasm following alcohol ingestion, suggesting that reduced magnesium intake or impaired magnesium metabolism potentiates the pro-arrhythmic effect of alcohol *(Altura)*.

Furthermore, magnesium deficiency is common among patients with acute medical conditions. For example, 20% of a group of 102 consecutive patients admitted into a medical intensive care unit had hypomagnesemia *(Reinhart)*, while 7% of patients in a coronary care unit were hypomagnesemic and 53% had low mononuclear cell magnesium *(Ryzen)*. Results of studies suggest that magnesium may be deficient in patients with ventricular arrhythmias *(Singh, 1994b)* and in those with symptomatic atrial fibrillation *(DeCarli)*.

Even in the absence of a magnesium deficit, magnesium supplementation may prevent and correct a wide variety of arrhythmias, including atrial tachyarrhythmias, supraventricular arrhythmias, and ventricular arrhythmias *(Dietch)*. This includes toxic arrhythmias caused by digitalis, perhaps because digitalis tends to produce a loss of intracellular potassium (which can be minimized by magnesium supplements) *(Cohen)* and torsade de pointes *(Tzivoni)*.

A 44 year-old health professional had noted a "change in heart rhythm" starting 5 hours earlier. In the past, he had very occasional random heart palpitations. Two years earlier, he had experienced a brief episode of tachycardia and a mitral murmur was detected. An echocardiogram demonstrated calcification of the mitral valve.

On examination, his cardiac rhythm was grossly irregular, consistent with atrial fibrillation, and he had a grade 1 to 2 (out of 6) diastolic mitral murmur. A 12-lead EKG showed indistinct P-waves and irregular QRS complexes averaging 120 per minute.

He was treated with magnesium chloride 1 gram IV and started on oral magnesium 500 mg twice daily. Two hours after the injection, the rhythm disturbance abruptly ceased, and his pulse became regular at 70 beats per minute.

One week later, he had a normal cardiac rhythm at 60 beats per minute, and a repeat EKG was normal. Over the subsequent two years, he has remained on oral magnesium and his heart rhythm has been normal (Anderson).

Potassium Deficiency

Potassium deficiency is associated with arrhythmias as well as decreased tolerance to cardiac medications and EKG alterations. In one study of 211 patients with an acute myocardial infarction, 17% were hypokalemic. Moreover, those with a serum potassium level of less than 4 mEq per liter (4 mmol/L) had an increased risk of ventricular arrhythmias *(Kafka)*.

Even when serum potassium is normal, potassium nutriture may still be so inadequate as to promote EKG abnormalities. Measurement of erythrocyte potassium levels may reveal the deficiency; if so, repletion has been shown to reverse the EKG abnormalities *(Sangiori)*.

Because of the inability of the heart muscle to hold onto potassium in the absence of magnesium, magnesium should be supplemented whenever potassium supplementation is provided to assure adequate magnesium nutriture *(Dychner)*.

Selenium

A subclinical selenium deficiency may cause subtle changes in myocardial contractility and excitability which could be reflected in altered responses to normal and abnormal stimuli *(Lehr)*.

Besides the repletion of a deficiency, selenium supplementation has been shown in animal studies to exert an antiarrhythmic effect. When pigs with experimentally induced myocardial infarction were supplemented with sodium selenite, ventricular extrasystoles and flutter developed less often, and "late potentials" in the peri-infarction area disappeared *(Keler)*.

Zinc to Copper Ratio

The zinc/copper antagonism has been postulated to be a factor in the pathogenesis of heart disease on the basis of experiments and the low copper content of human diets *(Klevay)*. Either excessive zinc ingestion, or low copper nutriture, may promote the development of cardiac arrhythmias *(Sandstead)*.

A man with premature ventricular contractions (PVCs) for 3 years had started taking supplemental zinc one year earlier. Hair mineral analysis showed a low normal zinc level with a very low level of copper.

He was placed on 30 mg zinc and 5 mg copper daily with disappearance of his PVCs in 1 month. After 6 months, repeat hair analysis showed a slight decrease in zinc but copper was nearly normal. He was placed on 50 mg zinc and 3 mg copper with no further PVCs reported (Wright).

OTHER NUTRITIONAL FACTORS

L-Carnitine

In controlled studies, L-carnitine supplementation has been found to reduce the incidence of extrasystolic ventricular multifocal arrhythmias in patients with ischemic heart disease *(Palazzuoli)*, including those with acute myocardial infarction *(Martina)*. Moreover, it potentiates the anti-arrhythmic effect of other drugs such as propafenone and mexiletine *(Mondillo)*.

Coenzyme Q_{10}

In a controlled study, coenzyme Q_{10} supplementation was shown to be helpful in reducing the incidence of ventricular arrhythmias in patients undergoing elective coronary bypass surgery *(Chello)*. It has also been found effective in open trials for patients with ventricular premature beats *(Fujioka)*. Even intractable supraventricular tachyarrhythmias have responded to CoQ_{10} supplementation after one to two weeks, although sometimes another drug had to be added *(Imanishi)*.

Omega-3 Fatty Acids

Results of a large number of human and animal studies leave little doubt of the efficacy of fish oil supplementation for the prevention of cardiac arrhythmias. Still unclear is whether the effects of omega-3 fatty acids in preventing arrhythmias are mediated by changes in the plasma or in vascular tissues, or if they directly affect the electrophysiology of cardiomyocytes. Fish oil supplementation may help decrease thrombin levels, thereby reducing myocardial repolarization and electrical abnormalities *(Nair)*.

Taurine

Much like magnesium, taurine affects membrane excitability by normalizing potassium flux in and out of the heart muscle cell *(Chazov)*. Arrhythmias characteristic of acute myocardial ischemia may be partly due to loss of intracellular taurine *(Crass)*.

In animal studies, taurine supplementation reduces ventricular arrhythmias following myocardial ischemia and increases the recovery of normal electrical and mechanical activity *(Franconi)*. The supplement may also prevent digitalis-induced arrhythmias *(Sebring)*. Controlled clinical trials are badly needed.

OTHER RELATED FACTORS

Food Sensitivities

Food and chemical sensitivities can sometimes trigger ventricular or atrial fibrillation. The arrhythmias can be reproduced with controlled, repeated double-blind incitant challenges.

When exposed to the incitant, before the arrhythmia develops, these patients usually exhibit a sequential progression of minor signs or symptoms such as rhinorrhea, mild confusion, nose or mouth irritations, nausea, vomiting or an uneasy feeling *(Rea,1978)*.

A 60- year-old male truck driver was resuscitated following ventricular fibrillation. On 3 occasions, he immediately developed bloating, premature ventricular contractions and hypotension upon eating. He noted that milk or eggs usually precipitated these symptoms as well as gasoline fumes (Rea,1980).

BIBLIOGRAPHY

Abraham R et al. Adipose fatty composition and the risk of serious ventricular arrhythmias in acute myocardial infarction. Am J Cardiol 63(5):269-72, 1989

Altura BM et al. Magnesium deficiency potentiates coronary arterial spasms induced by alcohol. Abstract. J Am Coll Nutr 8(5):456, 1989

Anderson S, Morris S. A Change in heart rhythm. Townsend Letter for Doctors, July, 1991:519

Charnock JS. Dietary fats and cardiac arrhythmia in primates. Nutrition 10(2):161-9, 1994a

Charnock JS. Lipids and cardiac arrhythmia. Prog Lipid Res 33(4):355-85, 1994b

Chazov EL et al. Taurine and electrical activity of the heart. Circ Res 35 Suppl. 3:11-21, 1974

Chello M et al. Protection by coenzyme Q_{10} from myocardial reperfusion injury during coronary bypass grafting. Ann Thorac Surg 58:1427-32, 1994

Cohen I, Kitzes R. Magnesium deficiency and digitalis toxicity. JAMA 251:730, 1984

Crass MF, Lombardini JB. Release of tissue taurine from the oxygen-deficient perfused rat heart. Proc Soc Exp Biol Med 157:486-8, 1978

DeCarli C et al. Serum magnesium levels in symptomatic atrial fibrillation and their relation to rhythm control by intravenous digoxin. Am J Cardiol 57:956, 1986

Dietch D. Magnesium is underused in acute atrial fibrillation. Letter. BMJ 312:1101, 1996

Dobmeyer DJ et al. The arrhythmogenic effects of caffeine in human beings. N Engl J Med 308(14):814-16, 1983

Dychner T, Wester PO. Magnesium and potassium in serum and muscle in relation to disturbances of cardiac rhythm, in Magnesium in Health and Disease. Spectrum Publishing Company, 1980:551-7

Franconi F et al. The protective effect of taurine on hypoxia (performed in the absence of glucose) and on reoxygenation (in the presence of glucose) in guinea-pig heart. Biochem Pharmacol 34(15):2611-15, 1985

Fuenmayor AJ et al. Vitamin E and ventricular fibrillation threshold in myocardial ischemia. Jpn Circ J 53:1229-32, 1989

Fuenmayor AJ, Fuenmayor AM. Cardiac arrest following holiday heart syndrome. Int J Cardiol 59(1):101-3, 1997

Fujioka T et al. Clinical study of cardiac arrhythmias using a 24-hour continuous electrocardiographic recorder (5th report): Antiarrhythmic action of coenzyme Q_{10} in diabetics. Tohuku J Exp Med 141(suppl):453-63, 1983

Hoffer A. Schizophrenia: an evolutionary defence against nerve stress. J Orthomol Psychiatry 9(4):205-21, 1994

Imanishi S et al. Jpn J Clin Exp Med 58:216-19, 1981) (in Japanese)

Kafka H et al. Serum magnesium and potassium in acute myocardial infarction. Influence on ventricular arrhythmias. Arch Intern Med 147(3):465-9, 1987

Keler KH et al. [Effect of sodium selenite on the course of acute experimental myocardial infarct]. Kardiologiia 25(9):72-6, 1985

Kessel L. Sick sinus syndrome cured by ... vitamin D? Geriatrics 45:83-5, 1990

Klevay L. The role of copper, zinc and other chemical elements in ischemic heart disease, in O Rennert, W Chan, Eds. Metabolism of Trace Metals in Man Vol 1, Boca Raton, FL, CRC Press, 1984:129-57

Lehr D. A possible beneficial effect of selenium administration in antiarrhythmic therapy. J Am Coll Nutr 14(5):496-8, 1994

Martina B et al. [Anti-arrhythmia treatment using L-carnitine in acute myocardial infarct.] Schweiz Med Wochenschr 122(37):1352-5, 1992

Mehta A et al. Caffeine and cardiac arrhythmias. An experimental study in dogs with review of literature. Acta Cardiol 52(3):273-83, 1997

Mondillo S et al. [Therapy of arrhythmia induced by myocardial ischemia. Association of L-carnitine, propafenone and mexiletine]. Clin Ter 146(12):769-74, 1995

Moushmoush B, Abi-Mansour P. Alcohol and the heart. The long-term effects of alcohol on the cardiovascular system. Arch Intern Med 151:36-42, 1991

Myers MG. Caffeine and cardiac arrhythmias. Ann Intern Med 114:147-50, 1991

Nair SS et al. Prevention of cardiac arrhythmia by dietary (n-3) polyunsaturated fatty acids and their mechanism of action. J Nutr 127:383-93, 1997

Otero-Anton E et al. Prolongation of the QTc interval during alcohol withdrawal syndrome. Acta Cardiol 52(3):285-94, 1997

Palazzuoli V et al. [The evaluation of the antiarrhythmic activity of L-carnitine and propafenone in ischemic cardiopathy.] Clin Ter 142(2):155-9, 1993 (in Italian)

Rea WJ. Environmentally triggered cardiac disease. Ann Allergy 40(4):243-51, 1978

Rea WJ, Suits CW. Cardiovascular disease triggered by foods and chemicals, in JW Gerrard, Ed. Food Allergy: New Perspectives. Springfield, Illinois, Charles C. Thomas, 1980

Reinhart R et al. Hypomagnesemia in patients entering the ICU. Critical Care Med 13(6):506, 1985

Robertson D et al. Effects of caffeine on plasma activity, catecholamines and blood pressure. N Engl J Med 298:181-6, 1978

Ryzen E et al. Low blood mononuclear cell magnesium in intensive cardiac care unit patients. Am Heart J 111:475-80, 1986

Sandstead HH. Requirements and toxicity of essential trace elements, illustrated by zinc and copper. Am J Clin Nutr 61(suppl):621S-4S, 1995

Sangiori GB et al. Serum potassium levels, red-blood-cell potassium and alterations of the repolarization phase of electrocardiography in old subjects. Age Ageing 13:309, 1984

Sebring LA, Huxtable RJ. Cardiovascular actions of taurine, in Sulfur Amino Acids: Biochemical & Clinical Aspects, 1983

Singh RB et al. Plasma levels of antioxidant vitamins and oxidative stress in patients with acute myocardial infarction. Acta Cardiol 49(5):441-52, 1994a

Singh RB et al. Dietary and serum magnesium levels in patients with acute myocardial infarction, coronary heart disease and noncardiac diagnoses. J Am Coll Nutr 13(2):139-43, 1994b

Singh RB et al. Usefulness of antioxidant vitamins in suspected acute myocardial infarction (The Indian Experiment of Infarct Survival-3). Am J Cardiol 77(4):232-6, 1996

Tzivoni D, Keren A. Suppression of ventricular arrhythmias by magnesium. Am J Cardiol 65(20):1397-9, 1990

Wright JV. Dr. Wright's Guide to Healing with Nutrition. Emmaus, PA, Rodale Press, 1984

CARDIOMYOPATHY

See Also: ALCOHOLISM
CONGESTIVE HEART FAILURE

NUTRITIONAL TREATMENT GUIDE

✓ = Efficacy generally accepted.
* = Efficacy *demonstrated* by controlled human trials.
[+] = Efficacy *suspected* from uncontrolled human trials.
[-] = Efficacy *suspected* from indirect data.
? = Efficacy *challenged* in a study of similar design.

DIETARY FACTORS

✓ avoid excessive **Alcohol** ingestion

NUTRITIONAL FACTORS

✓ **Thiamine deficiency:** 50 mg daily

* **L-carnitine deficiency:** 4 g daily (1 year trial)
* ? **Coenzyme Q_{10} deficiency:** 100 to 150 mg daily in divided doses (2 to 6 month trial)

[+] **Selenium deficiency:** 200 µg daily

[-] **Magnesium deficiency:** ≈ 400 mg daily (Consider IM or IV administration.)
[-] **Vitamin C deficiency:** 500 mg twice daily
[-] **Vitamin E deficiency:** D,L-alpha-tocopheryl acetate 200 to 2,000 mg or IU daily for 6 weeks; then maintenance levels as needed
[-] **Vitamin E:** *to protect against magnesium deficiency & alcohol excess:* ? 400 to 800 IU daily

DIETARY FACTORS

Alcohol

Excessive alcohol intake is a leading cause of cardiomyopathy and should be avoided. Chronic ethanol exposure leads to alterations in the contractile function of the heart and also has an acute negative inotropic effect mediated by direct interaction with cardiac muscle cells *(Thomas)*. Substances contained in alcoholic beverages, such as cobalt, may also contribute to its toxicity *(Burch,1974)*. Also, acute alcohol ingestion depresses myocardial contractility in patients with pre-existing cardiac disease *(Gould)*.

Although alcoholics are prone to malnutrition, the low prevalence of clinical nutritional deficiency in patients with alcoholic cardiomyopathy suggests that this disorder is usually not dependent upon malnutrition for its pathogenesis *(Regan)*.

NUTRITIONAL FACTORS

VITAMINS

Thiamine Deficiency

Cardiomyopathy may be a feature of beri-beri, the classic thiamine deficiency disease (*Djoenaidi*). The response to a thiamine supplement, such as thiamine tetrahydrofurfuryl disulfide, is often dramatic (*Djoenaidi*).

Vitamin C Deficiency

A report from India suggests that cardiomyopathy patients may have a reduced intake of vitamin C as well as lower plasma levels of the vitamin *(Singh)*. Whether vitamin C deficiency promotes the development of cardiomyopathy is unknown, although it has been theorized that oxidative stress promotes the disorder *(Romero-Alvira)* and ascorbic acid is central to water-soluble antioxidant defenses.

Vitamin E

Vitamin E is as important an antioxidant in the lipid-soluble milieu as vitamin C is in the water-soluble environment. Moreover, like vitamin C, a single report from India found that cardiomyopathy patients had a reduced intake of the vitamin as well as lower plasma levels *(Singh)*. Whether vitamin E deficiency is of causal importance awaits the results of further studies.

Even if the vitamin is not deficient, supplementation with vitamin E may be protective. Results of animal studies suggest that vitamin E supplementation may protect against the cardiotoxic effects of alcohol *(Redetzki)* as well as the cardiomyopathy caused by magnesium deficiency *(Freedman)*.

MINERALS

Copper

Rats *(Medeiros)* and pigs *(Wildman)* made copper-deficient develop a cardiomyopathy, and it has been suggested that P-type copper ATPase may be one of the obligatory factors contributing to cardiomyopathy in humans *(Nath)*.

Since the few studies of serum copper levels in cardiomyopathy have found elevated values *(Burguera;Oster)*, abnormal copper metabolism resulting in loss of myocardial copper could be more important in common forms of human cardiomyopathies than dietary copper deficiency.

There is no evidence to suggest that copper supplementation may be beneficial.

Magnesium Deficiency

Cardiac changes produced by experimental magnesium deficiency resemble those produced in mice fed large quantities of alcohol and are particularly prominent in myocardial mitochondriae *(Burch,1977)*. This cardiomyopathy appears to be the consequence of a pro-inflammatory condition leading to excessive free radical production *(Weglicki)*. Although myocardial magnesium should be repleted, supplementation with vitamin E and other antioxidants appears to be important *(Freedman; Weglicki)*.

A trial of providing physiologic levels of oral magnesium (15 mmol daily) to patients with idiopathic dilated cardiomyopathy failed to influence serum magnesium, left ventricular ejection fraction, or prognosis *(Fruhwald)*. These unfavorable results suggest that intramuscular or intravenous routes of magnesium administration should be attempted to see if they are more successful in producing beneficial changes.

Selenium Deficiency

Selenium deficiency is believed to be cause a cardiomyopathy *(Poley)*. Keshan disease, a dilated congestive cardiomyopathy occurring primarily in children living in rural China, is specifically attributed to a chronic deficiency of selenium *(Yang)*. This relationship has been observed in cases of low dietary intake *(Collipp)* and in alcoholic cardiomyopathy *(Goldman)*. Patients on total parenteral nutrition are especially at risk *(Huttenen)*.

A 2-year-old girl with dyspnea, congestive heart failure and cardiomegaly was found to have minimal selenium in her diet and a low serum selenium concentration.

Following selenium supplementation, her condition improved (Collipp).

OTHER NUTRITIONAL FACTORS

L-Carnitine Deficiency

Cardiomyopathy in infants and young children may be due to an inborn error of metabolism causing carnitine deficiency *(Winter)*. Moreover, there is growing evidence that reduced myocardial carnitine levels are a common finding in adult-onset cardiomyopathies *(Mortensen,1991;Regitz)*.

Supplementation

Carnitine supplementation has been shown to reverse cardiomyopathy in experimental animals *(Maresca)*, although it has been poorly studied in humans - with the exception of genetic disorders of carnitine metabolism *(Pepine;Tripp)*.

However, a randomized, controlled study has been published whose findings suggest that carnitine supplementation may reverse cardiomyopathy in patients with post-infarction ischemic myopathy: Half of a group of 160 patients aged 39 to 86 years with a recent myocardial infarction randomly received L-carnitine 4 g daily in addition to their usual drug treatment.

After 12 months, compared to controls, L-carnitine-treated patients showed statistically significant improvement in heart rate, systolic arterial pressure, and the frequency of anginal attacks, as well as improvement in the lipid pattern. These changes were accompanied by a significant reduction in mortality from 12.5% down to 1% *(Davini)*.

Carnitine supplementation should be especially considered whenever a patient presents with both cardiomegaly and progressive skeletal muscle weakness, as both may be due to a metabolic carnitine deficiency *(Hirata)*. Whether the efficacy of supplementation is purely due to repletion of a myocardial tissue deficiency is unknown

A 4-month-old male infant with a dilated cardiomyopathy secondary to renal tubular losses of carnitine was admitted to the hospital with severe congestive heart failure. An echocardiogram demonstrated normal anatomy. The left ventricular shortening fraction measured 10%. Total plasma carnitine level was only 25 mumol/ml, but the urine carnitine measured 434 nm/mg of creatinine.

He was begun on oral L-carnitine and weaned from mechanical ventilation and inotropic support 10 days later. Two years later he remained asymptomatic with normal left ventricular function (Zales).

Coenzyme Q_{10} (ubiquinone) Deficiency

In various cardiomyopathies, endomyocardial tissue levels of coenzyme Q_{10} may be reduced; moreover, the worse the stage of the disease, the lower the level of the coenzyme *(Folkers;Mortensen,1993)*. Also, in patients with dilated cardiomyopathy, blood ubiquinone levels may be reduced *(Langsjoen,1990)*.

Numerous studies have investigated the efficacy of supplementation with the coenzyme. Results of the controlled studies have been mixed; several, however, have documented significant benefits from oral supplementation. For example, the results of a double-blind double-crossover study of patients with advanced (New York Heart Association class III or IV) cardiomyopathies were reported in the *Proceedings of the National Academy of Sciences U S A*. At baseline, their condition was steadily worsening, and they were expected to die within 2 years if they simply continued to receive conventional therapy.

The patients received CoQ_{10} and placebo in either order. Those that first received CoQ_{10} showed significant increases in cardiac function during treatment that reversed during placebo treatment, while the other group was unchanged during the placebo period and showed improved cardiac function when switched to CoQ_{10}. Increases in blood levels of the coenzyme occurred during active treatment and were coincident with their objective responses *(Langsjoen, 1985)*.

BIBLIOGRAPHY

Burch GE, Giles TD. Alcoholic cardiomyopathy, in B Kissin, H Begleiter, Eds. The Biology of Alcoholism: Vol. 3: Clinical Pathology. New York, Plenum Press, 1974

Burch BE, Giles TD. The importance of magnesium deficiency in cardiovascular disease. Am Heart J 94:649-56, 1977

Burguera JL et al. Concentration changes of zinc, copper and iron in serum of chronic chagasic myocardiopathic patients. J Trace Elem Electrolytes Health Dis 2(4):215-19, 1988

Collipp PJ, Chen SY. Cardiomyopathy and selenium deficiency in a two-year-old girl. Letter. N Engl J Med 304:1304-5, 1981

Davini P et al. Controlled study on L-carnitine therapeutic efficacy in post-infarction. Drugs Exp Clin Res 18(8):355-65, 1992

Djoenaidi W et al. Beriberi cardiomyopathy. Eur J Clin Nutr 46(3):227-32, 1992

Folkers K et al. Biochemical rationale and myocardial tissue data on the effective therapy of cardiomyopathy with coenzyme Q10. Proc Natl Acad Sci U S A. 82(3):901-4, 1985

Freedman AM et al. Magnesium deficiency-induced cardiomyopathy: Protection by vitamin E. Biochem Biophys Res Commun 170:1102-6, 1990

Fruhwald FM et al. A physiological oral magnesium supplement does not influence total serum magnesium, left ventricular ejection fraction and prognosis in patients with dilated cardiomyopathy. Magnes Res 6(3):251-5, 1993

Goldman IS, Kantrowitz NE. Cardiomyopathy associated with selenium deficiency. Letter. N Engl J Med 305:701, 1982

Gould L et al. Cardiac effects of a cocktail. JAMA 218:1799-802, 1971

Hirata K et al. [Carnitine deficiency: a treatable cardiomyopathy.] J Cardiogr 16(1):217-25, 1986

Huttenen JK. Selenium and cardiovascular diseases – an update. Biomed Environ Sci 10(2-3):220-6, 1997

Langsjoen PH et al. Response of patients in classes III and IV of cardiomyopathy to therapy in a blind and crossover trial with coenzyme Q10. Proc Natl Acad Sci U S A 82(12):4240-4, 1985

Langsjoen PH, Folkers K. Long-term efficacy and safety of coenzyme Q_{10} therapy for idiopathic dilated cardiomyopathy. Am J Cardiol 65:521-3, 1990

Maresca P et al. Positive action of propionyl-L-carnitine on mechanical performance of papillary muscle from Syrian hamsters with hereditary dilated cardiomyopathy. Eur J Pharmacol 287(3):303-7, 1995

Medeiros DM. Copper and its possible role in cardiomyopathies. The Nutrition Report 11(12), December, 1993

Mortensen SA et al, in Folkers K, Y Yamamura, Eds. Biomedical and Clinical Aspects of Coenzyme Q_{10}, Volume 6, New York, Elsevier, 1991:269-81

Mortensen SA. Perspectives on therapy of cardiovascular diseases with coenzyme Q10 (ubiquinone). Clin Invest 71(8 suppl):S116-S123, 1993

Nath R. Copper deficiency and heart disease: molecular basis, recent advances and current concepts. Int J Biochem Cell Biol 29(11):1245-54, 1997

Oster O. Trace element concentrations (Cu, Zn, Fe) in sera from patients with dilated cardiomyopathy. Clin Chim Acta 214(2):209-18, 1993

Pepine CJ. The therapeutic potential of carnitine in cardiovascular disorders. Clin Ther 13(1):2-21, 1991

Poley JR et al. Selenium deficiency and cardiomyopathy. Abstract. J Am Coll Nutr 13(5):522, 1994

Regan TJ et al. The role of ethanol in cardiac disease. Annu Rev Med 28:393-409, 1977

Regitz V et al. Defective myocardial carnitine metabolism in congestive heart failure secondary to dilated cardiomyopathy and to coronary, hypertensive and valvular heart diseases. Am J Cardiol 65(11):755-60, 1990

Redetzki JE et al. Amelioration of cardiotoxic effects of alcohol by vitamin E. J Toxicol Clin Toxicol 20(4):319-31, 1983

Romero-Alvira D et al. Cardiomyopathies and oxidative stress. Med Hypotheses 47(2):137-44, 1996

Singh RB et al. Dietary intake and plasma levels of antioxidant vitamins in health and disease: a hospital-based case-control study. J Nutr Environ Med 5:235-42, 1995

Thomas AP et al. Effects of ethanol on the contractile function of the heart: a review. Alcohol Clin Exp Res 18(1):121-31, 1994

Tripp ME et al. Systemic carnitine deficiency presenting as familial endocardial fibroelastosis: A treatable cardiomyopathy. N Engl J Med 305:385, 1982

Weglicki WB et al. Antioxidants and the cardiomyopathy of Mg-deficiency. Am J Cardiovasc Pathol 4(3):210-15, 1992

Wildman RE et al. Aspects of cardiomyopathy in copper-deficient pigs. Electrocardiography, echocardiography, and ultrastructural findings. Biol Trace Elem Res 55(1-2):55-70, 1996

Winter S et al. The role of L-carnitine in pediatric cardiomyopathy. J Child Neurol [Canada] 10(suppl 2):2S45-2S51, 1995

Yang FY et al. Keshan disease–an endemic mitochondrial cardiomyopathy in China. J Trace Elem Electrolytes Health Dis 2(3):157-63, 1988

Zales VR, Benson DW Jr. Reversible cardiomyopathy due to carnitine deficiency from renal tubular wasting. Pediatr Cardiol 16(2):76-8, 1995

CARPAL TUNNEL SYNDROME

**See Also: MUSCLE CRAMPS (FUNCTIONAL)
NEURALGIA AND NEUROPATHY**

NUTRITIONAL TREATMENT GUIDE

✓ = Efficacy generally accepted.
* = Efficacy *demonstrated* by controlled human trials.
[+] = Efficacy *suspected* from uncontrolled human trials.
[-] = Efficacy *suspected* from indirect data.
? = Efficacy *challenged* in a study of similar design.

NUTRITIONAL FACTORS

* ? **Vitamin B_6 deficiency:** pyridoxal phosphate 50 mg daily (3 month trial)

- -

[+] rule out **Lithium** toxicity
[+] **Riboflavin deficiency:** *in addition to vitamin B_6 supplementation:* 50 mg daily (5 month trial)

NUTRITIONAL FACTORS

Vitamin B_6 Deficiency

Based initially on his clinical observations, John Ellis has argued for many years that a deficiency of vitamin B_6 may cause a carpal tunnel syndrome. There is evidence that changes in erythrocyte glutamic oxaloacetic transaminase activity levels may suggest B_6 deficiency (*Ellis, 1981*) as well as reduced plasma levels of pyridoxal phosphate (*Fuhr*). Moreover, in a study of 441 adult volunteers, there were significant relationships between plasma levels of pyridoxal 5'-phosphate and both the specific symptoms of carpal tunnel syndrome and median nerve slowing *(Keniston)*.

Many studies have investigated the efficacy of vitamin B_6 supplementation, although most of them suffer from the lack of proper controls or other design flaws. Perhaps the best group study to date reported on the treatment of 28 patients with pyridoxine hydrochloride. Based on the results of distal motor latency and conduction measurements of the median nerve, as well as on the judgment of their physicians, all but one patient were substantially improved after 5 to 18 weeks. By comparison, only one of four patients treated with placebo was improved after 15 to 36 weeks (*Driskell*).

A Warning

While poorly documented, there is the possibility that chronic megadoses of pyridoxine (over 100 mg daily) can *cause* a sensory neuropathy by exceeding the liver's ability to phosphorylate pyridoxine to the active coenzyme, pyridoxal phosphate. This would result in a high pyridoxine level which could either be directly neurotoxic or may compete with pyridoxal phosphate for binding sites; the result would be a relative deficiency of the active metabolite (*Parry*). Supplementing with pyridoxal phosphate instead of pyridoxine should thus avoid this danger while also eliminating treatment failures due to idiosyncratic problems in phosphorylating high supplementary doses of pyridoxine.

A man with severe carpal tunnel syndrome had markedly reduced basal specific activity of erythrocyte glutamic-oxaloacetic transaminase. Pyridoxal phosphate levels were also low.

He received 2 mg daily of pyridoxine. After 11 weeks, all but marginal symptoms were relieved, the EGOT activity deficiency was reduced from about 70% to 50%. Pyridoxal phosphate remained deficient. Vitamin B_6 was increased to 100 mg daily and, after 12 weeks, he had nearly achieved a "ceiling" EGOT level and the pyridoxal phosphate deficiency was eliminated. Placebo administration for 9 weeks led to worsened clinical symptoms and laboratory values.

After administration of vitamin B_6 100 mg daily for 12 weeks, the patient became asymptomatic and laboratory values normalized again (Folkers,1978).

Riboflavin Deficiency

There is preliminary evidence that a deficiency of riboflavin may promote the development of carpal tunnel syndrome, at least in association with a vitamin B_6 deficiency *(Folkers,1990)*.

To become the coenzyme pyridoxal-5'-phosphate, dietary pyridoxine is converted by a kinase to pyridoxine 5'-phosphate and then a riboflavin-containing enzyme oxidizes it. Thus a riboflavin deficiency may cause an identical syndrome to that caused by a vitamin B_6 deficiency.

A patient with a 3-year history of carpal tunnel syndrome (CTS) was found to be deficient in both vitamin B_6 and riboflavin as based on a reduction in the specific activities of erythrocyte glutamic-oxaloacetic transaminase (vitamin B_6) and erythrocyte glutathione reductase (riboflavin) to the 30% levels.

After 5 months of supplementation with riboflavin alone, there was nearly complete disappearance of the CTS without a change in the specific activity of erythrocyte glutamic-oxaloacetic transaminase. Combined riboflavin and pyridoxine significantly increased the specific activities of both enzymes to normal levels with total disappearance of the CTS. Objectively, the strength of pinch of both hands significantly increased on treatment with riboflavin and further increased on the combined treatment (Folkers,1984).

Lithium Toxicity: A Warning

High-dosage lithium treatment can cause carpal tunnel syndrome as a side effect of the medication. Therefore patients presenting with carpal tunnel syndrome should be asked if they are taking lithium for the treatment of bipolar disorder *(Deahl)*.

BIBLIOGRAPHY

Deahl MP. Lithium-induced carpal tunnel syndrome. Br J Psychiatry 153:250-1, 1988

Driskell JA et al. Effectiveness of pyridoxine hydrochloride treatment on carpal tunnel patients. Nutr Reports Int 34:1031-40, 1986

Ellis J et al. Therapy with vitamin B6 with and without surgery for treatment of patients having the idiopathic carpal tunnel syndrome. Res Commun Chem Path Pharm 33(2):331, 1981

Folkers K et al. Biochemical evidence for a deficiency of vitamin B6 in the carpal tunnel syndrome based on a crossover clinical study. Proc Natl Acad Sci USA 75(7):3410-2, 1978

Folkers K et al. Enzymology of the response of the carpal tunnel syndrome to riboflavin and to combined riboflavin and pyridoxine. Proc Natl Acad Sci U S A 81(22):7076-8, 1984

Folkers K, Ellis J. Successful therapy with vitamin B6 and vitamin B2 of the carpal tunnel syndrome and need for determination of the RDAs for vitamins B6 and B2 for disease states. Ann N Y Acad Sci 585:295-301, 1990

Fuhr JE et al. Vitamin B6 levels in patients with carpal tunnel syndrome. Arch Surg 124:1329-30, 1989

Keniston RC et al. Vitamin B6, vitamin C, and carpal tunnel syndrome. A cross-sectional study of 441 adults. J Occup Environ Med 39(10):949-59, 1997

Parry GJ, Bredesen DE. Sensory neuropathy with low-dose pyridoxine. Neurology 35:1466-8, 1985

CATARACT

See Also: DIABETES MELLITUS

NUTRITIONAL TREATMENT GUIDE

✓ = Efficacy generally accepted.
* = Efficacy *demonstrated* by controlled human trials.
[+] = Efficacy *suspected* from uncontrolled human trials.
[-] = Efficacy *suspected* from indirect data.
? = Efficacy *challenged* in a study of similar design.

DIETARY FACTORS

[+] eat **Yogurt** (*if* galactose metabolism is abnormal)

- -

[-] avoid excessive **Calorie** intake
[-] eat **Fruits and Vegetables**
[-] restrict **Lactose** (*if* galactose metabolism is abnormal)

NUTRITIONAL FACTORS

[+] **Riboflavin:** 15 mg daily
[+] **Vitamin C:** ? 350 mg daily
[+] **Zinc:** 30 mg daily (6 week trial)

- -

[-] **alpha-Lipoic acid:** ? 100 mg daily
[-] **mixed Carotenoids**
[-] **Flavonoids**
[-] **Folic acid:** ? 800 μg daily
[-] **Quercetin:** *for diabetics:* ? 300 mg 3 times daily
[-] **Selenium:** ? 200 μg daily
[-] **Vitamin E:** ? 400 IU daily

OTHER RELATED FACTORS

[-] rule out **Mercury** toxicity

DIETARY FACTORS

Avoid Excessive Calorie Intake

In an animal model, restricting calories by about 21% delayed the development of senile cataracts *(Taylor,1989)*, raising the question as to whether the same is true for humans. Indeed, the combination of obesity, hyperglycemia and hypertriglyceridemia is associated with posterior subcapsular cataract occurring at an early age *(Jahn)*. Elevated fat intake is also associated with increased cataract risk *(Tavani)*, perhaps because of its high caloric content.

Consume Fruits and Vegetables

A higher intake of fruits and vegetables seems to protect against cataract formation *(Mares-Perlman;Taylor,1993)*. In one study, people who consumed fewer than 3 ½ servings of fruit or vegetables daily had 5 times the risk of cortical cataract and 13 times the risk of subcapsular cataract *(Jacques,1991)*.

Restrict Lactose Intake

Lactose (milk sugar) is broken down to glucose and galactose. There is some evidence that a high lactose (and consequently galactose) intake may encourage cataract formation in predisposed people due to the accumulation of galactitol in the lens *(Couet;Simoons)*. Since sugar alcohols have slower rates of diffusion out of the lens than their parent sugars, they may accumulate and cause hypertonicity and osmotic swelling which, in turn, can eventually rupture the fiber cells.

One study found that subjects with a high intake of lactose had double the risk of cataracts. While this difference did not reach significance, if subjects had both a high lactose intake and low red cell levels of the enzyme galactokinase (suggesting inhibition of galactose metabolism), their increased risk of senile cataracts became significant *(Jacques,1988a)*. Another study of 22 patients under age 50 with presenile cataracts found that 5 of the patients were heterozygous for galactokinase deficiency, while 2 were heterozygous for galactose uridyl transferase deficiency *(Prchal)*.

While the intake of high-lactose-containing dairy products may increase cataract risk, there is early evidence that yogurt ingestion may *reduce* cataract risk in the subgroup with abnormal galactose metabolism. Free galactose in yogurt could stimulate intestinal galactokinase; moreover the greater insulin secretion after yogurt consumption could increase the rate of galactose and lactose utilization. Indeed, in a study of 240 elderly subjects, yogurt consumption was found to have a protective dose-response effect on cataract formation *(Birlouez-Aragon)*.

NUTRITIONAL FACTORS

ANTIOXIDANTS

With its continual exposure to light and ambient oxygen, the lens is at high risk of photooxidative damage. Oxygen free radicals cause cataracts by oxidizing the lens proteins while also impairing the proteolytic enzymes designed to eliminate the damaged proteins. Normal lenses of older people only show early evidence of oxidation which is confined to the intrinsic membrane fraction and membrane-related components; the development of cataract is associated with progressive oxidative changes in these components which eventually extends beyond them to also involve the soluble components of the lens proteins.

The lens has two lines of defense against oxygen free radicals. One is the antioxidant nutrients such as vitamins C and E, selenium and beta-carotene and glutathione. The other is the enzymatic defense system which includes glutathione peroxidase, glutathione reductase and superoxide dismutase.

VITAMINS

Folic Acid

At least two epidemiological studies have found that folic acid intake may be inversely associated with cataract risk *(Jacques,1987;Tavani)*. Whether this finding is due to a beneficial effect of folate, or whether it is because high-folate foods contain other nutrients which are beneficial, is not known.

Riboflavin

While the results of observational studies are contradictory, there is evidence of an association between riboflavin deficiency and increased risk of presenile and senile cataracts *(Skalka,1981a)*. The concentration of lenticular reduced glutathione is decreased in all forms of human cataract. Since riboflavin is a precursor of flavin adenine dinucleotide which is required as a coenzyme for glutathione reductase, a riboflavin deficiency may promote cataract formation by interfering with glutathione reductase activity *(Skalka, 1981b)*.

In an open trial of 18 patients with lens opacities and 6 with fully developed cataracts, after only 24 to 48 hours of supplementing them with riboflavin, there was a dramatic improvement. After 9 months, all lens opacities had disappeared *(Sydenstricker)*. These results need confirmation by controlled trials.

Galactose which, as noted above, may foster cataractogenesis, is also a riboflavin antagonist; thus a high lactose intake may promote the development of cataracts by causing a riboflavin deficiency *(Lerman)*.

Vitamin C

The concentration of ascorbic acid in the aqueous humor is among the highest of all the body fluids, and the intake of vitamin C supplements over at least the past decade is inversely correlated with cataract risk *(Jacques, 1997)*. Moreover, the blood level of the vitamin has been inversely correlated with cataract risk *(Jacques, 1988b)*.

Confirmation of its antioxidant effect comes from a study in which rat lenses were maintained in a solution designed to cause free radical damage as the addition of vitamin C protected them *(Varma, 1979)*. These results are consistent with those of animal models in which vitamin C protected against the development of selenite-induced cataracts in rats *(Devamanoharan)* and against the development of ultraviolet light-induced cataracts in guinea pigs *(Blondin)*.

In open trials, 60% to 90% of patients with incipient senile cataracts have had visual improvement following supplementation with the vitamin, improvement which was sometimes marked *(Bouton; Muhlmann)*. The results of controlled clinical trials will likely provide confirmation of ascorbate's protectiveness against cataractogenesis.

Vitamin E

As with vitamin C, vitamin E intake is inversely related to the risk of cataract *(Carson; Robertson)*. Furthermore, the same relationship has been noted in regard to blood levels of vitamin E *(Rouhiainen; Vitale)*.

Cataract-free subjects use significantly more supplemental vitamin E than matched subjects with cataracts *(Robertson)*. A recent longitudinal study found that, in regular users of multivitamin supplements, the risk of nuclear opacification was reduced about one third; in regular users of vitamin E supplements and persons with higher plasma levels of vitamin E, the risk was reduced by approximately half *(Leske)*.

Like vitamin C, the addition of vitamin E protected rat lenses from free radical damage when they were immersed in a solution designed to cause such damage *(Varma, 1982)*. In addition, when added to the perfusion solution, vitamin E doubled the survival time of isolated rabbit corneal endothelium *(Neuwirth-Lux)*.

Controlled clinical trials of vitamin E are badly needed to see if the vitamin does, in fact, help to protect the human lens from cataract formation.

MINERALS

Selenium Deficiency

The enzymatic antioxidant glutathione peroxidase requires selenium for its functioning. Serum selenium levels, which appear to be reduced in patients with senile cataracts *(Karakucuk)*, are positively correlated with aqueous humor levels of erythrocyte glutathione peroxidase *(Huang)*. Patients with senile cataracts may have decreased selenium levels in the aqueous humor *(Karakucuk)* and the selenium concentration of cataractous lenses may be only 15% of normal *(Swanson)*.

Controlled clinical trials of selenium supplementation, especially for patients with evidence of selenium deficiency, are needed.

Zinc

Compared to subjects of the same age with normal lenses, patients with senile cataract may have lower plasma zinc levels *(Bhat)*. Some studies have found lens zinc levels to be higher in patients with senile cataract *(Srivastava; Stanojevik-Paovik)*, possibly secondary to disturbed glucose utilization in the lens due to loss of activity of key zinc-dependent enzymes *(Heinitz)*. When, however, zinc levels in lenses with mature senile cataract were compared with those in lenses with traumatic cataract, those with senile cataract had the lower levels *(Jeru)*.

Zinc supplementation improves the impaired glucose metabolism occurring in old age *(Heinitz)*, and a rabbit study found that zinc stimulates mitotic activity of the lens epithelium *(Chuistova)*. Therefore, zinc supplementation may theoretically be beneficial for both prevention and treatment of senile cataract.

While controlled clinical trials are lacking, Todd has reported excellent results in his practice from zinc supplementation. His conviction that zinc supplementation reverses cataractogenesis began when a man presented with bilateral 20/200 cataracts. After one cataract was removed, he was placed on a multivitamin tablet and zinc in order to speed healing in preparation for surgery on the other eye. When his vision in the other eye improved to 20/25 over the next 6 months, surgery was canceled. Four years later, his visual acuity remained at 20/25. (Patients placed on the multivitamin alone had no improvement in vision; thus his improvement appeared to have been due to the addition of zinc.)

Subsequently, Todd began placing all cataract patients on the multivitamin and zinc supplement for a trial prior to considering cataract surgery. His results: 67% had improved vision, and over 50% of those who initially needed surgery improved to the point where surgery was no longer indicated. He notes that a response should be seen within 6 weeks; improvement may continue for a year or more and is usually 50% (enough to avoid surgery).

In his experience, cataracts most likely to respond to zinc are cortical cataracts and "opalescent" cataracts (i.e. cataracts in which there is a milky character to the cortex). Posterior subcapsular cataracts do sometimes respond after a period of many months, but zinc is ineffective for nuclear sclerotic cataracts *(Todd)*.

OTHER NUTRITIONAL FACTORS

Carotenoids

The intake of carotenoids, particularly alpha-carotene, lutein and lycopene, has been inversely correlated with cataract risk *(Hankinson;Mares-Perlman)*. Although two studies failed to find a relationship between beta-carotene intake and the risk of cataract *(Carson;Mares-Perlman)*, the blood level of beta-carotene has been inversely correlated with cataract risk *(Jacques,1988b)*. In fact, one study found that those with serum levels of beta-carotene in the lowest third of the distribution had almost a 3-fold risk of senile cataract *(Knekt)*.

Controlled clinical trials are needed to ascertain the efficacy of carotenoid supplementation.

Glutathione

Glutathione is the antioxidant substrate for two important antioxidant enzymes, glutathione peroxidase and glutathione reductase. In an article published in the *Journal of the American Medical Association*, it was proposed that increased cysteine or methionine (the rate-limiting amino acids in glutathione synthesis) would help to prevent cataract formation by retarding the age-related decline in glutathione levels *(Cole)*. In support of this suggestion, while glutathione levels decrease gradually in normal lenses with advancing age, cataractous lenses contain only about one-tenth as much glutathione. Moreover, as glutathione levels fall, lens oxidation increases *(Kamei)*.

There is a lack of human studies demonstrating whether increasing glutathione levels in the lens or aqueous humor protects against cataract formation. In rats, supplementation with alpha-lipoic acid (thioctic acid), a substance known to increase endogenous glutathione levels, did protect 60% of the animals from experimentally-induced cataract formation *(Maitra)*.

As with glutathione, levels of the enzyme superoxide dismutase (SOD)decrease in human lenses with senile cataracts as the cataract advance *(Fujiwara)*. SOD activity appears to act as a barrier against photooxidation. Glutathione levels are positively correlated with SOD activity in the human cataractous lens *(Fujiwara)*. Although it is not known how to increase lens SOD activity directly, animal work suggests that the levels of both SOD and glutathione reductase decrease as a result of vitamin E deficiency *(Cai)*.

COMBINED MICRONUTRIENT INTERVENTION

Five years after almost 18,000 male physicians completed questionnaires regarding dietary supplements, those who had taken multivitamins had only 73% of the relative risk of cataract and 79% of the relative risk of cataract extraction. This finding could not be attributed to their vitamin C and/or their vitamin E intake, as the small sub-group taking only one or both of these antioxidants showed no reduction in risk *(Seddon)*.

Ophthalmologist Robert Azar, whose clinic treats 25,000 patients annually, places cataract patients on a low-fat, complex-carbohydrate diet that stresses fish, fowl and fresh produce, and supplemented them with vitamin C, water-soluble vitamin E and zinc for 2 months. If improvement is noted, surgery is delayed. He reports that many people on the program improve enough so that surgery is unnecessary *(Azar)*.

Other authors have noted benefits from supplements of several micronutrients. For example, under double-blind conditions, more than 3,000 subjects from rural communities in Linxian, China received one of 4 different nutrient combinations. After 5 to 6 years, the prevalence of nuclear cataract was significantly lower in persons receiving the combination of riboflavin 3 mg and niacin 40 mg daily compared with those not receiving them, although the combination was also associated with a significant increase in the small number of posterior subcapsular cataracts *(Sperduto)*.

How these findings pertain to better nourished populations is not known.

Mrs. C.W. developed cloudy vision in both eyes at age 70 while supplementing her diet with ascorbic acid 1.5 g, thiamine 100 mg, pyridoxine 250 mg, niacinamide 1.5 g and vitamin E 800 IU daily. She was advised to add riboflavin 25 mg daily and cod liver oil capsules (for vitamins A and D) 3 daily.

One year later, her lenses were clear; 3 years later no evidence of cataract was seen on optometric examination (Hoffer).

MERCURY TOXICITY

Mercury accumulation may increase cataract risk. In a study of 414 eye patients, a strong association was found between heavy weekly consumption of large, carnivorous marine fish (a source of mercury), erythrocyte and hair methylmercury levels, abnormal erythrocyte levels of glutathione peroxidase (a selenium-dependent enzyme that defuses mercury), and precocious development of subcapsular and progressing nuclear cataracts. Subjects who were at least 42 years old who averaged three 3-ounce tuna servings per week had 3 times the risk for subcapsular cataractogenesis of persons consuming an average of less than one 3-ounce serving of tuna in 2 weeks *(Lane)*.

DIABETIC CATARACTS

Diabetics are particularly predisposed to developing premature cataracts. Hyperglycemia in the aqueous humor activates aldose reductase in the lens which converts glucose into sorbitol. Sorbitol tends to accumulate, increasing the osmotic pressure until the fluid from the aqueous humor diffuses into the lens. Swollen fibers eventually lead to disruption of the lens structure, causing it to lose its transparency.

Vitamin E

Vitamin E may offer protection against the destructive effects of prolonged hyperglycemia. When adult rats were pretreated with vitamin E before they were made diabetic, they were protected from cataractogenesis as the hyperglycemia continued *(Ross)*.

Flavonoids

Fortunately, it may be possible to inhibit aldose reductase by administration of flavonoids such as quercetin and naringin. When quercetin was given to diabetic rodents, there was a significant decrease in sorbitol accumulation in lens tissue and cataract onset was delayed *(Varma, 1977)*.

Human trials are needed for confirmation and to determine a safe and effective dosage.

BIBLIOGRAPHY

Azar R - interviewed in Prevention July, 1983, pp. 99-103

Bhat KS. Plasma calcium and trace minerals in human subjects with mature cataract. Nutr Rep Int 37:157-63, 1988

Birlouez-Aragon et al. Disturbed galactose metabolism in elderly and diabetic humans is associated with cataract formation. J Nutr 123:1370-6, 1993

Blondin J et al. Prevention of eye lens protein damage by dietary vitamin C. Abstract. Fed Proc 45:478, 1986

Bouton SM Jr. Vitamin C and the aging eye. Arch Intern Med 63:930-45, 1939

Cai QY et al. Biochemical and morphological changes in the lens of selenium and/or vitamin E deficient rats. Biomed Environ Sci 7(2):109-15, 1994

Carson C et al. Antioxidant intake and cataract in the Melbourne Visual Impairment project. Am J Epidemiol 139(11):S18, 1994

Chuistova IP et al. [Experimental morphologic foundation for the usage of zinc in the treatment of cataract.] Oftalmol Zh 7:396, 1985
Cole H. Enzyme activity may hold the key to cataract activity. JAMA 254(8):1008, 1985
Couet C et al. Lactose and cataract in humans: A review. J Am Coll Nutr 10(1):79-86, 1991
Devamanoharan P et al. Prevention of selenite cataract by vitamin C. Exp Eye Res 52:563-8, 1991
Fujiwara H et al. Superoxide dismutase activity in cataractous lenses. Jpn J Ophthalmol 36(3):273-80, 1992
Hankinson S et al. Nutrient intake and cataract extraction in women: A prospective study. BMJ 305:335-9, 1992
Heinitz M. [Clinical and biochemical aspects of the prophylaxis and therapy of senile cataract with zinc aspartate.] Klin Monatsbl Augenheilkd 172(5):778-83, 1978
Hoffer A. Cataracts and orthomolecular treatment. J Orthomol Med 3(2):61-62, 1988
Huang W et al. Extracellular glutathione peroxidase and ascorbic acid in aqueous humor and serum of patients operated on for cataract. Clin Chim Acta 261(2):117-30, 1997
Jacques PH et al. Vitamin intake and senile cataract. Abstract. J Am Coll Nutr 6(5):435, 1987
Jacques PF et al. Lactose intake and senile cataract. Abstract. J Am Coll Nutr 7(5):424, 1988a
Jacques PF et al. Antioxidant status in persons with and without senile cataract. Arch Ophthalmol 106(3):337-40, 1988b
Jacques PF, Chylack LT Jr. Epidemiologic evidence of a role for the antioxidant vitamins and carotenoids in cataract prevention. Am J Clin Nutr 53:352S-5S, 1991
Jacques PF et al. Long-term vitamin C supplement use and prevalence of early age-related lens opacities. Am J Clin Nutr 66:911-16 1997
Jahn CE et al. Identification of metabolic risk factors for posterior subcapsular cataract. Ophthalmic Res 18(2):112-16, 1986
Jeru I. [The role of zinc in the appearance of cataract.] Oftalmologia 41(4):329-32, 1997
Kamei A. Glutathione levels of the human crystalline lens in aging and its antioxidant effect against the oxidation of lens proteins. Biol Pharmacol Bull 16:870-5, 1993
Karakucuk S et al. Selenium concentrations in serum, lens and aqueous humor of patients with senile cataract. Acta Ophthalmol Scand 73:323-32, 1995
Knekt P et al. Serum antioxidant vitamins and risk of cataract. BMJ 305:1392-4, 1992
Lane BC. Fish methylmercury and human cataractogenesis. Abstract. J Am Coll Nutr 11(5):637, 1992
Lerman S. Arch Ophthalmol 65:181, 1961
Leske MC et al. Antioxidant vitamins and nuclear opacities: the longitudinal study of cataract. Ophthalmology 105(5):831-6, 1998
Maitra I et al. Alpha-lipoic acid prevents buthionine sulfoximine-induced cataract formation in newborn rats. Free Rad Biol Med 18(4):823-9, 1995
Mares-Perlman JA et al. Diet and nuclear lens opacities. Am J Epidemiol 141(4):322-34, 1995
Muhlmann V et al. Vitamin C therapy of incipient senile cataract. Arch Oftalmol B Aires 14:552-75, 1939
Neuwirth-Lux O, Billson F. Vitamin E and rabbit corneal endothelial cell survival. Aust N Z J Ophthalmol 15(4):309-14, 1987
Prchal JT et al. Association of presenile cataracts with heterozygosity for galactosaemic states and with riboflavin deficiency. Lancet i:12-13, 1978
Robertson JM et al. Vitamin E intake and risk of cataracts in humans. Ann N Y Acad Sci 570:372-82, 1989
Ross WM et al. Modelling cortical cataractogenesis: III. In vivo effects of vitamin E on cataractogenesis in diabetic rats. Can J Ophthalmol 17(2):61-6, 1982
Rouhiainen P et al. Association between low plasma vitamin E concentration and progression of early cortical lens opacities. Am J Epidemiol 144(5):496-500, 1996
Seddon J et al. The issue of vitamin supplements and the risk of cataract among US male populations. Am J Public Health 84(5):788-92, 1994
Simoons FJ. A geographic approach to senile cataracts: possible links with milk consumption, lactase activity, and galactose metabolism. Dig Dis Sci 27(3):257-64, 1982
Skalka HW et al. Riboflavin deficiency and cataract formation. Metab Pediatr Ophthalmol 5(1):17-20, 1981a
Skalka HW, Prchal JT. Cataracts and riboflavin deficiency. Am J Clin Nutr 34(5):861-3, 1981b
Sperduto RD et al. The Linxian Cataract Studies: two nutrition intervention trials. Arch Ophthalmol 111(9):1246-53, 1993
Srivastava VK et al. Role of trace elements in senile cataract. Acta Ophthalmol (Copenh) 70(6):839-41, 1992
Stanojevik-Paovic A et al. Macro- and microelements in the cataractous eye lens. Ophthalmic Res 19(4):230-4, 1987
Swanson A, Truesdale A. Elemental analysis and cataractous human lens tissue. Biochem Biophys Res Commun 45:1488-96, 1971
Sydenstricker, U. of Georgia and U. of Georgia Hospital - reported in Gerras C et al, Eds. The Encyclopedia of Common Diseases. Emmaus, PA, Rodale Press, 1976
Tavani A et al. Food and nutrient intake and risk of cataract. Ann Epidemiol 6:41-6, 1996
Taylor A et al. Moderate caloric restriction delays cataract formation in the Emory mouse. FASEB J 3(6):1741-6, 1989
Taylor A. Cataract: relationships between nutrition and oxidation. J Am Coll Nutr 12(2):138-46, 1993
Todd, GP - interviewed in Prevention March, 1985 pp. 74-80; Todd GP. Nutrition, Health & Disease. Norfolk, Virginia Beach, The Donning Company, 1985
Varma SD et al. Diabetic cataracts and flavonoids. Science 195:205-06, 1977
Varma SD, Richards RD. Light-induced damage to ocular lens cation pump: Prevention by vitamin C. Proc Natl Acad Sci U S A 76:3504-6, 1979
Varma SA et al. Photoperoxidation of lens lipids: prevention by vitamin E. Photochem Photobiol 36(6):623-36, 1982
Vitale S et al. Plasma antioxidants and risk of cortical and nuclear cataract. Epidemiology 4:195-203, 1993

CELIAC DISEASE

See Also: DERMATITIS HERPETIFORMIS

NUTRITIONAL TREATMENT GUIDE

✓ = Efficacy generally accepted.
* = Efficacy *demonstrated* by controlled human trials.
[+] = Efficacy *suspected* from uncontrolled human trials.
[-] = Efficacy *suspected* from indirect data.
? = Efficacy *challenged* in a study of similar design.

NUTRITIONAL FACTORS

* **Vitamin K deficiency:** phytonadione 10 mg intramuscularly as needed

- -

[+] **L-Carnitine deficiency:** 1 to 6 g daily
[+] **Copper deficiency:** 2 mg twice daily for up to 6 weeks *AND* **Zinc** 50 mg daily
[+] **Folic acid deficiency:** 800 μg daily
[+] **Iron deficiency:** 30 mg twice daily until repletion; then minimal possible dosage
[+] **Selenium deficiency:** 200 μg daily
[+] **Vitamin A deficiency:** 50,000 IU daily for 6 weeks (10,000 IU daily during pregnancy)
[+] **Vitamin B_6 deficiency:** 50 to 100 mg daily
[+] **Vitamin B_{12} deficiency:** 1,000 μg intramuscularly weekly initially and monthly afterwards
[+] **Vitamin D deficiency:** 50,000 to 100,000 IU 2 or 3 times during the first week; then if needed, either 100,000 IU of ergo- or cholecalciferol every 3 to 6 months *OR* 800 to 1,600 IU daily
[+] **Vitamin E deficiency:** D,L-alpha-tocopheryl acetate 200 to 2,000 mg or IU daily for 6 weeks; then maintenance levels as needed
[+] **Zinc deficiency:** zinc sulfate 220 mg twice daily *AND* **Copper** 2 mg daily

FOOD SENSITIVITIES

✓ rule out **Gluten sensitivity**

- -

[+] rule out **Lactose intolerance**
[+] rule out **Wheat Starch sensitivity**

A nutritional disease involving genetically induced sensitivity to gluten, celiac disease is induced in susceptible persons by dietary exposure to the food-grain antigens in wheat, rye, and barley.

Specific toxic amino acid sequences have been identified in alpha-gliadin, the alcohol-soluble extract of wheat gluten *(Goggins)*. This toxicity can be confirmed by measurement of alpha-gliadin antibodies, which are elevated in the vast majority of celiac patients *(Kelly)*. Unfortunately, avoidance of gluten-containing foods can lead to inadequate provision of energy as well as of a number of important nutrients, resulting in the promotion of other nutritionally-related disorders such as osteoporosis *(McFarlane)*. It has been suggested that the inadequacy of the diet may be because some patients find gluten-free products unpalatable, causing them to reduce their intake of all cereal products *(McFarlane)*.

NUTRITIONAL FACTORS

VITAMIN DEFICIENCIES

Fat-soluble Vitamin Deficiencies

Due to the malabsorption of fats, vitamins A, D, E and K may all be deficient *(Passmore,1986b)*.

Vitamin D Deficiency

Hypovitaminosis D is common, and secondary hyperparathyroidism is sometimes found. In one study of 43 patients, 88% of celiacs who were unresponsive to a gluten-free diet and immunosuppressive therapy were deficient in vitamin D. This compares to 58% of newly-diagnosed (untreated) celiacs and only 25% of celiacs who showed a histologic response to a gluten-free diet. Secondary hyperparathyroidism was found in 25% of the refractory patients, 19% of the diet-responsive patients, and 25% of the untreated patients. Moreover, bone reabsorption markers were significantly elevated in all groups *(Keaveny)*.

Vitamin E Deficiency

A number of case reports have suggested that, despite a gluten-free diet, vitamin E deficiency may occasionally produce neurological degenerative findings, including a cerebellar syndrome, posterior and lateral column abnormalities, and a neuromyopathy. While the responsible mechanisms are poorly understood, patients whose duodenal histology fails to improve on a gluten-free diet may be at greater risk *(Muller)*.

Vitamin K Deficiency

Changes in the prothrombin complex may be noted *(Benitez)*. Deficiency of vitamin K may even be serious enough to result in a bleeding disorder *(Graham)*. In fact, an unexplained hemorrhagic diathesis should arouse suspicion of occult celiac disease *(Mitterstieler)*.

A woman presented with adult-onset celiac disease complicated by a cerebellar syndrome which progressed on a gluten-free diet despite resolution of malabsorption. She was found to have a vitamin E deficiency. Following the institution of vitamin E supplementation, her cerebellar symptoms improved (Mauro).

Vitamin B Complex Deficiencies

Folic Acid Deficiency

Folic acid may be deficient in celiac disease patients due to malabsorption *(Halsted)*. This may lead not only to the development of a megaloblastic anemia *(Hoffbrand)*, but also to the development of epilepsy *(Bye)*.

While correction occurs coincidentally with the improvement in absorption resulting from a gluten-free diet, oral supplementation is recommended until recovery is complete *(Passmore,1986a)*.

Vitamin B_6 Deficiency

Malabsorption of vitamin B_6 may cause a deficiency of the vitamin *(Reinken)*.

The resolution of depression is among the positive effects of repleting a vitamin B_6 deficiency. In an open trial, supplementation was found effective in resolving depression in celiacs whose mood had failed to improve on a gluten-free diet despite histologic improvement in the small intestines *(Hallert)*.

Vitamin B_{12} Deficiency

Untreated celiacs have significantly lower serum vitamin B_{12} levels than patients in remission *(Kemppainen)*. The absorption defect in this vitamin may not become clinically significant until after a long duration of the disease *(Kokkonen)*.

MINERAL DEFICIENCIES

Calcium Deficiency

Malabsorption may result in calcium deficiency and its complications. Osteopenia, for example, is a common complication of celiac disease *(Mautalen)*. In one group of newly-diagnosed patients, 11 out of the 15 had hypocalcemia, 3 had skeletal disease, and 1 had both. Serum total alkaline phosphatase was elevated in 10 patients, while parathyroid hormone was low in all 15 patients. Bone mineral density was low in all patients tested.

Most importantly, from a diagnostic perspective, only 4 of the patients had persistent diarrhea, while 7 had mild, intermittent gastrointestinal symptoms. This finding suggests that celiac disease should be considered in all patients with unexplained metabolic bone disease or hypocalcemia - not just those with gastrointestinal symptoms *(Shaker)*.

Fortunately, bone mineral density can usually be rapidly improved with a calcium-rich, gluten-free diet. After one year of treatment, one group of patients averaged a 14.1% increase in bone mineral density at the lumbar spine *(Ciacci)*.

Tetany, a symptom of hypocalcemia, will sometimes be the presenting complaint, suggesting that celiac disease should be considered as a cause of unexplained tetany.

Three female patients with spontaneous episodes of tetany due to severe hypocalcemia and hypomagnesemia were diagnosed with celiac disease. The tetany was successfully reversed with intravenous calcium supplementation and a gluten-free diet (Cano).

Copper Deficiency

Malabsorption may cause a copper deficiency. Celiac disease causing copper deficiency should therefore be considered as a cause of unexplained anemia or neutropenia *(Jameson)*. Young children with severe celiac disease are particularly prone to copper deficiency, and its effects can be rapidly reversed with copper supplementation along with a gluten-free diet *(Goyens)*.

Iron Deficiency

Malabsorption causing an iron-deficient anemia may result in a deficiency of iron *(Kemppainen)*. Although iron supplementation is helpful for celiac patients *(Passmore, 1986a)*, the introduction of a gluten-free diet may, by itself, eliminate all evidence of iron deficiency, while the reintroduction of gluten causes the suboptimal iron balance to rapidly reappear *(Stahlberg)*. This finding suggests that the intestinal bleeding that may accompany the disease may be another cause of iron deficiency *(Fine)*.

Magnesium Deficiency

Deficiency impairs parathyroid secretion and action. In animal models, magnesium deficiency has been shown to result in osteopenia and increased skeletal fragility *(Rude)*.

Based on erythrocyte magnesium levels, 8 out of a group of 23 asymptomatic patients on a gluten-free diet had an intracellular magnesium deficiency. Five of them received oral magnesium supplementation. After 2 years, there was a significant increase in bone mineral density seen in the femoral neck and total proximal femur which correlated with a rise in red blood cell magnesium level and a rise in parathyroid hormone *(Rude)*.

Selenium Deficiency

Selenium may be deficient, again because of malabsorption *(Cortigiani)*. Even on a gluten-free diet, erythrocyte selenium levels may indicate deficiency *(Boda)*, a finding that has been attributed to inadequate selenium in the gluten-free diet *(Cortigiani)*.

Evidence of decreased activity of the selenium-containing antioxidant glutathione peroxidase, as well as of increased sensitivity of oxidative stress, suggests that supplemental selenium should be strongly considered *(Boda)*.

Zinc Deficiency

Concerning zinc, prior to gluten elimination, there is increased turnover and loss of endogenous zinc despite normal absorption at physiological intakes *(Crofton)*. In a group of 50 consecutive adult patients, for example, serum zinc concentration was found to be low in 31% *(Bode)*.

While the maintenance of a gluten-free diet should result in the restoration of normal zinc nutriture, zinc deficiency could inhibit the recovery of the intestinal mucosa, so repletion with a zinc supplement may be advisable during the first 2 to 4 weeks of treatment *(Henker)*.

OTHER NUTRITIONAL FACTORS

L-Carnitine Deficiency

Serum levels of carnitine may be reduced in celiac disease *(Lerner)*. This is understandable since absorption of exogenous carnitine takes place mainly at the duodenal-jejunal level by an active transport mechanism.

As with other nutrients, when patients follow a gluten-free diet, carnitine levels increase *(Ceccarelli)*.

A 47 year-old-man without a previous known illness presented with acute hematomas in both legs and malnutrition. He reported having large, foul-smelling stools once or twice daily. Hemoglobin concentration was 5.6 g/dl, serum iron was normal and ferritin was reduced. Quick value was less than 5%, while activated partial thromboplastin time was prolonged to 180 seconds. Vitamin A and E concentrations were reduced. Coumarin derivatives were not demonstrated in his blood.

He immediately received 4 units of erythrocyte concentration together with 2000 IU of factors II, VII, X and anti-hemophilic factor B (PPSB), and 10 mg vitamin K intravenously. Further investigation revealed vitamin A malabsorption; upper intestinal endoscopy revealed celiac disease which was confirmed by biopsy.

Supplementation with vitamins A, D, E, and K as well as a gluten-free diet quickly improved his condition (Heidinger).

FOOD SENSITIVITIES

Gluten

Gluten is found in wheat, rye, oats, barley (including malt) and buckwheat.

Even though celiac disease is clearly related to gluten sensitivity, it is not a typical allergic disorder for the following reasons:

(1) Oral gluten challenge usually is not as rapid or as acute as in the case of wheat allergy.
(2) Celiac disease is invariably permanent, whereas wheat allergy is usually temporary.
(3) Serum IgE levels are usually not elevated.
(4) Intradermal testing with gluten or wheat seldom causes an immediate wheal-and-flare response.
(5) Levels of specific IgE antibodies to wheat protein are not elevated. *(Bahna)*.

It appears that most patients can consume moderate amounts of oats on a daily basis without obvious adverse effects over the following year *(Schmitz)*. However, since celiac patients have a markedly increased cancer incidence related to the intake of even small quantities of gluten and its prolamins, and a gluten-free diet of at least 5 years decreases cancer incidence, some authorities believe it is too early to recommend eating even a moderate amount of oats *(Branski)*.

Wheat Starch

In a one-year open trial, 17 patients on a gluten-free diet who had never consumed wheat starch added it into their diets. When compared to control celiacs who tolerated wheat starch, the majority of these patients developed symptoms which resolved within weeks of discontinuing the product *(Chartrand)*.

Lactose

Intolerance to dairy products due to lactase deficiency may be present in celiac patients. This is probably due to reduced epithelial cells and alterations in the function of individual cells *(Plotkin)*.

BIBLIOGRAPHY

Bahna SL. Celiac disease: A food allergy? Contra! Highlights in Food Allergy 32:211-15, 1996

Benitez L et al. Changes in the prothrombin complex as clinical manifestation of celiac sprue in adults. Rev Clin Esp 196(7):492-3, 1996

Boda M, Nĕmeth I. [Selenium levels in erythrocytes of children with celiac disease.] Orv Hetil 130(39):2087-90, 1989

Bode S, Gudmand-Hoyer E. Symptoms and haematologic features in consecutive adult coeliac patients. Scand J Gastroenterol 31(1):54-60, 1996

Branski D, Shine M. Oats in celiac disease. Letter. N Engl J Med 334(13):865-6, 1996

Bye AM et al. Cortical vascular abnormalities in the syndrome of celiac disease, epilepsy, bilateral occipital calcifications, and folate deficiency. Ann Neurol 34(3):399-403, 1993

Ceccarelli M et al. [Plasma L-carnitine levels in children with celiac disease.] Minerva Pediatr 44(9):401-5, 1992 (in Italian)

Chartrand LJ et al. Wheat starch intolerance in patients with celiac disease. J Am Diet Assn 97(6):612-8, 1997

Ciacci C et al. Effects of dietary treatment on bone mineral density on adults with celiac disease: factors predicting response. Am J Gastroenterol 92(6):992-6, 1997

Cortigiani L et al. [Selenium in celiac disease.] Minerva Pediatr 41(11):539-42, 1989 (in Italian)

Crofton RW et al. Zinc metabolism in celiac disease. Am J Clin Nutr 52(2):379-82, 1990

Fine KD. The prevalence of occult gastrointestinal bleeding in celiac sprue. N Engl J Med 334:1163-7, 1996

Goggins M, Kelleher D. Celiac disease and other nutrient related injuries to the gastrointestinal tract. Am J Gastroenterol 89:Suppl:S2-S17, 1994

Goyens P et al. Copper deficiency in infants with active celiac disease. J Pediatr Gastroenterol Nutr 4(4):677-80, 1985

Graham DR et al. Celiac disease presenting as acute bleeding disorders. Postgrad Med J 58(677):178-9, 1982

Hallert C et al. Reversal of psychopathology in adult coeliac disease with the aid of pyridoxine (vitamin B6). Scand J Gastroenterol 18(2):299-304, 1983

Halsted CH et al. Jejunal perfusion of simple and conjugated folates in celiac sprue. J Clin Invest 59:933-40, 1977

Heidinger K et al. [Endemic sprue: its first diagnosis based on bleeding complications.] Dtsch Med Wochenschr 120(45):1543-6, 1995

Henker J, Gabsch HC. [Serum zinc levels in children with celiac disease.] Helv Paediatr Acta 40(1):47-53, 1985

Hoffgrand AV. Anaemia in adult coeliac disease. Clin Gastroenterol 3:71-89, 1974

Jameson S et al. Copper malabsorption in coeliac disease. Sci Total Environ 42(1-2):29-36, 1985

Keaveny AP et al. Bone remodeling indices and secondary hyperparathyroidism in celiac disease. Am J Gastroenterol 91(6):1226-31, 1996

Kelly J et al. Alpha-gliadin antibodies in childhood celiac disease. Letter. Lancet September 7, 1985, p. 558

Kemppainen T et al. Intakes of nutrients and nutritional status in celiac patients. Scand J Gastroenterol 30(6):575-9, 1995

Kokkonen J, Similä S. Gastric function and absorption of vitamin B12 in children with celiac disease. Eur J Pediatr 132(2):71-5, 1979

Lerner A et al. Serum carnitine concentrations in coeliac disease. Gut 34(7):933-5, 1993

Mauro A et al. Cerebellar syndrome in adult celiac disease with vitamin E deficiency. Acta Neurol Scand 84(2):167-70, 1990

Mautalen C et al. Effect of treatment on bone mass, mineral metabolism, and body composition in untreated celiac disease patients. Am J Gastroenterol 92(2):313-18, 1997

McFarlane XA et al. Subclinical nutritional deficiency in treated coeliac disease and nutritional content of the gluten free diet. J Hum Nutr Diet 8:231-7, 1995

Mitterstieler G, Zieglauer H. [Vitamin K deficiency bleeding as a leading symptom in celiac disease.] Padiatr Padol 13(2):175-82, 1978

Muller AF et al. Neurological complications of celiac disease: a rare but continuing problem. Am J Gastroenterol 91(7):1430-5, 1996

Passmore R, Eastwood MA. Davidson and Passmore: Human Nutrition and Dietetics. Edinburgh, Churchill Livingstone, 1986a:440

Passmore R, Eastwood MA. Davidson and Passmore: Human Nutrition and Dietetics. Edinburgh, Churchill Livingstone, 1986b:141

Plotkin GR, Isselbacher KJ. Secondary disaccharidase deficiency in adult celiac disease. N Engl J Med 271:1033-7, 1964

Reinken L, Zieglauer H. Vitamin B6 absorption in children with acute celiac disease and in control subjects. J Nutr 108:1562, 1978

Rude RK, Olerich MI. Magnesium deficiency: possible role in osteoporosis associated with gluten-sensitive enteropathy. Osteoporosis Int 6(6):453-61, 1996

Schmitz J. Lack of oats toxicity in coeliac disease. BMJ 314:159-60, 1997

Shaker JL et al. Hypocalcemia and skeletal disease as presenting features of celiac disease. Arch Intern Med 157(9):1013-16, 1997

Stahlberg MR et al. Iron deficiency in coeliac disease is mild and it is detected and corrected by gluten-free diet. Acta Paediatr Scand 80(2):190-3, 1991

CEREBROVASCULAR DISEASE

including

CEREBROVASCULAR ACCIDENT (STROKE)

See Also: **ATHEROSCLEROSIS**
DEMENTIA
HYPERTENSION
ORGANIC MENTAL DISORDERS

NUTRITIONAL TREATMENT GUIDE

✓ = Efficacy generally accepted.
* = Efficacy *demonstrated* by controlled human trials.
[+] = Efficacy *suspected* from uncontrolled human trials.
[-] = Efficacy *suspected* from indirect data.
? = Efficacy *challenged* in a study of similar design.

DIETARY FACTORS

[-] avoid **Obesity**
[-] minimize **Salt** intake
[-] **high Potassium diet**
[-] drink **Milk**
[-] ? eat **fresh Fruits and Vegetables**
[-] ? eat a moderate amount of fatty **Fish** and other food sources of omega-3 fatty acids
[-] ? moderate **Alcohol** consumption (Alcohol may reduce risk of *ischemic* stroke, but increase risk of *hemorrhagic* stroke.)

NUTRITIONAL FACTORS

* **Acetyl L-carnitine:** ? 1 to 3 g daily in divided doses
* **Coenzyme Q_{10}:** ? 30 to 100 mg daily
* **Folic acid deficiency:** *to reduce homocysteine:* 400 µg daily (6 week trial)
* **Glycosaminoglycans:** Mesoglycan 100 mg daily
* **Vitamin E:** ? 400 IU daily

- -

[+] **Magnesium:** *to treat acute non-hemorrhagic cerebrovascular disease:* 8 mmol magnesium sulfate IV
[+] **Vitamin B_6 deficiency:** *to normalize homocysteine metabolism:* 50 to 100 mg daily
[+] **Vitamin B_{12} deficiency:** *to normalize homocysteine metabolism:* 1,000 µg intramuscularly weekly initially and monthly afterwards

- -

[-] **Alpha-Lipoic acid:** 100 to 300 mg daily
[-] **Magnesium deficiency:** ≈ 400 mg daily
[-] **Vitamin A:** 50,000 IU daily for 6 weeks (10,000 IU during pregnancy)
[-] **Vitamin C:** 500 mg twice daily

OTHER RELATED FACTORS

[-] avoid **Obesity**

DIETARY FACTORS

Fresh Fruits and Vegetables

A number of studies have found a significant protective effect for the consumption of fresh fruits and vegetables *(Ness).* In one study, for example, the higher the quintile of daily servings of fruits and vegetables, the lower the age-adjusted risk of stroke *(Gillman).* While the reason(s) for their protective effective are not well understood, their flavonoid content is probably relevant, as flavonoid intake has been found to be inversely related to stroke risk *(Keli,1996).*

By contrast, a positive correlation was found between the total dietary intake of plant *proteins* - except for cereal-derived proteins - and cerebrovascular mortality rates *(Seely,1982).* The same author notes that the geographical distribution of cerebrovascular disease seems best matched by that of the consumption of soya beans as well as of other legumes *(Seely,1983).* These data are difficult to interpret until more data are collected for confirmation and to broaden our knowledge of the factors involved.

Meat and Fish

The effect of meat and fish intake upon the risk of cerebrovascular disease is unclear, at least partly because of the interaction of multiple factors. These include the relationship of the intake of meat and fish to the intake of fruits and vegetables, the relationship between intakes of saturated versus unsaturated fat, the differences between plant and animal proteins, and the relationship between the omega-3 and omega-6 essential fatty acids.

Several observational studies have specifically investigated the relationship between fish consumption and cerebrovascular disease. American *(Gillum),* Dutch *(Keli,1994)* and Japanese *(Hirai)* studies have found that frequent fish consumption reduced the risk of stroke by one-half. Another American study, however, found no relationship between fish consumption and stroke *(Morris),* while yet another found that men who consumed the greatest amount of fish (over 35 grams daily) actually had an *increased* risk of death from stroke *(Orencia).*

The weight of the evidence suggests that, despite the tendency of fish oils to reduce platelet aggregation *(Tremoli),* moderate fish intake helps to reduce stroke risk. In fact, the specific risk of hemorrhagic stroke appears to be reduced in areas with higher fish consumption *(Gerster).*

One study found the intake of animal protein to be inversely associated with the incidence of thromboembolic strokes *(Lee).* Since, as noted above, there is early evidence that vegetable *protein* intake could increase the risk of cerebrovascular mortality, this isolated finding should not be the basis of recommending higher meat intake.

Dietary Cholesterol

Because dietary cholesterol may influence serum cholesterol levels, yet another factor complicating and obscuring our understanding of the relationship between the intake of animal foods and stroke is the serum cholesterol level. While the picture is far from clear, it appears that there may be an inverse association between total serum cholesterol and the risk of *hemorrhagic* stroke, while there may be a direct association between total serum cholesterol and the risk of *ischemic* stroke *(Bronner).* The result is a U-shaped curve, with moderate serum cholesterol levels appearing to be preferable.

Dietary Fat

The amount and type of total fat intake is another variable whose relationship to cerebrovascular disease remains unclear. A recent 20-year follow-up study found that, among men, the higher the quintile of total fat, saturated fat, and monounsaturated fat (but not polyunsaturated fat), the lower the risk of ischemic stroke *(Gillman)*. Others, however, have noted an independent *positive* correlation between saturated fatty acid intake and stroke mortality ratios *(Sasaki)*. Still other investigators have found no relationship between saturated fat intake and the risk of stroke *(Lapidus;McGee)*.

Obviously, more work needs to be done to sort out the relationships between the various types of fat and stroke, ischemic versus hemorrhagic stroke, and the risk of stroke versus the risk of death from stroke. Until then, it seems premature to make dietary recommendations for fat intake in regard to protecting against the dangers of stroke.

Salt (sodium chloride)

Salt intake is positively associated with cerebrovascular mortality, and it may well be the most important dietary factor in determining stroke mortality *(Sasaki)*.

Since hypertension is known to be a major risk factor for stroke, and since dietary salt intake may be a substantial contributor to hypertension, the relationship between salt intake and stroke could be attributed to salt's promotion of hypertension. There is evidence from both animal work *(Tobian)* and a large epidemiological study *(Perry,1992)*, however, that the deleterious effect of a high salt intake may be independent of its effects on blood pressure.

Alcohol

The relationship of moderate alcohol intake to the risk of stroke has yet to become well clarified, in part because it seems to have a different relationship with ischemic stroke than it has with hemorrhagic stroke.

Moderate alcohol consumption appears to show a dose-response relationship with the risk of intracerebral and subarachnoid hemorrhage. The relative risk varies from 2 to 4, with some increased risk at all levels of intake *(Bronner)*.

In regard to ischemic stroke, moderate alcohol consumption of up to 2 drinks per day was *protective* in both younger and older groups, in men and women, and in whites, blacks, and Hispanics. However, *increased* risk was significant among those consuming 7 or more drinks per day *(Sacco)*.

Studies of predominantly white groups have also found an inverse relationship at low levels of intake with a relative risk of 0.3 to 0.5 for one to two drinks daily increasing to 2 for three or more drinks daily. This finding contrasts with studies of Japanese, for whom no association was present at low levels of intake, and increased risk was found at higher levels of consumption *(Bronner)*.

In a controlled study, 8 middle-aged men randomly received 40 grams alcohol as beer, wine or spirits or received mineral water on 4 different days over a period of 11 days along with the evening meal. The study's findings suggested that moderate drinking may reduce the risk of ischemic stroke by increasing local tissue type plasminogen activator activity to help prevent blood clot formation and stimulate the dissolution of existing clots *(Hendriks)*.

In contrast to moderate drinking, a single alcoholic binge may immediately cause a stroke and thus is clearly contraindicated *(Wilkins)*.

Milk

Milk intake appears to have a protective effect. In a 22-year study of more than 3,000 men older middle-aged men, those who did not drink milk experienced a thromboembolic stroke at twice the rate of men who consumed 16 ounces or more daily. Further analysis showed that this association could not be explained by the increased calcium intake, suggesting that, assuming a causal relationship, other factors in milk may explain its efficacy *(Abbott)*.

This finding is consistent with the results of an animal study in which the intake of two milk protein-rich diets, one containing casein and the other containing whey protein, attenuated the development of severe hypertension in stroke-prone spontaneously hypertensive rats and extended their life span. Moreover, a milk fat-rich diet reduced their incidence of cerebrovascular disease even though blood pressure was unchanged *(Ikeda)*.

HOMOCYSTEINE

[See Atherosclerosis for a full discussion.]

Several recent studies have confirmed that elevated levels of the toxic amino acid homocysteine is a major, independent risk factor for stroke *(Stampfer)*. Moreover, a meta-analysis found that the odds ratio for cerebrovascular disease goes up 50% for each 5 mmol/L increase in total plasma or serum homocysteine levels *(Boushey)*.

Heterozygous homocystinuria is especially common in patients with premature cerebrovascular disease. For example, of 25 patients who developed occlusive cerebrovascular disease before age 50, heterozygous homocystinuria was established in 7 (28%) *(Boers,1985)*.

Three B vitamins, namely folic acid, vitamin B_6, and vitamin B_{12}, are important cofactors in the detoxification of homocysteine, and their nutriture has been shown to relate to the risk of stroke. Of the 3, folic acid appears to be the most important *(Verhoef)* although, once the decision is made to supplement, it appears rational to supplement all 3 at once along with a general B complex mixture. (See Folic Acid Deficiency, Vitamin B_6 Deficiency, and Vitamin B_{12} Deficiency below.)

NUTRITIONAL FACTORS

VITAMINS

Folic Acid Deficiency

Serum levels of folic acid, a coenzyme for the conversion of homocysteine back to methionine, may be inversely associated with carotid artery stenosis and the risk of stroke *(Selhub;Stampfer)*.

Supplementation with this vitamin has been found to significantly reduce homocysteine levels both before and after methionine loading *(Brattström)*. Moreover, it appears to be the most important vitamin to supplement in order to normalize homocysteine metabolism *(Ubbink,1994)*.

Vitamin A

There is early evidence that the plasma or serum level of vitamin A bears an inverse relationship to stroke, although the preventive and therapeutic value of supplementation remains to be determined.

Specifically, in the day following a stroke, patients may have a significantly reduced plasma level of the vitamin *(Singh)*. Whether the reduced level promoted the stroke or is merely a result of the stroke is unknown. Another study, this time of patients with sudden focal neurological deficits due to acute ischemia in the middle cerebral artery, found that those patients who had higher mean vitamin A levels had a higher frequency of recovery within the first day, decreased mortality, and less of a permanent neurological deficit than those with lower levels of the vitamin *(De Keyser)*.

Vitamin B_6 Deficiency

Plasma levels of vitamin B_6, a coenzyme for the conversion of homocysteine to the non-toxic cystathionine, may be inversely associated with stroke risk *(Selhub)*. Moreover, deficiency of the vitamin is associated with abnormal homocysteine metabolism *(Ubbink,1996)*.

In a study of 11 patients with heterozygous homocystinuria and premature cerebral and peripheral arterial disease, abnormal homocysteine metabolism improved in all but one following pyridoxine supplementation *(Boers,1985)*. However, pyridoxine supplementation may not be as successful in preventing homocystinemia after methionine loading *(Boers,1983)*.

Although we do not yet have a terribly clear picture of the relative importance of vitamin B_6 nutriture in homocysteine metabolism, results of an animal study echo the findings of the above study in suggesting that vitamin B_6 alone may only be partially successful in ameliorating the adverse effects of homocysteine accumulation. Rabbits were given homocysteine and arteriosclerotic plaques developed. Pretreatment with pyridoxine failed to prevent plaque development; however, it did prevent both thrombosis and pulmonary embolism *(McCully)*.

Vitamin B_{12} Deficiency

As with vitamin B_6 and folic acid, plasma/serum levels of vitamin B_{12} may be inversely related to homocysteine levels and risk of stroke *(Clarke)*. In fact, the relationship between vitamin B_{12} deficiency and elevated homocysteine levels is now believed to be so intimate that a recent recommendation for evaluating vitamin B_{12} deficiency is to determine the serum cobalamin level as a screening test and, if it is low, then determine either serum or urine homocysteine levels, as well as methylmalonic acid levels, for confirmation *(Swain)*.

Vitamin C

Animal work suggests that the brain releases large amounts of ascorbic acid in response to cerebral ischemia,
perhaps to act as a scavenger of free radicals *(Oriot)* or to prevent glutamate toxicity due to its massive release *(Smythies)*.

Both the dietary intake *(Daviglus)* and plasma levels *(Gey)* of the vitamin may be inversely correlated with the risk of stroke. Rath and Pauling have theorized that a marginal ascorbate deficiency results in the accumulation of lipoprotein (a) and fibrinogen/fibrin in the vascular wall. This impairment, they claim, is unmasked mainly at sites of altered hemodynamic conditions, leading to stroke as well as to myocardial infarction *(Rath)*.

The value of vitamin C supplementation for this disorder remains to be explored.

Vitamin E

Plasma levels of vitamin E may be inversely related to stroke incidence *(Singh)*.

In an as-yet unpublished, controlled study, more than 2,000 patients who had suffered a cerebral infarction received either alpha-tocopherol supplementation or a conventional treatment. After 3 years, those patients who received alpha-tocopherol had a consistently lower cumulative incidence of cerebrovascular events, both fatal and non-fatal *(Anonymous)*. This finding is in keeping with the results of an animal study in which the effects of vitamin E on cerebral ischemia were investigated in dogs and supplementation was found to have a major protective effect *(Fujimoto)*.

Moreover, in a randomized, double-blind study published in the *American Journal of Clinical Nutrition*, 100 patients with transient ischemic attacks, minor strokes, or residual ischemic neurologic deficits randomly received either aspirin (a platelet anti-aggregating agent) 325 mg alone or aspirin plus vitamin E 400 IU daily for 2 years. Preliminary results showed a significant reduction in the incidence of ischemic events in patients in the aspirin plus vitamin E group as compared to patients taking only aspirin. In addition, based on measurements in a randomized sub-group of both populations, there was a highly significant reduction in platelet adhesiveness in patients taking aspirin plus vitamin E compared to patients taking only aspirin *(Steiner)*.

Reduction in platelet adhesiveness is not the only mechanism by which vitamin E may protect against cerebrovascular disease. It is a major lipid-soluble antioxidant, protecting vascular endothelial cells from polyunsaturated lipid-mediated oxidative stress *(Cockcroft)*. It is also a membrane stabilizer, stimulating endothelial cell proliferation to attempt to maintain endothelial integrity *(Boscobionik)*.

MINERALS

Magnesium Deficiency

Water hardness appears to be inversely related to mortality from stroke *(Nebrand)*. According to a recent analysis, although calcium is an important contributor to water hardness, this relationship is entirely due to the water's magnesium content *(Yang)*. Moreover, chronic magnesium deficiency has been implicated in some cases of transient ischemic attacks *(Fehlinger)*, and the serum magnesium level appears to be inversely correlated with the risk of hospitalization and death from vascular disease *(Gartside)*.

Experimentally, acute magnesium deficiency can produce cerebrovasospasm. The lower the extracellular concentration of magnesium ions, the greater the magnitude of cerebral arterial contraction *(Altura)*.

These findings suggest that avoidance of magnesium deficiency by providing adequate magnesium intake in the water and food supplies or through supplementation will decrease the risk of strokes related to cerebrovasospasm.

Once cerebrovasospasm and ischemia have occurred, intravenous magnesium may be highly effective. In one study, for example, half of a group of 34 patients with non-hemorrhagic cerebrovascular disease showed marked improvement within one to two minutes after intravenous injections of 8 mmol magnesium sulfate, often with dramatic recovery of function *(Browne)*.

Recent evidence suggests that magnesium may act by opposing calcium-dependent cerebral arterial vasoconstriction. It may also antagonize the increase in intracellular calcium caused by ischemia and thus prevent cell damage and death *(Sadeh)*.

Hypomagnesemia is of special importance in regard to hospitalized patients, for whom its overall incidence ranges from 7 to 52%. The greatest association of hypomagnesemia in these patients appears to be in hypokalemic states and in those confined to intensive care units *(Altura)*.

Because of its importance, magnesium nutriture should be routinely evaluated in all cases of transient ischemic attacks and non-hemorrhagic stroke.

A 57 year-old woman with congestive heart failure had a gradual onset of marked weakness and loss of sensation in her left arm, hand, leg and foot which failed to improve during 3 months of standard treatment.

Intramuscular magnesium sulfate produced slight improvement. After the rapid injection of 10 mmol of intravenous magnesium sulfate, her symptoms completely resolved for 12 hours and then relapsed. She was given a short course of rapid bolus injections of magnesium sulfate [daily to weekly IV injections of 8 mmol] and had a full recovery along with substantial improvement of her congestive heart failure (Browne).

Potassium Deficiency

Potassium intake appears to be negatively correlated with mortality from stroke *(Khaw)*. In fact, in stroke-prone hypertensive rats, a high intake of potassium almost abolishes the occurrence of stroke *(Luft)*.

Stroke patients at the time of hospital admission may be twice as likely to exhibit low potassium levels as normals, and a low serum potassium at that time increases the likelihood of mortality from the stroke *(Gariballa)*. Similarly, 24-hour urinary potassium levels are independently negatively correlated with stroke mortality *(Sasaki)*.

These findings suggest that a high potassium intake, which is best achieved by eating foods that are rich in potassium, helps to protect against stroke and stroke-associated mortality.

OTHER NUTRITIONAL FACTORS

Alpha-Lipoic Acid

In animal studies, the metabolic antioxidant alpha-lipoic acid protects against cerebral ischemic injury *(Cao; Panigrahi)*. It has been proposed as a useful intervention strategy for the treatment of stroke, although controlled human studies have yet to be published *(Packer)*.

Beta-carotene

As with cardiovascular disease, the relationship between beta-carotene nutriture and risk of stroke is highly controversial. Both the dietary intake and plasma levels of the nutrient are inversely related to the incidence of ischemic stroke *(Singh)*. However, supplementation with 50 mg every other day for 12 years failed to reduce the risk of stroke-related deaths in a group of more than 22,000 initially healthy American physicians *(Hennekens)*.

L-Carnitine

L-carnitine plays an essential role in fatty acid metabolism. Acetyl-L-carnitine is a patented derivative of L-carnitine and a naturally occurring ester.

Evidence from controlled studies suggests that the administration of acetyl-L-carnitine may improve cerebral blood flow in patients with cerebral ischemia and protect them against the adverse effects of the ischemia. In one study, 10 patients who suffered a stroke at least 6 months earlier received acetyl-L-carnitine intravenously while another 10 patients received a placebo. Forty-five minutes later, those patients who received the active treatment had improved cerebral blood flow in both hemispheres in the ischemic area, although not in the zone corresponding to the stroke *(Postiglione)*.

Data suggesting that this improvement in cerebral blood flow may be of clinical benefit comes from a double-blind crossover study of 12 patients who were undergoing rehabilitation for acute cerebral insufficiency. Testing revealed significant differences between the drug and placebo in regard to memory, number and word tests and in the responses to simple stimuli as well as in the performance of a maze test *(Arrigo)*.

While acetyl-L-carnitine has not been directly compared to L-carnitine, a study of mice who were exposed to ammonia found that pretreatment with carnitine suppressed the development of seizures as well as of changes in the concentrations of brain energy metabolites *(Igisu)*, suggesting that L-carnitine may have similar effects to those of its derivative.

Coenzyme Q_{10}

In a recent study of an animal model of cerebral vasospasm, untreated rabbits developed moderate to severe neurological deficits with focal ischemia in brain regions whose blood supply was compromised, while oral supplementation with coenzyme Q_{10} prevented these findings from developing *(Grieb)*. Similarly, gerbils with unilateral carotid ligation-induced stroke died within 28 hours, but when coenzyme Q_{10} was implanted subcutaneously, 45% of the animals lived for 4 weeks *(Ogawa)*.

Clinical studies, some of them double-blind, have been conducted in Japan using coenzyme Q_7 and coenzyme Q_9, both closely related to coenzyme Q_{10}. The substances were found to be beneficial for both acute and chronic stroke symptoms including mental disturbances and lower extremity performance *(Yamamura)*.

Glycosaminoglycans

Mesoglycan is a purified bovine-derived mixture of dermatan sulfate, heparin sulfate, hyaluronic acid, chondroitin sulfate, and related hexosaminoglycans. Although blood coagulation measures do not change, treatment may cause fibrinogen levels to decrease and erythrocyte filterability to improve *(Vecchio)*.

In several studies, its administration has been found to improve cognitive and behavioral parameters in patients with cerebrovascular insufficiency *(Ambrosio)*. Moreover, its effects were found to be superior to those of standard treatment in regard to both the occurrence of further ischemic episodes and the quality of life *(Abate)*. For the treatment of acute focal cerebral ischemia, however, it failed to improve the efficacy of intravenous dexamethasone *(Cazzato)*.

Omega-3 Fatty Acids

Earlier we noted that the results of epidemiological studies suggest that fish consumption may reduce stroke risk. When temporary cerebral ischemia was produced in gerbils by bilateral carotid occlusion, cerebral blood flow in the control animals was decreased after reperfusion and brain water was increased. By contrast, in animals that had been fed a diet supplemented with menhaden fish oil, cerebral blood flow did not fall during reperfusion and edema did not appear *(Black)*.

Fish oils may protect against stroke by improving the distensibility of cerebral arteries. In a double-blind study, both the large arteries and more peripheral vasculature of non-insulin-dependent diabetics who received fish oil supplements showed improved compliance as measured by pulse-contour analysis *(McVeigh)*.

In contrast to this evidence of beneficial effects, an autopsy study which compared perirenal adipose-tissue fatty acids in 26 Greenlanders with no cerebral pathology and 4 cases with fatal hemorrhagic strokes found that high adipose tissue levels of omega-3 fatty acids (which is believed to be representative of the long-term diet) was associated with an *increased* risk of hemorrhagic stroke, independent of age and hypertension *(Pedersen)*. This finding is consistent with that of a study discussed above in which men who consumed the greatest amount of fish had an increased risk of death from stroke *(Orencia)*.

Since the traditional Greenland diet contains high amounts of omega-3 fatty acids, these apparently contradictory findings could be because a moderate amount of omega-3 fatty acid intake is protective, while too high an intake increases the risk of hemorrhagic stroke, possibly because of its anti-thrombogenic effect. Until the ideal level of intake is known, it may be safer to encourage a greater intake of foods such as fish that are rich in omega-3 fatty acids than to provide concentrated supplements at a level that could be excessive.

OTHER RELATED FACTORS

Obesity

Many studies have observed a positive, independent association between obesity and stroke, with the risk of stroke ranging from 1½ to twice that of a person of normal weight *(Bronner)*. Moreover, for stroke of all types, obesity appears to account for 15 to 25% of total stroke risk *(Bronner)*.

BIBLIOGRAPHY

Abate G et al. [Controlled multicenter study on the therapeutic effectiveness of mesoglycan in patients with cerebrovascular disease.] Minerva Med 82(3):101-5, 1991

Abbott RD et al. Effect of dietary calcium and milk consumption on risk of thromboembolic stroke in older middle-aged men: the Honolulu Heart Program. Stroke 27(3):813-18, 1996

Altura BT, Altura BM. Interactions of Mg and K on cerebral vessels — aspects in view of stroke. Review of present status and new findings. Magnesium 3(4-6):195-211, 1984

Ambrosio LA et al. The effect of mesoglycan in patients with cerebrovascular disease: a psychometric evaluation. J Int Med Res 21(3):138-46, 1993

Anonymous. Japanese Cerebrovascular Prevention Study reported in: Secondary prevention tried in patients with cerebrovascular accident. Medical Tribune Meeting Focus Suppl, May 22, 1997:4

Arrigo A et al. Effects of acetyl-L-carnitine on reaction times in patients with cerebrovascular insufficiency. Int J Clin Pharmacol Res 10(1-2):133-7, 1990

Black KL et al. Eicosapentaenoic acid: Effect on brain prostaglandins, cerebral blood flow and edema in ischemic gerbils. Stroke 15(1):65-9, 1984

Boers GH et al. Pyridoxine treatment does not prevent homocystinemia after methionine loading in adult homocystinuria patients. Metabolism 32(4):390-7, 1983

Boers GH et al. Heterozygosity for homocystinuria in premature peripheral and cerebral occlusive arterial disease. N Engl J Med 313(12):709-15, 1985

Boscobionik D et al. Alpha-tocopherol (vitamin E) regulates vascular smooth muscle cell proliferation and protein kinase C activity. Arch Biochem 286:264-9, 1991

Boushey CJ et al. A quantitative assessment of plasma homocysteine as a risk factor for vascular disease: Probable benefits of increasing folic acid intakes. JAMA 274(13):1049-57, 1995

Brattström LE et al. Folic acid responsive postmenopausal homocysteinemia. Metabolism 34(11):1073-7, 1985

Bronner LL et al. Primary prevention of stroke. N Engl J Med 333(21):1392-400, 1995

Browne SE. The case for intravenous magnesium treatment of arterial disease in general practice: review of 34 years of experience. J Nutr Med 4:169-77, 1994

Cao X, Phillis JW. The free radical scavenger, alpha-lipoic acid, protects against cerebral ischemia-reperfusion injury in gerbils. Free Rad Res 23(4):365-70, 1995

Cazzato G et al. [Mesoglycan in acute focal cerebral ischemia.] Riv Neurol 59(3):121-6, 1989

Clarke R et al. Hyperhomocysteinemia: an independent risk factor for vascular disease. N Engl J Med 324(17):1149-55, 1991

Cockcroft J, Chowienczyk P. Beyond cholesterol reduction in coronary heart disease: Is vitamin E the answer? Heart 76:293-4, 1996

Daviglus M et al. Dietary vitamin C, B-carotene and 30-year risk of stroke: Results from the Western Electric Study. Neuroepidemiology 16(2):69-77, 1997

De Keyser J et al. Serum concentrations of vitamins A and E and early outcome after ischemic stroke. Lancet 339:1562-5, 1992

Fehlinger R et al. Hypomagnesemia and transient ischemic cerebral attacks. Magnesium Bull 6:100-4, 1984

Fujimoto S et al. The protective effect of vitamin E on cerebral ischemia. Surg Neurol 22(5):449-54, 1984

Gariballa SE et al. Serum potassium following stroke. Age Aging 24(Suppl 2):20, 1995

Gartside PS, Glueck CJ. The important role of modifiable dietary and behavioral characteristics in the causation and prevention of coronary heart disease hospitalization and mortality: the prospective NHANES I follow-up study. J Am Coll Nutr 14(1):71-9, 1995

Gerster H. n-3 fish oil polyunsaturated fatty acids and bleeding. J Nutr Environ Med 5:281-96, 1995

Gey KF et al. Poor plasma status of carotene and vitamin C is associated with higher mortality from ischemic heart disease and stroke: Basel Prospective Study. Clin Invest 71:3-6, 1993

Gillman MW et al. Protective effect of fruits and vegetables on development of stroke in men. JAMA 273(14):1113-17, 1995

Gillum RF et al. The relationship between fish consumption and stroke incidence: The NHANES I Epidemiologic Follow-Up Study. Arch Intern Med 156:537-42, 1996

Grieb P et al. Oral coenzyme Q10 administration prevents the development of ischemic brain lesions in a rabbit model of symptomatic vasospasm. Acta Neuropathol (Berl) 94(4):363-8, 1997

Hendriks HFJ et al. Effect of moderate dose of alcohol with evening meal on fibrinolytic factors. Br Med J 308:1003-7, 1994

Hennekens CH et al. Lack of effect of long-term supplementation with beta carotene on the incidence of malignant neoplasms and cardiovascular disease. N Engl J Med 334(18):1145-9, 1996

Hirai A et al. Clinical and epidemiological studies of eicosapentaenoic acid in Japan, in WEM Lands, Ed. Polyunsaturated Fatty Acids and Eicosanoids. Champaign, IL, American Oil Chemists' Society, 1987:9-24

Igisu H et al. Protection of the brain by carnitine. Sangyo Eiseigaku Zasshi 37(2):75-82, 1995

Ikeda K et al. Effect of milk protein and fat intake on blood pressure and the incidence of cerebrovascular diseases in stroke-prone spontaneously hypertensive rats (SHRSP). J Nutr Sci Vitaminol (Tokyo) 33(1):31-6, 1987

Keli SO et al. Fish consumption and risk of stroke: the Zutphen Study. Stroke 25:328-32, 1994

Keli SO et al. Dietary flavonoids, antioxidant vitamins, and incidence of stroke: the Zupthen study. Arch Intern Med 147:637-42, 1996

Khaw KT, Barrett-Connor E. Dietary potassium and stroke-associated mortality. A 12-year prospective population study. N Engl J Med 316(5):235-40, 1987

Lapidus L et al. Dietary habits in relation to incidence of cardiovascular disease and death in women: a 12-year follow-up of participants in the population study of women in Gothenburg, Sweden. Am J Clin Nutr 44:444-8, 1986

Lee CN et al. Dietary potassium and stroke. Letter. N Engl J Med 318(15):995-6, 1988

Luft F, Weinberger M. Potassium and blood pressure regulation. Am J Clin Nutr 45:1289-94, 1987

McCully KS, Wilson RB. Homocysteine theory of arteriosclerosis. Atherosclerosis 22(2):215-27, 1975

McGee D et al. The relationship of dietary fat and cholesterol to mortality in 10 years: the Honolulu Heart Program. Int J Epidemiol 14:97-105, 1985

McVeigh GE et al. Fish oil improves arterial compliance in non-insulin-dependent diabetes mellitus. Arterioscler Thromb 14(9):1425-9, 1994

Morris MC et al. Fish consumption and cardiovascular disease in the Physicians' Health Study: a prospective study. Am J Epidemiol 142:166-75, 1995

Nebrand C et al. Cardiovascular mortality and morbidity in seven counties in Sweden in relation to water hardness and geological settings. Eur Heart J 13:721-7, 1992

Ness AR, Powles JW. Fruit and vegetables, and cardiovascular disease: a review. Int J Epidemiol 26(1):1-13, 1997

Ogawa N et al. Survival effect of coenzyme Q10 and naloxone on experimental stroke gerbils. Pharmacol Biochem Behav 24(2):315-17, 1986

Orencia AJ et al. Fish consumption and stroke in men: 30-year findings of the Chicago Western Electric Study. Stroke 27(2):204-9, 1996

Oriot D et al. Ascorbic acid during cerebral ischemia in newborn piglets. Acta Paediatr 84:621-6, 1995

Packer L et al. Neuroprotection by the metabolic antioxidant alpha-lipoic acid. Free Radic Biol Med 22(1-2):359-378, 1997

Panigrahi M et al. α-Lipoic acid protects against reperfusion injury following cerebral ischemia in rats. Brain Res 717:184-8, 1996

Perry IJ, Beevers DG. Salt intake and stroke: a possible direct effect. J Hum Hypertens 6(1):23-5, 1992

Pedersen HS et al. N-3 fatty acids as a risk factor for haemorrhagic stroke. Research letter. Lancet 353:812-3, 1999

Postglione A et al. Effect of acute administration of L-acetyl carnitine on cerebral blood flow in patients with chronic cerebral infarct. Pharmacol Res 23(3):241-6, 1991

Rath M, Pauling L. Solution to the puzzle of human cardiovascular disease: its primary cause is ascorbate deficiency leading to the deposition of lipoprotein (a) and fibrinogen/fibrin in the vascular wall. J Orthomol Med 6(3-4):125-34, 1991

Sacco RL et al. The protective effect of moderate alcohol consumption on ischemic stroke. JAMA 281(1):53-60, 1999

Sadeh M. Action of magnesium sulfate in the treatment of preeclampsia-eclampsia. Stroke 20(9):1273-5, 1989

Sasaki S et al. Dietary sodium, potassium, saturated fat, alcohol, and stroke mortality. Stroke 26(5):783-9, 1995

Seely S. Diet and cerebrovascular disease: search for linkages. Med Hypotheses 9(5):509-15, 1982

Seely S. The changing face of cerebrovascular disease. Ecol Dis 2(2):125-8, 1983

Selhub J et al. Association between plasma homocysteine concentrations and extracranial carotid-artery stenosis. N Engl J Med 332(5):286-91, 1995

Singh RB et al. Dietary intake and plasma levels of antioxidant vitamins in health and disease: a hospital-based case-control study. J Nutr Environ Med 5:235-42, 1995

Smythies JR. The role of ascorbate in brain: therapeutic considerations. Editorial. J R Soc Med 89(5):241, 1996

Stampfer MJ, Malinow MR. Can lowering homocysteine reduce cardiovascular risk? Editorial. N Engl J Med 332(5):328-9, 1995

Steiner M, Div. of Hematology/Oncology, Memorial Hospital, Pawtucket, RI. Vitamin E enhances the benefits of aspirin in preventing or reducing the incidence of strokes. Abstract. Second Int. Conf. on Antioxidant Vitamins and Beta-carotene in Disease Prevention. Berlin, Germany, October 10-12, 1994

Swain R. An update of vitamin B12 metabolism and deficiency states. J Fam Pract 41(6):595-600, 1995

Tobian L, Hanlon S. High sodium chloride injure arteries and raise mortality without raising blood pressure. Hypertension 15:900-3, 1990

Tremoli E et al. Prolonged inhibition of platelet aggregation after n-3 fatty acid ethyl ester ingestion by healthy volunteers. Am J Clin Nutr 61:607-13, 1995

Ubbink J et al. Vitamin requirements for the treatment of hyperhomocysteinemia in humans. J Nutr 124:1927-33, 1994

Ubbink JB et al. The effect of a subnormal vitamin B-6 status on homocysteine metabolism. J Clin Invest 98(1):177-84, 1996

Vecchio F et al. Mesoglycan in treatment of patients with cerebral ischemia: effects on hemorrheologic and hematochemical parameters. Acta Neurol (Napoli) 15(6):449-56, 1993

Verhoef P et al. Homocysteine metabolism and risk of myocardial infarction: relation with vitamin B6, B12, and folate. Am J Epidemiol 143(9):845-59, 1996

Wilkins MR, Kendall MJ. Stroke affecting young men after alcoholic binges. Br Med J [Clin Res] 291:1342, 1985

Yamamura Y. A survey of the therapeutic use of coenzyme Q, in G Lenaz, Ed. Coenzyme Q. John Wiley & Son, Ltd., 1985:479-505

Yang CY. Calcium and magnesium in drinking water and risk of death from cerebrovascular disease. Stroke 29(2):411-14, 1998

CERVICAL DYSPLASIA

See Also: CANCER

NUTRITIONAL TREATMENT GUIDE

✓ = Efficacy generally accepted.
* = Efficacy *demonstrated* by controlled human trials.
[+] = Efficacy *suspected* from uncontrolled human trials.
[-] = Efficacy *suspected* from indirect data.
? = Efficacy *challenged* in a study of similar design.

NUTRITIONAL FACTORS

* **Selenium:** ? 200 µg daily
* ***Trans*-retinoic acid:** Apply using a cervical cap with a sponge containing 1.0 mL of 0.372% beta-*trans*-retinoic acid for 4 days initially, then for 2 days at months 3 and 6.
* ? **Folic Acid deficiency:** 5 mg twice daily (6 month trial)

- -

[+] **Beta-carotene deficiency:** 30 mg daily (6 month trial)

- -

[-] **Selenium deficiency:** ? 200 µg daily
[-] **Vitamin A deficiency:** 50,000 IU daily for 6 weeks (10,000 IU daily during pregnancy)
[-] **Vitamin C deficiency:** 500 mg twice daily
[-] **Vitamin E deficiency:** D,L-alpha-tocopheryl acetate 200 to 2,000 mg or IU daily for 6 weeks; then maintenance levels as needed

HOMOCYSTEINE

A recent survey found that total plasma levels of the toxic amino acid homocysteine were significantly higher in patients with cervical dysplasia than in healthy controls *(Thomson)*. Whether this elevation is simply a marker for deficiencies of nutrients required for homocysteine metabolism (most likely folate deficiency), or due to other mechanisms, is not yet known.

NUTRITIONAL FACTORS

VITAMINS

Folic Acid Deficiency

Low folate intake *(Liu,1993)* and folate deficiency *(Harper)* may be correlated with cervical dysplastic changes. Even when serum folate levels are normal, erythrocyte folate may provide the evidence of deficiency

(Lindenbaum). Both pregnancy and the use of oral contraceptives are associated with a macromolecule in the serum and leukocytes that binds folate; thus women in these categories are especially susceptible to folate deficiency *(Steiff)*.

When cervical biopsies were taken following the discovery of characteristic changes in cervicovaginal smears believed to be due to systemic B_{12} or folate deficiency, the biopsies showed that folic acid deficiency-like tissue changes were frequently associated with carcinoma-in-situ, and were usually in close proximity to papillomavirus cytopathic changes *(Fekete)*. The meaning of these findings is unclear. One possibility is that papillomavirus infection may be encouraged by localized folate deficiency and may promote the dysplastic tissue changes.

Supplementation

The efficacy of oral supplementation with folic acid has been investigated in several studies. While an earlier double-blind study found supplementation to be effective for women on combination-type birth control pills with mild or moderate dysplasia *(Butterworth,1982)*, more recent double-blind studies have had negative results *(Butterworth,1992;Childers;Zarcone)*. Reasons for the differing results are unclear, although the lack of efficacy reported in the later studies could be because the subjects were not folate-deficient.

Vitamin A Deficiency

Women with severe dysplasia or carcinoma-in-situ are likely to have a lower intake of vitamin A than matched normals, and a reduced intake nearly triples the risk of developing either condition *(Wylie-Rosett)*. Not only may plasma retinol levels be reduced *(Romney,1995)*, but they may be inversely related to the odds of regression of the lesion *(Liu,1995)*. Moreover, women with abnormal uterocervical cytology may have reduced retinol binding protein in both their blood and their cervical tissue *(Romney,1995;Wylie-Rosett)*.

While the efficacy of supplementation with vitamin A (retinol) in humans is unexplored, the vitamin was able to inhibit the induction of cervical tumors in hamsters by carcinogenic polycyclic hydrocarbons *(Chu)*. Moreover, cervical application of a retinyl acetate gel for one week was shown to increase plasma retinol and retinol binding protein *(Palan,1988)*, suggesting that it may be a method of normalizing vitamin A nutriture.

Using a cervical cap for topical application, *trans*-retinoic acid, a synthetic vitamin A derivative, appears to be somewhat effective in reversing the lesion. In a randomized study, topical retinoic acid increased the complete histologic remission rate of moderate dysplasia (CIN II) from 27% in the placebo group up to 43%, although it was ineffective in severe dysplasia *(Meyskens,1994a)*.

Vitamin C Deficiency

As with vitamin A, the intake of vitamin C appears to be inversely related to the risk of cervical dysplasia. In one study, for example, 29% of cases versus 3% of controls had a vitamin C intake of less than 50% of the US RDA *(Wassertheil-Smoller)*. Furthermore, plasma vitamin C levels are lower in patients than in matched controls *(Romney,1985)*.

Despite these correlations, the efficacy of supplementation with vitamin C to reverse cervical dysplasia has not been explored.

Vitamin E Deficiency

Both the intake and plasma levels of vitamin E may be reduced in women with cervical dysplasia *(Buckley;Palan,1996)*. However, as in regard to vitamins A and C, supplementation or topical application of vitamin E for the treatment of cervical dysplasia has not been investigated.

MINERALS

Selenium Deficiency

Selenium deficiency is known to increase the risk of epithelial cancers *(Prasad)*, and patients with cervical dysplasia have significantly lower plasma selenium levels than do normal controls *(Dawson)*. However, the efficacy of selenium supplementation is unknown.

OTHER NUTRITIONAL FACTORS

Carotenoid Deficiency

Women with severe dysplasia or carcinoma-in-situ are likely to have a lower intake of beta-carotene than matched normals, and a reduced intake triples the risk of severe dysplasia *(Romney,1995;Wylie-Rosett)*.

Compared to healthy controls, women with cervical dysplasia have reduced plasma levels of beta-carotene, lycopene and canthanxanthin *(Palan,1996)*. Moreover, they have lower levels of beta-carotene in exfoliated epithelial cells of cervical and vaginal tissues *(Palan,1992)*.

In a phase II trial of 30 women with stages I or II of cervical intraepithelial neoplasia, supplementation with beta-carotene was associated with the development of negative Pap smears with either negative colposcopy or a negative biopsy for 70% of the patients. Even after the supplement has been discontinued for 6 months, 30% of the patients continued to have negative findings *(Meyskens,1994b)*. However, a placebo-controlled study found that supplementation failed to reduce the risk of cervical carcinoma 9 months later *(Romney,1997)*.

While high consumption of carrots and green vegetables (which are high in beta-carotene) is associated with a low risk of cervical cancer, high consumption of milk, liver and meats (which are high in vitamin A) does not affect cervical cancer risk *(La Vecchia)*. This suggests that beta-carotene supplementation may be more effective than supplementation with vitamin A.

COMBINED NUTRITIONAL SUPPLEMENTATION

The Pap smear of a 26 year-old woman revealed moderate cervical dysplasia. A smear done 6 months earlier had shown only mild dysplasia, while a smear done 3 months earlier had also shown a moderate degree of dysplasia. Colposcopic examination was normal. She had been using birth control pills for 6 years but stopped after the second Pap smear. Since then she noted much heavier menstrual flow, with the last menses lasting 8 days.

She was given dietary counseling and supplemented with folic acid 5 mg 3 times daily, vitamin A 60,000 IU daily for 2 months followed by 25,000 IU daily, vitamin B complex "50" twice daily, vitamin C 1 gram daily and vitamin E 400 IU daily.

Two months later the Pap smear was entirely normal. At the 4-year follow-up visit, the Pap smear was still entirely normal (Wright).

BIBLIOGRAPHY

Buckley DI et al. Dietary micronutrients and cervical dysplasia in southwestern American Indian women. Nutr Cancer 17(2):179-85, 1992

Butterworth CE et al. Improvement in cervical dysplasia associated with folic acid therapy in users of oral contraceptives. Am J Clin Nutr 35:73-82, 1982

Butterworth CE Jr et al. Oral folic acid supplementation for cervical dysplasia: a clinical intervention trial. Am J Obstet Gynecol 166(30):803-9, 1992

Childers JM et al. Chemoprevention of cervical cancer with folic acid: a phase III Southwest Oncology Group Intergroup study. Cancer Epidemiol Biomarkers Prev 4(2):155-9, 1995

Chu EW, Malmgren RA. An inhibitory effect of vitamin A on the induction of tumors of forestomach and cervix in the Syrian hamster by carcinogenic polycyclic hydrocarbons. Cancer Res 25(6):884-95, 1965

Dawson E et al. Serum vitamin and selenium changes in cervical dysplasia. Fed Proc 43:612, 1984

Fekete PS, Hammami A. Folic acid deficiency-like changes in cervicovaginal smears: A possible manifestation of papillomavirus infection? Abstract. Acta Cytologica 31(5):679, 1987

Harper JM et al. Erythrocyte folate levels, oral contraceptive use, and abnormal cervical cytology. Acta Cytol 38(3):324-30, 1994

La Vecchia C et al. Dietary vitamin A and the risk of invasive cervical cancer. Int J Cancer 34:319-22, 1984

Lindenbaum J et al. Oral contraceptive hormones, folate metabolism, and the cervical epithelium. Am J Clin Nutr, April, 1975:346-53

Liu T et al. A case control study of nutritional factors and cervical dysplasia. Cancer Epidemiol Biomarkers Prev 2(6):525-30, 1993

Liu T et al. A longitudinal analysis of human papillomavirus 16 infection, nutritional status, and cervical dysplasia progression. Cancer Epidemiol Biomarkers Prev 4(4):373-80, 1995

Meyskens FL Jr et al. Enhancement of regression of cervical intraepithelial neoplasia II (moderate dysplasia) with topically applied all-trans-retinoic acid: a randomized trial. J Natl Cancer Inst 86(7):539-43, 1994a

Meyskens FL Jr, Clinical Cancer Center, U. of California, Irvine, CA. Prevention of cervical dysplasia. Abstract. Second Int. Conf. on Antioxidant Vitamins and Beta-carotene in Disease Prevention. Berlin, Germany, October 10-12, 1994b

Palan PR et al. Vaginal hydrolysis of retinyl acetate: increase in plasma retinol and retinol binding protein in women with cervical dysplasias. Biochem Med Metab Biol 40(3):282-90, 1988

Palan PR et al. Beta carotene levels in exfoliated cervicovaginal epithelial cells in cervical intraepithelial neoplasia and cervical cancer. Am J Obstet Gynecol 167:1899-903, 1992

Palan PR et al. Plasma-levels of beta-carotene, lycopene canthanxanthin, retinol, and alpha-tocopherol and tau-tocopherol in cervical intraepithelial neoplasia and cancer. Clin Cancer 2(1):181-5, 1996

Prasad K, Ed. Vitamins, Nutrition and Cancer. New York, Karger, 1984

Romney SL et al. Plasma vitamin C and uterine cervical dysplasia. Am J Obstet Gynecol 151(7):976-80, 1985

Romney SL et al. Nutrient antioxidants in the pathogenesis and prevention of cervical dysplasia and cancer. J Cell Biochem 23:96-103, 1995

Romney SL et al. Effects of beta-carotene and other factors on outcome of cervical dysplasia and human papillomavirus infection. Gynecol Oncol 65:483-92, 1997

Steiff R. Folate deficiency and oral contraceptives. JAMA 214:105-8, 1970

Thomson SW et al. Effect of total plasma homocysteine on cervical dysplasia risk. Abstract. Am J Clin Nutr 66:206, 1997

Wassertheil-Smoller S et al. Dietary vitamin C and uterine cervical dysplasia. Am J Epidemiol 114(5):714-24, 1981

Wright JV. Dr. Wright's Guide to Healing with Nutrition. Emmaus, Penn., Rodale Press, 1984

Wylie-Rosett JA et al. Influence of vitamin A on cervical dysplasia and carcinoma in situ. Nutr Cancer 6(1):49-57, 1984

Zarcone R et al. [Folic acid and cervix dysplasia.] Minerva Ginecol 48:397-400, 1996

CHRONIC FATIGUE SYNDROME

See Also: FATIGUE
FIBROMYALGIA

NUTRITIONAL TREATMENT GUIDE

✓ = Efficacy generally accepted.
* = Efficacy *demonstrated* by controlled human trials.
[+] = Efficacy *suspected* from uncontrolled human trials.
[-] = Efficacy *suspected* from indirect data.
? = Efficacy *challenged* in a study of similar design.

DIETARY FACTORS

[+] adequate **Salt** intake

NUTRITIONAL FACTORS

* **Essential Fatty Acids:** *example*: evening primrose oil containing 35 mg gamma linolenic acid *and* fish oil containing 17 mg eicosapentaenoic acid daily (15 week trial)
* **Magnesium deficiency:** 50% magnesium sulfate (1 g in 2 ml) [98.7 mg elemental magnesium] IM every week. Oral supplementation may also be effective for repletion, although its efficacy is unverified.
* ? **L-Carnitine:** 1 g daily in divided doses (2 month trial)

- -

[+] **Beta-carotene:** ? 60 mg daily (limit to 3 weeks to minimize skin pigmentation)
[+] **Coenzyme Q_{10} deficiency:** 100 mg daily (3 month trial)
[+] **Malic acid:** ? 1,200 to 2,400 mg daily *AND* oral magnesium hydroxide 300 to 600 mg daily. Taper dosage gradually. (6 month trial)
[+] **Vitamin B_{12}:** 2,500 to 5,000 µg daily subcutaneously or IM every 2 to 3 days as needed
[+] **Vitamin C:** ? regular intravenous infusions containing 15 g

- -

[-] **Folic acid deficiency:** 800 µg daily
[-] **Thiamine deficiency:** 50 mg daily
[-] **Zinc deficiency:** zinc sulfate 220 mg daily *AND* **Copper** 2 mg daily

OTHER RELATED FACTORS

[+] rule out **Food Sensitivities**

DIETARY FACTORS

Adequate Salt Diet

Sixty-one percent of a group of 23 patients fulfilling standard criteria for chronic fatigue syndrome (CFS) were found, by means of upright tilt-table testing, to have neurally mediated hypotension *(Bou-Holaigah)*. When interviewed, they reported that they usually or always tried to avoid salt and salty foods. Therefore, increasing sodium intake should ameliorate symptoms in this sub-group of patients *(Bou-Holaigah)*.

NUTRITIONAL FACTORS

VITAMINS

Vitamin B Complex Deficiencies

Certain B vitamins have been found to be deficient in CFS patients. These include folic acid *(Jacobson)*, thiamine *(Grant)*, and vitamin B_{12} *(Regland)*.

While research on the effects of folic acid and thiamine supplementation has not been published, the beneficial effects of massive-dosage vitamin B_{12} injections (much higher dosages than those needed to replete a B_{12} deficiency) have been noted in an informal report. Patients typically felt increased energy, stamina or well-being within 12 hours, an effect that wore off within 2-3 days. Roughly 50 to 80% of patients improved. Some noted immediate improvement in their overall condition; however the majority required weeks of therapy before they achieved a notable response *(Lapp)*.

While controlled clinical trials are needed to substantiate these preliminary results, they are consistent with reports of analgesia produced by massive vitamin B_{12} supplementation in patients with pain, including that of cancer *(Dettori)*, and with an animal model of inflammation which also found a considerable dose-dependent analgesic effect *(Hanck)*.

The subjective clinical benefit from massive vitamin B_{12} administration is also consistent with the objective observation that symptoms in CFS patients may sometimes be reflected by changes in blood rheology which could impair microcirculatory blood flow *(Simpson, 1993)*. Moreover, among the 5% of patients with increased nondiscocytic erythrocytes, one investigator found that the increased feelings of well-being in CFS patients following a vitamin B_{12} injection was reflected by a reduced percentage of nondiscocytic (abnormally shaped) erythrocytes. At the same time, patients who failed to perceive a beneficial response showed no change in red cell shape *(Simpson, 1991)*.

Vitamin C

There is no evidence that vitamin C is deficient in CFS. However, as in the case of vitamin B_{12}, erythrocyte deformities that could impair microcirculatory blood flow may respond to vitamin C supplementation *(Ali, 1990, 1993)*.

Since similar changes toward normalization of red cell rheology were accompanied by subjective improvement when the changes were induced by vitamin B_{12} supplementation, it is likely that vitamin C supplementation would also provide subjective benefit to patients with impaired microcirculation due to erythrocyte deformities. This hypothesis, however, is untested.

MINERALS

Magnesium Deficiency

Many of the symptoms of CFS are similar to those of magnesium deficiency *(Cox)* and, while not all studies are in agreement, there is evidence that magnesium nutriture is often deficient in CFS patients as assessed by erythrocyte or white blood cell levels *(Grant; Howard)*. Furthermore, CFS patients are commonly stressed, and the release of stress hormones (both catecholamines and corticoids) can promote reduction in tissue magnesium levels *(Seelig)*.

Several studies, some of which were double-blind, have found that magnesium supplementation, when administered by intravenous or intramuscular injection, significantly reduces CFS symptomatology in magnesium-deficient patients *(Cox; Durlach)*. Moreover, an informal report suggests that oral magnesium may be effective in at least half of patients who have evidence of deficiency on the basis of leukocyte or erythrocyte levels, or on the basis of a magnesium loading test *(Howard)*.

AND Malate

Since malate plays an important role in generating in generating mitochondrial ATP both under aerobic and hypoxic conditions, it has sometimes been added to magnesium supplementation in treating CFS patients. In a double-blind crossover study, the combination failed to improve upon placebo when given at a dosage of 600 mg twice daily of magnesium and 150 mg twice daily of malic acid for 4 weeks. This negative finding suggests that, if the combination is effective, a longer treatment period and/or a higher dosage would be needed *(Russell)*.

In open trials, about 40% of patients seem to respond to the combination. While fibromyalgia pain may respond in about 2 days, fatigue takes about 2 weeks to lessen *(Anonymous)*. Moreover, with escalation of the dosage up to 1,200 mg of magnesium and 300 mg of malic acid twice daily for up to 6 months, there were significant reductions in measure of pain and tenderness and improvement in functional and psychological measures *(Russell)*.

An 11 year-old boy with a 2 year history of myalgic encephalomyelitis had been absent from school for 9 months. Due to muscular weakness, he was confined to a wheelchair when outside of his home. On evaluation, his red cell magnesium level was 1.42 mmol/l (normal range: 1.7-2.6 mmol/l).

He was given 6 injections of magnesium sulfate at weekly intervals. By the end of that time, he was not using the wheelchair. Two weeks later, following physiotherapy, he was able to run and play football (Dowson).

Zinc Deficiency

Erythrocyte and blood zinc have been found to be low in some CFS patients *(Grant;Jessupt)*. However, whether repletion of a zinc deficiency is beneficial is unknown.

OTHER NUTRITIONAL FACTORS

Beta-carotene

Natural killer cells play a pivotal role in immune surveillance against virus-infected cells *(Toth)*. CFS patients often demonstrate a decrease in natural killer cell numbers or activity. In fact, this finding is the most consistent laboratory abnormality found in CFS *(Caligiuri)*.

In a informal study of CFS patients who also had low (less than 6%) natural killer cell counts and low serum levels of vitamin A, high-dosage beta-carotene supplementation increased the natural killer cell count in the majority of patients. Patients whose counts increased reported decreased fatigue. Cognitive function also seemed to improve, although not consistently. In patients with normal counts of natural killer cells, beta-carotene seemed less effective *(Cunha)*.

Controlled studies are needed to confirm these interesting preliminary findings.

Carnitine Deficiency

Carnitine plays an important role in energy production and in the modulation of the intramitochondrial coenzyme A to acyl-CoA ratio in skeletal muscle; thus a deficiency might induce an energy deficit and/or abnormality within the mitochondria resulting in general fatigue, myalgia, muscle weakness, and postexertional fatigue *(Kuratsune)*. Patients with CFS have demonstrated significant reductions in serum carnitine and/or acylcarnitine levels *(Plioplys,1995;Kuratsune)*.

In a controlled crossover study, supplementation with L-carnitine for at least 2 months was found to dramatically help some CFS patients, although at least two-thirds failed to respond, and others showed only a partial improvement *(Plioplys,1997)*.

Coenzyme Q_{10} Deficiency

Levels of CoQ_{10} may be reduced, and preliminary findings suggest that supplementation may be of some benefit. In a recent study, 20 female patients who had been ill for 2 to 5 years and required bed rest following mild exercise were compared to 20 healthy, matched controls. Compared to the controls, the patients had reduced blood and tissue levels of CoQ_{10} at baseline.

The patients received 100 mg daily of the supplement as a soft gel capsule in a liquid base. After 90 days, 90% of the patients had reductions in their complaints of mild fever, sore throat, and painful lymph nodes, suggesting immune enhancement.

Moreover, every patient had improved exercise tolerance, although they did not achieve pre-illness levels, and 85% of patients had decreased post-exercise fatigue. While, prior to supplementation, they were able to exercise for 208 seconds before complaints of fatigue and muscle cramps caused them to stop, after 90 days they were able to exercise for 460 seconds *(Judy)*. (At least some of this improvement was due to conditioning.)

Essential Fatty Acids

Both abnormal metabolism and deficiencies of essential fatty acids have been reported in CFS patients *(Gray;Horrobin;Howard)*. It has been hypothesized that these abnormalities may explain immune, endocrine and sympathetic nervous system abnormalities *(Gray)* as well as the relationship between the syndrome and viral infections *(Horrobin)*.

In one study, 63 patients with a good employment and mental health history who had suffered from post-viral fatigue for at least one year were found to have low levels of essential fatty acids. They randomly received 4 capsules twice daily of Efamol Marine (a mixture of 80% of evening primrose oil and 20% of concentrated fish oil containing about 35 mg GLA and 17 mg EPA per capsule) or an olive oil placebo. After 5 weeks, 74% of treated patients and 23% of those on placebo rated themselves as better than at baseline.

After 15 weeks, 85% of treated patients rated themselves as better than at baseline compared to only 17% of those on placebo, a highly significant difference. Without exception, all the individual symptoms, including fatigue, aches and pains and depression, showed a highly significantly greater improvement on the fatty acid supplement than on placebo. While placebo patients who improved at 5 weeks reverted to baseline by 15 weeks, treated patients showed progressive improvements. Although none of the patients was cured, many were able to return to work *(Behan)*.

OTHER RELATED FACTORS

Food Sensitivities

CFS patients sometimes report food sensitivities. In one survey, 13% of 200 consecutive patients reported intolerance to foods *(Manu)*. Because such patients are more likely to have more lifetime functional somatic complaints and a higher prevalence of somatization disorder, it has been suggested that these complaints could be simply a manifestation of somatization *(Manu)*.

However, in another 20 patients, an elimination diet remarkably improved the fatigue. Moreover, provocative testing found that specific foods appeared to be associated with specific symptoms. Fatigue was associated with sensitivity to sugar and refined grains including wheat, maize and rice, while myalgias and flu-like symptoms were associated with wheat, milk, beef, pumpkins, tomatoes, and pineapple *(Borok)*. Obviously, careful studies are needed to clarify the contribution of food sensitivities to the clinical picture.

BIBLIOGRAPHY

Ali M. Ascorbic acid reverses abnormal erythrocyte morphology in chronic fatigue syndrome. Abstract. Am J Clin Pathol 94:515, 1990

Ali M. Hypothesis: chronic fatigue is a state of accelerated oxidative molecular injury. J Advancement Med 6(2):83-96, 1993

Anonymous. A follow-up on malic acid: CFIDS Buyers Club. Health Watch, Spring, 1993

Behan PO et al. Effect of high doses of essential fatty acids on the postviral fatigue syndrome. Acta Neurol Scand 82(3):209-16, 1990

Borok G. Another answer to yuppie flu? S Afr Med J 76:176, 1989

Bou-Holaigah I et al. The relationship between neurally mediated hypotension and the chronic fatigue syndrome. JAMA 274(12):961-7, 1995

Caligiuri M et al. Phenotypic and functional deficiency of natural killer cells in patients with chronic fatigue syndrome. J Immunol 139:3306-13, 1987

Cox IM et al. Red blood cell magnesium and chronic fatigue syndrome. Lancet 337:757-60, 1991

Cunha BA. Beta-carotene stimulation of natural killer cell activity in adult patients with chronic fatigue syndrome. The CFIDS Chronicle Physicians' Forum, Fall, 1993, pp. 18-19

Dettori AG, Ponari O. Effetto antalgico della cobamamide in corso di neuropatie periferiche di diversa etiopatogenesi. Minerva Med 64:1077-82, 1973) (in Italian)

Dowson D. Lancet magnesium study. Interaction: The Journal of M.E. Action, No. 7, Spring, 1991

Durlach J. Chronic fatigue syndrome and chronic primary magnesium deficiency (CFS and CPMD). Magnes Res 5(1):68, 1992

Grant JE et al. Analysis of dietary intake and selected nutrient concentrations in patients with chronic fatigue syndrome. J Am Diet Assoc 96(4):383-6, 1996

Gray JB, Martinovic AM. Eicosanoids and essential fatty acid modulation in chronic disease and the chronic fatigue syndrome. Med Hypotheses 43(1):31-42, 1994

Hanck A, Weiser H. Analgesic and anti-inflammatory properties of vitamins. Int J Vitam Nutr Res (suppl)27:189-206, 1985

Horrobin DF. Post-viral fatigue syndrome, viral infections in atopic eczema, and essential fatty acids. Med Hypotheses 32(3):211-17, 1990

Howard JMcL et al. Magnesium and chronic fatigue syndrome. Letter. Lancet 340:426, 1992

Jacobson W et al. Serum folate and chronic fatigue syndrome. Neurology 43(12):2645-7, 1993

Jessop C - reported in the Fibromyalgia Network Newsletter compendium #2, October 1990-January 1992

Judy, William. Southeastern Institute of Biomedical Research, Bradenton, Florida. Presentation to the 37th Annual Mtg., American College of Nutrition, October 13, 1996

Kuratsune H et al. Acylcarnitine deficiency in chronic fatigue syndrome. Clin Infect Dis 18(suppl 1):S62-7, 1994

Lapp CW, Cheney PR. The rationale for using high-dose cobalamin (Vitamin B12). The CFIDS Chronicle Physicians' Forum Fall, 1993, pp. 19-20

Manu P et al. Food intolerance in patients with chronic fatigue. Int J Eat Disord 13(2):203-9, 1993

Plioplys AV, Plioplys S. Serum levels of carnitine in chronic fatigue syndrome: clinical correlates. Neuropsychobiology 32(3):132-8, 1995

Plioplys AV, Plioplys S. Amantadine and L-carnitine treatment of Chronic Fatigue Syndrome. Neuropsychobiology 35(1):16-23, 1997

Regland B et al. Increased concentrations of homocysteine in the cerebrospinal fluid in patients with fibromyalgia and chronic fatigue syndrome. Scand J Rheumatol 26(4):301-7, 1997

Russell IJ et al. Treatment of fibromyalgia syndrome with Super Malic: a randomized, double blind, placebo controlled, crossover pilot study. J Rheumatol 22(5):953-8, 1995

Seelig M. Presentation to the 37th Annual Meeting, American College of Nutrition, October 13, 1996

Simpson LO et al. Red cell shape changes following trigger finger fatigue in subjects with chronic fatigue tiredness and healthy controls. N Z Med J 106:104-7, 1993

Simpson LO. Myalgic encephalomyelitis. Letter. J Royal Soc Med 84(10):633, 1991

Toth J. [NK cells and their characteristics and immunogenetic aspects.] Bratisl Lek Listy 95(5):212-23, 1994

CONGESTIVE HEART FAILURE

See Also: ATHEROSCLEROSIS
CARDIOMYOPATHY
HYPERTENSION

NUTRITIONAL TREATMENT GUIDE

✓ = Efficacy generally accepted.
* = Efficacy *demonstrated* by controlled human trials.
[+] = Efficacy *suspected* from uncontrolled human trials.
[-] = Efficacy *suspected* from indirect data.
? = Efficacy *challenged* in a study of similar design.

DIETARY FACTORS

✓ restrict **Salt** intake.
✓ avoid heavy **Alcohol** intake.

NUTRITIONAL FACTORS

✓ **Potassium** deficiency: ? 80 to 100 mEq daily total intake, preferably from potassium-rich foods

- -

* **L-Arginine:** 5,600 to 12,600 mg per day (6 week trial)
* **L-Carnitine deficiency:** L-carnitine *OR* L-propionylcarnitine 500 mg 3 times daily (6 mo. trial)
* **Coenzyme Q_{10} deficiency:** 100 mg daily in divided doses (3 month trial)
* **Creatine deficiency:** 20 g daily (10 day trial)
* **Taurine:** 2 g 2 to 3 times daily
* **Vitamin C:** *to combat the development of nitrate intolerance:* Oral dosage unknown
* ? **Thiamine deficiency:** 50 mg daily

- -

[+] **Magnesium deficiency:** *initial trial:* 5 ml of an IV solution containing 17% magnesium chloride (100 mg; 4.8 mmol)
[+] **Magnesium & Potassium Aspartates:** 1 g of each twice daily
[+] **Vitamin D deficiency (in infants):** calcitriol 0.25 mg daily for 3 weeks; then calciferol 40 mg daily for 5 weeks
[+] **Vitamin E:** 400 IU daily

OTHER RELATED FACTORS

[+] rule out **Lead** toxicity

DIETARY FACTORS

Low Salt Diet

In patients with congestive heart failure (CHF), myocardial sodium tends to be elevated, while serum sodium may be reduced. Sodium retention is due to activation of the renin-angiotensin-aldosterone system, while the secondary hyperaldosteronism may give rise to elevated intracellular sodium through a direct permeability effect on the cell membrane *(Wester)*.

Activation of the renin-angiotensin-aldosterone system may also cause magnesium loss (see below). Since magnesium is necessary for the function of the sodium-potassium pump, this leads to further retention of intracellular sodium *(Wester)*.

For these reasons, it has been suggested that the sodium intake of patients with CHF should be restricted to 3 grams per day *(Dracup)*.

Alcohol

Ingestion of large amounts of alcohol should be avoided. Acute alcohol ingestion depresses myocardial contractility in patients with known cardiac disease *(Conway)*, while chronic ingestion for at least 80 grams almost everyday for at least 10 years is associated with the development of cardiac decompensation *(Burch)*.

NUTRITIONAL FACTORS

VITAMINS

Thiamine Deficiency

Congestive heart failure may be part of the presentation of beriberi, the classic disease of thiamine deficiency, in which case repletion of the deficiency is the specific treatment.

In addition, furosemide, a commonly used diuretic, may occasionally impair cardiac function *(Seligman)*. If so, thiamine supplementation has been shown to be beneficial under double-blind conditions *(Shimon)*. The frequency with which furosemide and other loop diuretics cause thiamine deficiency leading to cardiac decompensation is uncertain, with some studies finding no evidence of reduced thiamine nutriture *(Yue)*.

A 37-year-old male presented with peripheral edema of sudden onset. Other signs of heart failure were absent. Subsequent evaluation revealed that he was a schizophrenic whose diet consisted almost entirely of carbohydrates. A clinical diagnosis of beriberi heart disease was made and he improved dramatically within several days of thiamine supplementation (Danielson).

Vitamin C

The efficacy of nitroglycerin as a vasodilator for CHF patients is well established. While intolerance to nitrates may develop with regular use, a double blind study has shown that ascorbic acid may help to prevent the development of nitrate intolerance *(Watanabe)*.

Vitamin D Deficiency

In infants, vitamin D deficiency may cause CHF *(Brunvand)*. Whether the same is true in regard to adults has not been established. There is evidence, however, that low levels of activated (1,25-dihydroxy) vitamin D along with hyperparathyroidism and osteopenia are common findings among CHF patients, and that patients with more severe CHF have lower levels of vitamin D metabolites as well as higher bone turnover *(Shane)*.

Vitamin E

Animal studies have demonstrated that vitamin E supplementation may reduce the oxidative stress that is often found to be associated with poor ejection fractions and cardiac failure *(Li)*, and may even prevent or retard the development of cardiac failure *(Dhalla)*.

In a double-blind study, 20 patients and 10 matched healthy controls received 400 mg vitamin E or placebo for 4 weeks. Vitamin E supplementation significantly reduced levels of malonyldialdehyde and superoxide anion (suggesting reduced antioxidant stress), and elevated antioxidant enzymes *(Ghatak)*. These findings suggest that vitamin E supplementation may have a therapeutic role in CHF.

MINERALS

Magnesium Deficiency

During the last several years, numerous studies have demonstrated the importance of magnesium for proper cardiac function. In CHF, intracellular magnesium loss, along with elevation of intracellular sodium and reduction of intracellular potassium, is believed to be due to activation of the renin-angiotensin-aldosterone system. Magnesium deficiency may, in turn, may add to the sodium and potassium abnormalities since magnesium is necessary for the function of the sodium-potassium pump *(Wester)*.

Patients often present with low serum magnesium levels *(Altura;Gottlieb,1990)*, a finding associated with a worse one-year survival than patients with normal levels *(Gottlieb,1990)*. Myocardial magnesium (which, when available, is a much better indicator of cardiac nutriture) may also be low *(Gottlieb,1989;Wester)*. Furthermore, cardiac glycosides and diuretics (loop and distal types) often exacerbate or result in hypomagnesemia, a development which may lead to cardiac arrhythmias and sudden cardiac death *(Altura)*.

Intravenous magnesium supplementation has been shown to improve cardiac function, reversing diastolic dysfunction by lowering elevated left ventricular end-diastolic pressure *(Benzer)*. In addition to correcting the magnesium deficit, magnesium supplementation makes possible the correction of a myocardial potassium deficit *(Wester)*.

> *A woman with congestive heart failure and gross hepatic enlargement showed dramatic improvement in exercise tolerance and complete resolution of liver enlargement following a course of rapid bolus IV magnesium sulfate administration [an injection of 1 mmol delivered fairly slowly to accustom the patient to the feeling of warmth, followed in 10 seconds by 4 mmol; then 5 injections of 8 mmol given either daily or weekly] (Browne).*

Potassium Deficiency

CHF is often associated with hypokalemia as well as potassium tissue deficits *(Altura)*. Magnesium and potassium deficiencies are often interrelated. In addition to intracellular magnesium loss, activation of the renin-angiotensin-aldosterone system causes potassium losses, while the secondary hyperaldosteronism may give rise to low intracellular potassium through a direct permeability effect on the cell membrane. In addition, magnesium loss leads to further loss of intracellular potassium *(Wester)*.

Cardiac glycosides and diuretics (loop and distal types) often exacerbate, or result in, hypokalemia, which may lead to cardiac arrhythmias and sudden cardiac death. Moreover, there is often an increase in peripheral vascular resistance, and potassium deficits may be partly responsible *(Altura)*.

Because hypokalemia is known to predispose patients to ventricular arrhythmias, low serum potassium levels should be aggressively treated *(Francis)*.

Magnesium and Potassium Aspartates

Several open trials have administered magnesium and potassium together to CHF patients in the form of mineral aspartates and have reported good results. In addition to the effects of the two cations described above, the combination of the two salts is believed the speed the onset of the therapeutic effects of digitalis while reducing both its maintenance dosage and potential cardiotoxic effects. Hyperkalemia is the major contraindication *(Grujic)*.

OTHER NUTRITIONAL FACTORS

Arginine

Apparently by serving as a precursor for nitric oxide, a smooth muscle relaxant, L-arginine supplementation causes peripheral vasodilation and improves cardiac output. Nitric oxide may also promote vasodilation by inhibiting alpha receptor-mediated sympathetic vasoconstriction *(Ceremuzynski)*.

Under double-blind conditions, 15 patients with moderate to severe CHF received L-arginine for 6 weeks. Compared to placebo, L-arginine significantly reduced their number of physical limitations due to CHF, the distance they could walk in 6 minutes, and the rate of blood flow during exercise *(Rector)*.

Carnitine Deficiency

Primary carnitine deficiency is a rare metabolic disorder seen in early childhood which causes severe congestive heart failure *(Squarcia)*. In adults with CHF, myocardial free carnitine levels may be reduced, while the levels of the metabolite, long-chain acylcarnitine, may be elevated *(Kobayashi)*.

Supplementation with L-propionylcarnitine, a naturally-occurring derivative, was found to be effective under double-blind conditions *(Caponnetto)* while, in an open trial, supplementation with L-carnitine was followed by improvement *(Kobayaski)*.

Coenzyme Q_{10} Deficiency

The levels of coenzyme Q_{10} in blood and endomyocardial biopsies were found to be significantly decreased in various groups of patients with myocardial failure (dilated and restrictive cardiomyopathy and alcoholic heart disease). The deficiency was more pronounced with increasing symptoms *(Mortensen)*.

In numerous studies, some of which were double-blind, supplementation with CoQ_{10} has been shown to improve cardiac function in CHF patients who remained symptomatic following standard treatment resulting, for example, in significantly less hospitalizations for worsening heart failure and a reduced frequency of episodes of pulmonary edema and cardiac asthma *(Morisco)*.

While pregnant, a 24 year-old woman started having breathing problems and went into early labor. Ten days after delivery she was diagnosed with severe congestive heart failure due to treatment with Adriamycin for kidney and lung cancer during childhood. Evaluation by a second cardiologist revealed evidence of a severe cardiomyopathy with a cardiac ejection fraction of only 15% and a very poor prognosis.

She was initially started on CoQ_{10} 120 mg 3 times daily while staying with her mother, a registered nurse, and started to feel better within a month. After 3 months, she was strong enough to return home. Eleven years later, she is able to perform most activities of daily living. She continues to take the same dose of CoQ_{10}, but now takes a water-miscible form that has further improved her energy levels. In addition, she takes 10 gm of carnitine daily (Langsjoen).

Creatine Deficiency

Creatine levels in the myocardium are commonly depressed in CHF *(Field)*. Under double-blind conditions, supplementation has been shown to improve measures of cardiac function *(Ferraro)* as well as measures of physical strength and endurance *(Gordon)* in cardiac-impaired patients.

Taurine

Taurine supplementation has been demonstrated to reduce both signs and symptoms of CHF in double-blind crossover studies *(Azuma,1983,1985)*. When added to conventional treatment, taurine improved the New York Heart Association functional class, pulmonary crackles, and chest film abnormalities. Moreover, while heart-failure scores failed to change significantly on placebo, their decrease was highly significant on taurine *(Azuma,1985)*.

Taurine supplementation (3 grams daily) has been compared with coenzyme Q_{10} (30 mg daily) for a group of patients with an ejection fraction of less than 50%. After 6 weeks, only the taurine-treated group showed a significant treatment effect on systolic left ventricular function, suggesting that, at these dosages, taurine supplementation may be more effective *(Azuma,1992)*.

OTHER RELATED FACTORS

Lead Toxicity

Chronic lead intoxication from occupational exposure may cause a congestive cardiomyopathy. Diagnosis may be difficult because the patient may present without the typical signs and symptoms of lead poisoning such as foot or wrist drop, abdominal pain, gingival lead lines, microcytic anemia, gout or interstitial nephritis *(Balestra)*.

BIBLIOGRAPHY

Altura BM, Altura BT. Biochemistry and pathophysiology of congestive heart failure: Is there a role for magnesium? Magnesium 5(3-4):134-43, 1986

Azuma J et al. Double-blind randomized crossover trial of taurine in congestive heart failure. Curr Ther Res 34(4):543-57, 1983

Azuma J et al. Therapeutic effect of taurine in congestive heart failure: A double-blind crossover trial. Clin Cardiol 8:276-82, 1985

Azuma J et al. Usefulness of taurine in chronic congestive heart failure and its prospective application. Jpn Circ J 56(1):95-9, 1992

Balestra DJ. Adult chronic intoxication. Arch Intern Med 151:1718-20, 1991

Benzer W et al. Effects of intravenous magnesium chloride reverses left ventricular end-diastolic pressure in coronary artery disease. Am J Cardiol 77:638-40, 1996

Browne SE. The case for intravenous magnesium treatment of arterial disease in general practice: review of 34 years of experience. J Nutr Med 4:169-77, 1994

Brunvand L et al. Congestive heart failure caused by vitamin D deficiency? Acta Paediatr 84:106-8, 1995

Burch GE, Giles TD. Alcoholic cardiomyopathy: concept of the disease and its treatment. Am J Med 50:141-5, 1971

Caponnetto S et al. Efficacy of L-propionylcarnitine treatment in patients with left ventricular dysfunction. Eur Heart J 15(9):1267-73, 1994

Ceremuzynski L et al. Effect of supplemental oral l-arginine on exercise capacity in patients with stable angina pectoris. Am J Cardiol 80:331-3, 1997

Conway N. Hemodynamic effects of ethyl alcohol in coronary heart disease Am Heart J 76:581-2, 1968

Danielson C, Joyce SM. Beriberi heart disease in a schizophrenic with an unusual diet. J Emerg Med 8(6):705-7, 1990

Dhalla AK et al. Role of oxidative stress in transition of hypertrophy to heart failure. J Am Coll Cardiol 28(2):506-14, 1996

Dracup K et al. Management of heart failure. II. Counseling, education, and lifestyle modifications. JAMA 272(18):1442-6, 1994

Ferraro S et al. Hemodynamic effects of creatine phosphate in patients with congestive heart failure: a double-blind comparison trial versus placebo. Clin Cardiol 19(9):699-703, 1996

Field ML. Creatine supplementation in congestive heart failure. Cardiovasc Res 31:174-5, 1996

Francis GS. Interaction of the sympathetic nervous system and electrolytes in congestive heart failure. Am J Cardiol 65(10):24E-27E, 1990

Ghatak A et al. Oxy free radical system in heart failure and therapeutic role of oral vitamin E. Int J Cardiol 57(2):119-27, 1996

Gordon A et al. Creatine supplementation in chronic heart failure increases skeletal muscle creatine phosphate and muscle performance. Cardiovasc Res 30(3):413-18, 1995

Gottlieb SS. Importance of magnesium in congestive heart failure. Am J Cardiol 63(14):39G-42G, 1989

Gottlieb SS et al. Prognostic importance of the serum magnesium concentration in patients with congestive heart failure. J Am Coll Cardiol 16(4):827-31, 1990

Grujic M, Pernovic M. [Treatment of acute myocardial infarction and chronic heart failure with K-Mg aspartate.] Med Welt 25(50):2124-6, 1974 (in German)

Kobayashi A et al. L-carnitine treatment for congestive heart failure - experimental and clinical study. Jpn Cir J 56(1):86-94, 1992

Langsjoen P - as told to Jack Challem. Transformations: How nutritional therapy changes three lives. Let's Live, December 1998:32-5

Li RK et al. Vitamin E and oxidative stress in the heart of the cardiomyopathic Syrian hamster. Free Radic Biol Med 24(2):252-8, 1998

Morisco C et al. Effect of coenzyme Q10 in patients with congestive heart failure: a long-term multicenter randomized study. Clin Invest 71:S134-6, 1993

Mortensen SA. Coenzyme Q10: clinical benefits with biochemical correlates suggesting a scientific breakthrough in the management of chronic heart failure. Int J Tissue React 12(3):155-62, 1990

Rector TS et al. Randomized, double-blind, placebo-controlled study of supplemental oral L-arginine in patients with heart failure. Circulation 93:2135-41, 1996

Seligmann H et al. Thiamine deficiency in patients with congestive heart failure receiving long-term furosemide therapy: a pilot study. Am J Med 91(2):151-5, 1991

Shane E et al. Bone mass, vitamin D deficiency, and hyperparathyroidism in congestive heart failure. Am J Med 103:197-207, 1997

Shimon I et al. Improved left ventricular function after thiamine supplementation in patients with congestive heart failure receiving long-term furosemide therapy. Am J Med 98:485-90, 1995

Squarcia U et al. [Dilated cardiomyopathy due to primary carnitine deficiency.] Pediatr Med Chir 8(2):157-61, 1986) (in Italian)

Watanabe H et al. Randomized, double-blind, placebo-controlled study of ascorbate on the preventive effect of nitrate tolerance in patients with congestive heart failure. Circulation 97(9):886-91, 1988

Wester PO, Dyckner T. Intracellular electrolytes in cardiac failure. Acta Med Scand [Suppl] 707:33-6, 1986

Yue QY et al. No difference in blood thiamine diphosphate levels between Swedish Caucasian patients with congestive heart failure treated with furosemide and patients without heart failure. J Intern Med 242(6):491-5, 1997

CONSTIPATION

NUTRITIONAL TREATMENT GUIDE

✓ = Efficacy generally accepted.
* = Efficacy *demonstrated* by controlled human trials.
[+] = Efficacy *suspected* from uncontrolled human trials.
[-] = Efficacy *suspected* from indirect data.
? = Efficacy *challenged* in a study of similar design.

DIETARY FACTORS

✓ increase **Dietary Fiber**
Example: 1/2 cup of wheat bran (9 gm fiber) daily with increases by 1/2 cup increments as tolerated up to 2 to 3 cups daily.

- -

[+] **moderate Fat** diet
[+] **moderate Protein** diet

NUTRITIONAL FACTORS

✓ **Magnesium Hydroxide**: 25 ml daily

- -

* **Pantothenic Acid**: ? 250 to 500 mg daily

- -

[+] **Folic Acid deficiency**: 800 μg daily

OTHER RELATED FACTORS

* rule out **Food Sensitivities**

- -

[+] ***Lactobacillus Acidophilus***: (dosage depends upon preparation)
(trial may take weeks to months)

DIETARY FACTORS

In the absence of organic disease, inadequacy of dietary fiber in the modern Western diet is believed to be the primary cause for constipation *(Taylor)*. Undigested fiber absorbs water which increases the weight and bulk of the stool and makes it softer. The increased bulk reduces intraluminal pressure and activates propulsive motility, reducing intestinal transit time *(Corinaldesi)*.

Furthermore, fiber acts as a substrate for the growth of colonic microflora, increasing the production of gases such as hydrogen and methane which also augment the bulking effect. Corn bran appears to be significantly more effective than wheat bran *(Graham)*. Current recommendations for chronic constipation call for a trial of increasing dietary fiber first; then, it the trial fails, an evaluation to determine whether slow gastrointestinal transit and/or a disorder of defecation explains the poor outcome *(Voderholzer)*.

Excessive intake of protein or fat can also cause constipation *(Leung)*. Moreover, children switched from human milk or formula to whole cow's milk may sometimes develop constipation because of the higher protein to carbohydrate ratio *(Leung)*.

NUTRITIONAL FACTORS

VITAMINS

Folic Acid Deficiency

Folic acid deficiency, the most common of the vitamin deficiencies, may be associated with constipation. Accompanying neurologic signs and symptoms may suggest the diagnosis *(Botez)*.

Pantothenic Acid

Pantothenic acid deficiency, although rarely seen, may be associated with constipation. Even in the absence of deficiency, however, anecdotal reports suggest that supplementation with pantothenic acid stimulates peristalsis when given in adequate doses *(Williams)*; it has even been found to be effective in cases of paralytic ileus *(Jacques)*.

Moreover, dexpanthenol, the alcohol of pantothenic acid, (which is readily oxidized in the cells to pantothenic acid) has been found to be effective in two double-blind studies as well as in several open trials *(Hanck)*.

MINERALS

Osmotic laxatives such as magnesium hydroxide (milk of magnesia) may play a role in the treatment of chronic constipation in elderly patients confined to convalescent or nursing homes when other measures fail to produce adequate bowel evacuations *(Kinnunen)*.

They may, however, result in a watery stool, urgency in defecation and, occasionally, incontinence. Moreover, hypermagnesemia is a possible complication for patients with impaired renal function *(AMA)*.

OTHER RELATED FACTORS

BACTERIAL CULTURES

In an open trial, 27 patients with chronic constipation were treated with an antibiotic regimen to eliminate preexisting flora, then non-pathogenic anaerobes and aerobes were administered by colonic infusion. During the follow-up period, none of the patients required further laxatives *(Andrews)*.

Lactobacillus acidophilus

A stable and important member of the normal bacterial flora, successful implantation of *Lactobacillus acidophilus* by oral administration has been found effective in relieving constipation due to a variety of causes *(Rettger)*.

In contrast to the action of the laxatives, it may take weeks or even months before the full benefits of *L. acidophilus* administration are realized. If acidophilus succeeds in relieving constipation, however, it has probably been successfully implanted; it may then be possible to discontinue it without experiencing the return of symptoms.

FOOD SENSITIVITIES

Cow's milk protein allergy appears to be the most frequent manifestation of food sensitivity-related constipation. In a double-blind crossover study published in the *New England Journal of Medicine*, cow's milk was compared with soy milk in 65 children with chronic constipation who had been treated with laxatives without success. Six-eight percent improved on soy milk, while none improved on cow's milk *(Iacono, 1998)*.

The pediatric gastroenterologists who conducted this study hypothesize that constipation in these infants is due to anal and perianal lesions that cause pain which intensifies during the passing of stools and eventually inhibits their evacuation. They found similar manifestations, though less frequently, with other food antigens, especially eggs, tomatoes, fish and citrus. An elimination diet was the best means of assessment as about one-third of infants had no increase in IgE or IgG anti-beta-lactoglobulin *(Iacono, 1995)*.

While poorly researched, adults are also reported to develop constipation as a symptom of food sensitivity *(Rinkel)*. The presence of other symptoms suggestive of food sensitivities should raise the suspicion of this diagnosis. In one early study, a group of adult patients with gastrointestinal reactions to foods presented with constipation as well as gas, bloating and abdominal pain. All showed evidence of hypothyroidism, and x-rays most frequently showed evidence of a spastic colon *(Gay)*.

A 2-month-old boy suffered from chronic constipation, abdominal distension, vomiting, and irritability. He was unable to defecate without the use of laxatives and drugs that stimulate intestinal contraction.

On 3 separate occasions, the symptoms disappeared when cow's milk was eliminated from his diet, but ingestion of milk caused the symptoms to return each time. The constipation resolved when the child was fed an extensively hydrolyzed cow's milk formula (Arreguin).

BIBLIOGRAPHY

AMA Drug Evaluations, Fifth Edition. Chicago, American Medical Association, 1983

Andrews PJ et al. Abstract Gastroenterology 106(4):A459, 1994

Arreguin L, Ortiz I. Chronic constipation as a manifestation of allergy to cow's milk. Ann Allergy Asthma Immunol 78:147, 1997

Botez MI et al. Neurologic disorders responsive to folic acid therapy. Can Med Assoc J 15:217, 1976

Corinaldesi F et al. Dietary fibers and intestinal transit times. Curr Ther Res 31:173-80, 1983

Gay LP. Gastrointestinal allergy. J Missouri Med Assoc 29:7-10, 1932

Graham DY et al. The effect of bran on bowel function in constipation. Am J Gastroenterol 77(9):599-603, 1982

Hanck AB, Goffin H. Dexpanthenol (Ro 01-4709) in the treatment of constipation. Acta Vitaminol Enzymol 4(1-2):87-97, 1982

Iacono G, Carroccio A - interviewed in Clinical Pearls News 5(6), June, 1995b

Iacono G et al. Intolerance of cow's milk and chronic constipation in children. N Engl J Med 339:1100-4, 1998

Jacques JE. Pantothenic acid in paralytic ileus. Lancet 2:861-2, 1951

Kinnunen O, Salokannel J. Constipation in elderly long-stay patients: Its treatment by magnesium hydroxide and bulk-laxative. Ann Clin Res 19(5):321-3, 1987

Leung AK et al. Constipation in children. Am Fam Physician 5(2):611-18, 1996

Rettger LF et al. Lactobacillus Acidophilus. Its Therapeutic Application. New Haven, Conn., Yale U. Press, 1935

Rinkel HJ et al. Food Allergy. Springfield, Illinois, Charles C. Thomas, 1951

Taylor R. Management of constipation: High fiber diets work. Br Med J 300:1063-4, 1990

Voderholzer WA et al. Clinical response to dietary fiber treatment of chronic constipation. Am J Gastroenterol 92(1):95-8, 1997

Williams RJ. The expanding horizon in nutrition. Texas Rep Biol Med 19(2):245-58, Summer, 1961

CROHN'S DISEASE

See Also: ULCERATIVE COLITIS

NUTRITIONAL TREATMENT GUIDE

✓ = Efficacy generally accepted.
* = Efficacy *demonstrated* by controlled human trials.
[+] = Efficacy *suspected* from uncontrolled human trials.
[-] = Efficacy *suspected* from indirect data.
? = Efficacy *challenged* in a study of similar design.

DIETARY FACTORS

✓ **Elemental (protein-free) or Polymeric (protein-containing) liquid diets**

- -

* **high Fiber, low Refined Carbohydrate diet**

- -

[+] **low Disaccharide diet**

- -

[-] restrict **Animal Protein**
[-] avoid **Chemically-Hardened Fats**

NUTRITIONAL FACTORS

* **Zinc deficiency:** zinc sulfate 220 mg twice daily *AND* **Copper** 2 mg daily
* ? **Omega-3 fatty acid deficiency:** 3 grams daily (enteric-coated capsules from fish oil) (1 yr. trial)

- -

[+] **Calcium deficiency:** ≈ 1 g daily
[+] **Folic acid deficiency:** 800 µg daily
[+] **Glycosaminoglycans** (dosage depends upon preparation)
[+] **Iron deficiency:** 30 mg twice daily until repletion; then minimal possible dosage
[+] **Magnesium deficiency:** ≈ 400 mg daily (Consider IM or IV administration, especially in hypomagnesemia.)
[+] **Riboflavin deficiency:** 5 to 10 mg daily
[+] **Selenium deficiency:** 200 µg daily
[+] **Thiamine deficiency:** 50 mg daily
[+] **Vitamin A deficiency:** 50,000 IU daily for 6 weeks (10,000 IU during pregnancy)
[+] **Vitamin B_6 deficiency:** 50 to 100 mg daily
[+] **Vitamin B_{12} deficiency:** 1,000 µg intramuscularly weekly initially and monthly afterwards
[+] **Vitamin C deficiency:** 500 mg twice daily
[+] **Vitamin D deficiency:** 50,000 to 100,000 IU 2 or 3 times during the first week; then, if needed, either 100,000 IU of ergo- or cholecalciferol every 3 or 6 months *OR* 800 to 1,600 IU daily
[+] **Vitamin E:** ? 2,000 to 16,000 IU daily in divided doses (4 week trial)
[+] **Vitamin K deficiency:** phytonadione 10 mg intramuscularly as needed

[-] **Lactobacillus casei GG:** 10^{10} colony-forming units twice daily (10 day trial)

OTHER RELATED FACTORS

✓ rule out **Food Sensitivities**

DIETARY FACTORS

Patients may be grossly malnourished, due both to dietary inadequacies secondary to anorexia and to nutrient malabsorption secondary to impairment in the function of absorptive surfaces by the disease process.

DIETARY FIBER AND REFINED CARBOHYDRATES

It has become increasingly obvious that reactions to dietary constituents have a major effect on the course of the disease. Refined sugar has been shown to alter colonic activity in ways which increase the risk of Crohn's disease *(Kruis,87)*, and sugar intake increases with the duration of the illness *(Persson)*. Moreover, epidemiological studies suggest that patients with Crohn's disease eat more sugar than either normal controls or patients with ulcerative colitis, another inflammatory bowel disease *(Penny)*. This difference in intake, however, appears to develop well after the disease is diagnosed *(Järnerot)*.

A diet rich, not only in sugar, but also in other refined carbohydrates, is likely to be low in dietary fiber. Consistent with the research on sugar, a low intake of dietary fiber intake is also associated with an increased risk of the disease *(Persson;Thornton)*. Even when the disease is in remission, patients with long-standing disease often have a lower dietary intake of fiber than normals *(Geerling)*.

Conversely, there is evidence from controlled studies is that Crohn's patients may benefit from a diet which is high in fiber and low in refined carbohydrates. In a study reported in the *British Medical Journal*, for example, 32 patients received a fiber-rich unrefined carbohydrate diet in addition to their usual treatments and were followed for a average of four and one-third years. Compared with 32 matched patients who had received no dietary instruction, diet-treated patients had only 111 days in the hospital while controls had 533 hospital days. Moreover, while 5 of the controls required intestinal surgery, only one diet-treated patient needed it *(Heaton)*.

THE ELEMENTAL DIET

Numerous studies have found that patients often respond dramatically to defined-formula, elemental diets whose short-term efficacy appear to be similar to that of treatment with steroids but without the serious adverse effects of the latter. Moreover, these diets may be superior to steroids in improving the patients' nutritional status, probably by more rapidly restoring normal intestinal permeability *(Zoli)*.

Once remission has been achieved with an elemental diet, foods need to be returned slowly in order to avoid provoking an exacerbation of the disease. In a study reported in the *Lancet*, half of a group of patients who had successfully achieved remission on an elemental diet were instructed to introduce one new food daily, excluding any that precipitated symptoms. They were compared with the other half of the group which received corticosteroids along with advice on healthy eating. Physicians who were unaware of group assignment assessed their progress for up to 2 years.

Intention-to-treat analysis showed median lengths of remission of 3.8 months in the corticosteroid group compared to 7.5 months in the diet group. Relapse rates at 2 years, adjusted for withdrawals, were 79% in the steroid group and 62%, in the diet group, a statistically significant difference *(Riordan)*.

The mechanism(s) by which elemental diets induce remission in Crohn's disease is unclear. Hypotheses include bowel rest, reduced antigenic load, nutritional effects, the substitution of protein with trophic amino acids, modification of gut flora, normalization of intestinal permeability, changes in fecal pH, and a fat profile which modifies disease activity by reducing proinflammatory eicosanoid synthesis *(O'Sullivan)*.

For example, epidemiologic studies have shown that a high intake of animal protein is a strong risk factor for development of Crohn's disease *(Shoda)*. Moreover, ingestion of partially hydrogenated fats containing high levels of *trans* fats have been implicated in the development of Crohn's disease in both animal and human studies *(Heckers;Nagel)*.

A low disaccharide diet has been proposed based on the premise that disaccharide digestion may be impaired in some patients either as a primary problem or as the result of the intestinal disorder, resulting in colonization of certain harmful bacteria and further damage to the intestinal tract. Carbohydrates are restricted to fruits, honey, properly-prepared yogurt, and specific vegetables and fruit. All cereal grains are forbidden. In an informal clinical setting, many patients went into long-term remission after 2 years on the diet *(Gottschall)*.

Also, the contribution of specific food sensitivities to the activity of the disease has been demonstrated in numerous studies. Perhaps the most careful study to date induced remission in 28 patients by a 4-week elemental diet and then introduced single foods over 5 days. While 20 patients complained of food reactions, only 10 consistently identified the same foods as causing their symptoms, and for only 3 of these 10 patients were the sensitivities confirmed by double-blind challenge *(Pearson)*.

Foods implicated as incitants tend to be common in the diet. Wheat, dairy products, yeast, and corn are some of the more frequently implicated *(Workman)*.

NUTRITIONAL FACTORS

Supplies of several important nutrients may be low. As repleting nutritional deficiencies is important for strengthening the body's defenses and preventing complications due to the deficiencies, an attempt should be made to restore adequate nutriture. Unfortunately, scientific investigation of the effect of nutritional treatment on the course of the disease has been minimal; thus it is not even known whether nutritional deficiencies play a causal role in the progress of the disease.

FAT-SOLUBLE VITAMINS

Vitamin A Deficiency

It is not uncommon for Crohn's patients to ingest less than the US RDA for vitamin A *(Hodges)*. Serum levels may be reduced, and there is a marked inverse correlation between these levels and disease activity *(Schoelmerich)*.

While supplementation is indicated to replete a deficiency, it is usually ineffective in changing the manifestations of the illness *(Noorby)*.

Vitamin D Deficiency

Mild deficiency of vitamin D is common among patients with gastrointestinal and liver disorders, especially in those with active disease, and plasma 25-OH vitamin D levels are inversely correlated with both hemoglobin and erythrocyte sedimentation rate. Severe deficiency will sometimes be seen, as well as secondary hyperparathyroidism and osteomalacia *(Dibble)*. Even when in remission, patients with long-standing disease may have reduced serum vitamin D concentrations *(Geerling)*. As with vitamin A, deficiencies should be repleted to prevent the development of manifestations of vitamin D deficiency.

Vitamin E

Even when the disease is clinically in remission, patients with long-standing Crohn's disease may have reduced serum vitamin E concentrations *(Geerling)*.

While controlled clinical trials have yet to be performed, there are case studies in the literature suggesting dramatic responses by patients who received either large dosages of D-alpha tocopherol *(Hood)*, or alpha-tocopherylquinone (which is poorly absorbed from the gut) along with a low fat diet *(Bennet)*.

A woman diagnosed as suffering from Crohn's experienced up to 10 diarrheal movements daily and violent abdominal cramps. Findings included rectal hemorrhages and 4 large perianal and perineal openings which had been left open since 4 abscesses had been surgically incised. Medication was unsuccessful in inducing a remission, although 50 mg prednisone every other day helped for 2 months.

She was given 40 capsules of 400 IU alpha tocopherol daily. By the end of 4 weeks, the diarrhea had stopped and the fistulas were reduced to ½ of their previous size. Subsequently the cramps became increasingly rare and the patient felt good for first time since the disease-onset years previously.

By 5½ months after starting supplementation, 2 fistulas had reduced to very small openings and 2 had closed completely. X-rays of the lower bowel failed to reveal signs of acute colitis or ulceration, either in the section of the ileum left after surgery or in the colon or rectum. She reported one solid bowel movement daily and no cramps (De Liz).

Vitamin K Deficiency

A deficiency of vitamin K is common with disease of the terminal ileum treated with sulfasalazine or antibiotics *(Krasinski)*. After repletion, abnormal prothrombin times return toward normal *(Krasinski)*.

WATER-SOLUBLE VITAMINS

Vitamin B Complex Deficiencies

Folic Acid Deficiency

Serum folate levels may be low, not only due to insufficient intake, malabsorption and chronic drug-induced low-grade hemolysis *(Elsborg,1979)*, but also to antifolate actions of sulfasalazine *(Baum)*.

In about 10% of patients, oral folate will fail to increase serum folate levels. For this group, parenteral folate supplementation should be considered *(Steger)*.

A 33-year-old man developed severe sensory peripheral neuropathy associated with low serum folate levels. No systemic disease was identified on the initial evaluation, but 2 ½ years later he developed clinical and radiological features of Crohn's disease, confirmed by intestinal biopsy. Thus, sensory polyneuropathy may occur as the first manifestation of Crohn's disease (Lossos).

Riboflavin, Thiamine & Vitamin B_6 Deficiencies

Not infrequently, patients fail to ingest the US RDA of thiamine, vitamin B_6, and/or vitamin B_{12} *(Hodges)*. When patients' serum, blood and erythrocyte concentrations of these vitamins were compared with those of healthy controls, they were found to be lower in patients than in the controls *(Kuroki)*.

Vitamin B_{12} Deficiency

Since vitamin B_{12} is absorbed in the terminal ileum (a common site for disease activity), it may not be properly absorbed and may require supplementation by injection *(Elsborg,1982)*.

Most patients with ileorectal anastomoses have vitamin B_{12} malabsorption, particularly those who have lost more than 60 cm of ileum *(Behrend)*. Malabsorption of the vitamin is not limited to these patients, however, as up to three-fifths of patients who have not had surgery are also B_{12} malabsorbers *(Barton)*.

Vitamin C Deficiency

Although vitamin C intake appears to be similar to that of normals *(Linaker)*, leukocyte vitamin C may be reduced *(Hughes)*. Moreover, patients with fistulas may have lower vitamin C levels than those without *(Gerson)*.

Ascorbic acid is known to concentrate at sites of disease activity. Since patients with fistulas do not have as great an increase in vitamin C at such sites, it has been suggested that an inability to concentrate ascorbate may somehow be related to fistula formation *(Pettit,1987)*.

Other work by the same team suggests that vitamin C absorption is normal in Crohn's patients, regardless of whether there are fistulas *(Pettit,1989)*. It now appears that a marginal vitamin C deficiency may result from its consumption as it defends against oxidant stress produced by the inflammatory process *(Buffinton)*.

MINERALS

Calcium Deficiency

Calcium nutriture is often deficient, thus increasing the risk of osteoporosis *(Andreassen)*. While corticosteroid treatment is a major contributor, other factors include inadequate dietary intake, malabsorption, and vitamin D deficiency *(Rosenberg;Silvennoinen)*.

Fortunately, bone loss can usually be prevented by providing supplementation with vitamin D *(Vogelsang)* and assuring an adequate calcium intake.

Copper

The body distribution of copper is abnormal in active Crohn's disease. Serum copper levels may be elevated, *(Ringstad)*, while tissue copper levels may be reduced *(Lih-Brody)*.

Following the institution of an elemental diet, low serum copper levels increase towards normal *(Teahon)*.

Iron Deficiency

Women and children with Crohn's disease frequently ingest less than the US RDA of iron *(Hendricks,1994; Hodges)*. Chronic blood loss through the gut also contributes to vulnerability to iron deficiency *(Rosenberg)* which, like calcium deficiency, is one of the most common deficiencies seen in the disorder *(Rath)*.

Magnesium Deficiency

A high intake of magnesium is negatively associated with the risk of Crohn's disease *(Reif)*.

Magnesium deficiency is common due to decreased intake, malabsorption and increased intestinal losses *(Galland;Hendricks,1994)*. Serum magnesium levels may be reduced compared to normal controls *(Geerling)*. Intracellular levels are frequently low and may be associated with anorexia, hypotension, confusion, hyperirritability, tetany, convulsions, and EKG or EEG abnormalities *(Rosenberg)*. Clinically important deficiency should be especially suspected in patients with small bowel resections exceeding 75 cm *(Hessov)*.

Selenium Deficiency

Whole blood *(Penny)* and serum *(Ringstad)* levels of selenium are reduced as compared to normal controls. Furthermore, plasma and erythrocyte levels of glutathione peroxidase, a selenium-dependent, antioxidant enzyme, may be reduced *(Rannem)*.

Zinc Deficiency

Zinc deficiency appears to be related to accelerated turnover *(Nakamura)*, although there is also evidence of impaired absorption *(Sturniolo)*. Plasma *(Ainley; Hendricks,1994)*, serum and red cell zinc *(Sjögren)* may be reduced. Intracellular zinc, as measured from percutaneous muscle biopsies, may also be reduced *(Sjögren)*. The various zinc parameters may fail to correlate with one another *(Sjögren)*; however, a zinc-loading test usually reveals a decreased rise in serum zinc and decreased urinary zinc excretion *(Nishi)*.

Also of interest, patients with fistulas may have lower serum zinc levels than those without fistulas. This finding suggests that there may be a relationship between zinc nutriture and fistula formation *(Kruis,1985)*.

Even severe zinc deficiency is rapidly responsive to oral supplementation *(Hendricks,1988)*. However, if a patient without clinical evidence of zinc deficiency is hypozincemic, serum zinc may fail to increase even with intravenous infusions, suggesting that zinc is inefficiently transported in the tissues *(Main)*.

OTHER NUTRITIONAL FACTORS

Essential Fatty Acid Deficiencies

Research has shown that Crohn's disease patients have imbalances in plasma fatty acid ratios, including decreased percentages and concentrations of saturated, monounsaturated and polyunsaturated fatty acids *(Siguel)*. Based on plasma essential fatty acid composition, at least 25% of patients may be deficient *(Siguel)*, although this high percentage has been contested *(Kuroki)*.

Omega-3 Fatty Acid Deficiency

There is an inverse correlation between the total serum omega-3 fatty acid concentration and the Crohn's Disease Activity Index *(Kuroki)*.

Supplementation of omega-3 polyunsaturated fatty acids in the form of enteric-coated fish oil capsules has been shown to be effective under double-blind conditions in reducing the risk of relapse when evaluated after one year *(Belluzzi)*. These results are consistent with those of a study of patients receiving parenteral nutrition who received a fish oil-containing lipid emulsion. After 2 weeks, there was evidence of an anti-inflammatory effect based on an increase in the ratio of leukotriene B5 to leukotriene B4 *(Ikehata)*.

However, other studies which employed non-enteric-coated fish oil capsules have failed to find a reduction in the clinical activity of the disease, even though the extent and severity of macroscopic bowel involvement was moderately improved *(Lorenz; Lorenz-Meyer)*. It is therefore possible that the enteric coating of fish oil supplements is particularly important in inflammatory bowel disease due to associated disturbances in lipid digestion and absorption *(Ikehata)*.

The anti-inflammatory effect of fish oils may be due to the reduced production of inflammatory prostaglandins in the form of leukotriene B4 and thromboxane A2, which are elevated in inflamed intestinal mucosa, or to inhibition of cytokine synthesis *(Belluzzi)*. Fish oil may also induce enterocyte hyperplasia, thereby increasing the mucosal surface area with a corresponding increase in enteral absorption of nutrients *(Vanderhoof)*.

Omega-6 Fatty Acids

An increased ratio of omega-6 to omega-3 fatty acids in the diet, generally due to a high intake of animal protein, may a strong risk factor for the development for Crohn's disease *(Shoda)*. Moreover, the plasma levels of dihomogammalinolenic acid (DGLA), an omega-6 fatty acid which is the immediate precursor to anti-inflammatory PGE_1, may be reduced *(Esteve-Comas)*.

Glycosaminoglycans

Glycosaminoglycans are part of the ground substance of connective tissue and consist of long unbranched chains made up of disaccharide repeating units, usually in combination with protein. Except for hyaluronic acid, they contain sulfate groups. Inflammatory disruption of vascular and connective tissue glycosaminoglycans may be an important pathogenic mechanism of Crohn's disease, contributing to the leakage of protein and fluid, thrombosis, and tissue remodeling *(Murch)*. Their therapeutic value is thought to be due to the chondroitin sulfates, of which chondroitin-4-sulfate is thought to be the most important.

In a preliminary study, 4 patients with inadequate results from traditional treatments received subcutaneous injections of an activated acid-pepsin-digested calf tracheal cartilage preparation ("Catrix-S") rich in glycosaminoglycans. The injections were given over 10 to 35 days followed by booster injections every 3 to 4 weeks. All 4 patients improved; 3 had an "excellent" response, while 1 had a "good" response *(Prudden)*.

Assuming that the efficacy of the preparation is due to the presence of the chondroitin sulfates, there is evidence that chondroitin-4-sulfate is well absorbed from the gut intact; thus oral administration may be equally effective. In any event, controlled studies with more subjects are needed to better assess this treatment.

OTHER RELATED FACTORS

Intestinal Microflora

Digestive bacterial flora are said to play a major role in the pathogenesis of Crohn's disease *(Favier)*, and lactobacilli counts are significantly reduced *(Giaffer)*.

In an open trial, supplementation of *Lactobacillus casei* GG to children with Crohn's disease significantly increased secretory IgA, a major factor in the immunological barrier of the gut mucosa *(Malin)*. This may be important in reducing Crohn's disease symptoms, since increases in intestinal permeability precede clinical relapses *(Wyatt)*.

Bifidobacteria counts are also reduced *(Favier;Giaffer)*. These bacteria are known to be beneficial to the host, and their reduction in Crohn's disease is responsible for decreased activity of the bacterial enzyme beta-D-galactosidase *(Favier)*. However, therapeutic trials of providing supplementation with bifidobacteria have yet to be conducted.

COMBINED NUTRITIONAL TREATMENT REGIMEN

A.C. first began nutritional treatment 3 years earlier. At that time he responded to the Specific Carbohydrate Diet and nutritional supplements. He was asymptomatic and was able to discontinue all medications. However, he gradually discontinued the treatment program and returned to his former pattern of eating "junk food." This was followed by a severe exacerbation during which he required intestinal surgery resulting in the loss of 18 inches of his intestines.*
He was restarted on the Specific Carbohydrate Diet, a general vitamin/mineral supplement in capsules, MaxEPA (fish oil) about 5 grams daily, vitamin A 50,000 IU daily, L-glutamine 1 gram twice daily for a few weeks and then 1 gram daily, zinc picolinate 30 mg elemental twice daily for 6 weeks and then 30 mg daily, vitamin E 400 IU, vitamin C, folic acid (Folirinse) 5 drops daily, and a lactobacillus preparation. He was also started on intramuscular vitamin B_{12} injections with vitamin B complex. In addition, as previous testing had revealed almost no stomach acid as well as undigested food in his stool, he was placed on a combination of hydrochloric acid and pepsin with meals and pancreatic enzymes afterwards. Finally, he was given a few intravenous drips containing high levels of nutrients.

After 4 months he felt entirely well. After another 2 months, the dosages of his supplements were reduced. Five years later, he remains almost entirely symptom-free (Wright).

** The Specific Carbohydrate Diet is a low-disaccharide diet (see discussion above). Carbohydrates are restricted to fruits, honey, properly-prepared yogurt, and specific vegetables and fruit. All cereal grains are forbidden (Gottschall).*

BIBLIOGRAPHY

Ainley CC et al. Zinc status in inflammatory bowel disease. Clin Sci 75(3):277-83, 1988

Andreassen H et al. Inflammatory bowel disease and osteoporosis. Scand J Gastroenterol 32(12):1247-55, 1997

Barton R. Macrocytic anaemias. Three fifths of patients with Crohn's disease that has not been operated on have vitamin B12 malabsorption. Letter. BMJ 314:1552, 1997

Baum CL et al. Antifolate actions of sulfasalazine on intact lymphocytes. J Lab Clin Med 97(6):779-84, 1981

Behrend C et al. Vitamin B12 absorption after ileorectal anastomosis for Crohn's disease: effect of ileal resection and time span after surgery. Eur J Gastroenterol Hepatol 7(5):397-400, 1995

Belluzzi A et al. Effect of an enteric-coated fish-oil preparation on relapses in Crohn's disease. N Engl J Med 334(24):1557-60, 1996

Bennet JD. Use of alpha-tocopherylquinone in ulcerative colitis. Gut 27(6):695-97, 1986

Buffinton GD, Doe WF. Altered ascorbic acid status in the mucosa from inflammatory bowel disease patients. Free Radic Res 22(2):131-43, 1995

De Liz AL - reported in Shute WE. Dr. Wilfrid E. Shute's Complete Updated Vitamin E Book. New Canaan, CT, Keats Publishing Inc., 1975, pp. 238-9

Dibble JB et al. A survey of vitamin D deficiency in gastrointestinal and liver disorders. Quart J Med 53:119-34, 1984

Elsborg L, Larsen L. Folate deficiency in chronic inflammatory bowel disease. Scand J Gastroenterol 14:1019-24, 1979

Elsborg L. Vitamin B12 and folic acid in Crohn's disease. Dan Med Bull 29(7):362-5, 1982

Esteve-Comas M et al. Plasma polyunsaturated fatty acid pattern in inflammatory bowel disease. Gut 33(10):1365-9, 1992

Favier C et al. Fecal beta-D-galactosidase production and Bifidobacteria are decreased in Crohn's disease. Dig Dis Sci 42(4):817-22, 1997

Galland L. Magnesium and inflammatory bowel disease. Magnesium 7(2):78-83, 1988

Geerling BJ et al. Comprehensive nutritional status in patients with long-standing Crohn disease currently in remission. Am J Clin Nutr 67:919-26, 1998

Gerson CD, Fabry EM. Ascorbic acid deficiency and fistula formation in regional enteritis. Gastroenterology 67:428, 1974

Giaffer MH et al. The assessment of faecal flora in patients with inflammatory bowel disease by a simplified bacteriological technique. J Med Microbiol 35(4):238-43, 1991

Gottschall E. Breaking the Vicious Cycle. Ontario, Kirkton Press, 1994

Heaton KW et al. Treatment of Crohn's disease with an unrefined-carbohydrate, fibre-rich diet. Br Med J 2:764-66, 1979

Heckers H et al. [Chemically prepared fats and Crohn disease. A pilot study of the occurrence of trans-fatty acids in the subcutaneous tissue of Crohn patients in comparison with healthy controls as a parameter of long-term fat intake.] Z Gastroenterol 26(5):259-64, 1988 (in German)

Hendricks KM, Walker WA. Zinc deficiency in inflammatory bowel disease. Nutr Rev 46(12):401-8, 1988

Hendricks KM et al. Dietary intake of adolescents with Crohn's disease. J Am Diet Assoc 94(4):441-4, 1994

Hessov I et al. Magnesium deficiency after ileal resections for Crohn's disease. Scand J Gastroenterol 18:643-49, 1983

Hodges P et al. Vitamin and iron intake in patients with Crohn's disease. J Am Diet Assoc 84(1):52-8, 1984

Hood RP. Nonspecific ulcerative colitis: successful treatment with D-alpha tocopherol. Digest of Chiropractic Economics Sept.-Oct. 1984

Hughes RG, Williams N. Leukocyte ascorbic acid in Crohn's disease. Digestion 17:272, 1978

Ikehata A et al. Effect of intravenously infused eicosapentaenoic acid on the leukotriene generation in patients with active Crohn's disease. Am J Clin Nutr 56:938-42, 1992

Järnerot G et al. Consumption of refined sugar by patients with Crohn's disease, ulcerative colitis, or irritable bowel syndrome. Scand J Gastroenterol 18(8):999-1002, 1983

Krasinski SD et al. The prevalence of vitamin K deficiency in chronic gastrointestinal disorders. Am J Clin Nutr 41(3):639-43, 1985

Kruis W et al. Zinc deficiency as a problem in patients with Crohn's disease and fistula formation. Hepatogastroenterology 32(3):133-4, 1985

Kruis W et al. Influence of diets high and low in refined sugar on stool qualities, gastrointestinal transit time and fecal bile acid excretion. Gastroenterology 92:1483, 1987

Kuroki F et al. Serum n3 polyunsaturated fatty acids are depleted in Crohn's disease. Dig Dis Sci 42(6):1137-41, 1997

Lih-Brody L et al. Increased oxidative stress and decreased antioxidant defenses in mucosa of inflammatory bowel disease. Dig Dis Sci 41(10):2078-86, 1996

Linaker BD. Scurvy and vitamin C deficiency in Crohn's disease. Postgrad Med J 55:26-9, 1979

Lorenz R et al. Supplementation with n-3 fatty acids from fish oil in chronic inflammatory bowel disease: a randomized, placebo-controlled, double-blind cross-over trial. J Intern Med Suppl 225(731):225-32, 1989

Lorenz-Meyer H et al. Omega-3 fatty acids and low carbohydrate diet for maintenance of remission in Crohn's disease: A randomized controlled multicenter trial. Scand J Gastroenterol 31:778-85, 1996

Lossos A et al. Peripheral neuropathy and folate deficiency as the first sign of Crohn's disease. J Clin Gastroenterol 13(4):442-4, 1991

Main AN et al. Clinical experience of zinc supplementation during intravenous nutrition in Crohn's disease: value of serum and urine zinc measurements. Gut 23(11):984-91, 1982

Malin M et al. Promotion of IgA immune response in patients with Crohn's disease by oral bacteriotherapy with Lactobacillus GG. Ann Nutr Metab 40:137-45, 1996

Murch SH et al. Disruption of sulphated glycosaminoglycans in intestinal inflammation. Lancet 341:711-14, 1993

Nagel E et al. [Animal experiment studies of ultrastructural changes in the lamina propria of the ileum caused by dietary fats and comparison with cytopathology in Crohn disease.] Z Gastroenterol 31(12):727-34, 1993 (in German)

Nakamura T et al. Zinc clearance correlates with clinical severity of Crohn's disease. A kinetic study. Dig Dis Sci 33(12):1520-4, 1988

Nishi Y et al. Zinc status and its relation to growth retardation in children with chronic inflammatory bowel disease. Am J Clin Nutr 33(12):2613-21, 1980

Noorby S et al. Ineffectiveness of vitamin A therapy in severe Crohn's disease. Acta Chir Scand 151:465-8, 1985

O'Sullivan MA, O'Morain CA. Nutritional therapy in Crohn's disease. Inflamm Bowel Dis 4(1):45-53, 1998

Pearson M et al. Food intolerance and Crohn's disease. Gut 34:783-7, 1993

Penny WJ et al. Relationship between trace elements, sugar consumption, and taste in Crohn's disease. Gut 24(4):288-92, 1983

Persson PB et al. Diet and inflammatory bowel disease: a case-control study. Epidemiol 3(1):47-51, 1992

Pettit SH, Irving MH. Does intestinal ascorbate deficiency predispose to fistula formation in Crohn's disease? Dis Colon Rectum 30(7):552-57, 1987

Pettit SH et al. Ascorbic acid absorption in Crohn's disease. Studies using L-[carboxyl-14C]ascorbic acid. Dig Dis Sci 34(4):559-66, 1989

Prudden JF, Balassa LL. The biological activity of bovine cartilage preparations. Sem Arthritis Rheum 3(4):287-321, 1974

Rannem T et al. Selenium status in patients with Crohn's disease. Am J Clin Nutr 56:933-7, 1992

Rath HC et al. [Nutritional deficiencies and complications in chronic inflammatory bowel diseases]. Med Klin 93(1):6-10, 1998) (in German).

Reif S et al. Pre-illness dietary factors in inflammatory bowel disease. Gut 40(6):754-60, 1997

Ringstad J et al. Serum selenium, copper, and zinc concentrations in Crohn's disease and ulcerative colitis. Scand J Gastroenterol 28:605-8, 1993

Riordan AM et al. Treatment of active Crohn's disease by exclusion diet: East Anglian Multicentre Controlled Trial. Lancet 342:1131-4, 1993

Rosenberg IH et al. Nutritional aspects of inflammatory bowel disease. Ann Rev Nutr 5:463-84, 1985

Schoelmerich J et al. Zinc and vitamin A deficiency in patients with Crohn's disease is correlated with activity but not with localization or extent of the disease. Hepatogastroenterology 32(1):34-8, 1985

Shoda R et al. Epidemiologic analysis of Crohn disease in Japan: increased dietary intake of n-6 polyunsaturated fatty acids and animal protein relates to increased incidence of Crohn disease in Japan. Am J Clin Nutr 63:741-5, 1996

Siguel E, Lerman R. Prevalence of essential fatty acid deficiency in patients with chronic gastrointestinal disorders. Metabolism 45(1):12-23, 1996

Silvennoinen J et al. Dietary calcium intake and its relation to bone mineral density in patients with inflammatory bowel disease. J Intern Med 240:285-92, 1996

Sjögren A et al. Evaluation of zinc status in subjects with Crohn's disease. J Am Coll Nutr 7(1):57-60, 1988

Steger GG et al. Folate absorption in Crohn's disease. Digestion 55(4):234-8, 1994

Sturniolo GC et al. Zinc absorption in Crohn's disease. Gut 21(5):387-91, 1980

Teahon K et al. Alterations in nutritional status and disease activity during treatment of Crohn's disease with elemental diet. Scand J Gastroenterol 30(1):54-60, 1995

Thornton JR et al. Diet and Crohn's disease: Characteristics of the pre-illness diet. Br Med J 2:762-4, 1979

Vanderhoof JA et al. Effects of dietary menhaden oil mucosal adaptation after small bowel resection in rats. Gastroenterology 106:94-9, 1994

Vogelsang H et al. Prevention of bone mineral loss in patients with Crohn's disease by long-term oral vitamin D supplementation. Eur J Gastroenterol Hepatol 7(7):609-14, 1995

Workman EM et al. Diet in the management of Crohn's disease. Hum Nutr Appl Nutr 38A:469-73, 1985

Wright JV. Treating Crohn's disease. Healing with Nutrition 5(1), January, 1998

Wyatt J et al. Intestinal permeability and the prediction of relapse in Crohn's disease. Lancet 341:1437-9, 1993

Zoli G et al. A randomized controlled study comparing elemental diet and steroid treatment in Crohn's disease. Aliment Pharmacol Ther 11(4):735-40, 1997

DEMENTIA

(including MILD MEMORY IMPAIRMENT)

See Also: ACQUIRED IMMUNODEFICIENCY SYNDROME
CEREBROVASCULAR DISEASE
ORGANIC MENTAL DISORDERS

NUTRITIONAL TREATMENT GUIDE

✓ = Efficacy generally accepted.
* = Efficacy *demonstrated* by controlled human trials.
[+] = Efficacy *suspected* from uncontrolled human trials.
[-] = Efficacy *suspected* from indirect data.
? = Efficacy *challenged* in a study of similar design.

DIETARY FACTORS

[-] minimize **Fat** consumption
[-] consume **Fish** regularly
[-] drink **Wine** moderately (3 to 4 glasses daily)

NUTRITIONAL FACTORS

✓ rule out **Copper** toxicity (Wilson's disease)
✓ **Iron deficiency:** *to treat mild memory impairment:* 30 mg twice daily until repletion; then minimal possible dosage
✓ **Vitamin B_{12} deficiency:** 100 µg IM daily for 1 week; then reduce to a maintenance level

- -

* **Carnitine:** acetyl-L-carnitine 1.5 to 3 g daily (3 month trial)
* **Choline:** citicoline (CDP-choline) 1,000 mg daily (3 month trial)
* **Folic acid:** 5'-methyltetrahydrofolic acid 50 mg daily (8 week trial)
* **Inositol:** 6 g daily (1 month trial)
* **Phosphatidylserine:** 300 mg daily (3 month trial)
* **S-adenosyl-L-methionine:** 1,200 mg daily (3 month trial)
* **Vitamin B_6:** *to improve memory in the healthy elderly:* 20 mg daily (3 month trial)
* **Vitamin E:** *to treat Alzheimer's dementia:* 2,000 IU daily
* ? **Thiamine:** *to treat Alzheimer's dementia:* 3 to 8 g daily (3 month trial)

- -

[+] **Folic Acid deficiency:** 10 to 20 mg daily for 1 week; then 2.5 to 10 mg daily
[+] **Niacin deficiency:** 300 to 500 mg niacinamide for the first few days; then 100 mg daily (several week trial)
[+] **Niacin:** *to stimulate dopamine synthesis:* nicotinamide adenine dinucleotide sodium 10 mg daily 30 min. before breakfast (8-12 wk. trial)

[+] **Zinc**: ? 30 mg daily

- -

[-] **Calcium deficiency:** ≈ 1 g daily
[-] **Magnesium deficiency:** ≈ 400 mg daily
[-] rule out **Manganese** toxicity
[-] **Selenium deficiency:** 200 μg daily
[-] **Vitamin C**: 500 mg twice daily

OTHER RELATED FACTORS

* ? minimize **Aluminum** exposure

- -

[+] rule out **Gluten sensitivity** (celiac disease)
[+] rule out **Manganese** toxicity
[+] rule out **Mercury** toxicity
[+] rule out **Hydrochloric Acid** deficiency

MALNUTRITION

About 10 to 20% of dementias in the elderly are believed to be reversible, and some of these dementias are caused by nutritional deficiencies. Even among a group of elderly subjects with no significant cognitive impairment, subjects who performed best on two mental status questionnaires were better nourished *(Ortega)*.

It is theorized that impaired nutrient absorption through the gut lining and perhaps impaired transport of nutrients across the blood/brain barrier contribute to deficient nutriture of brain tissue *(Abalan;Evans)*. Moreover, when severely demented patients were compared to normal controls, their poorer nutritional status could not be explained satisfactorily by reduced intake, suggesting that they were less able to utilize ingested nutrients *(Thomas)*.

DIETARY FACTORS

Dietary Fat

When regression analyses were performed on the prevalence of Alzheimer's dementia in the elderly population for 11 countries, fat and total caloric supply had the highest correlations with prevalence rates. Rates of Alzheimer's dementia increased by 0.3% with every 100-calorie increase in the average daily diet. Moreover, most of the tests generally applied to determine causality seemed to be satisfied, strongly supporting the hypothesis that fat consumption, with assistance from total caloric consumption, is the primary cause of Alzheimer's dementia *(Grant)*.

These findings are consistent with those of a study of elderly subjects who had no significant cognitive impairment. Those who made no errors on Pfeiffer's Mental Status Questionnaire had lower intakes of saturated fatty acids, while those with adequate results on the Mini-Mental State Exam had lower intakes of monounsaturated fatty acids, saturated fatty acids and cholesterol compared with those with less satisfactory results *(Ortega)*. Moreover, another recent study of the elderly found that a high intake of linoleic acid (an omega-6 essential fatty acid) was associated with cognitive impairment *(Kalmijn)*.

Fish

High fish consumption is inversely correlated with cognitive impairment and cognitive decline in the elderly *(Kalmijn)*. In fact, when the prevalence of Alzheimer's dementia was related to foods eaten in 11 countries, fish was the only food whose intake was inversely associated with risk in regions with relatively high-fat diets such as Europe and the United States *(Grant)*.

Alcohol

In a large group of elderly subjects, moderate drinkers (3 to 4 glasses of wine daily), as compared to nondrinkers, had only 19% of the risk for dementia and 28% of the risk of Alzheimer's disease after adjusting for confounding variables *(Orgogozo)*.

While moderate drinking appears to be protective, heavy drinking, by fostering the development of hypertension and hepatic injury, results in a dementia that is far more frequent in elderly alcoholics than in aged people in general *(Kasahara)*.

HOMOCYSTEINE

Higher serum concentrations of homocysteine, a toxic amino acid, have been shown to be directly associated with the presence of Alzheimer's dementia *(Joosten)*. Among older subjects without dementia, higher plasma homocysteine concentrations were associated with poorer spatial copying skills *(Riggs)*.

NUTRITIONAL FACTORS

VITAMINS

Folic Acid

A deficiency of folic acid is known to be associated with apathy, disorientation, poor concentration and memory deficits in addition to pyramidal tract damage. Although even the healthy elderly may fail to ingest adequate folate, serum and red cell folate is more likely to be low in patients with dementia *(Riggs;Thomas)*.

When folate deficiency is the cause of the dementia, the dementia as well as the neurologic symptoms may be at least partly reversible with folate supplementation *(Crellin;Melamed)*.

Even if serum folate levels are normal, folate supplementation may be beneficial. In a double-blind study, normofolatemic patients with mild to moderate senile dementia and depression were either supplemented with 5'-methyltetrahydrofolic acid or treated with an antidepressant (trazodone) for 8 weeks. By the end of the fourth week, both groups showed similar improvements in immediate and delayed recall as well as in depression. Furthermore, similar improvements were noted by the end of the study *(Passeri)*.

> *A 75 year-old epileptic female with severe dementia demonstrated reversal of the dementia and regression of spastic tetraparesis following folate supplementation. Serial EEG's recorded improvements, and her abnormal extensor plantar responses normalized (Melamed).*

Niacin

Deficiency

Dementia is one of the three cardinal signs of pellagra, the classical niacin deficiency disease; diarrhea and dermatitis are the other two. In a group of 18 pellagrins, 28% presented with dementia but without diarrhea or dermatitis, suggesting that the diagnosis could readily be missed if blood work is not performed *(Spivak)*. Other common findings include steatorrhea, alopecia, anemia and lymphopenia. The dementia may be reversible, with full recovery in several weeks.

Niacin deficiency is not uncommon in the elderly, even despite adequate dietary intake and oral supplementation *(Frank)*. Among patients with senile dementia, it appears to be fairly common *(Thomas)*, and repletion of a niacin deficiency should be beneficial.

Nicotinamide Adenine Dinucleotide (NADH)

Even when vitamin B_3 nutriture is adequate, supplementation of the vitamin in the form of the coenzyme nicotinamide adenine dinucleotide (NADH) may be efficacious. The enzyme tyrosine hydroxylase catalyzes the conversion of tyrosine to dopa, the precursor to the neurotransmitter dopamine. In senile dementia of the Alzheimer type, the activity of tyrosine hydroxylase is decreased in key regions of the brain *(Sawada)*, while *in vitro* work has shown that NADH can increase the activity of tyrosine hydroxylase and dopamine production in the cells up to 6 times *(Vrecko)*.

Because of its potential to stimulate endogenous L-dopa synthesis, patients with symptoms ranging from mild cognitive decline to severe dementia received oral NADH as the disodium salt. All showed notable improvements in mental function within 8 to 12 weeks and there were no side effects *(Birkmayer)*.

Mr. C, age 76, had serious short-term memory loss and was starting to have problems with long-term memory. He was started on a comprehensive vitamin program including niacinamide 1.5 g daily and began to improve within a month. Niacin 3 g daily was added and, by 5 months after starting treatment, he was normal.

Two months later, he revealed that he felt so well that he had decreased the dosage of niacin to 1.5 grams daily while remaining on the rest of the program. Soon, however, he noted the return of short-term memory problems (Hoffer).

Thiamine Deficiency

Like the drug tacrine, high dosages of thiamine have a central cholinergic effect *(Meador, 1993a)*, although there is no literature on its efficacy other than to replete a thiamine deficiency.

Marginal thiamine deficiency is not uncommon in the elderly in general *(Thomas)* and specifically in patients with Alzheimer's disease *(Gold)*. Even though their dietary intake may not be low compared to that of healthy people, Alzheimer's patients may still have lower functional values for thiamine *(Aghayewa)*. Their level of thiamine diphosphate may be reduced which, although mild, could result in impaired brain function *(Mastrogiacomo)*. Moreover, there is evidence of reduced brain activity of thiamine-dependent enzymes *(Eisinger; Gibson)*.

While the memory deficit associated with thiamine deficiency rarely disappears, adequate supplementation can mildly reduce symptoms and prevent further deterioration in cases of Alzheimer's dementia. Two out of 3 randomized controlled trials have reported benefit *(Blass; Meador, 1993b; Nolan)*.

Vitamin B_6

Perhaps one-third of the elderly population is marginally deficient in vitamin B_6 *(Rall)*. Higher plasma levels do appear to be associated with better memory in older subjects without dementia *(Riggs)* although, compared to the healthy elderly, the intake and nutriture of vitamin B_6 does not appear to be lower in Alzheimer patients *(Aghayewa)*.

In a double-blind study, healthy elderly men were randomly divided into 2 groups matched for age, plasma pyridoxal-5'-phosphate concentrations and IQ, and received either pyridoxine HCl 20 mg daily or placebo. After 3 months, vitamin B_6 supplementation was found to be associated with a modest, but significant, improvement in memory, especially long-term memory *(Deijen)*. Controlled studies are needed to clarify the protective and therapeutic effects of vitamin B_6 supplementation for various other groups.

Vitamin B_{12} Deficiency

The most common cause of vitamin B_{12} deficiency in the elderly is not malnutrition; it is degenerative changes in the mucous membrane of the gut causing B_{12} malabsorption *(Geland)*.

It is standard practice to evaluate serum B_{12} levels in patients who present with new-onset dementia, as a deficiency of the vitamin, which is associated with confusion, memory deficits, depression and mental slowness in addition to neurologic deficits, is not uncommon among patients with dementia *(Teunisse)*. While vitamin B_{12} deficiency is obvious in pernicious anemia, the vitamin may be deficient even in the absence of any hematologic findings *(Stott)*.

Supplementation of patients presenting with B_{12} deficiency is beneficial and may occasionally reverse the dementia *(Martin)*. Neurologic improvement is usually evident within a few days of initiating therapy and is often complete after one month. Supplementation may even be effective despite normal serum B_{12} levels and the lack of suspicious findings, probably due to low cerebrospinal fluid B_{12} levels *(Ikeda)*.

An 85-year-old Caucasian man presented with normal serum vitamin B_{12} values and dementia. He was started on IM injections of vitamin B_{12} 1,000 μg daily for 3 days, then 1,000 μg weekly for 1 month and then monthly thereafter. By the fifth injection, he showed improvement in the Mini-Mental Status Examination, his neurocognitive assessment deficits had disappeared, vibratory sensation in the lower extremities was improving, and his lethargy and cognitive slowing had disappeared. His serum vitamin B_{12} level was 368 pg/ml, which was well within the normal range (Goodman).

Vitamin C

While not all studies agree, there is evidence that, in the elderly, vitamin C intake is inversely related to cognitive function *(Ortega;Gale)*. Moreover, in the same age group, low plasma *(Perrig)* and cerebrospinal fluid *(Barabas)* ascorbate levels may be associated with poorer cognitive functioning.

In a prospective study, 633 persons 65 years or older were followed for an average of 4.3 years. Ninety-one of them developed Alzheimer disease. While between 3.2 and 3.3 cases were predicted among the 23 patients who used vitamin C supplements, none of them had developed the disease *(Morris)*.

In senile dementia of the Alzheimer's type, supplementation may theoretically be beneficial by reducing lipid peroxidative damage in the brain *(Barabas)*, although the clinical effects of high dosage ascorbate supplementation remain to be studied.

Vitamin E

Although a relationship between vitamin E intake and cognitive decline has been difficult to demonstrate *(Kalmijn;Jama)*, plasma/serum levels may be reduced in Alzheimer's patients *(Zaman)*.

It has been postulated that Alzheimer's dementia may be due to damage caused by the release of free radicals *(Clausen)*. If so, vitamin E, the major lipid-soluble antioxidant, would theoretically be important in reducing their effects. The results of both animal *(Meydani)* and *in vitro (Behl)* work confirm the importance of the vitamin in protecting the brain against oxidative damage and free radical degeneration.

The New England Journal of Medicine recently published a double-blind study of Alzheimer patients with moderately severe impairment who received either vitamin E or placebo. Compared to placebo, vitamin E was effective in increasing the time to occurrence of death, institutionalization, loss of the ability to perform basic activities of daily living, or severe dementia from a median time of 440 days to 670 days *(Sano)*.

In a prospective study, 633 persons 65 years or older were followed for an average of 4.3 years. Ninety-one of them developed Alzheimer disease. While between 2.5 and 3.9 cases were predicted among the 27 patients who used vitamin E supplements, none of them had developed the disease *(Morris)*.

MINERALS

Calcium Deficiency

Cognitive impairment in the elderly may be inversely related to calcium intake *(Jacqmin-Gadda)*. Inadequate intake could increase the bioavailability of aluminum, and thereby play a role in the etiology of Alzheimer's disease *(Foster;West)* (see Aluminum below). This hypothesis was tested by maintaining monkeys for 41 to 46 months on a low-calcium diet with supplemental aluminum. Mild calcium and aluminum deposition and degenerative changes were found in motor neurons of the substantia nigra, cerebrum, brain stem and spinal cord. The magnitude and extent of these lesions far exceeded those found in normal aged monkeys *(Garruto)*.

In Alzheimer's dementia, there are alterations in cellular calcium regulation throughout the body which are greater than the alterations found in normal aging *(Peterson)*. Calcium absorption may be reduced *(Ferrier)*. In the brain tissue, total calcium levels may be elevated *(Ward)* while ionized calcium may be reduced *(Pavlova)*. Cerebrospinal fluid *(Subhash)*, serum *(Ogihara)*, and hair calcium levels *(Kobayashi)* may all be reduced.

Either chronic low levels of brain calcium or frequent changes in the calcium flux have been theorized to increase the likelihood of plaque and neurofibrillary tangle formation, both typical of Alzheimer's dementia, suggesting that calcium supplementation may provide some protection against cognitive decline *(Deary)*. However, there is also an argument that calcium toxicity in the brain fosters the degenerative process in ischemic brain lesions such as vascular dementia as well as possibly Alzheimer's dementia *(Fritze)*.

Human trials investigating the effect of calcium supplementation on the risk of dementia have not been reported.

Copper Toxicity

Wilson's disease, an inborn error of metabolism characterized by abnormal copper accumulation, can cause mental deterioration if left untreated *(Wilson)*. The initial treatment consists of chelating drugs. (See below for the use of zinc supplementation in Wilson's disease.)

Iron

In the healthy elderly, iron intake has been directly related to cognitive function *(Ortega)*, perhaps because iron deficiency is associated with impaired cognition *(Darnell)*. However, in the brains of Alzheimer patients, iron and iron-regulating proteins may be abnormally distributed *(Connor,1992a)* and transferrin, an iron-binding protein, may malfunction and transport aluminum to the brain *(Connor,1992b)*. Moreover, in these patients, iron may accumulate in specific brain regions, regions where there are severe histopathologic alterations *(Deibel)*.

Iron accumulation in these specific regions may serve as a source of the highly reactive hydroxyl radical. Evidence for this is the finding of redox-active iron in association with the senile plaques and neurofibrillary tangles that are characteristic for the disease *(Smith)*.

Until further research clarifies the relationship between iron intake and the development of dementia, iron supplementation appears contraindicated except to replete a deficiency.

Magnesium Deficiency

In Alzheimer's dementia, both serum *(Lemke)* and hair *(Kobayashi)* levels of magnesium may be reduced and there may be a relative insufficiency of brain tissue magnesium *(Durlach;Glick)*.

Low brain tissue magnesium may be due to low intake or retention of magnesium, high intake of a neurotoxic metal (such as aluminum which inhibits the activity of magnesium-requiring enzymes), or impaired magnesium transport and/or enhanced transport of the neurotoxic metal into brain tissue *(Glick)*; thus magnesium supplementation will not necessarily correct it and has yet to be tested in controlled clinical trials.

Manganese Toxicity

Chronic excessive manganese exposure of manganese is associated with an increased risk of dementia *(Mena)*. However, in Alzheimer's dementia, brain manganese levels appear to be similar to those of non-demented elderly controls *(Markesbery)*.

Selenium Deficiency

Both brain *(Ward)* and blood *(Simonoff)* levels of selenium may be decreased in dementia. This may increase oxidative damage due to reduced activity of the selenium-dependent enzyme glutathione peroxidase *(Castano)*.

While there are no clinical studies, it has been suggested that selenium supplementation may theoretically be helpful *(Clausen)*.

Silicon

The relationship between silicon ingestion and dementia is poorly understood. Silicon has been found in association with aluminum in senile plaques in the form of aluminosilicates, suggesting that they may be involved in the initiation or early stages of senile plaque formation *(Candy)* (see Aluminum below). Moreover, elevated cerebrospinal fluid silicon levels are frequently found in Alzheimer disease *(Hershey)*.

Despite these findings, there is evidence that silicon ingestion reduces the gastrointestinal absorption of aluminum *(Jacqmin-Gadda)* and increases urinary aluminum excretion *(Bellia)*. Although a recent study failed to find an association between lower silicon concentration in drinking water and Alzheimer's disease *(Martyn)*, another noted that high levels of aluminum in the drinking water were only associated with cognitive impairment in the elderly when silica concentrations were low *(Jacqmin-Gadda)*.

Zinc

In the healthy elderly, zinc intake appears to be directly related to cognitive function *(Ortega)* while, in Alzheimer's disease, zinc deficiency appears to enhance the formation of neurofibrillary tangles *(Nachev)*.

Alzheimer patients may have reduced zinc concentrations in the brain tissue *(Corrigan,1989)*. Reduced brain zinc appears to cause a rise in brain aluminum which, in turn, may have an etiologic role in Alzheimer's *(Ward)* (see Aluminum below). Also, it has been theorized that, since most of the enzymes concerned with DNA replication, repair and transcription are zinc metallo-enzymes, decreased incorporation of zinc into those enzymes could lead to neuronal loss *(Burnet)*. Moreover, in a post-mortem study of elderly Nuns, serum zinc levels were negatively correlated with senile plaque counts *(Tully)*.

There are reasons to believe that the role of zinc in dementia is complex. While some studies show that total zinc is significantly reduced in several brain regions in Alzheimer victims, zinc has been shown to enhance the aggregation of beta-amyloid protein, the main component of the senile plaques found in the brains of patients with the disease *(Cuajungco)*. It has also been found to be elevated in the hair and nails of Alzheimer patients *(Vance)*.

Due to its nutritional importance, however, zinc is considered unlikely to promote the development of the disorder *(Cuajungco)*. In fact, in 2 small open trials, Alzheimer patients given zinc supplementation showed modest cognitive improvement over time *(Constantinidis; Potocnik)*.

Also, in cases of Wilson's disease that have already been treated with a copper-chelating agent, maintenance therapy with zinc acetate, by preventing the intestinal absorption of copper, has been found to be a safe and effective treatment *(Anderson)*.

An 82-year-old woman had become increasingly confused and forgetful and was having increasing difficulty looking after her 84-year-old husband who had recently suffered a disabling stroke. The quality of her diet had been deteriorating.

On examination, she was in good health but her memory was impaired. Blood testing revealed no evidence of anemia, kidney, liver or thyroid disease, but her alkaline phosphatase was depressed, a finding that could be due to zinc deficiency, and her blood zinc concentration was only two-thirds of normal.

She was placed on a multivitamin supplement along with additional zinc. This was followed by a marked improvement in mental function. She became better able to care for her husband and noted how much less confused and more mentally alert she now was (Davies).

OTHER NUTRITIONAL FACTORS

Beta-carotene

A low intake of beta-carotene is related to cognitive impairment among the elderly *(Ortega)*. Moreover, plasma beta-carotene levels are correlated with memory performance is this age group *(Perrig)*. Multi-infarct dementia is associated with low plasma levels, while plasma beta-carotene levels in Alzheimer's dementia have been both reported to be both higher *(Singh)* and lower *(Zaman)* than those of age-matched normals.

The efficacy of carotenoid supplementation in dementia has not been tested.

Carnitine

Carnitine is required for mitochondrial transport of long-chain fatty acids for beta-oxidation and may also have a role in neurotransmitter metabolism. Alzheimer's disease patients have decreased brain content of acetylcholine, and choline is structurally related to carnitine *(Bowman)*.

Acetyl-carnitine is a patented natural derivative of L-carnitine formed by acetylation. In dementia, is appears to be reduced in erythrocytes, although not in brain tissue *(Corrigan, 1995)*. The results of numerous double-blind studies have suggested that supplementation of acetyl-carnitine may be beneficial *(Thal)* and may slow the natural course of Alzheimer's dementia *(Carta)*. Elderly patients with just mild mental impairment have shown improvements in memory as well as in mental, emotional, behavioral and depression test scores which last at least one month after the supplement is discontinued *(Salvioli)*.

The benefits of acetyl-carnitine appear to be due, not only to its cholinergic properties, but also to its ability to support physiological cellular functioning at the mitochondrial level. It is thought to exhibit restorative and even protective actions against aging processes and neurodegeneration *(Carta)*.

Choline

Cholinergic mechanisms are involved in normal memory functioning and age-related memory loss, and a decline in the functioning of the cholinergic system in the brain is related to Alzheimer's dementia. For example, in a study of Alzheimer's patients, the theoretical choline uptake into choline-depleted red blood cells was strongly correlated with the severity of the dementia *(Kanof)*, and choline acetyl-transferase activity (which normally declines with aging) is lower in Alzheimer's patients than in age-matched controls *(White)*.

Supplementation with choline, phosphatidylcholine or lecithin has demonstrated only modest success at best in affecting the illness *(Dysken)*. However, the results of more recent studies utilizing *citicoline* (cytidine 5'-diphosphocholine), an essential intermediate in the biosynthesis of the structural phospholipids of cell membranes, have been more promising.

Citicoline increases noradrenaline and dopamine levels in the CNS and has improved learning and memory performance in animal models of brain aging. In patients with cognitive impairment due to chronic cerebral ischemia, it improves scores on cognitive evaluation scales, while in patients with senile dementia of the Alzheimer's type, it slows the disease's evolution *(Secades)*.

Inositol

In a double-blind crossover study, the response of Alzheimer patients to inositol versus a glucose placebo was studied. After one month, there were significant improvements in orientation and language with inositol, and an insignificant improvement in cognition. Higher dosages given for a longer period of time may possibly be more effective *(Barak)*.

Phosphatidylserine

Supplementation with phosphatidylserine, the major acidic phospholipid in the brain, has generated much interest in the treatment of Alzheimer's disease. In the elderly, supplementation appears to increase dopamine release from the striatum and stimulate acetylcholine release from the cerebral cortex. It may also prevent age-induced loss of dendritic spines in the hippocampal pyramidal neurons and atrophy of cholinergic cells in the basal forebrain *(Crook)*.

The initial studies were done with a product derived from the brain cortex of cows. In numerous double-blind studies, bovine brain-derived phosphatidylserine was shown to improve both behavior and cognition in elderly patients with moderate to severe cognitive decline *(Cenacchi)*. However, as the greatest improvements were after 2 and 4 months, it appeared that they were largely short-term *(Heiss)*.

More recently, the bovine product has been taken off the market and a soy-derived product has become available. Due to differences in their composition, there is some question as to whether the two products are equivalent, although it is likely that they are equally effective *(Kidd)*.

S-Adenosyl-L-Methionine

The major methyl donor of the brain, S-adenosyl-L-methionine (SAMe) may be reduced in the cerebrospinal fluid of dementia patients *(Bottiglieri)*.

Although an open trial was unsuccessful *(Cohen)*, a small double-blind study of SAMe supplementation found improved measures of mood, cognitive function and the speed of mental processing *(Reynolds)*.

OTHER RELATED FACTORS

Heavy Metal Toxicity

Aluminum

The role of aluminum in causing dementia is highly controversial, although evidence for a pathogenic role is growing *(Lukiw)*. While the presence of aluminum in neurofibrillary tangles is well established, it is the question of whether aluminum contributes to the development of the lesions which has not been fully answered.

Among the several lines of evidence suggesting that aluminum exposure may promote the development of dementia, there are epidemiologic studies which have found an association between aluminum in drinking water, especially when the silica concentrations are low, and the prevalence of Alzheimer's dementia *(Jacqmin-Gadda)*. In an animal model, aluminum produces neurofibrillary degeneration in the brain that resembles Alzheimer's disease *(Beal)* and, in humans, aluminum is found in association with neurofibrillary tangles *(Good)*.

In addition, serum levels of aluminum have been reported to be higher in Alzheimer's disease patients than in healthy controls *(Zapatero)* and the use of desferrioxamine, an aluminum chelator, reduced the rate of decline of Alzheimer's patients by one-half *(McLachlan)*.

Other studies have refuted the aluminum-dementia connection. For example, in one study, no relationship was found between aluminum and silica in drinking water and Alzheimer risk *(Martyn)*. Using improved analytic techniques, no evidence was found of the presence of aluminum in brain lesions from Alzheimer patients *(Makjanic;Landsberg)*, suggesting that conventional techniques may have produced artifactual results.

Until the question of whether aluminum is causative is answered, it would seem prudent to reduce aluminum exposure. Insuring adequate zinc nutriture may also be protective, since sub-optimal zinc status may facilitate a increase in brain aluminum *(Wenk)*.

Mercury

An increased body mercury burden appears to be related to Alzheimer's dementia. For example, brain mercury concentrations in patients were found to be almost double that of age-matched controls *(Grant)*. One study found blood mercury concentrations to be more than double *(Hock)* - although another failed to confirm this difference *(Fung)*. Both selenium and zinc protect against mercury toxicity, while in isolated subcellular fractions of temporal lobe tissue, there were increased ratios of mercury to selenium and of mercury to zinc, suggesting that selenium and zinc were being utilized to detoxify mercury *(Wenstrup)*.

Still controversial is whether the increased mercury load is causative, or whether it is a secondary phenomenon of the disease process.

Gluten Sensitivity

Gluten sensitivity should be especially considered as a possible etiologic agent in presenile dementia, since the neurologic manifestations of celiac disease include dementia *(Cooke)*. Notable is the finding that celiac patients who develop presenile dementia usually have only mild gastrointestinal symptoms *(Collin)*.

Hydrochloric Acid Deficiency

As many as 30% of people over age 65 are deficient, primarily related to atrophic gastritis, and the prevalence increases with age *(Russell,1986)*. Such patients have significantly reduced ability to absorb both folic acid and protein-bound vitamin B_{12} *(Russell,1987)* and, as discussed above, the resulting deficiencies may promote the development of dementia.

BIBLIOGRAPHY

Abalan F. Alzheimer's disease: The nutritional hypothesis. J Orthomol Med 3(1):13-17, 1988

Aghayewa MO et al. Pyridoxine, ascorbic acid and thiamine in Alzheimer and comparison subjects. Can J Psychiatry 37(9):661-2, 1992

Anderson LA et al. Zinc acetate treatment in Wilson's disease. Ann Pharmacother 32(1):78-87, 1998

Barabas J et al. Ascorbic acid in cerebrospinal fluid - a possible protection against free radicals in the brain. Arch Gerontol Geriatr 21:43-8, 1995

Barak Y et al. Inositol treatment of Alzheimer's disease a double-blind, cross-over placebo controlled trial. Prog Neuro-Psychopharmacol Biol Psychiatry 20:729-35, 1996

Beal MF et al. Neurochemical characteristics of aluminum-induced neurofibrillary degeneration in rabbits. Neuroscience 29(2):339-46, 1989

Behl C et al. Vitamin E protects nerve cells from amyloid B protein toxicity. Biochem Biophys Res Commun 186:944-50, 1992

Bellia JP et al. The role of silicic acid in the renal excretion of aluminum. Ann Clin Lab Sci 26:227-33, 1996

Birkmayer JGD. Coenzyme nicotinamide adenine dinucleotide`: new therapeutic approach for improving dementia of the Alzheimer type. Ann Clin Lab Sci 26(1):1-9, 1996

Blass JP et al. Thiamine and Alzheimer's disease. A pilot study. Arch Neurol 45:833-35, 1988

Bottiglieri T et al. Cerebrospinal fluid S-adenosylmethionine in depression and dementia: effects of treatment with parenteral and oral S-adenosylmethionine. J Neurol Neurosurg Psychiatry 53(12):1096-8, 1990

Bowman BAB. Acetyl-carnitine and Alzheimer's disease. Nutr Rev 50(5):142-4, 1992

Burnet FM. A possible role of zinc in the pathology of dementia. Lancet i:186-88, 1981

Candy JM et al. Aluminosilicates and senile plaque formation in Alzheimer's disease. Lancet i:354-7, 1986

Carta A, Calvani M. Acetyl-L-carnitine: a drug able to slow the progress of Alzheimer's disease? Ann N Y Acad Sci 640:228-32, 1991

Castano A et al. Low selenium diet affects monoamine turnover differentially in substantia nigra and striatum. J Neurochem 61:1302-7, 1993

Cenacchi T et al. Cognitive decline in the elderly: a double-blind placebo-controlled multicenter study on the efficacy of phosphatidylserine administration. Aging Clin Exp Res 5:123-33, 1993

Clausen J. Demential syndromes and the lipid metabolism. Acta Neurol Scand 70(5):345-55, 1984

Cohen BM et al. S-adenosyl-L-methionine in the treatment of Alzheimer's disease. J Clin Psychopharmacol 8(1):43-7, 1988

Collin P et al. Celiac disease, brain atrophy, and dementia. Neurology 41(3):372-5, 1991

Connor JR et al. A histochemical study of iron, transferrin, and ferritin in Alzheimer's diseased brains. J Neurosci Res 31(1):75-83, 1992a

Connor JR, Benkovic SA. Iron regulation in the brain: histochemical, biochemical, and molecular considerations. Ann Neurol 32:34-44, 1992b

Constantinidis J. [Alzheimer's dementia and zinc.] Schweiz Arch Neurol Psychiatr 141(6):523-56, 1990 (in German)

Cooke WT. Neurologic manifestations of malabsorption, in Handbook of Clinical Neurology, Volume 28, Metabolic and Deficiency Diseases of the Nervous System, Part II. Amsterdam: North-Holland Publishing Co. 1976:225-41

Corrigan FM et al. Aluminium and Alzheimer's disease. Letter. Lancet ii:268-9, 1989

Corrigan FM et al. Carnitine and acetyl-L-carnitine content of human hippocampus and erythrocytes in Alzheimer's disease. J Nutr Environ Med 5:35-9, 1995

Crellin R et al. Folates and psychiatric disorders. Clinical potential. Drugs 45(5):623-36, 1993

Crook T et al. Effects of phosphatidylserine in Alzheimer's disease. Psychopharmacol Bull 28(1):61-6, 1992

Cuajungco Math P, Lees GJ. Zinc and Alzheimer's disease: is there a direct link? Brain Res Rev 23:219-36, 1997

Darnell LS, Sandstead HH. Iron, zinc and cognition of women. Abstract. Am J Clin Nutr 53:P-16, 1991

Davies S, Stewart A. Nutritional Medicine. London, Pan Books, 1987

Deary IJ, Hendrickson AE. Calcium and Alzheimer's disease. Letter. Lancet i:1219, 1986

Deibel MA et al. Copper, iron, and zinc imbalances in severely degenerated brain regions in Alzheimer's disease: possible relation to oxidative stress. J Neurol Sci 143(1-2):137-42, 1996

Deijen JB et al. Vitamin B6 supplementation in elderly men. Effects on mood, memory, performance, and mental effort. Psychopharmacology 109:489-96, 1992

Durlach J. Magnesium depletion and pathogenesis of Alzheimer's disease. Letter. Magnes Res 3(3):217-8, 1990

Dysken M. A review of recent clinical trials in the treatment of Alzheimer's disease. Psychiatric Annals 17(3):178, 1987

Eisinger J et al. Erythrocyte transketolase in Alzheimer's disease: the thiamin hypothesis. J Adv Med 7(2):69-75, 1994

Evans JR. Alzheimer's dementia: Some possible mechanisms related to vitamins, trace elements and minerals, suggesting a possible treatment. J Orthomol Med 1(4):249-54, 1987

Ferrier IN et al. Reduced gastrointestinal absorption of calcium in dementia. Age Ageing 19(6):368-75, 1990

Foster HD. Health, Disease and the Environment. Boca Raton, CRC Press, 1992:311-16

Frank O et al. Superiority of periodic intramuscular vitamins over daily oral vitamins in maintaining normal vitamin titers in a geriatric population. Am J Clin Nutr 30:630, 1977

Fritze J, Walden J. Clinical findings with nimodipine in dementia: test of the calcium hypothesis. J Neural Transm Suppl 46:439-53, 1995

Fung YK et al. Brain mercury in neurodegenerative disorders. J Toxicol Clin Toxicol 35(1):49-54, 1997

Gale CR et al. Cognitive impairment and mortality in a cohort of elderly people. BMJ 312:608-11, 1996

Garruto RM et al. Low-calcium, high-aluminum diet-induced motor neuron pathology in cynomolgus monkeys. Acta Neuropathol (Berl) 78(2):210-9, 1989

Geland B. Presentation to the European College of Neuropsychopharmacology - reported in Clin Psychiatry News, September, 1989

Gibson GE et al. Reduced activities of thiamine-dependent enzymes in the brains and peripheral tissues of patients with Alzheimer's disease. Arch Neurol 45:836-40, 1988

Glick JL. Dementias: the role of magnesium deficiency and an hypothesis concerning the pathogenesis of Alzheimer's disease. Med Hypotheses 31(3):211-25, 1990

Gold M et al. Plasma and red blood cell thiamine deficiency in patients with dementia of the Alzheimer's type. Arch Neurol 52(11):1081-6, 1995

Good PF et al. Selective accumulation of aluminum and iron in the neurofibrillary tangles of Alzheimer's disease: a laser microprobe (LAMMA) study. Ann Neurol 31:286-92, 1992

Goodman M et al. Are U.S. lower normal B12 limits too low? J Am Geriatr Soc 44(10):1274-5, 1996

Grant WB. Dietary links to Alzheimer's disease. Alzheimer's Dis Rev 2:42-55, 1997

Heiss WD et al. Long-term effects of phosphatidylserine, pyritinol, and cognitive training in Alzheimer's disease. A neuropsychological, EEG, and PET investigation. Dementia 5(2):88-98, 1994

Hershey CO et al. Cerebrospinal fluid trace element content in dementia: Clinical, radiologic, and pathologic correlations. Neurology 33(10):1350-3, 1983

Hock C et al. Increased blood mercury levels in patients with Alzheimer's disease. J Neural Transm 105(1):59-68, 1998

Hoffer A. Vitamin B-3: niacin and its amide. Townsend Letter for Doctors and Patients October, 1995:30-9

Ikeda T et al. Vitamin B12 levels in serum and cerebrospinal fluid of people with Alzheimer's disease. Acta Psychiatr Scand 82(4):327-9, 1990

Jacqmin-Gadda H et al. Silica and aluminum in drinking water and cognitive impairment in the elderly. Epidemiology 7(3):281-5, 1996

Jama JW et al. Dietary antioxidants and cognitive function in a population-based sample of older persons. The Rotterdam study. Am J Epidemiol 144:275-9, 1996

Joosten E et al. Is metabolic evidence for vitamin B-12 and folate deficiency more frequent in elderly patients with Alzheimer's disease? J Gerontol A Biol Sci Med Sci 52(2):M76-M79, 1997

Kalmijn S et al. Polyunsaturated fatty acids, antioxidants, and cognitive function in very old men. Am J Epidemiol 145(1):33-41, 1997

Kanof P. Red blood cell choline. Biol Psychiatry 20:375-83, 1985

Kasahara H et al. Alcohol dementia and alcohol delirium in aged alcoholics. Psychiatry Clin Neurosci 50(3):115-23, 1996

Kidd P. Phosphatidylserine: membrane nutrient for memory. A clinical and mechanistic assessment. Altern Med Rev 1(2):70-84, 1996

Kobayashi S et al. Hair aluminum in normal aged and senile dementia of Alzheimer type. Prog Clin Biol Res 317:1095-109, 1989

Landsberg JP et al. Absence of aluminum in neuritic plaque cores in Alzheimer's disease. Nature 360:65-8, 1992

Lemke MR. Plasma magnesium decrease and altered calcium/magnesium ratio in severe dementia of the Alzheimer type. Biol Psychiatry 37:341-3, 1995

Lukiw WJ. Alzheimer's disease and aluminum, in Mineral and Metal Neurotoxicology. CRC Press, 1997:113-26

Makjanic J et al. Absence of aluminium in neurofibrillary tangles in Alzheimer's disease. Neurosci Lett 240(3):123-6, 1998

Markesbery WR et al. Brain manganese concentrations in human aging and Alzheimer's disease. Neurotoxicology 5(1):49-57, 1984

Martin DC et al. Time dependency of cognitive recovery with cobalamin replacement: report of a pilot study. J Am Geriatr Soc 40(2):168-72, 1992

Martyn CN et al. Aluminum concentrations in drinking water and risk of Alzheimer's disease. Epidemiology 8(3):281-86, 1997

Mastrogiacomo F et al. Brain thiamine, its phosphate esters, and its metabolizing enzymes in Alzheimer's disease. Ann Neurol 39:585-91, 1996

McLachlan DRC et al. Intramuscular desferrioxamine in patients with Alzheimer's disease. Lancet 337:1304-8, 1991

Meador KJ et al. Evidence for a central cholinergic effect of high-dose thiamine. Ann Neurol 34(5):724-6, 1993a

Meador K et al. Preliminary findings of high-dose thiamine in dementia of Alzheimer's type. J Geriatr Psychiatry Neurol 6(4):222-9, 1993b

Melamed E et al. Reversible central nervous system dysfunction in folate deficiency. J Neurol Sci 25:93-98, 1975

Mena I. Manganese, in F. Bronner, JW Coburn Eds. Disorders of Mineral Metabolism. I. Trace Minerals. New York, Academic Press, 1981:233-70

Meydani M et al. Effect of vitamin E, selenium and age on lipid peroxidation events in rat cerebrum. Nutr Res 5:1227-36, 1985

Morris MC et al. Vitamin E and vitamin C supplement use and risk of incident Alzheimer disease. Alzheimer Dis Assoc Disord 12(3):121-6, 1998

Nachev PC, Larner AJ. Zinc and Alzheimer's disease. Trace Elem Electrolytes 13(2):55-9, 1996

Nolan KA et al. A trial of thiamine and Alzheimer's disease. Arch Neurol 48(1):81-3, 1991

Ogihara T et al. Possible participation of calcium-regulating factors in senile dementia in elderly female subjects. Gerentology 36 Suppl 1:25-30, 1990

Orgogozo JM et al. Wine consumption and dementia in the elderly: a prospective community study in the Bordeaux area. Rev Neurol (Paris) 153(3):185-92, 1997

Ortega RM et al. Dietary intake and cognitive function in a group of elderly people. Am J Clin Nutr 66:803-09 1997

Passeri M et al. Oral 5'-methyltetrahydrofolic acid in senile organic mental disorders with depression: results of a double-blind multicenter study. Aging (Milano) 5(1):63-71, 1993

Pavlova GA. [Content of amino acids, ionized forms of calcium and acetylcholinesterase in the cerebral cortex in senile dementia.] Zh Nevropatol Psikhiatr 84(7):1012-6, 1984

Perrig WJ et al. The relation between antioxidants and memory performance in the old and very old. J Am Geriatr Soc 45:718-24, 1997

Peterson C, Goldman JE. Alterations in calcium content and biochemical processes in cultured skin fibroblasts from aged and Alzheimer donors. Proc Natl Acad Sci USA 83(8):2758-62, 1996

Potocnik FC et al. Zinc and platelet membrane microviscosity in Alzheimer's disease. The in vivo effect of zinc on platelet membranes and cognition. S Afr Med J 87(9):1116-9, 1997

Rall L, Meydani S. Vitamin B6 and immune competence. Nutr Rev 51:217-25, 1993

Reynolds EH et al. S-adenosylmethionine and Alzheimer's disease. Abstract. Neurology 39(Suppl):397, 1989

Riggs KM et al. Relations of vitamin B-12, vitamin B-6, folate, and homocysteine to cognitive performance in the Normative Aging Study. Am J Clin Nutr 63:306-14, 1996

Russell RM et al. Folic acid malabsorption in atrophic gastritis: possible compensation by bacterial folate synthesis. Gastroenterology 91:1476-82, 1986

Russell RM et al. Decreased bioavailability of protein bound vitamin B-12 in mild atrophic gastritis: reversal by antibiotics. Abstract. Gastroenterology 92:1606, 1987

Salvioli G, Neri M. L-acetylcarnitine treatment of mental decline in the elderly. Drugs Exp Clin Res 20(4):169-76, 1994

Sano M et al. A controlled trial of selegiline, alpha-tocopherol, or both as treatment for Alzheimer's disease. N Engl J Med 336:1216-22, 1997

Sawada M et al. Tyrosine hydroxylase, tryptophan hydroxylase, biopterin, and neopterin in the brains of normal controls and patients with senile dementia of Alzheimer type. J Neurochem 48(3):760-4, 1987

Secades JJ, Frontera G. CDP-choline: pharmacological and clinical review. Methods Find Exp Clin Pharmacol 17 Suppl B:2-54, 1995

Simonoff M et al. Serum and erythrocyte selenium in normal and pathological states in France. Trace Elem Med 5:64-9, 1988

Singh S et al. Carotenaemia in Alzheimer's disease. Br Med J 297:458-9, 1988

Smith MA et al. Iron accumulation in Alzheimer disease is a source of redox-generated free radicals. Proc Natl Acad Sci U S A 94(18):9866-8, 1997

Spivak JL, Jackson DL. Pellagra: an analysis of 18 patients and a review of the literature. Johns Hopkins Med J 140(6):295-309, 1977

Stott DJ et al. Prevalence of hemopoietic effects of low serum vitamin B12 levels in geriatric medical patients. Br J Nutr 78:57-63, 1997

Subhash MN et al. Calcium and phosphorus levels in serum and CSF in dementia. Neurobiol Aging 12(4):267-9, 1991

Tenisse S et al. Dementia and subnormal levels of vitamin B12: Effects of replacement therapy on dementia. J Neurol 243:522-9, 1996

Thal LJ et al. A 1-year multicenter placebo-controlled study of acetyl-L-carnitine in patients with Alzheimer's disease. Neurology 47:705-11, 1996

Thomas DE et al. Tryptophan and nutritional status of patients with senile dementia. Psychol Med 16(2):297-305, 1986

Tully CL et al. Serum zinc, senile plaques, and neurofibrillary tangles: findings from the Nun study. Aging 13:6(16):2105-8, 1995

Vance DE et al. Trace element imbalances in hair and nails of Alzheimer's disease patients. Neurotoxicology 9(2):197-208, 1988

Vrecko K et al. Stimulation of dopamine biosynthesis in cultured PC 12 phaeochromocytoma cells by the coenzyme nicotinamide adeninedinucleotide (NADH). J Neurol Transm Park Dis Dement Sect 5(2):147-56, 1993

Ward NI, Mason JA. Neutron activation analysis techniques for identifying elemental status in Alzheimer's disease. J Radioanalyt Nucl Chem 113(2):515-26, 1987

Wenk GI. Stemmer KL. Sub-optimal dietary zinc increases aluminum accumulation in the rat brain. Brain Res 288:393-95, 1983

Wenstrup D et al. Trace element imbalances in isolated subcellular fractions of Alzheimer's disease brains. Brain Res 533(1):125-31, 1990

West BD. Aluminosilicates and Alzheimer's disease. Letter. Lancet ii:682, 1985

White P et al. Neocortical cholinergic neurons in elderly people. Lancet i:668-71, 1977

Wilson SA. Progressive lenticular degeneration: A familial nervous disease associated with cirrhosis of the liver. Brain 34:296, 1912

Zaman Z et al. Plasma concentrations of vitamins A and E and carotenoids in Alzheimer's disease. Age Aging 21:91-4, 1992

Zapatero MD. Serum aluminum levels in Alzheimer's disease and other senile dementias. Biol Trace Elem Res 47:235-40, 1995

DEPRESSION

See Also: BIPOLAR DISORDER
CELIAC DISEASE
'HYPOGLYCEMIA'
INSOMNIA
ORGANIC MENTAL DISORDERS
PREMENSTRUAL SYNDROME

NUTRITIONAL TREATMENT GUIDE

✓ = Efficacy generally accepted.
* = Efficacy *demonstrated* by controlled human trials.
[+] = Efficacy *suspected* from uncontrolled human trials.
[-] = Efficacy *suspected* from indirect data.
? = Efficacy *challenged* in a study of similar design.

DIETARY FACTORS

* avoid **Caffeine**
* avoid **simple Sugars**

- -

[+] **low Fat, high Complex Carbohydrate diet**
[+] Consume **Fish** (to increase omega-3 fatty acid intake)
[+] avoid **Alcohol**

- -

[-] consume **Soluble Fiber**

NUTRITIONAL FACTORS

✓ **Lithium (pharmacologic dosage):** lithium carbonate 900-1800 mg daily (by prescription)

- -

* **Calcium:** 1000 mg twice daily *AND*
Vitamin D: 600 IU twice daily (4 week trial)
* **Carnitine:** acetyl-L-carnitine 500 mg 4 times daily
* **Folic acid deficiency:** 800 µg daily
* **L-5-Hydroxytryptophan:** start with 25 mg daily and increase as tolerated over 10-14 days to 75mg 3 times daily with meals (14 day trial)
* **Inositol:** 12 g daily (2 tsp in juice twice daily) (1 month trial)
* **Iron deficiency:** ferrous sulfate 300 mg 3 times daily
* **Lithium (nutritional dosage):** 400 µg daily
* **D-, L-, or D,L-Phenylalanine:** Start with 100 mg twice daily. Increase gradually if needed as tolerated up to 2 g 3 times daily. Combine each dose with **Vitamin B_6** 50 mg. (14 day trial)

* **Phosphatidylserine:** 300 mg daily (1 month trial)
* **S-Adenosyl-L-Methionine:** 800 mg twice daily (14 day trial)
* **Selenium deficiency:** 200 µg daily
* **Thiamine:** 50 mg daily
* **L-Tryptophan:** 2 g 3 times daily (14 day trial)
* **Vitamin B_6:** *for women on oral contraceptives:* 40 mg daily
* **Vitamin B_{12}:** ? 1000 µg by injection repeated as needed
* **Vitamin C deficiency:** 500 mg twice daily
* **Vitamin C:** ? 1 g daily
* ? **L-Tyrosine:** 2 g 3 times daily (100 mg/kg) in 3 divided doses (14 day trial)

- -

[+] avoid **Choline**
[+] **Magnesium deficiency:** ≈ 400 mg daily
[+] **Niacin deficiency:** 50 to 100 mg daily
[+] **Niacin:** nicotinamide adenine dinucleotide (NADH) 5 mg daily
[+] **Omega-3 fatty acid deficiency:** *example:* MaxEPA 1 g caps [180 mg EPA; 120 mg DHA] 10 to 20 daily
[+] **Potassium deficiency:** 20 to 80 mEq daily in excess of losses, preferably from potassium-rich foods
[+] **Riboflavin deficiency:** 5 to 10 mg daily
[+] **Rubidium:** rubidium chloride 180 mg 3 times daily
[+] **Thiamine deficiency:** 50 mg daily
[+] **Vitamin B_6 deficiency:** 50 to 100 mg daily
[+] **Vitamin B_{12} deficiency:** 1,000 µg intramuscularly weekly initially and monthly afterwards
[+] **Zinc deficiency:** zinc sulfate 220 mg twice daily *AND* **Copper** 2 mg daily

OTHER RELATED FACTORS

* rule out **Food Sensitivities**

- -

[+] rule out **Aluminum** toxicity
[+] rule out **Hydrochloric Acid** deficiency
[+] rule out **Lead** toxicity

DIETARY FACTORS

Low Fat, High Complex Carbohydrate Diet

There is some evidence that the composition of the diet may affect mood. While controlled trials are lacking, it appears that a low fat, high complex carbohydrate diet may be associated with a better emotional state than the typical high fat, high refined carbohydrate Western diet. In one study, for example, people who switched from a Western diet to a low fat, high complex carbohydrate diet for the goal of reducing plasma cholesterol levels demonstrated significant improvements in depression and aggressive hostility *(Weidner)*.

The results of a few epidemiological studies have suggested the same conclusion. In a study of dietary habits in 16 Western European nations, suicide rates were associated with the total fat supply *per capita* as well as the fat supply *per capita* from meats and offals, while neither the total calorie intake nor the protein intake was related to the risk of suicide *(Lester)*. Also, compared to apparently healthy controls, a group of patients with a 2 to 5 month history of depression was found to have a significantly lower dietary intake of soluble fiber *(Singh)*.

Mood-Altering Dietary Substances

Simple sugars (especially sucrose), caffeine and alcohol share some of the same complex characteristics in regard to their effects on depression. They are used by people to improve mood when they feel depressed; yet there is evidence that their use may increase depression. We will discuss each substance separately.

Sugar

Simple sugars, especially sucrose, are often attractive to people feeling "low" because of their mood-enhancing qualities *(Willner)*. When the diets of depressed patients were compared with those of normals, carbohydrate consumption was higher in the depressed group, primarily from increased sucrose consumption *(Christensen,1996)*. This may be related to the finding that depressed patients have an impaired rate of glucose utilization with insulin resistance *(Wright JH)*, while sucrose rapidly increases serum glucose levels *(Charles)*.

Despite sugar's mood-enhancing effects, some individuals experience amelioration of depression following the elimination of sugar from their diet, and a worsening mood when sugar is returned *(Christensen,1991)*. This effect has been demonstrated in a double-blind case report *(Christensen,1985)*. The frequency that sugar intake promotes depression is unknown.

Caffeine

Caffeine is well recognized as a psychostimulant. It quickens reaction time, enhances vigilance, and improves mood *(Rogers)*. At the same time, caffeine deprivation may rapidly produce a withdrawal syndrome which is adverse enough to cause the victim to seek relief by imbibing more caffeine. In fact, one of the major factors motivating caffeine consumption appears to be "withdrawal relief" *(Rogers)*. This syndrome starts within hours and may occur in people who drink less than average amounts of caffeine *(Strain)* and may be sufficiently intense to make people depressed *(Silverman)*.

In addition, chronic caffeine ingestion may contribute to a chronically depressed mood state, as higher levels of regular caffeine intake have repeatedly been shown to be associated with depression *(Gilliland)*. An example is a study of hospitalized psychiatric patients who consumed in excess of 750 mg of caffeine daily. Half of them scored in the severely depressed range on the Beck Depression Inventory. This was a significantly greater percentage of patients than either moderate or low caffeine users in the same population *(Greden)*.

Sugar and Caffeine Elimination Diet

Investigators asked 23 people experiencing unexplained depression to consume a caffeine- and refined-sucrose-free diet for one week. Those whose symptoms improved were challenged double-blind with caffeine, cellulose (placebo), a sucrose-sweetened Kool-Aid drink, and an aspartame-sweetened Kool-Aid drink (placebo) in random order, each for 6 consecutive days. About half of the subjects experienced a return of their mood disturbance and symptoms when challenged with caffeine and sucrose, but not when challenged with the placebos, suggesting that both caffeine and sucrose may be frequent contributors to depression and related complaints *(Kreitsch)*.

Alcohol

While people often drink alcoholic beverages to improve their mood, alcohol may promote depression by reducing brain levels of serotonin *(Goodwin)* and catecholamines *(Cottereau)*. People with genetically low serotonin levels may crave alcohol because it transiently increases serotonin turnover. However, once its immediate effects are gone, serotonin levels will be lower than before imbibing the alcoholic beverage *(Goodwin)*.

Moreover, alcohol abuse is associated with a well-defined withdrawal syndrome that includes depression *(Winokur)*.

NUTRITIONAL FACTORS

NEUROTRANSMITTER PRECURSORS

Since neurotransmitters are derived from dietary precursors, supplementation with selected precursors of neurotransmitters known to relate to mood regulation has met with some success.

Serotonin Precursors

L-Tryptophan

The neurotransmitter serotonin (5-hydroxytryptamine) is derived from L-tryptophan following conversion to 5-hydroxytryptophan. There is evidence from a variety of sources that inadequate dietary intake of the amino acid promotes depression. A tryptophan-depleted diet may lower mood in people with a history *(Smith)* - or even with a family history *(Benkelfat)* - of affective illness. When dietary intakes of L-tryptophan from several English-speaking countries were compared, a low tryptophan intake was associated with a high suicide rate *(Kitahara,1987a)*. Furthermore, a decreased ratio of tryptophan to other amino acids competing for brain transport may be associated with depression *(Maes,1996a)*.

Hospitalized patients with primary unipolar depressions may have decreased free plasma tryptophan levels which improve upon recovery *(Coppen)*, while a low-tryptophan diet may cause relapse in recovering depressives *(Delgado)*. A low concentration of 5-HIAA (the major metabolite of serotonin) in the cerebrospinal fluid is positively correlated with strong suicidal thoughts, suicidal attempts and self-aggressivity *(Lopez-Ibor)*.

Supplementation

Double-blind studies have found L-tryptophan supplementation to be similar in efficacy to imipramine, amitriptyline and mianserin. However, because of their small sample size, and the mixed results of studies comparing tryptophan to placebo, some doubt remains about its efficacy *(Young)*. It has been suggested that there may be a therapeutic window, as the negative studies have tended to use daily doses above 6 grams *(Walinder)*.

Tryptophan should be given with a carbohydrate (as insulin lowers peripheral levels of amino acids competing for transport across the blood-brain barrier), and no protein should be eaten for 90 minutes either before or after its ingestion.

L-5-Hydroxytryptophan

Supplementation with L-5-hydroxytryptophan, the metabolite of tryptophan and immediate precursor of serotonin, also appears promising, and may be superior to L-tryptophan *(van Praag,1984)*. There is evidence that the transport of 5-hydroxytryptophan is compromised in major depression *(Agren)*. The results of controlled studies suggest that it may have antidepressant properties which are roughly equal to those of antidepressant medications *(van Praag,1986)*. Since the most common side effects are gastrointestinal, supplementation should be taken at mealtimes.

The efficacy of the serotonin precursors appears to be due to their ability to treat the anxiety/aggressive component of depressive syndromes *(van Praag,1987)*. They appear to be most effective for depressed patients presenting with anxiety and/or agitation, and for patients with acute endogenous depressions *(Zmilacher)*.

Norepinephrine Precursors

Phenylalanine

The neurotransmitter norepinephrine is derived from L-phenylalanine following conversion to L-tyrosine. L-phenylalanine can also be decarboxylated to 2-phenylethylamine (PEA) in a reaction which requires vitamin B_6. PEA is an amphetamine-like neurotransmitter that may affect both mood and attention, and a deficit of brain PEA is believed to lead to certain forms of depression. Since phenylacetic acid (PAA) is a metabolite of PEA, urinary PAA levels are used as a measure of brain PEA. Urinary phenylacetic acid levels are reduced in depression, and the more severe the depression, the lower the levels. Moreover, in studies of antidepressant drugs, urinary PAA levels rise towards normal when the drug is effective.

In a study reported in the *Journal of Clinical Psychiatry*, patients with major depression had significantly lower plasma and 24-hour urinary PAA levels than normals. When 40 of these patients were supplemented with L-phenylalanine, 31 of them (almost 80%) improved almost immediately, and PAA levels rose concomitantly. Side effects consisted of slight, transient headaches, constipation, transient nausea, insomnia and increased anxiety *(Sabelli)*.

D-phenylalanine, since it can be converted by the liver into L-phenylalanine, the natural form in humans, has similar effects to those of its stereoisomer and has been found to be as effective as imipramine under double-blind conditions *(Heller)*. D,L-phenylalanine, the synthetic form, has also been found to be as effective as imipramine under double-blind conditions *(Beckmann)*.

Short-term side effects include elevation of blood pressure, headache, irritability, aggressiveness and insomnia, while long-term side effects have not been studied *(Simonson)*. Phenylalanine treatment is believed to be contraindicated for schizophrenics *(Yarayura-Tobias)*.

Tyrosine

The results of small double-blind studies have suggested that L-tyrosine supplementation may be effective for some unipolar depressives *(Gelenberg,1980;Gibson)*. As with phenylalanine, tyrosine supplementation may cause stimulant-type side effects.

A 22 year-old woman was suffering from sleepiness, lethargy and loss of appetite. Her weight had fallen to 92 pounds. A nursing student, her depression had caused her work to deteriorate so badly that she was forced to leave the university. Her blood tyrosine level was low, while her phenylalanine level was normal.

She was started on tyrosine with doses up to 6 grams daily. Her depression slowly remitted. Eventually she was able to return to school on a maintenance dose of 1500 mg 3 times daily (Braverman).

Combined Precursor Supplementation

Since there is no definitive method for predicting which neurotransmitter may require boosting via precursor therapy, it is possible that a combination of serotonin and norepinephrine precursors may be more effective. One investigator found L-tryptophan alone to be no better than placebo, while the combination of L-5-hydroxytryptophan (which he believes to be superior to L-tryptophan) and L-tyrosine was effective *(van Praag,1984).*

VITAMINS

Vitamin B Complex Deficiencies

Deficiencies of certain members of the vitamin B complex will cause depression as part of their respective deficiency syndromes. While the efficacy of B vitamin repletion in a clinically depressed population has been poorly studied, studies in which normal volunteers became depressed following diets which were severely restricted in one or more B vitamins have found no evidence of irreversibility following repletion *(Sterner).*

Folic Acid Deficiency

Folic acid deficiency is the most common vitamin deficiency, and depression is the most common neuropsychiatric symptom of folate deficiency *(Alpert).* (Other manifestations, which are seen in the more overt neuropsychiatric syndrome, include organic mental changes and a polyneuropathy.)

Borderline low or deficient serum or red blood cell folate levels are found in between 15 and 38 percent of adults diagnosed with depressive disorders *(Alpert)*, and the severity of the deficiency may correlate with the severity of the depression *(Abou-Saleh).* Even if folate stores appear adequate, and serum and erythrocyte folate are elevated, abnormal folate metabolism may cause a functional folate deficiency which results in depression *(Coleman;Lietha).*

An important example is homozygosity for thermolabile methylenetetrahydrofolate reductase. These patients, who have elevated plasma homocysteine levels *(Jacques)*, may require folate supplementation to prevent or treat major depression *(Arinami).* Routine screening for hyperhomocysteinemia would help to identify this sub-population.

While contributing to depression, folate deficiency often occurs secondary to depressions caused by such factors as poor diet and the use of alcohol and drugs *(Reynolds).* Not surprisingly, folate-deficient patients have a poorer response to antidepressant medication *(Fava).*

According to one authority, folate-deficient patients for whom the depression is secondary to easy fatigability comprise the group most likely to respond to supplementation with folic acid *(Botez).*

An 81 year-old man ate poorly after the death of his wife. Initially depressed by his wife's death, he seemed cheerful and was making plans several months later. Gradually, however, he became increasingly apathetic and confused and began to complain of sharp, stabbing leg pains, easy fatigability, blurred vision, and weakness. He was found to have rare bowel movements. Oral supplementation with vitamin B complex was unsuccessful. Serum folic acid, red blood cell folic acid and neutrophilic segmentation tests were consistent with folate deficiency.

He was started on folic acid 5 mg 3 times daily. After 2 months, his folic acid levels normalized; however, neutrophilic segmentation took longer to decrease to normal. By the end of the second month, his symptoms had cleared (Wright JV,1984).

Niacin

While depression is one of the possible manifestations of niacin deficiency *(Gelenberg,1988)*, little has been done to assess the efficacy of niacin for various types of depression. Half a century ago, an open trial of 15 patients with different types of depression reported rapid subjective and objective improvement following high-dosage supplementation in all but one patient. Most relapsed following discontinuation of the supplement and responded again when the supplement was restarted. The usual side effects of high-dosage niacin were noted *(Washburne)*.

This study was soon following by a placebo-controlled trial in which the same protocol was followed as in the earlier study. Three of the 11 patients given nicotinic acid had a full remission and, as in the first study, all of them experienced an exacerbation when the supplement was stopped and another remission when it was restarted. One of the 5 patients who received placebo also had a complete remission.

The author of this latter study concluded that there was no evidence that niacin was better than placebo *(Tonge)* and, in subsequent years, the efficacy of niacin does not appear to have been investigated any further - despite the fact that the design of the second study was so poor that it did little to clarify the possible efficacy of the nutrient.

However, the efficacy of nicotinamide adenine dinucleotide (NADH), the coenzyme form of niacin, has started to be investigated. In an open trial of more than 200 patients suffering from various types of depressions, 93% of the patients improved *(Birkmayer)*.

Properly controlled clinical trials of both niacin and NADH are needed to better assess their efficacy.

Riboflavin Deficiency

Depression is part of the riboflavin deficiency syndrome *(Sterner)*. Using erythrocyte glutathione reductase activity as a measure of riboflavin adequacy, even healthy subjects who are chronically riboflavin-deficient show evidence of significantly more depression *(Heseker)*. Moreover, riboflavin deficiency is common among patients suffering from depression *(Carney,1982)*.

While little has been done to investigate the efficacy of riboflavin supplementation in treating clinical depressions, a double-blind study of healthy university students found that, following one year of multivitamin supplementation at 10 times the RDA, improvement in blood riboflavin levels was associated with increased self-rated agreeableness in males and females. Moreover, females were more composed and slept better *(Benton,1995)*.

Thiamine

Depression, which often presents as a neurasthenic syndrome, is common in the earliest stage of thiamine deficiency. For example, when 9 normal volunteers were placed on a thiamine-deficient diet, 5 of them (56%) developed marked depression and irritability along with muscle weakness, paresthesias and peripheral nerve involvement *(Brozek)*.

Megadose thiamine supplementation (400 mg daily) has been shown to significantly inhibit platelet monoamine oxidase activity *(Connor)*. This action is the basis of the efficacy of the MAO inhibitors, a class of antidepressant drugs. Moreover, there is evidence from double-blind studies that megadose supplementation (50 mg daily) improves mood in healthy university students *(Benton,1997)*. Its efficacy in clinical depressions, however, remains to be investigated in controlled clinical trials.

Vitamin B_6

Vitamin B_6 in an important coenzyme in the production of monamine neurotransmitters and is required for the conversion of dietary tryptophan into serotonin, a neurotransmitter important in mood regulation. Laboratory evidence of vitamin B_6 deficiency is common in depression *(Russ)* and, among hospitalized patients, correlates specifically with endogenous depression versus other psychiatric diagnoses *(Carney,1979)*. The presence of mild neurologic symptoms such as numbness, paresthesias or "electric shock" sensations should increase suspicion of the diagnosis *(Stewart)*.

Two sub-groups with both depression and vitamin B_6 deficiency have been shown to be responsive so far to supplementation:

1. Estrogen supplementation can cause depression by blocking vitamin B_6 activity and accelerating tryptophan metabolism (making it less available for conversion into serotonin). Supplementation with vitamin B_6 therefore benefits depressed women with B_6 deficiencies secondary to the administration of estrogenic agents or other causes of estrogen excess *(Bermond)*.

2. Supplementation may be beneficial to adult celiacs who have remained depressed long after gluten withdrawal *(Hallert)*.

In addition, in a double-blind study of healthy university students, after one year of multivitamin megadose supplementation (10 times the RDA), improvement in blood vitamin B_6 concentrations was associated with improvement in specific aspects of mood as well as with a reduction in sleep disturbance - but in female subjects only *(Benton, 1995)*.

Vitamin B_{12}

Depression may be due to a vitamin B_{12} deficiency *(Levitt)*. While this deficiency is commonly associated with a macrocytic anemia, hematologic indices are normal in up to 30% of patients with B_{12} deficiency, and the results of the Schilling test may be normal *(Fine)*.

Among patients admitted to a psychiatric hospital, perhaps 6 percent are vitamin B_{12}-deficient while another 10 percent are subnormal *(Edwin)*, and those with lower B_{12} levels are more likely to have affective disorders than those with adequate levels *(Bell)*.

The efficacy of vitamin B_{12} supplementation in relieving depression has not been well studied. A group of patients complaining of tiredness (which could be a manifestation of depression) noted a significant improvement in general well-being following a course of vitamin B_{12} (hydroxycobalamin) injections, but not following a course of placebo injections, in a double-blind crossover study *(Ellis)*.

Another study used the Minnesota Multiphasic Personality Inventory (MMPI) as a measure of emotional distress for studying the efficacy of vitamin B_{12} (hydroxocobalamin) injections in a mixed group of patients with normal serum B_{12} levels. The patients received both B_{12} and placebo injections at different times. Those who felt better with vitamin B_{12} received additional injections to establish the dosage that gave the maximum feeling of well-being, and serum B_{12} levels were measured and the MMPI was administered the same day. Then the injections were discontinued for 5 to 7 days and both measures were repeated. With lower serum vitamin B_{12} levels, MMPI patterns showed more emotional distress than with higher serum vitamin B_{12} levels *(Newbold)*.

While these preliminary results appear promising, a double-blind study found oral vitamin B_{12} (cyanocobalamin) ineffective in treating patients with seasonal affective disorder *(Oren)*.

On the basis on their clinical experience, Wright and Gaby recommend that patients over the age of 70 who are experiencing fatigue, depression, poor appetite, or bowel complaints receive a therapeutic trial of a series of 4 to 8 injections of the vitamin, usually over 2 to 4 weeks. Afterwards, they suggest the injections be given as needed. They note that some patients find the effect to last a month or longer, while others seem to need them once a week *(Gaby)*.

Vitamin C

Depression is the first clinical symptom of experimental scurvy *(Hodges)*, and a sub-scorbutic state is marked by chronic depression, tiredness, irritability and vague ill-health *(Heseker)*.

When the diets of 12 depressed women who subsequently attempted suicide were compared to the diets of 12 other women who were not depressed and had no history of suicide attempts, the only significant difference found was a lower intake of ascorbic acid *(Kitahara, 1987b)*. Similarly, a group of 58 patients with a 2 to 5 month history of depression was found to have a significantly lower plasma vitamin C level than a group of apparently healthy controls *(Singh)*.

Among hospitalized psychiatric patients, plasma vitamin C levels may be lower than those of healthy controls *(Schorah)*. Ascorbic acid saturation (as measured by urinary excretion curves following supplementation) may be delayed *(Leitner)*, suggesting borderline or frank scurvy. However, the prevalence of ascorbic acid deficiency among various populations of depressives remains to be explored.

Supplementation

The results of two controlled studies suggest that megadose vitamin C supplementation may improve mood. In a study of more than 1000 healthy young men aged 17 to 29, administration of ascorbic acid, but not of placebo, to those with a suboptimal ascorbate status led to less depression along with decreased nervousness and emotional lability *(Heseker)*.

In the other study, 40 male chronic psychiatric patients, most of whom were schizophrenic, randomly received either ascorbic acid or placebo. Three weeks later, there was a significant decline in the MMPI "D" (depression) scale only in the supplemented group. When the mean

24-hour urinary excretion of ascorbic acid was measured in the control group, it was found to be at the lowest limit of normal *(Milner)*.

MINERALS

Calcium

In hypercalcemia (high serum calcium levels), which is commonly due to a pathologic process (such as hyperparathyroidism) causing excessive bone resorption, depression may be a prominent symptom *(Joborn)*. There are also preliminary data which suggest that, in depressive states, serum calcium concentrations may be elevated. For example, in a group of patients with chronic depression, most of whom were taking lithium, both 8 AM and mean diurnal (24-hour) serum calcium levels were significantly higher than those of depressed patients in remission and normal controls, and depressive symptoms were positively correlated with the serum calcium level *(Linder)*. The fact that serum calcium tends to decline following successful electroconvulsive therapy is supportive of this hypothesis *(Carman)*.

Depression may also be seen in patients with *hypo*calcemia (low serum calcium levels) *(Reiser)*. One cause is magnesium deficiency, which is found in about one in five patients with hypocalcemia *(Whang)*. In this case, magnesium supplementation should normalize serum calcium levels. Hypoparathyroidism, another cause of hypocalcemia, may require supplemental calcium and vitamin D until the underlying abnormality is corrected.

In depressive states, *plasma* calcium levels may be reduced. For example, in a group of acutely depressed patients, depressive symptoms were negatively correlated with the 8 AM plasma calcium level *(Linder)*, and plasma calcium was lower in a group of 29 unipolar depressed patients than in 10 healthy controls *(Bowden)*. The differences between serum and plasma calcium levels have been attributed to a change in a calcium-binding factor present in plasma but not in serum *(Linder)*.

Cerebrospinal fluid calcium concentrations appear to be elevated in depression. For a group of 32 drug-free women with major depression, CSF calcium was higher than in controls *(Banki, 1983)* while, after electro-convulsive therapy, cerebrospinal fluid calcium levels in other groups of depressed patients declined *(Carman; Jimerson)*.

Supplementation

Studies investigating the efficacy of calcium supplementation for the treatment of depression are lacking. However, two double-blind studies of healthy student volunteers examined the effect of calcium and vitamin D supplements upon mood.

After 4 weeks, there were significant improvements in the Beck Depression Inventory for the calcium-supplemented groups in both studies. Also, while improvements in the Depression Adjective Check List and the Zung Depression Scales failed to reach significance, the mean decreases in both of these scales were greater for the calcium-supplemented groups than for the placebo groups *(Arasteh)*.

A 45 year-old female was admitted to a hospital because of depression. She had a history of depressive moods since the birth of her child 15 years ago and a history of thyroid disease with thyroid replacement in 1991. She did not take calcium or "vitamin" supplements.

Laboratory testing revealed hypercalcemia which, upon further evaluation, was found to be due to the presence of a parathyroid adenoma (Anonymous).

Iron Deficiency

Depression may appear as part of the syndrome caused by chronic iron deficiency. Once it has developed, it may take months to resolve, even after supplementation has normalized hemoglobin levels *(Parker)*.

As menstruating women are a high-risk group for iron deficiency, the results of a double-blind study of healthy female adolescents who received an iron-containing syrup are particularly interesting. After 2 months, girls whose serum iron levels had been low now had normal serum iron levels. Compared to the controls, supplemented subjects reported statistically significant improvements in mood, energy and the ability to concentrate in school. Two-thirds of the subjects who were hypoferremic initially reported improvement in mood and energy, while all of the girls who initially were hypoferremic reported improved concentration *(Ballin)*.

While these results are promising, serum iron concentrations are usually normal in clinically depressed patients *(Heinze)*, raising the question of the relevance of iron supplementation to the treatment of clinical depressions. Clearly, further studies are needed to clarify the importance of iron supplementation.

Lithium

The use of pharmacologic dosages of lithium is well known as a treatment for depression. While it is most effective for the treatment of bipolar depression, acute unipolar depression sometimes responds *(Lieberman)*. In addition, pharmacologic dosages of lithium augment the efficacy of essentially all antidepressant medications *(Kramlinger)*. The downside, however, is that the danger of serious side effects is so great that blood levels need to be regularly monitored to prevent toxicity.

By contrast, the use of lithium supplementation in a range similar to that derived from foods and the water supply has been poorly studied. The findings of an intriguing study suggest, however, that nutritional lithium supplementation may be a useful therapeutic strategy. Twenty-four former drug users, some with a history of violence, randomly received either naturally lithium-rich brewer's yeast or normal, lithium-free, brewer's yeast placebo for 4 weeks. In the lithium group, total mood test scores increased steadily and significantly during supplementation. Based on these results, and the analysis of written comments of study participants, lithium supplementation appeared to have a mood-improving and mood-stabilizing effect *(Schrauzer)*.

Magnesium

Depression, often with irritability and agitation, may be part of the magnesium deficiency syndrome *(Hall)*. Evidence of magnesium deficiency calls for determining the cause and providing adequate supplementation until the underlying problem is corrected.

Compared to controls, cerebrospinal fluid magnesium may be reduced in hospitalized depressed patients, especially in those who are suicidal *(Banki,1986)*. Plasma magnesium levels vary widely, especially in the more disturbed, excitable patients, suggesting that they may have some abnormality of magnesium metabolism *(Kirow)*.

Potassium

Hypokalemia is frequently associated with a dysphoric mood along with fatigue and weakness. Not uncommonly, patients may also present with an organic brain syndrome *(Webb)*. The underlying cause of the hypokalemia should be ascertained and treated.

Among depressed patients, intracellular potassium levels may be low, even though serum and plasma potassium levels are likely to be normal *(Cox)*. Among patients who suicided, cerebral potassium levels may be reduced *(Webb)*.

Normokalemic patients have not been shown to respond to potassium supplementation.

Rubidium

An alkali metal which resembles potassium physiologically, rubidium elevates mood and enhances the sense of well-being in normals *(Fieve,1971)*. It appears to exert several biologic and pharmacologic effects that are similar if not identical to those of many of the classic antidepressant drugs *(Williams)*.

When given orally as rubidium chloride, it appears to be nontoxic and therapeutically effective in several types of depressive disorders *(Williams)*. Moreover, several open trials have reported that rubidium chloride was at least as effective in depression as were antidepressant medications *(Carolei)*, and it was frequently effective in patients who were refractory to standard treatments *(Fieve,1973)*.

Patients with retarded endogenous depressions appear to be the best candidates *(Placidi)*. No major adverse effects have been reported, although mild diarrhea, polyuria, excitement *(Placidi)* and skin rashes *(Torta)* have been noted.

In order to maintain electrolyte balance, it has been suggested that patients on rubidium should be supplemented with 5 g sodium and 60 to 80 mmol potassium daily. Daily plasma and urine electrolyte levels and EKG monitoring are also recommended *(Fieve,1971)*.

Selenium Deficiency

Marginal selenium status is not uncommon *(Neve)*. The results of a double-blind crossover study suggest that a marginal selenium intake may affect mood. Moreover, a moderate increase in selenium intake may reverse the adverse effect of marginal selenium status on mood *(Benton,1991)*.

Zinc Deficiency

A deficiency of zinc may cause anorexia, loss of libido and fatigue, all of which suggest depression and respond to zinc replacement *(Tasman-Jones)*. In depressed populations, serum zinc levels may be reduced *(McLoughlin)*. Moreover, the more severe the depression *(Maes,1994)*, and the more resistant the depression is to standard treatment *(Maes,1997)*, the lower the serum zinc concentration.

Other than to replete a zinc deficiency, zinc supplementation for the treatment of depression remains to be studied.

OTHER NUTRITIONAL FACTORS

Carnitine

Acetyl-L-carnitine, a patented derivative of L-carnitine, is a naturally occurring ester. In several controlled studies, it has been found effective for the treatment of both major *(Gecele)* and minor *(Bella)* depressions in the elderly.

Choline: A Warning

The administration of choline has been reported to *induce* depression in psychiatric patients with a depressive diathesis *(Tamminga)*.

Essential Fatty Acids

It has been suggested that the increasing prevalence of depression in this past century may be influenced by increased consumption of omega-6 fatty acids and saturated fatty acids, and decreased consumption of omega-3 fatty acids *(Hibbeln,1995)*. There is also evidence from observational studies that an elevated ratio of omega-6 fatty acids to omega-3 fatty acids in both serum cholesteryl esters and phospholipids may be associated with depression *(Maes,1996b)*. Moreover, low plasma concentrations of docosahexaenoic acid (an omega-3 fatty acid), predict low concentrations of cerebrospinal fluid 5-hydroxyindolacetic acid (a marker of brain serotonin turnover), and such low concentrations are strongly associated with depression and suicide *(Hibbeln,1996)*.

Consistent with these findings, long-term supplementation of omega-3 fatty acids in the form of a high fish diet was followed by significant reductions in measures of depression and aggressive hostility for a group of roughly 300 participants in a 5-year cholesterol-lowering study *(Weidner)*. Controlled clinical trials are needed to confirm these promising results.

Inositol

A naturally occurring isomer of glucose, inositol is a key intermediate of the phosphatidyl-inositol cycle, a second-messenger system used by several noradrenergic, serotonergic and cholinergic receptors *(Benjamin)*. Moreover, in both unipolar and bipolar depressed patients, inositol levels in the cerebrospinal fluid have been found to be reduced *(Barkai)*.

Supplementation has been shown to be effective under double-blind conditions as the sole therapy for depression *(Benjamin)*. Moreover, again under double-blind conditions, inositol was effective in treating antidepressant-resistant depression *(Levine,1995a)*.

Although supplementation increases cerebrospinal fluid levels *(Levine,1993)*, baseline levels fail to predict who will respond *(Levine,1996)*. It has been used safely in dosages of up to 20 grams daily with minimal side effects *(Benjamin)*. Relapse is common, however, within the year following discontinuation *(Levine,1995b)*.

Phosphatidylserine

Phosphatidylserine is the major acidic phospholipid in the brain. Supplementation in the elderly appears to increase dopamine release from the striatum and stimulate acetylcholine release from the cerebral cortex *(Crook)*.

When 10 elderly women with depressive disorders received placebo for 15 days followed by bovine cortex phosphatidylserine 300 mg daily for 30 days, they had consistent improvement of depressive symptoms, memory and behavior *(Maggioni)*. It is not known whether the supplement is effective for depressions that are not related to aging.

More recently, the bovine product has been taken off the market and a soy-derived product has become available. Due to differences in their composition, there is some question as to whether the two products are equivalent, although it is likely that they are equally effective *(Kidd)*.

S-Adenosyl-L-Methionine

S-Adenosyl-L-methionine (SAMe) is an important methyl group donor. SAMe and folate metabolism are intimately related, and experimental folate deficiency has been shown to lower SAMe levels *(Ordonez)*. For its synthesis, 5,10-methylenetetrahydrofolate is reduced to 5-methyltetrahydrofolate; then a methyl group is transferred from it to homocysteine in a reaction which requires both vitamin B_{12} and SAMe, and methionine is converted to SAMe by the enzyme methionine adenosyl transferase.

In depressive states, the activity of this enzyme may be reduced. Moreover, clinical improvement is usually associated with normalization of its activity *(Tolbert)*.

Supplementation with SAMe has been found to be effective in a number of studies, some of which were controlled. For example, it was significantly more effective than placebo in a double-blind study of inpatients with a diagnosis of Major Depression, Unipolar, without Psychotic Features *(Kagan)*. Also, when added to an antidepressant, it may shorten the time to treatment response *(Spillmann)*.

Side effects are mild and transient; however it is contraindicated in bipolar depressives as they may develop mania from its administration *(Kagan)*.

OTHER RELATED FACTORS

Hydrochloric Acid Deficiency

Insufficient gastric acidity may reduce intestinal absorption of many of the nutrients we have discussed above. Concerning the vitamin B complex, current evidence is that vitamin B_6 and folic acid nutriture should be unimpaired due to compensatory bacterial overgrowth in the small bowel; however, there are several mechanisms by which vitamin B_{12} deficiency may occur, and there is objective evidence which suggests the possibility that niacin, riboflavin and thiamine deficiencies can develop.

As to mineral absorption, the situation is not yet entirely clear. For example, absorption of ferric iron is known to be impaired, although absorption of heme iron is not, while recent studies on the effect of hydrochloric acid upon calcium absorption have had conflicting results. We can state that reduced hydrochloric acid production is most likely to impair mineral nutriture in patients who consume diets which are low in animal protein and high in phytate and fiber.

The efficacy of hydrochloric acid supplementation in treating depression in cases of hydrochloric acid deficiency remains to be studied scientifically. However, clinicians have reported cases where supplementation, along with the vitamin B complex seemed to be effective. For example, a patient with a 17-year history of endogenous depression was found to show clinical signs of vitamin deficiency. This individual improved dramatically following supplementation with hydrochloric acid before meals along with vitamin B complex *(Keuter)*.

A 36-year-old woman had depression for many years which was resistant to antidepressants, tranquilizers and psychotherapy. She reported excess gas and chronic constipation. Lab testing suggested hypochlorhydria and reactive hypoglycemia along with deficient mineral absorption. Serum vitamin B_{12} was in the normal range, but on the low side.

She was treated with vitamin B_{12} 100 µg intramuscularly twice weekly, folic acid 1 mg twice daily, and betaine hydrochloride 15 gr before meals along with pancreatin 1,300 to 2,600 milligrams. The B_{12} injections gave dramatic relief within 24 hours lasting 2 to 3 days, and were gradually tapered successfully (Wright JV, 1979).

Food Sensitivities

Various foods, was well as chemicals and molds, may provoke depression in susceptible individuals. Thirty patients complaining of depression, confusion, difficulty concentrating or other psychological symptoms were double-blind tested sub-lingually with common foods, auto exhaust, chlorine and *Alternaria*. They noted significantly greater cognitive-emotional symptoms when tested with the antigens than when tested with placebos (which failed to increase symptoms above baseline) *(King)*.

However, complaints of depression which patients believe to be food-related will sometimes fail to be substantiated by objective testing procedures *(Pearson)*.

Heavy Metal Toxicity

Toxicity due to chronic exposure to either aluminum *(White)* or lead *(Balestra)* frequently results in depression. Depression due to lead intoxication may include symptoms of fatigue, irritability and poor concentration. However, the diagnosis is easily missed, as it may occur without the typical signs and symptoms of lead toxicity such as foot or wrist drop, abdominal pain, gingival lead lines, microcytic anemia, gout or interstitial nephritis *(Balestra)*.

BIBLIOGRAPHY

Abou-Saleh MT, Coppen A. Serum and red blood cell folate in depression. Acta Psychiatr Scand 80(1):78-82, 1989

Agren H et al. Low Brain uptake of L-[^{11}C]5-hydroxytryptophan in major depression: a positron emission tomography study on patients and healthy volunteers. Acta Psychiatr Scand 83:449-55, 1991

Alpert JE, Fava M. Nutrition and depression: the role of folate. Nutr Rev 55(5):145-9, 1997

Anonymous. Depression and hypercalcemia. Am J Med 101:111-17, 1996

Arasteh K. A beneficial effect of calcium intake on mood. J Orthomol Psychiatry 9(4):199-204, 1994

Arinami T et al. Methylenetetrahydrofolate reductase variant and schizophrenia/depression. Am J Med Genet 74(5):526-8, 1997

Balestra DJ. Adult chronic intoxication. Arch Intern Med 151:1718-20, 1991

Ballin A et al. Iron state in female adolescents. Am J Dis Child 146(7):803-5, 1992

Banki CM et al. Cerebrospinal fluid biochemical examination. Do they reflect clinical or biological differences? Biol Psychiatry 18(9):1033-44, 1983

Banki CM et al. Aminergic studies and cerebrospinal fluid cations in suicide. Ann N Y Acad Sci 487:221-30, 1986

Barkai AI et al. Reduced myo-inositol levels in cerebrospinal fluid from patients with affective disorder. Biol Psychiatry 13(1):65-72, 1978

Beckmann H et al. DL-phenylalanine versus imipramine: A double-blind controlled study. Arch Psychiatr Nervenkr 227:49-58, 1979

Bell I et al. Vitamin B12 and folate status in acute geropsychiatric inpatients: Affective and cognitive characteristics of a vitamin nondeficient population. Biol Psychiatry 27(2):125-37, 1990

Bella R et al. Effect of acetyl-L-carnitine on geriatric patients suffering from dysthymic disorders. Int J Clin Pharmacol Res 10(6):355-60, 1990

Benjamin J et al. Inositol treatment in psychiatry. Psychopharmacol Bull 31(1):167-75, 1995

Benkelfat C et al. Mood-lowering effect of tryptophan depletion. Arch Gen Psychiatry 51:687-97, 1994

Benton D, Cook R. The impact of selenium supplementation on mood. Biol Psychiatry 29(11):1092-8, 1991

Benton D et al. Vitamin supplementation for 1 year improves mood. Neuropsychobiology 32(2):98-105, 1995

Benton D et al. Thiamine supplementation, mood and cognitive functioning. Psychopharmacology 129(1):66-71, 1997

Bermond P. Therapy of side effects of oral contraceptive agents with vitamin B6. Acta Vitaminol Enzymol 4(1-2):45-54, 1982

Birkmayer JGD, Birkmayer W. The coenzyme nicotinamide adenine dinucleotide (NADH) as a biological antidepressive agent. Experience with 205 patients, in New Trends in Neuropharmacology 6:1-7,1992

Botez MI et al. Neuropsychological correlates of folic acid deficiency: Facts and hypotheses, in MI Botez MI, EH Reynolds, Eds. Folic Acid in Neurology, Psychiatry and Internal Medicine. New York, Raven Press, 1979

Bowden CL et al. Calcium function in affective disorders and healthy controls. Biol Psychiatry 23(4):367-76, 1988

Braverman ER. The Healing Nutrients Within. New Canaan CT, Keats Publishing, 1987:51

Brozek J. Psychologic effects of thiamine restriction and deprivation in normal young men. Am J Clin Nutr 5(2):109-20, 1957

Carman JS et al. Calcium and electroconvulsive therapy of severe depressive illness. Biol Psychiatry 12(1):5-17, 1977

Carney MW et al. Thiamin and pyridoxine lack in newly-admitted psychiatric patients. Br J Psychiatry 135:249-54, 1979

Carney MW et al. Thiamine, riboflavin and pyridoxine deficiency in psychiatric in-patients. Br J Psychiatry 141:271-72, 1982

Carolei A et al. [Pharmacological action of rubidium chloride - anti-depressant effect: Comparison with imipramine.] Clin Ter 75:469-78, 1975

Charles MA et al. Comparison of oral glucose tolerance tests and mixed meals in patients with apparent idiopathic postabsorptive hypoglycemia: Absence of hypoglycemia after meals. Diabetes 30:465-70, 1981

Christensen L et al. Impact of a dietary change on emotional distress. J Abnorm Psychol 94(4):565-79, 1985

Christensen L. The roles of caffeine and sugar in depression. Nutr Rep 9(3), March, 1991

Christensen L, Somers S. Comparison of nutrient intake among depressed and nondepressed individuals. Int J Eat Disord 20(1):105-9, 1996

Coleman N. Laboratory assessment of folate status. Clin Lab Med 12:775-96, 1981

Connor DJ. Thiamine intake and monoamine oxidase activity. Biol Psychiatry 16(9):869-72, 1981

Coppen A, Wood K. Tryptophan and depressive illness. Psychological Med 8:49-57, 1978

Cottereau MJ et al. [Alcoholism and depression.] Encephale 6(3):209-26, 1980

Cox JR et al. Changes in sodium, potassium and fluid spaces in depression and dementia. Gerontology Clin 13:232-45, 1971

Crook T et al. Effects of phosphatidylserine in Alzheimer's disease. Psychopharmacol Bull 28(1):61-6, 1992

Delgado PD et al. Serotonin function and the mechanism of antidepressant action. Arch Gen Psychiatry 47:411-18, 1990

Edwin E et al. Vitamin B12 hypovitaminosis in mental diseases. Acta Med Scand 177:689-99, 1965

Ellis FR, Nasser S. A pilot study of vitamin B12 in the treatment of tiredness. Br J Nutr 30:277-83, 1973

Fava M et al. Folate, vitamin B12, and homocysteine in major depressive disorder. Am J Psychiatry 154(3):426-8, 1997

Fieve RR et al. Rubidium chloride ingestion by volunteer subjects: Initial experience. Psychopharmacologia 20:307-14, 1971

Fieve RR et al. Rubidium: Biochemical, behavioral, and metabolic studies in humans. Am J Psychiatry 130:55-61, 1973

Fine EJ, Soria ED. Myths about vitamin B12 deficiency. South Med J 84(12):1475-8, 1991

Gaby AR. The story of vitamin B12: Is vitamin B12 a panacea or placebo? Nutrition & Healing 2(7), July, 1995

Gecele M et al. Acetyl-L-carnitine in aged subjects with major depression: clinical efficacy and effects on the circadian rhythm of cortisol. Dementia 2:333-7, 1991

Gelenberg AJ et al. Tyrosine for the treatment of depression. Am J Psychiatry 137:622-3, 1980

Gelenberg AJ. Psychiatric disorders, in DM Paige, Ed. Clinical Nutrition. Second Edition. St. Louis, C.V. Mosby, 1988

Gibson CJ, Gelenberg A. Tyrosine for the treatment of depression. Adv Biol Psychiatry 10:148-59, 1983

Gilliland K, Bullick W. Caffeine: A potential drug of abuse. Adv Alcohol Subst Abuse 3(1-2):53-73, 1984

Goodwin FK. Alcoholism research: delivering on the promise. Public Health Rep 103(6):569-74, 1988

Greden J. Caffeine and tobacco dependence, in Comprehensive Textbook of Psychiatry. Baltimore, Williams & Wilkins, 1985:1026-33

Hall RCW, Joffe JR. Hypomagnesemia: physical and psychiatric symptoms. JAMA 224(13):1749-51, 1973

Hallert C et al. Reversal of psychopathology in adult coeliac disease with the aid of pyridoxine (vitamin B6). Scand J Gastroenterol 18(2):299-304, 1983

Heinze G et al. Serum iron levels in depressed patients. Pharmakopsychiatr Neuropsychopharmakol 10(4):239-42, 1977

Heller B. Pharmacological and clinical effects of D-phenylalanine in depression and Parkinson's disease, in Mosnaim, Wolf, Eds. Noncatecholic Phenylethylamines, Part I. New York, Marcel Dekker, 1978:397-417

Heseker H et al. Psychological disorders as early symptoms of a mild-moderate vitamin deficiency. Ann N Y Acad Sci 669:352-7, 1992

Hibbeln JR, Salem N Jr. Dietary polyunsaturated acids and depression: when cholesterol does not satisfy. Am J Clin Nutr 62:1-9, 1995

Hibbeln JR et al. Do plasma polyunsaturates predict hostility and violence? World Rev Nutr Diet 82:175-86, 1996

Hodges RE et al. Clinical manifestations of ascorbic acid deficiency in man. Am J Clin Nutr 24:432-3, 1971

Jacques PF et al. Relation between folate status, a common mutation in methylenetetrahydrofolate reductase, and plasma homocysteine concentrations. Circulation 93(1):7-9, 1996

Jimerson DC et al. CSF calcium: clinical correlates in affective illness and schizophrenia. Biol Psychiatry 14(1):37-51, 1979

Joborn C et al. Psychiatric symptomatology in patients with primary hyperparathyroidism. Ups J Med Sci 91(1):77-87, 1986

Kagan BL et al. Oral S-adenosylmethionine in depression: A randomized, double-blind, placebo-controlled trial. Am J Psychiatry 147(5):591-95, 1990

Keuter EJW. Nutr Abstr Rev 29:273, 1959

Kidd P. Phosphatidylserine: membrane nutrient for memory. A clinical and mechanistic assessment. Altern Med Rev 1(2):70-84, 1996

King DS. Can allergic exposure provoke psychological symptoms? A double-blind test. Biol Psychiatry 16(1):3-19, 1981

Kirow GK et al. Plasma magnesium levels in a population of psychiatric patients: correlation with symptoms. Neuropsychobiology 30(2-3):73-8, 1994

Kitahara M. Dietary tryptophan ratio and suicide in the United Kingdom, Ireland, the United States, Canada, Australia, and New Zealand. Omega J Death Dying 18:71-6, 1987a

Kitahara M. Insufficient ascorbic acid uptake from the diet and the tendency for suicide. J Orthomol Med 2(4):217-18, 1987b

Kramlinger K, Post R. The addition of lithium to carbamazepine. Arch Gen Psychiatry 46:794-800, 1989

Kreitsch K et al. Prevalence, presenting symptoms, and psychological characteristics of individuals experiencing a diet-related mood disturbance. Behav Ther 19:593-604, 1988

Leitner ZA, Church IC. Nutritional studies in a mental hospital. Lancet i:565-7, 1956

Lester D. Fat consumption and suicide. J Orthomol Med 5(1):20-1, 1990

Levine J et al. Inositol treatment raises CSF inositol levels. Brain Res 627(1):168-70, 1993

Levine J et al. Double-blind, controlled trial of inositol treatment of depression. Am J Psychiatry 152(5):792-4, 1995a

Levine J et al. Follow-up and relapse analysis of an inositol study of depression. Isr J Psychiatry Relat Sci 32(1):14-21, 1995b

Levine J et al. CSF inositol does not predict antidepressant response to inositol. Short communication. J Neural Transm 103(12):1457-62, 1996

Levitt AJ, Joffe RT. Folate, B12 and thyroid function in depression. Biol Psychiatry 33:52-3, 1993

Lieberman JA et al. Acute antidepressant effect of lithium in unipolar depression. Psychosomatics 25(12):932-3, 1984

Lietha R, Zimmerman M. Neuropsychiatric disorders associated with functional folate deficiency in the presence of elevated serum and erythrocyte folate: a preliminary report. J Nutr Med 4:441-7, 1994

Linder J et al. Calcium and magnesium concentrations in affective disorder: Difference between plasma and serum in relation to symptoms. Acta Psychiatr Scand 80:527-37, 1989

Lopez-Ibor JJ Jr et al. Biological correlations of suicide and aggressivity in major depressions (with melancholia). Neuropsychobiology 14(2):67-74, 1985

Maes M et al. Hypozincemia in depression. J Affect Disord 31(2):135-40, 1994

Maes M et al. Lower serum L-tryptophan availability in depression as a marker of a more generalized disorder in protein metabolism. Neuropsychopharmacology 15(3):243-51, 1996a

Maes M et al. Fatty acid composition in major depression: decreased ω-3 fractions in cholesteryl esters and increased c20:4ω6/c20:5ω3 ratio in cholesteryl esters and phospholipids. J Affect Dis 38:35-46, 1996b

Maes M et al. Lower serum zinc in major depression is a sensitive marker of treatment resistance and of the immune/inflammatory response in that illness. Biol Psychiatry 42(5):349-58, 1997

Maggioni M et al. Effects of phosphatidylserine therapy in geriatric patients with depressive disorders. Acta Psychiatr Scand 81:264-70, 1990

McLoughlin IJ, Hodge JS. Zinc in depressive disorder. Acta Psychiatr Scand 82(6):451-3, 1990

Milner G. Ascorbic acid in chronic psychiatric patients: A controlled trial. Br J Psychiatry 109:294-9, 1963

Neve J et al. Selenium deficiency. Clin Endocrinol Metab 14(3):629-56, 1985

Newbold HL. Vitamin B-12: placebo or neglected therapeutic tool? Med Hypotheses 28(3):155-64, 1989

Ordonez LA, Wurtman RJ. Folic acid deficiency and methyl group metabolism in rat brain: effects of L-dopa. Reversal effect of S-adenosyl-L-methionine. Arch Biochem Biophys 160:372-6, 1974

Oren DA et al. A controlled trial of cyanocobalamin (vitamin B12) in the treatment of winter seasonal affective disorder. J Affect Disord 32(3):197-200, 1994

Parker SD. Depression and nutrition: Anemia and glucose imbalances. Anabolism Jan.-Feb., 1984

Pearson DJ et al. Food allergy: How much in the mind? Lancet i:1259-61, 1983

Placidi G et al. Exploration of the clinical profile of rubidium chloride in depression: a systematic open trial. J Clin Psychopharmacol 8(3):184-8, 1988

Reiser LE, Reiser MF. Endocrine disorders, in HI Kaplan, BJ Sadock, Eds. Comprehensive Textbook of Psychiatry/IV. Baltimore, Williams & Wilkins, 1985:1167-78

Reynolds EH et al. Methylation and mood. Lancet ii:196-8, 1984

Rogers PJ, Dernoncourt C. Regular caffeine consumption: a balance of adverse and beneficial effects for mood and psychomotor performance. Pharmacol Biochem Behav 59(4):1039-45, 1998

Russ CS et al. Vitamin B6 status of depressed and obsessive-compulsive patients. Nutr Rep Int 27(4):867-73, 1983

Sabelli HC et al. Clinical studies on the phenylethylamine hypothesis of affective disorder: Urine and blood phenylacetic acid and phenylalanine dietary supplements. J Clin Psychiatry 47(2):66-70, 1986

Schorah CJ et al. Plasma vitamin C concentration in patients in a psychiatric hospital. Hum Nutr Clin Nutr 37C:447-52, 1983

Schrauzer GN, de Vroey E. Effects of nutritional lithium supplementation on mood: A placebo-controlled study with former drug users. Biol Trace Elem Res 40(1):89-101, 1994

Silverman K et al. Withdrawal syndrome after the double-blind cessation of caffeine consumption. N Engl J Med 327:1109-14, 1992

Simonson M. L-phenylalanine. Letter. J Clin Psychiatry 46(8):355, 1985

Singh RB et al. Dietary intake and plasma levels of antioxidant vitamins in health and disease: a hospital-based case-control study. J Nutr Environ Med 5:235-42, 1995

Smith KA et al. Relapse of depression after rapid depletion of tryptophan. Lancet 349:915-19, 1997

Spillmann M, Fava M. S-Adenosylmethionine (Ademetionine) in psychiatric disorders: historical perspective and current status. CNS Drugs 6(6):416-25, 1996

Sterner RT, Price WR. Restricted riboflavin: within-subject behavioral effects in humans. Am J Clin Nutr 26:150-60, 1973

Stewart JW et al. Low B6 levels in depressed outpatients. Biol Psychiatry 19(4):613-16, 1984

Strain EC et al. Caffeine dependence syndrome: evidence from case histories and experimental evaluations. JAMA 272(13):1043-8, 1994

Tamminga CA et al. Cholinergic influences in tardive dyskinesia. Am J Psychiatry 134:769-74, 1977

Tasman-Jones C. Zinc deficiency states. Adv Intern Med 26:97-114, 1980

Tolbert LC et al. Clinical correlations of one-carbon metabolism abnormalities. Prog Neuropsychopharmacol Biol Psychiatry 12(4):491-502, 1988

Tonge WL. Nicotinic acid in the treatment of depression. Ann Intern Med 38:551-3, 1953

Torta R et al. [Rubidium chloride in the treatment of major depression]. Minerva Psichiatr 34(2):101-10, 1993 (in Italian)

van Praag HM. Studies in the mechanism of action of serotonin precursors in depression. Psychopharmacol Bull 20:599-602, 1984

van Praag HM, Lemus C. Monamine precursors in the treatment of psychiatric disorders, in RJ Wurtman, JJ Wurtman, Eds. Nutrition and the Brain, Volume 7. New York, Raven Press, 1986

van Praag HM et al. Therapeutic indications for serotonin-potentiating compounds: a hypothesis. Biol Psychiatry 22(2):205-12, 1987

Walinder J. Combination of tryptophan with MAO inhibitors, tricyclic antidepressants and selective 5-HT reuptake inhibitors. Adv Biol Psychiatry 10:82-93, 1983

Washburne AC. Nicotinic acid in the treatment of certain depressed states: a preliminary report. Ann Intern Med 32:261-9, 1950

Webb WL, Gehi M. Electrolyte and fluid imbalance: Neuropsychiatric manifestations. Psychosomatics 22(3):199-203, 1981

Weidner G et al. Improvements in hostility and depression in relation to dietary change and cholesterol lowering. The Family Heart Study. Ann Intern Med 117(10):820-3, 1992

Whang R et al. Predictors of clinical hypomagnesemia. Arch Intern Med 144:1794-96, 1984

White DM et al. Neurologic syndrome in 25 workers from an aluminum smelting plant. Arch Intern Med 152(7):1442-8, 1992

Williams RH et al. Pharmacologic role of rubidium in psychiatric research. Compr Ther 13(9):46-54, 1987

Willner P. "Depression" increases "craving" for sweet rewards in animal and human models of depression and craving. Psychopharmacology (Berl) 136(3):272-83, 1998

Winokur G. Alcoholism and depression. Subst Alcohol Actions Misuse 4(2-3):111-19, 1983

Wright JH. Glucose metabolism in unipolar depression. Br J Psychiatry 132:386-93, 1978

Wright JV. Dr. Wright's Book of Nutritional Therapy. Emmaus, Penn., Rodale Press, 1979

Wright JV. A case of apathy and depression. Prevention June, 1984

Yaryura-Tobias JA, Neziroglu F. Phenylethylamine and glucose in true depression. Orthomol Psychiatry 5(3):199-202, 1976

Young SN. The clinical psychopharmacology of tryptophan, in RJ Wurtman, JJ Wurtman, Eds. Nutrition and the Brain Volume 7. New York, Raven Press, 1986:49-88

Zmilacher K et al. L-5-hydroxytryptophan alone and in combination with a peripheral decarboxylase inhibitor in the treatment of depression. Neuropsychobiology 20(1):28-35, 1988

DERMATITIS HERPETIFORMIS

See Also: CELIAC DISEASE

NUTRITIONAL TREATMENT GUIDE

✓ = Efficacy generally accepted.
* = Efficacy *demonstrated* by controlled human trials.
[+] = Efficacy *suspected* from uncontrolled human trials.
[-] = Efficacy *suspected* from indirect data.
? = Efficacy *challenged* in a study of similar design.

NUTRITIONAL FACTORS

[+] **Para-amino Benzoic acid:** 18 g daily (Potassium salt is better tolerated.)

- -

[-] rule out **Hydrochloric Acid** deficiency
[-] rule out **Iron** deficiency
[-] **Selenium deficiency:** 200 μg daiily
[-] **Vitamin B_{12} deficiency:** 1000 μg intramuscularly weekly initially and monthly afterwards
[-] **Zinc deficiency:** zinc sulfate 220 mg twice daily *AND* **Copper** 2 mg daily

OTHER RELATED FACTORS

✓ rule out **Food Sensitivities**

Most patients with this skin disorder have celiac disease, an illness that is associated with numerous nutrient deficiencies (see Celiac Disease). As dermatitis herpetiformis has been much less studied, it is likely that only a few of the nutrient deficiencies that patients may demonstrate have been identified.

NUTRITIONAL FACTORS

VITAMINS

Para-amino Benzoic Acid

In an open trial, supplementation with para-amino benzoic acid, a member of the vitamin B complex, was an effective treatment for all of a group of 16 patients. Particularly intriguing was the finding that even patients who were not avoiding gluten responded *(Zarafonetis).* Para-amino benzoic acid has potential side effects that include skin rash, anorexia, nausea and fever *(Physician's Desk Reference)*, vitiligo *(Hughes)*, and rarely, liver toxicity *(Kantor).* Administration of the potassium salt (Potaba; Glenwood) is preferable as it is easier to tolerate *(Grace).*

Vitamin B_{12} Deficiency

Low serum vitamin B_{12} levels were found in 21% of a group of 129 patients, almost all of whom showed evidence of functional or morphological involvement of the small intestine. Moreover, evidence of pernicious anemia (atrophic gastritis resulting in defective secretion of intrinsic factor) was not uncommon within this patient group, suggesting that patients found to have low serum vitamin B_{12} levels should be further evaluated *(Kastrup, 1986)*.

MINERALS

Iron Deficiency

Although they had adequate absorption of ferrous iron, 4 out of a group of 20 patients were iron-deficient (defined as lack of hemosiderin in bone marrow smears). This suggests that iron deficiency is not only fairly common, but is often caused by factors other than malabsorption *(Kastrup, 1977)*.

Selenium Deficiency

Patients may be deficient in selenium, as suggested by a reduced blood level of the selenium-dependent enzyme glutathione peroxidase *(Juhlin)*.

In a double-blind study, patients with low blood glutathione peroxidase levels were supplemented with selenium and vitamin E for 5 months. Glutathione peroxidase levels rose; however, no evidence of clinical improvement was found *(Ljunghall)*.

Zinc Deficiency

The intestinal absorption of zinc may be reduced *(Crofton)*, and epidermal zinc concentrations may be low *(Michäelsson)*.

Whether zinc supplementation improves the lesions is not known.

OTHER RELATED FACTORS

Food Sensitivities

While gluten sensitivity is common, only 50 to 60% of patients were completely controlled after 5 years on a gluten-free diet *(Reunala)*. Sensitivity to bovine milk has also been noted *(Barnes)*.

A 74 year-old man with dermatitis herpetiformis had characteristic skin lesions, upper abdominal pain and loose stools for 10 years.

He was treated with a milk-free diet. His dermatitis improved in less than a week, although his dyspepsia was only slightly better. Both the dermatitis and the dyspepsia were completely controlled with a gluten and milk-free diet, while reintroduction of milk and milk proteins caused recurrence of the dermatitis.

After 4 months of a gluten-free diet, reintroduction of gluten no longer provoked recurrence of the dermatitis (Engquist).

Hydrochloric Acid Deficiency

As mentioned earlier, atrophic gastritis is fairly common in this patient group. It is therefore not surprising that hydrochloric acid deficiency is a frequent finding. Back in 1929, Ayres tested 4 patients following a standard test meal and found 3 of them to have gastric hypoacidity, while one had hyperacidity. Moreover, for 3 patients, the severity of the eruption correlated with the abnormal levels of gastric secretion *(Ayres)*.

A more recent investigation found achlorhydria in 30 out of a group of 116 patients (26%) following pentagastrin stimulation *(Kastrup, 1986)*. Whether acid supplementation reduces the skin lesions has not been reported.

BIBLIOGRAPHY

Ayres S. Gastric secretion in psoriasis, eczema and dermatitis herpetiformis. Arch Dermatol Syphilol 20:854-7, 1929

Barnes RM, Lewis-Jones MS. Isotype distribution and serial levels of antibodies reactive with dietary protein antigens in dermatitis herpetiformis. J Clin Lab Immunol 30(2):87-91, 1989

Crofton RW et al. Zinc absorption in celiac disease and dermatitis herpetiformis: a test of small intestinal function. Am J Clin Nutr 38(5):706-12, 1983

Engquist A, Pock-Steen OC. Dermatitis herpetiformis and milk-free diet. Lancet ii:438, 1971

Grace WJ et al. Therapy of scleroderma and dermatomyositis. N Y State J Med 63(1):140-4, 1963

Hughes CG. Oral PABA and vitiligo. J Am Acad Dermatol 9:770, 1983

Juhlin L. Blood glutathione-peroxidase levels in skin diseases: Effect of selenium and vitamin E treatment. Acta Dermatovener (Stockholm) 62:211-14, 1982

Kantor GR, Ratz JL. Liver toxicity from potassium para-aminobenzoate. Letter. J Am Acad Dermatol 13(4):671-72, 1985

Kastrup W et al. Iron absorption in patients with dermatitis herpetiformis. Acta Derm Venereol 57(5):407-12, 1977

Kastrup W et al. Malabsorption of vitamin B12 in dermatitis herpetiformis and its association with pernicious anaemia. Acta Med Scand 220(3):261-8, 1986

Ljunghall K et al. Selenium, glutathione-peroxidase and dermatitis herpetiformis. Acta Derm Venereol 64(6):546-7, 1984

Michäelsson G, Ljunghall K. Patients with dermatitis herpetiformis, acne, psoriasis and Darier's disease have low epidermal zinc concentrations. Acta derm Venereol (Stockholm) 70(4):304-8, 1990

Physicians' Desk Reference Oradell, NJ, Med. Economics Co., Inc. 1989

Reunala T, Nuutinen T. Control of dermatitis herpetiformis with totally gluten-free dietary products. Scand J Gastroenterol 28(Suppl 197), 1993

Zarafonetis CJD et al. Paraaminobenzoic acid in dermatitis herpetiformis. Arch Dermatol Syphilol 63:115-32, 1951

DIABETES MELLITUS

See Also: **ATHEROSCLEROSIS**
CATARACTS
NEURALGIA and NEUROPATHY

NUTRITIONAL TREATMENT GUIDE

✓ = Efficacy generally accepted.
* = Efficacy *demonstrated* by controlled human trials.
[+] = Efficacy *suspected* from uncontrolled human trials.
[-] = Efficacy *suspected* from indirect data.
? = Efficacy *challenged* in a study of similar design.

DIETARY FACTORS

✓ avoid **Obesity**
✓ **low Fat, low Cholesterol, high Carbohydrate diet**
✓ **high Soluble Fiber intake** (up to 40 g daily *OR* 15 to 25 g/1,000 calories)
✓ choose high-carbohydrate foods with a **low Glycemic Index**
✓ avoid **Alcohol**
✓ moderate **Protein** restriction (to combat nephropathy)
✓ eat **Frequent Small Meals**

- -

* **high Monounsaturated Fat, low Carbohydrate diet**
* **Vegetarian diet**
* avoid **Partially Hydrogenated Vegetable Oils**
* ? moderate **Sucrose** and **Fructose** restriction

- -

[-] avoid **Coffee** and **Tea** in children's diets
[-] avoid **Nitrates** and **Nitrosamines** in children's diets
[-] ? restrict **Cow's Milk** in infancy

NUTRIENTS TO IMPROVE GLYCEMIC RESPONSE

* **Biotin:** 9 to 16 mg daily (one month trial)
* **Calcium deficiency:** ≈ 1 g daily
* **Glucose Tolerance Factor:** *in type II diabetes:* brewer's yeast 9 g daily (2 month trial)
* **Magnesium deficiency:** *in type II diabetes:* ≈ 400 mg daily
* **Pyridoxine Alpha-ketoglutarate:** 600 mg 3 times daily (1 month trial)
* **Vitamin C:** 0.5 to 1 g twice daily
* ? **Chromium deficiency:** *in type II or gestational diabetes:* 200 μg daily
* ? **Niacin:** *in type I diabetes, to preserve residual beta-cell function:* nicotinamide 200 mg to 1 g daily
* ? **Vitamin E:** ? 800 IU daily (6 month trial)

* ? **Zinc deficiency**: zinc sulfate 220 mg twice daily *AND* **Copper** 2 mg daily (only if there are signs or symptoms of deficiency)

- -

[+] **Calcium:** calcium lactate 3 g daily
[+] **Coenzyme Q_{10}:** 60 mg daily
[+] **Copper deficiency:** 2 mg twice daily for up to 6 weeks *AND* **Zinc** 50 mg daily
[+] **Manganese deficiency:** 3 to 5 mg daily
[+] **Phosphorus deficiency:** dibasic calcium phosphate 2 g 3 times daily with meals
[+] **Potassium deficiency:** ? 80 to 100 mEq daily total intake, preferably from potassium-rich foods
[+] **Vitamin B_6 deficiency:** 50 to 100 mg daily

NUTRIENTS TO PREVENT AND TREAT DIABETIC COMPLICATIONS

* **Carnitine:** *to combat neuropathy:* acetyl-L-carnitine ? 1 to 3 g daily
* **alpha-Lipoic acid:** *to combat peripheral and autonomic neuropathy:* 600 to 1,200 mg daily
* **Omega-6 Fatty Acids:** *to combat neuropathy: example:* evening primrose oil 6 g daily
* **Selenium:** *to combat neuropathy:* sodium selenite 100 µg daily (3 month trial)
* **Taurine:** *to combat platelet hyperaggregability:* 500 mg 3 times daily
* **Vitamin B_{12}:** *to combat neuropathy:* methylcobalamin 500 µg 3 times daily
* **Vitamin E:** *to combat neuropathy, platelet hyperaggregability and atherosclerosis:* ? 1,200 to 1,600 IU daily

- -

[+] **Biotin:** *to combat neuropathy:* 10 mg IM daily for 6 weeks; then 10 mg 3 times weekly for 6 weeks; then 5 mg daily orally
[+] **Chromium deficiency:** *to combat neuropathy:* ? 250 µg daily
[+] **Omega-3 Fatty Acids:** *to combat neuropathy:* purified EPA 600 mg 3 times daily (3 mo. trial)
[+] **Phosphorus:** *to combat microangiopathy:* dibasic calcium phosphate 2 g 3 times daily with meals
[+] **Pycnogenol®:** *to combat retinopathy:* 60 to 120 mg daily
[+] **Rutin:** *to combat retinopathy:* 250 to 500 mg daily
[+] **Thiamine:** *to combat neuropathy:* ? 50 mg daily (especially if deficient)
[+] **Vitamin B_6:** *to combat macular edema:* 300 mg daily
[+] **Vitamin B_{12}:** *to combat retinopathy:* 100 to 1,000 µg daily by injection

- -

[-] **L-Arginine:** *to combat microangiopathy:* ? 1 g twice daily
[-] **Daflon:** *to combat microangiopathy:* 3 g daily
[-] **Magnesium deficiency:** *to combat retinopathy and atherosclerosis:* ≈ 400 mg daily
[-] **Niacin:** *to combat nephropathy:* nicotinamide
[-] **Taurine:** *to combat macro- and microangiopathy:* ? 500 mg to 5 g daily
[-] **Vitamin C:** *to combat microangiopathy:* ? 500 mg twice daily
[-] **Vitamin E:** *to combat gangrene and necrobiosis lipoidica diabeticorum:* 400 IU daily

OTHER RELATED FACTORS

✓ avoid **Obesity**

- -

* rule out **Hydrochloric Acid** deficiency

In diabetes mellitus, nutritional interventions may be efficacious both in improving glucose metabolism and in combating the complications of the disease. Since diabetics are prone to developing atherosclerosis, the chapter of this book on atherosclerosis should also be consulted.

DIETARY FACTORS

Results of a fascinating study of Australian aborigines underscore the intimate relationship between diabetes mellitus and the diet. Until the 1930s, the aborigines ate few processed foods. Since meat from wild animals is lean, their diet was high in protein but low in fat. Dietary fiber was high.

That diet began to change when missionaries introduced flour and sugar. Soon urbanization radically changed their lifestyle and they adopted a typical Western diet. Diabetes mellitus, which had been virtually unknown, quickly increased in prevalence to 20% of the adult population.

For the study, 10 urbanized type II diabetic aborigines, with an average age of 54, agreed to return to the hunter-gatherer existence of their ancestors and to only eat what they could hunt, fish or collect for 7 weeks. All were overweight and exercised little. Most ate a diet high in fatty meat and several suffered from hypertension. Five of the 10 drank moderately to heavily.

During the 7 weeks of the study, their activity levels increased, and food intake was reduced to 1,200 kcal/day. Despite a high contribution of animal food to their total energy intake (64%), the diet was low in total fat (13%).

All lost weight steadily and their blood pressures and triglyceride levels fell. As to their diabetes, glucose tolerance markedly improved due to both a fall in fasting glucose (from an average of 200 mg/dl to 120 mg/dl) and an improvement in postprandial glucose clearance *(O'Dea)*.

Meal Frequency

Frequent nibbling appears preferable to 3 meals and one snack. In experiments with both normals *(Jenkins, 1989)* and non-insulin-dependent diabetics *(Jenkins, 1992)*, a nibbling diet significantly reduced serum insulin and 24-hour urinary C peptide levels. Moreover, for the diabetics, mean blood glucose was reduced *(Jenkins, 1992)*.

High Carbohydrate, Low Fat, Low Cholesterol Diet

Current thinking emphasizes a diet which is high in carbohydrates and low in fat and cholesterol. Protein should be between 10 and 20% of calories. Of the remaining calories, less than 10% may be from saturated fats and up to 10% may be from polyunsaturates, leaving 60 to 70% of total calories to be derived from monounsaturates and carbohydrates *(Am. Diabetes Assn., 1998)*.

However, some studies on type II diabetics have reported deterioration in glycemic control and increased serum lipids from such a diet. It is therefore questionable as to whether this diet should be used routinely *(Parillo; Reaven)*.

Dietary Fats

Saturated fats should clearly be minimized; dietary fat should come primarily from mono- and polyunsaturates *(Reaven)*. *Trans* fats act much like saturated fats; their intake should also be minimized since higher consumption promotes higher insulin levels in response to glucose load *(Christiansen)*.

Although a diet emphasizing monounsaturated fats may result in a more desirable plasma glucose, lipid and insulin profile *(Sheard)*, a diet too high in fat, no matter what the type, may worsen insulin sensitivity *(Mayer-Davis)*. Furthermore, a high fat diet is particularly atherogenic for diabetics *(Steiner)*.

Protein

Protein restriction is clearly beneficial for patients who have developed diabetic nephropathy *(Khan)*. Evidence that protein restriction may retard or even reverse the development of nephropathy comes from an open trial of 22 patients with insulin-dependent diabetes who randomly received either an unrestricted protein diet or a moderately protein-restricted diet for 6 months. While patients on the unrestricted diet showed a progressive decline in glomerular filtration rate with no change in proteinuria, patients on the protein-restricted diet showed a marked decrease in proteinuria and a stabilization of glomerular filtration rate independently of changes in blood pressure or glycemic control *(Raal)*.

Fruits and Vegetables

Fruits and vegetables which are high in fiber, particularly *soluble* fiber, should be emphasized since, due to its physical viscosity, soluble fiber slows gastric emptying time and the intestinal absorption of glucose *(Maki)*. High fiber diets may worsen diabetic control, however, in Type II diabetics who are poorly controlled with oral agents *(Scott AR)*.

Vegetarian Diet

A vegetarian diet (which is likely to automatically follow the above guidelines) is preferable. Not only is such a diet associated with a reduced risk of developing diabetes *(West)*, but it is also associated with a reduced risk of diabetes as an underlying or contributing cause of death *(Snowdon)*. Moreover, results of an open trial suggest that a vegan (total vegetarian) diet of unrefined foods, when combined with a program of conditioning exercises, may rapidly reduce the pain and numbness of diabetic neuropathy *(Crane)*.

Glycemic Index

The glycemic index is a measure of the ability of a high carbohydrate food to raise blood glucose. The concept has revolutionized the dietary treatment of diabetes, as starchy foods may have a lower glycemic index than sugary ones. For example, the glycemic response to ice cream is lower than the response to mashed potatoes.

In long-term trials, low-glycemic-index diets result in modest improvements in overall blood glucose control in patients with both insulin-dependent and non-insulin-dependent diabetes. Moreover, low-glycemic-index diets reduce insulin secretion and lower blood lipid concentrations in patients with hypertriglyceridemia *(Wolever)*. This may explain why a low-glycemic-index diet has been shown to be associated with a decreased risk of diabetes *(Salmeron)*.

Dietary Sugar

Sucrose intake should be somewhat restricted. When added to the diet of laboratory animals *(Storlien)*, or increased in the diet of healthy volunteers *(Reiser,1986)*, glucose tolerance may be impaired and the tissues may become less insulin sensitive.

Diabetic retinopathy and nephropathy also appear to be encouraged by a high sucrose intake *(Cohen AM)*. Moreover, chromium deficiency is associated with glucose intolerance (see below), and a high sucrose diet (35% of calories) increases the likelihood of developing chromium deficiency by increasing urinary chromium excretion *(Kozlovsky)*.

However, factors such as differences in the background diet and individual variations in sucrose sensitivity have caused the results of studies on the effects of sucrose on diabetics to be mixed. In fact, surprisingly, both insulin-dependent and non-insulin-dependent diabetics seem to be protected from alterations in plasma lipid concentrations brought about by large amounts of dietary sugars *(Frayn)*. Therefore, most diabetics can tolerate modest amounts of dietary sucrose with no adverse effects *(Frayn;Malerbi)*.

Fructose

It is debatable whether the use of fructose is advisable, since glycemic responses in insulin-dependent diabetics appear to be largely determined by the glucose moiety of sucrose *(Hughes)*. Indeed, fructose is clearly superior to sucrose, and may be similar to starch, in regard to glycemic control *(Thorburn)*. However, it is the fructose moiety of the sucrose molecule which appears to be responsible for the adverse effects of sucrose upon serum lipids *(Reiser,1989)*, and the addition of fructose may increase insulin resistance *(Hallfrisch)*. Finally, when used as a major source of dietary carbohydrate, fructose may induce a copper deficiency *(Reiser,1985)* which, in turn, can adversely affect glucose tolerance (see below).

Alcohol

In diabetics, single bouts of alcohol ingestion not only do not worsen, but may even improve, glucose tolerance. However, moderate daily drinking in the same range as that associated with a decreased risk of myocardial infarction and cardiovascular mortality in the general population (see Atherosclerosis) clearly worsens diabetic control and increases the prevalence of impotence, retinopathy, and possibly peripheral neuropathy *(Swade)*.

Foods as Diabetogens

Whether the early ingestion of <u>cows' milk</u> (before 3 to 4 months of age) can increase the risk of later development of insulin-dependent (Type I) diabetes is currently uncertain *(Atkinson)*. <u>Wheat</u> and <u>soy</u> as diabetogens are both more potent and consistent than cows' milk *(Scott FW)* so it is likely that, if more conclusive evidence that certain foods provoke pancreatic beta cell destruction through immunologic mechanisms, they will also be implicated. Increased risk of insulin-dependent diabetes has also been associated with the childhood intake of <u>coffee</u> and <u>tea</u> *(Virtanen)*, as well as with the intakes <u>nitrates</u> *(Kostraba)* and <u>nitrosamines</u> *(Dahlquist)*.

When admitted to the hospital, a type I diabetic male was receiving 28 units of insulin daily. Initial fasting plasma glucose was 204 mg/dL; serum cholesterol, 280 mg/dL; and fasting serum triglycerides, 1485 mg/dL.

After 10 days on a traditional diabetic diet, he was given a high-carbohydrate, high-fiber diet providing 70% of energy as carbohydrate, 18% protein, 12% fat, 50 mg cholesterol, and 70 g plant fiber daily. Insulin requirements dropped steadily to 16 units/day with no alterations in weight or activity level. After 30 days, fasting blood glucose fell to 143 mg/dL, cholesterol to 131 mg/dL, and triglycerides to 306 mg/dL (Anderson,1989).

NUTRITIONAL FACTORS

Glucose Tolerance Factor

Glucose tolerance factor (GTF) is a micronutrient which differs from typical vitamins and trace elements. It occurs preformed in certain foods (especially *brewer's yeast*), and humans have a varying ability to synthesize it. In response to acute increases of insulin in the blood, GTF is released and potentiates insulin at the target organs *(Mertz,1975)*. Unfortunately, its exact biochemical structure is still not identified.

In a study of elderly non-insulin-dependent diabetics, supplementation with brewer's yeast, but not with tortula yeast, improved glucose tolerance, increased insulin sensitivity and lowered blood lipid levels *(Offenbacher)*. A problem with commercial "GTF" preparations, however, is that their GTF activity is uncertain unless the specific preparation has actually been laboratory-tested.

VITAMINS

Niacin

Since niacin is believed to be a component of glucose tolerance factor, a deficiency will interfere with GTF synthesis and thus may reduce glycemic control *(Mertz,1975)* and should be corrected.

In addition, megadose supplementation with vitamin B_3 has been explored. A recent meta-analysis of the data from 10 randomized, controlled trials concluded that, if *insulin-dependent* diabetics receive high-dose niacinamide when first diagnosed in addition to insulin, the supplement will help to preserve residual beta-cell function *(Pozzilli)*. Moreover, results of a study which employed an animal model of diabetes suggest that nicotinamide supplementation may retard the development of diabetic nephropathy *(Wahlberg)*.

The results of two reports of small open trials of niacin supplementation for *non-insulin-dependent* diabetics were dramatically different. The positive report, published in the *Journal of Nutritional Medicine*, was an informal presentation of 4 males who received niacin 500 to 750 mg daily. (One patient also received a multivitamin, vitamin C and zinc; another also received a multivitamin, vitamin C and linseed oil.) Blood sugar levels fell to normal in all 4 patients, and 2 of the 3 patients on oral hypoglycemic agents were able to discontinue them. Two patients suffered from gout which remitted on niacin, in one case only 4 days after niacin was started *(Cleary)*.

The negative report, published in the *Journal of the American Medical Association*, was a randomized crossover trial of 13 patients who received either 1,500 mg of niacin 3 times daily or no therapy for 8 weeks each. Niacin supplementation resulted in the deterioration of glycemic control, with increased mean plasma glucose concentrations, increased glycosylated hemoglobin levels, a consistent increase in plasma uric acid levels and, in some patients, marked glycosuria *(Garg)*. As the design of this study was clearly superior to that of the positive study, and treatment may be associated with numerous side effects, niacin supplementation should not be attempted with non-insulin-dependent diabetics unless the relevant laboratory parameters are closely followed until further data becomes available.

Thiamine

Thiamine may be marginally deficient *(Saito)*. Since acute thiamine deficiency may cause a neuropathy which responds to supplementation *(Skelton)* while, in a an informal clinical setting, about 80% of patients with diabetic neuropathy improved with thiamine supplementation *(Mirsky)*, it is possible that the diabetics who responded had a marginal thiamine deficiency.

Vitamin A

In insulin-dependent diabetes, plasma concentrations of vitamin A and its carrier proteins are decreased, while hepatic vitamin A is increased. This is due to an impaired transport mechanism from its hepatic storage to the target site, an abnormality that is corrected by insulin treatment.

Therefore, in poorly controlled patients, vitamin A supplementation may fail to increase plasma levels while promoting hepatotoxicity due to vitamin A overload *(Basu)*; it is thus contraindicated for this population.

Vitamin B_6

In normals, a subclinical deficiency of vitamin B_6 may cause insulin resistance *(Ribaya-Mercado)*, while both insulin-dependent *(Hollenbeck)* and non-insulin-dependent *(Rao)* diabetics sometimes have marginal vitamin B_6 nutriture. As deficiency of the vitamin may cause abnormal glucose tolerance, reduced serum and pancreatic insulin levels, degeneration of the pancreatic beta cells and reduced insulin response to glucose *(Rogers)*, repletion is important. Moreover, gestational diabetics with biochemical evidence of a subclinical vitamin B_6 deficiency show a tendency toward normalization of glucose tolerance following supplementation *(Coelingh Bennink)*.

Initial hope that vitamin B_6 supplementation would benefit diabetic neuropathy has been dimmed by later studies. A finding that diabetics with neuropathy had lower serum pyridoxal concentrations than other diabetics *(McCann,1978)* was not confirmed by others *(Rieder;Straub)*. Furthermore, positive results of an open trial of supplementation for diabetics with neuropathy and vitamin B_6 deficiency *(Jones)* were not replicated in subsequent controlled trials *(Cohen KL;Levin; McCann,1983)*.

While controlled trials are lacking, two case reports suggest that megadosage pyridoxine supplementation may be effective in treating diabetic macular edema *(Folkers)*:

Case One: *A 38 year-old diabetic female with macular edema started a multivitamin formula containing 2 mg pyridoxine. After 22 months the dosage of pyridoxine was increased to 300 mg. Four months later, the macular edema had disappeared, visually and by fluorescein angiogram.*

Case Two: *A 74 year-old diabetic male with cystoid macular edema had been taking 50 mg of pyridoxine daily for 1 year. When his dosage of pyridoxine was increased to 300 mg daily, the macular edema disappeared in about 3 months, as evidenced by a fluorescein angiogram.*

Vitamin B_{12}

Vitamin B_{12} is another member of the vitamin B complex which may be beneficial in treating neuropathy. It is known that impaired tissue availability or utilization of cobalamins may cause neurological disorders. Studies utilizing animal models of diabetes have suggested that tissue cobalamin metabolism may be abnormal and that methylcobalamin may ameliorate the development of neuropathy *(Bhatt)*.

In open trials, diabetic neuropathy has shown dramatic subjective improvement with vitamin B_{12} injected intramuscularly *(Sancetta)* or intrathecally *(Ide)*. These results were subsequently confirmed in a randomized double-blind study in which there was significant improvement in somatic and autonomic symptoms and a reduction in neuropathic signs. However, after 4 months, motor and sensory nerve conduction studies showed no significant improvements *(Yaqub)*.

Other studies on diabetic neuropathy have combined vitamin B_{12} with thiamine and vitamin B_6 with excellent results. In contrast to the study just cited, two of these studies reported significant increases in nerve conduction velocities that coincided with clinical progress *(Stracke;Tong)*.

There are also a few studies from the 1950s that reported limited success in treating diabetic retinopathy with vitamin B_{12} injections. In the most positive study, 10 patients received IM cobalamin daily for 14 days. The degree of retinal exudate, as based on photographs, diminished in 3 patients, while 5 patients had clinical improvement, some of which was maintained at 6-month follow-up. By comparison, none of the 10 control patients improved, and 5 of them showed further deterioration *(Cameron)*.

Following the completion of 2 studies, another investigating group concluded that the "curative" effect of treatment was limited to incipient hemorrhagic retinopathy in young diabetics whose disease started before age 15 *(Kornerup)*.

Vitamin C

The intake of vitamin C may be reduced in diabetic patients compared to apparently healthy controls *(Singh)*. Even when vitamin C intake is in the range normally considered to be adequate, ascorbic acid levels are frequently depressed in both the plasma *(Sinclair)* and leukocytes *(Cunningham,1991)*; in fact, most studies have found that diabetics have at least 30% lower circulating ascorbic acid levels than normals *(Will)*. Results of studies employing animal models of diabetes suggest that these low levels, when not due to low intake, are caused by increased urinary excretion *(Zebrowski)* and defective transport across cell membranes *(Cunningham,1988)*, as well as increased oxidation of ascorbic acid to dehydroascorbic acid (DHAA) *(Som)*.

Defective cell membrane transport of ascorbic acid into vascular epithelial cells during hyperglycemia may promote the development of atherosclerosis and angiopathies *(Kapeghian)*, while the accumulation of DHAA may not only promote the diabetic process *(Patterson)* but also oxidative damage *(Jennings)*.

Also, the antioxidant *glutathione* reduces DHAA to vitamin C in red blood cells *(Banerjee)*. As it is frequently depressed in diabetics *(Banerjee)*, inadequate glutathione nutriture could be a cause of increased DHAA levels.

While diabetes causes these disorders in ascorbic acid metabolism, a vitamin C deficiency may provoke disorders in glycoregulation resembling diabetes. Thus a vicious circle may occur which requires an increased supply of ascorbic acid in order to be terminated *(Ginter,1983)*.

Supplementation

There is substantial evidence that diabetics may require supplemental ascorbic acid in order to achieve tissue saturation and maximal physiologic function *(Cunningham,1998)*. Vitamin C supplementation has been shown to improve glucose tolerance *(Eriksson)* and lipid profiles *(Ginter,1978)* in non-insulin-dependent diabetics, and to reduce cutaneous capillary fragility *(Cox)*. There is some evidence that supplementation may reduce the nonenzymatic glycosylation of proteins *(Vinson)*, a process that plays an important role in the development of diabetic complications, although its efficacy in this regard is still uncertain *(Cunningham,1998)*. Moreover, DHAA disappears after continued ascorbic acid administration *(Banerjee)*.

Finally, vitamin C supplementation may lower erythrocyte *sorbitol* levels independent of changes in diabetic control *(Cunningham,1994a)*. Tissue sorbitol accumulation is associated with the development of diabetic complications including cataracts, retinopathy and neuropathy. Hyperglycemia causes the accumulation of sorbitol in tissues due to the action of the enzyme aldose reductase on glucose. Intracellular sorbitol draws in water by osmosis while low molecular weight compounds are lost in an attempt to maintain osmotic equilibrium. *(Cogan)*.

For an insulin-dependent diabetic, each gram of oral vitamin C taken daily permitted a 2 unit reduction in daily insulin requirements (Dice).

Vitamin E

Diabetics appear to have an increased requirement for vitamin E *(Lubin)*, yet their intake may be reduced *(Singh)*. Research on plasma/serum levels of the nutrient has been conflicting, with some studies finding reduced levels *(Singh)*, others finding elevations *(Martinoli)*, and still others finding normal levels *(Granado)*.

Of interest is a 4 year prospective study of almost 1000 men which found a strong independent association between low plasma vitamin E at baseline and an excess risk of diabetes at follow-up. Specifically, a standardized plasma vitamin E concentration below the mean was associated with a 3.9-fold greater risk of diabetes *(Salonen)*.

Supplementation

There are several reasons why supplementation with vitamin E should be routinely considered for diabetics. Several double-blind studies have found that supplementation may improve glycemic control in type I *(Duntas)* and type II *(Paolisso,1993)* diabetes. Moreover, under double-blind conditions, supplementation may decrease platelet hyperaggregability which may contribute to microvascular complications and atherogenesis *(Ginsinger;Jain,1996a)*, a process that it also combats in diabetics by decreasing lipid peroxidation *(Jain,1996b)* and LDL oxidation *(Fuller)*.

In a randomized controlled study, vitamin E improved both temperature and vibratory sensitivity in distal symmetric neuropathy *(Kahler)*. In uncontrolled studies, supplementation appeared to be beneficial in treating diabetic gangrene *(Block)* and necrobiosis lipoidica diabeticorum *(Ayres)*.

Finally, studies of animal models of spontaneous diabetes have found evidence that vitamin E supplementation may reduce the risk, or delay the onset, of insulin-dependent diabetes *(Beales)*.

MINERALS

Calcium

In a study of almost 85,000 women, calcium intake was found to be inversely related with the risk of non-insulin-dependent diabetes. Women in the highest quintile had 70% of the risk of those in the lowest quintile *(Colditz)*. Moreover, among a small group of similar patients, only 30% of them met the RDA for calcium *(Schmidt)*, although another small study found normal levels of intake *(Kawagishi)*.

Numerous studies have shown diabetes to be associated with abnormal regulation of intracellular calcium. Increased calcium has been found in cardiac, renal, aortic, hepatic and neural tissues of insulin-dependent and non-insulin-dependent diabetics *(Levy)*. In a large epidemiological study, total serum calcium levels were found to be correlated with serum glucose levels as well as with blood pressures and serum cholesterol levels *(Lind)*.

These findings and others have led to the suggestion that changes in calcium metabolism resulting in elevation of total serum calcium levels may be related, not only to glycoregulation, but also to lipid metabolism and blood pressure regulation *(Levy)*. Serum ionized calcium levels, by contrast, tend to be depressed *(Fogh-Anderson)*.

Supplementation

The hypothesis that low calcium intake causes insulin resistance was tested on 20 non-diabetics with essential hypertension. They were placed on a 4-week trial of a low calcium diet (500 mg daily) and then randomly assigned to receive 1,500 mg of calcium daily or placebo. Only in the supplemented group, mean fasting plasma insulin levels went down and the insulin sensitivity index increased *(Sanchez)*.

In a small open trial, an oral calcium load appeared to augment glucose-induced insulin secretion in diabetics but not in normals *(Fujita)*. Controlled trials are needed to better evaluate the efficacy of high-dosage calcium supplementation in treating diabetes, although calcium deficiency should clearly be repleted.

Chromium Deficiency

Glucose intolerance is one of the first signs of chromium deficiency *(Freund)*, in which case glucose uptake in insulin-sensitive tissues is impaired *(Mertz,1969)*. Moreover, serum chromium levels are positively correlated with serum insulin levels *(Liu)*.

Supplementation

Several double-blind studies have found chromium supplementation to improve the glycemic response in non-insulin-dependent *(Anderson,1997)* and gestational *(Jovanovic-Peterson)* diabetics, although 4 studies failed to confirm its efficacy when given either as elemental chromium or as brewer's yeast *(Finney)*. Anderson notes that the large majority of patients with marginally impaired glucose tolerance respond to supplementation with 200 μg of inorganic chromium, while diabetic subjects may require greater levels of chromium in a biologically active form *(Anderson,1992)*.

In addition, case reports suggest that, in diabetics who are chromium-deficient, peripheral neuropathy may respond to supplementation *(Chatfield;Jeejeebhoy)*. Controlled trials are needed for confirmation.

Although the beneficial effects of chromium are usually attributed to its role as a component of glucose tolerance factor *(Haylock)* (see Glucose Tolerance Factor above), the essentiality of chromium to GTF has come into question following studies in which fractions of extracts of brewer's yeast were purified and GTF activity was found in fractions that contained no chromium *(Davies; Simonoff)*.

A 51-year-old type I diabetic female presented with large vessel disease (atherosclerosis), microvascular disease (glomerular nephritis, retinitis), peripheral neuropathy, discoloration and ulceration of the anterior portion of the left first toe, mood swings and anxiety. Disease onset was at age 27; microvascular retinal changes were noted at age 39. At age 46, bilateral distal sensory polyneuropathy of the feet and hands ("glove and stocking" distribution) began and subsequently had slowly progressed. At age 50, atherosclerosis and discoloration and ulceration of the first toe were diagnosed. Mood swings and anxiety had existed as long as the patient could remember.

Dietary history revealed a high complex carbohydrate diet with adequate protein and limited refined sugar. Hair chromium and manganese were depressed. Urinalysis revealed proteinuria, hematuria and RBC casts.

She was placed on trivalent chromium as glucose tolerance factor 200 μg twice daily and micellized vitamin E 400 IU twice daily. Follow-up visits at 3, 6 and 9 weeks showed gradual improvement. By 6 months, her insulin requirement had decreased from 140 units to 40 units daily. Her glomerular nephritis was in remission. There was a moderate reduction in her peripheral neuropathy. Her extremities showed no signs of discoloration or ulceration and her mental state was excellent (Chatfield).

Copper Deficiency

A copper deficiency may be associated with glucose intolerance *(Klevey)*. Also, when copper-deficient animals receive sucrose or fructose rather than starch as their source of dietary carbohydrate, sorbitol accumulates in their tissues *(Fields)*. (See the discussion of sorbitol under Vitamin C above).

Therefore, copper status should be evaluated and any deficiency treated.

Magnesium Deficiency

Magnesium intake appears to be inversely related to the risk of diabetes *(Colditz)* as well as fasting serum insulin levels *(Ma)*. Moreover, a study of 50 non-insulin-dependent diabetics found that only 20% of them met the RDA for magnesium *(Schmidt)*.

Magnesium nutriture is frequently depressed in diabetics *(Durlach),* especially those with coronary heart disease *(Wen-gang)* or proliferative retinopathy *(McNair,1978)*. Hypomagnesemia is a common finding and may result from increased urinary magnesium excretion as a consequence of glycosuria *(Tosiello)*. Reduced erythrocyte and platelet magnesium concentrations are also common *(Corica)*.

A consensus panel of the American Diabetes Association has suggested that "magnesium deficiency may play a role in insulin resistance, carbohydrate intolerance, and hypertension" *(Am. Diabetes Assn.,1992)*. While insulin enhances magnesium uptake *(Lostroh)*, when a dietary magnesium deficiency was induced in normal male volunteers, they developed insulin resistance *(Nadler)*.

There is evidence that magnesium activates the key enzymes of glycolysis *(Elamin),* and results of controlled studies suggest that chronic magnesium supplementation may improve glycoregulation by improving insulin response and action *(Paolisso,1989)*.

Another consensus panel of the American Diabetes Association has suggested that diabetic patients with documented magnesium deficiency should receive "oral magnesium chloride of dependable potency and bioavailability" *(Am. Diabetes Assn.,1995)*. No matter which magnesium salt is provided, it may take a minimum of 3 months to correct hypomagnesemia *(Eibl)*.

Manganese Deficiency

Manganese is an important cofactor in the key enzymes of glycolysis *(Wimhurst)*, yet its levels may be only half those of normals *(Kosenko)*. Animal studies have found that manganese deficiency is associated with impaired glycoregulation due to impaired insulin synthesis and secretion *(Baly)*.

Supplementation has been poorly studied. While manganese supplementation dramatically improved glucose tolerance in a type I diabetic *(Rubenstein),* it is likely that it is only effective when repleting a deficiency.

Phosphorus

A deficiency of phosphorus is associated with an impaired response to insulin *(DeFronzo),* which suggests that repleting a deficiency may improve insulin sensitivity. Also, insulin-dependent diabetics appear to have a fluctuating disorder in the oxygen-releasing capacity of their erythrocytes which may contribute to the development of angiopathy *(Ditzel).* The position of the oxyhemoglobin dissociation curve is positively correlated with 2,3-diphosphoglycerate levels in the red blood cells; these levels, in turn, vary in response to inorganic phosphate levels in the plasma *(Ditzel).*

Supplementation with inorganic phosphate salts may therefore improve erythrocyte oxygen-releasing capacity (and reduce the development of angiopathy) by preventing the inhibitory effect of a low inorganic phosphorus concentration on red cell oxygen delivery *(Freyler).* In one study, insulin-dependent diabetics received dibasic calcium phosphate 2 gm 3 times daily with meals. After 2 years, diabetic control was improved, the patients felt less tired, and there were no adverse effects *(Ditzel).*

Controlled clinical trials are needed to better assess the efficacy of this treatment.

Potassium Deficiency

Potassium intake may be inversely associated with the risk of diabetes *(Colditz).* Moreover, potassium depletion is common in diabetics and may cause a decrease in peripheral insulin levels and insulin resistance *(Norbiato).*

However, there is a potential of hyperkalemia developing immediately following the administration of potassium salts in diabetics with hypoaldosteronism *(Perez)*; thus, until the effects of potassium supplementation are better established, it would be advisable to avoid it as a routine measure. Of course, in diabetic ketoacidosis, hypokalemia should be aggressively treated *(Fish).*

Selenium

While plasma selenium appears to be normal, erythrocyte selenium levels may be markedly decreased in insulin-dependent diabetics. These low levels appear to contribute to increased whole blood viscosity *(Osterode).*

Few human trials of selenium supplementation have been reported. However, selenium administration to diabetics under controlled conditions has been found to combat free radical oxidation and to reduce the symptoms of diabetic neuropathy *(Kahler).*

Vanadium

Vanadium salts mimic most of the effects of insulin on the main target tissues of the hormone *in vitro. In vivo* they induce a sustained fall in blood glucose levels in insulin-deficient diabetic rats, and improve glucose homeostasis in obese, insulin-resistant diabetic rodents *(Brichard).*

For non-insulin-dependent diabetics, recent short-term clinical trials with vanadium salts also seem promising for reducing liver and peripheral insulin resistance *(Brichard).* Under controlled conditions, supplementation has been shown to reduce fasting glucose and glycosylated hemoglobin concentrations *(Halberstam).*

Given that insulin hypersecretion increases the risk of diabetes, while inhibition of insulin secretion helps to prevent it, vanadium may act by preventing hyperinsulinemia, partly because of its own insulin activity *(Sprietsma).*

If vanadium supplementation is utilized, it will likely need to be lifelong. Toxicity in that case may be an issue, since studies of diabetic rats treated with vanadyl (4+) or vanadate (5+) to improve glucose homeostasis found tissue accumulation and serious toxicity at the dosages utilized *(Domingo)*, while human studies have yet to be reported proving the long-term safety of pharmacologic dosages. Long-term vanadium supplementation is not recommended until it is shown to be safe.

Zinc

Zinc nutriture is another important factor in glycoregulation. Normals on a low-zinc diet develop a significant increase in fasting blood glucose *(Solomon).* In a small study, only 14% of non-insulin-dependent diabetics were found to meet the RDA for zinc *(Schmidt),* while another study found low groundwater levels of zinc to be directly related to the risk of insulin-dependent diabetes *(Haglund).*

Moreover, zinc metabolism in diabetes appears to be abnormal. Non-insulin-dependent diabetics may show evidence of zinc malabsorption *(Kinlaw)*. Hyperzincuria is common in both insulin-dependent *(Cunningham,1994b)* and non-insulin-dependent *(Chen)* diabetics and may correlate with serum glucose levels *(Kinlaw)* and the degree of glycosuria *(McNair,1981)*. Tissue *(Sjogren)* and blood *(Chen)* zinc levels are frequently depressed.

Zinc plays a role in the synthesis, storage and secretion of insulin as well as conformational integrity of insulin in the hexameric form *(Chausmer)*; thus a deficiency is likely to contribute to the problems with insulin regulation. Furthermore, several diabetic complications may be related to increased cellular oxidants and free radicals associated with decreases in intracellular zinc and zinc-dependent antioxidant enzymes *(Chausmer)*.

Following plasma or serum zinc levels is probably not useful. Poor indicators of tissue stores *(Solomons)*, they have been found to be both elevated *(Mateo)* and depressed *(Kinlaw)* in various studies.

Supplementation

Repletion of a zinc deficiency would be an obvious goal. Indeed, normal volunteers who received zinc supplements the evening before and prior to glucose tolerance testing showed increased glucose assimilation and efficacy *(Brun)*. However, the issue of whether diabetics should routinely receive zinc supplementation is unresolved.

When, for example, insulin-dependent diabetics were supplemented with 50 mg of zinc for 28 days, fasting plasma glucose levels were unchanged, while mean glycosylated hemoglobin levels *increased* from 6.5% at baseline to 9.4% compared to an increase from 4.4% to 5.3% in normal controls *(Cunningham,1994b)*. This result is consistent with that of an earlier study in which non-insulin-dependent diabetics received 50 mg of zinc 3 times daily for 7 to 8 weeks. Glucose disposal *decreased* significantly while fasting glucose levels were significantly *increased (Raz)*.

In addition to these worrisome findings, there is the question of whether zinc supplementation, due to its poor absorption and increased excretion, is able to effectively replete a tissue deficiency *(Thompson)*. Thus, until further controlled trials are completed, zinc supplementation cannot be recommended for diabetics unless there are signs and symptoms of classic zinc deficiency which are confirmed by appropriate laboratory testing and then followed by repeat laboratory studies.

ANTIOXIDANT COMBINATIONS

The value of a combination of antioxidants nutrients in treating diabetic retinopathy was demonstrated in study in which 20 diabetics with retinal changes were treated with vitamin A 10,000 IU, vitamin C 1 gram, vitamin E 800 IU and selenium 500 μg daily. After several years, all but one exhibited improvement or no progression of the lesions *(Crary)*.

OTHER NUTRITIONAL FACTORS

Arginine

Nitric oxide is a powerful vasodilator released from the vascular endothelium. In non-insulin-dependent diabetes, either the activity of nitric oxide synthase is increased, or nitric oxide sensitivity is decreased, resulting in endothelial dysfunction, a factor which contributes to the pathogenesis of diabetic vascular disorders *(Schmetterer)* and which is associated with increased oxidative stress *(Chowienczyk)*.

The results of early studies of arginine supplementation appear promising. In an open trial, intravenous administration of L-arginine, the nutritional precursor of nitric oxide, not only restored impaired vasodilation, but improved insulin sensitivity in non-insulin-dependent diabetics *(Wascher)*. Moreover, in a placebo-controlled study, oral supplementation with L-arginine significantly reduced the levels of malondialdehyde, a measure of lipid peroxidation, in diabetic patients *(Lubec)*.

More studies are needed to better assess the efficacy of L-arginine in this disorder.

Biotin

At least in insulin-dependent diabetics, tissue biotin levels may be increased *(Coggeshall)*. Plasma/serum levels, which may be in the normal range *(Coggeshall)* or low *(Maebashi)*, may be inversely correlated with blood glucose levels *(Coggeshall;Maebashi)*.

Supplemental biotin, while poorly studied, may improve glycoregulation. When a group of insulin-dependent diabetics were taken off of insulin and treated with biotin for one week, they showed a significant drop in fasting blood sugar, while a control group that was given placebo showed the expected rise *(Coggeshall)*. Similarly, one month after non-insulin-dependent diabetics were supplemented with biotin (along with an antibiotic to retard biotin degradation by microflora), mean blood sugar levels were significantly decreased, although serum insulin levels were unchanged *(Maebashi)*.

There is also evidence from an open trial that biotin supplements may be an effective treatment for diabetic neuropathy. Within 4 to 8 weeks of starting supplementation, 3 patients with severe peripheral neuropathy had marked improvement of clinical and laboratory findings. After one year, there was nearly complete symptom remission *(Kousikos)*.

The authors of this report speculate that, in diabetes, biotin may be deficient, inactive or unavailable, causing disordered activity of the biotin-dependent enzyme pyruvate carboxylase. This would lead to the accumulation of pyruvate and/or the depletion of aspartate, both of which play an important role in nervous system metabolism *(Kousikos)*.

Further studies are needed to clarify the safety and efficacy of biotin supplementation.

Carnitine

Acetyl-L-carnitine, a patented derivative of L-carnitine and a naturally occurring ester, has been investigated for its effects on diabetic neuropathy. Several studies have been performed in experimental animal models of diabetes. They have found that, in diabetes, acetyl-L-carnitine depletion may affect nerve intermediary and energy metabolism and impulse conduction *(Stevens)*. Moreover, treatment with acetyl-L-carnitine restored depleted nerve myo-inositol content and decreased elevated nerve malondialdehyde content (a measure of lipid peroxidation) to normal *(Lowitt)*, suggesting that the nutrient may protect against the development of neuropathy.

Under double-blind conditions, patients with symptomatic diabetic neuropathy who received acetyl-L-carnitine by intramuscular injection showed highly significant improvements *(Quatraro)*.

Coenzyme Q_{10} (ubiquinone)

Coenzyme Q_{10} is more commonly deficient in diabetics, especially those on oral hypoglycemic agents, than in normals *(Kishi)*. It has been found in open trials to stimulate insulin synthesis and secretion, peripheral glucose utilization, and blood sugar control *(Shimura)*.

In one study utilizing CoQ_7 (which is interchangeable in the body for CoQ_{10}), fasting blood sugar was reduced by at least 20% in 36% of 39 stable patients, and by at least 30% in 31% of the patients, while ketone bodies fell by at least 30% in 59% *(Shigeta)*.

Flavonoids

Sorbitol Reduction

It was noted above that tissue sorbitol accumulation is associated with the development of diabetic complications. The results of studies with animal models suggest that sorbitol accumulation and its consequences can be combated by administering certain flavonoids such as *quercetin* and *naringin* (from the flowers, fruit and rind of grapefruit) which inhibit aldose reductase, an enzyme involved in the synthesis of sorbitol from glucose *(Varma)*. *Sorbinol*, a drug known to be a potent aldose reductase inhibitor, has been shown to benefit neuropathy and amyopathy *(Jaspan)*, suggesting that natural aldose reductase inhibitors may have a similar effect.

Clinical trials are needed to assess the efficacy of flavonoids for this application.

Reduced Erythrocyte Aggregation

Vascular complications of diabetes may be due to rheological disorders such as hypoviscosity, red cell hyperaggregation or hypodeformity. Since flavonoids have been shown to improve blood rheology in venous thrombosis, *Daflon*, a micronized flavonoid mixture of 90% *diosmin* and 10% *hesperidin*, was given to diabetics in a clinical trial. Hemorheological improvement was found due to a decrease in erythrocyte aggregation. This could theoretically lead to clinical benefits due to a decrease in blood flow resistance and a reduction in stasis and resulting ischemia *(Lacombe)*.

Basement Membrane Damage

Flavonoids have also been shown to strengthen capillary basement membranes *(Gabor)*. In diabetes, administration of certain flavonoids such as *quercetin* or *rutin* may prevent ascorbic acid from being oxidized in the jejunum to dehydroascorbic acid which is damaging to these membranes *(Clemetson)*.

Controlled trials are needed to ascertain whether this effect is clinically relevant.

Retinopathy

Certain flavonoids have shown efficacy in treating diabetic retinopathy in open trials. These include *hesperidin (Beardwood)*, *pycnogenol® (Magnard)* and *rutin (Palmer)*.

Inositol

Inositol is a 6-carbon, cyclic polyalcohol present in all mammalian cells. Concentrations within peripheral nerves are extremely high, suggesting a role in peripheral nerve function. There is evidence from some, but not all, studies of diabetic polyneuropathy that patients may have decreased *myo*-inositol concentrations in the afflicted nerves *(Mayhew)*. Moreover, it has been suggested that the adverse effects of sorbitol accumulation upon peripheral nerves may be a direct effect of *myo*-inositol loss *(Greene)*.

In open trials, diabetics with neuropathy demonstrated improved sensory nerve function with increased evoked nerve action potential amplitude following supplementation *(Clements;Salway)*, although 2 double-blind studies failed to find objective evidence of improvement *(Gregersen,1978,1983)*.

alpha-Lipoic Acid

alpha-Lipoic acid (thioctic acid) plays an important role as an enzyme cofactor in energy metabolism. In diabetes, cellular sugar uptake is impaired, and thioctic acid stimulates glucose carriers to increase sugar uptake in cells, thus improving insulin action. An antioxidant, thioctic acid can regenerate other antioxidants such as vitamin C, vitamin E and glutathione *(Barbirolly)*.

Supplementation has been found to increase insulin action *(Jacob)* and improve energy metabolism *(Barbiroli)*. Under double-blind conditions, supplementation has reduced the pain, burning, paresthesia and numbness of diabetic peripheral neuropathy, and reduced the heart rate variability of diabetic autonomic neuropathy, in non-insulin dependent diabetics *(Ziegler)*.

Omega-3 Essential Fatty Acids

alpha-linolenic acid → EPA → 3 series prostaglandins
└→ DHA

In non-insulin-dependent diabetics, plasma levels of alpha-linolenic acid and docosahexaenoic acid (DHA), both members of the omega-3 family of essential fatty acids, may be decreased *(Das)*.

Red blood cell membranes in diabetics may be less fluid than in normals, thus making them less able to change shape in order to travel through smaller capillaries and stenotic areas, and thus more liable to symptoms such as intermittent claudication. In a controlled study, dietary sardine oil rich in omega-3 fatty acids increased membrane fluidity in both diabetics and normals, and the difference in membrane fluidity between diabetics and normals disappeared *(Kamada)*. Moreover, supplementation with fish oils has been found to augment nitric oxide production or release in non-insulin-dependent diabetics to improve vasodilator response *(McVeigh)*.

Omega-3 fatty acid supplementation has been shown in open trials to increase insulin sensitivity in non-insulin-dependent diabetics *(Popp-Snijders)*. However, double-blind studies have shown that it may also impair insulin secretion, elevate basal hepatic glucose *(Glauber)*, and raise fasting glucose levels *(Puhakainen)*.

Although these latter findings are worrisome, a double-blind crossover study of normal volunteers found significant increases in fasting blood glucose levels when 30 ml of fish oil was accompanied by 1.5 IU per gram of vitamin E, but no increase when the fish oil was accompanied with 6 IU per gram of the vitamin *(Luostarinen)*. It appears that the vitamin E acts as an antioxidant and prevents the adverse effects of increased lipid peroxidation from fish oil supplementation *(McGrath)*.

Other studies on insulin-dependent diabetics have found supplementation with MaxEPA (a standardized fish oil preparation) *(Vandongen)* and with cod liver oil *(Jensen)* to be associated with an increase in HDL cholesterol. MaxEPA, however, also caused a rise in LDL cholesterol *(Vandongen)*. This finding appears to be because it contains 30% saturated fats, while cod liver oil contains only 15% of saturated fats *(Jensen)*. Also, with non-insulin-dependent diabetics, an open trial of a marine lipid concentrate found decreases in both total cholesterol and triglycerides *(Friday).*

In an open trial, 21 patients with chronic diabetic neuropathy received purified eicosapentaenoic acid for 48 weeks. After the first 12 weeks they showed improvements in the signs and symptoms of peripheral neuropathy and foot circulation, benefits which were maintained throughout the trial *(Okuda).*

Omega-6 Essential Fatty Acids

linoleic acid → GLA → DGLA → 1 series prostaglandins

Prostaglandin E1, derived from linoleic acid, has insulin-like actions and potentiates insulin effects *(Haessler).* The first step in its conversion requires the enzyme delta-6-desaturase whose activity, as suggested by animal models of diabetes, may be inhibited *(Mercuri).*

A controlled study has found that a linoleic acid-enriched diet was associated after 5 years with decreased microangiopathy, cardiac ischemia and risk of death from myocardial infarction *(Houtsmuller),* while a crossover study of non-insulin-dependent diabetics found a linoleic-enriched diet (polyunsaturated to saturated fat ratio of 1 versus 0.3 in the control diet) was associated after 30 weeks with significant declines in total and LDL cholesterol *(Heine).*

The benefits of evening primrose oil, which has a high content of the PGE1 precursor gamma-linolenic acid (GLA), in the treatment of diabetic neuropathy has been demonstrated in double-blind studies. When, for example, 111 patients received 12 caps of evening primrose oil daily for one year, 13 out of 16 objective parameters showed statistically significant improvements *(Keen).*

Pyridoxine Alpha-ketoglutarate

The complex of pyridoxine and alpha-ketoglutaric acid (pyridoxine alpha-ketoglutarate; PAK) appears to be more effective for certain applications that either component alone, perhaps because it may cross the mitochondrial membrane to enhance the oxidative process more easily than its separate components.

The results of a double-blind study suggest that PAK may potentiate the effects of both insulin and oral hypoglycemic agents: Both type I and type II diabetics received either PAK or placebo. After 4 weeks, both groups receiving PAK showed significant decreases in fasting glucose, glycosylated hemoglobin, lactate and pyruvate compared to pretreatment levels. There were no adverse effects *(Passariello).*

Taurine

Taurine has a hypoglycemic effect that is mediated through potentiation of insulin action by interaction with the insulin receptor *(Kulakowski).* Plasma and platelet taurine levels may be reduced in insulin-dependent diabetics *(Franconi).*

In vitro and *in vivo*, taurine supplementation may normalize the increased tendency for platelets to aggregate in diabetes *(Franconi).* Since altered platelet function in diabetes appears to contribute to the pathogenesis of micro- and macrovascular complications *(Mustard),* this finding suggests that taurine supplementation may retard the development of these complications, an hypothesis that remains to be tested.

OTHER RELATED FACTORS

Obesity

Obesity should be avoided or, if present, treated. The exaggerated serum insulin levels seen after glucose administration in type II diabetics correlate with the degree of obesity, and the risk of type II diabetes correlates with the degree and duration of obesity *(Karam).*

In fact, there is a higher risk of diabetes in people with "beer bellies" (excess upper body fat) than in those with excess fat in the hips and thighs *(Nat. Inst. Health).* Although type II diabetes is fairly uncommon among thin people *(Williams),* it remains unknown whether weight control can prevent development of the disease *(Nat. Inst. Health).*

Hydrochloric Acid Deficiency

There is evidence from several studies that diabetics have decreased hydrochloric acid secretion following feeding, a finding that is not due to hyperglycemia *(Richardson).*

In an informal report dating from 1949, a large group of diabetics with severe neuritis who were under good control but who failed to benefit from thiamine supplementation (see Thiamine above) were placed on hydrochloric acid supplements. Their neuritis markedly improved, suggesting that the hydrochloric acid deficiency prevented them from absorbing the thiamine supplements *(Rabinowich).*

The effects of repleting a hydrochloric acid deficiency in diabetics needs further study.

BIBLIOGRAPHY

American Diabetes Association. Consensus statement. Magnesium supplementation in the treatment of diabetes. Diabetes Care 15(8):1065-7, 1992

American Diabetes Association. Consensus panel. Magnesium supplementation in the treatment of diabetes. Diabetes Care 18(Suppl 1):83-5, 1995

American Diabetes Association. Clinical Practice Recommendations 1998. Position Statement: Nutrition recommendations and principles for people with diabetes mellitus. Diabetes Care 21:Suppl 1, 1998

Anderson JW. Recent advances in carbohydrate nutrition and metabolism in diabetes mellitus. J Am Coll Nutr 8(Suppl):61S-67S, 1989

Anderson RA. Chromium, glucose tolerance, and diabetes. Biol Trace Elem Res 32:19-24, 1992

Anderson RA et al. Elevated intakes of supplemental chromium improve glucose and insulin variables in individuals with type 2 diabetes. Diabetes 46(11):1786-91, 1997

Atkinson MA, Ellis TM. Infants diets and insulin-dependent diabetes: evaluating the "cows' milk hypothesis" and a role for anti-bovine serum albumin immunity. J Am Coll Nutr 16(4):334-40, 1997

Ayers S Jr, Mihan R. Vitamin E and dermatology. Cutis 16:1017-21, 1975

Baly D et al. Effect of manganese deficiency on insulin binding, glucose transport and metabolism of rat adipocytes. J Nutr 120:1075-9, 1990

Banerjee S. Physiological role of dehydroascorbic acid. Indian J Physiol Pharmacol 21(2):85-93, 1977

Barbiroli B - summarized in Conference Report: Thioctic acid - a rational remedy for the treatment of diabetic polyneuropathy. Exp Clin Endocrinol Diabetes 104:126-7, 1995

Basu TK, Basualdo C. Vitamin A homeostasis and diabetes mellitus. Nutrition 13(9):804-6, 1997

Beales PE et al. Vitamin E delays diabetes onset in the non-obese diabetic mouse. Metab Res 26:450-2, 1994

Beardwood et al quoted in Shils ME, Goodhart RS. The Flavonoids in Biology and Medicine. National Vitamin Foundation, Inc., 1956:34-69

Bhatt HR et al. Can faulty vitamin B12 (cobalamin) metabolism produce diabetic neuropathy? Letter to the Editor. Lancet ii:572, 1983

Block MT. Vitamin E in the treatment of diseases of the skin. Clin Med 60:31, 1953

Brichard SM, Henquin JC. The role of vanadium in the management of diabetes. Trends Pharmacol Sci 16(8):265-70, 1995

Brun J-F et al. Effects of oral zinc gluconate on glucose effectiveness and insulin sensitivity in humans. Biol Trace Elem Res 47:385-91, 1995

Cameron AJ, Ahern GJ. Diabetic retinopathy and cyanocobalamin (vitamin B12). A preliminary report. Br J Ophthalmol 42:686-93, 1958

Chatfield K. Preventive medicine clinics: A case of diabetes. Townsend Letter for Doctors March, 1985, p. 105

Chausmer AB. Zinc, insulin and diabetes. J Am Coll Nutr 17(2):109-15, 1998

Chen M-D et al. Selected metals status in patients with noninsulin-dependent diabetes mellitus. Biol Trace Elem Res 50:119-24, 1995

Chowienczyk P, Ritter J. Arginine: NO more than a simple amino acid? Lancet 250:901-2, 1997).

Christiansen E et al. Intake of a diet high in *trans* monounsaturated fatty acids or saturated fatty acids. Effects on postprandial insulinemia and glycemia in obese patients with NIDDM. Diabetes Care 20(5):881-7, 1997

Cleary JP. Vitamin B3 in the treatment of diabetes mellitus: Case reports and review of the literature. J Nutr Med 1:217-25, 1990

Clements RS et al. Dietary myo-inositol intake and peripheral nerve function in diabetic neuropathy. Metabolism 28:477, 1979

Clemetson AB. Ascorbic acid and diabetes mellitus. Med Hypotheses 2:193-4, 1976

Coelingh Bennink HJT, Schreurs WHP. Improvement of oral glucose tolerance in gestational diabetes by pyridoxine. Br Med J 3:13-15, 1975

Cogan DG et al. Aldose reductase and complications of diabetes. Ann Intern Med 101:82-91, 1984

Coggeshall JC et al. Biotin status and plasma glucose in diabetics. Ann N Y Acad Sci 447:389-92, 1985

Cohen AM et al. Experimental models in diabetes, in Sugars in Nutrition. San Francisco, Academic Press, 1974:483-511

Cohen KL et al. Effect of pyridoxine (vitamin B6) on diabetic patients with peripheral neuropathy. J Am Podiatry Assoc 74(8):394-7, 1984

Colditz GA et al. Diet and risk of clinical diabetes in women. Am J Clin Nutr 55:1018-23, 1992

Corica F et al. Magnesium levels in plasma, erythrocyte, and platelets in hypertensive and normotensive patients with non-insulin-dependent diabetes mellitus. Biol Trace Elem Res 51:130-2, 1996

Cox BD, Butterfield WJH. Vitamin C supplements and diabetic cutaneous capillary fragility. Br Med J 3:205, 1975

Crane MG, Sample C. Regression of diabetic neuropathy with total vegetarian (vegan) diet. J Nutr Med 4:431-9, 1994

Crary EJ, McCarty MF. Potential clinical applications for high-dose nutritional antioxidants. Med Hypotheses 13:77-98, 1984

Cunningham JJ. Altered vitamin C transport in diabetes mellitus. Med Hypotheses 26:263-5, 1988

Cunningham JJ et al. Reduced mononuclear leukocyte ascorbic-acid content in adults with insulin-dependent diabetes mellitus consuming adequate dietary vitamin C. Metabolism 40:146-9, 1991

Cunningham JJ et al. Vitamin C: an aldose reductase inhibitor that normalizes erythrocyte sorbitol in insulin-dependent diabetes mellitus. J Am Coll Nutr 13(4):344-50, 1994a

Cunningham JJ et al. Hyperzincuria in individuals with insulin-dependent diabetes mellitus: concurrent zinc status and the effect of high-dose zinc supplementation. Metabolism 43:1558-62, 1994b

Cunningham JJ. The glucose/insulin system and vitamin C: implications in insulin-dependent diabetes mellitus. J Am Coll Nutr 17(2):105-8, 1998

Dahlquist GG et al. Dietary factors and the risk of developing insulin dependent diabetes in children. Br Med J 300:1302-6, 1990

Das UN et al. Lipid peroxides and essential fatty acids in patients with diabetes mellitus and diabetic nephropathy. J Nutr Med 4:149-55, 1994

Davies DM et al. The isolation of glucose tolerance factors from brewer's yeast and their relationship to chromium. Biochem Med 33(3):297-311, 1985

DeFronzo RA, Lang R. Hypophosphatemia and glucose intolerance: Evidence for tissue insensitivity to insulin. N Engl J Med 303(22):1259-63, 1980

Dice JF, Daniel CW. The hypoglycemic effect of ascorbic acid in a juvenile-onset diabetic. J Int Res Commun 1(1):41, 1973

Ditzel J. Oxygen transport in diabetes. Diabetes 25:832-8, 1976

Domingo JL et al. Oral vanadium administration to streptozotocin-diabetic rats has marked negative side-effects which are independent of the form of vanadium used. Toxicology 66:279-87, 1991

Duntas L et al. Administration of d-alpha tocopherol in patients with insulin-dependent diabetes mellitus. Curr Ther Res 57:682-90, 1996

Durlach J, Collery P. Magnesium and potassium in diabetes and carbohydrate metabolism. Review of the present status and recent results. Magnesium 3(4-6):315-23, 1984

Eibl NL et al. Hypomagnesemia in non-insulin-dependent diabetes: effect of a 3-month replacement therapy. Diabetes Care 18(2):188-92, 1995

Elamin A, Tuvemo T. Magnesium and insulin-dependent diabetes mellitus. Diabetes Res Clin Pract 10:203-9, 1990

Eriksson J, Kohvakka A. Magnesium and ascorbic acid supplementation in diabetes mellitus. Ann Nutr Metab 39(4):217-23, 1995

Fields M et al. Accumulation of sorbitol in copper deficiency: Dependency on gender and type of dietary carbohydrate. Metabolism 38(4):371-75, 1989

Finney LS, Gonzalez-Campoy M. Dietary chromium and diabetes: is there a relationship? Clin Diabetes 15(1), 1997

Fish LH. Diabetic ketoacidosis. Treatment strategies to avoid complications. Postgrad Med 96(3):75-8, 1994

Fogh-Andersen N et al. Lowered serum ionized calcium in insulin treated diabetic subjects. Scand J Clin Lab Invest Suppl 165:93-7, 1983

Folkers K. Evidence for a clinically significant deficiency of vitamin B6 in populations. J Optimal Nutr 2(4):239-43, 1993

Franconi F et al. Plasma and platelet taurine are reduced in subjects with insulin-dependent diabetes mellitus: effects of taurine supplementation. Am J Clin Nutr 61:1115-9, 1995

Frayn KN, Kingman SM. Dietary sugars and lipid metabolism in humans. Am J Clin Nutr 62(suppl):250S-63S, 1995

Freund H et al. Chromium deficiency during total parenteral nutrition. JAMA 241(5):496-8, 1979

Freyler H. [Modern trends in the treatment of diabetic retinopathy.] Wien Klin Wochenschr 89(4):101-6, 1977

Friday KE et al. Omega-3 fatty acid supplementation has discordant effects on plasma glucose and lipoproteins in type II diabetes. Abstract. Diabetes 36(Suppl 1):12A, 1987

Fujita T et al. Insulin secretion after oral calcium load. Endocrinol Jpn 25(6):645-8, 1978

Fuller CJ et al. RRR-α-tocopheryl acetate supplementation at pharmacologic doses decreases low-density-lipoprotein oxidative susceptibility but not protein glycation in patients with diabetes mellitus. Am J Clin Nutr 63:753-9, 1996

Gabor M. Pharmacologic effect of flavonoids on blood vessels. Angiologica 9:355-74, 1972

Garg A, Grundy SM. Nicotinic acid as therapy for dyslipidemia in non-insulin-dependent diabetes mellitus. JAMA 264(6):723-6, 1990

Ginter E et al. Hypocholesterolemic effect of ascorbic acid in maturity-onset diabetes mellitus. Int J Vitam Nutr Res 48(4):368-73, 1978

Ginter EM, Chorvathova V. Vitamin C and diabetes mellitus. Nutr Health 2:3-11, 1983

Gisinger C et al. Vitamin E and platelet eicosanoids in diabetes mellitus. Prostaglandins Leukot Essent Fatty Acids 40:169-76, 1990

Glauber H et al. Adverse metabolic effect of omega-3 fatty acids in non-insulin-dependent diabetes mellitus. Ann Intern Med 108(5):663-8, 1988

Granado F et al. Carotenoids, retinol and tocopherols in patients with insulin-dependent diabetes mellitus and their immediate relatives. Clin Sci (Colch) 94(2):189-95, 1998

Greene DA et al. Are disturbances of sorbitol, phosphoinositide, and Na^+-K^+-ATPase regulation involved in pathogenesis of diabetic neuropathy? Diabete

Gregersen G et al. Myoinositol and function of peripheral nerves in human diabetics. A controlled clinical trial. Acta Neurol Scand 58(4):241-8, 1978

Gregersen G et al. Oral supplementation of myoinositol: Effects on peripheral nerve function in human diabetics and on the concentration in plasma, erythrocytes, urine and muscle tissue in human diabetics and normals. Acta Neurol Scand 67:164-72, 1983

Haessler HA, Crawford JD. Insulin-like inhibition of lipolysis and stimulation of lipo-genesis by prostaglandin E1. J Clin Invest 46:1065-70, 1967

Haglund B et al. Evidence of a relationship between childhood-onset type I diabetes and low groundwater concentration of zinc. Diabetes Care 19(8):873-5, 1996

Halberstam M. Oral vanadyl sulfate improves insulin sensitivity in NIDDM but not in obese diabetic subjects. Diabetes 45:659-66, 1996

Hallfrisch J et al. Effects of dietary fructose on plasma glucose and hormone responses in normal and hyperinsulinemic men. J Nutr 113:1819-26, 1983

Haylock SJ et al. Separation of biologically active chromium-containing complexes from yeast extracts and other sources of glucose tolerance factor (GTF) activity. J Inorg Biochem 18(3):195-211, 1983

Heine RJ et al. Linoleic-acid-enriched diet: Long-term effects on serum lipoprotein and apolipoprotein concentrations and insulin sensitivity in noninsulin-dependent diabetic patients. Am J Clin Nutr 49:448-56, 1989

Hollenbeck CB et al. The composition and nutritional adequacy of subject-selected high carbohydrate, low fat diets in insulin-dependent diabetes mellitus. Am J Clin Nutr 38(1):41-51, 1983

Houtsmuller AJ et al. Favourable influences of linoleic acid on the progression of diabetic micro- and macroangiopathy. Nutr Metab 24(Suppl 1):105-18, 1980

Hughes TA et al. Glycemic responses in insulin-dependent diabetic patients: effect of food composition. Am J Clin Nutr 49:658-66, 1989

Ide H et al. Clinical usefulness of intrathecal injection of methylcobalamin in patients with diabetic neuropathy. Clin Ther 9(2):183-92, 1987

Jacob S et al. Improvement of insulin-stimulated glucose-disposal in type 2 diabetes after repeated parenteral administration of thioctic acid. Exp Clin Endocrinol Diabetes 104(3):284-8, 1996

Jain SK et al. Vitamin E (E) supplementation (placebo-controlled double-blind) lowers blood thromboxane and malondialdehyde (MDA) levels in type-1 diabetics (D). Abstract. J Am Coll Nutr 15(5):536, 1996a

Jain SK et al. The effect of modest vitamin E supplementation on lipid peroxidation products and other cardiovascular risk factors in diabetic patients. Lipids 31(suppl):S87-S90, 1996b

Jaspan J et al. Treatment of severely painful diabetic neuropathy with an aldose reductase inhibitor: Relief of pain and improved somatic and autonomic nerve function. Lancet 2:758-62, 1983

Jeejeebhoy KN et al. Chromium deficiency, glucose tolerance, and neuropathy reversed by chromium supplementation, in a patient receiving long-term parenteral nutrition. Am J Clin Nutr 30(4):531-8, 1977

Jenkins DJ et al. Nibbling versus gorging: metabolic advantages of increased meal frequency. N Engl J Med 321(14):929-34, 1989

Jenkins DJ et al. Metabolic advantages of spreading the nutrient load: effects of increased meal frequency in non-insulin-dependent diabetes. Am J Clin Nutr 55:461-7, 1992

Jennings PE et al. Vitamin C metabolites and microangiopathy in diabetes mellitus. Diabetes Res 6(3):151-4, 1987

Jensen T et al. Partial normalization by dietary cod-liver oil of increased microvascular albumin leakage in patients with insulin-dependent diabetes and albuminuria. N Engl J Med 321:1572-7, 1989

Jones CL, Gonzales V. Pyridoxine deficiency: A new factor in diabetic neuropathy. J Am Podiatry Assoc 68(9):646-53, 1978

Jovanovic-Peterson L et al. Chromium supplementation for gestational diabetic women improves glucose tolerance and decreases hyperinsulinemia. Abstract. J Am Coll Nutr 14(5):530, 1995

Kahler W et al. [Diabetes mellitus: a free radical-associated disease. Results of adjuvant antioxidant supplementation.] Z Gesamte Inn Med 48(5):223-32, 1993 (in German)

Kamada T et al. Dietary sardine oil increases erythrocyte membrane fluidity in diabetic patients. Diabetes 35:604-11, 1986

Kapeghian JC, Verlangieri AJ. The effects of glucose on ascorbic acid uptake in heart endothelial cells: Possible pathogenesis of diabetic angiopathies. Life Sci 34(6):577-84, 1984

Karam JH et al. The relationship of obesity and growth hormone to serum insulin levels. Ann N Y Acad Sci 131(1):374-87, 1965

Kawagishi T et al. Calcium metabolism in diabetes mellitus. J Nutr Sci Vitaminol (Tokyo) 37 Suppl:S51-S56, 1991

Keen H et al. Treatment of diabetic neuropathy with gamma-linolenic acid. Diabetes Care 16(1):8-15, 1993

Khan MA. Nutritional therapy of the patient with diabetes mellitus. Abstract. J Am Coll Nutr 13(5):520, 1994

Kinlaw WB et al. Abnormal zinc metabolism in type II diabetes mellitus. Am J Med 75(2):273-7, 1983

Kishi T et al. Bioenergetics in clinical medicine. IX. Studies on coenzyme Q and diabetes mellitus. J Med 7:307, 1976

Klevey LM et al. Diminished glucose tolerance in two men due to a diet low in copper. Abstract. Am J Clin Nutr 37:717, 1983

Kornerup T, Strom L. Vitamin B12 and retinopathy in juvenile diabetes. Acta Paediatr 47:646-51, 1958

Kosenko LG. Klin Med 42:113, 1964

Kostraba JN et al. Nitrate levels in community drinking waters and risk of IDDM. An ecological analysis. Diabetes Care 15(11):1505-8, 1992

Koutsikos D et al. Biotin for diabetic peripheral neuropathy. Biomed Pharmacother 44(10):511-14, 1990

Kozlovsky AS et al. Effects of diets high in simple sugars on urinary chromium losses. Metabolism 35(6):515-18, 1986

Kulakowski EC, Maturo J. Hypoglycemic properties of taurine not mediated by enhance insulin release. Biochem Pharmacol 33:2835-8, 1984

Lacombe C et al. Hemorheological improvement after Daflon 500 mg treatment in diabetes. Int Angiol 7(2 Suppl):21-24, 1988

Levin ER et al. The influence of pyridoxine in diabetic peripheral neuropathy. Diabetes Care 4 (6):606-9, 1981

Levy J et al. Diabetes mellitus: a disease of abnormal cellular calcium metabolism? Am J Med 260-71, 1994

Lind L et al. Relation of serum calcium concentration to metabolic risk factors for cardiovascular disease. Br Med J 297:960-3, 1988

Liu VJ, Abernathy RP. Chromium and insulin in young subjects with normal glucose tolerance. Am J Clin Nutr 25(4):661-7, 1982

Lostroh AJ, Krahl. Magnesium, a second messenger for insulin: Ion translocation coupled to transport activity. Adv Enz Regul 12:73-81, 1974

Lowitt S et al. Acetyl-L-carnitine corrects the altered peripheral nerve function of experimental diabetes. Metabolism 44(5):677-80, 1995

Lubec B et al. L-arginine reduces lipid peroxidation in patients with diabetes mellitus. Free Rad Biol Med 22(1-2):355-7, 1997

Lubin B, Machlin L. Biological aspects of vitamin E. Ann N Y Acad Sci 1982, p. 393

Luostarinin R et al. Vitamin E supplementation counteracts the fish oil-induced increase of blood glucose in humans. Nutr Res 15:953-68, 1995

Ma J et al. Associations of serum an dietary magnesium with cardiovascular disease, hypertension, diabetes, insulin and carotid artery wall thickness: the ARIC study. J Clin Epidemiol 48(7):927-40, 1995

Maebashi M et al. Therapeutic evaluation of the effect of biotin on hyperglycemia in patients with non-insulin dependent diabetes mellitus. J Clin Biochem Nutr 14:211-18, 1993

Magnard G et al. [Value of tetrahydroxy flavan-diol in ophthalmology, especially in chronic retinopathy (40 cases).] Lyon Med 223(4):259-63, 1970 (in French)

Maki KC et al. Fiber intake and risk of developing non-insulin-dependent diabetes mellitus. Letter. JAMA 277(22):1761, 1997

Malerbi DA et al. Metabolic effects of dietary sucrose and fructose in type II diabetic subjects. Diabetes Care 19(11):1249-56, 1996

Martinoli L et al. Plasma retinol and alpha-tocopherol concentrations in insulin-dependent diabetes mellitus: their relationship to microvascular complications. Int J Vitam Nutr Res 63(2):87-92, 1993

Mateo MC et al. Serum zinc, copper and insulin in diabetes mellitus. Biomedicine 29(2):56-8, 1978

Mayer-Davis EJ et al. Dietary fat and insulin sensitivity in a triethnic population: the role of obesity. The Insulin Resistance Atherosclerosis Study (IRAS). Am J Clin Nutr 65:79-87, 1997

Mayhew JA et al. Free and lipid inositol, sorbitol and sugars in sciatic nerve obtained post-mortum from diabetic and control subjects. Diabetologia 24:13-15, 1983

McCann VJ, Davis RE. Serum pyridoxal concentrations in patients with diabetic neuropathy. Aust N Z J Med 8:259-61, 1978

McCann VJ, Davis RE. Pyridoxine and diabetic neuropathy: a double-blind controlled study. Letter. Diabetes Care 6(1):102-3, 1983

McGrath LT et al. Effect of dietary fish oil supplementation on peroxidation of serum lipids in patients with non-insulin dependent diabetes mellitus. Atherosclerosis 121:275-83, 1996

McNair P et al. Hypomagnesemia, a risk factor for diabetic retinopathy. Diabetes 27:1075-7, 1978

McNair P et al. Hyperzincuria in insulin treated diabetes mellitus: Its relation to glucose homeostasis and insulin administration. Clin Chim Acta 112:343-8, 1981

McVeigh GE et al. Dietary fish oil augments nitric oxide production or release in patients with type 2 (non-insulin-dependent) diabetes mellitus. Diabetologica 36(1):33-8, 1993

Mercuri O et al. Depression of microsomal desaturation of linoleic to gamma-linolenic acid in the alloxan-diabetic rat. Biochim Biophys Acta 116:409-11, 1966

Mertz W. Chromium occurrence and function in a biological system. Physiol Rev 49:163-230, 1969

Mertz W. Effects and metabolism of glucose tolerance factor. Nutr Rev 33(5):129-35, 1975

Mirsky, Stanley. Diabetes: Controlling It the Easy Way. New York, Random House, 1981

Mustard JF, Packam MA. Platelets and diabetes mellitus. N Engl J Med 311:665-7, 1994

Nadler JL et al. Magnesium deficiency produces insulin resistance and increased thromboxane synthesis. Hypertension 21:1024-9, 1993

National Institutes of Health Consensus Development Conference (USA), December 8-10, 1986

Norbiato G et al. Effects of potassium supplementation on insulin binding and insulin action in human obesity: Protein-modified fast and refeeding. Europ J Clin Invest 44:414-9, 1984

O'Dea K. Marked improvement in carbohydrate and lipid metabolism in diabetic Australian aborigines after temporary reversion to traditional lifestyle. Diabetes 33(6):596-603, 1984

Offenbacher E, Stunyer F. Beneficial effect of chromium-rich yeast on glucose tolerance and blood lipids in elderly patients. Diabetes 29:919-25, 1980

Okuda Y et al. Long-term effects of eicosapentaenoic acid on diabetic peripheral neuropathy and serum lipids in patients with type II and diabetes mellitus. J Diabetic Complications 10:280-7, 1996

Osterode W et al. Nutritional antioxidants, red cell membrane fluidity and blood viscosity in type I (insulin dependent) diabetes mellitus. Diabetic Med 13:1044-50, 1996

Palmer LJ et al. The influence of rutin upon diabetic retinitis. Northwest Med 50:669-71, 1951

Paolisso G et al. Improved insulin response and action by chronic magnesium administration in aged NIDDM subjects. Diabetes Care 12:265-69, 1989

Paolisso G et al. Daily vitamin E supplements improve metabolic control but not insulin secretion in elderly non-insulin-dependent diabetic patients. Diabetes Care 16:1433-7, 1993

Parillo M et al. Does a high-carbohydrate diet have different effects in NIDDM patients treated with diet alone or hypoglycemic drugs? Diabetes Care 19(5):498-500, 1996

Passariello N et al. Effects of pyridoxine alpha-ketoglutarate on blood glucose and lactate in type I and type II diabetics. Int J Clin Pharmacol Ther Toxicol 21:252-56, 1983

Patterson JW. The diabetogenic effect of dehydroascorbic acid and dehydroisoascorbic acids. J Bio Chem 183:81, 1950

Perez GO et al. Potassium homeostasis in chronic diabetes mellitus. Arch Intern Med 137(8):1018-22, 1977

Popp-Snijders C et al. Dietary supplementation of omega-3 polyunsaturated fatty acids improves insulin sensitivity in non-insulin-dependent diabetes. Diabetes Res 4:141-7, 1987

Pozzilli P et al. Meta-analysis of nicotinamide treatment in patients with recent-onset IDDM. The Nicotinamide Trialists. Diabetes Care 19(12):1357-63, 1996

Puhakainen I et al. Dietary supplementation with n-3 fatty acids increases gluconeogenesis from glycerol but not hepatic glucose production in patients with non-insulin-dependent diabetes mellitus. Am J Clin Nutr 61:121-6, 1995

Quatraro A et al. Acetyl-L-carnitine for symptomatic diabetic neuropathy. Diabetalogica 38:123, 1995

Raal FJ et al. Effect of moderate protein restriction on the progression of overt diabetic nephropathy: a 6-mo prospective study. Am J Clin Nutr 60:579-85, 1994

Rabinowich IM. Achlorhydria and its clinical significance in diabetes mellitus. Am J Dig Dis 16:322-32, 1949

Rao RH et al. Failure of pyridoxine to improve glucose tolerance in diabetics. J Clin Endocrinol Metab 50(1):198-200, 1980

Raz I et al. The influence of zinc supplementation on glucose homeostasis in NIDDM. Diabetes Res 11(2):73-9, 1989

Reaven GM. Dietary therapy for non-insulin-dependent diabetes mellitus. Editorial. N Engl J Med 319(13):862-64, 1988

Reiser S et al. Indices of copper status in humans consuming a typical American diet containing either fructose or starch. Am J Clin Nutr 42:242-51, 1985

Reiser S et al. Effects of sugars on indices of glucose tolerance in humans. Am J Clin Nutr 43(1):151-9, 1986

Reiser S et al. Blood lipids, lipoproteins, apoproteins, and uric acid in men fed diets containing fructose or high-amylose cornstarch. Am J Clin Nutr 49:832-9, 1989

Ribaya-Mercado J et al. Vitamin B6 deficiency elevates serum insulin in elderly subjects. Ann N Y Acad Sci 585:531-3, 1990

Richardson CT et al. Diabetics have reduced acid secretion and delayed digestion. Am Family Physician June, 1978, p. 143

Rieder HP et al. [Vitamin status in diabetic neuropathy (thiamine, riboflavin, pyridoxine, cobalamin and tocopherol).] Z Ernahrungswiss 19(1):1-13, 1980

Rogers KS, Mohan C. Vitamin B6 metabolism and diabetes. Biochem Med Metab Biol 52:10-17, 1994

Rubenstein AH. Hypoglycemia induced by manganese. Nature 194:188-89, 1962

Saito N et al. Blood thiamine levels in outpatients with diabetes mellitus. J Nutr Sci Vitaminol (Tokyo) 33(6):421-30, 1987

Salmeron J et al. Dietary fiber, glycemic load, and risk of non-insulin-dependent diabetes mellitus in women. JAMA 277(6):472-7, 1997

Salonen JT et al. Increased risk of non-insulin diabetes mellitus at low plasma vitamin E concentrations: a four year follow-up study in men. BMJ 311:1124-7, 1995

Salway JG et al. Effect of myo-inositol on peripheral-nerve function in diabetes. Lancet ii:1282, 1978

Sancetta SM et al. The use of vitamin B12 in the management of the neurological manifestations of diabetes mellitus, with notes on the administration of massive doses. Ann Intern Med 35:1028-48, 1951

Sanchez M. Oral calcium supplementation reduces intraplatelet free calcium concentration and insulin resistance in essential hypertensive patients. Hypertension 29(2):531-6, 1992

Schmetterer L et al. Nitric oxide and ocular blood flow in patients with IDDM. Diabetes 46(4):653-8, 1997

Schmidt LE et al. Evaluation of nutrient intake in subjects with non-insulin-dependent diabetes mellitus. J Am Diet Assoc 94(7):773-4, 1994

Scott AR et al. Comparison of high fibre diets, basal insulin supplements, and flexible insulin treatment for non-insulin dependent (type II) diabetics poorly controlled with sulphonylureas. Br Med J 297:707-10, 1988

Scott FW et al. Milk and type I diabetes, Examining the evidence and broadening the focus. Diabetes Care 19(4):379-83, 1996

Sheard NF. The diabetic diet: evidence for a new approach. Nutr Rev 53(1):16-18, 1995

Shigeta Y et al. Effect of coenzyme Q7 treatment on blood sugar and ketone bodies of diabetics. J Vitaminol 12:293, 1966

Shimura Y, Hogomoto S. Jpn J Clin Exp Med 58:1349-532, 1981

Simonoff M et al. The isolation of glucose tolerance factors from brewer's yeast and their relation to chromium. Biol Trace Elem Res 32:25-8, 1992

Sinclair AJ et al. Low plasma ascorbate levels in patients with type 2 diabetes mellitus consuming adequate dietary vitamin C. Diabetic Med 11:893-8, 1994

Singh RB et al. Dietary intake and plasma levels of antioxidant vitamins in health and disease: a hospital-based case-control study. J Nutr Environ Med 5:235-42, 1995

Sjogren A et al. Magnesium, potassium and zinc deficiency in subjects with type II diabetes mellitus. Acta Med Scand 224:461-3, 1988

Skelton WP III, Skelton NK. Thiamine deficiency neuropathy: It's still common today. Postgrad Med 85(8):301-6, 1989

Snowdon DA, Phillips RL. Does a vegetarian diet reduce the occurrence of diabetes? Am J Public Health 75(5):507-12, 1985

Solomon SJ, King JC. Effect of low zinc intake on carbohydrate and fat metabolism in men. Fed Proc 42:391, 1983

Solomons NW. On the assessment of zinc and copper nutriture in man. Am J Clin Nutr 32:856-71, 1979

Som S et al. Ascorbic acid metabolism in diabetes mellitus. Metabolism 30(6):572-7, 1981

Spreitsma JE, Schuitemaker GE. Diabetes can be prevented by reducing insulin production. Med Hypotheses 42(1):15-23, 1994

Steiner G. Editorial: From an excess of fat, diabetics die. JAMA 262(3):398-9, 1989

Stevens MJ et al. Acetyl-L-carnitine deficiency as a cause of altered nerve myo-inositol content, Na,K-ATPase activity, and motor conduction velocity in the streptozotocin-diabetic rat. Metabolism 45(7):865-72, 1996

Storlien LH et al. Effects of sucrose vs starch diets on in vivo insulin action, thermogenesis, and obesity in rats. Am J Clin Nutr 47:420-7, 1988

Stracke H et al. A benfotiamine-vitamin B combination in treatment of diabetic polyneuropathy. Exp Clin Endocrinol Diabetes 104(4):311-16, 1996

Straub RH et al. No evidence of deficiency of vitamins A, E, beta-carotene, B1, B2, B6, B12 and folate in neuropathic non-insulin-dependent diabetic women. Int J Vitam Nutr Res 63(3):239-40, 1993

Swade TF, Emanuele NV. Alcohol & diabetes. Compr Ther 23(2):135-40, 1997

Thompson DH, Godin DV. Micronutrients and antioxidants in the progression of diabetes. Nutr Res 15:1377-410, 1995

Thorburn AW et al. Fructose-induced in vivo insulin resistance and elevated plasma triglyceride levels in rats. Am J Clin Nutr 49:1155-63, 1989

Tong HI. Influence of neurotropic vitamins on the nerve conduction velocity in diabetic neuropathy. Ann Acad Med Singapore 9(1):65-70, 1980

Tosiello L. Hypomagnesemia and diabetes mellitus. Arch Intern Med 156:1143-8, 1996

Vandongen R et al. Hypercholesterolaemic effect of fish oil in insulin-dependent diabetic patients. Med J Aust 148:141-3, 1988

Varma SD et al. Diabetic cataracts and flavonoids. Science 195:205-6, 1977

Vinson JA, Howard TB III. Inhibition of protein glycation and advanced glycation end products by ascorbic acid and other vitamins and nutrients. J Nutr Biochem 7:659-63, 1996

Virtanen SM et al. Is children's or parents' coffee or tea consumption associated with the risk for insulin-dependent diabetes mellitus in children? Eur J Clin Nutr 48:279-85, 1994

Wahlberg G et al. Protective effect of nicotinamide against nephropathy in diabetic rats. Diabetes Res 2:307, 1985

Wascher TC et al. Effects of low-dose L-arginine on insulin-mediated vasodilation and insulin sensitivity. Eur J Clin Invest 27:690-5, 1997

Wen-gang Z et al. Hypomagnesemia and heart complications in diabetes mellitus. Chin Med J 100:719-22, 1987

West KM, Kalbfleisch JM. Influence of nutritional factors on prevalence of diabetes. Diabetes 20:99-108, 1971

Will JC, Byers T. Does diabetes mellitus increase the requirement for vitamin C? Nutr Rev 54(7):193-202, 1996

Williams G. Management of non-insulin-dependent diabetes mellitus. Lancet 343:95-100, 1994

Wimhurst JM, Manchester KL. Comparison of ability of Mg and Mn to activate the key enzymes of glycolysis. FEBS Letters 27:321-6, 1972

Wolever TM et al. The glycemic index: methodology and clinical implications. Am J Clin Nutr 54(5):846-54, 1991

Yaqub BA et al. Effects of methylcobalamin on diabetic neuropathy. Clin Neurol Neurosurg 94(2):105-11, 1992

Zebrowski EJ, Bhatnagar PK. Urinary excretion pattern of ascorbic acid in streptozotocin diabetic and insulin treated rats. Pharm Res Commun 11(2):95-103, 1979

Ziegler D, Gries FA. α-lipoic acid in the treatment of diabetic peripheral and cardiac autonomic neuropathy. Diabetes 46(Suppl. 2):S62-S66, 1997

DOWN'S SYNDROME

See Also: DEMENTIA

NUTRITIONAL TREATMENT GUIDE

✓ = Efficacy generally accepted.
* = Efficacy *demonstrated* by controlled human trials.
[+] = Efficacy *suspected* from uncontrolled human trials.
[-] = Efficacy *suspected* from indirect data.
? = Efficacy *challenged* in a study of similar design.

DIETARY FACTORS

[+] **low Protein, high Carbohydrate, high Potassium diet with Serotonin-containing foods:** *to reduce self- injurious behavior*

NUTRITIONAL FACTORS

* **L-Tryptophan:** *to treat infantile hypotonia:* 10 to 50 mg/kg
* **Vitamin A deficiency:** *to reduce infections and improve absorption:* repletion (monthly oral dose of water-miscible form) (5 month trial)
* **Vitamin B_6:** *to improve brain function* (when given between age 8 weeks and 3 years)

- -

[+] **Carnitine:** *to improve attention and visual memory:* L-acetyl-carnitine (90 day trial)
[+] **Choline:** *to improve brain function: example:* phosphatidylcholine (plus related nutrients)
[+] **5-Hydroxytryptophan:** *to treat infantile hypotonia:* 0.5 to 1.5 mg/kg initially; increase stepwise to 5 mg/kg
[+] **Selenium:** *to reduce infections:* 10 to 25 μg/kg
[+] **Zinc deficiency:** *to reduce infections, improve thyroid and thymus function, and accelerate growth:* repletion (20 mg/kg)

- -

[-] **Folic Acid deficiency:** adult dosage: 800 μg daily
[-] **Iron deficiency:** adult dosage: 30 mg twice daily until repletion; then minimal possible dosage
[-] **Magnesium deficiency:** adult dosage ≈ 400 mg daily (Consider IM or IV administration, especially in hypomagnesemia)
[-] **Manganese deficiency:** adult dosage: 3 to 5 mg daily
[-] **Selenium deficiency:** adult dosage: 200 μg daily
[-] **Thiamine deficiency:** adult dosage: 50 mg daily
[-] **Vitamin B_{12} deficiency:** adult dosage 1000 μg IM weekly initially and monthly afterwards
[-] **Vitamin C deficiency:** adult dosage: 500 mg twice daily
[-] **Vitamin E deficiency:** adult dosage: D,L-alpha-tocopheryl acetate 200 to 2,000 IU daily for 6 weeks; then maintenance levels as needed

OTHER RELATED FACTORS

[+] avoid **Aluminum** exposure

[-] rule out **Food Sensitivities**

A LINK BETWEEN GENETICS AND FREE RADICAL CHEMISTRY

One of the dictums in clinical nutrition over the last few years has been the beneficial role of the antioxidant enzyme superoxide dismutase. In Down's syndrome, however, overexpression of the gene for superoxide dismutase is believed to cause excessive production of hydrogen peroxide and other free radicals causing increased oxidative stress *(Brugge)*.

Normal superoxide dismutase activity is sometimes found in patients with the clinical features of Down's syndrome. Thus, the segment of chromosome 21 which is responsible for encoding copper/zinc superoxide dismutase may not be the critical region responsible for the genetic disorder *(De La Torre)*.

MALABSORPTION

Malabsorption appears to be prevalent in Down's syndrome patients *(Abalan)*. The malabsorption may be secondary to gluten-gliadin sensitivity or to multiple food sensitivities causing a celiac disease-like picture *(Reading,1984a)*. (See Food Sensitivities below.)

It is highly likely that malabsorption contributes to a number of the vitamin and mineral deficiencies found in Down's patients *(Williams)*. Moreover, it could lead to the neuropathologic signs of Alzheimer's disease which occurs at or slightly before the fourth decade *(Abalan)*.

DIETARY FACTORS

Other than avoiding foods to which patients are reactive, there is little evidence that a particular diet is specifically indicated for Down's patients. An exception is the following case study, the results of which suggest that self-injurious behavior may be reduced if the appropriate patients are placed on a low protein, high carbohydrate, high potassium diet with serotonin-containing foods *(Gedye)*.

A 26-year-old profoundly mentally handicapped woman with Down's syndrome exhibited severe self-injurious behavior. Treatment consisted of regular institutional entrees, supplemented with serotonin-containing foods, and modified to ensure dietary sources of potassium each meal and a low protein intake relative to carbohydrate. Dramatic benefit was evident the first day and, after 6 months, self-hitting was still close to 90% lower than baseline rates (Gedye).

NUTRITIONAL FACTORS

VITAMINS

Folic Acid Deficiency

The evidence is that children and younger adolescents, with Down's syndrome have normal erythrocyte and serum folate levels. However, mean corpuscular volume of erythrocytes is increased *(David)*, a finding also noted by other investigators *(Ibarra; Wachtel)*.

As Down's patients age, serum folate levels decline while macrocytosis increases. Moreover, in a group of patients of mixed ages, erythrocyte folate levels were very low *(Gericke)*, suggesting that they may also decline with aging, and that folate deficiency may develop in adult patients.

Thiamine Deficiency

In a study of 90 patients up to 16 years of age, measurement of erythrocyte transketolase activity suggested a marginal thiamine deficiency *(Schmid)*.

Vitamin A Deficiency

A group of 23 Down's children, when compared to their normal siblings and age-matched controls, had a significantly higher incidence of respiratory and gastrointestinal infections, impaired absorption of vitamin A from a oily medium, and clinical symptoms of vitamin A deficiency. After 5 months of supplementation with water-miscible vitamin A, there was a significant decrease in the incidence of infection, improvement in plasma vitamin A levels *(Palmer)*.

Vitamin B_6

There is suggestive evidence that the metabolism of vitamin B_6 may be abnormal *(McCoy,1969)*. Moreover, levels in leukocytes may be decreased *(Coburn)*.

In a double-blind study, 19 patients received either vitamin B_6 or placebo starting at age 8 weeks and continuing for 3 years. As previous work had found that cortical auditory evoked potentials were abnormally elevated in Down's patients, they were recorded at 1 and 3 years of age.

At age 3, peak-to-peak amplitudes of prominent components were significantly lower in the vitamin B_6-treated patients, and latencies for several prominent evoked peaks were significantly longer, suggesting that brain function in treated patients may be closer to normal *(Frager)*. However, no significant differences were found between the 2 groups in mental age, height, weight, cranial circumference or tongue protrusion *(Coleman,1985)*.

Although the differences in cortical auditory evoked potentials are provocative, the lack of significant differences between the other measures raises the question as to whether they are clinically relevant. Further studies are clearly indicated, including a follow-up study of these patients.

Vitamin B_{12} Deficiency

While some studies have found reduced blood levels of vitamin B_{12} in Down's patients *(Hestnes)*, others have found normal values *(David)*.

We previously noted, in discussing folic acid, that the patients' erythrocytes may be macrocytic. As red cell survival half-time is often substantially shorter, erythrocytes may have a younger mean age, and their increased turnover may indicate an accelerated aging process in these cells *(Wachtel)*; thus the macrocytosis may be unrelated to folate and vitamin B_{12} nutriture. An alternate hypothesis is that the macrocytosis may not be an expression of reduced red cell survival but rather of an altered folate remethylation pathway secondary to enhanced activity of cystathionine beta-synthase, the gene for which is present on chromosome 21 *(David)*.

Vitamin C Deficiency

In one study, many Down's children had evidence of a blood ascorbic acid deficiency which, in this case, seemed to be diet-related. Children who showed evidence of vitamin C deficiency in the blood also had an increased incidence of infections, suggesting that the deficiency was sufficient to produce clinically relevant findings *(Colombo,1989a)*.

Vitamin E Deficiency

While cortical brain tissue levels of vitamin E in Down's syndrome fetuses appear to be normal *(Metcalfe)*, patients may have reduced plasma levels of vitamin E *(Shah)*. Moreover, those with dementia have lower plasma levels than those who do not *(Jackson)*. Cortical brain tissue levels of vitamin E in children and adults with Down's syndrome have not been assessed.

It has been suggested that vitamin E supplementation may reduce superoxide dismutase-generated oxidative damage in Down's syndrome patients *(Sylverster)* and the associated dementia that is also common in this population *(Burns; Wisniewski)*.

MINERALS

Calcium

Decreased intracellular *(McCoy,1984)* and hair *(Barlow)* calcium levels have been noted. By contrast, erythrocyte levels have been found to be elevated *(Anneren,1985a)*.

Copper

Elevations in copper levels have been found in erythrocytes *(Purice)*, neutrophils *(Anneren,1985a)*, platelets *(Anneren,1985a)*, and serum *(Anneren,1987; Kadrabova)*.

Iron Deficiency

In one study, levels of erythrocyte, neutrophil, and serum iron were found to be reduced in children with Down's syndrome *(Anneren,1985a)*. However, another study of patients aged 2 to 15 years found both serum iron and ferritin levels to be similar to those of age-matched controls *(David)*.

Magnesium Deficiency

Magnesium levels in erythrocytes and thrombocytes, but not those in neutrophils, were lower in Down's children than in controls in one study *(Anneren,1985a)*. Another study, however, found serum magnesium levels in Down's patients of mixed ages to be similar to those of age- and sex-matched controls *(Kadrabova)*.

Manganese Deficiency

Depressed amounts of erythrocyte and neutrophil manganese have been noted in children with Down's syndrome *(Anneren,1985a)*. Hair manganese levels also appear to be reduced *(Barlow)*.

Selenium

Low levels of serum selenium have been noted *(Kadrabova)* as well as decreased whole blood, erythrocyte, and plasma selenium levels *(Gromadzinska)*. One study, however, found similar mean plasma and erythrocyte selenium levels in adult patients, and higher erythrocyte levels in pediatric patients *(Anneren,1985b)*.

Supplementation

It has been suggested that selenium supplementation could enhance glutathione peroxidase activity in erythrocytes, possibly improving protection against oxygen radicals which might cause damage by lipid peroxidation *(Anneren,1989)*.

Indeed, when a group of patients of mixed ages was given selenium for up to one and one-half years in a placebo-controlled study, the supplemented group showed a 25 percent increase in erythrocyte glutathione peroxidase levels *(Antila)*. In another study, however, when a group of affected children received a lower dosage of selenium for 6 months, erythrocyte glutathione peroxidase levels *decreased* and remained reduced from pre-supplementation levels 12 months after supplementation was stopped, even though plasma and erythrocyte selenium levels had almost dropped to their initial values *(Anneren,1989)*.

The reason for these disparate findings is not known. Moreover, since erythrocyte glutathione peroxidase levels may already be elevated in Down's patients *(Neve)*, the value of a further elevation is questionable.

The hypothesis that selenium supplementation may augment immune responses in Down's patients is on firmer ground. Following 6 months of supplementation, parents of children with Down's syndrome reported that their children had a reduced rate of infections *(Anneren,1989)*. When the 4 immunoglobulin G subclasses of 29 of these children were measured, selenium was found to have a significant augmentative effect on the serum concentrations of IgG2 and 4 *(Anneren,1990)*.

Until we have more data from controlled trials, the value of selenium supplementation must remain questionable.

Zinc

Several studies have found plasma or serum zinc levels to be reduced *(Kadrabova)*, and one study reported reduced zinc in platelets *(Anneren,1985a)*. While one study found erythrocyte zinc to be reduced *(Anneren,1985)*, others have found this measure to be elevated *(Neve;Purice)*, suggesting that there may be an abnormality in zinc metabolism.

Evidence that low blood zinc is correlated with immune deficits comes from a study of 35 Down's infants aged 6 to 20 months. Blood zinc levels of the whole group were in the normal range; however, 16 of the infants had below normal values, and 69% were particularly vulnerable to infections, 63% had a complete lymphocyte deficit (compared to 42% with normal zinc levels), and 56% had an abnormal T helper/T suppressor cell ratio *(Colombo,1989b)*.

In Downs' patients, moreover, low plasma zinc levels have been related to the presence of immature myeloid cells in the peripheral blood which are less able to fight infections *(Trubiani)*, and low serum zinc with high zinc levels in blood clots have been related to depressed neutrophil chemotaxis, delayed skin reactivity and *in vitro* lymphocyte responses to PHA *(Bjorksten)*.

Supplementation

There have been a number of studies which have investigated whether zinc supplementation benefits patients with Down's syndrome. In general, the results are impressive, and are consistent with those seen following repletion of a zinc deficiency in non-Down's patients. Depressed neutrophil chemotaxis normalized, and delayed skin reactivity and *in vitro* responses to PHA improved *(Bjorksten;Licastro,1994;Stabile)*. The absolute number of circulating T-lymphocytes increased *(Franceschi)*, depressed *in vitro* lymphocyte proliferation and polymorphonuclear activity increased to normal *(Licastro,1994)*, the presence of immature myeloid cells in the blood (which are less able to fight infection) was eliminated *(Trubiani)*, and the number of apoptotic peripheral blood cells declined *(Antonucci)*.

DNA synthesis increased *(Stabile)* and the rate of DNA damage decreased *(Chiricolo)*. Elevated TSH levels and low rT3 levels normalized *(Licastro,1993)*, and the incidence of subclinical hypothyroidism declined *(Napolitano,1990a)*. Low thymulin *(Licastro,1993)* and Serum Thymic Factor *(Franceschi)* levels normalized.

Clinically, growth accelerated *(Napolitano,1990b)*, the incidence of infectious disease was reduced and school attendance increased *(Licastro,1992,1994)*,

OTHER NUTRITIONAL FACTORS

Amino Acids

Abnormal levels of amino acids have been noted in several studies on Down's syndrome patients. Brain cortical levels of alanine, cystine, isoleucine, leucine, phenylalanine, and threonine may be elevated *(Abasheva)*.

Plasma levels of cysteine *(Lejeune)*, cystine and phenylalanine *(Watkins)* may be high. In contrast, plasma/serum levels of histidine may be reduced *(Abasheva)* as well as plasma/serum levels of serine *(Lejeune)*, tryptophan *(Abasheva)*, and tyrosine *(Abasheva)*. Plasma levels of isoleucine, leucine and phenylalanine were elevated in one study *(Watkins)*, but depressed in another *(Abasheva)*, while plasma lysine levels were elevated in 3 studies *(Heggarty;Lejeune; Mircher)*, but depressed in one *(Abasheva)*.

There is also evidence that degradation of phenylalanine to tyrosine may be impaired. Theoretically, this abnormality could be related to the development of mental retardation *(Shaposhnikov)*.

Results of attempts to normalize amino acid concentrations have not been reported, and the effects of these abnormal findings are not well understood. Of the various findings, only elevated plasma lysine has been reported in multiple studies (although one study found plasma lysine levels to be depressed). Hyperlysinemia, despite serum lysine concentrations which are usually much higher than those found in Down's syndrome, is usually a benign disorder; thus the lysine elevation is unlikely to have a notable clinical effect by itself *(Heggarty)*.

Carnitine

Blood levels of carnitine may be deficient. Thirty-nine percent of one group of children had below average levels, while 4 of them had a severe deficiency *(Columbo,1989c)*.

In an open trial, Down's patients who were supplemented with L-acetyl-carnitine for 90 days demonstrated statistically significant improvements in visual memory as well as in attention both in absolute terms and when compared to untreated patients with Down's syndrome.

Supplementation had no effect on patients who were mentally retarded due to other causes, suggesting that the benefits are specific to Down's patients. The investigators theorize that the benefits may be due to the substance's direct and indirect cholinomimetic effect *(DeFalco)*.

Choline

Down's syndrome, as in Alzheimer's dementia and Parkinson's disease, is associated with a presynaptic cortical cholinergic deficit reflected by an extensive loss of choline acetyltransferase *(Perry)*. While little has been done to investigate the efficacy of cholinergic agents, the following case report is suggestive:

A 2½ year-old Down's syndrome boy was given 150 mg/kg of a phosphatidylcholine compound (Supercholine; Cardiovascular Res., USA) (which also contains phosphatidylinositol, phosphatidylethanolamine, pyridoxine, manganese, methionine and serine) for 7 months starting 3 weeks after initiating supplementation with a multivitamin (GTC No. 2; Bronson Pharm., USA).

His pre-treatment language skills, which were 12 months behind normal, improved to 6 months behind normal post-treatment, and he also showed improvements in motor and social skills. Objectively, his EEG pattern showed normalization during the treatment period with minor reoccurrence of abnormalities during a 2-month placebo period at the end of the 7 months (Cantor).

5-Hydroxytryptophan

Open trials have reported that, when hypotonic infants with Down's syndrome were supplemented with L-5-hydroxytryptophan, muscle tone improved *(Weise;Petre-Quadens)*. One of these studies also noted that there was a longlasting improvement in motor behavior *(Weise)*.

In a double-blind study, 89 Down's children were given 5-hydroxytryptophan, pyridoxine hydrochloride or the combination in the first 3 years of life. Each supplement raised blood levels of 5-hydroxyindole equally well in 40% of the children, and there were no significant differences in muscle tone between the 3 groups *(Pueschel)*, suggesting that vitamin B_6 supplementation may be as effective as 5-hydroxytryptophan in improving muscle tone.

A Warning

In Down's infants, supplementation may cause myoclonus and infantile spasms *(Coleman,1971)*.

Tryptophan

There appears to be an abnormality of tryptophan metabolism in Down's syndrome. Not only is plasma free tryptophan reduced in children with Down's *(Abasheva)* but, following a tryptophan load, these children appear to excrete a lesser amount of xanthurenic acid, a tryptophan metabolite, than normal controls *(O'Brien)*.

In older Down's patients, there was a marked increase of kynurenic acid, another tryptophan metabolite, in both the frontal and temporal cortex. As kynurenic acid blocks all 3 classical excitatory amino acid receptors, and these receptors are central to brain physiology and play important roles in learning and memory processes, this finding may help to explain defects in central nervous system function *(Baran)*.

When infants with Down's syndrome were supplemented with L-tryptophan during the first 2 years of life, muscle tone improved over that of untreated infants, although not to the level of normal infants. The effect resembled that of L-5-hydroxytryptophan (see above); in fact, one of the 9 treated infants developed infantile spasms, the same side effect to which infants receiving L-tryptophan are liable *(Airaksinen)*. It is not known whether L-tryptophan supplementation has other benefits when given over a longer time period.

COMBINED NUTRITIONAL SUPPLEMENTS

In 1981, Harrell published the exciting results of a exploratory double-blind study in the *Proceedings of the National Academy of Sciences*. Sixteen mentally retarded children, 4 of whom had Down's syndrome, received either a multivitamin/multimineral supplement or placebo. Three of the 4 Down's children in the experimental group gained 10 to 25 IQ units; moreover they showed physical changes towards normal *(Harrell)*.

Unfortunately, virtually every study on combined nutrient supplementation in Down's patients since then has failed to demonstrate statistically significant positive effects *(Kleijnen;Menolascino)*.

Rather than limit supplementation to nutrients, Turkel, starting in the 1930s, developed empirically a treatment regimen consisting of a large number of supplemental nutrients including digestive enzymes, along with thyroid supplementation, an antihistamine and a diuretic *(Turkel,1985)*. He named it the "U" series, adopting the name from the Greek prefix "eu'" (which means well) and claimed that its components "act synergistically to remove accumulations due to storage of overproduced enzymes, which in turn decrease space for transportation of nutrient and elimination of wastes. . . . The "U" series accelerates development of all organs simultaneously *(Turkel,1982)*."

An effort to replicate his work using a double-blind design found no evidence of benefit *(Bumbalo)*.

A young girl began the "U" series at age 5, with bone age of 3, height 38.25 inches, IQ of 49 and attention span of 10 to 15 seconds. Results of the treatment were quickly apparent with an increase in attention span to 10 minutes within 2 weeks. Within 3 months, she began speaking in complete sentences for the first time. Her growth rate increased by 3 times her pretreatment rate. After 1 year, her IQ had increased 23 points. At 3 years, her IQ was measured at 85.

Physical changes included palate development from greatly raised to nearly normal. Bone growth was 50% prior to treatment and 94% after 8 years of treatment (Turkel,1985).

OTHER RELATED FACTORS

Food Sensitivities

Down's patients appear prone to multiple food reactions *(Bade)*. Those with recurrent diarrhea and weight loss may have increased IgG and IgA antibodies to gluten, casein and ovalbumin, as well as reduced serum zinc levels, suggesting zinc deficiency may have caused a defect in immune regulation which led to intestinal malfunction (see Zinc above) *(Kanavin)*.

Gluten-gliadin sensitivity or intolerance could cause a celiac disease-like picture which may explain nutrient malabsorption and autoimmune disease *(Reading,1984a)*. In a group of 26 patients, for example, gluten antibodies were found in 47% and alpha-gliadin antibodies in 43% *(Reading,1984b)*.

Another study found the prevalence of actual celiac disease in a group of institutionalized Down's patients to be between 4 and 14% *(Gale)*. It is particularly clear that celiac disease should be strongly considered in Down's children with either persistent diarrhea or failure to thrive *(Hilhorst)*.

Aluminum Toxicity

Down's patients may have higher levels of unbound aluminum than normals. This unbound aluminum can move readily into the brain where it has neurotoxic effects *(Farrar)*. Moreover, gastrointestinal absorption of aluminum may be enhanced in Down's patients *(Moore)*.

It may thus be wise to make special efforts to reduce dietary aluminum in addition to reducing exposure to aluminum from other sources.

BIBLIOGRAPHY

Abalan F et al. A study of digestive absorption in four cases of Down's syndrome. Down's syndrome, malnutrition, malabsorption, and Alzheimer's disease. Med Hypotheses 31(1):35-8, 1990

Abasheva GK. [Free plasma and cerebral amino acids in children with Down's syndrome.] Zh Nevropatol Psikhiatr 81(7):1068-70, 1981 (in Russian)

Airaksinen EM. Tryptophan treatment of infants with Down's syndrome. Ann Clin Res 6(1):33-9, 1974

Anneren G et al. Trace element profiles in individual blood cells from patients with Down's syndrome. Acta Paediatr Scand 74(2):259-63, 1985a

Anneren G et al. Selenium in plasma and erythrocytes in patients with Down's syndrome and healthy controls. Variation in relation to age, sex and glutathione peroxidase activity in erythrocytes. Acta Paediatr Scand 74(4):508-14, 1985b

Anneren G, Gebre-Medhin M. Trace elements and transport proteins in serum of children with Down syndrome and of healthy siblings living in the same environment. Hum Nutr Clin Nutr 41(4):291-9, 1987

Anneren G et al. Increased plasma and erythrocyte selenium concentrations but decreased erythrocyte glutathione peroxidase activity after selenium supplementation in children with Down syndrome. Acta Paediatr Scand 78(6):879-84, 1989

Anneren G et al. Increase in serum concentrations of IgG2 and IgG4 by selenium supplementation in children with Down's syndrome. Arch Dis Child 65(12):1353-5, 1990

Antila E et al. Selenium therapy in Down syndrome (DS): a theory and a clinical trial. Adv Exp Med Biol 264:183-6, 1990

Antonucci A et al. Detection of apoptosis in peripheral blood cells of 31 subjects affected by Down syndrome before and after zinc therapy. Ultrastruct Pathol 21(5):449-52, 1997

Bade MA et al. [Symptoms of disease and food allergy in children with Down syndrome.] Ned Tijdschr Geneeskd 139(33):1680-4, 1995 (in Dutch)

Baran H et al. Increased kynurenic acid levels and decreased brain kynurenine aminotransferase I in patients with Down syndrome. Life Sci 58(21):1891-9, 1996

Barlow PJ et al. Hair trace metal levels in Down syndrome patients. J Ment Defic Res 25 (Pt 3):161-8, 1981

Bjorksten B et al. Zinc and immune function in Down's syndrome. Acta Paediatr Scand 69(2):183-7, 1980

Brugge KL et al. The role of alterations in free radical metabolism in mediating cognitive impairments in Down's syndrome. EXS 62:190-8, 1992

Bumbalo TS et al. Negative results - treatment of Down's syndrome with the "U" series. JAMA 187:361, 1964

Burns A, Holland T. Vitamin E deficiency. Letter. Lancet i:805-6, 1986

Cantor DS et al. A report on phosphatidylcholine therapy in a Down's syndrome child. Psychol Rep 58:207-17, 1986

Chiricolo M et al. Enhanced DNA repair in lymphocytes of Down syndrome patients: The influence of zinc nutritional supplementation. Mutat Res 295:105-11, 1993

Coburn SP, Seidenburg M. Leucocyte pyridoxal phosphate level in Down's syndrome and other retardates. Fed Proc 27:554, 1968

Coleman M. Infantile spasms associated with 5-hydroxytryptophan administration in patients with Down's syndrome. Neurology 21(9):911-19, 1971

Coleman M et al. A double blind study of vitamin B6 in Down's syndrome infants. part 1--Clinical and biochemical results. J Ment Defic Res 29(Pt 3):233-40, 1985

Colombo ML et al. [Vitamin C in children with trisomy 21.] Minerva Pediatr 41(4):189-92, 1989a (in Italian)

Columbo ML et al. [Blood zinc in patients with Down's syndrome and its relations with their immune status.] Minerva Pediatr 41(2):71-5, 1989b (in Italian)

Columbo ML et al. [Carnitine and Down's syndrome.] Minerva Pediatr 41(4):173-6, 1989c (in Italian)

David O et al. Hematological studies in children with Down syndrome. Pediatr Hematol Oncol 13(3):271-5, 1996

De Falco FA et al. [Effect of the chronic treatment with L-acetylcarnitine in Down's syndrome.] Clin Ter 144(2):123-7, 1994 (in Italian)

De La Torre et al. Overexpression of copper-zinc superoxide dismutase in trisomy 21. Experientia 52(9):871-3, 1996

Farrar G et al. Defective gallium-transferrin binding in Alzheimer disease and Down syndrome: possible mechanism for accumulation of aluminum in brain. Lancet 335:747-50, 1990

Frager J et al. A double blind study of vitamin B6 in Down's syndrome infants. Part 2--Cortical auditory evoked potentials. J Ment Defic Res 29(Pt 3):241-6, 1985

Franceschi C et al. Oral zinc supplementation in Down's syndrome: restoration of thymic endocrine activity and of some immune defects. J Ment Defic Res 32(Pt 3):169-81, 1988

Gale L et al. Down's syndrome is strongly associated with coeliac disease. Gut 40(4):492-6, 1997

Gedye A. Dietary increase in serotonin reduces self-injurious behavior in a Down's syndrome adult. J Ment Defic Res 34(2):195-203, 1990

Gericke GS et al. Leucocyte ultrastructure and folate metabolism in Down's syndrome. S Afr Med J 51(12):369-74, 1977

Gromadzinska J et al. Glutathione peroxidase activity, lipid peroxides and selenium status in blood in patients with Down's syndrome. J Clin Chem Clin Biochem 26(5):255-8, 1988

Harrell RF et al. Can nutritional supplements help mentally retarded children? An exploratory study. Proc Natl Acad Sci USA 78(1):574-8, 1981

Heggarty HJ et al. Amino acid profile in Down's syndrome. Arch Dis Child 74:347-9, 1996

Hestnes A et al. Hormonal and biochemical disturbances in Down's syndrome. J Ment Defic Res 35(Pt 3):179-93, 1991

Hilhorst MI et al. Down syndrome and celiac disease: five new cases with a review of the literature. Eur J Pediatr 152(11):884-7, 1993

Ibarra B et al. Hematological and biochemical studies in children with Down syndrome. Ann Genet 33(2):84-7, 1990

Jackson CV et al. Vitamin E and Alzheimer's disease in subjects with Down's syndrome. J Ment Defic Res 32(6):479-84, 1988

Kadrabova J et al. Changed serum trace element profile in Down's Syndrome. Biol Trace Elem Res 54(3):201-6, 1996

Kanavin O et al. Immunological studies of patients with Down's syndrome. Measurements of autoantibodies and serum antibodies to dietary antigens in relation to zinc levels. Acta Med Scand 224(5):473-7, 1988

Kleijnen J, Knipschild P. Niacin and vitamin B6 in mental functioning: a review of controlled trials in humans. Biol Psychiatry 29(9):931-41, 1991

Lejeune J et al. Amino acids and trisomy 21. Ann Genet 35(1):8-13, 1992

Licastro F et al. Zinc affects the metabolism of thyroid hormones in children with Down's syndrome: normalization of thyroid stimulating hormone and of reversal triiodothyronine plasmic levels by dietary zinc supplementation. Int J Neurosci 65(1-4):259-68, 1992

Licastro F et al. Modulation of the neuroendocrine system and immune functions by zinc supplementation in children with Down's syndrome. J Trace Elem Electrolytes Health Dis 7(4):237-9, 1993

Licastro F et al. Oral zinc supplementation in Down's syndrome subjects decreased infections and normalized some humoral and cellular immune parameters. J Intellect Disabil Res 38(Pt 2):149-62, 1994

McCoy EE et al. The metabolism of vitamin B6 in Down's syndrome. Ann N Y Acad Sci 166(1):116-25, 1969

McCoy EE, Sneddon JM. Decreased calcium content and $45Ca2^+$ uptake in Down's syndrome blood platelets. Pediatr Res18(9):914-16, 1984

Menolaascino FJ et al. Vitamin supplements and purported learning enhancement in mentally retarded children. J Nutr Sci Vitaminol 35(3):181-92, 1989

Metcalfe T et al. Vitamin E concentrations in human brain of patients with Alzheimer's disease, fetuses with Down's syndrome, centenarians, and controls. Neurochem Res 14(12):1209-12, 1989

Mircher C et al. [Variation of amino acids in relation to age in Down syndrome subjects]. Arch Pediatr 4(11):1093-9, 1997) (in French)

Moore PB et al. Gastrointestinal absorption of aluminum is increased in Down's syndrome. Biol Psychiatry 41(4):488-92, 1997

Napolitano G et al. Is zinc deficiency a cause of subclinical hypothyroidism in Down syndrome? Ann Genet 33(1):9-15, 1990a

Napolitano G et al. Growth delay in Down syndrome and zinc sulphate supplementation. Am J Med Genet Suppl 7:63-5, 1990b

Neve J et al. Selenium, zinc and copper in Down's syndrome (trisomy 21): blood levels and relations with glutathione peroxidase and superoxide dismutase. Clin Chim Acta 133(2):209-14, 1983

O'Brien D, Grashek A. The abnormality of tryptophan metabolism in children with mongolism. Arch Dis Child 37:17, 1962

Perry EK et al. Cholinergic receptors in cognitive disorders. Can J Neurol Sci 13(4 Suppl):521-7, 1986

Petre-Quadens O, De Lee C. 5-Hydroxytryptophan and sleep in Down's syndrome. J Neurol Sci 26(3):443-53, 1975

Pueschel SM et al. 5-hydroxytryptophan and pyridoxine. Their effects in young children with Down's syndrome. Am J Dis Child 134(9):838-44, 1980

Purice M et al. Zinc and copper in plasma and erythrocytes of Down's syndrome children. Endocrinologie 26(2):113-17, 1988

Reading CM. Down's syndrome: nutritional intervention. Nutr Health 3(1-2):91-111, 1984a

Reading CM. Down's syndrome: is gluten/alpha-gliadin sensitivity/coeliac disease the cause? Int J Biosoc Res 6(1):62-5, 1984b

Schmid F et al. [Studies on the state of vitamins B1, B2, and B6 in Down's syndrome.] Fortschr Med 3(25):1170-2, 1975 (in German)

Shah SN et al. Antioxidant vitamin (A and E) status of Down's syndrome subjects. Nutr Res 9:709-15, 1989

Shaposhnikov AM et al. [Disorders of phenylalanine and tyrosine metabolism in Down's syndrome.] Vopr Med Khim 25(1):15-19, 1979) (in Russian)

Stabile A et al. Immunodeficiency and plasma zinc levels in children with Down's syndrome: a long-term follow-up of oral zinc supplementation. Clin Immunol Immunopathol 58(2):207-16, 1991

Sylverster PE. Ageing in the mentally retarded, in J Dobbing et al. Eds. Scientific Studies in Mental Retardation. London, Macmillian, for the Royal Society of Medicine, 1984, 259-77

Trubiani O Programmed cell death of peripheral myeloid precursor cells in Down patients: effect of zinc therapy. Ultrastruct Pathol 20(5):457-62, 1996

Turkel H, Nusbaum I. Rationale of components of the "U" series. Txu 106-93, July, 14 1982

Turkel H and Nusbaum I. Medical Treatment of Down Syndrome and Genetic Diseases, Fourth Edition, Ubiotica, Southfield, MI, 1985 (available from the Autism Research Institute, 4182 Adams Ave., San Diego, CA 92116, USA)

Wachtel TJ, Pueschel SM. Macrocytosis in Down syndrome. Am J Ment Retard 95(4):417-20, 1991

Watkins SE et al. Plasma amino acids in patients with senile dementia and in subjects with Down's syndrome at an age vulnerable to Alzheimer changes. J Ment Defic Res 33(Pt 2):159-66, 1989

Weise P. The use of 5-HTP in the treatment of Down's syndrome. Pediatrics 54(2):165-8, 1974

Williams CA et al. Xylose absorption in Down's syndrome. J Ment Defic Res 29(Pt 2):173-7, 1985

Wisniewski KE et al. Occurrence of neuropathological changes and dementia of Alzheimer's disease in Down's syndrome. Ann Neurol 17:270-82, 1985

DYSMENORRHEA

NUTRITIONAL TREATMENT GUIDE

✓ = Efficacy generally accepted.
* = Efficacy *demonstrated* by controlled human trials.
[+] = Efficacy *suspected* from uncontrolled human trials.
[-] = Efficacy *suspected* from indirect data.
? = Efficacy *challenged* in a study of similar design.

DIETARY FACTORS

[-] consume a diet rich in **Green Vegetables** and **Fatty Fish**

NUTRITIONAL FACTORS

* **Magnesium:** ? 100 mg 4 times daily; increase as needed during menses.
Consider adding **Vitamin B_6** ? 25 mg 4 times daily
* **Omega-3 fatty acids:** fish oil 6 g daily (1,080 mg EPA, 720 mg DHA, 1.5 mg vitamin E) (2 month trial)
* **Thiamine:** 100 mg daily (90 day trial)
* **Vitamin E:** alpha-tocopherol 50 mg 3 times daily for 14 days starting 10 days prior to menses

- -

[+] **Iron deficiency:** 30 mg twice daily until repletion; then minimal possible dosage
[+] **Niacin:** 100 mg twice daily. Increase to 100 mg every 2 to 3 hours during menses.
(Consider adding **Vitamin C** 300 mg and **Rutin** 60 mg daily.)

DIETARY FACTORS

Little has been reported concerning dietary influences on menstrual pain. However, a Danish epidemiological study found that women with dysmenorrhea characteristically ate a limited diet which was low in green vegetables and almost totally lacking in fatty fish *(Deutch).*

While the relationship of green vegetables to dysmenorrhea is difficult to analyze in regard to specific nutrients, the lack of fatty fish most likely resulted in an inadequate intake of omega-3 fatty acids (see below).

NUTRITIONAL FACTORS

VITAMINS

Niacin

In the 1950s, Hudgins reported the results of open trials which suggested that niacin supplementation provided relief of menstrual cramps for about 90% of women whose cramps had been severe enough to require bed rest, heavy sedation or loss of time from work *(Hudgins).*

He believed that the dosage should to be adequate to produce flushing - although he found in a preliminary trial that niacinamide (which does not produce flushing) seemed to work as well. He also believed that the efficacy of niacin was enhanced by the addition of ascorbic acid and rutin, and suggested that, by improving capillary permeability, they enhanced the vasodilating effect of the niacin.

Unfortunately, his work has yet to be confirmed by controlled studies, although his high rate of success makes it likely that the response to niacin was more than a placebo effect.

Thiamine

A group of 556 young women aged 12 to 21 with moderate to very severe primary spasmodic dysmenorrhea randomly received thiamine hydrochloride and placebo in random order for 90 days each. When the results of the 2 treatment groups were combined, it was found that 87% of the women were completely cured, while for 8% the pain was reduced to almost gone. Only 5% noted no relief from the treatment. Moreover, 2 months after the treatment ended, the improvements remained, causing the investigator to believe that the treatment was curative *(Gokhale)*.

While these findings need independent confirmation, they are consistent with those of open trials which found thiamine to have an analgesic effect, although those studies employed much higher dosages (see Pain).

Vitamin E

In 1955, the *Lancet* published a placebo-controlled study in which 100 young women with spasmodic dysmenorrhea received either alpha-tocopherol or placebo for 10 days premenstrually and for the next 4 days. After 2 cycles, 68% of women in the supplemented group improved compared to only 18% of the controls *(Butler)*.

A recent Russian study confirmed the analgesic effect of vitamin E in dysmenorrhea, but noted that its efficacy seemed dependent upon the cause of the dysmenorrhea. Also, treatment with naloxone blocked the ability of vitamin E to induce analgesia in some patients, suggesting that the effect was related to endorphin release *(Kryzhanovskii)*.

Beta-endorphin-like immunoreactivity was increased only 15 minutes after vitamin E administration *(Kryzhanovskii)*, suggesting that vitamin E supplementation may be effective when given after the start of menstrual pain. However, the vitamin is also known to inhibit thromboxane A2 release and to stimulate prostacyclin synthesis *(Gisinger)*, so supplementation is likely to be more effective if started at least several days prior to menses.

MINERALS

Iron Deficiency

Iron deficiency, as marked by low ferritin levels or low transferrin saturation, may be associated with an increased risk of dysmenorrhea *(Penland)*.

In 1965, Nathaniel Shafer of the department of medicine, New York Medical College, learned from 2 patients receiving iron supplementation for iron deficiency anemia that their severe symptoms of dysmenorrhea had disappeared. He proceeded to question another 4 patients whom he had treated for iron-deficiency anemia, and to treat another 6 patients complaining of dysmenorrhea (several of whom also had iron deficiency anemia) with iron, without informing them that the treatment may relieve their pain. (None of these patients had endometriosis or other organic pelvic disease to account for the dysmenorrhea.)

All reported diminution or complete disappearance of menstrual pain following iron supplementation *(Shafer)*. Unfortunately, these preliminary findings have yet to be confirmed by other investigators.

Magnesium

There is some evidence that magnesium nutriture may be reduced *(Henrotte)*.

Double-blind studies have reported that magnesium supplementation may be effective for treating primary dysmenorrhea *(Fontana-Klaiber;Seifert)*. In addition to its vasodilatory and muscle relaxant effects, it inhibits the synthesis of prostaglandin F2 alpha *(Seifert)*

Since vitamin B_6 increases the influx of ionic magnesium into the myometrial cell, it may increase magnesium's efficacy *(Abraham)*. Indeed, the combination of magnesium and pyridoxine given every 2 hours as needed during menses and 4 times daily during the rest of the cycle was followed, in the next 4 to 6 months, by a progressive decrease in the intensity and duration of menstrual cramps *(Abraham)*. It is not known, however, if the addition of pyridoxine added to the efficacy of the treatment.

OTHER NUTRITIONAL FACTORS

Omega-3 Fatty Acids

A study of the dietary habits of Danish women aged 20 to 45 who were not pregnant and did not use oral contraceptives found that their diet was almost totally lacking in fatty fish. A low intake of omega-3 fatty acids, and a low dietary omega-3 to omega-6 ratio was inversely associated with dysmenorrhea *(Deutch).*

Supplementation with omega-3 fatty acids from fish oils was studied in a group of 42 adolescents with dysmenorrhea who had a low dietary intake of fish. In a double-blind crossover study, one-half of the group received fish oil daily for 2 months followed by a placebo for an additional 2 months, while the other half of the group took placebo followed by fish oil. While there were no baseline differences in menstrual symptoms between the 2 sub-groups, following the 2 months of treatment with fish oil, each of the sub-groups had a marked reduction in menstrual symptoms *(Harel).*

BIBLIOGRAPHY

Abraham GE. Primary dysmenorrhea. Clin Obstet Gynecol 21(1):139-45, 1978

Butler EB, McKnight E. Vitamin E in the treatment of primary dysmenorrhoea. Lancet i:844-7, 1955

Deutch B. Menstrual pain in Danish women correlated with low n-3 polyunsaturated fatty-acid intake. Eur J Clin Nutr 49(7):508-16, 1995

Fontana-Klaiber H, Hogg B. [Therapeutic effects of magnesium in dysmenorrhea.] Schweiz Rundsch Med Prax 79(16):491-4, 1990

Gisinger C et al. Vitamin E and platelet eicosanoids in diabetes mellitus. Prostaglandins Leukot Essent Fatty Acids 40:169-76, 1990

Gokhale LB. Curative treatment of primary (spasmodic) dysmenorrhoea. Indian J Med Res 103:227-31, 1996

Harel Z et al. Supplementation with omega-3 polyunsaturated fatty acids in the management of dysmenorrhea in adolescents. Am J Obstet Gynecol 174(4):1335-8, 1996

Henrotte JG et al. Les variations de la magnesemie liee au sexe, leurs relations avec l'excitabilite et la fatigue. CR Soc Biol 167:843-7, 1973

Hudgins AP. Vitamins P, C and niacin for dysmenorrhea therapy. West J Surg Gynecol 62:610-11, 1954

Kryzhanovskii GN et al. [Endogenous opioid system in the realization of the analgesic effect of alpha-tocopherol.] Biull Eksp Biol Med 105(2):148-50, 1988

Penland J, Hunt J. Nutritional status and menstrual-related symptomology. Abstract. FASEB J 7:A379, 1993

Seifert B et al. [Magnesium - a new therapeutic alternative in primary dysmenorrhea.] Zentralbl Gynakol 111(11):755-60, 1989

Shafer N. Iron in the treatment of dysmenorrhea: A preliminary report. Curr Ther Res 7(6):365-6, 1965

EATING DISORDERS

See Also: OBESITY

NUTRITIONAL TREATMENT GUIDE

✓ = Efficacy generally accepted.
* = Efficacy *demonstrated* by controlled human trials.
[+] = Efficacy *suspected* from uncontrolled human trials.
[-] = Efficacy *suspected* from indirect data.
? = Efficacy *challenged* in a study of similar design.

DIETARY FACTORS

✓ consume a **Nutrient-Dense** diet

* avoid **Sugar** ingestion

NUTRITIONAL FACTORS

* **Carnitine deficiency:** ? 90 mg daily *AND*
Cobamamide ? 1 mg daily
* **L-Tryptophan:** 3 g daily *AND*
Vitamin B_6: pyridoxine 45 mg daily (1 month trial)
* **Zinc deficiency:** zinc sulfate 220 mg twice daily *AND* **Copper** 2 mg daily

[+] **Folic acid deficiency:** 800 μg daily
[+] **Niacin deficiency:** 50 to 100 mg daily
[+] **Thiamine deficiency:** 50 mg daily

[-] **Calcium deficiency:** ≈ 1 g daily
[-] **Omega-3 Essential Fatty Acid deficiency:** *example:* MaxEPA 1 g caps [180 mg EPA; 120 mg DHA] 10 to 20 daily
[-] **Omega-6 Essential Fatty Acid deficiency:** *example:* evening primrose oil 500 mg caps [7-10% GLA] 6 to 8 daily
[-] **Potassium deficiency:** ? 80 to 100 mEq daily total intake, preferably from potassium-rich foods
[-] **Riboflavin deficiency:** 5 to 10 mg daily
[-] **Vitamin B_6 deficiency:** 50 to 100 mg daily
[-] **Vitamin B_{12} deficiency:** 1,000 μg intramuscularly weekly initially and monthly afterwards
[-] **Vitamin D deficiency:** 50,000 to 100,000 IU 2 or 3 times during the first week; then, if needed, either 100,000 IU ergo- or cholecalciferol every 3 to 6 months *OR* 800 to 1,600 IU daily

DIETARY FACTORS

General

Due to their grossly inadequate food intake, patients with anorexia nervosa require a diet designed to promote weight gain through increased energy intake and expansion of their dietary choices *(Rock,1995).*

Patients with bulimia nervosa, even though anthropometry may show no signs of malnutrition, also need a nutrient-dense diet, since the results of immune function studies suggest that they may be subclinically malnourished *(Marcos).*

Sugar

The results of animal studies suggest that sugar is the nutrient that most affects opiate-mediated feeding behavior. Moreover, clinical experience with humans suggests that carbohydrates, particularly sugar, play a role in binge eating *(Fullerton).*

In a double-blind study, bulimic women and matched controls randomly received injections of glucose or placebo. Throughout the entire monitoring period, bulimics reported more symptoms of distressed mood than controls. Blood glucose levels were correlated with mood in the bulimic group, but not in the control group, and these levels were lower than those of the control group. Furthermore, the glucose injection induced a heightened urge to binge in the bulimic group, while it reduced food cravings in the controls *(Blouin).*

NUTRITIONAL FACTORS

VITAMINS

Folic Acid Deficiency

Folate intake may be lower than that of normals, not only in anorexia nervosa, but also in bulimia *(Howat).* In fact, a case of bulimia nervosa with profound folate deficiency has been reported which responded well to folate repletion *(Eedy).*

In anorexia nervosa, total plasma homocysteine concentrations have been found to be increased, probably due to subclinical folate deficiency, even though blood folate levels are usually in the reference range *(Moyano).*

Niacin Deficiency

Since anorexia is one of the first symptoms of pellagra, it has been suggested that anorexia nervosa is simply sub-clinical pellagra, a disease of niacin deficiency *(Cleary).* In support of this theory, supplementation of niacin has been helpful in improving appetite and mental state in anorexic patients *(Cleary).*

> *A 20-year-old woman was seen with the associated disorders of pellagra and anorexia nervosa, both of which had been present for approximately 6 months. Treatment with niacin induced resolution of the pellagra skin changes (Rapaport).*

Riboflavin Deficiency

Patients with anorexia nervosa may have a low intake of riboflavin *(Thibault).* Based on erythrocyte enzyme activity, patients with either anorexia nervosa or bulimia nervosa are often riboflavin-deficient; in fact, body weight is positively associated with riboflavin status *(Rock,1996).*

Thiamine Deficiency

Thiamine intake may be low in anorexia nervosa *(Thibault).* Moreover, thiamine nutriture may be deficient, and the deficiency may contribute to the lack of appetite *(Smith).*

Vitamin A

Plasma concentrations of vitamin A have been found to be normal *(Rock,1995)*, high *(Mira,1989a)* and low *(Vaisman)* in eating disorder patients. The reason is such disparate results is unknown. Vitamin A metabolism appears to be normal *(Vaisman)*.

Vitamin B_6 Deficiency

Patients with low body weight may have a subclinical deficiency of vitamin B_6, putting them in the upper quartile of erythrocyte aspartate transaminase activation *(Mira,1989a).*

Vitamin B_{12} Deficiency

In anorexia nervosa, vitamin B_{12} nutriture usually appears to be adequate *(Van Binsbergen)*. However, on rare occasions, a deficiency severe enough to produce a neurologic syndrome can occur *(Patchell)*.

Vitamin D Deficiency

Bone mineral density is often decreased in patients with anorexia nervosa *(Jornod)*. This measure is significantly lower in these patients than in patients with anorexia/bulimia or bulimia for whom overt osteopenia is uncommon *(Carmichael)*.

Vitamin D intake may be low *(Jornod)*. Moreover, serum levels of 25-hydroxyvitamin D and 1,25-dihydroxy-vitamin D are sometimes low *(Aarskog;Fonseca)*.

However, bone mineral density does not appear to correlated with serum vitamin D levels *(Carmichael)* and vitamin D deficiency is believed unlikely to be a primary contributor to bone loss in these patients *(Kiriike)*.

Vitamin E

As with vitamin A, vitamin E levels may be normal *(Van Binsbergen)*, high *(Mira,1989a)* or low *(Vaisman)* in patients with eating disorders. One study found plasma alpha-tocopherol concentrations to be inversely correlated to body mass index *(Rock,1995)*, suggesting that emaciated patients may have higher plasma levels of the vitamin.

MINERALS

Calcium Deficiency

As already noted, bone mineral density is often decreased in patients with anorexia nervosa. This finding is partly due to low calcium intake, especially in adolescent patients who have yet to reach peak bone mass *(Jornod; Salisbury)*.

In addition, calcium absorption is decreased in anorexia nervosa, and urinary calcium excretion may be 4 times as high as in normals *(Abrams)*. Calcium kinetics data reveal increased bone resorption and decrease bone formation rates, probably due to abnormal calcium metabolism *(Abrams)*; thus increased calcium and vitamin D intake may not be enough by themselves to restore normal bone metabolism.

Copper

Compared to normals, plasma/serum copper levels are frequently depressed in patients with anorexia nervosa *(Casper)*, while patients with bulimia nervosa have copper levels that are intermediate between the two groups *(McClain,1993)*. Whether this finding indicates a deficiency is not known. Ceruloplasmin and hair copper levels, by contrast, appear to be normal *(Casper)*.

Potassium Deficiency

In both anorexia nervosa and bulimia nervosa, serum potassium concentration may occasionally be low *(Greenfield)*. Hypokalemic patients have a lower mean weight and body mass index, and more of them purge by abusing laxatives, either alone or with vomiting *(Greenfield)*.

In a group of 25 hospitalized patients with anorexia nervosa, 7 of them vomited, usually surreptitiously. Hypokalemia was detected in 5 of them compared to none of the other 18 patients *(Koh)*.

Also useful in detecting surreptitious vomiting is a low urinary chloride to sodium ratio *(Koh)*.

Zinc Deficiency

Zinc deficiency is well known to be detrimental to taste and smell. Anorexia nervosa can thus be a manifestation of zinc deficiency which, in turn, can be caused by such factors as inadequate intake, the use of oral contraceptives, vomiting, diarrhea or impaired absorption. Bulimia nervosa may also be associated with evidence of zinc deficiency *(Birmingham;McClain,1992)*.

When zinc is deficient, placebo-controlled studies have found that supplementation improves appetite, taste sensitivity *(Ward)*, and emotional state *(Katz)*.

An emaciated 16-year-old female with anorexia nervosa was hospitalized due to vomiting, epigastric pain and diarrhea. A taste disorder, low serum alkaline phosphatase activity and a relatively low serum zinc concentration suggested a zinc deficiency.

Zinc was initially administered intravenously (40 mmol/d) for 7 days, then orally (15 mg elemental zinc daily) for about 60 days. Digestive symptoms disappeared after the second day of intravenous zinc administration, and she rapidly regained her normal weight after one month of oral zinc supplementation. Also, both exocrine pancreatic function and intestinal absorption were improved by prolonged supplementation with oral zinc (Yamaguchi).

OTHER NUTRITIONAL FACTORS

Carnitine Deficiency

When patients with anorexia nervosa have severe liver damage, they may develop a deficiency of carnitine causing progressive weakness and muscle atrophy. A muscle biopsy or muscle carnitine levels will establish the diagnosis *(Fukusako)*.

Studies have reported beneficial effects in treating cachectic patients with anorexia nervosa with carnitine along with cobamamide (adenosylcobalamin, the activated form of vitamin B_{12}), as vitamin B_{12} appears to stimulate hepatic carnitine synthesis by activating methylation *(Podlepa)*.

Following supplementation, patients have shown weight gain, normalization of gastrointestinal function, reduction in latent fatigue and improvement in mental work capacity *(Korkina,1989,1992)*, probably due to repletion of a subclinical carnitine deficiency.

Carotenoids

Patients with either anorexia nervosa or bulimia nervosa frequently have elevated serum carotenoid levels *(Curran-Celenano,1985)*. Liver abnormalities do not appear to be the cause of this finding *(Sherman)*. Its etiology is unknown *(Curran-Celenano,1993)*.

Essential Fatty Acid Deficiencies

Anorexia nervosa patients have selected deficiencies of both omega-3 and omega-6 essential fatty acids *(Holman)*. While human trials are lacking, animal studies suggest that supplementation with omega-3 fatty acids may increase appetite *(Dinerello)*.

Also, we have already noted the importance of repleting zinc deficiency, and Horrobin has argued for combining zinc and essential fatty acid supplements, noting that there is substantial evidence that anorexia nervosa may be due to a combined deficiency of the two. Many of the features of zinc deficiency are similar to those of essential fatty acid deficiency. Essential fatty acids are important in zinc absorption, and zinc seems necessary in at least 2 stages in essential fatty acid metabolism *(Horrobin)*.

Tryptophan

In women, even moderate dieting appears to lower brain serotonin levels, leading to compensatory changes *(Cowen)*. It is therefore not surprising that both anorexia nervosa *(Goodwin)* and bulimia nervosa *(Weltzin)* are marked by alterations in brain serotonin function. Men appear to be less liable to develop these changes *(Goodwin)*, a finding that may help to explain why eating disorders are so much less common in men.

Patients with anorexia nervosa, including those with bulimic features, appear to have reduced blood *(Askenazy)* and cerebrospinal fluid *(Kaye)* tryptophan levels.

Earlier we noted that sugar ingestion increases the urge to binge. Sugar promotes serotonin release from brain neurons by stimulating insulin secretion. Insulin, in turn, increases the brain uptake of L-tryptophan, the nutritional precursor of serotonin, relative to the other large, neutral amino acids *(Wurtman)*.

Supplementation

Despite the theoretical rationale for supplementation with L-tryptophan (or L-5-hydroxytrypophan), few studies have been published. In a double-blind crossover study, young normal-weight bulimic women received L-tryptophan and pyridoxine (which increases serotonin synthesis from L-tryptophan). After about one month, the supplements significantly improved mood, eating behavior, and feelings about eating *(Mira,1989b)*. However, a similar study noted no benefit from L-tryptophan supplementation alone *(Krahn)*.

Jessica, age 17, had a sallow face with dark rings around her eyes. For the past year she had been bulimic. Almost every other day she experienced severe carbohydrate cravings and gorged on 2 or 3 boxes of heavily sugared breakfast cereal. Then she would usually stick her finger down her throat to regurgitate. Her grades in school had plummeted and she had withdrawn from most of her activities.

She had been discharged from an inpatient treatment center just a few weeks earlier after participating in an intensive 30-day program. Her doctors had prescribed Zoloft, a serotonin reuptake inhibitor, but she soon stopped it due to agitation and nausea. She was having individual psychotherapy twice a week and her family was also seeing a counselor. The day before her visit, her mother found her unconscious on the bathroom floor.

Following evaluation, she was told to start a food diary and to make a concerted effort to avoid high-sugar foods. In addition, she was started on 5-hydroxytryptophan 100 mg 3 times daily 20 minutes before meals. One week later, she reported that she noticed results almost immediately. By the fourth day, she was feeling more in control, had fewer and less intense food cravings, and was sleeping better. By the end of three months of follow-up, she remained in good spirits and had had only one episode of bingeing and purging (Murray).

COMBINED NUTRITIONAL TREATMENT

The efficacy of nutritional treatment for bulimia was demonstrated in a study of 20 bulimic women. Half of the group was placed on a nutrient-dense diet containing no fewer than 1400 kcal and free of suspected blood sugar-insulin level destabilizers for 6 weeks. Alcohol, caffeine, refined sugar, white flour, flavor enhancers, most salt, cigarettes and medications were eliminated, and they were supplemented with vitamin C 1 g, vitamin B complex '50', and a multivitamin/multimineral daily. Simultaneously, the other half of the group was placed on a sham food plan which allowed unknowing duplications of their pre-study food patterns. After 3 weeks they were switched to the nutrient-rich diet for another 3 weeks.

The treatment group ceased to binge, while the control group binged steadily until switched to the nutrient-dense diet, after which all bingeing ceased. Subjects lost weight effortlessly or maintained weight by choice, and remained binge-free for up to 2.5 years of observation *(Dalvit-McPhillips).*

BIBLIOGRAPHY

Aarskog D et al. Plasma concentrations of 25-hydroxyvitamin D metabolites in pubertal girls with anorexia nervosa. Acta Endocrinol Suppl (Copenh) 279:458-67, 1986

Abrams S et al. Mineral balance and bone turnover in adolescents with anorexia nervosa. J Pediatr 123:326-31, 1993

Askenazy F et al. Whole blood serotonin content, tryptophan concentrations, and impulsivity in anorexia nervosa. Biol Psychiatry 43(3):188-95, 1998

Birmingham CL et al. Controlled trial of zinc supplementation in anorexia nervosa. Int J Eat Disord 15:251-5, 1994

Blouin AG et al. A double-blind placebo-controlled glucose challenge in bulimia nervosa: psychological effects. Biol Psychiatry 33(3):160-8, 1993

Carmichael KA, Carmichael DH. Bone metabolism and osteopenia in eating disorders. Medicine (Baltimore) 74(5):254-67, 1995

Casper RC et al. An evaluation of trace metals, vitamins and taste function in anorexia nervosa. Am J Clin Nutr 33:1801-9, 1980

Cleary MJ, Cleary JP. Anorexia nervosa: A form of subclinical pellagra. Int Clin Nutr Rev 9(3):137-43, 1989

Cowen PJ et al. Moderate dieting causes 5-HT2C receptor supersensitivity. Psychol Med 26(6):1155-9, 1996

Curran-Celentano J et al. Alternations in vitamin A and thyroid hormone status in anorexia nervosa and associated disorders. Am J Clin Nutr 42(6):1183-91, 1985

Curran-Celenano J, Erdman JW. A case study of carotenemia in anorexia nervosa may support the interrelationship of vitamin A and thyroid hormone. Nutr Res 13:379-86, 1993

Dalvit-McPhillips S. A dietary approach to bulimia treatment. Physiol Behav 33(5):769-75, 1984

Dinarello CA et al. Interleukin-1, anorexia, and dietary fatty acids. Ann NY Acad Sci 587:332-8, 1990

Eedy DJ et al. A patient with bulimia nervosa and folate deficiency. Postgrad Med J 62:853-4, 1986

Fonseca VA et al. Vitamin D deficiency and low osteocalcin concentrations in anorexia nervosa. J Clin Pathol 41(2):195-7, 1988

Fukusako T et al. [A case of secondary carnitine deficiency due to anorexia nervosa and severe liver damage]. Rinsho Shinkeigaku 35(1):34-7, 1995) (in Japanese)

Fullerton DT et al. Sugar, opioids and binge eating. Brain Res Bull 14(6):673-80, 1985

Goodwin GM et al. Dieting changes serotonergic function in women, not men: implications for the aetiology of anorexia nervosa? Psychol Med 17(4):839-42, 1987

Greenfield D et al. Hypokalemia in outpatients with eating disorders. Am J Psychiatry 152(1):60-3, 1995

Holman RT et al. Patients with anorexia nervosa demonstrate deficiencies of selected essential fatty acids, compensatory changes in nonessential fatty acids and decreased fluidity of plasma lipids. J Nutr 125(4):901-7, 1995

Horrobin DF, Cunnane SC. Interactions between zinc, essential fatty acids and prostaglandins. Med Hypotheses 6(3):277-96, 1980

Howat PM et al. The effect of bulimia upon diet, body fat, bone density, and blood components. J Am Diet Assoc 89(7):929-34, 1989

Jornod P, Ruedi B. [Osteopenia: a consequence of anorexia nervosa]. Rev Med Suisse Romande 117(6):485-94, 1997) (in French)

Katz RL et al. Zinc deficiency in anorexia nervosa. J Adolesc Health Care 8(5):400-6, 1987

Kaye WH et al. CSF 5-HIAA concentrations in anorexia nervosa: reduced values in underweight subjects normalize after weight gain . Biol Psychiatry 23:102-5, 1988

Kiriike N et al. Reduced bone density and major hormones regulating calcium metabolism in anorexia nervosa. Acta Psychiatr Scand 86(5):358-63, 1992

Koh E et al. Clinical evaluation of hypokalemia in anorexia nervosa. Jpn J Med 28(6):692-6, 1989

Korkina MV et al. [Clinico-experimental substantiation of the use of carnitine and cobalamin in the treatment of anorexia nervosa.] Zh Nevropatol Psikhiatr 89(2):82-7, 1989) (in Russian)

Korkina MV et al. [Effects of carnitine and cobamamide on the dynamics of mental work capacity in patients with anorexia nervosa.] Zh Nevropatol Psikhiatr Im S S Korsakova 92(2):99-102, 1992 (in Russian)

Krahn D, Mitchell J. Use of L-tryptophan in treating bulimia. Letter. Am J Psychiatry 142(9):1130, 1985

Marcos A et al. Evaluation of immunocompetence and nutritional status in patients with bulimia nervosa. Am J Clin Nutr 57:65-9, 1993

McClain CJ et al. Zinc status before and after zinc supplementation of eating disorder patients. J Am Coll Nutr 11(6):694-700, 1992

McClain CJ et al. Gastrointestinal and nutritional aspects of eating disorders. J Am Coll Nutr 12(4):466-74, 1993

Mira M et al. Vitamin and trace element status of women with disordered eating. Am J Clin Nutr 50:940-4, 1989a

Mira M, Abraham S. L-tryptophan as an adjunct to treatment of bulimia nervosa. Letter. Lancet ii:1162-3, 1989b

Moyano D et al. Plasma total-homocysteine in anorexia nervosa. Eur J Clin Nutr 52(3):172-5, 1998

Murray MT. 5-HTP: The Natural Way to Overcome Depression, Obesity, and Insomnia. New York, Bantam Books, 1998

Patchell RA et al. Neurologic complications of anorexia nervosa. Acta Neurol Scand 89(2):111-16, 1994

Podlepa EM et al. [The effect of methylation on the carnitine synthesis]. Prikl Biokhim Mikrobiol 26(2):179-83, 1990) (in Russian)

Rapaport MJ. Pellagra in a patient with anorexia nervosa. Arch Dermatol 121(2):255-7, 1985

Rock C, Vasantharajan S. Vitamin status of eating disorder patients - relationship to clinical indexes and effect of treatment. Int J Eating Disorders 18(3):257-62, 1995

Rock CL, Curran-Celentano J. Nutritional management of eating disorders. Psychiatr Clin North Am 19(4):701-13, 1996

Salisbury JJ, Mitchell JE. Bone mineral density and anorexia nervosa in women. Am J Psychiatry 148(6):768-74, 1991

Sherman P et al. Hypercarotenemia and transaminitis in female adolescents with eating disorders: a prospective, controlled study. J Adolesc Health 15(3):205-9, 1994

Smith DK et al. Hypothermia in a patient with anorexia nervosa. Metabolism 32(12):1151-4, 1983

Thibault L, Roberge AG. The nutritional status of subjects with anorexia nervosa. Int J Vitam Nutr Res 57(4):447-52, 1987

Vaisman N et al. Vitamin A metabolism in plasma of normal and anorectic women. Eur J Clin Nutr 46:873-8, 1992

Van Binsbergen CJ et al. Nutritional status in anorexia nervosa: clinical chemistry, vitamins, iron and zinc. Eur J Clin Nutr 42(11):929-37, 1988

Ward NI. Assessment of zinc status and oral supplementation in anorexia nervosa. J Nutr Med 1:171-7, 1990

Weltzin TE et al. Serotonin and bulimia nervosa. Nutr Rev 52:399-408, 1994

Wurtman RJ, Wurtman JJ. Brain serotonin, carbohydrate-craving, obesity and depression. Obes Res 3 Suppl 4:477S-480S, 1995

Yamaguchi H et al. Anorexia nervosa responding to zinc supplementation: a case report. Gastroenterol Jpn 27(4):554-8, 1992

ECZEMA
(ATOPIC DERMATITIS)

NUTRITIONAL TREATMENT GUIDE

✓ = Efficacy generally accepted.
* = Efficacy *demonstrated* by controlled human trials.
[+] = Efficacy *suspected* from uncontrolled human trials.
[-] = Efficacy *suspected* from indirect data.
? = Efficacy *challenged* in a study of similar design.

DIETARY FACTORS

[+] **low Salt diet**

NUTRITIONAL FACTORS

* **Vitamin C:** 50 to 75 mg/kg (3 month trial)
* ? **Omega-3 Fatty Acids:** fish oil extract 10 g daily (containing 1.8 g EPA) (3 month trial)
* ? **Omega-6 Fatty Acids:** evening primrose oil 3 to 6 g daily (4 week trial)

- -

[+] **Selenium deficiency:** repletion (sodium selenate 200 μg daily)
WITH **Vitamin E:** tocopheryl succinate 10 mg daily (2 month trial)
[+] **Vitamin A:** vitamin A palmitate 20,000 to 200,000 IU daily
[+] **Zinc deficiency:** repletion (50 mg 3 times daily) (3 to 8 month trial)

OTHER RELATED FACTORS

✓ rule out **Food Sensitivities**

- -

[+] rule out **Hydrochloric acid** deficiency: betaine *or* glutamic HCl 10 to 50 gr at the end of meals as tolerated
[+] ***Lactobacillus acidophilus*:** dosage unknown

DIETARY FACTORS

Back in 1912, it was reported that reducing salt intake was beneficial to certain patients, primarily those with a major secretory component to their rash. Responding patients noted a lessening of lesions and improvement in pruritus within 3 to 4 days. A major improvement occurred in about 3 weeks *(Finkelstein)*.

Recently, in a letter to the editor, a preschool girl was described whose eczema improved following a change to low-salt table water *(Barthel)*. While the possible benefit of sodium restriction is unexplained, sweat sodium is reported to be increased in the disorder *(Liebke)*.

Controlled trials are needed to validate the efficacy of salt restriction.

NUTRITIONAL FACTORS

VITAMINS

Vitamin A

Experiences with treating 10 allergic children with chronic eczema by supplementing them with oral vitamin A palmitate at varying dosages for between 3 and 21 months were published in 1952. Three of the 9 children who tolerated the preparation showed some improvement, and 6 had marked improvement. There was no evidence of adverse effects, although the possibility of vitamin A toxicity must be kept in mind when using such high dosages, particularly in children.

The authors concluded that vitamin A is of value in the treatment of the "dryness and ichthyotic skin, which so often underlies infantile eczema *(Strosser)*." This finding is somewhat surprising as dry, scaly skin is one of the adverse effects of hypervitaminosis A.

Formal controlled trials are needed to validate these preliminary results.

Vitamin C

At the 1989 meeting of the American Academy of Allergy and Immunology, the results of a randomized, double-blind, crossover study conducted by faculty of the University of California at San Francisco were reported. Significant symptomatic improvement were found in 10 severely affected patients aged 3 to 21 years following supplementation with vitamin C.

Treated patients required half as many courses of antibiotics for skin infections as those given placebo. Improvements in lymphocyte transformation and neutrophil chemotaxis were also seen, suggesting that vitamin C may act may boosting the immune response *(Kline)*.

Unfortunately, this study does not appear to have been published, and its findings have yet to be replicated.

MINERALS

Selenium Deficiency

Patients sometimes have reduced erythrocyte levels of glutathione peroxidase, a selenium-containing enzyme *(Fairris)*. Since the level of this enzyme is a sensitive index of selenium nutriture *(Ganther)*, this suggests the possibility of a marginal selenium deficiency.

In an open trial, patients who had low levels of glutathione peroxidase compared to normal controls showed "encouraging" improvements as enzyme levels rose over 6 to 8 weeks following supplementation with selenium along with vitamin E *(Juhlin)*. (Deficiency syndromes of both vitamin E and selenium overlap and most can be treated successfully with either nutrient due to their closely-related mechanisms of action *[Combs]*). When, however, an unselected group of patients were given similar supplementation in a double-blind study, the supplement was found to be ineffective *(Fairris)*.

Since it is possible that the double-blind study failed to find benefit from supplementation because it was not limited to patients with reduced glutathione peroxidase levels, controlled studies limited to such patients are needed to ascertain if selenium supplementation is of benefit for that sub-group.

Zinc Deficiency

A sub-group of patients appears to be hypozincemic *(David, 1984)*. It appears that reduced serum zinc levels are correlated with the severity of the lesions *(Endre)* and a tendency towards recurrent skin infections *(David, 1984)*.

There is also evidence that both serum *(David, 1990)* and hair *(DiToro)* copper may be elevated in children with eczema. Since elevated copper would decrease zinc absorption and increase its urinary excretion *(Scott)*, it is possible that it contributes to a tendency towards reduced zinc nutriture.

An anecdotal report suggests that zinc supplementation may be strikingly effective, with full remission occurring in 3 to 8 months in most patients *(Wright)*. However, an 8-week double-blind trial using less than one-third the dosage failed to find evidence of beneficial effects *(Ewing)*. Obviously, a longer double-blind study using a larger dosage of zinc is needed to resolve the issue of its efficacy. (A study limited to patients with evidence of marginal zinc deficiency would be preferable.)

OTHER NUTRITIONAL FACTORS

Essential Fatty Acids

Patients who present with atopic eczema and allergic illnesses appear to have impairment of the enzyme delta-6-desaturase causing defective desaturation of alpha-linolenic (omega-3) and linoleic (omega-6) acids. The resulting changes in the production of prostaglandins and leukotrienes may theoretically account for the variety of clinical symptoms reported to be due to their effects on the immune response *(Galland)*.

Omega-3 Fatty Acids

In a double-blind study, patients supplemented with fish oil rich in eicosapentaenoic acid (EPA), an omega-3 fatty acid, had reduced scaling, itching, and overall subjective severity of skin lesions compared to olive oil-treated controls *(Bjorneboe)*. Another double-blind study, which used a mixture of saturated fatty acids as the placebo, failed to confirm these findings. However, the study was only published in abstract form and the dosage of EPA was unstated *(Kunz)*.

Omega-6 Fatty Acids

Consistent with the hypothesis that there is a defect in the enzyme delta-6-desaturase, patients may have increased levels of linoleic acid and reduced levels of its metabolites *(Manku)*. It is possible to compensate for the defect by supplementation with evening primrose oil (EPO) as it is rich in gamma-linolenic acid, the metabolite formed by the action of the defective enzyme *(Manku)*.

In a meta-analytic study which investigated the results of 9 placebo-controlled studies, EPO was significantly more effective than placebo, especially in reducing itching *(Morse)*. Since then, however, additional placebo-controlled studies have failed to confirm the efficacy of gamma-linolenic acid *(Borrek;Hederos;Whitaker)*, leaving the issue unresolved.

A 44 year-old postman developed itchy red patches on his arms and legs which were diagnosed as eczema. He was found to have a very low level of sweat zinc (90 parts/billion; normal range 360-910) and was treated with zinc sulfate 220 mg twice daily together with evening primrose oil 500 mg 6 times daily and multivitamins.

His intense itching improved markedly over the next 4 weeks, and disappeared almost completely after 8 weeks (Davies).

OTHER RELATED FACTORS

Food Sensitivities

In several double-blind studies, reactions to foods have been shown to provoke rashes in about one out of two people with a history of atopic eczema *(Sampson,1986)*, and evidence of increased gut absorption of food antigens has been found *(Caffarelli)*.

Histamine is an important mediator of these responses. Atopic dermatitis patients who are found to have food sensitivities also have an elevated spontaneous release of histamine from basophils that is reduced following the elimination of the inciting foods *(Sampson,1989)*. Moreover, a positive food challenge is followed by a rise in plasma histamine level *(Sampson,1984)*.

Milk, egg and peanut are three of the biggest offenders *(Sampson,1985)*, but many other foods have also been implicated *(Steinman,1994)*.

A suggested protocol is to remove egg, fish, milk, nuts, wheat, tomatoes, oranges, pineapple, peaches, bananas, chocolate, potato chips and foods containing preservatives and additives such as soft drinks for 2 to 4 weeks. If improvement occurs, reintroduce the foods singly to discover which, if any, produces a skin reaction *(Steinman,1995)*.

A 53-year-old male presented with cortisone-dependent eczema on the trunk and the thighs.

He was placed on a lactose-free diet. The eczema completely disappeared and he was successfully able to discontinue corticosteroid treatment (Grimbacher).

Hydrochloric Acid Deficiency

Studies conducted many years ago found reduced baseline levels of hydrochloric acid to be common in this patient population, and the severity of the eczema correlated with the extent of the reduction as well as the presence of gastrointestinal symptoms *(Allison;Ayers)*. In an open trial, supplementation of hydrochloric acid and vitamin B complex was reported to be an effective treatment for those patients with reduced baseline hydrochloric acid *(Allison)*.

However, it is not known whether such patients are able to secrete normal amounts of hydrochloric acid following administration of a potent parietal-cell stimulant, and this latter measure is now accepted as the one which is clinically relevant *(Rappaport)*. Moreover, controlled trials of supplementation with hydrochloric acid have not been done.

A 52 year-old patient with a 46-year history of eczema as well as a history of gas in the stomach and bowels for at least one year presented with a red, lichenified face and a less severe eruption on the hand and thigh. The patient was found to be achlorhydric following a standard (Ewalt) test meal, and was treated with dilute hydrochloric acid with dramatic improvement. For nearly one year of follow-up, the patient's skin condition has been practically normal (Ayers).

Lactobacillus acidophilus

Compared to normals, patients may often be found to have a low number of lactobacilli on stool analysis along with reduced counts of bifidobacteria and enterococci and increased counts of pathogenic strains of bacteria.. When such findings are present, administration of *Lactobacillus acidophilus* may be helpful in alleviating pruritus as well as in reducing gastrointestinal symptoms such as obstipation, flatulence or abdominal discomfort *(Ionescu,1988,1990)*.

COMBINED INTERVENTIONS

A 13 year-old pre-menarchal girl presented with red, rough, cracked and peeling skin in her hands, with additional patches in her forearms, by her elbows and behind her knees. In addition, her fingernails had over 40 white spots. A trial of corticosteroid cream had been unsuccessful.

She had been breast-fed until age 6 months. Within one to two months afterwards, she broke out in the same locations and developed a bad diaper rash. Switching to goat's milk was unsuccessful, although she improved slightly on soy milk. Some eczema remained until age 6. Afterwards the rash was intermittent.

She was taken off of dairy products and placed on chelated zinc 50 mg 3 times daily, vitamin C 1000 mg twice daily, cod liver oil [a source of omega-3 fatty acids] 1 tbsp daily, vegetable oil [a source of omega-6 fatty acids] 1 tbsp daily and pancreatic enzymes [to improve intestinal absorption of nutrients] 2 with meals.

On follow-up 11 weeks later, her hands were nearly clear with only a few deeper fissures remaining and the other involved areas were substantially smaller. A few weeks later, her skin was almost completely clear. Zinc was then reduced to 25 mg daily. At the 2-year follow-up, her skin was still almost completely clear.

The author notes that, out of 40 cases, zinc supplementation was followed by full remission in all except one case which showed a partial response. Improvement may take up to 6 weeks and full remission from 3 to 8 months (Wright).

BIBLIOGRAPHY

Allison JR. The relation of deficiency hydrochloric acid and vitamin B complex in certain skin diseases. South Med J 38:235-41, 1945
Ayers S. Gastric secretion in psoriasis, eczema and dermatitis herpetiformis. Arch Dermatol Syph 20:854-57, 1929
Barthel HR, Stuhlmuller B. Improvement in atopic dermatitis with change in low-salt table water. Letter. Lancet 344:1089, 1994
Bjorneboe A et al. Effect of dietary supplementation with eicosapentaenoic acid in the treatment of atopic dermatitis. Br J Dermatol 117(4):463-69, 1987
Borrek S et al. [Gamma-linolenic-acid-rich borage seed oil capsules in children with atopic dermatitis. A placebo-controlled double-blind study]. Klin Padiatr 209(3):100-4, 1997
Caffarelli C et al. Elimination diet and intestinal permeability in atopic eczema: a preliminary study. Clin Exp Allergy 23:28-31, 1993
Combs GF. Assessment of vitamin E status in animals and man. Proc Nutr Soc 40:187-94, 1981
David TJ et al. Low serum zinc in children with atopic eczema. Br J Dermatol 111(5):597-601, 1984
David TJ et al. Serum levels of trace metals in children with atopic eczema. Br J Dermatol 122(4):485-9, 1990
Davies S, Stewart A. Nutritional Medicine. London, Pan Books, 1987
Di Toro R et al. Zinc and copper status of allergic children. Acta Paediatr Scand 76(4):612-17, 1987
Endre L et al. [Incidence of food allergy and zinc deficiency in children treated for atopic dermatitis.] Orv Hetil 130(46):2465-9, 1989
Ewing CI et al. Failure of oral zinc supplementation in atopic eczema. Eur J Clin Nutr 45(10):507-10, 1991
Fairris GM et al. The effect on atopic dermatitis of supplementation with selenium and vitamin E. Acta Derm Venereol (Stockh) 69(4):359-62, 1989
Finkelstein H. Lehrbuch der Säuglingkrankheiten: Fischer's medicin. Berlin, Buchhandlung h Kornfeld, 1912) (in German)
Galland L. Increased requirements for essential fatty acids in atopic individuals: A review with clinical descriptions. J Am Coll Nutr 5(2):213-28, 1986
Ganther HE et al. Selenium and glutathione peroxidase in health and disease - a review, in AS Prasad, D Overleas, Eds. Trace Elements in Human Health and Disease, Volume II. New York, Academic Press, 1976:165
Grimbacher B et al. Lactose-intolerance may induce severe chronic eczema. Int Arch Allergy Immunol 113:516-18, 1997
Hederos CA, Berg A. Epogam evening primrose oil treatment in atopic dermatitis and asthma. Arch Dis Child 75:494-7, 1996
Ionescu G, Spezialklinik Neukirchen - reported in Dermatology News International 21(3), March, 1988
Ionescu G et al. Immunobiological significance of fungal and bacterial infections in atopic eczema. J Advance Med 3:47-58, 1990
Juhlin L et al. Blood glutathione-peroxidase levels in skin diseases: Effect of selenium and vitamin E treatment. Acta Derm Venereol (Stockh) 62:211-14, 1982
Kline G. Presentation to the Annual Meeting, American Academy of Allergy and Immunology, 1989
Kunz B et al. Eicosapentaenoic acid (EPA) treatment in atopic eczema (AE): a prospective double-blind trial. Abstract. J Allergy Clin Immunol 83:196, 1989
Liebke C et al. Sweat electrolyte concentrations in children with atopic dermatitis. Letter. Lancet 350:1678-9, 1997
Manku MS et al. Reduced levels of prostaglandin precursors in the blood of atopic patients. Defective delta-6-desaturase function as a biochemical basis for atopy. Prostaglandins Leukotrienes Med 9(6):615-28, 1982
Morse PF et al. Meta-analysis of placebo-controlled studies of the efficacy of Epogram in the treatment of atopic eczema: relationship between plasma essential fatty changes and treatment response. Br J Dermatol 121:75-90, 1989
Rappaport EM. Achlorhydria: Associated symptoms and response to hydrochloric acid. New Engl J Med 252(19):802-5, 1955
Sampson HA, Jolie PL. Increased plasma histamine concentrations after food challenges in children with atopic dermatitis. N Engl J Med 311:371-6, 1984
Sampson HA, McCaskill CC. Food hypersensitivity and atopic dermatitis: evaluation of 113 patients. J Pediatr 107:669-75, 1985
Sampson HA. Food hypersensitivity as a pathogenic factor in atopic dermatitis. N Engl Reg Allergy Proc 7(6):511-19, 1986
Sampson HA et al. Spontaneous release of histamine from basophils and histamine-releasing factor in patients with atopic dermatitis and food hypersensitivity. N Engl J Med 321(4):228-32, 1989
Scott KC, Turnlund JR. A compartmental model of zinc metabolism in adult men used to study effects of three levels of dietary copper. Am J Physiol 267(1 Pt 1):E165-73, 1994
Steinman HA, Potter PC. The precipitation of symptoms by common foods in children with atopic dermatitis. Allergy Proc 15(4):203-10, 1994
Steinman HA - interviewed in Clinical Pearls News, 5(6), June, 1995
Strosser AV, Nelson LS. Synthetic vitamin A in the treatment of eczema in children. Ann Allergy 10:703-4, 1952
Whitaker DK et al. Evening primrose oil (Epogam) in the treatment of chronic hand dermatitis: Disappointing therapeutic results. Dermatology 193:115-20, 1996
Wright JV. Dr. Wright's Book of Nutritional Therapy. Emmaus, Penn., Rodale Press, 1979

EPILEPSY

NUTRITIONAL TREATMENT GUIDE

✓ = Efficacy generally accepted.
* = Efficacy *demonstrated* by controlled human trials.
[+] = Efficacy *suspected* from uncontrolled human trials.
[-] = Efficacy *suspected* from indirect data.
? = Efficacy *challenged* in a study of similar design.

DIETARY FACTORS

✓ **Ketogenic diet** (A low carbohydrate, high fat diet reserved for intractable seizures in children.)

- -

[+] avoid **Alcohol**

- -

[-] avoid **Caffeine**
[-] avoid consumption of **Soft Drinks** (if serum calcium levels are low)

NUTRITIONAL FACTORS

I. TO REDUCE SEIZURES

✓ **Vitamin B_6**: *for vitamin B_6-dependent infantile seizures and seizures secondary to infectious diseases:* pyridoxine 5 to 50 mg/kg in divided doses

- -

* ? **Folic acid:** *to augment anticonvulsants:* ? 5 mg daily (1 year trial)
* ? **Vitamin E:** *to augment anticonvulsants:* D-alpha tocopherol acetate 400 IU/d

- -

[+] **Biotin deficiency:** *to treat biotinidase deficiency:* 5 to 10 mg daily
[+] **Choline:** *for complex partial seizures:* Start with 4 g/d. Increase to 12-16 g/d by the 3rd month.
[+] **Copper deficiency:** 2 mg twice daily for up to 6 weeks *AND* **Zinc** 50 mg daily
[+] **Dimethylglycine:** 90 mg twice daily
[+] **Magnesium:** *for grand mal or petit mal seizures (not status epilepticus):* 450 mg or more daily
[+] **Magnesium deficiency:** ≈ 400 mg daily
[+] **Manganese deficiency:** 3 to 5 mg daily
[+] **Niacin:** *to augment anticonvulsants:* niacinamide 1 g 3 times daily
[+] avoid **Omega-6 Fatty Acid** supplements in temporal lobe epilepsy
[+] **Phosphatidylserine** *AND*
Gamma-aminobutyric Acid (GABA): *for absence seizures*
[+] **Selenium deficiency:** *for childhood seizures:* repletion
[+] **Thiamine deficiency:** 50 mg daily
[+] **L-Tryptophan:** ? 750 mg daily (3 week trial)
[+] **Vitamin B_6 deficiency**: 50 to 100 mg daily
[+] **Vitamin B_{12} deficiency:** 1,000 μg intramuscularly weekly initially and monthly afterwards
[+] **Zinc deficiency**: zinc sulfate 220 mg twice daily *AND* **Copper** 2 mg daily

[-] **Iron deficiency:** 30 mg twice daily until repletion; then minimal possible dosage
[-] **Vitamin C deficiency:** 500 mg twice daily

II. TO PREVENT GINGIVAL HYPERPLASIA FROM PHENYTOIN

* **Folic Acid (topical):** Add 5 mg folic acid to 5 ml water. Use as a mouthwash for 2 min. twice daily.
* ? **Folic Acid (oral):** 5 mg daily (1 year trial)

- -

[-] **Biotin deficiency:** add vitamin B complex, preferably to the diet
[-] **Vitamin C deficiency:** 500 mg twice daily

III. TO PREVENT BONE LOSS FROM ANTICONVULSANT DRUGS

[+] **Calcium deficiency:** ≈ 1 g daily
[+] **Vitamin D deficiency:** 400 to 4000 IU daily (usually 2400 IU daily)

IV. TO IMPROVE NEUROPSYCHOLOGICAL FUNCTION IN PHENYTOIN-TREATED PATIENTS

* **Thiamine** 50 mg daily

V. TO PREVENT HYPERAMMONEMIA IN VALPROATE-TREATED PATIENTS

[+] **L-Carnitine deficiency:** 1 to 6 g daily

OTHER RELATED FACTORS

* rule out **Food Sensitivities**
* ? avoid **Aspartame**

- -

[+] rule out **Reactive Hypoglycemia**

DIETARY FACTORS

In general, patients should have normal, well-balanced meals eaten at regular intervals. Excessive water consumption, or eating an unusually large meal, may provoke a seizure *(Passmore).*

The Ketogenic Diet

The ketogenic diet, which has been used since the early 1920s, is a low carbohydrate, high fat diet which may reduce seizures by 50 to 70% in children who fail to respond to anticonvulsants *(Freeman).* About one-third of these children become seizure-free *(Tallian).* It is particularly helpful in treating intractable absence-type seizures *(De Vivo).*

However, since the diet is unhealthy for growing children *(Passmore)*, and since about one-third of children are unable to tolerate it due to side effects such as diarrhea and dehydration *(Freeman),* its use should be restricted to children whose seizures cannot be adequately controlled by medications. The diet, which is initiated by a 24 to 36 hour fast, should be introduced during a hospitalization by personnel trained in its preparation.

Alcohol

Regular alcohol consumption can cause occasional seizures in otherwise normal people, usually only once or twice yearly. The degree of risk is directly related to the amount of alcohol consumption and returns to normal once the person abstains from drinking *(Baulac).*

Alcohol withdrawal can also trigger seizures. These seizures are often multiple and occur 10 to 48 hours after discontinuing or reducing alcohol intake. Alcohol-provoked seizures are usually tonic-clonic seizures with a normal EEG and CT-scan *(Baulac)*.

Seizures appear to occur in alcoholics because of a long-term kindling effect of recurrent detoxifications and a shorter-term effect of ethanol exposure *(Lechtenberg)*, although patients who have partial seizures usually have a history of brain damage, head trauma or stroke *(Baulac)*. Alcohol abuse is also a common cause of status epilepticus; in fact, status epilepticus may be the first presentation of alcohol-related seizures *(Alldredge)*.

Caffeine

Caffeine, a methylxanthine, is a known stimulant and proconvulsant *(Marangos)*; thus epileptics consuming caffeine-containing beverages may be more prone to seizures. In a study of patients who underwent neurosurgery for medically intractable complex seizures, 23% consumed 400 mg or more of caffeine (3 or more cups of coffee) daily, a dosage that is clearly above the intoxication threshold *(Krahn)*.

Soft Drinks

Heavy consumption of phosphoric acid-containing soft drinks appears to be a risk factor for seizures due to hypocalcemia. In a group of children with hypocalcemia (<8.8 mg/dl), two-thirds were found to drink more than 1.5 liters per week of soft drinks compared to only 28% of normocalcemic children. In other terms, the children with the high intake of soft drinks had more than 5 times the risk of hypocalcemia.

Moreover, 7% of the hypocalcemic children had at least one seizure in the previous 3 months compared to only 0.6% of normal children. Once the soft drinks were stopped for 30 days, serum calcium levels rose into the normal range *(Mazariegos-Ramos)*.

NUTRITIONAL FACTORS

VITAMINS

Folic Acid

Folate metabolism appears to be intimately involved in the epileptogenic process. Experimentally induced seizures deplete brain folate *(Smith)*. Certain anticonvulsants (such as phenytoin, primidone and phenobarbital) reduce both blood and cerebrospinal folate levels *(Smith)*, while folate supplementation may lower serum barbiturate and anticonvulsant levels *(Mattson)*.

Reduced folate nutriture in these patients may result in psychological disturbances *(Bäckman)*. Organic psychological syndromes are more likely in patients on 3 or more drugs and in those who have megaloblastosis *(del Ser)*. However, even in the presence of subnormal serum and erythrocyte folate levels, there does not appear to be an increase in clinically-significant peripheral neuropathy *(Nimmo)*.

Supplementation

The results of studies investigating the effect of folate supplementation upon seizures have been mixed. Several uncontrolled studies have suggested that it could even have an epileptogenic effect, although controlled studies have failed to confirm this finding *(Smith)*. Of 2 placebo-controlled studies, one found a significant improvement in seizure frequency after one year *(Givverd)*, while the other found folate to be ineffective after 6 months *(Botez)*. Since these studies have generally been done on patients receiving anticonvulsants, it is unclear what influence the anticonvulsants had upon their results.

Folate supplements have also been used to prevent gingival hyperplasia, a common side-effect from phenytoin administration. In a placebo-controlled study, gingival hyperplasia was inhibited by the regular use of a folic acid mouthwash *(Drew)*. In other placebo-controlled studies, the efficacy of oral folic acid supplementation is less clear *(Brown)*, although it may be effective for the sub-group of patients with reduced folate levels and high phenytoin levels *(Bäckman)*.

Niacin

The results of animal studies suggest that supplementary niacin in the form of niacinamide has a weak anticonvulsant effect *(Krzhanovskii)*. While it does not appear to be powerful enough to be used alone, it may potentiate the effect of anticonvulsants without potentiating their toxicity, and could thus reduce the unpleasant and sometimes intolerable side effects frequently associated with anticonvulsant therapy *(Bourgeois, 1983)*. It appears to do so by inhibiting the metabolism of anticonvulsant drugs, probably by inhibiting the cytochrome P-450 system *(Bourgeois, 1982)*.

Several patients were unable to achieve good control with anticonvulsants as the required dosages made them so drowsy and sluggish that they were unable to function normally. They were supplemented with vitamin B_3 1 gram 3 times daily. After they were on the supplement for several months, the anticonvulsant dose could be slowly reduced while monitoring them carefully for an increase in seizure frequency (Hoffer).

Thiamine Deficiency

Blood levels may be low in epileptics, possibly due to the ingestion of anticonvulsants *(Krause,1988)*. Moreover, thiamine deficiency may provoke seizures in predisposed patients *(Keyser)*.

In a double-blind crossover study, patients who had been on phenytoin alone or in combination with phenobarbital for several years (31% of whom had subnormal blood thiamine levels), received 50 mg thiamine daily. After 6 months, thiamine improved neuropsychological functions in both verbal and non-verbal IQ testing *(Botez)*.

Vitamin B_6

Deficiency

Experimentally-induced deficiency of vitamin B_6 is known to cause seizures in humans and experimental animals *(Coursin,1969)*. When infants were inadvertently placed on a formula that was deficient in the vitamin, many of them developed epileptic seizures that disappeared when they were given a vitamin B_6 supplement *(Coursin,1954)*.

Similarly, when healthy young women were fed a vitamin B_6-deficient diet, 2 of them exhibited abnormal EEG tracings within 12 days which rapidly reverted to normal following repletion of the vitamin *(Kretsch)*. Furthermore, adult epileptics on anticonvulsants may have reduced blood vitamin B_6 levels *(Krause,1986, 1988)*, suggesting that repletion could be beneficial *(Nakagawa)*.

For a female epileptic, red cell glutamic oxaloacetic transaminase (EGOT), a measure of vitamin B_6 nutriture, was found to be 34 units (deficient). She was supplemented with 200 mg pyridoxine daily which was raised to 300 mg daily after one month. EGOT rose to 68 units (normal) and seizure activity decreased from an average of 2.1 seizures per month to 0.5 seizures per month.

After 7 months, she stopped pyridoxine. Two months later, she was averaging 6 seizures per month (Sholer).

Pharmacotherapy

High-dose pyridoxine may benefit patients with recurrent seizures due to acute infectious diseases. In a recent study, 40 infants and children with recurrent convulsions primarily due to acute infections were randomly treated with high-dose pyridoxine by intravenous infusion, while 50 others served as controls. Antiepileptic drugs and other therapies were similar in the 2 groups except for pyridoxine. Clinical efficacy criteria were based on the frequency of convulsions per day and on the duration of individual seizures after therapy was initiated. Total response rates in the pyridoxine and control groups were 92.5% and 64%, respectively, a highly significant difference. After initiation of therapy, seizures resolved after 2.4 ± 1.4 days in the pyridoxine group and after 3.7 ± 2.0 days in the control group, again a highly significant difference. No adverse effects of pyridoxine were apparent during the observation period *(Jiao)*.

Dependency

Pyridoxine-dependent epilepsy is a rare autosomal recessive disorder which should be considered in any infant with recurrent seizures. Pyridoxine binds to glutamate decarboxylase which converts glutamic acid to the inhibitory neurotransmitter gamma-amino butyric acid (GABA). Defective binding of pyridoxine may reduce GABA levels, causing a lowering of the seizure threshold. This binding defect can be compensated for by large doses of pyridoxine *(Baumeister,1996;Crowell).*

A 3-month-old male infant with pyridoxine-dependent seizures responded to pyridoxine 5 mg/kg daily but still had elevated levels of glutamate (which can be neurotoxic). However, at a daily dosage of 10 mg/kg, glutamate levels normalized, suggesting that optimal treatment may be the dosage that reduces glutamate levels to normal (Baumeister,1994).

Vitamin B_{12} Deficiency

Even in the absence of hematological abnormalities, seizures may occur in vitamin B_{12} deficiency states, although subtle laboratory abnormalities may be noted. Depression, dementia, myelopathy and neuropathy may be other findings *(Karnaze).*

Among epileptics on anticonvulsant medications, there is a tendency for a reduction in serum vitamin B_{12} levels. In one study, although the mean serum levels were in the normal range, they were lower in patients with an earlier age of disease onset, frequent seizures and higher drug dosages *(Rosciszewska).*

Vitamin C Deficiency

Plasma levels of vitamin C may be reduced *(Singh).* In one study of 500 patients, although the blood vitamin C concentration of group as a whole was normal, the dosage and length of time that a patient received anticonvulsant therapy seemed to have a negative influence on blood levels.

Moreover, lower vitamin C levels were associated with poorer results in tests of central and peripheral nervous system function including cerebellar disturbances. The incidence of gingival hyperplasia was also possibly linked to vitamin C adequacy, and both males and females with lower vitamin C levels showed a tendency towards macrocytic anemia *(Krause,1988).*

Vitamin D Deficiency

As a result of anticonvulsant treatment, serum levels of both 25-hydroxyvitamin D and 1,25-dihydroxyvitamin D may be depressed, at least in females *(Valimaki).* Marked elevation of serum alkaline phosphatase, particular when in concert with hypercalcemia, would suggest anticonvulsant-induced bone disease. This should be followed up with bone density scans *(Alderman).*

In a prospective study, 78% of a group of epileptic patients taking carbamazepine, phenytoin and/or phenobarbitol required 2,400 IU daily of vitamin D3 to maintain normal serum 25-hydroxyvitamin D levels. The range of dosages required varied widely however, from 400 IU to 4,000 IU daily *(Collins).*

Vitamin E

Epileptics on anticonvulsant therapy may have reduced plasma alpha tocopherol levels *(Ogunmekan,1985; Krause,1988).* This finding may be due, at least in part, to the use of anticonvulsants *(Ogunmekan,1985)*, and the results of one study suggests that it may be limited to males *(Krause,1988).*

Under double-blind conditions, vitamin E supplementation has been shown to reduce seizures. In a small study, epileptics on anticonvulsants with markedly reduced serum vitamin E levels compared to age-matched controls randomly received either alpha-tocopherol or placebo. After 9 months, 2 of the 3 adults receiving vitamin E showed between an 11% and a greater than 50% reduction in seizures, while 2 out of 6 children improved *(Sullivan).*

Another study concerned 24 epileptic children who were refractory to anticonvulsants. They randomly received D-alpha-tocopherol acetate or placebo in addition to their anticonvulsants. After 3 months 83% of the 12 treated children had a greater than 60% reduction in seizures (and half of these children had a 90 to 100% reduction) compared to none of the controls. When the controls were switched to vitamin E, seizure frequency was reduced 70 to 100% in all of them *(Ogunmekan,1989).*

By contrast, a more sophisticated double-blind crossover study of 43 anticonvulsant-refractory patients found no significant change in seizure frequency following 3 months of vitamin E treatment *(Raju)*.

Lipid peroxidation could foster the development of epileptic seizures. If so, the antioxidant effect of vitamin E may theoretically combat seizures by reducing lipid peroxidation. When animals were exposed to either hyperbaric oxygen or hyperoxia, they developed epileptiform activity along with a decrease in the brain level of alpha-tocopherol and the accumulation of lipid peroxidation products. Pretreatment with vitamin E (or other antioxidants) both decreased the frequency of the seizures and prevented lipid peroxidation *(Kagan; Jerrett)*.

Similarly, a group of anticonvulsant-resistant epileptics showed a 2- to 10-fold increase in plasma levels of lipid peroxidation products. One month after receiving alpha-tocopherol supplementation, the plasma levels of these products had decreased *(Kovalenko)*.

MINERALS

Calcium Deficiency

Serum calcium levels are rarely of value in the work-up of an adult seizure patient. While seizures may be the presenting symptom of hypocalcemia, they occur primarily in neonates and rarely in patients with hypoparathyroidism, in whom other clinical signs (such as tetany) are usually present *(Bohr)*. Moreover, during idiopathic generalized tonic-clonic seizures, serum and cerebrospinal fluid calcium levels may be elevated and remain so for at least 24 hours *(Sood)*.

Anticonvulsants interfere with calcium metabolism in a poorly understood manner, causing depressed blood calcium levels. Occasionally, rickets or osteomalacia may develop *(Flodin)*.

Copper Deficiency

Seizures can be caused by copper deficiency *(Sorenson, 1979)*. However, serum copper and ceruloplasmin concentrations are often elevated. These findings appear to be at least partly due to the effects of anticonvulsants, perhaps through hepatic enzyme induction *(Motta)*.

A 21-month-old boy was admitted to the hospital because of repeated seizures and failure to thrive. He had blonde, curly hair, spurring of the femora and tibiae, and mild anemia. The mother and maternal uncle had copper deficiency with mild symptoms.

Oral copper supplementation was followed by general improvement, but as soon as it was reduced or stopped, hypocupremia and seizures resumed (Mëhes).

Iron Deficiency

Iron deficiency does not appear to be related to most types of seizures. However, a case-control study of children with febrile convulsions suggests that it may be common in this population. In a group of 156 children, 30% of the patients were iron-deficient (based on low serum, low hemoglobin and low erythrocyte MCV) compared to 14% of hospitalized control children and 12% of normal controls *(Pisacane)*.

Whether repletion reduces the risk of future seizures is not known.

Magnesium

Magnesium depletion is known to cause marked irritability of the nervous system which eventually results in epileptic seizures *(Nuytten)*. While an uncommon cause of epilepsy, hypomagnesemia may be cause grand mal or multifocal seizures *(Hall)*.

Among a group of patients with idiopathic generalized tonic-clonic seizures, cerebrospinal fluid magnesium levels were low. Moreover, they were lower within 24 hours of a seizure than 4 weeks afterwards, and low levels correlated with increased frequency, poor control and longer duration of seizures. Status epilepticus and EEG abnormalities were also related to low cerebrospinal fluid magnesium levels *(Sood)*. By contrast, a group of epileptic children had significantly *higher* cerebrospinal fluid magnesium levels than controls *(Benga)*. The reason for these contrasting findings is unknown.

Among epileptics, serum and erythrocyte magnesium levels are reduced *(Sood)*, and there is evidence of a negative correlation between the serum magnesium level and the severity of the epilepsy *(Benga;Gupta)*, with the lowest levels seen in status epilepticus *(Gupta)*. Serum magnesium levels appear to be unrelated to serum concentrations of anticonvulsants *(Shoji)*.

Hair magnesium levels may be elevated *(Shrestha)* while, at least in patients with idiopathic generalized tonic-clonic seizures, 24-hour urinary magnesium levels appear to be normal *(Sood)*.

Supplementation

Supplementation to correct magnesium deficiency is clearly indicated *(Galland)*. Less certain is the efficacy of magnesium supplementation when serum and erythrocyte magnesium levels are within the normal range. However, magnesium supplementation in an animal model of epilepsy directly suppressed neuronal burst firing and interictal EEG spike generation at serum levels below those producing paralysis *(Gorges)*.

Moreover, 29 out of 30 epileptic children with grand mal or petit mal seizures who received magnesium and stopped their anticonvulsants showed marked improvement. One of the patients was a 13-year-old boy with a 10-year history of drug-resistant epilepsy who was severely depressed and showed signs of mental retardation. His seizures stopped and he became mentally alert after starting magnesium *(Barnet)*. In another study, however, high-dose intravenous magnesium sulfate was unable to control myoclonic status epilepticus *(Fisher)*.

Further studies are badly needed to clarify the therapeutic role of magnesium supplementation.

A 16-year-old girl with acute intermittent porphyria presented with abdominal pain, generalized tonic-clonic and simple partial seizures, and inappropriate antidiuretic hormone secretion. Because most antiepileptic drugs are contraindicated in porphyria, she was treated with intravenous magnesium sulfate. Soon after starting treatment, seizures stopped. Her seizures were restarted and stopped again with discontinuation and reinstitution of magnesium sulfate (Sadeh).

Manganese Deficiency

Blood and hair manganese levels, and often tissue manganese levels, are reduced in epileptics *(Papavasiliou)*. Since whole blood manganese levels correlate poorly with the amount of anticonvulsant medication *(Carl)*, it is likely that the reduction is related to the presence of the seizure disorder.

When manganese-deficient animals were given manganese, their seizure threshold was raised *(Hurley)*. Similarly, the results of human trials suggest that manganese supplementation may be beneficial *(Pfeiffer;Tanaka)*, but controlled studies are lacking.

Whether supplementation is only beneficial when manganese is deficient is not yet known. Until further studies are completed, it is probably best to restrict manganese supplementation to the repletion of a manganese deficiency.

A middle-aged woman developed increasing shoulder pain. X-rays suggested that the pain was due to osteoarthritis and she was placed on a nonsteroidal anti-inflammatory drug. The pain gradually worsened until it became severe, and she developed frequent unexplained grand mal seizures.

Hair mineral analysis revealed a markedly low manganese level. Oral manganese supplementation was started and the seizures rapidly disappeared. Repeat radiographic studies later showed evidence of a Pancoast tumor as the actual cause of her pain.

Selenium Deficiency

Several case reports have appeared describing the successful treatment of early childhood seizures with selenium supplementation. The children were found to be deficient in selenium as well as in glutathione peroxidase activity, suggesting that brain selenium depletion may trigger seizures and subsequent neural damage due to its important role in the defense of neuronal cells against oxygen radical formation and peroxidative processes *(Calomme;Ramaekers;Weber)*.

Zinc Deficiency

Zinc deficiency is known to cause seizures *(Prasad)*. Serum and cerebrospinal fluid levels of zinc appear to be reduced in *febrile convulsions (Gunduz)*, while studies in *epileptic* patients have found lower *(Shoji)* normal *(Altunbasak)*, and higher *(Davidson)* concentrations.

Among anticonvulsant-treated epileptics, serum zinc levels appear to be lower than those of both untreated epileptics and normal controls *(Sozuer)*, even though they do not appear to correlate with the anticonvulsants' serum levels *(Kuzuya)*. Anticonvulsants can cause zinc deficiency either by reducing zinc absorption in the gut through chelation or by causing diarrhea *(Lewis-Jones)*.

Supplementation

In chronic alcoholics, seizures can be caused by dietary zinc deficiency; these may respond to zinc supplementation *(Sullivan)*. Little has been done to ascertain the efficacy of zinc supplementation in treating seizures in other situations, including when there is evidence of deficiency.

We do know that zinc ions limit the excitatory responses in the dentate granule cells of patients with medial temporal lobe epilepsy, probably by blocking the N-methyl-D-aspartate (NMDA) receptors *(Williamson)*. Furthermore, zinc supplementation protects against the development of seizures in at least 3 different animal models of epilepsy, suggesting that zinc may be an essential component of a natural, anticonvulsant tissue response to abnormal excitation *(Sterman)*.

OTHER NUTRITIONAL FACTORS

Biotin Deficiency

While uncommon, biotin deficiency is frequently associated with epileptic seizures, and the results of an animal study suggest that it facilitates convulsive disorders *(Bregola)*. The deficiency can be caused by the excessive ingestion of avidin from eggs, although this occurs quite rarely. Also, biotinidase deficiency is an autosomal recessive inherited disorder causing biotin deficiency characterized by neurologic abnormalities including seizures *(Salbert)*.

Treatment with anticonvulsants appears to increase biotin catabolism. Over time, this can lead to reduced biotin status *(Mock)*. Among anticonvulsant-treated epileptics, lower plasma biotin levels are associated with cerebellar symptoms, a well-known side effect of the drugs *(Krause,1982)*. There also appears to be a correlation between reduced biotin status and gingival hyperplasia *(Krause, 1988)*.

Supplementation

Whether biotin repletion is indicated for epileptics receiving long-term anticonvulsant treatment is uncertain, especially as reduced biotin status could be related to the clinical actions of the medications *(Krause,1986)*. By contrast, biotin repletion is strongly indicated for infants and children with biotinidase deficiency. It should be included in the differential diagnosis of an infant or child with unexplained seizures, and a trial of biotin should be considered for infants less than 1 year of age with poorly controlled seizures *(Salbert)*.

Carnitine Deficiency

Numerous studies have found that patients taking valproate have lower plasma carnitine levels than controls *(Coulter)*. Although serum carnitine levels do not correlate with valproic acid levels, they do correlate with the duration of valproate treatment *(Chung)*. Carnitine deficiency in epilepsy may also be caused by underlying metabolic diseases or nutritional inadequacy *(Coulter)*.

The relationship between carnitine deficiency and valproate-induced hepatotoxicity is unclear. Carnitine supplementation can alleviate valproate-induced hyperammonemia, but it does not always prevent the emergence of serious hepatotoxicity. It is indicated in high-risk, symptomatic patients and those with free carnitine deficiency *(Coulter)*.

Choline

A member of the vitamin B complex, choline serves as a precursor to acetylcholine. In a preliminary study, 4 patients with intractable complex partial seizures were supplemented with oral choline. Three of the patients considered themselves much improved; they had shorter seizure durations and less post-seizure fatigue, although there was a slight increase in seizure frequency. The fourth patient failed to improve. When plasma choline in the other 3 patients increased 75 to 300%, plasma choline only increased 21% in this patient, suggesting that a greater increase in plasma choline than was achieved by the treatment regimen could still prove effective *(McNamara)*.

The fact that patients with seizures which were intractable to standard medications improved with choline is impressive; however, controlled studies are needed for confirmation. Whether other types of seizures respond to choline supplementation is unknown.

Also, in an animal model of epilepsy, there is evidence that the cholinergic system may play a role in generating or maintaining complex partial seizures. Theoretically, if this is so, then *anticholinergic*, rather than cholinergic, agents would be indicated in seizure management *(Olney)*.

Dimethylglycine

A precursor of glycine, a neuroinhibitory amino acid. In an animal model, dimethylglycine produced a dose-dependent decrease in seizure incidence and an increase in the latency to the first seizure *(Freed)*. Although a placebo-controlled study of 19 patients failed to find evidence of its efficacy *(Gascon)*, a case report suggests that it may occasionally reduce seizure frequency in anticonvulsant-resistant patients:

A 22 year-old man with long-standing mental retardation and mixed complex, partial and grand mal seizures had been having 16 to 18 generalized seizures per week despite phenobarbitol and carbamazepine for the previous 6 months.

Within one week of starting dimethylglycine 90 mg twice daily, his seizure frequency dropped to 3 per week. Two attempts to withdraw the supplement caused dramatic increases in seizure frequency (Roach).

Omega-6 Fatty Acids: A Warning

There is evidence that supplementation with omega-6 fatty acids may exacerbate temporal lobe epilepsy *(Holman)*. In fact, this adverse effect has been put to use as a means of differentiating between temporal lobe epilepsy and schizophrenia, as worsening of "schizophrenia" following administration of evening primrose oil suggests that temporal lobe epilepsy may be the true diagnosis *(Vaddadi)*.

Phosphatidylserine

In an animal model of generalized seizures, phosphatidylserine exerted substantial anti-seizure activity *(Pasqui)*. An open trial explored combining phosphatidylserine with GABA, a neuroinhibitory amino acid, for treating 42 patients with drug-resistant epilepsy. While patients with simple or complex partial seizures failed to benefit, there was a remarkable decrease in absence seizures which was linearly related to drug dosages. Nine of the patients had side effects; however, these were usually mild *(Loeb)*.

These exciting preliminary findings have yet to be followed up with more sophisticated studies.

Taurine

Low brain concentrations of this neuroinhibitory amino acid have been found at the site of maximal seizure activity *(Sturman)*. In epileptics, urinary taurine excretion is decreased *(Hartley)* as are platelet taurine levels *(Goodman)*. Furthermore, plasma taurine may be reduced in children with seizure disorders *(Ko)*.

Taurine supplementation has been shown to be effective in animal models of epilepsy *(Mantovani)*. However, perhaps due to its limited diffusibility across the blood-brain barrier, the results of clinical trials have not been very encouraging, since the positive responses seen in short-term trials are not found in trials with longer follow-up periods *(Durelli)*.

Tryptophan

There is some evidence that both cerebrospinal fluid and plasma tryptophan levels are reduced in patients with seizure disorders *(Ko;Marion)*. Moreover, epileptics, and especially those with frequent seizures and with longstanding epilepsy, may have reduced blood serotonin levels *(Avanesova)*. Whether these findings are related to the effects of anticonvulsive medication is not known.

An open trial of tryptophan supplementation found "suggestive changes in the clinical picture" of epileptics in as little as one week. These changes paralleled an increase in their blood serotonin levels *(Avanesova)*. Also, 3 children with drug-resistant Lennox-Gastaut epilepsy showed a positive, but transient, improvement following supplementation *(Prusinski)*.

Better studies are obviously needed to ascertain the efficacy of tryptophan in treating seizure disorders.

OTHER RELATED FACTORS

Food Sensitivities

Reactions to foods have been shown under double-blind conditions to initiate seizures. In one study, 45 epileptic children who also suffered from recurrent headaches, abdominal symptoms or hyperkinetic behavior were placed on a food exclusion diet. When foods were reintroduced singly, some of them appeared to produce the presenting symptoms.

Foods found to provoke seizures or other symptoms were removed, and 36 of the children (80%) recovered or improved. Sixteen of these 36 children were then tested in a double-blind manner. All but one had recurrence of symptoms when supposedly reactive foods were tested, while none had symptoms when the placebo was given.

The same testing was performed with another 18 epileptic children who did not have additional symptoms suggestive of food sensitivities. Food re-introductions failed to elicit reactions in them *(Egger)*.

A 19 year-old woman developed grand mal seizures 2 years earlier which were treated unsuccessfully with carbamazepine, primidone and dilantin. Her EEG revealed paroxysmal 3 to 5 per second slow-wave activity and occasional temporal spikes. She reported that several of the seizures followed food ingestion by 1 to 2 hours.

After a 4-day elimination diet, individual foods were tested and she showed strong reactions (tachycardia, cutaneous hypothermia and seizures) when given beef or substances derived from beef and several other foods. As chicken was one of the foods which failed to elicit a reaction, she was tested to beef and chicken (which were chopped up and placed in gelatin capsules) in a double-blind manner. Beef, but not chicken, precipitated seizures; however, there was no clear EEG evidence of seizure activity during the seizures (Crayton).

Aspartame

Anecdotal reports that the use of aspartame, an artificial sweetener, may provoke seizures have been followed by double-blind experiments to investigate their validity. In a study of 10 children with untreated generalized absence seizures, aspartame appeared to exacerbate the amount of EEG spike wave activity *(Camfield)*. Two subsequent crossover studies, however, failed to substantiate an adverse effect of the substance either in epileptic children *(Shaywitz)* or in 18 individuals who believed that aspartame provoked their seizures *(Rowan)*.

Reactive Hypoglycemia

Brain function is highly dependent upon adequate glucose levels, so a drop in brain glucose would be expected to cause neurological signs and symptoms. Moreover, various medical conditions causing a large enough decline in peripheral blood sugar levels produce a similar picture, most likely because blood glucose drops are reflecting a drop in brain glucose levels.

Whether otherwise normal people may develop seizures following the ingestion of carbohydrates due to a reactive drop in brain sugar levels (neuroglycopenia) as measured by blood glucose levels (hypoglycemia) is more controversial. In one study of 185 women and 115 men who had a drop of 20 mg% or more below their fasting blood glucose level during a 6-hour glucose tolerance test, 4% had convulsions. Eighty-five percent of these patients appeared to respond to a high protein, low carbohydrate, caffeine-free diet along with snacking every 2 hours *(Gyland)*.

Further studies are needed to validate these observations.

BIBLIOGRAPHY

Alderman CP, Hill CL. Abnormal bone mineral metabolism after long-term anticonvulsant treatment. Ann Pharmacother 28(1):47-8, 1994

Alldredge BK, Lowenstein DH. Status epilepticus related to alcohol abuse. Epilepsia 34(6):1033-7, 1993

Altunbasak S et al. Serum and hair zinc levels in epileptic children taking valproic acid. Biol Trace Elem Res 58(1-2):117-25, 1997

Avanesova TS, Sviridova EI. [Therapeutic activity of tryptophan and its effect on serotonin metabolism in epilepsy patients]. Zh Nevropatol Psikhiatr 80(6):857-63, 1980) (in Russian)

Bäckman N et al. Folate treatment of diphenylhydantoin-induced gingival hyperplasia. Scand J Dent Res 97(3):222-32, 1989

Barnet LB. J Clin Physiol 1:25, 1959

Baulac M, Laplane D. [Alcohol and epilepsy.] Rev Prat 40(4):307-11, 1990

Baumeister F et al. Glutamate in pyridoxine-dependent epilepsy: neurotoxic glutamate concentration in the cerebrospinal fluid and its normalization by pyridoxine. Pediatrics 94(3):318-21, 1994

Baumeister FAM, Egger J. Diagnosis and therapy of vitamin B6 dependent epilepsy. Monatsschr Kinderheilkd 144:534-5, 1996

Benga I et al. Plasma and cerebrospinal fluid concentrations of magnesium in epileptic children. J Neurol Sci 67(1):29-34, 1985

Bohr T. Evaluation and treatment of seizures. Letter. N Engl J Med 324(17):1213-14, 1991

Botez MI et al. Thiamine and folate treatment of chronic epileptic patients: a controlled study with the Wechsler IQ scale. Epilepsy Res 16(2):157-63, 1993

Bourgeois BF et al. Interactions between primidone, carbamazepine, and nicotinamide. Neurology 32(10):1122-6, 1982

Bourgeois BFD et al. Potentiation of the antiepileptic activity of phenobarbital by nicotinamide. Epilepsia 24:238-44, 1983

Bregola G et al. Biotin deficiency facilitates kindling hyperexcitability in rats. Neuroreport 7(11):1745-8, 1996

Brown RS. The administration of folic acid to institutionalized epileptic adults with phenytoin-induced gingival hyperplasia. A double-blind, randomized, placebo-controlled, parallel study. Oral Surg Oral Med Oral Pathol 71(5):565-8, 1991

Calomme MR et al. Selenium deficiency triggering intractable seizures. Therapeutic Uses Trace Elements 62:359-64, 1996

Camfield PR et al. Aspartame exacerbates EEG spike-wave discharge in children with generalized absence epilepsy: a double-blind controlled study. Neurology 42(5):1000-1003, 1992

Carl GF et al. Association of low blood manganese concentration with epilepsy. Neurology 36:1584-7, 1986

Chung S et al. Alterations in the carnitine metabolism in epileptic children treated with valproic acid. J Korean Med Sci 12(6):553-8, 1997

Collins N et al. A prospective study to evaluate the dose of vitamin D required to correct low 25-hydroxyvitamin D levels, calcium, and alkaline phosphatase in patients at risk of developing antiepileptic drug-induced osteomalacia. Q J Med 78(286):113-22, 1991

Coulter DL. Carnitine deficiency in epilepsy: Risk factors and treatment. J Child Neurol 10 Suppl 2:S32-S39, 1995

Coursin DB. Convulsive seizures in infants with pyridoxine-deficient diet. JAMA 154:406-8, 1954

Coursin DB. Vitamin B6 and brain function in animals and man. Ann N Y Acad Sci 166:7-15, 1969

Crayton JW et al. Epilepsy precipitated by food sensitivity: report of a case with double-blind placebo-controlled assessment. Clin Electroencephalography 12(4):192-8, 1981

Crowell GF, Roach ES. Pyridoxine-dependent seizures. Am Fam Physician 27(3):183-7, 1983

Davidson DL, Ward NI. Abnormal aluminium, cobalt, manganese, strontium and zinc concentrations in untreated epilepsy. Epilepsy Res 2(5):323-30, 1988

del Ser Quijano T et al. Psychological disturbances and folic acid in chronic epileptic outpatients. Epilepsia 24(5):588-96, 1983

De Vivo DC. How to use other drugs (steroids) and the ketogenic diet, in PL Morselli, CE Pippenger and JK Penry, Eds. Antiepileptic Drug Therapy in Pediatrics. New York, Raven Press, 1983:283-92

Drew HJ et al. Effect of folate upon phenytoin hyperplasia. J Clin Periodontol 14:350, 1987

Durelli L, Mutani R. The current status of taurine in epilepsy. Clin Neuropharmacol 6(1):37-48, 1983

Egger J et al. Oligoantigenic diet treatment of children with epilepsy and migraine. J Pediatr 114:51-58, 1989

Fisher RS et al. Failure of high-dose intravenous magnesium sulfate to control myoclonic status epilepticus. Clin Neuropharmacol 11(6):537-44, 1988

Flodin NW. Pharmacology of Micronutrients. New York, Alan R. Liss, Inc., 1988

Freed WJ. N,N-dimethylglycine, betaine, and seizures. Letter. Arch Neurol 41(11):1129-30, 1984

Freeman JM. The Epilepsy Diet: An Introduction to the Ketogenic Diet. New York, Demos Pub, 1994

Galland L. Magnesium, stress and neuropsychiatric disorders. Magnes Trace Elem 10(2-4):287-301, 1991-2

Gascon G et al. N,N dimethylglycine and epilepsy. Epilepsia 30(1):90-3, 1989

Givverd FB et al. The influence of folic acid on the frequency of epileptic attacks. Europ J Clin Pharm 19(1):57-60, 1981

Goodman HO et al. Antiepileptic drugs and plasma and platelet taurine in epilepsy. Epilepsia 30(2):201-7, 1989

Gorges LF, G:ucer G. Effect of magnesium on epileptic foci. Epilepsia 19(1):81-91, 1978

Gunduz Z et al. Serum and cerebrospinal fluid zinc levels in children with febrile convulsions. Acta Paediatr Jpn 38:237-41, 1996

Gupta SK. Serum magnesium levels in idiopathic epilepsy. J Assoc Physicians India 42(6):4567, 1994

Gyland SP. Possibly neurogenic hypoglycemia. JAMA 152:1184, 1953

Hall RCW, Joffe, JR. Hypomagnesemia: physical and psychiatric symptoms. JAMA 224(13):1749-51, 1973

Hartley SG et al. Urinary excretion of taurine in epilepsy. Neurochem Res 14(2):149-52, 1989

Hoffer A. Niacin Therapy in Psychiatry. Springfield, Ill., Charles C. Thomas, 1962

Holman CP, Bell AFJ. A trial of evening primrose oil in the treatment of chronic schizophrenia. J Orthomol Psychiatry 12:302-04, 1983

Hurley LS et al. Proc Soc Exp Biol Med 106:343-6, 1963

Jerrett SA et al. H2O2 formation and lipid peroxides in brain during exposure to oxygen under high pressure. Aerosp Med 40-44, 1973

Jiao FY, et al. Randomized, controlled trial of high-dose intravenous pyridoxine in the treatment of recurrent seizures in children. Pediatr Neurol 17(1):54-7, 1997

Kagan VE et al. Role of lipid peroxidation in damage to serotonin receptors and development of epileptiform seizures during hyperoxia. Biull Eksp Biol Med 96(12):16-18, 1983

Karnaze DS, Carmel R. Neurologic and evoked potential abnormalities in subtle cobalamin deficiency states, including deficiency without anemia and with normal absorption of free cobalamin. Arch Neurol 47(9):1008-12, 1990

Keyser A. Epileptic manifestations and vitamin B1 deficiency. Eur Neurol 31:121-5, 1991

Ko FJ et al. Alteration of amino acid in plasma and cerebrospinal fluid of children with seizure disorders. Ko Hsiung I Hsueh Ko Hsueh Tsa Chih 9(3):131-42, 1993

Kovalenko VM et al. [Alpha-tocopherol in the complex treatment of several forms of epilepsy.] Zh Neuropathol Psikhitv 6:892-7, 1984) (in Russian)

Krahn LE et al. Use of caffeine in medically refractory seizure patients. Neuropsychiatr Neuropsychol Behav Neurol 7(2):136-7, 1994

Krause KH et al. [Reduction of biotin level as a possible factor in the mode of action of anticonvulsants]. Arch Psychiatr Nervenkr 231(2):141-8, 1982) (in German)

Krause KH et al. B vitamins in epileptics. Bibl Nutr Dieta 38:154-67, 1986

Krause KH et al. Effect of long-term treatment with antiepileptic drugs on the vitamin status. Drug Nutr Interact 5(4):317-43, 1988

Kretsch MJ et al. Electroencephalographic changes and periodontal status during short-term vitamin B-6 depletion of young, non-pregnant women. Am J Clin Nutr 53:1266-74, 1991

Kryzhanovskii GN, Shandra AA. [Effect of diazepam and nicotinamide on convulsive activity of various types]. Farmakol Toksikol 48(4):21-5, 1985) (in Russian)

Kuzuya T et al. Effect of anti-epileptic drugs on serum zinc and copper concentrations in epileptic patients. Int J Clin Pharmacol Ther Toxicol 31(2):61-5, 1993

Lechtenberg R, Worner TM. Total ethanol consumption as a seizure risk factor in alcoholics. Acta Neurol Scand 85(2):90-4, 1992

Lewis-Jones MS et al. Cutaneous manifestations of zinc deficiency during treatment with anticonvulsants. Br Med J 290:603-4, 1985

Loeb C et al. Preliminary evaluation of the effect of GABA and phosphatidylserine in epileptic patients. Epileptic Res 1:209-12, 1987

Mantovani J et al. Effects of taurine on seizures and growth hormone release in epileptic patients. Arch Neurol 35:672, 1979

Marangos PJ et al. The benzodiazepines and inosine antagonize caffeine-induced seizures. Psychopharmacology (Berlin) 72(3):269-73, 1981

Marion JL et al. [Alcoholic epilepsy. Decrease of tryptophan levels in the blood and cerebrospinal fluid.] Presse Med 14(12):681-3, 1985) (in French)

Mattson R et al. Folate therapy in epilepsy. Arch Neurol 29:78, 1973

Mazariegos-Ramos E et al. Consumption of soft drinks with phosphoric acid as a risk factor for the development of hypocalcemia in children: a case-control study. J Pediatr 126:940-2, 1995

Mëhes K, Petrovicz E. Familial benign copper deficiency. Arch Dis Child 57(9):716-18, 1982

Mock DM, Dyken ME. Biotin catabolism is accelerated in adults receiving long-term therapy with anticonvulsants. Neurology 49(5):1444-7, 1997

Motta E. [Concentration of copper and ceruloplasmin in serum of patients treated for epilepsy]. Wiad Lek 51(3-4):156-161, 1998) (in Polish)

Nakagawa E et al. Efficacy of pyridoxal phosphate in treating an adult with intractable status epilepticus. Neurology 48:1468-9, 1997

McNamara JO et al. Effects of oral choline on human complex partial seizures. Neurology 30(12):1334-6, 1980

Mëhes K, Petrovicz E. Familial benign copper deficiency. Arch Dis Child 57(9):716-18, 1982

Motta E et al. [Concentration of copper and ceruloplasmin in serum of patients treated for epilepsy]. Wiad Lek 51(3-4):156-161, 1998) (in Polish)

Nimmo GR et al. The clinical importance of subnormal folate levels in epileptic patients on anticonvulsant therapy. Scott Med J 32(6):171-2, 1987

Nuytten D. Magnesium deficiency as a cause of acute intractable seizures. J Neurol 238(5):262-4, 1991

Ogunmekan AO. Plasma vitamin E levels in normal children and in epileptic children with and without anticonvulsant therapy. Trop Geog Med 37:175-7, 1985

Ogunmekan AO, Hwang PA. A randomised double blind, placebo-controlled, clinical trial of D-alpha-tocopherol acetate (vitamin E) as add-on therapy for epilepsy in children. Epilepsia 30(1):84-9, 1989

Olney JW et al. Excitotoxic mechanisms of epileptic brain damage. Adv Neurol 44:857-77, 1986

Papavasiliou PS et al. Seizure disorders and trace metals: Manganese tissue levels in treated epileptics. Neurology 29:1466, 1979

Pasqui L et al. [Effects of phosphatidylserine in an experimental model of generalized epilepsy]. Riv Neurol 54(2):128-38, 1984) (in Italian)

Passmore R, Eastwood MA. Davidson and Passmore: Human Nutrition and Dietetics. Edinburgh, Churchill Livingstone, 1986:471

Pfeiffer CC, LaMola S. Zinc and manganese in the schizophrenias. J Orthomol Psychiatry 12:215-34, 1983

Pisacane A et al. Iron deficiency anemia and febrile convulsions: case-control study in children under 2 years. BMJ 313:343, 1996

Prasad AS et al. Determination of zinc in biological fluids by atomic absorption spectrophotometry in normal and cirrhotic subjects. J Lab Clin Med 66:508-16, 1965

Prusinski A, Stepien-Barcikowska A. [Use of tryptophan in the treatment of epilepsy of the Lennox-Gastaut type]. Neurol Neurochir Pol 18(3):287-9, 1984) (in Polish)

Ramaekers VT. Selenium deficiency triggering intractable seizures. Neuropediatrics 25(4):217-23, 1994

Raju GB et al. Randomized, double-blind, placebo-controlled, clinical trial of D-alpha-tocopherol (vitamin E) as add-on therapy in uncontrolled epilepsy. Epilepsia 35(2):368-72, 1994

Roach ES, Carlin L. N,N-dimethylglycine for epilepsy. Letter. N Engl J Med 307:1081-2, 1982

Rosciszewska D et al. [Serum levels of vitamin B12 in epileptic patients treated with carbamazepine]. Neurol Neurochir Pol 27(5):671-5, 1993) (in Polish)

Rowan AJ et al. Aspartame and seizure susceptibility: results of a clinical study in reportedly sensitive individuals. Epilepsia 36(3):270-5, 1995

Sadeh M et al. Treatment of porphyric convulsions with magnesium sulfate. Epilepsia 3295):712-15, 1991

Salbert BA et al. Characterization of seizures associated with biotinidase deficiency. Neurology 43(7):1351-5, 1993

Shaywitz BA et al. Aspartame has no effect on seizures or epileptiform discharges in epileptic children. Ann Neurol 35(1):98-103, 1994

Shoji Y. Serum magnesium and zinc in epileptic children. Brain Dev 5(2):200, 1983

Sholer A, Pfeiffer CC. Vitamin B6 and the treatment of mental disease. Int Clin Nutr Rev 8(3), 1988

Shrestha KP, Oswaldo A. Trace elements in hair of epileptic and normal subjects. Sci Total Environ 67(2-3):215-25, 1987

Singh RB et al. Dietary intake and plasma levels of antioxidant vitamins in health and disease: a hospital-based case-control study. J Nutr Environ Med 5:235-42, 1995

Smith DB, Obbens EAMT. Anti-folate-antiepileptic relationships, in MI Botez, EH Reynolds, Eds. Folic Acid in Neurology, Psychiatry and Internal Medicine. New York, Raven Press, 1979

Sood AK et al. Serum, CSF, RBC & urinary levels of magnesium & calcium in idiopathic generalised tonic clonic seizures. Indian J Med Res 98:152-4, 1993

Sorenson JRJ. Therapeutic uses of copper, in JO Nriagu, Ed. Copper in the Environment. Part II: Health Effects. New York, John Wiley & Sons, 1979:83-162

Sozuer DT, et al. The effects of antiepileptic drugs on serum zinc and copper levels in children. J Basic Clin Physiol Pharmacol 6(3-4):265-9, 1995

Sterman MB et al. Zinc and seizure mechanisms, in J Morley, MB Sterman, Eds. Nutritional Modulation of Neural Function. New York, Academic Press, 1988, pp. 307-19

Sturman J. Taurine in nutrition. Compr Ther 3:64, 1977

Sullivan JF, Lankford HG. Zinc metabolism and chronic alcoholism. Am J Clin Nutr 17:57-72, 1965

Tallian KB et al. Role of the ketogenic diet in children with intractable seizures. Ann Pharmacother 32(3):349-61, 1998

Tanaka Y. Low manganese may trigger epilepsy. JAMA 238:1805, 1977

Vaddadi KS. The use of gamma-linolenic acid and linoleic acid to differentiate between temporal lobe epilepsy and schizophrenia. Prostaglandins Med 6:375-79, 1981

Valimaki MJ et al. Bone mineral density measured by dual-energy x-ray absorptiometry and novel markers of bone formation and resorption in patients on antiepileptic drugs. J Bone Miner Res 9(5):631-7, 1994

Weber GF et al. Glutathione peroxidase deficiency and childhood seizures. Lancet 337:1443-4, 1991

Williamson A, Spencer D. Zinc reduces dentate granule cell hyperexcitability in epileptic humans. Neuroreport 6(11):1562-4, 1995

FATIGUE

See Also: **ANEMIA**
CHRONIC FATIGUE SYNDROME
DEPRESSION
EATING DISORDERS
'HYPOGLYCEMIA' (FUNCTIONAL)
ORGANIC MENTAL DISORDERS

NUTRITIONAL TREATMENT GUIDE

✓ = Efficacy generally accepted.
* = Efficacy *demonstrated* by controlled human trials.
[+] = Efficacy *suspected* from uncontrolled human trials.
[-] = Efficacy *suspected* from indirect data.
? = Efficacy *challenged* in a study of similar design.

DIETARY FACTORS

* avoid regular **Caffeine** ingestion
* avoid regular refined **Sugar** ingestion

- -

[+] avoid **high Carbohydrate, low Protein meals**

NUTRITIONAL FACTORS

* **Iron deficiency:** 30 to 60 mg daily to 3 times daily
* **Pantothenic acid deficiency:** 100 to 200 mg daily
* **Potassium/Magnesium Aspartate**: 1 g twice daily (10 day trial)
* **Selenium deficiency:** 200 μg daily
* **Thiamine deficiency:** 50 mg daily
* **Tyrosine:** *to counteract acute fatigue due to overwork:* 75 mg/kg body weight twice daily
* **Vitamin B_6:** pyridoxine 20 mg twice daily (one week trial)
* **Vitamin B_{12}:** 1000 μg IM once weekly or as needed
* **Vitamin C deficiency:** 500 mg twice daily
* **Zinc deficiency:** zinc sulfate 220 mg twice daily *AND* **Copper** 2 mg daily

- -

[+] **Coenzyme Q_{10}:** ? 90 mg daily
[+] **Folic Acid deficiency:** 800 μg daily
[+] **Magnesium deficiency:** ≈ 400 mg daily
[+] **Potassium deficiency:** 60 mmol daily - preferably by increasing dietary intake

OTHER FACTORS

[+] rule out **Food Sensitivities**
[+] rule out **'Reactive Hypoglycemia'**

DIETARY FACTORS

Effects of a High Carbohydrate Meal

Fatigue may be increased following the consumption of a high carbohydrate, low protein meal. Carbohydrates trigger insulin production which elevates the plasma tryptophan ratio, enhancing serotonin synthesis from tryptophan *(Spring)*. While this is not a basis for reducing carbohydrate consumption, patients complaining of fatigue should be aware that carbohydrates may temporarily worsen their fatigue.

Caffeine

In a study of hospitalized psychiatric patients, 61% of those ingesting at least 750 mg of caffeine daily complained of tiring easily, compared to 54% of those ingesting 250 to 749 mg daily, and 24% of those ingesting less than 250 mg daily *(Greden)*.

Although the acute ingestion of caffeine can relieve fatigue and increase endurance *(Costill)*, double-blind studies have found that chronic caffeine use, at least at higher levels of ingestion, may cause fatigue during withdrawal periods *(Hughes;Silverman)*. A vicious cycle may therefore be created in which the patient drinks increasing amounts of caffeine to prevent fatigue and other withdrawal symptoms.

Further evidence that caffeine may cause fatigue comes from an animal study which tested the swimming capacity of mice under different conditions. In contrast to a single dose of caffeine, 6 weeks of treatment with caffeine greatly reduced their swimming capacity. These findings suggested that chronic caffeine ingestion may interfere with the ability to mobilize and spend metabolic substrates for the energy requirements of skeletal muscle *(Estler)*.

A middle-aged physician complained of constant fatigue and difficulty falling asleep. Physical examination and laboratory testing were normal.

He was found to be drinking 15 cups of coffee daily while in the hospital to "perk him up." Once weaned away from coffee, he was soon feeling fine (Fox).

Sugar

It appears that the initial energy increase following sugar ingestion is soon followed by the opposite reaction. Based on self-ratings by normal volunteers who compared eating a candy bar with brisk walking on each of 12 separate days, the sugar snack increases energy and reduces tiredness in the first hour, and then reduces energy and increases tiredness one hour later *(Thayer)*.

Caffeine-free, Sugar-free Diet

Regardless of its effects in the first few hours after ingestion, chronic, large intakes of refined sugar have long been suspected of having a similar effect to that of caffeine in promoting fatigue.

In one study, 16 people complaining of such symptoms as fatigue, depression, headaches and moodiness were placed on a caffeine-free and refined-sucrose-free diet for up to two weeks. Those who improved were sequentially challenged double-blind with caffeine, cellulose placebo, sucrose-sweetened Kool-Aid, and aspartame-sweetened Kool-Aid for 6 days each. Seven out of the 16 subjects (44%) demonstrated a return of symptoms and mood disturbance when challenged with caffeine or refined sucrose, but not with cellulose or aspartame *(Christensen)*.

NUTRITIONAL FACTORS

VITAMINS

Folic Acid Deficiency

Folates play an important role in the synthesis of neurotransmitters and elements of neuron structure *(Ortega)*. In patients with folate deficiency and only minor neurological signs, fatigue is a prominent symptom along with depression and lassitude *(Botez;Heseker)*.

Folate deficiency is the most common of the vitamin deficiencies. Adolescent and pregnant women, the elderly, and people with malabsorption syndromes are particularly prone to become folate-deficient. While a megaloblastic anemia is often present, folate deficiency may occur in its absence *(Matthews)*.

An 81 year-old man ate poorly after the death of his wife. Initially depressed by his wife's death, he seemed cheerful and was making plans several months following her demise. Gradually, however, he became increasingly apathetic and confused and began to complain of sharp, stabbing leg pains, easy fatigability, blurred vision, and weakness. Bowel movements were rare. Oral supplementation with vitamin B complex was ineffective, so laboratory tests for nutritional deficiencies were performed. Serum folic acid, red blood cell folic acid and neutrophilic segmentation tests were consistent with folate deficiency.

He was started on folic acid 5 mg three times daily. After two months, his folic acid levels normalized; however, neutrophilic segmentation took longer to decrease to normal. By the end of the second month, his symptoms had cleared (Wright, 1984a).

Pantothenic Acid Deficiency

Fatigue is the most prominent pantothenic acid deficiency symptom, along with listlessness, insomnia, sullenness, and depression *(Fry)*.

A sub-clinical deficiency decreases energy availability by shifting the major portion of energy production from the tricarboxylic acid cycle to glycolysis alone, a process that is much less efficient *(Early)*.

Thiamine Deficiency

A mild thiamine deficiency may present with fatigue *(Heseker)*. Correction of a marginal deficiency has been shown under double-blind conditions to decrease fatigue and increase the general sense of well-being *(Smidt)*.

A deficiency of thiamine would inhibit the body's ability to use pyruvate in the tricarboxylic acid cycle, forcing it to utilize acetate derived from fatty acid breakdown, a source that cannot increase when energy demands are higher. Moreover, a deficiency could cause heme to decrease, which would decrease the oxygen-carrying capacity of the blood *(Early)*.

Vitamin B_6

A controlled crossover study examined the effects of vitamin B_6 supplementation on a group of 19 patients who complained of chronic exhaustion, some of whom had not been helped by a wide variety of treatments. They received pyridoxine 20 mg twice daily and placebo, each for 7 days. All but one was better on vitamin B_6, and most remarked that they felt considerably better while on vitamin B_6 than while on placebo *(Annand)*.

Whether these patients were marginally B_6-deficient is not known.

Vitamin B_{12}

Fatigue or generalized weakness is an early manifestation of vitamin B_{12} deficiency, which suggests that B_{12} deficiency should be a diagnostic consideration whenever neuropsychiatric signs or symptoms are unexplained *(Goodwin)*.

Also, vitamin B_{12} supplementation by injection has long been used empirically for the treatment of fatigue in patients with no evidence of vitamin B_{12} deficiency. Proof of its efficacy comes from a double-blind crossover study in which 28 patients who complained of tiredness but had normal serum B_{12} levels and no physical findings were given injections of hydroxycobalamin 5 mg or placebo twice daily for 2 weeks followed by a 2-week rest period and 2 weeks of the crossover treatment.

Based on the sum of daily subjective scores, those who received placebo first felt significantly better in regard to "general well being" during the second period when they received vitamin B_{12}. However, those who initially received vitamin B_{12} noted no differences between the vitamin B_{12} and placebo periods. The authors suggest that the effects of the vitamin may persist for at least 4 weeks *(Ellis)*.

Moreover, in a study involving 5 healthy volunteers, intravenous injections of methylcobalamin 10 mg/kg produced greater alertness than the saline placebo *(Uchizyama)*.

A 44 year-old male university professor complained of an inadequate energy level. A thorough work-up had failed to find any abnormality. He exercised regularly and ate a healthy diet. There was no evidence of depression.

He began injections of vitamin B_{12} 300 µg three times a week for two weeks and his tiredness left. Two or three weeks after stopping the injections, however, his energy level lowered again. He repeated the trial. As the results were identical, he decided to continue to take the injections on a regular schedule (Wright, 1979).

Vitamin C Deficiency

When 5 prisoners underwent controlled ascorbic acid deprivation, they reported increased fatigue, lassitude and depression *(Kinsman)*. Conversely, there is evidence that repletion of a longstanding marginal ascorbate deficiency increases energy *(Schorah)*.

Also, studies concerning the effect of vitamin C upon physical performance have found that a marginal vitamin C deficiency may impair a person's ability to work, while the performance deficit usually disappears following supplementation *(Gerster)*.

Another perspective on the issue of fatigue as related to vitamin C nutriture comes from a survey of 411 dentists and their wives. The average number of fatigue-related symptoms among the low vitamin C users was found to be double that among the relatively high users of vitamin C *(Cheraskin)*. Since this finding could easily be explained by confounding variables, it is premature to draw definite conclusions, although it does suggest that fatigue due to marginal vitamin C nutriture may be fairly common.

MINERALS

Iron Deficiency

Iron deficiency may be associated with fatigue and a diminished work capacity *(Schultz)*. Often forgotten is the fact that iron may be deficient despite the lack of anemia and a normal serum iron *(Finch)*.

Moreover, iron supplementation is often effective in relieving fatigue in women. For example, in a double-blind study, about two-thirds of a group of chronically fatigued non-anemic women improved following iron supplementation *(Buetler)*.

A Warning

Iron should not be supplemented unless there is evidence of a deficiency. In fact, iron overload may even be the *cause* of disabling fatigue. For example, in hereditary hemochromatosis (an iron storage disease), fatigue, the most common symptom, is reported by over 80% of patients *(Niederau)*.

A 34-year-old woman with constant tiredness for 20 years had normal complete blood count and thyroid function studies, but serum ferritin was very low.

She was started on 40 to 50 mg of iron daily. Four months later, her ferritin had risen into the normal range and she no longer felt tired (Wright, 1984b).

Magnesium Deficiency

Magnesium is required for the synthesis of ATP and enhances potassium transport into cells. Fatigue is one of the central symptoms of chronic magnesium deficiency. Others, which may occur simultaneously, include anxiety, hyperemotionality, headaches, insomnia, lightheadedness, dizziness, and nervous fits.

Peripheral signs of magnesium deficiency include acroparesthesias, cramps, muscle fasciculations and myalgias. Dysautonomic disturbances are common and may involve both the sympathetic and parasympathetic systems *(Durlach)*.

Potassium Deficiency

Malaise, along with muscle weakness, is the most common symptom of chronic potassium deficiency *(Snively)*. The elderly, who are often potassium-deficient *(Abdulla)*, have been shown to suffer from muscle weakness (as measured by grip strength) when they fail to ingest adequate potassium in their diets *(Judge)*. Supplementation, preferably in the form of fresh fruit and vegetables, should restore strength and energy.

Magnesium deficiency is an important cause of potassium depletion, and potassium deficiency may be refractory in the presence of magnesium depletion *(Rude)*. Moreover, potassium supplementation may increase urinary magnesium excretion *(Saito)*. Patients presenting with evidence of a potassium deficit should therefore have their magnesium nutriture evaluated.

A 78 year-old man complaining of increasing generalized muscle weakness and rapid fatigue had a normal serum potassium but a low whole blood potassium.

Fresh fruit and vegetable juice were added to his diet. Three months later, his energy and muscle strength had returned to normal (Wright,1974).

Selenium Deficiency

A marginal selenium deficiency - which is not uncommon in areas of the world with low soil and water selenium content - may cause tiredness.

In a double-blind crossover study of 50 unselected subjects, initial reports of tiredness were found to be negatively correlated with the subjects' dietary selenium content. They then received a daily selenium supplement or a placebo for 5 weeks each in random order. Selenium, but not placebo, supplementation was associated with improvement in reports of tiredness *(Benton)*.

Zinc Deficiency

Perhaps half of the population of industrialized societies consumes less than the US RDA for zinc. A marginal zinc deficiency may be associated with decreased muscle strength and endurance *(Cordova;Krotkiewski)* as well as with mental lethargy *(Prasad)*.

Leukonychia (white spots on fingernails) is thought to be an indicator of zinc nutriture; it is said to disappear within a few months following zinc supplementation *(Wright,1989)*. In a study of college students, 74% of 28 students who reported themselves to be "very often drowsy" had leukonychia compared to 46% of 11 students who reported themselves as "never drowsy." These students were also significantly more likely to report longer sleep times *(Bakan)*.

When marginally deficient, zinc supplementation has been shown under double-blind conditions to decrease fatigue by increasing isokinetic strength and isometric endurance in striated muscles *(Krotkiewski)*.

OTHER NUTRITIONAL FACTORS

Aspartic Acid salts

Aspartic acid is converted intracellularly into oxaloacetate, an important substrate in the energy-producing Krebs cycle. It is also a carrier molecule for the transport of potassium and magnesium into the cell.

Supplementation with potassium/magnesium aspartate has been investigated in several double-blind studies. Between 75% and 91% of treated patients experienced pronounced relief of fatigue compared to between 5% and 25% of the controls. Side effects, which were mild and uncommon, included mild gastrointestinal distress and dryness of the mouth. Patients usually continued treatment for 4 to 6 weeks; afterwards fatigue frequently did not return. Side effects, which were mild and uncommon, included mild gastrointestinal distress and dryness of the mouth *(Gaby)*.

Coenzyme Q_{10}

Supplementation with coenzyme Q_{10}, which can increase work output in normal sedentary individuals *(Zeppilli)*, may be effective in improving impaired aerobic function in people complaining of fatigue with no medical origin *(Yamabe)*.

Tyrosine

In animals, brain norepinephrine levels are closely related to stress-induced performance decrements. Experimental data suggest that supplementation with tyrosine, precursor to norepinephrine, may counteract stress-related performance decrements and mood deterioration *(Owasoyo)*. In a placebo-controlled study, supplementation with L-tyrosine delayed the onset of performance fatigue following sleep deprivation and continuous nighttime work *(Neri)*.

However, the efficacy of tyrosine in treating fatigue which is unrelated to overwork is unknown.

COMBINED NUTRITIONAL TREATMENT

A woman, who was both a mother and a student, on a vegetarian diet developed increasing fatigue over several years. She noted that she could function for about 3 hours in the morning, but was never really awake and clearheaded and always felt in need of more sleep. She quit her part-time job and took a long nap each afternoon. She drank coffee and took over-the-counter stimulants to energize her so that she could go jogging, but afterwards she would feel even more exhausted and take another nap.

In addition, she increasingly developed odd and inexplicable injuries and ailments. Her toenails would fall out, and her teeth and gums would ache. One day, she grabbed her pet dog as he ran into the street and broke a finger. Several weeks later, x-rays revealed that this injury had not even begun to heal.

A nutritional evaluation revealed that her diet consisted mostly of pastas, fast foods and packaged foods. Blood tests revealed marked deficiencies of vitamin C and selenium as well as many other nutrient deficiencies.

She was given vitamin C intravenously and placed on oral supplements of vitamin C, vitamin E, selenium, vitamin B complex and essential fatty acids. In addition to starting supplements, she improved her diet. While continuing to avoid meat and fish, she began to avoid packaged and processed food while relying on eggs and milk as her primary protein sources. She also began to eat a lot of fresh vegetables and fruits, some organically grown.

During the next month, she gradually started to feel better, although her improvement was erratic. After about 2 months, her energy level was up and she went on vacation without becoming fatigued. Sleep, which previously had been disturbed, now had become peaceful.

Currently, despite taking more classes and working long hours at two research labs, she has enough energy for evening activities and no longer needs afternoon naps (Riordan).

OTHER RELATED FACTORS

Food Sensitivities

Food sensitivities have been accused of causing an "allergic tension-fatigue syndrome" characterized by sensory and motor hyperactivity and/or sensory and motor fatigue in conjunction with more classical allergy symptoms.

Most of the literature, which goes back half a century, is anecdotal. However, in one study of 44 patients with a history of the syndrome, laboratory studies showed lymphocyte stimulation to a series of food extracts and additives in all but 2 patients. Elimination diets based on the *in vitro* results produced remissions in 86% and partial remissions in 5% *(Valverde)*.

Furthermore, there is recent evidence suggesting that the allergic tension-fatigue syndrome, as well as other examples of non-IgE-mediated food sensitivities, may be associated with ileal-lymphoid-nodular hyperplasia *(Sabra; Wakefield)*. This finding suggests that a reactive inflammatory response in the adjacent lymphoid tissue of Peyer's patches may result in the entry of antigens across the inflamed mucosa of the bowel *(Sabra)*.

A 13 year-old boy with severe bronchial asthma was strikingly pale with dark circles under his eyes. He was morose, listless and lethargic and complained of musculoskeletal pains, headache and abdominal pain. He drank two pints of milk daily and ate chocolate or drank a cola-type beverage daily.

Within 48 hours of starting milk and chocolate elimination, the facial pallor and the dark circles under his eyes almost completely disappeared. Most remarkable was the improvement in his mood and behavior. He became alert, cheerful and interested in his surroundings. His physical complaints ceased and his asthma was easily controlled.

After three weeks, milk was added to his diet. Within one week his pallor and the dark circumorbital circles returned and he became morose, listless and behaved badly. He was returned to the therapeutic diet with the same satisfactory result as before (Weinberg).

'Reactive Hypoglycemia'

(Also see the 'Hypoglycemia' chapter.)

A series of 300 patients has been described who experienced a drop of 20 mg% or more below their fasting blood sugar level during a 6-hour glucose tolerance test. Two-thirds of these patients complained of exhaustion or fatigue. Previous treatments with tranquilizers, sedatives and/or electroconvulsive therapy had been ineffective.

About 85% of the patients responded to a high protein, low carbohydrate, caffeine-free diet during which they ate between meals and every 2 hours throughout the evening. In addition, nearly 70% of them received 6 to 12 injections of calcium-glycerophosphate 10 cc intragluteally *(Salzer)*.

Better studies are needed to better ascertain whether this pattern of blood glucose responses to a glucose challenge is an objective indicator of subjective feelings of fatigue, as well as whether the efficacy of this particular treatment regimen is more than a placebo effect.

BIBLIOGRAPHY

Abdulla M et al. Dietary intake of potassium in the elderly. Lancet ii:562, 1975

Annand JC. Pyridoxine and magnesium in the treatment of shock. Lancet ii:340-1, 1957

Bakan P. Confusion, lethargy and leukonychia. J Orthomol Med 5(4):198-202, 1990

Benton D, Cook R. The impact of selenium supplementation on mood. Biol Psychiatry 29:1092-8, 1991

Botez MI. Neuropsychological correlates of folic acid deficiency: facts and hypotheses, in MI Botez, EH Reynolds, Eds. Folic Acid in Neurology, Psychiatry and Internal Medicine. New York, Raven Press, 1979

Buetler E et al. Iron therapy in chemically fatigued non-anemic women: A double-blind study. Ann Intern Med 52:378, 1960

Cheraskin E et al. Daily vitamin C consumption and fatigability. J Am Geriatr Soc 2493):136-7, 1976

Christensen L. Psychological distress and diet - effects of sucrose and caffeine. J Appl Nutr 40(1):44-50, 1988

Cordova A, Alvarez-Mon M. Behaviour of zinc in physical exercise: a special reference to immunity and fatigue. Neurosci Biobehav Rev 19(3):439-45, 1995

Costill DL et al. Effects of caffeine ingestion on metabolism and exercise performance. Med Sci Sports 1093):155-8, 1978

Durlach J et al. Magnesium and therapeutics. Magnes Res 7(3/4):313-28, 1994

Early RG, Carlson BR. Water-soluble vitamin therapy in the delay of fatigue from physical activity in hot climatic conditions. Int Z angew Physiol 27:43-50, 1969

Ellis FR, Nasser S. A pilot study of vitamin B12 in the treatment of tiredness. Br J Nutr 30:277-83, 1973

Estler CJ et al. Swimming capacity of mice after prolonged treatment with psychostimulants. I. Effects of caffeine on swimming performance and cold stress. Psychopharmacology (Berlin) 58(2):161-6, 1978

Finch CA. Editorial: Evaluation of iron status. JAMA 251(15):2004, 1984

Fox A. Caffeine - unexpected cause of fatigue! Let's Live April, 1982, pp. 16-20

Fry PC et al. Metabolic response to a pantothenic acid deficient diet in humans. J Nutr Sci Vitaminol 22:339-46, 1976

Gaby AR. Aspartic acid salts and fatigue. Curr Nutr Therapeut, November, 1982

Gerster H. The role of vitamin C in athletic performance. J Am Coll Nutr 8(6):636-43, 1989

Goodman KI, Salt WB 2nd. Vitamin B12 deficiency. Important new concepts in recognition. Postgrad Med 88(3):147-50, 153-8, 1990

Greden JF et al. Anxiety and depression associated with caffeinism among psychiatric inpatients. Am J Psychiatry 135(8):963-6, 1978

Heseker H et al. Psychological disorders as early symptoms of a mild-moderate vitamin deficiency. Ann N Y Acad Sci 669:352-7, 1992

Hughes JR et al. Caffeine self-administration, withdrawal, and adverse effects among coffee drinkers. Arch Gen Psychiatry 48:611-17, 1991

Judge TG, Cowan NR. Dietary potassium intake and grip strength in older people. Gerontologia Clinica 13:221-6, 1971

Kinsman RA, Hood J. Some behavioral effects of ascorbic acid deficiency. Am J Clin Nutr 24(4):455-64, 1971

Krotkiewski M et al. Zinc and muscle strength and endurance. Acta Physiol Scand 116(3):309-11, 1982

Matthews J et al. Effect of therapy with vitamin B12 and folic acid on elderly patients with low concentrations of serum vitamin B12 or erythrocyte folate but normal blood counts. Acta Haematologica 79:84-7, 1988

Neri DF et al. The effects of tyrosine on cognitive performance during extended wakefulness. Avit Space Environ Med 66:313-19, 1995

Niederau C et al. Survival and causes of death in cirrhotic and noncirrhotic patients with primary hemochromatosis. N Engl J Med 313:1256-62, 1985

Ortega TM et al. [The role of folates in the diverse biochemical processes that control mental function]. Nutr Hosp 9(4):251-6, 1994 (in Spanish)

Owasoyo JO et al. Tyrosine and its potential use as a countermeasure to performance decrement in military sustained operations. Aviat Space Environ Med 63(5):364-9, 1992

Prasad A. Clinical manifestation of zinc deficiency. Nutr Rev 41(7):197, 1983

Riordan, Hugh - told to Jack Challem. Transformations: How nutritional therapy changed three lives. Let's Live December, 1998:32-5

Rude RK. Physiology of magnesium metabolism and the important role of magnesium in potassium deficiency. Am J Cardiology 63:31G-34G, 1989

Sabra A et al. Ileal-lymphoid-nodular hyperplasia, non-specific colitis, and pervasive developmental disorder in children. Letter. Lancet 352:234-5, 1998

Saito N, Kuchiba A. The changes of magnesium under high salt diets and by administration of antihypertensive diuretics. Magnesium Bull 9:53, 1987

Salzer HM. Relative hypoglycemia as a cause of neuropsychiatric illness. J Natl Med Assoc 58(1):12-17, 1966

Schorah CJ et al. Clinical effects of vitamin C in elderly inpatients with low blood-vitamin C levels. Lancet i:403-5, 1979

Schultz BM, Freedman ML. Iron deficiency in the elderly. Baillieres Clin Haematol 1(2):291-313, 1987

Silverman K et al. Withdrawal syndrome after the double-blind cessation of caffeine consumption. N Engl J Med 327:1109-14, 1992

Smidt LJ et al. Influence of thiamin supplementation on the health and general well-being of an elderly Irish population with marginal thiamin deficiency. J Gerontol 46(1):M16-M22, 1991

Snively WD, Westerman RL. Minn Med June, 1965

Spring B et al. Psychobiological effects of carbohydrates. J Clin Psychiatry 50 Suppl:27-33, 1989

Thayer RE. Energy, tiredness, and tension effects of a sugar snack versus moderate exercise. J Pers Soc Psychol 52(1):119-25, 1987

Uchizyama M et al. Effects of vitamin B12 on human circadian body temperature rhythm. Neurosci Lett 192:1-4, 1995

Valverde E et al. In vitro response of lymphocytes in patients with allergic tension-fatigue syndrome. Ann Allergy 4593):185-8, 1980

Wakefield AJ et al. Ileal-lymphoid-nodular hyperplasia, non-specific colitis, and pervasive developmental disorder in children. Lancet 351:637-41, 1988

Weinberg EG, Tuchinda M. Allergic tension-fatigue syndrome. Ann Allergy 31:209-11, 1973

Wright JV. A case of weak muscles. Prevention October, 1974, pp. 113-20

Wright JV. A case of tiredness. Prevention September, 1979, pp. 68-72

Wright JV. A case of apathy and depression. Prevention June, 1984a

Wright JV. A case of iron deficiency without anemia. Prevention November, 1984b

Wright JV. The healing powers of zinc. Let's Live, March, 1989

Yamabe H, Fukuzaki H, in K Folkers, GP Littarru, Y Yamagami, Eds. Biochemical and Clinical Aspects of Coenzyme Q, Volume 6. Amsterdam, Elsevier Science Pub., 1991:535-40

Zeppilli P et al, in K Folkers, GP Littarru, Y Yamagami, Eds. Biochemical and Clinical Aspects of Coenzyme Q, Volume 6. Amsterdam, Elsevier Science Pub., 1991:541-5

FIBROMYALGIA

(MUSCULAR RHEUMATISM)

See Also: MUSCLE CRAMPS (FUNCTIONAL)
PAIN

NUTRITIONAL TREATMENT GUIDE

✓ = Efficacy generally accepted.
* = Efficacy *demonstrated* by controlled human trials.
[+] = Efficacy *suspected* from uncontrolled human trials.
[-] = Efficacy *suspected* from indirect data.
? = Efficacy *challenged* in a study of similar design.

NUTRITIONAL FACTORS

* **L-5-Hydroxytryptophan:** 100 mg 3 times daily (30 day trial)
* **Selenium deficiency:** 90 to 200 μg daily *AND*
Vitamin E: 20 to 100 mg daily
* ? **Magnesium:** 600 mg daily *AND*
Malic acid: 2400 mg daily (8 week trial)
* ? **S-adenosyl-L-Methionine:** 600-1,200 mg daily (Full benefits may take several wks. or months.)

- -

[+] **Lithium:** lithium carbonate 300 mg 2 to 4 times daily as an adjunct to antidepressant drugs
[+] **Thiamine:** thiamine pyrophosphate 50 mg IM 3 times weekly *AND*
Vitamin B_6 (6 week trial)
[+] **Vitamin E:** mixed tocopherols 100 mg 3 times daily initially, then reduce dose as tolerated.

- -

[-] **L-Tryptophan:** 1 to 6 g daily

OTHER RELATED FACTORS

[+] rule out **Food Sensitivities** (especially member of the nightshade family)

Fibromyalgia is a chronic, painful, musculoskeletal condition characterized by widespread aching and points of tenderness associated with:

1) changed perception of pain, abnormal sleep patterns and reduced brain serotonin, and

2) abnormalities in the microcirculation and muscle energy metabolism *(Eisinger, 1994a)*.

NUTRITIONAL FACTORS

VITAMINS

Thiamine

Based on the mean transketolate activity coefficient, thiamine nutritional status may be impaired. This impairment does not appear to be due to the experience of pain, as patients with osteoarticular pain do not show a similar abnormality *(Eisinger,1992)*.

In an open trial, all but one of 21 patients had good results following intramuscular administration of thiamine, while 5 out of 13 patients reported good results following intramuscular administration of thiamine hydrochloride. The authors speculate that the better clinical response to thiamine pyrophosphate may mean that patients have an abnormality in thiamine metabolism rather than a dietary thiamine deficiency *(Eisinger,1988)*. Controlled studies are needed to confirm these findings.

As vitamin B_6 supplementation helps to normalize erythrocyte transketolase activity (a functional measure of thiamine status) in this patient group, it may be of additional value *(Eisinger,1994b)*.

Vitamin E

While blood vitamin E level is usually normal, the utilization curve is a plateau pattern, indicating difficulty in utilization *(Steinberg)*. Moreover, fibromyalgia is particularly common among menopausal women. The need for vitamin E is tremendously increased in this population, especially if estrogen replacement is given *(Anonymous)*.

Back in 1949, vitamin E supplementation was reported to be helpful in alleviating fibromyalgic symptoms in a clinical setting. Three hundred middle-aged patients with generalized primary fibrositis who had failed to respond to a barbiturate sedative received mixed natural tocopherols. The vast majority were said to respond. After clinical cure was obtained, most patients required a maintenance dose *(Steinberg)*.

These promising findings have yet to be confirmed in a controlled clinical trial.

MINERALS

Lithium

Patients with fibromyalgia who are ingesting trycyclic antidepressants may benefit from pharmacologic doses of lithium in the form of lithium carbonate. In one report, 3 patients on tricyclic antidepressants experienced prompt and marked reduction of pain and stiffness when lithium carbonate was added *(Tyber)*.

Whether a pharmacologic dosage of lithium is effective by itself, as well as whether a nutritional dosage of lithium is effective, is unknown.

Magnesium Deficiency

Several studies have linked magnesium deficiency with fibromyalgia, as both are associated with myalgias, fatigue, sleep disturbance and anxiety *(Romano)*. The magnesium loading test may show evidence of low magnesium status *(Moorkens)*. Erythrocyte magnesium levels may be decreased *(Romano)*, although leukocyte levels may be elevated *(Eisinger,1994c)*. Plasma magnesium concentrations, which are less sensitive indicators of magnesium status, appear to be normal, however *(Romano)*.

Fibromyalgia has been theorized to result from a defect in ATP synthesis. Magnesium deficiency could contribute to this defect by creating a sluggish respiratory chain and a decreased efficiency in the transfer of reducing equivalents from the cytosol to the mitochondria *(Abraham)*.

Supplementation: Magnesium & Malic Acid

While the efficacy of magnesium supplementation is not known, magnesium has been combined with malic acid in several studies, as malate plays an important role in generating mitochondrial ATP. Results of controlled trials have been mixed. When patients were treated for an average of 8 weeks, their tender point index scores were reduced by more than half. They were switched to placebo. Within 48 hours, they experienced worsening of muscle pain and, after 2 weeks, the tender point index scores had returned to baseline *(Abraham)*.

These findings contrast with those of a double-blind crossover study in which patients received magnesium and malic acid at the lower end of the dosage range used in the previous study for 4 weeks each with a 2-week washout in between. Magnesium malate was no more effective than placebo as assessed by pain, tenderness, and functional and psychological measures *(Russell)*.

A future trial will hopefully further examine whether a larger dosage and longer trial period lead to a significant treatment effect.

Selenium Deficiency

While selenium nutriture in fibromyalgia is uncertain, selenium deficiency appears to be associated with muscle pain *(van Rij)*. For example, middle-aged women with sustained pains in the back and shoulder had reduced serum selenium levels *(James)*.

Further evidence that selenium nutriture may be relevant to fibromyalgia comes from a study of residents of areas of New Zealand where soil selenium levels are low who presented with fibromuscular rheumatism. They were treated with selenium as selenomethionine or with placebo under double-blind conditions. After 12 weeks 58% of the patients in the selenium group improved compared to 36% of the controls. While these results failed to reach statistical significance, they are suggestive of an effect *(Robinson)*.

Selenium deficiency syndromes overlap with those of vitamin E and, because of their closely related mechanisms of action, most can be treated successfully with either nutrient *(Combs)*. Therefore the combination of selenium and vitamin E has been explored. The results of two such studies, both double-blind, suggest that the selenium supplement is beneficial. One of these studies involved patients with chronically disabling muscular pain, stiffness and aching. Following supplementation, mean pain score reduction was significantly more frequent and more marked among patients whose (selenium-dependent) glutathione peroxidase levels increased than among those whose levels decreased *(Jameson)*.

In the other study, middle-aged women with sustained pains in the back and shoulder received supplementation along with physiotherapy. Women whose initial serum selenium was high, or whose serum selenium rose, were more often improved by physiotherapy than the other women *(James)*.

OTHER NUTRITIONAL FACTORS

L-5-Hydroxytryptophan

Supplementation with the tryptophan metabolite, 5-hydroxytryptophan, has been shown to be beneficial. In a double-blind study, 30 days after supplementation there were significant declines in the number of tender points and in the intensity of subjective pain, as well as significant improvements in morning stiffness, sleep patterns, anxiety and fatigue *(Caruso)*.

A 42-year-old homemaker had gone from doctor to doctor for 5 years looking for a cure for chronic pain. Ibuprofen severely upset her stomach, and she had tried antidepressants, special diets, and supplements. She reported having strong cravings for sweets, suffered from frequent headaches, and had trouble falling and staying asleep.

She was placed on 50 mg 5-hydroxytryptophan (5-HTP) 3 times daily for the first 2 weeks and 100 mg 3 times daily thereafter. In addition, she was prescribed St. John's wort extract 300 mg 3 times daily, a high-potency multiple vitamin and mineral formula, an additional 400 IU of vitamin E, and 500 mg 3 times daily of vitamin C, plus magnesium 250 mg 3 times daily and a daily tablespoon of flaxseed oil.

After 6 weeks, her mood was better and her sleep had improved, but she hadn't noticed much improvement in her pain. After 3 months of treatment, she said she was cured. She was told to continue the program for 3 more months and then to stop the St. John's wort and the extra magnesium and to reduce the 5-HTP dosage to 150 mg at bedtime.

After another 3 months, she tried to gradually taper off of the 5-HTP over the course of a month. However, a few days after she stopped it completely, her fibromyalgia returned "with a vengeance." She again started on 5-HTP 150 mg at bedtime and experienced complete relief after only 3 nights. Later she was able to reduce her dosage to 50 mg each night without any change in symptoms (Murray).

L-Tryptophan

Plasma tryptophan levels have been reported to be reduced in fibromyalgia *(Yunus)*. Moreover, in one study of patients severe fibrositis syndrome, plasma free tryptophan levels were inversely related to the severity of subjective pain *(Moldofsky)*.

While the efficacy of supplementation in fibromyalgia has not been explored, there is evidence that L-tryptophan has an analgesic effect (see Pain).

S-Adenosyl-L-Methionine

The efficacy of S-adenosyl-L-methionine (SAMe) has been explored in double-blind studies. In one of the studies, the number of trigger points plus painful anatomic sites decreased, and both depression scales improved, only after SAMe supplementation *(Tavoni)*. In another, improvements were seen for clinical disease activity, pain during the last week, fatigue, morning stiffness and mood in the SAMe group versus placebo, although the tender point scores, isokinetic strength and mood scores were similar in the 2 groups *(Jacobsen)*.

The third study found a trend towards statistical significance in favor of SAMe for pain at rest and upon movement, as well as for overall well-being; however, there were no significant findings *(Volkmann)*.

OTHER RELATED FACTORS

Food Sensitivities

Food sensitivities have long been reported to cause aching and soreness in muscles, usually along with fatigue and mental symptoms *(Rowe)*. One particular family of foods that has been accused of causing muscle spasms, pain, stiffness and inflammation are the nightshades *(Childers)*. Member of this genus (Solanaceae) include the white potato, the tomato, eggplant, all peppers (except black) and tobacco.

Unfortunately, although there are numerous anecdotal reports of improvement in musculoskeletal complaints after following a nightshade-free diet for several months, research exploring this hypothesis is yet to be reported.

BIBLIOGRAPHY

Abraham GE, Flechas JD. Hypothesis: Management of fibromyalgia: rationale for the use of magnesium and malic acid. J Nutr Med 3:49-59, 1992

Anonymous. Editorial. JAMA 167:1896, 1958

Caruso I et al. Double-blind study of 5-hydroxytryptophan versus placebo in the treatment of primary fibromyalgia syndrome. J Int Med Res 18(3):201-9, 1990

Childers NF, Margoles MS. An apparent relation of nightshades (Solanacceae) to arthritis. J Neurol Orthop Med Surg 14:227-31, 1993

Combs GF. Assessment of vitamin E status in animals and man. Proc Nutr Soc 40:187-94, 1981

Eisinger J et al. Donnees actuelles sur les fibromyalgies: traitment des fibromyalgies primitives par la cocarboxylase. Lyon Med Med 24:11585-6, 1988 (in French)

Eisinger J et al. Studies of transketolase in chronic pain. J Adv Med 5(2):105-13, 1992

Eisinger J et al. Glycolysis abnormalities in fibromyalgia. J Am Coll Nutr 13(2):144-8, 1994a

Eisinger J et al. Effects of magnesium, high energy phosphates, piracetam and thiamin on erythrocyte transketolase. Magnes Res 7(1):59-61, 1994b

Eisinger J et al. Selenium and magnesium status in fibromyalgia. Magnes Res 7(3-4):285-8, 1994c

Jacobsen S et al. Oral S-adenosylmethionine in primary fibromyalgia. Double-blind clinical evaluation. Scand J Rheumatol 20(4):294-302, 1991

James S et al. Effekter av selenvitamin E-behandling till kvinnor med lang variga arbetsrelaterade nack-och skuldersmartor. En dubbelblindstudie. Lakaresallskapets Riksstamma, 1985 (in Swedish)

Jameson S et al. Pain relief and selenium balance in patients with connective tissue disease and osteoarthrosis: A double-blind selenium tocopherol supplementation study. Nutr Res Suppl:391-7, 1985

Moldofsky H, Warsh JJ. Plasma tryptophan and musculoskeletal pain in non-articular rheumatism ('fibrositis syndrome'). Pain 5(1):65-71, 1978

Moorkens G et al. Magnesium deficit in a sample of the Belgian population presenting with chronic fatigue. Magnes Res 10(4):329-37, 1997

Murray MT. 5-HTP: The Natural Way to Overcome Depression, Obesity, and Insomnia. New York, Bantam Books, 1998

Robinson MF et al. Effect of daily supplements of selenium on patients with muscular complaints in Otago and Canterbury. N Z Med J 289-92, 1981

Romano TJ, Stiller JW. Magnesium deficiency in fibromyalgia syndrome. J Nutr Med 4:165-7, 1994

Rowe AH. Allergic fatigue and toxemia. Ann Allergy 17:9-18, 1959

Russell IJ et al. Treatment of fibromyalgia syndrome with Super Malic®: a randomized, double blind, placebo controlled, crossover pilot study. J Rheumatol 22:953-8, 1995

Steinberg CL. Vitamin E and collagen in the rheumatic diseases. Ann NY Acad Sci 52:380-9, 1949

Tavoni A et al. The evaluation of S-adenosylmethionine in primary fibromyalgia. A double-blind crossover study. Am J Med 83(SA):107-10, 1987

Tyber M. Lithium augmentation therapy in fibromyalgia. Can Med Assoc J 143(9):902-4, 1990

van Rij Am et al. Selenium deficiency in total parenteral nutrition. Am J Clin Nutr 32:2076-85, 1979

Volkmann H et al. Double-blind, placebo-controlled cross-over study of intravenous S-adenosyl-L-methionine in patients with fibromyalgia. Scand J Rheumatol 26(3):206-11, 1997

Yunus B et al. Plasma tryptophan and other amino acids in primary fibromyalgia: a controlled study. J Rheumatol 19(1):90-4, 1992

GALLBLADDER DISEASE

NUTRITIONAL TREATMENT GUIDE

✓ = Efficacy generally accepted.
* = Efficacy *demonstrated* by controlled human trials.
[+] = Efficacy *suspected* from uncontrolled human trials.
[-] = Efficacy *suspected* from indirect data.
? = Efficacy *challenged* in a study of similar design.

I. *TO REDUCE THE RISK OF GALLSTONES*

DIETARY FACTORS

[-] **Do not skip meals**
[-] **Vegetarian** diet
[-] avoid **dietary Cholesterol**
[-] moderate **Fat** intake
[-] avoid **Legumes**
[-] ? moderate **Alcohol** consumption
[-] ? avoid high **Animal Fat** intake
[-] ? moderate **Coffee** consumption
[-] ? minimize **Sugar**

NUTRITIONAL FACTORS

[-] **Calcium:** ≈ 1 g daily
[-] rule out **Essential Fatty Acid** deficiency
[-] **Iron deficiency:** 30 mg twice daily until repletion; then minimal maintenance dosage
[-] **Taurine**: 40 μmol/kg daily
[-] **Vitamin C**: 500 mg 4 times daily
[-] **Vitamin E**: D-alpha tocopherol 200 mg 3 times daily

OTHER RELATED FACTORS

[+] avoid **Obesity**

- -

[-] rule out **Hydrochloric Acid deficiency**

II. *TO AVOID GALLBLADDER COLIC*

[+] rule out **Food Sensitivities**
[+] avoid **Chili**
[+] avoid **Coffee**
[+] minimize **Fatty Foods**
[+] avoid **Oranges**

III. *TO REDUCE SECONDARY SYMPTOMS OF FLATULENT DYSPEPSIA*

[+] **Betaine Hydrochloride:** dosage uncertain. Suggestion: Take one to five 10 mg capsules per meal as needed at the end of the meal. (Reduce dosage in the event of gastric irritation.)

DIETARY FACTORS

Diet appears to have a major influence on the development and course of cholelithiasis. In fact, the frequency and regularity of meals appears to influence risk. Gallstone patients may have longer periods of fasting than normals. As food stimulates gallbladder contractions, the resulting gallbladder stasis would favor the formation and growth of gallstones *(Hoffmann;Ortega)*.

In one study, women who skipped breakfast or had only coffee were found to have a much greater incidence of gallstones than those who ate a morning meal *(Capron)*. In another study, gallstone patients were found to eat fewer meals per day than normals (*Ortega*). However, in a study of more than 1,000 blood donors, gallstone prevalence was unrelated to both the regularity and number of daily meals *(Kratzer)*.

Dietary Fat

Both a high intake of total calories and a high intake of fat are directly related to the risk of gallstones *(Ortega)*. Moreover, among patients with biliary disease and chronic upper abdominal pain, the ingestion of fatty foods often causes acute pain *(Kang)*.

Animal Fat

The type of fat ingested may make a difference. When a group of patients with cholelithiasis were compared to age- and sex-matched controls with regard to the frequency of consumption of over 100 food items, the only ones that correlated positively with the disease was the consumption of animal fat and using butter on the table, while high consumption of olive oil was protective *(Linos)*.

Similarly, when the incidence of gallstones found at autopsy was compared to diets, so long was the total daily energy intake was below 3,000 calories there was a striking correlation between the intake of animal fats and the incidence of gallstones, while vegetable fat intake was only slightly correlated with gallstone incidence *(Sarles)*.

Not all evidence implicates animal fat intake in the etiology of gallstones, however, as a study of almost 90,000 middle-aged women failed to find a significant association between the energy-adjusted intake of animal fat and the relative risk of symptomatic gallstones *(Maclure)*.

Dietary Cholesterol

Findings concerning dietary cholesterol are similar to those concerning animal fat. A review by the Committee on Diet and Health under the auspices of the National Academy of Sciences (US) concluded that, despite the obvious logic relating cholesterol intake to cholesterol gallstones, the variability in results suggests that only a relatively few persons are sensitive to the lithogenic effects of dietary cholesterol *(Comm. on Diet & Health)*.

Since then, while observational studies have continued to have opposing findings *(Moerman;Ortega)*, there has been new experimental evidence implicating dietary cholesterol in cholesterol gallstone formation. A group of women were studied both on regular diets and on the same diet supplemented with 5 eggs daily for 15 to 18 days. In the sub-group of women who had gallstones, increasing dietary cholesterol was found to increase biliary cholesterol secretion and to decrease bile acid synthesis and pool, changes known to be associated with cholesterol gallstone formation *(Kern)*.

Dietary Fiber

Several observational studies have found an inverse correlation between dietary fiber intake and cholelithiasis *(Ortega)*, although the evidence is conflicting. Also, experimental studies have found a higher fiber intake to decrease the bile saturation index *(Thornton,1983; McDougall)*. However, in a double-blind study of high-risk patients, the risk of gallstone recurrence was not reduced by a high fiber, low refined carbohydrate diet as compared to placebo *(Hood)*.

If dietary fiber is beneficial, its efficacy may be related to its effect on intestinal transit time. Women with gallstones but without known risk factors (such as obesity) appear to have slow intestinal transit times, a condition that may promote gallstones by encouraging high biliary proportions of the secondary bile salt deoxycholate. This bile salt promotes hepatic cholesterol secretion more strongly than other bile salts and favors the nucleation of cholesterol crystals *(Heaton)*.

Vegetarian Diet

A vegetarian diet, low in animal fat and cholesterol and high in fiber, appears to be protective. Vegetarians have roughly half the incidence of gallstones of omnivores *(Maclure;Pixley)*. However, increasing fruit, vegetables and fiber in an omnivorous diet appears to confer the same benefit *(Nair)*.

Legumes

Legumes are one source of dietary fiber which appears to be contraindicated in cholesterol gallstone patients. Chileans and North American Indians have one of the highest prevalence rates of cholesterol gallstones in the world, and legumes are common foods consumed by both populations *(Nervi)*. Legume intake has now been shown to promote the saturation of bile by cholesterol in two controlled studies *(Duane;Nervi)*.

Their consumption appears to lower LDL cholesterol levels by partially interrupting the enterohepatic circulation of bile acids. By increasing hepatic cholesterol secretion, they increase biliary cholesterol saturation *(Duane)*.

Sugar

Numerous observational studies have found sugar intake to be directly correlated with the risk of gallstones *(Montalto;Ortega)*. Experimental studies have shown that, when sugar is chronically consumed in high amounts, biliary cholesterol secretion is enhanced through elevation of triglyceride levels and reduction of HDL-lipoprotein levels *(Moerman)*.

Moreover, excess sugar consumption would theoretically increase gallstone risk by increasing the risks of obesity and hyperinsulinemia. These conditions would tend to increase cholesterol saturation of the bile and decrease bile acid synthesis *(Ortega)*.

Alcohol

The majority of observational studies have found alcohol consumption to be associated with a reduced risk of cholelithiasis *(Kratzer;La Vecchia)*. While the mechanism is unclear, this effect may be due to reduced secretion of bile cholesterol *(LaVecchia)*.

However, due to its many adverse effects at higher levels of intake, alcohol consumption should be limited.

Caffeine and Coffee

In an animal study, caffeine administration resulted in changes, such as increased hepatic bile flow, which should inhibit gallstone formation *(Lillemoe)*. Coffee, however, regardless of caffeine content, may cause gallbladder colic in gallstone patients *(Kang)* due to stimulation of gallbladder contractions *(Douglas)*.

Specific Foods and the Frequency of Colic

We have already noted that the intake of fatty foods and coffee may provoke gallbladder colic. In one study, fatty foods provoked pain in 40% of patients, chili in 25 to 50% of patients, orange in 17% of patients and coffee in 14% of patients *(Kang)*.

NUTRITIONAL FACTORS

VITAMINS

Vitamin C

When given a high cholesterol diet, animals made vitamin C-deficient are prone to developing gallstones *(Jenkins,1978)*. This may be due to lower ratios of bile acids to cholesterol, and of phospholipids to cholesterol in the bile *(Jenkins,1980)*.

There is early evidence that ascorbic acid supplementation may reduce the risk of gallstones in humans. When gallstone patients scheduled for cholecystectomy were treated with the vitamin for 2 weeks before surgery, nucleation time, while shorter than for gallstone-free subjects, was longer than in the untreated controls. (A short nucleation time is strongly correlated with cholesterol crystal and gallstone formation.) Moreover, the percentage of cholic acid was lower and the percentages of deoxycholic acid, ursodeoxycholic acid, and lithocholic acid were higher in the bile of the vitamin C-treated patients compared to the controls *(Gustafsson)*.

In a cross-sectional analysis involving 2744 postmenopausal women, ascorbic acid supplement use was associated with a decreased prevalence of gallbladder disease and a trend toward a decreased prevalence of cholecystectomy. Further analysis, however, showed these correlations to be limited to drinkers *(Simon)*, possibly because they are more likely to be ascorbate-deficient.

Vitamin E

Like vitamin C, a deficiency of vitamin E is associated, at least in animals, with gallstone formation. While adequate vitamin E nutriture protects against the formation of gallstones in animals given large amounts of cholesterol or fat *(Christensen)*, vitamin E-deficient animals develop cholesterol stones even while on a fat-free, cholesterol-free diet *(Dam,1956)*.

In one study, cholesterol stones which developed when the animals were given a vitamin E-deficient diet dissolved when vitamin E was given *(Dam,1952)*. The results of these studies suggest that vitamin E nutriture may be more relevant in the etiology of cholesterol gallstones than are dietary fat and cholesterol.

Five patients with cholesterol gallstones who were supplemented with D-alpha tocopherol 200 mg three times daily had reduced biliary cholesterol levels and increased glycine-conjugated bile acids, with a corresponding improvement in the lithogenic index *(Saito)*. Further trials are needed to confirm these intriguing findings.

MINERALS

Calcium

The dietary intake of calcium is inversely associated with the risk of gallstone formation *(Moerman,1994;Ortega)*. Cholesterol saturation of the bile is known to promote gallstone formation. Calcium appears to reduce risk by binding secondary bile acids (chenodeoxycholic acid and deoxycholic acid) in the colon that are then subsequently excreted with the feces, thus reducing biliary saturation with cholesterol *(Moerman,1995)*.

Iron Deficiency

Animals receiving an iron-deficient diet have been shown to be more likely to have cholesterol crystals in their bile than controls. This finding may explain why cholesterol gallstones occur most commonly in multiparous women, a population that is prone to chronic iron deficiency anemia *(Johnston)*.

OTHER NUTRITIONAL FACTORS

Essential Fatty Acid Deficiency

Animal work has shown that a dietary deficiency of essential fatty acids results in gallstone formation *(Robins)*.

Omega-3 Fatty Acids

Both animal and human studies have explored the efficacy of omega-3 essential fatty acids in preventing cholelithiasis. Animals studies have found that both fish oils *(Magnuson)* and an ethyl ester of eicosapentaenoic acid *(Mizuguchi)* reduced gallstone formation.

The results of human trials have been less conclusive. In healthy males *(Wechsler)*, and in patients with gallstones *(Berr)*, supplementation reduced the cholesterol saturation index. However, the *in vitro* nucleation time of duodenal bile not prolonged in the gallstone patients, suggesting that the decrease in cholesterol saturation was insufficient to prevent nucleation of cholesterol crystals in bile *(Berr)*.

The results of another study are of greater concern. In this study, following the daily administration of fish oil, nucleation time was unchanged in cholesterol gallstone patients, and was *decreased* from an average of 12.1 days to 2 days in normal subjects, suggesting that fish oil could actually promote gallstone formation in normals *(Janowitz)*.

Further studies are clearly needed before omega-3 fatty acid supplementation should be recommended for the prevention of gallstones.

Taurine

Bile acids are often conjugated with taurine *(Vessey)*. In animal studies, taurine supplementation inhibits the formation of cholesterol gallstones due to a lithogenic diet by increasing the synthesis of bile acids *(Nakamura-Yamanaka)*. In humans, taurine supplementation has been shown to enhance the secretion and conjugation of bile acids under controlled conditions *(Wang)*, thus suggesting that it may inhibit cholesterol gallstone formation.

OTHER RELATED FACTORS

Obesity

Obesity increases the risk of symptomatic gallstones *(Maclure)*. The loss of excess weight may thus be beneficial. However, excessively rapid loss due to ingestion of very-low-calorie diets can actually increase the rate of gallstone formation, probably because of gallbladder stasis due to the lack of a fat challenge to the gallbladder *(Klawansky)*. This complication appears to be preventable by restricting weight loss to less than 1.5 kg (3.3lb) per week *(Weinsier)*.

A 41-year-old woman who was 55 pounds overweight had a large gallstone. She went on a 1,000 calorie diet and, after 15 months, she had lost 42 pounds and her gallstone had disappeared. Four months later, she was down to her ideal weight and her gallbladder was functioning normally (Thornton, 1979).

Food Sensitivities

Food sensitivities are an often unrecognized cause of gallbladder symptoms. In an open trial, 69 patients with gallstones or a post-cholecystectomy syndrome were placed on an elimination diet consisting of beef, rye, soy, rice, cherry, peach, apricot, beet and spinach. After one week, additional foods were added systematically, and each symptom-provoking food was re-tested several times. *All* patients were relieved of their symptoms, with improvements usually occurring in 3 to 5 days. Egg was by far the most frequent offender (93%), followed by pork (64%) and onion (52%) *(Brennerman)*.

There is also evidence from a 1940 study that gallbladder spasm may be associated with classical atopic symptoms. When offending foods were ingested, gallbladder emptying was disturbed usually within 2 hours, as evidenced by measurements of its size. This was associated with both typical symptoms of gallbladder colic and allergic symptoms such as shortness of breath, sneezing, headaches and hives *(Necheles)*.

A woman presented with a 10-year history of indigestion after some meals which gradually worsened until she was having right-sided pain under her ribs. She reduced her fat intake which helped slightly. Two years prior to evaluation, she awoke in the middle of the night after an unusually large meal with intense pain which was diagnosed as cholecystitis. The symptoms continued to worsen until she was bedridden 4 to 5 days each month. She eliminated all fats, oils and spices from her diet without improvement. X-rays revealed 2 gallbladder stones.

She began a food elimination diet which restricted her to beef, rye, soy, rice, cherry, peach, apricot, beet and spinach. One week later, she reported that she had had no pain for three days. She was told to reintroduce foods singly and found that ingestion of eggs, chicken, coffee, peanuts, onions, carrots and wheat provoked gallbladder pain. Two years later, she reported that she had remained fully asymptomatic (Wright).

Hydrochloric Acid Deficiency

The formation of gallstones appears to be associated with the reflux of bile and pancreatic juices into the stomach. These juices can destroy the oxyntic cells, causing gastric hyposecretion. The result is flatulent dyspepsia as well as other symptoms of hydrochloric acid deficiency. About half of all patients with gallstones are deficient in hydrochloric acid as evidenced by the augmented histamine test *(Capper)*.

In an open trial, hydrochloric acid supplementation occasionally relieved symptoms of flatulence, epigastric fullness and burning, diarrhea and urticaria in patients with histamine-fast achlorhydria. It had no effect, however, on food sensitivities or such symptoms as nausea, abdominal pain, constipation, bad breath, burning tongue or metallic taste *(Rappaport)*.

Because hypochlorhydria has adverse effects on nutrient metabolism, and increases both susceptibility to and severity of bacterial enteric infections, hydrochloric acid supplementation is suggested for all patients with histamine-fast hypochlorhydria.

BIBLIOGRAPHY

Berr F et al. Dietary N-3 polyunsaturated fatty acids decrease biliary cholesterol saturation in gallstone disease. Hepatology 16(4):960-7, 1992

Brenneman JC. Allergy elimination diet as the most effective gallbladder diet. Ann Allergy 26:83, 1968

Capper WM et al. Gallstones, gastric secretion, and flatulent dyspepsia. Lancet i:413-15, 1967

Capron JP et al. Meal frequency and duration of overnight fast: A role in gall-stone formation? Br Med J 283:1435, 1981

Christensen F et al. Acta Physiol Scand 27:315, 1952

Committee on Diet and Health, Food and Nutrition Board, National Research Council. Diet and Health: Implications for Reducing Chronic Disease Risk. Washington, D.C., National Academy Press, 1989

Dam H et al. Acta Pathol Microbiol Scand 30:256, 1952

Dam H et al. Acta Physiol Scand 36:329, 1956

Douglas BR et al. Coffee stimulation of cholecystokinin release and gallbladder contraction in humans. Am J Clin Nutr 52:553-6, 1990

Duane WC. Effects of legume consumption on serum cholesterol, biliary lipids, and sterol metabolism in humans. J Lipid Res 38(6):1120-8, 1997

Gustafsson U et al. The effect of vitamin C in high doses on plasma and biliary lipid composition in patients with cholesterol gallstones: prolongation of the nucleation time. Eur J Clin Invest 27:387-91, 1997

Heaton KW et al. An explanation for gallstones in normal-weight women: slow intestinal transit. Lancet 341:8-10, 1993

Hoffmann AF. Primary and secondary prevention of gallstone disease: implications for patient management and research priorities. Am J Surg 165(4):541-8, 1993

Hood KA et al. Gall stone recurrence and its prevention: the British/Belgian Gall Stone Study Group's post-dissolution trial. Gut 34(9):1277-88, 1993

Janowitz P et al. Fish oil, enriched with polyunsaturated fatty acids of the omega-3-type accelerates the nucleation time in healthy subjects. Klin Wochenschr 69(7):289-93, 1991

Jenkins SA. Biliary lipids, bile acids and gallstone formation in hypovitaminotic C guinea-pigs. Br J Nutr 40:317-22, 1978

Jenkins SA. Vitamin C status, serum cholesterol levels and bile composition in the pregnant guinea-pig. Br J Nutr 43(1):95-100, 1980

Johnston SM et al. Iron deficiency enhances cholesterol gallstone formation. Surgery 122(2):354-61, 1997

Kang JY et al. Chronic upper abdominal pain: site and radiation in various and functional disorders and the effect of various foods. Gut 33(6):743-8, 1992

Kern F Jr. Effects of dietary cholesterol on cholesterol and bile acid homeostasis in patients with cholesterol gallstones. J Clin Invest 93(3):1186-94, 1994

Klawansky S, Chalmers TC. Fat content of very-low-calorie diets and gallstone formation. Letter. JAMA 268(7):873, 1992

Kratzer W et al. Gallstone prevalence in relation to smoking, alcohol, coffee consumption, and nutrition. The Ulm Gallstone Study. Scand J Gastroenterol 32(9):953-8, 1997

La Vecchia C et al. Alcohol drinking and prevalence of self-reported gallstone disease in 1983 Italian National Health Survey. Epidemiology 5:533-6, 1994

Lillemoe KD et al. Caffeine prevents cholesterol gallstone formation. Surgery 106(2):400-07, 1989

Linos AD et al. Dietary and other risk factors in the aetiology of cholelithiasis: a case control study. HPB Surg 1(3):221-7, 1989

Maclure KM et al. Dietary predictors of symptom-associated gallstones in middle-aged women. Am J Clin Nutr 52:916-22, 1990

Magnuson TH et al. Dietary fish oil inhibits cholesterol monohydrate crystal nucleation and gallstone formation in the prairie dog. Surgery 118(3):517-23, 1995

McDougall RM et al. Effect of wheat bran on serum lipoproteins and biliary lipids. Can J Surg 21:433, 1978

Mizuguchi K et al. [Preventive effects of eicosapentaenoic acid (EPA) on cholesterol gallstone formation in hamsters]. Nippon Yakurigaku Zasshi 110 Suppl 1:50P-55P, 1997) (in Japanese)

Moerman CJ et al. Dietary risk factors for clinically diagnosed gallstones in middle-aged men. A 25-year follow-up study (The Zutphen Study). Ann Epidemiol 4(3):248-54, 1994

Moerman CJ et al. Consumption of foods and micronutrients and the risk of cancer of the biliary-tract. Prev Med 24(6):591-602, 1995

Montalto G et al. Diet and gallstones in women of a rural town of Sicily. J Nutr Environ Med 7:101-6, 1997

Nair P, Mayberry JF. Vegetarianism, dietary fibre and gastro-intestinal disease. Dig Dis 12(3):177-85, 1994

Nakamura-Yamanaka Y et al. Effect of dietary taurine on cholesterol 7 alpha-hydroxylase activity in the liver of mice fed a lithogenic diet. J Nutr Sci Vitaminol (Tokyo) 33(3):239-43, 1987

Necheles H et al. Allergy of the gallbladder: A study using the Graham-Cole test and the leukopenic index. Am J Dig Dis 7:238, 1940

Nervi F et al. Influence of legume intake on biliary lipids and cholesterol saturation in young Chilean men. Gastroenterology 96:825-30, 1989

Ortega RM et al. Differences in diet and food habits between patients with gallstones and controls. J Am Coll Nutr 16(1):88-95, 1997

Pixley F et al. Effect of vegetarianism on development of gall stones in women. Br Med J 291:11-12, 1985

Rappaport EM. Achlorhydria: Associated symptoms and response to hydrochloric acid. N Engl J Med 252:802-05, 1955

Robins SJ, Fasulo J. Mechanism of lithogenic bile production: studies in the hamster fed an essential fatty acid-deficient diet. Gastroenterology 65:104-14, 1973

Saito T, Tanimura H. The preventive effect of vitamin E on gallstone formation. (3). A study of the biliary lipids in patients with gallstones. Arch Jpn Chir 56(3):276-88, 1987

Sarles H et al. Diet and cholesterol gallstones: A multicenter study. Digestion 17(2):121-7, 1978

Simon JA et al. Ascorbic acid supplement use and the prevalence of gallbladder disease. Heart & Estrogen-Progestin Replacement Study (HERS) Research Group. J Clin Epidemiol 1(3):257-65, 1998

Thornton JR. Gallstone disappearance associated with weight loss. Letter. Lancet ii:478, 1979

Thornton JR et al. Diet and gallstones: Effects of refined carbohydrates on bile cholesterol saturation and bile acid metabolism. Gut 24:2-6, 1983

Vessey DA. The biochemical basis for the conjugation of bile acids with either glycine or taurine. Biochem J 174:621-6, 1978

Wang WY, Liaw KY. Effect of a taurine-supplemented diet on conjugated bile acids in biliary surgical patients. JPEN J Parenter Enteral Nutr 15(3):294-7, 1991

Wechsler JG et al. [Effect of omega-3-fatty acids on biliary lipids and lithogenicity]. Z Gastroenterol 1989 May;27(5):254-7, 1989) (in German)

Weinsier R et al. Medically safe rate of weight loss for the treatment of obesity: A guideline based on risk of gallstone formation. Am J Med 98:115-17, 1995

Wright JV. A case of gallbladder pain and allergy. Prevention September, 1980, pp. 67-71

GLAUCOMA

NUTRITIONAL TREATMENT GUIDE

✓ = Efficacy generally accepted.
* = Efficacy *demonstrated* by controlled human trials.
[+] = Efficacy *suspected* from uncontrolled human trials.
[-] = Efficacy *suspected* from indirect data.
? = Efficacy *challenged* in a study of similar design.

DIETARY FACTORS

* ? avoid **Caffeine**

[+] avoid **rapid ingestion of large volumes of fluid**

NUTRITIONAL FACTORS

* **Vitamin C**: 100 to 150 mg/kg 3-5 times daily *OR* topical application using a 10% aqueous solution.

[+] **alpha-Lipoic acid**: 150 mg daily (1 month trial)
[+] **Chromium deficiency**: 200 μg daily
[+] **Magnesium deficiency**: ≈ 400 mg daily
[+] **Thiamine deficiency**: 50 mg daily
[+] **Vitamin A deficiency**: 50,000 IU daily for 6 weeks (10,000 IU daily during pregnancy) (several month trial)
[+] **Vitamin B_{12}**: 5000 μg daily

[-] **Omega-3 fatty acids**: *example:* MaxEPA 1 g caps [180 mg EPA; 120 mg DHA] 10 to 20 daily

OTHER RELATED FACTORS

[+] rule out **Food Sensitivities**

DIETARY FACTORS

The rapid ingestion of large volumes of fluid will increase aqueous fluid production and cause a temporary elevation in intraocular pressure *(Lichter)*. For example, after patients with an ocular pressure greater than 18 mm Hg drank a half liter of water in 5 minutes, there was a pressure rise between 3 and 4 points in 28.5%, a rise of 5 to 6 points in 13.5%, and a rise of more than 6 points in 8% *(Warter)*. This sort of transitory rise might aggravate glaucoma-induced nerve head ischemia *(Warter)*.

Caffeine

There is a report of 2 patients with open-angle glaucoma who responded to caffeinated, but not to decaffeinated, expresso with clinically significant increases in intraocular pressure one hour later *(Davis)*. In a single-blind crossover study, acute caffeine ingestion significantly increased intraocular pressure in patients 90 minutes after ingestion - although this change was not clinically significant *(Higginbotham)*. Also, a subsequent double-blind study failed to find a significant difference in aqueous flow from 1 to 4 hours after caffeine administration *(Adams)*.

Further studies are needed to clarify whether any adverse effect of caffeine becomes clinically relevant over the long term.

NUTRITIONAL FACTORS

VITAMINS

Thiamine Deficiency

There is preliminary evidence that patients with chronic open-angle glaucoma may have impaired absorption of thiamine, causing reduced blood thiamine levels *(Asregadoo)*.

It has been theorized that thiamine deficiency, which is associated with degeneration of the ganglion cells of the brain and spinal cord in experimental animals, may also be associated with degeneration of the ganglion cells of the optic nerve. Also, there is reason to believe that chronic open angle glaucoma may be more common in populations suffering from thiamine deficiency. In such a population, treatment with thiamine along with vitamin B complex improves optic atrophy and, to a lesser extent, glaucoma *(Asregadoo)*.

Thiamine supplementation has not been shown to be beneficial other than to correct at least a marginal deficiency. Controlled clinical trials are needed to more fully assess the value of thiamine supplementation.

Vitamin A Deficiency

A deficiency of vitamin A is known to be associated with night blindness and loss of color vision. Although it has not been shown to produce glaucoma, one author has noted normalization of intraocular tension in several patients (believed to be vitamin A-deficient due to objective loss of color vision) following supplementation *(Todd)*.

Vitamin B_{12}

While a deficiency of vitamin B_{12} does not cause glaucoma, it may cause visual field defects and optic atrophy (the end-stage appearance of glaucoma).

In an open trial, glaucoma patients were supplemented with high doses of the vitamin. Even though intraocular fluid pressure was not reduced, progression of peripheral vision loss did not occur during 5 years of follow-up *(Sakai)*.

Vitamin C

When a group of 31 adult subjects whose mean daily intake of vitamin C was 75 mg was compared to a matched group with a mean daily intake of 1,200 mg, a lower vitamin C intake was associated with a significantly higher intraocular pressure (22.33 mm Hg vs. 15.15 mm Hg) *(Lane, 1980)*. Moreover, a case-control study involving 52 patients with ocular hypertension and/or glaucoma found that primary open-angle glaucoma was strongly associated with an inadequate daily ascorbic acid intake *(Lane, 1991)* - although another investigator has failed to confirm this finding *(Asregadoo)*.

In primary open-angle glaucoma, one study found ascorbic acid to be decreased in the aqueous humor while secondary products of lipid peroxidation were increased. In fact, in patients whose glaucoma was in stages III or IV, these two changes were correlated, suggesting that primary glaucoma may be caused by lipid peroxidation fostered by inadequate ascorbate *(Aleksidze)*. However, other studies have failed to find a deficiency of aqueous humor ascorbate in the majority of open-angle glaucomatous eyes *(Lee)*, or evidence of ascorbate deficiency in the blood *(Asregadoo)*.

Supplementation

Several studies, some of which were controlled, have investigated the efficacy of high dosages of ascorbate supplementation in reducing intraocular pressure in glaucoma and ocular hypertension. Most found the supplement to successfully reduce intraocular pressure.

In one report, a single dose of 500 mg/kg ascorbic acid reduced intraocular pressure in *all* of 39 patients with chronic open-angle glaucoma by an average of 16 mm Hg, although it usually caused gastrointestinal symptoms. Also, ascorbic acid 100 to 150 mg/kg 3 to 5 times daily resulted in almost normal intraocular pressures in 15 out of 16 patients by 45 days, some of whom were uncontrollable with acetazolamide and 2% pilocarpine, with only 3 to 4 days of gastrointestinal symptoms initially *(Virno)*.

Vitamin C has also been found to be effective in reducing intraocular pressure when administered by topical application in a 10% aqueous solution *(Linner)*. The advantage of topical application is that gastrointestinal symptoms are avoided.

Supplementation with the vitamin is believed to increase aqueous humor drainage by reducing the viscosity of hyaluronic acid *(Liu)*.

MINERALS

Chromium Deficiency

Chromium is a glucose-uptake insulin-receptor potentiator which is thought to enable sustained strong ciliary-muscle eye-focusing activity. A deficiency is associated with elevated intraocular pressure which tends to stretch the eye to reduce the need for focusing power *(Lane)*.

Primary open-angle glaucoma appears to be strongly associated with erythrocyte chromium deficiency. In fact, the most significant biochemical differentiator between normals and persons with primary open-angle glaucoma is erythrocyte chromium *(Lane)*.

Based on informal clinical observations, patients who are likely to respond to chromium repletion are likely to have undrugged intraocular pressures of more than 20 mm Hg as well as erythrocyte chromium levels of no more than 150 ng/ml *(Lane)*. These observations need confirmation with formal controlled trials.

Magnesium Deficiency

Six patients with primary open angle glaucoma and 4 with normal-tension glaucoma, all of whom had cold-induced digital vasospasm, received magnesium supplementation. After 4 weeks, visual field defects improved almost to the point of statistical significance, while digital temperature and nailfold capillaroscopic parameters significantly improved *(Gaspar)*.

Presumably, the cold-induced vasospasm was a sign of systemic magnesium deficiency. This promising early report has yet to be followed by further studies.

OTHER NUTRITIONAL FACTORS

Alpha-lipoic Acid

Levels of the antioxidant glutathione have been found to be low in lacrimal fluid *(Filina, 1993)*, anterior chamber humor, and red cells *(Bunin)* in patients with chronic open-angle glaucoma.

Based on measurements in lacrimal fluid, supplementation with alpha-lipoic acid appears to be an effective means of providing antioxidant therapy of chronic open-angle glaucoma by increasing glutathione levels *(Filina, 1993)*. Moreover, in a controlled study, supplementation improved visual function in patients with stage I or II open-angle glaucoma *(Filina, 1995)*.

Omega-3 Essential Fatty Acids

The Eskimos, whose diet is high in fish (a rich source of omega-3 fatty acids) have a low incidence of open-angle glaucoma *(Prasad)*. Furthermore, in studies on rabbits, cod liver oil supplementation was found to lower intraocular pressure dramatically, while lard and safflower oil had no effect *(Mancio)*.

Controlled human trials are needed to ascertain whether glaucoma patients would benefit from supplementation.

COMBINED NUTRITIONAL INTERVENTIONS

In West Africa, hundreds of patients with primary glaucoma were successfully treated with a combination of vitamin A 180,000 IU, vitamin C 3 gm and vitamin E 200 IU daily. Since many patients were protein-deficient, a 20 gm protein supplement was also provided daily. In most cases, ocular tension was reduced to normal within one week *(Evans)*.

It is likely that these protein-deficient patients were vitamin-deficient as well. Since vitamin C supplementation does not require a deficiency to be effective, these results are consistent with the theory that a deficiency of vitamin A can cause glaucoma.

Also, one study placed subjects with normal intraocular tension, but with hypertension and various degrees of hypertensive retinopathy, on a 2,000 kcal Kempner rice-fruit diet - essentially a low protein, low salt diet - and supplemented them with vitamins and calcium. Within 2 days, intraocular pressure fell dramatically. Reductions of 5 to 7 mm Hg in eye fluid pressure were not uncommon and lasted over long periods of time *(Stocker,1948,1949).* Whether glaucoma patients have a similar response is not known.

OTHER RELATED FACTORS

Food Sensitivities

Food sensitivities *(Berens),* as well as atopic allergies *(Raymond),* may increase intraocular pressure in some cases of chronic simple glaucoma. Patients with other signs and symptoms of food sensitivities or atopic allergies, especially those who have responded poorly to conventional treatments, should be properly evaluated.

Mrs. I.E., age 46, had been treated for 4 years for glaucoma of her right eye. She complained of sharp pain over that eye as well as of severe gastrointestinal distress and chronic constipation. The right eyelids were edematous and red and the conjunctiva was deeply congested. There was typical glaucomatous cupping of the optic disc and pallor of the nerve. Tension with the Schiötz tonometer was 30 mg Hg in the right eye compared to 12 mm Hg in the left. There was also evidence of sinusitis.

Drug treatment was unsuccessful and surgical procedures only reduced her intraocular tension, which rose at times to 60 mm Hg, temporarily. After almost two years, her tension began to rise again, this time in both eyes. She was tested for food sensitivities and eliminated reactive foods. Two weeks later, while continuing on the same dose of pilocarpine, her tension had reduced to the normal range and her gastrointestinal symptoms had disappeared for the first time in her memory. One year after starting the diet, despite stopping pilocarpine two months earlier, her tension was still lower (Berens).

BIBLIOGRAPHY

Adams BA, Brubaker RF. Caffeine has no clinically significant effect on aqueous humor flow in the normal human eye. Ophthalmology 97(8):1030-1, 1990

Aleksidze AT et al. [Effect of the ascorbic acid of the aqueous humor on the lipid peroxidation process in the eye in primary open-angle glaucoma]. Oftalmol Zh 2:114-16, 1989) (in Russian)

Asregadoo ER. Blood levels of thiamine and ascorbic acid in chronic open-angle glaucoma. Ann Ophthalmol 11(7):1095-1100, 1979

Berens C et al. Allergy in glaucoma. Ann Allergy 5:526-35, 1947

Bunin A et al. [A glutathione deficiency in open-angle glaucoma and the approaches to its correction.] Vestn Oftalmol 108(4-6):13-15, 1992 (in Russian)

Davis RH. Does caffeine ingestion affect intraocular pressure? Letter. Ophthalmology 96(11):1680-1, 1989

Evans SC. Ophthalmic nutrition and prevention of eye disorders and blindness. Nutr Metab 21(suppl 1):268-72, 1977

Filina AA et al. [The effect of lipoic acid on the components of the glutathione system in the lacrimal fluid of patients with open-angle glaucoma.] Vestn Oftalmol 109(5):5-7, 1993 (in Russian)

Filina AA et al. [Lipoic acid as a means of metabolic therapy of open-angle glaucoma.] Vestn Oftalmol 111:6-8, 1995) (in Russian)

Gaspar AZ et al. The influence of magnesium on visual field and peripheral vasospasm in glaucoma. Ophthalmologica 209:11-13, 1995

Higginbotham EJ et al. The effect of caffeine on intraocular pressure by glaucoma patients. Ophthalmology 96(5):624-26, 1989

Lane BC. Evaluation of intraocular pressure with daily, sustained closework stimulus to accommodation, lowered tissue chromium and dietary deficiency of ascorbic acid. Doc Ophthalmol 28:149-55, 1980

Lane BC. Diet and the glaucomas. Abstract. J Am Coll Nutr 10(5):536, 1991

Lee P et al. Aqueous humor ascorbate concentration and open-angle glaucoma. Arch Ophthalmol 95(2):308-10, 1977

Lichter RR. Caffeine and other prescriptions for patients with glaucoma. Editorial. Ophthalmology 97(8):965-6, 1990

Linner E. Intraocular pressure regulation and ascorbic acid. Acta Soc Med Upsal 69:225-32, 1964

Liu KM et al. Inhibition of oxidative degradation of hyaluronic acid by uric acid. Curr Eye Res 3(8):1049-53, 1984

Mancio M et al. A comparative study between cod liver oil and liquid lard intake on intraocular pressure on rabbits. Prostaglandins Leukot Essent Fatty Acids 45:239-43, 1992

Prasad SK, U. of Kentucky at Lousiville - reported in Medical Tribune August 19, 1991, p. 25

Raymond LF. Allergy and chronic simple glaucoma. Ann Allergy 22:146-50, 1964

Sakai T et al. Effect of long-term treatment of glaucoma with vitamin B12. Glaucoma 14:167-70, 1992

Stocker FW et al. Clinical experiments with new ways of influencing intraocular tension. 1. Effect of rice diet. Arch Ophthalmol 40:46-55, 1948

Stocker FW. New ways of influencing intraocular pressure. N Y State Med J 49:58-63, 1949

Todd, GP. Nutrition, Health & Disease. Norfolk Beach, Virginia, The Donning Company, 1985

Virno M et al. Oral treatment of glaucoma with vitamin C. Eye, Ear, Nose, Throat Monthly 46:1502-08, 1967

Warter G, Jeannenot N. [Increased intraocular pressure provoked by a water test]. Ophthalmologica 202(2):75-80, 1991) (in French)

GOUT

NUTRITIONAL TREATMENT GUIDE
✓ = Efficacy generally accepted. * = Efficacy *demonstrated* by controlled human trials. [+] = Efficacy *suspected* from uncontrolled human trials. [-] = Efficacy *suspected* from indirect data. ? = Efficacy *challenged* in a study of similar design.
DIETARY FACTORS ✓ low **Purine** diet (meats, seafood, lentils, beans, and peas) - [+] restrict **Alcohol** [+] eat **Cherries** [+] avoid **Fructose**
NUTRITIONAL FACTORS [+] ? **Folic acid:** 800 μg daily [+] ? **Vitamin C:** Start with 0.5 g twice daily and increase gradually over 1 to 2 months to the minimal dosage with maximal efficacy. (Avoid in cases of impaired renal function.) - [-] avoid **Niacin** supplementation [-] avoid **Vitamin A** supplementation (especially in cases of impaired renal function or gouty arthritis)

DIETARY FACTORS

Low Purine Diet

It is generally accepted that purine-containing foods should be avoided, since uric acid is formed by the catabolism of purine nucleotides *(Garcia Puig)*. These include meats (especially organ meats), seafood, lentils, beans, and peas.

Alcohol

Alcohol intake should be restricted - particularly beer, which has a higher purine content than wine or spirits. In fact, when the diets of men with gout were compared to those of normals, the major difference was that 41% of the afflicted men drank more than seven 12-ounce cans of beer daily compared to 17% of the healthy men. This difference was associated with a significantly higher intake of purine nitrogen, half of which was derived from beer *(Gibson)*.

In addition to serving as a source of purines, alcohol increases lactate production, and lactate competes with uric acid for renal clearance. Finally, alcohol increases the degradation of purine nucleotides in the liver, increasing oxypurine and thus uric acid production *(Emmerson)*.

Fructose

Fructose increases urate production. As this could lead to hyperuricemia, its intake should be avoided *(Henry)*.

Upon fructose challenge, patients with hereditary fructose intolerance are prone to develop gout and produce a significantly larger increment in the concentration of serum urate than normal. There is early evidence that this enzyme defect may be a fairly common cause of the disorder *(Seegmiller).*

Cherries

In an open trial, 12 patients on a non-restricted diet ate about one pound of fresh or canned cherries daily. Blood uric acid was reduced to normal in *all* of them, and no attacks of gouty arthritis occurred. Moreover, 4 of the patients reported greater freedom of movement in the joints of their fingers and toes.

Cherry juice seems to be as effective as the pulp. Sweet yellow and red sour cherries seem to be as effective as dark colored cherries. While the active ingredient is unknown, keracyanin, the coloring pigment, is suspected to be the beneficial agent *(Blan).*

NUTRITIONAL FACTORS

VITAMINS

Folic Acid

Because of its ability to inhibit the enzyme xanthine oxidase, a key enzyme in uric acid synthesis, folic acid supplementation has been investigated as a method of reducing uric acid production *(Kalckar).*

One clinical study did find that high doses of folic acid reduced elevated serum uric acid levels, and that discontinuation was followed by a rise of serum uric acid almost to the pretreatment level *(Oster).* However, two later studies were unable to replicate these findings *(Blouvier;Boss).*

It has been suggested that much of the inhibitory effect ascribed to folate in regard to xanthine oxidase was actually due to trace contamination by pterin-6-aldehyde, a potent inhibitor of the enzyme *(Boss).*

Niacin: A Warning

As uric acid competes with nicotinic acid for renal excretion, niacin supplementation could precipitate an attack of gout *(Scott).*

Vitamin A: A Warning

The enzyme xanthine oxidase is involved not only in the conversion of xanthine to uric acid but also in the conversion of retinol to its more toxic metabolite, retinoic acid. Several lines of indirect evidence implicate vitamin A intoxication, associated mainly with impaired renal function, in the pathogenesis of gouty arthritis. *(Mawson).*

Vitamin C

Vitamin C is a mild uricosuric agent. Supplementation has been shown to increase renal uric acid excretion in both normals and in patients with impaired uric acid excretion and hyperuricemia. When taken regularly, it can result in normalization of uric acid homeostasis and normalization of its serum concentration *(Neshyba).*

A Warning

Ascorbic acid supplementation is contraindicated in patients with kidney disease, since an abrupt increase in uric acid excretion can theoretically lead to the formation of uric acid kidney stones. Furthermore, rapid reduction in tissue uric acid levels has been known to have the paradoxic effect of precipitating gouty attacks. Therefore, vitamin C administration should be started slowly and built up gradually over a period of one to two months *(Gaby).*

MINERALS

Zinc

Plasma levels of zinc may be decreased during periods of disease activity *(Matarian).* Whether this is due to inadequate zinc nutriture, and whether zinc supplementation is beneficial, is not known.

A 74-year-old woman had a 4-year history of severe gout in her hands and knees. In addition, she had a cardiac arrhythmia for which she required a pacemaker, and a significant degree of kidney failure. Medications for these latter two disorders caused intolerable side effects.

She was placed on a low protein, low purine, low carbohydrate, alcohol-free diet. In addition to multivitamins, she received vitamin C 4 grams daily and a high dose of zinc.

Her gout improved dramatically, her kidney function improved, and she became better able to tolerate her medications (Davies).

BIBLIOGRAPHY

Blan LW. Cherry diet control for gout and arthritis. Texas Rep Biol Med 8:309-12, 1950

Blouvier B, Duvulder B. Folic acid, xanthine oxidase, and uric acid. Letter. Ann Intern Med 88(2):269, 1978

Boss GR et al. Failure of folic (pteroylglutamic acid) to affect hyperuricemia. J Lab Clin Med 96:783, 1980

Davies S, Stewart A. Nutritional Medicine. London, Pan Books, 1987

Emmerson BT. Therapeutics of hyperuricaemia and gout. Med J Aust 141:31-6, 1984

Gaby AR. Vitamin C, Part I. Nutrition & Healing, April, 1997

Garcia Puig J, Mateos FA. Clinical and biochemical aspects of uric acid overproduction. Pharm World Sci 16(2):40-54, 1994

Gibson T et al. A controlled study of diet in patients with gout. Ann Rheum Dis 42(2):123-7, 1983

Henry RR et al. Current issues in fructose metabolism. Annu Rev Nutr 11:21-39, 1991

Kalckar HM, Klenow H. Milk xanthopterin oxidase and pteroylglutamic acid. J Biol Chem 172:349-50, 1948

Mataran Perez L et al. [Zinc in arthrosis and microcrystalline arthritis.] Rev Clin Esp 189(2):60-2, 1991 (in Spanish)

Mawson AR, Onor GI. Gout and vitamin A intoxication: is there a connection? Semin Arthritis Rheum 20(5):297-304, 1991

Neshyba P, Hudec J. [Effects of hypersaturation with ascorbic acid in patients with impaired renal elimination of uric acid with hyperuricaemia.] Cas Lek Ces 124(11):335-40, 1985 (in Czech)

Oster KA. Evaluation of serum cholesterol reduction and xanthine oxidase inhibition in the treatment of atherosclerosis, in Recent Adv Stud Cardiac Struct Metab 3:73-80, 1973

Scott JT. Diet-induced gout. Baillieres Clin Rheumatol 5(1):39-60, 1991

Seegmiller JE et al. Fructose-induced aberration of metabolism in familial gout identified by 31P magnetic resonance spectroscopy. Proc Natl Acad Sci U S A 87(21):8326-30, 1990

HEADACHE (MIGRAINE)

See Also: **'HYPOGLYCEMIA' (FUNCTIONAL)**
PAIN
PREGNANCY-RELATED ILLNESS
PREMENSTURAL SYNDROME

NUTRITIONAL TREATMENT GUIDE

✓ = Efficacy generally accepted.
* = Efficacy *demonstrated* by controlled human trials.
[+] = Efficacy *suspected* from uncontrolled human trials.
[-] = Efficacy *suspected* from indirect data.
? = Efficacy *challenged* in a study of similar design.

DIETARY FACTORS

[+] **high Carbohydrate diet**
[+] **low Carbohydrate (or low Sucrose) diet** (in type II diabetes or reactive hypoglycemia)
[+] **low Tryptophan diet** (if history of flushing, urticaria or pruritus)

NUTRITIONAL FACTORS

* **Chromium:** 83 µg daily as chromium orotate
* **Omega-3 Fatty Acids:** fish oil containing eicosapentaenoic acid (EPA) 2.7 g daily and docosahexaenoic acid (DHA) 1.8 g daily (2 month trial)
* **Riboflavin:** 400 mg daily (3 month trial)
* **Vitamin C:** 500 mg twice daily
* ? **L-5-Hydroxytryptophan:** ? 400 mg daily (3 month trial)
* ? **Magnesium:** 600 mg daily (2 month trial) *OR* 1 to 3 g IV given over 10-minutes

- -

[+] **Calcium:** 1,200 mg daily
AND **Vitamin D** 1,200 to 1,600 IU daily
[+] avoid **Copper** supplementation
[+] **Thiamine:** 100 to 300 mg daily
[+] **Vitamin B_6:** 50 to 100 mg daily

OTHER RELATED FACTORS

* rule out **Food Sensitivities**

- -

[+] rule out **Reactive Hypoglycemia**

Research in the area of headache has essentially been confined to migraine headache, which suggests that tension-type headaches may be primarily psychophysiologic in origin. While migraines may also be influenced by psychophysiologic factors in susceptible people, many biological influences can serve as triggers.

DIETARY FACTORS

High Carbohydrate Diet

An essential amino acid, tryptophan is the nutritional precursor of serotonin which, in the brain, appears to have an anti-nociceptive effect *(Ferrari;Lance)*. A high carbohydrate diet may thus benefit some migraineurs due to its ability to increase brain serotonin levels. It does so by provoking insulin secretion which, in turn, increases the uptake of competing amino acids into the peripheral tissues *(Sicuteri)*.

Low Tryptophan Diet

While increasing brain serotonin may be beneficial, disturbances in serotonin metabolism in the peripheral blood may *facilitate* headaches in patients with disturbed 5-hydroxytryptamine uptake kinetics in their platelets (where most blood serotonin is concentrated) *(Crook)*.

By normalizing disturbed platelet serotonin uptake, a low tryptophan diet may be beneficial. Flushing is related to peripheral serotonin levels *(Medina)* and exacerbations of several pruritic skin disorders are associated with elevated serotonin levels in blood and skin *(Demis)*. Thus migraine patients who experience flushing, urticaria or itching excoriations in addition to their headaches are those most likely to improve on a low tryptophan diet.

Indeed, in an open trial, 10 female migraineurs with this symptom constellation, most of whom required ergotamine several times a month, were put on a mostly vegetarian diet in which the intake of foods with a high tryptophan to protein ratio was strongly restricted (which made the diet low in protein) and serotonin-rich foods were excluded. Symptoms improved in *all* patients within as little as 7 to 10 days and they no longer had need for medication. After one month, migraine-like symptoms and skin manifestations were reduced in 9 of the 10 patients and, in parallel, their severely disturbed serotonin uptake kinetics in platelets were normalized *(Unge)*

High Carbohydrate, Low Tryptophan Diet

A high carbohydrate diet can be combined with a low tryptophan diet in order to minimize *blood* serotonin levels while maximizing *brain* serotonin levels. In an open trial, 3 out of 4 patients with classic migraine, but none of 3 with common migraine, noted a marked improvement within 4 weeks of starting a such a diet *(Hasselmark)*. More studies are needed to confirm the value of this diet before it can be generally recommended:

HIGH CARBOHYDRATE, LOW TRYPTOPHAN DIET

- Restrict foods with a high tryptophan to protein ratio (examples: meat, fish, eggs, dairy products, soya beans).
- Emphasize vegetables, root vegetables, and tryptophan-poor cereals (ex. rye, corn, buckwheat).
- Exclude serotonin-rich foods (ex. bananas, tomatoes, walnuts).
- Consume fat, sugar, and honey *ad libitum*.

Low Carbohydrate (or Low Sucrose) Diet

A contrasting diet which has also shown some evidence of efficacy is a low carbohydrate, or even specifically a low sucrose, diet. Headaches developed in about 45% of a group of patients with relative hypoglycemia, defined as a drop of 20 mg% or more below the fasting blood sugar level during a 6-hour glucose tolerance test *(Salzer)*. Moreover, some type II diabetic migraineurs have a marked reduction of migraines with the onset of diabetic control, some develop migraines from nocturnal hypoglycemia, and some develop migraines when they miss a meal *(Blau,1970)*.

Data concerning the results of a low carbohydrate diet (which may be low in sucrose), and specifically of a low sucrose diet, are restricted to the results of a few open trials. In one study, *all* of 11 migraineurs with spontaneous hypoglycemia who were placed on a low carbohydrate diet improved or had complete symptom relief *(Wilkinson)*.

Another study of 135 headache patients with relative hypoglycemia placed them on a low carbohydrate, caffeine-free diet and told them to eat between meals and every 2 hours throughout the evening. In addition, the majority received injections of calcium glycerophosphate. Roughly 85% responded *(Salzer)*.

A low sucrose diet was utilized in another study. Migraineurs who associated their attacks with fasting or with the mid-morning or mid-afternoon fasting state were placed on a low sucrose, 6-meal regimen (protein:fat: carbohydrate ratio = 20:45:35). *All* 11 patients with a diabetic glucose tolerance curve showed an improvement of more than 75%, and 3 of them became headache-free. Forty percent of patients with reactive hypoglycemic curves showed more than a 75% improvement, while 9% showed a 25 to 50% improvement *(Dexter)*.

NUTRITIONAL FACTORS

VITAMINS

Riboflavin

In a randomized, controlled study, 55 migraineurs received either pharmacologic dosages of riboflavin or placebo for 3 months. Riboflavin was superior to placebo in reducing attack frequency and headache days *(Schoenen,1998)*. These findings confirm those of an earlier open trial which found that 80% of migraineurs treated with riboflavin had a 50% or greater reduction of monthly migraine days *(Schoenen,1994)*.

Thiamine

Pharmacologic dosages of thiamine are known to cause vasodilation, neuromuscular relaxation, central damping, synaptic blockade and suppression of nerve impulse transmission. Whether these effects are useful in the treatment of migraine headaches was examined in an open trial of 69 patients. Sixty-four percent were said to respond to treatment *(Hotzel)*.

This study has yet to be replicated under controlled conditions.

Vitamin B_6

Pain Medication-induced Headaches

Chronic use of ergotamine, opiate analgesics, or aspirin and other medications used for pain relief, may cause medication-induced chronic headache due to depletion of central nervous system endorphins with downregulating of receptor sites. A review article published in the *Annals of the New York Academy of Sciences* notes that, for this condition, one of the most successful treatments is vitamin B_6 supplementation to increase serotonin levels via vitamin B_6-mediated pathways in order to raise the pain threshold when given concurrently with an extremely gradual detoxification from the offending agent *(Bernstein)*.

Histamine-intolerance Headaches

Headaches due to histamine intolerance, an illness characterized by impaired histamine degradation based on reduced diamine oxidase activity, may also be helped by supplementation with vitamin B_6 (see Food Sensitivities below). This is because pyridoxal phosphate, the activated form of the vitamin, seems to be crucial for diamine oxidase activity *(Jarisch)*.

Vitamin C

While the results of the following double-blind case report suggest that vitamin C supplementation may be a highly effective treatment for migraine headaches, confirmatory data of its efficacy are lacking:

A 32-year-old male with a 6-year history of migraine headaches believed that vitamin C controlled his headaches. In order to ascertain if he was correct, he was asked to consume vitamin C 6 g daily or a citric acid placebo in random order under double-blind conditions for 15 consecutive days.

On each of the placebo days, he experienced severe headaches, while on the vitamin C days, headaches were absent or very minor (Bali).

MINERALS

Calcium

Four female migraineurs responded to supplementation of calcium along with vitamin D. Two of the women were postmenopausal; one had a history of a stroke while the other was on estrogen therapy *(Thys-Jacob,1994a)*. The other two women had menstrual migraines *(Thys-Jacob,1994b)*.

Controlled studies are needed to verify these findings.

Chromium

In the following double-blind case report, chromium supplementation relieved migraine-like headaches in a young woman. No further studies have been published to help ascertain when chromium supplementation may be effective:

A 26-year-old female with regular migraine-like headaches since childhood received active and placebo tablets in an A-B-A-B single case design. A highly significant reduction in headache frequency and intensity was reported when taking a multivitamin/multimineral tablet compared to placebo.

In subsequent open trials, it appeared that the benefit from the combination supplement was due to chromium which, as a single ingredient, was supplied as chromium orotate containing 83 μg chromium (compared to 1-2 mg in the combination supplement). Dietary analysis failed to reveal low chromium intake, suggesting a problem with chromium absorption or metabolism (Cook).

Copper: A Warning

Dietary copper, which is involved in the metabolism of vasoneuroactive amines, may be a migraine stimulus, especially when copper metabolism is abnormal. Avoidance of foods that increase copper availability as well as copper-containing nutritional supplements may thus be beneficial *(Harrison)*. Also, alcoholic drinks that are distilled in copper stills, such as red wine, beer or whisky, may bring on a migraine attack *(Leira)*.

FOODS AFFECTING COPPER NUTRITURE

High Copper Content

chocolate, nuts, wheat germ, shellfish

Increase Intestinal Copper Absorption

citrus

Bind and Transport Copper

monosodium glutamate

Magnesium Deficiency

Magnesium has a fundamental role in establishing the threshold for migraine attacks and the psychophysiologic mechanisms related to their onset *(Gallai,1992)*. Its concentration affects serotonin receptors, nitric oxide synthesis and release, n-methyl-D-aspartate (NMDA) receptors, and a variety of other migraine-related receptors and neurotransmitters *(Mauskop,1998)*. Furthermore, the action of prostanoids on smooth muscle (fostering contraction) is magnesium-dependent, and tissue levels of prostanoids have been shown to be higher in magnesium-deficient rats *(Fantidis)*.

In patients experiencing migraine headaches, serum ionized magnesium levels are often depressed. In one study, for example, a low serum ionized magnesium and a high ionized calcium to magnesium ratio were found in 42% of migraineurs during an attack compared to only 23% of patients with a severe continuous headache. These findings would be expected to cause promote cerebral vasospasm, reduced blood flow to the brain and changes in the activity of serotonin receptors *(Mauskop,1993)*.

Other studies have reported reductions in brain *(Ramadan)*, mononuclear *(Gallai,1994)*, erythrocyte *(Gallai,1993)*, serum *(Sarchielli)*, and salivary *(Sarchielli)* magnesium levels. Women who are perimenstrual *(Abraham)* or pre-eclamptic *(Weaver)*, are especially prone to migraines associated with decreased blood magnesium.

Supplementation

Several clinical trials, some conducted under controlled conditions, have found magnesium supplementation to be effective. For example, in a double-blind, randomized study, migraineurs with a mean attack frequency of 3.6 per month received magnesium as trimagnesium dicitrate or a placebo daily for 12 weeks. Between weeks 9 and 12, the attack frequency was reduced by 41.6% in the magnesium group compared to 15.8% in the placebo group, and there was a significant decrease in days with migraine and in drug use in the magnesium-treated patients *(Peikert)*.

Patients with low ionized serum magnesium levels are more likely to respond *(Mauskop,1996)*. Intravenous administration appears to be more effective than oral prophylaxis. In one study of almost 1,000 patients, up to 90% of those with low serum ionized magnesium levels improved following a single infusion of intravenous magnesium, and some remained migraine-free for up to 5 months. By contrast, only 40% of similar patients given prophylactic oral magnesium responded *(Altura)*.

L. A. suffered from severe headaches for about 20 years. Despite seeing numerous physicians, the cause of the headaches remained unknown. Medications were taken on a daily basis and "everything and anything" was tried to get some relief, even doubling doses of aspirin and prescription drugs, without any success in reducing the headaches.

However, within one hour of taking 800 mg of magnesium, the headache disappeared. Magnesium supplementation was then continued on a daily basis. Four weeks later, despite being off of all medications, headaches had not returned (Almanza).

OTHER NUTRITIONAL FACTORS

L-5-Hydroxytryptophan

Several controlled studies have found supplementation with 5-hydroxytryptophan, the precursor to serotonin, to be effective in both adults *(De Benedittis)* and children *(Longo)*. One double-blind study compared it to methysergide. The two substances were roughly equally effective, although side effects were more frequent in the methysergide group *(Titus)*. Another double-blind study compared it to propanolol. While propanolol was more effective, the efficacy of 5-hydroxytryptophan was good enough to be recommended as a possible alternative for many patients *(Maissen)*.

Omega-3 Fatty Acids

Small controlled trials published only in abstract form have reported excellent results from the administration of fish oils rich in omega-3 fatty acids *(Glueck,1986a; McCarren)*. The efficacy of these fatty acids appears to be due to a reduction in vasoconstriction and an increase in vasodilation, as well as to a reduction in platelet aggregation *(Glueck,1986b)*. Larger studies are needed for confirmation of its efficacy.

OTHER RELATED FACTORS

Food Sensitivities

The best-validated area of nutritional research regarding migraine treatment concerns the role of foods as triggering agents. Several double-blind studies have confirmed the numerous early reports that a wide variety of foods, most of which are commonly eaten, can provoke migraine headaches *(Ulrich)*. Results of food eliminations have been so impressive that a conservative estimate is that one out of three migraineurs will benefit markedly from food avoidance *(Mansfield)*. If fact, in one double-blind study *(Egger)*, 93% of 88 children with severe, frequent migraine did so well that the authors titled their study, "Is migraine food allergy?"

Without question, certain foods are more likely than others to provoke migraine. Some of most commonly-eaten foods in a person's diet may prove to trigger headaches following a common-food elimination diet and food provocation. Also, a number of substances in foods have been shown to be capable of causing a migraine-like headache:

1. Tyramine, a vasoneuroactive amine which is found in a number of foods (see below), has long been implicated as a causative agent *(Hanington)* and has been shown to provoke the release of both serotonin and norepinephrine.

Sources:
- Aged cheese (some)
- Chicken liver
- Dry, fermented sausage (some)
- Pickled herring
- Red wine (some) (especially Chianti)
- Sour Cream

2. Phenylethylamine, another vasoactive amine known to provoke headaches *(Sandler)*.

Sources:
- Chocolate
- Cheese

3. Nitrates, which are added to meats as preservatives and turn them red, may cause headaches *(Graham)*.

Sources:
- Salami
- Bologna
- Sausage
- Hot dogs

4. Lactose (milk sugar) can cause migraine headaches in lactase-deficient patients *(Ratner)*.

Sources:
- Milk and certain dairy products
- (cheese and yogurt usually OK)

5. Caffeine intake is correlated with headache prevalence. In one study, for people consuming 240 mg daily (about 4-5 cups of coffee), the relative risk of headaches was 1.3 for males and 1.2 for females *(Shirlow)*. When a habitual coffee drinker abstains, a caffeine-withdrawal headache may start in about 18 hours and peak 3 to 6 hours later. The headache typically starts with a feeling of "cerebral fullness" and quickly develops into a diffuse, throbbing pain which is exacerbated by exercise *(Greden)*.

Sources:
- Coffee
- Tea
- Caffeinated soft beverages

6. Histamine in food and wine causes a worsening of symptoms in atopics and headache patients and plays a major role in food and wine intolerance *(Wantke)*.

Sources:

- Beer
- Cheese
- Fish
- Hardcured sausage
- Pickled cabbage
- Wine

7. Dopamine, a neurotransmitter, appears to be involved in the pathophysiology of certain subtypes of migraine. Most migraine symptoms can be induced by dopaminergic stimulation. Moreover, migraineurs display dopamine hypersensitivity *(Peroutka)*.

Source:

- Fava beans
- (Italian green beans)

8. Aspartame, an artificial dipeptide sweetener produced from phenylalanine and aspartic acid, has been shown in double-blind studies to provoke migraine headache in susceptible people *(Van den Eeden)*.

A longstanding, common-migraine sufferer kept detailed records of the frequency of his headaches and of the medication taken. An aspirin-induced gastrointestinal bleed caused him to begin a bland oligoantigenic diet. Shortly thereafter, he became headache-free.

Single food challenges revealed sensitivities to banana, citrus, and cheese, all of which contain vasoactive amines. Headaches would occur up to 72 hours following ingestion of provoking foods.

The year prior to his discovery, he had headache on 326 days and took 1,316 aspirin tablets. The year following it, in which he eliminated offending foods, he had headache on 8 days and took 16 aspirin (Gettis).

Reactive Hypoglycemia

It is well documented that some migraineurs experience an attack during fasting *(Dalton)*. Surprisingly, administering glucose to fasting migraineurs may either prevent or precipitate an episode *(Blau, 1966)*.

The findings of a study of women who were disabled with classical migraine headaches suggest that either pattern may be related to food sensitivities. Based on the results of glucose tolerance testing, they were divided into groups according to the change in symptoms.

Patients whose symptoms increased reported that migraines were brought on by combinations of alcohol, cheese and chocolate. The mean curve for blood glucose levels had a 'flatter' appearance for this group than for the other patients, and this was substantiated statistically at 90 minutes. It is speculated that these patients may have a defect in glucose utilization (slow glucose absorption; fast liver uptake from the portal circulation; fast degradation or fast storage).

Symptoms fell for those patients who reported sensitivities to combinations of fat and pork or who denied food sensitivities, suggesting defective gluconeogenesis. The response pattern of patients who reported sensitivities to foods in both groups was intermediate to that of the other patients *(Marsters)*.

BIBLIOGRAPHY

Abraham GE, Lubran MM. Serum and red cell magnesium levels in patients with premenstrual tension. Am J Clin Nutr 34(11):2364-6, 1981

Almanza L. Headache-free with magnesium. Letter. Let's Live, March, 1996

Altura B, professor of physiology and medicine, New York Health Science Center, Brooklyn, NY USA - quoted in Monson N. Can vitamins and minerals cure migraines? Alternative & Complementary Therapies July/August 1996:217-19

Bali L et al. Vitamin C and migraine: a case report. N Engl J Med 299:364, 1978

Bernstein AL. Vitamin B6 in clinical neurology. Ann NY Acad Sci 585:250-60, 1990

Blau JN, Cumings JN. Method of precipitating and preventing some migraine attacks. Br Med J 11:1242, 1966

Blau JN, Pike DA. Effect of diabetes on migraine. Lancet ii:241-3, 1970

Cook R, Benton D. Chromium supplementation improves chronic headaches: a case-study. J Nutr Med 3:61-4, 1992

Crook M. Migraine: A biochemical headache? Biochem Soc Trans 9(4):351-7, 1981

Dalton K. Food intake prior to a migraine attack - study of 2,313 spontaneous attacks. Headache 15:188, 1975

De Benedittis G, Massei R. Serotonin precursors in chronic primary headache. A double-blind cross-over study with L-5-hydroxytryptophan vs. placebo. J Neurosurg Sci 29(3):239-48, 1985

Demis DJ et al. A study of the cutaneous effects of serotonin. J Invest Dermatol 34:43-50, 1960

Dexter JD et al. The five hour glucose tolerance test and the effect of low sucrose diet in migraine. Headache 18:91-94, 1978

Egger J et al. Is migraine food allergy? A double-blind controlled trial of oligoantigenic diet treatment. Lancet ii:865-9, 1983

Fantidis P et al. Intracellular (polymorphonuclear) magnesium content in patients with bronchial asthma between attacks. J R Soc Med 88(8):441-5, 1995

Ferrari MD, Saxena PR. On serotonin and migraine: a clinical and pharmacological review. Cephalalgia 13(3):151-65, 1993

Gallai V et al. Serum and salivary magnesium levels in migraine. Results in a group of juvenile patients. Headache 32(3):132-5, 1992

Gallai V et al. Red blood cell magnesium in migraine patients. Cephalalgia 113(2):94-81; discussion 73, 1993

Gallai V et al. Magnesium content of mononuclear blood cells in migraine patients. Headache 34(3):160-5, 1994

Gettis A. Serendipity and food sensitivity: A case study. Headache 27:73-75, 1987

Glueck CJ et al. Amelioration of severe migraine with omega-3 fatty acids: A double-blind, placebo-controlled clinical trial. Abstract. Am J Clin Nutr 43:710, 1986a

Glueck C, U. of Cincinnati College of Medicine - interviewed in Prevention, January, 1986b:122

Graham JR. Headache related to a variety of medical disorders, in O Appenzeller, Ed. Pathogenesis and Treatment of Headache. New York, Spectrum Publications, 1976

Greden JF et al. Caffeine-withdrawal headache: A clinical profile. Psychosomatics 21:411-18, 1980

Haningtron E. Preliminary report on tyramine headache. Br Med J 2:550-1, 1967

Harrison DP. Copper as a factor in the dietary precipitation of migraine. Headache 26(5):248-50, 1986

Hasselmark L et al. Effect of a carbohydrate-rich diet, low in protein-tryptophan, in classic and common migraine. Cephalalgia 7:87-92, 1987

Hotzel D. [Vitamins-an overview.] Nieren-Und Hochdruckkrankheiten 21(Suppl 1):S3-S9, 1992 (in German)

Jarisch R, Wantke F. Wine and headache. Int Arch Allergy Immunol 110(1):7-12, 1996

Lance JW. Current concepts of migraine pathogenesis. Neurology 43(6 Suppl 3):S11-15, 1993

Leira R, Rodriguez R. [Diet and migraine]. Rev Neurol 24(129):534-8, 1996) (in Spanish)

Longo G et al. [Treatment of essential headache in developmental age with L-5-HTP (cross over double-blind study versus placebo).] Pediatr Med Chir 6(2):241-5, 1984) (in Italian)

Maissen CP, Ludin HP. [Comparison of the effect of 5-hydroxytryptophan and propranolol in the interval treatment of migraine.] Schweiz med Wochenschr 121(43):1585-90, 1991) (in German)

Mansfield LE. Food allergy and migraine: Whom to evaluate and how to treat. Postgrad Med 83(7):46-55, 1988

Marsters JB et al. Glucose and diet in the fasting migraineur. Headache 26:243-7, 1986

Mauskop A et al. Deficiency in serum ionized magnesium but not total magnesium in patients with migraines. Possible role of $ICa2^{+}/IMg2^{+}$ ratio. Headache 33(3):135-8, 1993

Mauskop A et al. Intravenous magnesium sulfate rapidly alleviates headaches of various types. Headache 36 (3): 154-60, 1996

Mauskop A, Altura BM. Role of magnesium in the pathogenesis and treatment of migraines. Clin Neurosci 5(1):24-7, 1998

McCarren T et al. Amelioration of severe migraine by fish oil (ω-3) fatty acids. Abstract. Am J Clin Nutr 41:874a, 1985

Medina JL, Diamond S. The role of diet in migraine. Headache 18:31-4, 1978

Peikert A et al. Prophylaxis of migraine with oral magnesium: Results from a prospective, multi-center, placebo-controlled and double-blind randomized study. Cephalalgia 16:257-63, 1996

Peroutka SJ. Dopamine and migraine. Neurology 49(3):650-6, 1997

Ramadan NM et al. Low brain magnesium in migraine. Headache 29(9):590-3, 1989

Ratner D et al. Milk protein-free diet for nonseasonal asthma and migraine in lactase-deficient patients. Isr J Med Sci 19:806-9, 1983

Salzer HM. Relative hypoglycemia as a cause of neuropsychiatric illness. J Natl Med Assoc 58(1):12-17, 1966

Sandler M et al. A phenylethylamine oxidising defect in migraine. Nature 250:335, 1974

Sarchielli P et al. Serum and salivary magnesium levels in migraine and tension-type headache. Results in a group of adult patients. Cephalalgia 21(1):21-7, 1992

Schoenen J et al. High-dose riboflavin as a prophylactic treatment of migraine: results of an open pilot study. Cephalalgia 14:328-9, 1994

Schoenen J et al. Effectiveness of high-dose riboflavin in migraine prophylaxis. A randomized controlled trial. Neurology 50(2):466-70, 1998

Shirlow MJ, Mathers CD. A study of caffeine consumption and symptoms: Indigestion, palpitations, tremor, headache and insomnia. Int J Epidemiol 14(2):239-48, 1985

Sicuteri F. Endorphins, opiate receptors and migraine headaches. Headache 17:253-6, 1978

Thys-Jacob S. Alleviation of migraines with therapeutic vitamin D and calcium. Headache 34:590-2, 1994a

Thys-Jacob S. Vitamin D and calcium in menstrual headache. Headache 34:544-6, 1994b

Titus F et al. 5-Hydroxytryptophan versus methysergide in the prophylaxis of migraine. Randomized clinical trial. Eur Neurol 25(5):327-9, 1986

Ulrich V et al. A comparison of tension-type headache in migraineurs and in non-migraineurs: a population-based study. Pain 67(2-3:501-6, 1996

Unge G et al. Effects of dietary protein-tryptophan restriction upon 5-HT uptake by platelets and clinical symptoms in migraine-like headache. Cephalgia 3(4):213-18, 1983

Van den Eeden SK et al. Aspartame ingestion and headaches: a randomized crossover trial. Neurology 44(10):1787-93, 1994

Wantke F et al. [The histamine free diet.] Hautarzt 44(8):512-16, 1993

Weaver K. Magnesium in Health and Disease. Jamaica, NY, Spectrum Publications, 1980:833

Wilkinson CF. Return of migrainoid headaches associated with spontaneous hypoglycemia. Am J Med Sci 281:209-12, 1949

HERPES SIMPLEX

See Also: INFECTION

NUTRITIONAL TREATMENT GUIDE

✓ = Efficacy generally accepted.
* = Efficacy *demonstrated* by controlled human trials.
[+] = Efficacy *suspected* from uncontrolled human trials.
[-] = Efficacy *suspected* from indirect data.
? = Efficacy *challenged* in a study of similar design.

DIETARY FACTORS

* Avoid high-**Arginine** foods, especially **chocolate**, **nuts** and **seeds**.

NUTRITIONAL FACTORS

* **Lithium:** lithium carbonate 150-900 mg daily (ave. dosage 437 mg/d; ave. serum Li 0.56 mmol/L)
* **L-Lysine:** 1 g 3 times daily between meals until healed; then 500 mg daily to prevent recurrences
* **Vitamin C** 200 mg daily *AND*
Flavonoids (mixed) 200 mg 3 times daily

- -

[+] **Adensine-5'-Monophosphate:** 1.5 to 2 mg/kg body wt. by IM injection on alternate days for 9 to 12 doses
[+] **Vitamin C:** 250 mg twice daily *AND*
Zinc (sulfate) 100 mg twice daily (6 week trial)

- -

[-] **Iron deficiency:** 30 mg twice daily until repletion; then minimal possible dosage

TOPICAL APPLICATION

* **Vitamin C:** Apply as a paste for 2 minutes 3 times daily.
* **Vitamin E, Lithium, and Zinc:** lithium succinate 8%, zinc sulfate 0.05% and D,L alpha-tocopherol 0.1%. Apply as an ointment 4 times daily.

- -

[+] **Vitamin E:** Apply liquid soaked in cloth or cotton for 15 minutes 3 times daily
[+] **Zinc:** zinc sulfate 0.01-0.25% ointment or solution. Apply every 30 to 60 minutes when lesions first appear; then several times daily.

NUTRITIONAL FACTORS

VITAMINS

Vitamin C

Ascorbic acid has long been known to inactivate the herpes virus *(Holden)*. The results of an open trial suggest that supplementation with the vitamin may improve the clinical course of an eruption and prevent recurrences. Four years after starting daily supplementation, 30 out of 38 patients with recurrent cold sores remained free of recurrences, while the rest were able to inhibit the infection by increasing vitamin C intake at the first appearance of symptoms *(Lewin)*.

Vitamin C may also be helpful when applied topically. In a randomized, double-blind study, patients with recurrent mucocutaneous herpes were instructed to treat their lesions with a cotton wool pad soaked in an ascorbic acid solution or in a placebo solution and to apply it regularly. Those who applied the ascorbic acid solution had significantly fewer days with scabs and fewer occasions of worsening symptoms. Moreover, the nurses noted that the scabs did not last as long and the virus cultures yielded herpes simplex less frequently *(Hovi)*.

A paste can be made of either ascorbic acid or sodium ascorbate and water which can be covered by a bandage. Clinical experience suggests that one or more applications when made to intact skin where the patient perceives an outbreak is about to occur will completely abort the attack, although several applications may be necessary to penetrate through intact skin. For the eyes, a 20% sodium ascorbate solution may be effective *(Cathcart)*.

Vitamin E

Animal studies suggest that vitamin E supplementation may speed healing of gingival wounds *(Kim)*. For topical application, the liquid from capsules can be squeezed onto a cotton roll.

A group of 50 patients applied the vitamin to their lesions every 4 hours. They *all* experienced prompt and sustained relief, and the lesions healed more rapidly than expected *(Fink)*.

In another open trial, patients with gingivostomatitis applied vitamin E topically for 15 minutes. The pain was nearly always eliminated in less than 8 hours and lesions frequently disappeared in 12 to 24 hours. Larger or multiple lesions responded best when the treatment was administered 3 times daily for 3 days. Treatment was less effective if the vitamin was applied for less than 15 minutes *(Nead)*.

Controlled studies are needed to confirm these findings.

MINERALS

Iron Deficiency

People with a history of recurrent herpes simplex labialis are more often iron-deficient than are controls matched for age and sex *(Chandra)*. For example, when a group of patients with recrudescent herpes labialis were compared to matched controls, the ferritin level in the patients was significantly lower than in the controls, although only one patient was anemic *(Lamey)*.

It remains to be shown whether repletion of an iron deficiency reduces herpetic episodes.

Lithium

In vitro studies have shown that lithium administration suppresses replication of herpes simplex virus and allows synthesis of host proteins *(Ziaie)*. In a retrospective study, the mean rate of recurrent labial herpes infections in patients receiving pharmacologic dosages of lithium for the treatment of psychiatric illness was significantly reduced compared to before treatment *(Amsterdam)*.

The positive results of open trials have now been confirmed under controlled conditions. In a randomized, double-blind study, 11 healthy subjects who had at least 4 recurrent herpes simplex virus infections in the previous year received lithium carbonate at pharmacologic dosages or placebo.

Overall, lithium treatment resulted in a consistent reduction in the mean number of episodes per month, the average duration of each episode, the total number of infection days/month, and the maximum symptom severity. In contrast, treatment with placebo resulted in an increase in 3 out of the 4 severity measures. Although the comparisons between the treatment groups did not achieve statistical significance due to the limited sample size, there was a clear trend for a reduction in the total monthly duration of all HSV infections with lithium. Lithium treatment was well tolerated *(Amsterdam)*.

Because of the potential of pharmacologic dosages of lithium for adverse effects, interest has focused on using lithium topically. It has yet to be shown to be effective when used alone as a topical ointment. However, in a double-blind study of 73 patients with recurrent genital herpes, an ointment containing lithium along with zinc and vitamin E significantly reduced the median duration of pain and discomfort from 7 to 4 days and reduced viral shedding *(Skinner)*.

A 43-year-old woman was started on lithium treatment (900-1200 mg lithium carbonate daily) for bipolar disorder 10 years ago which was stopped 8 months ago because of renal complications. She reported that, before starting lithium, she had had frequent severe outbreaks of herpetic lesions around the mouth, while she had been almost completely free from these lesions since then.

About 5 months after stopping lithium, she was treated with chlorpromazine and haloperidol for an acute psychotic episode. Two months later she reported a severe outbreak of herpes labialis and stated that the frequency of her herpes attacks had reverted to that experienced prior to lithium therapy (Gillis).

Zinc

Like ascorbic acid, zinc is believed to play a role in protecting against infection. *In vitro*, it inhibits herpes simplex virus replication *(Gordon)*. An open trial combined vitamin C with zinc sulfate to treat patients with recurrent genital herpes. So long as supplementation was continued, the eruptions were completely suppressed in some patients. In other patients, a violent eruption would occur after which the eruptions were completely suppressed, or a local tingling sensation would occur but without an eruption or with local swelling and limited vesiculation which receded within 24 hours *(Fitzherbert)*.

Topical zinc sulfate has also been used successfully in open trials for the treatment of both type I and type II herpes simplex when applied to orolabial or genital lesions as an ointment *(Eby)* or as a solution *(Brody)*. Concentrations have ranged from 0.01% (for the mucus membrane) to 4% (for the skin). Applications every 30 to 60 minutes of the 0.25% solution usually stops the itching, burning, stinging and pain within 2 to 3 hours *(Finnerty)*. For skin lesions, crusting occurs in 1 to 3 days *(Wahba)*. With long-term application, recurrences may be greatly reduced or eliminated *(Eby)*.

OTHER NUTRITIONAL FACTORS

Adenosine-5'-Monophosphate (AMP)

AMP is a naturally occurring purine nucleotide that is an intermediate in cellular metabolism and nucleic acid synthesis. Reduced levels of AMP, along with elevated levels of adenosine triphosphate (ATP), have been noted in blood samples of patients with herpetic infections *(Sklar,1977)*.

In an open trial, 36 patients with recurrent herpes labialis received 9 to 12 intramuscular injections of AMP on alternate days. The lesions usually began to dry up in 24 to 36 hours, and pain disappeared within 48 hours. In follow-ups ranging from 1 month to more than 2 years, 64% of the patients remained free of recurrences, while the remainder had a single recurrence that was less severe *(Sklar,1979)*.

Occasionally, especially if more than 75 mg is injected at once, the injection can cause non-cardiac chest pain. This can be prevented by giving half of the full dose and then waiting 20 minutes before giving the other half *(Gaby;Sklar,1989)*.

There is also the theoretical danger over the ready conversion of AMP into adenosine, a substance which can cause immunodepression. Although recommended dosages appear to be too small to significantly affect systemic AMP levels, the possibility of immune suppression has not been ruled out by scientific studies *(Anonymous)*.

A woman had an 8-year history of at least one herpes simplex lesion on some part of her body daily. Within 48 hours of receiving the first of a series of 10 intramuscular injections of adenosine 5'-monophosphate, her lesions disappeared and did not return for more than 18 months (Gaby).

Flavonoids

Naturally occurring flavonoids possess a variable spectrum of antiviral activity against herpes simplex virus *(Kaul)*. Quercetin, for example, has been found effective in several *in vitro* studies *(Amoros;Mucsi)*.

Although flavonoid supplementation has not been tested on patients as the single treatment, mixed flavonoids were combined with vitamin C in a double-blind study. Thirty-eight patients with recurrent herpes labialis received either the combination or placebo for 3 days starting within 48 hours after symptom-onset. While 100% of patients on placebo developed blisters, only 37% of treated patients developed them. Moreover, the vesicular membrane was disrupted in only 26% of treated patients compared to all of the controls, and the interval from initial onset to complete remission was significantly shorter *(Terezhalmy)*.

L-Lysine

The amino acid arginine promotes the growth of herpes simplex virus, while lysine antagonizes its action. Supplementation with lysine, along with increasing the lysine/arginine ratio of the diet, has been shown to reduce the recurrence rate and symptom severity in double-blind studies *(Griffith;McCune;Thein)*. Other double-blind studies *(DiGiovanna;Milman)* have found it to be ineffective, however. The conflicting findings may be due to differences in serum lysine levels, as one study found that the recurrence rate decreased when serum lysine exceeded 165 nmol/ml, and increased when serum lysine fell below that value *(Thein)*.

A Warning

Since the results of animal studies have suggested that lysine may stimulate the liver to increase cholesterol synthesis *(Schmeisser)*, patients taking lysine supplementation for a period of time should have their cholesterol levels monitored.

LYSINE/ARGININE RATIOS OF FOODS

good	bad
meat	chocolate (1:2)
potatoes	peanuts (1:3)
milk	other nuts
brewer's yeast	seeds
fish	cereal grains
chicken	gelatin
beans	carob
eggs	raisins

M. Z. usually had 3 to 4 weeks of pain following an eruption of herpes simplex labialis. Lysine 1,300 milligrams daily was started after lesions appeared on and above the upper lip. This time the lesions did not spread after the second day, and began "drying up." After the fourth day, they were completely dried up and the pain was gone (Bricklin).

BIBLIOGRAPHY

Amoros M et al. Synergistic effect of flavones and flavonols against herpes simplex virus type 1 in cell culture. Comparison with the antiviral activity of propolis. J Nat Prod 55(12):1732-40, 1992

Amsterdam JD et al. Suppression of herpes simplex virus infections with oral lithium carbonate--a possible antiviral activity. Pharmacotherapy 16(6):1070-5, 1996

Anonymous. AMP for herpes infections Med Sci Bull 7(12), August, 1985

Bricklin M, Executive Editor. Rodale's Encyclopedia of Natural Home Remedies. Emmaus, PA, Rodale Press, 1982, p. 61

Brody I. Topical treatment of recurrent herpes simplex and post-herpetic erythema multiforme with low concentrations of zinc sulphate solution. Br J Dermatol 104(2):191-94, 1981

Cathcart RF III. Vitamin C in the treatment of acquired immune deficiency syndrome (AIDS). Med Hypotheses 14(4):423-33, 1984

Chandra RK. 1990 McCollum Award Lecture: Nutrition and immunity: lessons from the past and new insights into the future. Am J Clin Nutr 53:1087-101, 1991

DiGiovanna J, Blank H. Failure of lysine in frequently recurrent herpes simplex infection. Arch Dermatol 120:48-51, 1984

Eby G. Use of topical zinc to prevent recurrent herpes simplex infection: Review of literature and suggested protocols. Med Hypotheses 17:157-65, 1985

Fink M, Fink J. Treatment of herpes simplex by alpha-tocopherol (Vitamin E). Br Dent J 148:246, 1980

Finnerty EF. Topical zinc in the treatment of herpes simplex. Cutis 37(2):130-31, 1986

Fitzherbert J. Genital herpes and zinc. Letter. Med J Aust 1:399, 1979

Gaby AR. Herpes simplex, herpes zoster. Commentary. Nutrition & Healing, 3(10), October, 1996

Gillis A. Lithium in herpes simplex. Letter. Lancet ii:516, 1983

Gordon YJ et al. Irreversible inhibition of herpes simplex virus replication in BSC-1 cells by zinc ions. Antimicrob Agents Chemother 8(3):377-80, 1975

Griffith RS et al. Success of L-lysine therapy in frequently recurrent herpes simplex infection. Dermatologica 175:183-90, 1987

Holden M et al. Further experiments on the inactivation of herpes virus by vitamin C (l-ascorbic acid). J Immunol 33:251-7, 1937

Hovi T et al. Topical treatment of recurrent mucocutaneous herpes with ascorbic acid-containing solution. Antivi Res 27(3):263-70, 1995

Kaul TN et al. Antiviral effect of flavonoids on human viruses. J Med Virol 15(1):71-9, 1985

Kim JE, Shklar G. The effect of vitamin E on the healing of gingival wounds in man. J Periodontol 54:305, 1983

Lamey PJ, Biagioni PA. Relationship between iron status and recrudescent herpes labialis. Eur J Clin Microbiol Infect Dis 14(7):604-5, 1995

Lewin S. Vitamin C: Its Molecular Biology and Medical Potential. New York, Van Norstrand Reinhold Co., 1973

McCune MA et al. Treatment of recurrent herpes simplex infections with L-lysine monohydrochloride. Cutis 34(4):366-73, 1984

Milman N et al. Failure of lysine treatment in recurrent herpes simplex labialis. Lancet ii:942, 1978

Mucsi I et al. Combined effects of flavonoids and acyclovir against herpesviruses in cultures. Acta Microbiol Hung 39(2):137-47, 1992

Nead DE. Effective vitamin E treatment for ulcerative herpetic lesions. Dent Survey 52(7):50-1, 1976

Schmeisser DD et al. Effect of excess dietary lysine on plasma lipids of the chick. J Nutr 113(9):1777-83, 1983

Skinner GR. Lithium ointment for genital herpes. Letter. Lancet ii:288, 1983

Sklar SH. Herpesvirus infection. Letter. JAMA 237(9):871-72, 1977

Sklar SH, Buimovici-Klein E. Adenosine in the treatment of recurrent herpes labialis. Oral Surg Oral Med Oral Pathol 48(5):416-17, 1979

Sklar SH - reported in CFS Forum 2(3), April 15, 1989

Terezhalmy GT et al. The use of water-soluble bioflavonoid-ascorbic acid complex in the treatment of recurrent herpes labialis. Oral Surg 45:56-62, 1978

Thein DJ, Hurt WC. Lysine as a prophylactic agent in the treatment of recurrent herpes simplex labialis. Oral Surg Oral Med Oral Pathol 58(6):659-6, 1984

Wahba A. Topical application of zinc-solutions: a new treatment for herpes simplex infections of the skin? Acta Derm Venereol 60(2):175-7, 1980

Ziaie Z et al. Lithium chloride suppresses the synthesis of messenger RNA for infected cell protein-4 and viral deoxyribonucleic acid polymerase in herpes simplex virus-1 infected endothelial cells. Lab Invest 70(1):29-38, 1994

HERPES ZOSTER

including POST-HERPETIC NEURALGIA

See Also: INFECTION
PAIN

NUTRITIONAL TREATMENT GUIDE

✓ = Efficacy generally accepted.
* = Efficacy *demonstrated* by controlled human trials.
[+] = Efficacy *suspected* from uncontrolled human trials.
[-] = Efficacy *suspected* from indirect data.
? = Efficacy *challenged* in a study of similar design.

NUTRITIONAL FACTORS

* **Adenosine-5'- Monophosphate:** 100 mg in a gelatin base IM 3 times weekly for up to 4 weeks

- -

[+] **Vitamin B_{12}:** ? 1 mg IM daily *AND*
Thiamine: 250 to 500 mg orally daily. After 6 days, reduce vitamin B_{12} injections to once weekly for 6 weeks.
[+] **Vitamin C:** ? 10 g daily (1 g per hour) until lesions dry up
[+] ? **Vitamin E:** 400 to 1,600 IU daily orally with topical application

OTHER RELATED FACTORS

[+] **Proteolytic enzymes:** 160 mg trypsin, 160 mg chymotrypsin, and 400 mg papainases 5 times daily

VITAMINS

Vitamin B_{12}

Pharmacologic dosages of vitamin B_{12} have been shown in animal studies and in uncontrolled human trials to have an analgesic effect in patients with very painful conditions *(Dettori;Hanck)*. In an open trial, injections of vitamin B_{12} have also seemed to be dramatically effective in relieving the pain of herpes zoster and accelerating the disappearance of vesicles. Moreover, none of the group of 21 patients developed post-herpetic neuralgia *(Gupta)*. However, it is not known whether vitamin B_{12} reduces the risk of the illness.

AND Thiamine

Like vitamin B_{12}, pharmacologic dosages of thiamine have seemed to have an analgesic effect in open trials involving patients with very painful conditions *(Charonnat;Quinn)*. In an informal clinical setting, the combination of vitamin B_{12} injections with oral thiamine seemed beneficial in reducing the pain of herpes *(Ropert)*.

Controlled trials are needed to confirm the efficacy of this treatment and to ascertain whether the addition of thiamine confers additional potency to any pain-relieving effect of vitamin B_{12}.

Vitamin C

The administration of pharmacologic dosages of ascorbic acid is another method of achieving pain relief which has been found effective in both animal and human studies of other painful conditions (see Pain). The results of open trials suggest that intravenous injections of the vitamin not only relieve the pain of shingles, but also speed healing.

In one study, 7 out of 8 patients reported cessation of pain within 2 hours after the first injection. Seven also showed drying of blisters within one day and complete clearing in 3 days *(Klenner)*. This small study was followed by a larger trial involving 327 patients. All were "cured" following 3 days of intravenous administration of the vitamin *(Zureick)*.

Controlled clinical trials have yet to be performed.

Vitamin E

Vitamin E is yet another vitamin which appears to reduce pain in a number of conditions. Its efficacy seems to be due to its ability to activate the endorphin system (see Pain). In an open trial, 13 patients with chronic post-herpes zoster neuralgia received between 400 and 1,600 IU vitamin E daily before meals and also applied the vitamin topically at the area of discomfort. Nine of the 13 experienced complete or almost complete control of pain, 2 were moderately improved, and 2 were slightly improved. Two of those who experienced complete or almost complete pain relief had had neuralgia for 13 and 19 years, respectively *(Ayres, 1973)*.

A subsequent open trial of 8 patients with post-herpetic neuralgia, 2 of whom also used vitamin E cream, found that, after 10 weeks, only one of the patients was improved *(Cochrane)*. The authors of the earlier study attribute this poor outcome to two factors. First, they found that at least 6 months of treatment was necessary to achieve results. Second, they believe that, for the treatment to be effective, patients need to avoid any medication or foods (including mixed vitamins containing inorganic iron, white flour, vitamin-enriched cereals, and conjugated estrogens) which may inactivate vitamin E *(Ayres, 1975)*.

OTHER NUTRITIONAL FACTORS

Adenosine Monophosphate (AMP)

AMP is a naturally occurring purine nucleotide that is an intermediate in cellular metabolism and nucleic acid synthesis. Patients with herpes zoster have been found to have abnormally low levels of AMP and abnormally high levels of adenosine triphosphate (ATP) *(Sklar, 1977)*.

Occasionally, especially if more than 75 mg is injected at once, the injection can cause non-cardiac chest pain. This can be prevented by giving half of the full dose and then waiting 20 minutes before giving the other half *(Gaby; Sklar, 1989)*.

There is also the theoretical danger over its ready conversion of AMP into adenosine, a substance which can cause immunodepression. Although recommended dosages appear to be too small to significantly affect systemic AMP levels, the possibility of immune suppression has not been ruled out by scientific studies *(Anonymous)*.

In a double-blind study, 32 adult patients with an acute vesicular rash randomly received intramuscular injections of either AMP or placebo 3 times a week for up to 4 weeks. AMP moderately reduced the pain soon after the start of treatment, decreased desquamation time, and promoted faster healing of the skin than placebo. It also reduced virus shedding and cleared the virus faster than in placebo-treated subjects.

Following 4 weeks, 88% of AMP-treated patients were pain-free, compared to 43% of placebo patients. All patients who had not recovered from pain then started receiving AMP without breaking the code. All these patients recovered from pain within 3 weeks after initiation of treatment. No recurrence of pain or lesions was experienced from 3 to 18 month following termination of treatment. There were no side effects during or after treatment *(Sklar, 1985)*.

While tantalizing, the results of this study are preliminary, both because the number of patients was small and because the groups were not comparable at the onset of therapy with respect to factors known to influence the natural history of varicella zoster infections (such as severity of disease at initiation of therapy) *(Sherlock)*.

OTHER RELATED FACTORS

Proteolytic Enzymes

The administration of proteolytic enzymes may be beneficial. In multiple studies, a mixture of proteolytic enzymes has been found to be as effective as acyclovir *(Billingmann;Kleine,1987,1996)*.

Also, in a Russian study, 150 patients with herpetic infections received trypsin alone. Compared to 200 similar patients who received routine treatment, trypsin was highly effective. In addition to reducing the pathological signs and symptoms during the acute period, none of the trypsin-treated patients had recurrences or developed postherpetic neuralgia during 3 years of follow-up *(Sichko)*.

COMBINED NUTRIENT THERAPY

A woman had open sores on her face with severe intractable pain for several months which had been diagnosed as herpes zoster. Several physicians were unable to treat her illness successfully.

She was treated with ascorbic acid 6 g/d, L-lysine 1 g/d, and vitamin B_{12} 1 mg intramuscularly twice weekly. Twenty-four hours later all her pain was gone and the open sores had begun to heal (Hoffer).

BIBLIOGRAPHY

Anonymous. AMP for herpes infections. Med Sci Bull 7(12), August 1985

Ayres S, Mihan R. Post-herpes zoster neuralgia: Response to vitamin E therapy. Arch Dermatol 108:855-6, 1973

Ayres S, Mihan R. Letter. Arch Dermatol 111:396, 1975

Billingmann P. [Enzyme therapy: an alternative in treatment of herpes zoster. A controlled study of 92 patients.] Fortschr Med 113(4):43-8, 1995) (in German)

Charonnat R, Lechat P. Sur le phénomène de réveil de l'anesthésie cornéenne. Thérapie 8:704, 1953 (in French)

Cochrane T. Post-herpes zoster neuralgia: Response to vitamin E therapy. Letter. Arch Dermatol 111:396, 1975

Dettori AG, Ponari O. Effetto antalgico della cobamamide in corso di neuropatie periferiche di diversa etiopatogenesi. Minerva Med 64:1077-82, 1973) (in Italian)

Gaby AR. Herpes simplex, herpes zoster. Commentary. Nutrition & Healing, 3(10), October, 1996

Gupka AK, Mital HS. Cyanocobalamin (vitamin B12) in the management of herpes zoster. Indian Pract 20(7):457-9, 1967

Hanck A, Weiser H. Analgesic and anti-inflammatory properties of vitamins. Int J Vitam Nutr Res (suppl)27:189-206, 1985

Hoffer A. Orthomolecular Medicine for Physicians. New Canaan, CT, Keats Publishing, Inc., 1989

Klenner F. The treatment of poliomyelitis and other virus diseases with vitamin C. South Med Surg 111:209-14, 1949

Kline M-W. Therapie des Herpres Zoster Mit Proteolytische Enzymen. Therapiewoche 37:1108-12, 1987

Kline M-W et al. the intestinal absorption of orally administered hydrolytic enzymes and their effects in the treatment of acute herpes zoster as compared with those of oral acyclovir therapy. Phytomedicine 2(1):7-15, 1996

Quirin H. Pain and vitamin B1 therapy. Bibl Nutr Dieta 38:110-11, 1986

Ropert R. Utilisation de la vitamine B1 fortes doses dans le traitement de divers syndromes douloureux facio-cephaliques. Sem Hôp 34:508-9, 1958 (in French)

Sherlock CH, Corey L. Adenosine monophosphate for the treatment of varicella zoster infections: A large dose of caution. Editorial. JAMA 253(10):1444-5, 1985

Sichko ZhV, Kozlova OL. [Experience in treating a herpetic infection with trypsin.] Vrach Delo 3:86-9, 1991) (in Russian)

Sklar SH. Herpesvirus infection. Letter. JAMA 237(9):871-72, 1977

Sklar SH - reported in CFS Forum 2(3), April 15, 1989

Zureick M. Treatment of shingles and herpes with vitamin C intravenously. J des Praticiens 64:586, 1950

HYPERTENSION

See Also: PREGNANCY AND ILLNESS

NUTRITIONAL TREATMENT GUIDE

✓ = Efficacy generally accepted.
* = Efficacy *demonstrated* by controlled human trials.
[+] = Efficacy *suspected* from uncontrolled human trials.
[-] = Efficacy *suspected* from indirect data.
? = Efficacy *challenged* in a study of similar design.

DIETARY FACTORS

✓ **Vegetarian diet**

- -

* high **dietary Fiber** intake
* minimize **Sugar** (sucrose, fructose and glucose)
* avoid **Alcohol**
* ? **low Salt diet** (maximum 2 g daily) (1 month trial)
* ? low **Fat** intake (especially **Saturated Fat**)
* ? avoid **Caffeine**

NUTRITIONAL FACTORS

* **Calcium deficiency:** 800 mg to 1,000 mg daily (2 month trial)
* **Potassium deficiency:** 60 mmol daily (or increase intake of dietary sources of potassium)
* **Coenzyme Q_{10}:** 100 mg daily (12 week trial)
* **Taurine:** 6 g daily (1 week trial)
* **L-Tryptophan:** 3 g daily (3 week trial)
* **Vitamin C:** 500 mg twice daily (4 week trial)
* ? **Magnesium deficiency:** 400 to 600 mg daily (2 month trial)
* ? **Omega-3 Fatty Acids:** EPA and DHA 3 to 4 g daily (2 month trial)

- -

[+] **Omega-6 Fatty Acids:** gamma-linolenic acid (ex. blackcurrant seed oil 6 g daily) (2 mo. trial)
[+] **Selenium deficiency:** 200 μg daily
[+] **Vitamin D:** ? 1,25-dihydroxycholicalciferol 0.68 μg daily

- -

[-] **Vitamin A deficiency:** 50,000 IU daily for 6 weeks (10,000 IU during pregnancy)
[-] **Vitamin B_6:** 5 mg/kg body weight daily
[-] **Vitamin E deficiency:** D,L-alpha-tocopheryl acetate 200 to 2,000 mg or IU daily for 6 weeks
[-] **Zinc:** *to treat cadmium-induced hypertension* (dosage unknown)

OTHER RELATED FACTORS

✓ treat **Obesity**

- -

[+] rule out **Food Sensitivities**
[+] rule out **Cadmium** toxicity
[+] rule out **Mercury** toxicity
[+] ? rule out **Lead** toxicity

DIETARY FACTORS

High Protein Diet

Historically, dietary protein has been thought to raise blood pressure. This hypothesis has been increasingly questioned by newer research. In fact, there is increasing data suggesting the opposite; namely that a high intake of dietary protein *decreases* blood pressure. An inverse relationship between protein intake and blood pressure was found, for example, in two recent large observational studies *(Stamler,1996a,b)*.

However, intervention studies have mostly found no significant effects of protein on blood pressure, so better controlled and adequately powered studies are needed before firm conclusions can be drawn *(Obarzanek)*.

Vegetarian Diet

A vegetarian diet is clearly beneficial *(Belin)*. Vegetarians are less likely to be hypertensive *(Melby)*. Moreover, hypertensive omnivores placed on a vegetarian diet demonstrate a decline in systolic blood pressure, with a corresponding rise on returning meat to the diet *(Margetts)*.

Several features of the vegetarian diet are themselves known to be beneficial to blood pressure regulation. These include its high content of fiber, potassium and magnesium as well as its low content of saturated fat and cholesterol *(Margetts;Ophir;Rouse)*.

Dietary Fiber

Increasing dietary fiber tends to decrease blood pressure in both hypertensive and normotensive subjects. For example, in a double-blind study, the average systolic blood pressure of a group of mildly hypertensive patients was significantly reduced following the addition of a dietary fiber supplement *(Eliasson)*. Tablets consisting of fiber from grains, citrus and vegetables have also been found to be effective under double-blind conditions with a similar population *(Schlamowitz)*. Moreover, populations with high-fiber intakes do not have the age-associated increase in blood pressure seen in Western populations with low fiber intakes *(Anderson,1986)*.

Some specific dietary fibers have been investigated. For example, the intake of oats has been associated with lower systolic and diastolic blood pressures, as well as with a lower body mass index *(He,1995)*. Konjac glucomannan reduced systolic blood pressure in healthy men in a double-blind crossover study *(Arvill)*, and guar gum reduced both systolic and diastolic blood pressure under double-blind conditions, again in a group of healthy men *(Landin)*.

Dietary Fat

The results of most, but not all, studies, suggest that an excess intake of fat - and particularly saturated fat - may cause hypertension *(Preuss,1993a)*. Conversely, blood pressure reduction has been repeatedly observed during low-fat diets which have a high-polyunsaturated fat to saturated fat ratio *(Iacono,1989)*.

Sugar

The results of numerous animal studies suggest that excessive intake of certain dietary sugars (sucrose, glucose and fructose) may cause blood pressure to rise *(Preuss,1994)*. Controlled clinical trials have had similar findings.

When, for example, normotensive men ingested a sugar solution following an overnight fast, water, lactose or galactose did not produce a change in blood pressure one hour later, while sucrose produced a 9 mm Hg increase, and glucose produced a 10 mm increase, in systolic blood pressure *(Rebello)*.

Perhaps one-third of normotensives are believed to be sucrose-sensitive *(Ahrens)*.

Alcohol

Alcohol ingestion has been repeatedly shown under controlled conditions to raise blood pressure, and is a significant contributor to the prevalence of hypertension *(Beilin)*. One to two drinks a day appear to slightly increase blood pressure, while higher levels of daily alcohol intake result in greater increases *(Klatsky)*.

Its effects in essential hypertensives appear to be partly reversible over 2 to 4 weeks following moderation of ethanol intake *(Puddey)*.

Caffeine

While acute caffeine ingestion in a non-coffee drinker may well raise blood pressure, much evidence suggests that, with continued frequent ingestion, adaptation develops to its pressor effect so that blood pressure gradually returns towards baseline levels *(Myers)*.

There is evidence, however, from a double-blind crossover study that habitual consumption may only diminish the acute pressor effect of caffeine *(James)*. Also, caffeine consumption may increase the blood pressure response to exercise in hypertensive men *(Sung)*, and may potentiate their stress-related rise in blood pressure *(Lovallo)*.

Not all the evidence regarding the relationship of caffeine to blood pressure is consistent. Some studies have found little or no relationship between the two *(Lancaster)*. In fact, in one study, coffee consumption was *negatively* correlated with both systolic and diastolic blood pressure in a dose-dependent manner *(Periti)*.

COMBINED DIETARY INTERVENTION

Several controlled studies have examined the benefits of placing patients on a diet based on the research we have summarized. For example, in a study published in the *New England Journal of Medicine*, 133 hypertensive patients were fed a control diet low in fruits, vegetables, and diary products with a fat content typical of the average American diet. After 3 weeks they were randomly assigned to receive the control diet or a diet rich in fruits, vegetables, and low-fat dairy products, and with reduced saturated and total fat. The latter diet reduced systolic and diastolic blood pressure by 11.4 and 5.5 mm Hg more, respectively, than the control diet *(Appel,1997)*.

HOMOCYSTEINE

Homocysteine is a toxic amino acid whose levels are commonly affected by B vitamin nutriture (see Homocysteine in Atherosclerosis). In a study of 175 older patients with a systolic blood pressure of at least 160 mm Hg and a diastolic pressure of less than 90 mm Hg, homocysteine levels were directly correlated with the risk of systolic hypertension (*Sutton-Tyrrell*), suggesting that improvement in B vitamin nutriture may combat systolic hypertension by reducing homocysteine levels.

NUTRITIONAL FACTORS

VITAMINS

Vitamin A Deficiency

In a study of the intake of 17 nutrients in over 10,000 Americans who denied a history of hypertension, a significant decrease in vitamin A intake was one of the 4 nutritional factors that distinguished hypertensive from normotensive subjects *(McCarron,1984)*. Furthermore, when 105 newly diagnosed essential hypertensives were compared with age-matched controls, the patients had significantly lower plasma vitamin A concentrations *(Russo,1998)*.

Whether improved vitamin A nutriture combats hypertension is not yet known.

Vitamin B_6

The relationship of vitamin B_6 nutriture to hypertension has been poorly researched. However, 4 weeks after 20 essential hypertensives received supplementation of the vitamin, mean systolic blood pressure fell from 167 to 153 mm Hg, and mean diastolic blood pressure fell from 108 to 98 mm Hg. Plasma epinephrine and norepinephrine levels fell concomitantly *(Aybak)*.

Vitamin C

As a group, hypertensives tend to have a reduced dietary intake of ascorbic acid *(McCarron,1984;Singh)*. Moreover, numerous observational studies have found both systolic and diastolic blood pressures to inversely correlate with plasma vitamin C levels *(Ness)*, sometimes in a step-wise manner *(Jacques)*.

Several experimental studies, including a double-blind crossover study, have shown that supplementation with one gram of vitamin C daily may reduce blood pressure in both borderline hypertensives and normotensives *(Osilesi)*. A small double-blind study of elderly hypertensives failed to find vitamin C effective; however, the patients only received 500 mg daily *(Ghosh)*.

Vitamin D

In a study of 290 consecutive patients on a medical ward, 57% were vitamin D-deficient. Hypertension, as well as reduced serum ionized calcium concentrations, were two of the significant univariate predictors of hypovitaminosis D *(Thomas)*. In another observational study, young women who consumed at least 400 IU daily of vitamin D had significantly lower systolic blood pressures than those who did not *(Sowers MF)*.

Hypertension appears to improve with vitamin D supplementation whether or not the vitamin is deficient *(Boucher)*. This hypotensive effect has been noted in hypertensives undergoing hemodialysis for whom the effect has been found to be reversible *(Mak)*.

Vitamin E Deficiency

Patients with essential hypertension have been found to have reduced erythrocyte levels of alpha-tocopherol, although lipid-standardized plasma levels may be normal *(Wen)*.

The efficacy of normalizing diminished vitamin E levels has not been reported.

MINERALS

Hard versus Soft Water

While the results of studies are mixed, most show that hard water is associated with lower blood pressure levels than soft water. Since absorption of elements in drinking water is usually twice that of foods (as there are no chelating agents present), they may have a greater influence, even though the concentrations of these elements is usually small in relation to that in the food.

Water hardness is usually caused by dissolved calcium and magnesium although, in a few areas, hardness may also result from iron or aluminum salts. The beneficial influence of water hardness may be from alkalinity or from competition between divalent ions. Toxic elements, such as cadmium and lead (see Cadmium and Lead below), may be leached from pipes in soft water areas because of low pH. Also, the intestinal absorption of cadmium and lead may be retarded by the presence of competing ions in hard water, i.e. calcium and magnesium *(Borgman)*.

Salt (sodium chloride)

Even though public health policy emphasizes sodium restriction as its principal recommendation, experts continue to debate sodium's role in arterial blood pressure control *(McCarron,1988)*. A large meta-analysis of randomized controlled trials recently concluded that the evidence in the normotensive population does not support current recommendations for universal sodium restriction *(Midgley)*. Moreover, salt intake cannot usually be restricted successfully below 5 g daily on a long-term basis *(Staessen,1997)*.

It does appear that moderate salt restriction (2 to 5 g daily) may result in about a 5 mm Hg decline, on average, in both systolic and diastolic blood pressures for perhaps half of the total population *(Egan,1985;Luft)*. Another estimate is that 30% of the general public, and 40 to 50% of hypertensives, are salt-sensitive *(McCarron,1991; Preuss,1997)*. Conversely, in a small minority of people, moderate sodium restriction may actually *increase* blood pressure *(Luft)*.

Other research suggests that certain populations, such as African-Americans, the elderly, and diabetics, may have a relatively high prevalence of salt sensitivity. However, the salt sensitivity noted in these groups appears to be more related to decreased ingestion of calcium and potassium than to excessive salt intake *(Sowers JR)*. Low magnesium intake may also be a cause of salt sensitivity *(McCarron,1997)*.

Short-term, very-low-salt diets appear to be contraindicated in patients at risk for hypertension along with hyperinsulinemia/insulin resistance ("syndrome X"). Such patients have raised concentrations of renin and aldosterone, and salt restriction results in further increases in these variables *(Egan,1997)*. Since most of the data suggesting a link between salt intake and blood pressure comes from epidemiologic studies, long-term, large-scale clinical trials are still needed to resolve this lingering controversy

Salt intake, however, is believed to be primarily responsible for determining how much calcium is excreted. In fact, within the usual ranges of salt and calcium intake, salt intake is more important than calcium intake in determining urinary calcium excretion. Increased urinary calcium excretion due to a high salt intake may not be adequately compensated for by increased calcium absorption; thus calcium may be resorbed from bone in order to maintain calcium homeostasis *(Antonios;Massey).*

Because of the importance of calcium in blood pressure regulation (see Calcium below), excess sodium intake may contribute to hypertension via its effect on calcium levels. This suggests that decreasing a high sodium intake is most likely to be effective when accompanied by an increase in a low calcium intake *(Levey).*

Potassium Deficiency

In contrast to dietary sodium, dietary potassium may have an *inverse* correlation with blood pressure *(Gelijnse; Khaw).* Many of the benefits of reduced sodium intake may actually reflect increased dietary potassium, since potassium intake usually increases when sodium intake is reduced (as when natural foods are substituted for processed foods).

In fact, the evidence is that the dietary sodium/potassium ratio correlates better with blood pressure than either sodium or potassium intake alone *(Smith).* Furthermore, in hypertensives, dietary potassium depletion has been shown to decrease sodium excretion and to increase blood pressure *(Krishna,1994).*

Another benefit of high potassium intake is its association with low calcium excretion *(He,1992)*, as adequate calcium nutriture appears important to blood pressure regulation (see Calcium below).

Also, erythrocyte potassium levels have been inversely correlated with blood pressure *(Trevisian),* while potassium depletion has been shown in a double-blind crossover study to increase blood pressure in hypertensives *(Krisna,1991).*

Supplementation

Two meta-analyses have concluded that potassium supplementation lowers blood pressure (*Cappuccio; Whelton)*, at least partly by increasing the dietary sodium/potassium ratio and by increasing calcium nutriture through decreased calcium excretion *(Bell).*

From a dietary standpoint, a reasonable approach would be to replace high-sodium, low-potassium processed foods with low-sodium, high-potassium natural foods.

Calcium Deficiency

Although the influence of calcium on hypertension is less widely appreciated than that of sodium and potassium, it is of at least equal importance. Calcium is the original calcium channel blocker, controlling its own influx across the cell membrane *(Hurwitz).* Alterations in its metabolism may be a primary factor in the development of hypertension, leading to changes in vascular smooth muscle function and peripheral vascular resistance - they may even determine sodium sensitivity *(McCarron,1985).*

Reduced dietary calcium appears to be the most consistent nutritional correlate of hypertension; the correlation is stronger than either high dietary sodium or low dietary potassium *(Harlan).*

Both serum calcium concentration *(Lind)* and urinary calcium excretion *(Medeiros;Quereda)* have been directly correlated with blood pressure, while plasma ionized calcium has shown an inverse correlation *(Hvarfner).*

Supplementation

Two meta-analyses of randomized clinical trials have found that, although calcium supplementation lowers blood pressure, the effect for the general population is too small to be clinically meaningful for people with an adequate baseline calcium intake *(Allender;Bucher).*

Similar to the situation in regard to sodium, about one-third to one-half of hypertensives are believed to be calcium-sensitive and can be expected to respond well to calcium supplementation *(Resnick,1986).* Calcium-sensitive patients can be identified by measuring serum ionized calcium levels; low levels of ionized calcium suggest that blood pressure will respond to calcium supplementation - and that the patient is also likely to be sodium-sensitive *(Resnick,1986).*

Magnesium Deficiency

Magnesium is a potent vasodilator *(Altura,1981).* A low magnesium concentration reduces production of prostacyclin (a vasodilating, anti-aggregating prostanoid), and increases release of thromboxane (a vasoconstricting, platelet-aggregating prostanoid). Other endothelial derivatives (endothelium-derived relaxing factor [nitric oxide], endothelin, and fibronectin) may also be affected *(Seelig).*

Dietary magnesium intake is inversely related to both systolic and diastolic blood pressure *(Ma).* In one study, low magnesium intake was the strongest of 61 dietary variables in predicting hypertension *(Joffres).* In fact, half of all patients suffering from magnesium depletion are hypertensive and, once their deficiency is corrected, blood pressure returns to normal *(Anonymous,1983).*

Although the results are conflicting, serum *(Ma)*, urinary *(Fischer)*, ionized *(Seelig)*, lymphocyte *(Kisters)*, and erythrocyte free *(Resnick,1984)* magnesium have all been reported to be low in hypertensives.

Supplementation

The findings have not been entirely consistent, yet magnesium supplementation has repeatedly been demonstrated to lower blood pressure in hypertensives under double-blind conditions *(Sanjuliani; Witteman)*. Moreover, supplemental magnesium can reduce blood pressure in normotensives with type I *(Eriksson)* or type II *(Purvis)* diabetes. Also, potassium and magnesium supplementation together have been found to be more effective than potassium alone in restoring the anti-hypertensive efficacy of diuretics *(Wester)*.

Inconsistent results from clinical trials may be because supplementation only appears to be of value when the patient is magnesium-deficient *(Moore)*. Since magnesium deficiency is associated with the loss of cellular potassium *(Altura,1984)*, it may be wise to increase potassium intake when evidence of magnesium deficiency is found.

Copper

The results of animal studies suggest that excessive copper intake *(Lui)*, or elevated serum copper concentrations *(Ahmed)*, may cause primary pulmonary hypertension due to a marked increase in pulmonary vascular resistance. Moreover, in a group of 7 patients with primary pulmonary hypertension, the mean serum copper level was significantly increased *(Ahmed)*.

The situation in essential hypertension is less clear. While serum copper levels have been reported to be elevated *(Bergomi; Vijaya)*, a recent study found plasma copper levels to be reduced *(Russo,1998)*. These inconsistent findings may be because plasma and serum copper may fail to reflect either copper intake or organ copper. In fact, the results of animal studies suggest that high serum copper may actually reflect low copper nutritional status *(Klevay)*. As to copper excretion, both systolic and diastolic blood pressures have been directly correlated with urinary copper excretion in early hypertensives *(Vivoli)*.

It is not yet known if hypertension can be treated by changing copper metabolism or nutriture.

Selenium Deficiency

In hypertensives, whole blood and plasma selenium levels, as well as plasma selenium-dependent glutathione peroxidase levels, may be depressed *(Mihailovic)*. Serum selenium levels are inversely correlated with both systolic and diastolic blood pressures. Similarly, higher serum selenium levels have been found to be associated with lower blood pressures, both systolic and diastolic, with a marked elevation in blood pressure at the lowest levels of serum selenium *(Salonen)*.

Zinc

Also see Cadmium below.

For unknown reasons, both animal *(Henrotte)* and human *(Frithz)* studies have found erythrocyte zinc to be elevated in hypertension. Essential hypertensives may also have higher plasma zinc concentrations *(Russo,1998)*; in fact, an inverse correlation between serum zinc and blood pressure has been observed in this population *(Bergomi)*.

OTHER NUTRITIONAL FACTORS

Essential Fatty Acids

Fatty acid metabolism appears to be altered in essential hypertension. Specifically, the activity of the desaturase enzymes, which are responsible for the conversion of essential fatty acids to the longer-chain eicosanoid precursors, appear to be increased. This results in greater bioavailability of eicosanoid precursors, especially arachidonic acid. These changes could affect vascular functioning and thus play a role in the pathogenesis or complications of hypertension *(Russo,1997)*.

Omega-3 Fatty Acids

alpha-linolenic acid → EPA → 3 series prostaglandins
↳ DHA

There is early evidence of an inverse association between the dietary intake of alpha-linolenic acid, precursor of the omega-3 essential fatty acid series, and mean resting blood pressure *(Salonen)*. In fact, one study found that a one percent increase in the adipose tissue content of alpha-linolenic acid was associated with a 5 mm Hg decrease in systolic, diastolic and mean arterial blood pressures *(Berry)*.

While the findings are not entirely consistent, several controlled studies of patients with essential hypertension have confirmed a blood pressure-lowering effect of eicosapentaenoic acid (EPA) and docosahexaenoic acid (DHA) - which are found in fish oil or derived from alpha-linolenic acid *(Appel,1993).*

Omega-6 Fatty Acids

linoleic acid → GLA → DGLA → prostaglandin E_1

Two out of 3 studies have found adipose tissue levels of linoleic acid to be inversely correlated with blood pressure *(Oster;Singer)*, while the other found no association *(Berry).* Similarly, there is evidence that serum linoleic acid levels may be inversely correlated with blood pressure in essential hypertensives *(Prabha)*, although a recent study found a direct correlation between serum levels of cholesterol ester DGLA and blood pressure levels in a group of men at high risk for coronary heart disease *(Simon).*

While there is substantial evidence that supplementation with omega-6 polyunsaturates may fail to affect blood pressure *(Morris),* there is some evidence that supports the use of sources of gamma-linolenic acid. For example, a group of borderline hypertensives were supplemented with blackcurrant seed oil (BSO), a rich source of gamma-linolenic acid, or with safflower oil. While the safflower oil group only had a slight inhibition of blood pressure reactivity resulting from the stress of a mental arithmetic test, blood pressure reactivity was inhibited by more than 40% in the BSO-treated patients *(Deferne).*

The results of certain animal studies have also suggested that supplementation with sources of gamma-linolenic acid may be beneficial. For example, in the spontaneously hypertensive rat, borage oil supplementation lowers systolic blood pressure, an effect that appears to be at least partly mediated by interference with the renin-angiotensin-aldosterone system *(Engler).*

The results of early studies suggest that supplementation with linoleic acid *(Iacono,1983)*, an omega-6 essential fatty acid, or its metabolites, i.e., gamma-linolenic acid *(Appel,1993;Engler)* may be beneficial.

Comparing and Combining

A proper balance between the two families of essential fatty acids, the omega-3 and omega-6 families, is essential for homeostasis. The proper balance to prevent and treat hypertension remains in dispute. Studies on the animal models of hypertension showed that the omega-6 family is more effective than the omega-3 family in lowering and normalizing the blood pressure of these animals, probably through the production of tissue prostaglandins, which favor vasodilation *(Lee).*

The comparative results of human trials have not been so clear. In fact, findings from double-blind studies have tended to favor oils from the omega-3 family as a means of lowering blood pressure in mild hypertension *(Bønaa;Radack).* However, since balance is important, further research may find it to be preferable to supplement with both families concurrently. There is already epidemiological evidence that too high an intake of omega-6 fatty acids may actually *promote* hypertension and the other manifestations of hyperinsulinemia and insulin resistance - possibly because of a relative deficiency of the omega-3 fatty acids *(Simon;Yam).*

Studies have already shown that essential fatty acids that do not require delta-6-desaturase for their metabolism appear to be more effective than those that do. A double-blind crossover study compared the combination of evening primrose oil (a rich source of gamma-linolenic acid) and marine oils (rich in EPA and DHA) to the combination of sunflower seed oil (rich in linoleic acid) and linseed oil (rich in alpha-linolenic acid) for a group patients with mild to moderate essential hypertension. Only the combination of evening primrose and fish oils significantly lowered mean systolic blood pressure *(Venter).* Similar findings were noted when these same 6-desaturated essential fatty acids were compared to sunflower seed oil, another oil that is rich in linoleic acid but a poor source of gamma-linolenic acid *(Deferne).*

Amino Acids

Sulfur Amino Acids

One study found an inverse correlation between the dietary intake of the sulfur amino acids (taurine and methionine) and blood pressure in a population with an unusually high incidence of stroke *(Yamori).* Similarly, serum levels of the sulfur amino acids appear to be lower in essential hypertensives and are inversely correlated with systolic blood pressure *(Ogawa)*, and their urinary excretion may be decreased *(Kohashi).*

Under double-blind conditions, both systolic and diastolic blood pressures fell significantly in a group of young patients with borderline hypertension following taurine supplementation, probably due to a reduction in sympathetic tone *(Fujita).*

L-Tryptophan

Results of studies using animal models of hypertension suggest that tryptophan supplementation may prevent the development of hypertension *(Lark)*. Whether the same is true in regard to human essential hypertension has not been explored.

However, there is experimental data suggesting that supplementation with L-tryptophan may reduce blood pressure in hypertensives. In an open trial, single oral doses lowered blood pressure 90 to120 minutes later in essential hypertensives *(Feltkamp)*. This was followed by the publication of a double-blind study which confirmed the finding and attributed the lowering of blood pressure to enhancement of central serotonin synthesis *(Lehnert)*.

Coenzyme Q_{10} (ubiquinone)

Ubiquinone nutriture may often be deficient in essential hypertension. In one group of 59 patients, enzymatic assays found that coenzyme Q_{10} was deficient in 39% compared to only 6% of the controls *(Yamagami)*.

Numerous open trials of patients with essential hypertension have found that supplementation with the coenzyme was following by blood pressure reduction *(Langsjoen)*. These results were confirmed by a double-blind crossover study in which essential hypertensives received CoQ_{10} and placebo in either order for 10 weeks each with a 2-week washout period in between. Mean systolic and diastolic pressures fell significantly by 10.6 and 7.7 mm Hg, respectively, during CoQ_{10} treatment and failed to change during placebo treatment *(Digiesi)*.

OTHER RELATED FACTORS

Obesity

Although it is not known how weight gain induces increased blood pressure, it is well-established that obesity is associated with an increased risk of hypertension *(Richards)*. Postulated mechanisms as to why hypertension is promoted in overweight individuals include insulin resistance/hyperinsulinemia, augmented sympathetic nervous system activity, and/or increased sodium retention *(Preuss,1993a)*. For example, in a screening of over one million persons, the frequency of hypertension in self-reported overweight individuals, ages 20 to 39 was 2 to 3 times higher than in persons of average to below average weight in the same age group *(Anonymous,1982)*.

Weight reduction in overweight hypertensives has been shown to be associated with a substantial reduction in blood pressure, even without a change in sodium intake *(Anderson,1994)*. In fact, weight control is probably the single most important lifestyle change that lowers blood pressure *(Preuss,1993a)*. Furthermore, even a small weight loss will often lower blood pressure; this, in turn, can be a powerful motivator for an obese patient to continue a weight reduction diet.

Heavy Metal Toxicity

Cadmium

Elevated blood levels of cadmium are associated with an increased risk of hypertension *(Bakshi)*. In one study, for example, untreated hypertensives were found to have 3 to 4 times the level of blood cadmium of matched normotensives *(Glauser)*. While other epidemiological studies have failed to confirm this relationship *(Staessen,1996)*, rats with long-term exposure to cadmium develop both systolic and diastolic hypertension *(Carmignani)*.

These rats exhibit increased renal excretion of zinc. Similarly, in humans, elevated blood cadmium levels are associated with reduced plasma zinc levels *(Arora)*. The results of an animal study suggest that zinc supplementation may reverse cadmium-induced hypertension *(Schroeder)*, while another animal study found that hard water (which is rich in calcium and magnesium) protected rats against cadmium-induced hypertension *(Perry)*.

Lead

Hypertension is a cardinal feature of lead nephropathy, and epidemiologic studies have shown an association between blood lead levels and blood pressure (*Loghman-Adham)*. For example, in a group of children, for every 10 microgram per deciliter increase in blood lead levels, there was a half a millimeter of mercury (mm Hg) increase in systolic, and four-tenths of a millimeter increase in diastolic, blood pressure *(Factor-Litvak)*.

Acute, symptomatic lead toxicity is well-established. However, the harmful effects of persistent, low-grade exposure without obvious symptomatology are uncertain. Some believe that lead-induced hypertension has a renal basis, others suggest that its effect is through the vasculature, and still others suggest that it causes a defect in the renin-angiotensin system *(Preuss,1993b)*.

Mercury

Mercury toxicity *(Henningsson;Petronio)* is another cause of hypertension which can be missed unless the examiner becomes suspicious while doing a careful history and considers laboratory testing.

Food Sensitivities

Hypertension may be due to a non-atopic reaction to specific foods. When this occurs, removal of those foods results in normalization of blood pressure *(Grant;Price).*

In one study, 10 patients were selected who were thought to be suffering from a wheat-related syndrome due to symptoms involving multiple organ systems. Six of the 10 had a diastolic BP of ≥95 mm Hg, while 4 had a diastolic BP of 90 mm Hg.

They were placed on a wheat-free diet. After 3 months, all 4 patients with slightly elevated blood pressures had become normal, and 3 of the 6 with higher blood pressures had improved, including one patient who was able to discontinue diuretics. The authors speculate that, since the 'wheat-related syndrome' is similar to pesticide and herbicide poisoning, and wheat may be sprayed with chemicals more than other grains due to its longer period of storage, the contamination of wheat with pesticide and/or herbicide residues may produce toxic effects *(Gibson).*

Unfortunately, it is not known how often food reactions contribute to the development of hypertension.

A 51-year-old hypertensive woman had lost 70 pounds over 18 months on a salt-free, low-protein diet and thyroid pills but her blood pressure failed to improve. She noted that fruits made her skin itch.

She was placed on a diet restricted to foods that were found on testing to be safe. Her blood pressure came down to the normal range, but it rose again after she began taking large, regular doses of cascara for constipation. Wheat products were also found to increase her blood pressure. Once these items were removed, her blood pressure again became normal (Price).

COMBINED NUTRITIONAL INTERVENTIONS

A 46 year-old industrial painter had a 3-year history of hypertension, with his blood pressure ranging from 156/100 to 180/110. There was no family history of hypertension, and all laboratory tests as well as an IVP were normal. His diet was free of sugar, refined flour, methylxanthines and added salt, and potassium chloride was used as a salt substitute. Fish and chicken were eaten rarely, and red meats even less often. He exercised regularly by playing tennis twice weekly, swimming or skiing. His usual supplementation consisted of vitamin C 1 gm and vitamin E 200 IU daily. Pubic hair mineral analysis revealed elevations of lead, cobalt and cadmium, with the cadmium level especially high.

He was treated with zinc gluconate 50 mg 3 times daily (copper levels were normal), up to 5 to 6 g vitamin C 3 times daily as tolerated, vitamin B complex with 100 mg B_6 daily (to prevent kidney stones), selenium 100 µg daily, linseed oil 1 tbsp daily, and an increase in vitamin E to 400 IU daily.

Six months later his average blood pressure had dropped to 154/96. Twelve months later, blood pressure was 142/90 and, 18 months later, blood pressure was 134/80 and hair cadmium had dropped to a much more acceptable level. The level of nutritional supplementation was decreased, although zinc and vitamin C were continued at relatively high levels to prevent recurrence (Wright).

BIBLIOGRAPHY

Ahmed I, Sackner M. Increased serum copper in primary pulmonary hypertension: A possible pathogenic link? Respiration 47:243-6, 1985

Ahrens RA. National Academy of Sciences, 1975 - summarized in Preuss HG, Fournier RD. Minireview: Effects of sucrose ingestion on blood pressure. Life Sci 30:879-86, 1982

Allender PS et al. Dietary calcium and blood pressure: A meta-analysis of randomized clinical trials. Ann Intern Med 124(9):825-31, 1996

Altura BM, Altura BT. Magnesium ions and contraction of vascular smooth muscles: Relationship to some vascular diseases. Fed Proc 40(12):2672-9, 1981

Altura BM, Altura BT. Interactions of Mg and K on blood vessels: Aspects in view of hypertension. Magnesium 3(4-6):175-94, 1984

Anderson JW, Tietyen-Clark J. Dietary fiber: hyperlipidemia, hypertension, and coronary heart disease. Am J Gastroenterol 81(10):907-19, 1986

Anderson JW et al. Relationship of weight loss to cardiovascular risk factors in morbidly obese individuals. J Am Coll Nutr 14(3):256-61, 1994

Anonymous. Nutrition and blood pressure: The effect of diet on hypertension. The Salt Institute, 1982

Anonymous. Hypomagnesemia and hypertension. Anabolism 2(6), June, 1983

Antonios TFT, MacGregor GA. Salt - more adverse effects. Essay. Lancet 348:250-1, 1996

Appel LJ et al. Does supplementation of diet with 'fish oil' reduce blood pressure? A meta-analysis of controlled clinical trials. Arch Intern Med 153(12):1429-38, 1993

Appel LJ et al. A clinical trial of the effects of dietary patterns on blood pressure. N Engl J Med 336(16):1117-24, 1997

Arora RB et al. Role of elements in pathophysiology of hypertension and antihypertensive drug development. Acta Pharmacol Toxicol (Copenh) 59 Suppl 7:344-7, 1986

Arvill A, Bodin L. Effect of short-term ingestion of konjac glucomannan on serum cholesterol in healthy men. Am J Clin Nutr 61:585-9, 1995

Aybak M et al. Effect of oral pyridoxine hydrochloride supplementation on arterial blood pressure in patients with essential hypertension. Arzneimittelforsch 45:1271-3, 1995

Bakshi SK et al. Cadmium and hypertension. J Assoc Physicians India 42(6):449-50, 1994

Beilin LJ. Alcohol and hypertension. Clin Exp Pharmacol Physiol 22(3):185-8, 1995

Belin LJ. Vegetarian and other complex diets, fats, fiber, and hypertension. Am J Clin Nutr 59(suppl):1130S-5S, 1994

Bell R et al. The influence of NaCl and KCl on urinary calcium excretion in healthy young women. Nutr Res 12:17-26, 1992

Bergomi M et al. Zinc and copper status and blood pressure. J Trace Elem Med Biol 11(3):166-9, 1997

Berry EM, Hirsch J. Does dietary linolenic acid influence blood pressure? Am J Clin Nutr 44(3):336-49, 1986

Bønaa KH et al. Effect of eicosapentaenoic and docosahexaenoic acids on blood pressure in hypertension. N Engl J Med 322:795-801, 1990

Borgman RF. Dietary factors in essential hypertension. Prog Food Nutr Sci 9:109-47, 1985

Boucher BJ. Inadequate vitamin D status: does it contribute to the disorders comprising syndrome 'X'? Br J Nutr 79(4):315-17, 1998

Bucher HC et al. Effects of dietary calcium supplementation on blood pressure. JAMA 275(13):1016-22, 1996

Cappuccio FP et al. Does potassium supplementation lower blood pressure? A meta-analysis of published trials. J Hypertens 9:465-73, 1991

Carmignani M, Boscolo P. Cardiovascular responsiveness to physiological agonists of male rats made hypertensive by long-term exposure to cadmium. Sci Total Environ 34(1-2):19-33, 1984

Deferne JL, Leeds AR. The antihypertensive effect of dietary supplementation with a 6-desaturated essential fatty acid concentrate as compared with sunflower seed oil. J Hum Hypertens 6(2):113-19, 1992

Digiesi V et al. Effect of coenzyme Q10 on essential arterial hypertension. Curr Ther Res 47:841-5, 1990

Egan B. Nutritional and lifestyle approaches to the prevention and mangaement of hypertension. Comprehen Therapy 11(8):15-20, 1985

Egan BM, Stepniakowski KT. Adverse effects of short-term, very-low-salt diets in subjects with risk-factor clustering. Am J Clin Nutr 65(suppl):671S-7S, 1997

Eliasson K et al. A dietary fibre supplement in the treatment of mild hypertension. A randomized, double-blind, placebo-controlled trial. J Hypertens 10(2):195-9, 1992

Engler MM et al. Effects of dietary gamma-linolenic acid on blood pressure and adrenal angiotensin receptors in hypertensive rats. Proc Soc Exp Biol Med 218(3):234-7, 1998

Eriksson J. Magnesium and ascorbic acid supplementation in diabetes mellitus. Ann Nutr Metab 39:217-23, 1995

Factor-Litvak P et al. Blood lead and blood pressure in young children. Epidemiology 7:633-7, 1996

Feltkamp H et al. Tryptophan-induced lowering of blood pressure and changes of serotonin uptake by platelets in patients with essential hypertension. Klin Wochenschr 62(23):1115-9, 1984

Fischer PWF et al. Magnesium status and excretion in age-matched subjects with normal and elevated blood pressures. Clin Biochem 26:207-11, 1993

Frithz G Ronquist G. Increased red cell content of zinc in essential hypertension. Acta Med Scand 205:647-9, 1979

Fujita T et al. Effects of increased adrenomedullary activity and taurine in young patients with borderline hypertension. Circulation 75:525, 1987

Gelijnse JM et al. Sodium and potassium intake and blood pressure change in childhood. Br Med J 300:899-902, 1990

Ghosh S et al. A double-blind, placebo-controlled parallel trial of vitamin C treatment in elderly patients with hypertension. Gerontology 40:268-72, 1994

Gibson SLM et al. A clinical evaluation of a wheat-free diet. J Nutr Environ Med 5:243-53, 1995

Glauser SC. Blood cadmium levels in normotensive and untreated hypertensive humans. Lancet i:717-18, 1976

Grant ECG. Food allergies and migraine. Lancet i:966-9, 1979

Harlan WK et al. Blood pressure and nutrition in adults. The National Health and Nutrition Examination Survey. Am J Epidemiol 120:17-24, 1984

He J et al. Effect of dietary electrolytes upon calcium excretion: the Yi People Study. J Hypertens 10:671-6, 1992

He J et al. Oats and buckwheat intakes and cardiovascular disease risk factors in an ethnic minority of China. Am J Clin Nutr 61:366-72, 1995

Henningsson C et al. Acute mercury poisoning (acrodynia) mimicking pheochromocytoma in an adolescent. J Pediatr 122(2):252-3, 1993

Henrotte JG et al. Blood and tissue zinc levels in spontaneously hypertensive rats. J Am Coll Nutr 9(4):340-43, 1990

Hurwitz L et al. Specific inhibition of calcium channels by calcium ions in smooth muscle. J Pharmacol Exp Ther 220:382-88, 1982

Hvarfner A et al. Indices of mineral metabolism in relation to blood pressure in a sample of a healthy population. Acta Med Scand 219(5):461-8, 1986

Iacono JM et al. Effect of dietary fat on blood pressure in a rural Finnish population. Am J Clin Nutr 38:860, 1983

Iacono JM et al. Dietary polyunsaturated fat and hypertension. Ann Med 21(3):251-4, 1989

Jacques PF. Effects of vitamin C on high-density lipoprotein cholesterol and blood pressure. J Am Coll Nutr 11(2):139-44, 1992

James JE. Chronic effects of habitual caffeine consumption on laboratory and ambulatory blood pressure levels. J Cardiovasc Res 1:159-64, 1994

Joffres MR et al. Relationship of magnesium intake and other dietary factors to blood pressure: the Honolulu heart study. Am J Clin Nutr 45(2):469-75, 1987

Khaw KT, Barrett-Connor E. The association between blood pressure, age, and dietary sodium and potassium: A population study. Circulation 77(1):53-61, 1988

Kisters K et al. Plasma magnesium and total intracellular magnesium ion content of lymphocytes in untreated normotensive and hypertensive patients. Trace Elem Electrolytes 13(4):163-6, 1996

Klatsky AL et al. The relationships between alcoholic beverage use and other traits to blood pressure: A new Kaiser Permanente study. Circulation 73(4):628-36, 1986

Klevay LM. Re: serum copper and the risk of acute myocardial infarction: a prospective population study in men in eastern Finland. Letter. Am J Epidemiol 135(7):832-4, 1992

Kohashi N et al. Decreased urinary taurine in essential hypertension. Prog Clin Biol Res 125:73-87, 1983

Krishna GG, Kapoor SC. Potassium depletion exacerbates essential hypertension. Ann Intern Med 115(2):77-83, 1991

Krishna GG. Role of potassium in the pathogenesis of hypertension. Am J Med Sci 307 Suppl 1:S21-5, 1994

Lancaster T et al. The effects of coffee on serum lipids and blood pressure in a UK population. J R Soc Med 87:506-7, 1994

Landin K et al. Guar gum improves insulin sensitivity, blood lipids, blood pressure, and fibrinolysis in healthy men. Am J Clin Nutr 56:1061-5, 1992

Langsjoen H et al. Usefulness of coenzyme Q10 in clinical cardiology: a long-term study. Mol Aspects Med 15(Suppl):S165-S175, 1994

Lark LA et al. Prevention of Dahl salt-induced hypertension by chronic dietary tryptophan. Can J Physiol Pharmacol 68(11):1432-6, 1990

Lee RM. Fish oil, essential fatty acids, and hypertension. Can J Physiol Pharmacol 72(8):945-53, 1994

Lehnert H et al. Effecdts of L-tryptophan on blood pressure in essential hypertensives. Abstract. Clin Exp Theory Pract A9(1):208, 1987

Levey WA et al. Blood pressure responses of white men with hypertension in two low-sodium metabolic diets with different levels of dietary calcium. J Am Diet Assoc 95(11):1280-7, 1995

Lind L et al. Relation of serum calcium concentration to metabolic risk factors for cardiovascular disease. Br Med J 297:960-3, 1988

Loghman-Adham M. Renal effects of environmental and occupational lead exposure. Environ Health Perspect 105(9):928-39, 1997

Lovallo WR et al. Caffeine may potentiate adrenocortical stress responses in hypertension-prone men. Hypertension 14(2):170-6, 1989

Luft FC. Salt and hypertension at the close of the millenium. Wien Klin Wochenschr 110(13-14):459-66, 1998

Lui CF, Medeiros D. Excess diet copper increases systolic blood pressure in rats. Biol Trace Element Res 9:15, 1986

Ma J et al. Associations of serum and dietary magnesium with cardiovascular disease, hypertension, diabetes, insulin and carotid artery wall thickness: the ARIC study. J Clin Epidemiol 48(7):927-40, 1995

Mak R. Amelioration of hypertension and insulin resistance by 1,25-dihydroxycholecalciferol in hemodialysis patients. Pediatr Nephrol 6:345-8, 1992

Margetts RM et al. Vegetarian diet in mild hypertension: A randomized controlled trial. Br Med J 293:1468-71, 1986

Massey LK, Whiting SJ. Dietary salt, urinary calcium, and bone loss. J Bone Miner Res 11(6):731-6, 1996

McCarron DA et al. Blood pressure and nutrient intake in the United States. Science 224(4656):1392-8, 1984

McCarron DA. Is calcium more important than sodium in the pathogenesis of essential hypertension? Hypertension 7(4):607-27, 1985

McCarron DA. Importance of dietary calcium in hypertension. Letter. J Am Coll Nutr 17(1):97-9, 1988

McCarron DA, Reusser ME. The integrated effects of electrolytes on blood pressure. The Nutrition Report 9(8), August, 1991

McCarron DA. Role of adequate dietary calcium intake in the prevention and management of salt-sensitive hypertension. Am J Clin Nutr 65(suppl): 712S-6S, 1997

Medeiros DM et al. Blood pressure in young adults as influenced by diet, anthropometrics, calcium status and serum lipids. Nutr Res 6:359-68, 1986

Melby CL et al. Blood pressure and blood lipids among vegetarian, semivegetarian, and nonvegetarian African Americans. Am J Clin Nutr 59:103-9, 1994

Midgley JP et al. Effect of reduced dietary sodium on blood pressure. A meta-analysis of randomized controlled trials. JAMA 275(20):1590-7, 1996

Mihailovic MB et al. Blood and plasma selenium levels and GSH-Px activities in patients with arterial hypertension and chronic heart disease. J Environ Pathol Toxicol Oncol 17(3-4):285-9, 1998

Moore TJ. The role of dietary electrolytes in hypertension. J Am Coll Nutr 8 Suppl S:68S-80S, 1989

Morris MC. Dietary fats and blood pressure. J Cardiovasc Risk 1(1):21-30, 1994

Myers MG. Effects of caffeine upon blood pressure. Arch Intern Med 148(5):1189-93, 1988

Ness AR et al. Vitamin C status and blood pressure. J Hypertens 14(4):503-8, 1996

Obarzanek E et al. Dietary protein and blood pressure. JAMA 275(20):1598-603, 1996

Ogawa M et al. Decrease of plasma sulfur amino acids in essential hypertension. Jpn Circ J 49(12):1217-24, 1985

Osilesi O et al. Blood pressure and plasma lipids during ascorbic acid supplementation in borderline hypertensive and normotensive adults. Nutr Res 11:405-12, 1991

Ophir O et al. Low blood pressure in vegetarians: The possible role of potassium. Am J Clin Nutr 37:755-62, 1983

Oster P et al. Blood pressure and adipose tissue linoleic acid. Res Exp Med (Berl) 175:287, 1979

Periti M et al. Coffee consumption and blood pressure: An Italian study. Clin Sci 72(4):443-7, 1987

Perry HM et al, in DD Hemphill, Ed. Trace Substances in Environmental Health-VIII. Columbia, MO, U. of Missouri Press, 1974:51

Petronio L. Chemical and physical agents of work-related cardiovascular diseases. Eur Heart J (Suppl 1):26-34, 1988

Prabha PS et al. Free radical generation, lipid peroxidation and essential fatty acids in uncontrolled essential hypertension. Prostaglandins Leukot Essent Fatty Acids 41(1):27-33, 1990

Preuss HG. Association of macronutrients (calories, carbohydrates, fat, proteins) with hypertension. Abstract. J Am Coll Nutr 12:595, 1993a

Preuss HG. A review of persistent, low-grade lead challenge: neurological and cardiovascular consequences. J Am Coll Nutr 12(3):246-54, 1993b

Preuss HG et al. Effects of high sugar diets on renal fluid, electrolyte and mineral handling in rats: relationship to blood pressure. J Am Coll Nutr 13(1):73-82, 1994

Preuss HG. Diet, genetics and hypertension. J Am Coll Nutr 16(4):296-305, 1997

Price AS. The role of food allergy in hypertension: An experimental study. Rev Gastroenterol 10(5):233-45, 1943

Puddey IB et al. Regular alcohol use raises blood pressure in treated hypertensive subjects. Lancet i:647-51, 1987

Purvis JR et al. Effect of oral magnesium supplementation on selected cardiovascular risk factors in non-insulin-dependent diabetics. Arch Fam Med 3:303-8, 1994

Quereda C. Urinary calcium excretion in treated and untreated essential hypertension. J Am Soc Nephrol 7(7):1058-65, 1996

Radack K et al. The effects of low doses of N-3 fatty acid supplementation on blood pressure in hypertensive subjects: a randomized controlled trial. Arch Intern Med 151:1173-80, 1991

Rebello T et al. Short-term effects of various sugars on antinatriuresis and blood pressure changes on normotensive young men. Am J Clin Nutr 38(1):84-94, 1983

Resnick LM et al. Intracellular free magnesium in erythrocytes of essential hypertension: Relationship to blood pressure and serum divalent cations. Proc Natl Acad Sci USA 81(2):6511-5, 1984

Resnick LM. Alterations of dietary calcium intake as a therapeutic modality in essential hypertension. Can J Physiol Pharmacol 64(6):803-7, 1986

Richards RJ et al. Obesity-related hypertension: its physiological basis and pharmacological approaches to its treatment. J Hum Hypertens 10 Suppl 3:S59-64, 1996

Rouse IL et al. Blood pressure lowering effects of a vegetarian diet: Controlled trial in normotensive subjects. Lancet i:5-9, 1983

Russo C et al. Increased membrane ratios of metabolite to precursor fatty acid in essential hypertension. Hypertension 29(4):1058-63, 1997

Russo C et al. Anti-oxidant status and lipid peroxidation in patients with essential hypertension. J Hypertens 16(9):1267-71, 1998

Salonen JT et al. Blood pressure, dietary fats, and antioxidants. Am J Clin Nutr 48:1226-32, 1988

Sanjuliani AF et al. Effects of magnesium on blood pressure and intracellular ion levels of Brazilian hypertensive patients. Int J Cardiol 56:177-83, 1996

Schlamowitz P et al. Treatment of mild to moderate hypertension with dietary fibre. Letter. Lancet ii:622-3, 1987

Schroeder HA, Buckman J. Cadmium hypertension: Its reversal in rats by a zinc chelate. Arch Environ Health 14:693, 1967

Seelig MS et al. Low magnesium: a common denominator in pathologic processes in diabetes mellitus, cardiovascular disease and eclampsia. Abstract. J Am Coll Nutr 11(5):597-637, 1992

Simon JA et al. Serum fatty acids and blood pressure. Hypertension 27(2):303-7, 1996

Singer P et al. Inverse relationship between linoleic acid in serum and in adipose tissue of patients with essential hypertension. Prostaglandins Leukot Med 9(6):603-13, 1982

Singh RB et al. Dietary intake and plasma levels of antioxidant vitamins in health and disease: a hospital-based case-control study. J Nutr Environ Med 5:235-42, 1995

Smith WCS et al. Urinary electrolyte excretion, alcohol consumption, and blood pressure in the Scottish heart study. Br Med J 297:329-30, 1988

Sowers MF et al. The association of intakes of vitamin D and calcium with blood pressure among women. Am J Clin Nutr 42:135-42, 1985

Sowers JR. Dietary cation (micronutrient) effects in salt-sensitive hypertension. Abstract. J Am Coll Nutr 12:594, 1993

Staessen JA et al. Public health implications of environmental exposure to cadmium and lead: an overview of epidemiological studies in Belgium. Working Groups. J Cardiovasc Risk 3(1):26-41, 1996

Staessen JA et al. Salt and blood pressure in community-based intervention trials. Am J Clin Nutr 65(suppl):661S-70S, 1997

Stamler J et al. Inverse relation of dietary protein markers with blood pressure. Findings for 10,020 men and women in the INTERSALT Study. Circulation 94(7):1629-34, 1996a

Stamler J et al. Relationship to blood pressure of combinations of dietary macronutrients: findings of the multiple risk factor intervention trial (MRFIT). Circulation 94(10):2417-23, 1996b

Sung BH et al. Caffeine elevates blood pressure response to exercise in mild hypertensive men. Am J Hypertens 8:1184-8, 1995

Sutton-Tyrrell K et al. High homocysteine levels are independently related to isolated systolic hypertension in older adults. Circulation 96(6):1745-9, 1997

Thomas MK et al. Hypovitaminosis D in medical inpatients. N Engl J Med 338(12):777-83, 1998

Trevisian M et al. Red blood cell sodium and potassium concentration and blood pressure. Ann Epidemiol 5:44-51, 1994

Venter CP et al. Effects of essential fatty acids on mild to moderate hypertension. Prostaglandins Leukot Essent Fatty Acids 33(1):49-51, 1988

Vijaya J et al. Serum copper levels and lipid profile of ischemic heart disease patients and hypertensives. Trace Elem Electrol 13(3):147-50, 1996

Vivoli G et al. Zinc and copper levels in serum, urine and hair of humans in relation to blood pressure. Sci Total Environ 66:55-64, 1987

Wen Y et al. Lipid peroxidation and antioxidant vitamins C and E in hypertensive patients. Irish J Med 165(3):210-12, 1996

Wester PO, Dyckner T. Magnesium and hypertension. J Am Coll Nutr 6(4):321-8, 1987

Whelton PK et al. Effects of oral potassium on blood pressure. Meta-analysis of randomized controlled clinical trials. JAMA 277(20):1624-32, 1997

Wittemen JCM et al. Reduction of blood pressure with oral magnesium supplementation in women with mild to moderate hypertension. Am J Clin Nutr 60:129-35, 1994

Wright JV. A case of cadmium-related high blood pressure, in Wright JV. Dr. Wright's Guide to Healing with Nutrition. Emmaus, Penn., Rodale Press, 1984

Yam D et al. Diet and disease - the Israeli paradox. Is J Med Sci 32:1134-43, 1996

Yamagami T et al. Bioenergetics in clinical medicine. Studies on coenzyme Q10 and essential hypertension. Res Commun Chem Pathol Pharmacol 11:273, 1975

Yamori Y et al. Studies on stroke prevention in animal models, and their supportable epidemiological evidence, in H Barnett et al, Eds. Cerebrovascular Diseases: New Trends in Surgical and Medical Aspects. Amsterdam, Elsevier/North Holland, 1981:47-62

'HYPOGLYCEMIA' (FUNCTIONAL)

See Also: **ALCOHOLISM**
HEADACHE (MIGRAINE)
INNER EAR DISORDERS
MUSCLE CRAMPS

NUTRITIONAL TREATMENT GUIDE

✓ = Efficacy generally accepted.
* = Efficacy *demonstrated* by controlled human trials.
[+] = Efficacy *suspected* from uncontrolled human trials.
[-] = Efficacy *suspected* from indirect data.
? = Efficacy *challenged* in a study of similar design.

DIETARY FACTORS

* avoid **Caffeine**

- -

[+] **low Protein, high Unrefined Carbohydrate diet**
[+] increase **meal frequency**
[+] increase **Soluble Fiber** intake
[+] substitute **Fructose** for Glucose or Sucrose
[+] avoid **Alcohol**

NUTRITIONAL FACTORS

* **Chromium:** 125 to 200 μg daily (3 month trial)
* **Magnesium deficiency:** ≈ 400 mg daily (6 week trial)

- -

[+] **Niacin:** 100 mg before meals

OTHER RELATED FACTORS

[+] rule out **Food Sensitivities**

The prevalence of idiopathic reactive or functional hypoglycemia is highly controversial. While mainstream physicians consider it to be a rare finding *(Snorgaard)*, other practitioners believe it to be common in their patient population.

Other objective measures suggest that, whether or not hypoglycemia is central to the syndrome, the syndrome does exist. For example, there is evidence that, in patients exhibiting 'hypoglycemic' symptoms, the glucose nadir is coincident with a dramatic rise in adrenaline and cortisol levels *(Chalew)*. Also, EEG abnormalities have been found during glucose tolerance testing that are coincident with measurements of disturbed physiologic function as well as with the well-known subjective symptoms of distress; however, these disturbances tended to occur when blood glucose levels were either elevated or well after the glucose nadir *(Hudspeth).*

It has been suggested that true reactive hypoglycemia must meet all of the following diagnostic criteria *(Anderson JW, 1987)*:

1. Recurring symptoms after meals compatible with hypoglycemia
2. Plasma glucose values less than 45 mg/dL after meals or glucose intake
3. Symptoms of hypoglycemia at the time of chemical hypoglycemia

DIETARY FACTORS

Several dietary modifications have been suggested to combat reactive hypoglycemia. Increasing the frequency of meals, for example, has been claimed to prevent the onset of symptoms by assisting in the maintenance of stable blood sugar levels *(Bell).*

Refined Carbohydrates

Avoidance of sugars has long been held to be central to dietary planning *(Karlan).* With the discovery of the concept of the glycemic index, this dictum has been supplanted by a broader, but less extreme, reduction in all carbohydrates which have been stripped of their fiber content by refining *(Oettle; Wolever).*

In one study, for example, 8 patients with glucose nadirs less than 55 mg/dL accompanied by symptoms of reactive hypoglycemia, a peak plasma cortisol of more than 18 μg/ml, and at least a 5 μg/ml rise in plasma cortisol from its value at the glucose nadir, were placed on a low refined carbohydrate diet. All but one became asymptomatic and the other was substantially improved. When total grams of refined carbohydrate increased, symptoms returned *(Sanders).*

A 56-year-old woman had attacks of faintness after meals containing sugar. Postprandial hypoglycemia was found and her condition was diagnosed as idiopathic reactive hypoglycemia.

After sugar was eliminated from her diet, she had no further attacks (Weiss).

Fructose *versus* Glucose or Sucrose

Compared to glucose and sucrose, fructose causes substantially less stimulation of plasma glucose and insulin responses and is thus less likely to provoke reactive hypoglycemia *(Crapo; Schwarz).*

Soluble Fiber

In open trials, several soluble dietary fibers have been shown to reduce the occurrence of the hypoglycemic syndrome. One study found apple pectin and oat bran to be the most effective of the fibers tested *(Langseth).* Another study found glucomannan to be highly effective *(Hopman).*

Low Protein, High Unrefined Carbohydrate Diet

The ideal balance between protein and carbohydrates for these patients has long been a hotly debated topic. Historically, a high protein, low carbohydrate was advised. This diet was believed to be beneficial as the blood sugar response to protein ingestion in both normals and functional hypoglycemics is flatter than for glucose, suggesting that there may be a smaller subsequent hypoglycemic swing *(Conn).* However, when patients with impaired glucose tolerance were switched from a low protein, high carbohydrate diet to a high protein, low carbohydrate diet, there was a significant deterioration in glucose tolerance *(Anderson JW, 1975).*

A more modern approach is a diet which is high in unrefined carbohydrates (50-55% of energy), and relatively low in protein (15-20% of energy), leaving about 30 to 35% of energy from fat. High in plant fiber

(50 g), the diet contains less than 50 grams of simple carbohydrate. Patients must usually limit the intake of milk and fruit (especially fruit juices) to achieve these dietary parameters.

This diet increases insulin sensitivity and facilitates glucose uptake. In addition, the soluble fiber delays gastric emptying, slows glucose absorption, and minimizes blood glucose swings. Extensive clinical experience suggests that almost all patients with reactive hypoglycemia will respond to this diet *(Anderson JW,1987)*.

Alcohol

Alcohol ingestion has been shown to contribute to the onset of hypoglycemic symptoms *(Halmos;Nikkila)*. It is known to inhibit gluconeogenesis and promote a fall in plasma glucose *(Rabin)*. Moreover, the increase in gastric acidity which follows alcohol ingestion might cause excessive release of gut secretagogues which augment beta-cell responsiveness to glucose fluctuations, leading to excessive insulin release *(Freinkel)*.

Hypoglycemia is rarely seen in ethanol-intoxicated patients, however *(Sucov)*, and does not appear to occur any more frequently in an ethanol-intoxicated population than in a population without elevated ethanol levels *(Sporer)*. These findings suggest that alcohol need only be avoided by patients who are known to be prone to the syndrome.

Caffeine

Patients should avoid caffeine because it stimulates the adrenal gland; then liberated adrenalin causes glycogenolysis in the liver, and an elevation of the blood sugar occurs, only to be followed by a drop *(Salzer)*.

Under double-blind conditions, caffeine increased the sensitivity of healthy subjects to lower levels of plasma glucose. At glucose levels of 2.8 mmol/L and 3.8 mmol/L, only those subjects given caffeine experienced symptoms of hypoglycemia (trembling, sweating, palpitations). At that glucose level, the concentrations of epinephrine, norepinephrine, cortisol, and growth hormone were all significantly higher after caffeine than after placebo *(Kerr)*.

Not surprisingly, glucose ingestion appears to increase the hypoglycemic effect of caffeine. A recent study gave healthy subjects either caffeine (the amount in 2 cups of coffee), glucose, or both together. Only those in the caffeine plus glucose group acted as if they were hypoglycemic, becoming nervous, shaky and sweating and reacting to hunger much worse than those in the other two groups - even though they did not actually develop hypoglycemia. In addition, cerebral blood flow decreased in the two caffeine groups, and the caffeine-plus-glucose group had the greatest increases in insulin, epinephrine and cortisol levels *(Watson)*.

NUTRITIONAL FACTORS

VITAMINS

Niacin

There are no controlled clinical trials supporting the use of niacin supplementation. In an informal clinical setting, however, when 350 patients with relative hypoglycemia received niacin before meals, the results seemed to be highly beneficial *(Buehler)*. Similarly, niacin was found to be effective in normalizing blood sugar for a group of 507 patients with alcoholism accompanied by hypoglycemia *(Shansky)*.

MINERALS

Chromium

Chromium is well-known to have important effects on glucose regulation (see Diabetes Mellitus). It improves insulin binding, insulin receptor number, insulin internalization, beta-cell sensitivity and insulin receptor enzymes, and it increases insulin sensitivity *(Anderson RA,1997)*.

While the effects of chromium supplementation have only been reported for a small number of patients, dramatic improvements have been noted. In a double-blind crossover study, patients with symptoms of reactive hypoglycemia were supplemented with chromium or placebo for 3 months. Hypoglycemic symptoms (including severe shaking, blurred vision, sleepiness and abnormal sweating) improved dramatically.

Objectively, the glucose nadir following a glucose load was raised at 2 to 4 hours, and insulin binding to red blood cells and insulin receptor number improved significantly. All subjects, when asked to predict in which part of the study they had received chromium or placebo, were able to predict correctly *(Anderson RA,1987)*. Similar results were found in a 3-month open trial during which, in addition to subjective improvement, about three-quarters of the patients demonstrated a decrease in the area of the negative part of the glucose tolerance curve *(Clausen)*.

Magnesium Deficiency

It appears that magnesium may reduce glucose-induced insulin secretion *(Curry)*. A deficiency could therefore contribute to reactive hypoglycemia by enhancing glucose-induced insulin secretion. Evidence that some reactive hypoglycemics may be magnesium-deficient comes from a small group of 14 female and 8 male patients in which the women were found to have lower erythrocyte, plasma and hair magnesium levels than the controls, although magnesium nutriture in the men was normal *(Stebbing)*.

Six weeks after these 14 women were supplemented with magnesium, blood glucose no longer dropped below fasting levels during glucose tolerance testing and, for 3 of the women, glucose tolerance was much improved. Half of the group felt better as compared to only one-quarter of a group of similar women who had received placebo. Non-responders tended to either have an elevated hair calcium to magnesium ratio, or urinary magnesium excretion failed to increase with supplementation *(Stebbing)*.

OTHER RELATED FACTORS

Food Sensitivities

While some clinicians believe that functional hypoglycemia may be due to food sensitivities, scientific evidence is lacking. One author has suggested that, in his experience, three-quarters of the cases of functional hypoglycemia may be caused by such sensitivities *(Breneman)*.

COMBINED TREATMENT PROGRAM

A 36 year-old television company executive had become so fatigued that it affected his performance at work. Nutritional supplementation, food allergy treatments and relaxation techniques had been unsuccessful. He felt worse mid-morning, late morning, mid-afternoon and during his trip home in the evening, while a cup of tea with sugar, a sweet biscuit or a piece of chocolate resulted in a temporary lift. Glucose tolerance testing revealed a profound drop in blood sugar between one and four hours after the glucose load.

Refined carbohydrates were eliminated from his diet and he was told to keep his intake of high carbohydrate foods within moderation and to eat small frequent meals. Extra magnesium and chromium were added to his nutritional supplement program.

Symptoms remarkably improved; later they totally resolved when he changed his job for one he enjoyed more (Davies).

BIBLIOGRAPHY

Anderson JW, Herman RH. Effects of carbohydrate restriction on glucose tolerance of normal men and reactive hypoglycemic patients. Am J Clin Nutr 28:748, 1975

Anderson JW, Gustafson NJ. Dietary fiber in disease prevention and treatment. Compr Ther 13(1):43-53, 1987

Anderson RA et al. Effects of supplemental chromium on patients with symptoms of reactive hypoglycemia. Metabolism 36(4):351-5, 1987

Anderson RA. Nutritional factors influencing the glucose/insulin system: chromium. J Am Coll Nutr 16(5):404-10, 1997

Bell LS et al. Dietary strategies in the treatment of reactive hypoglycemia. J Am Diet Assoc 85(9):1141-3, 1985

Breneman JC. Basics of Food Allergy. Springfield, Illinois, Charles C. Thomas, 1978

Buehler MS. Relative hypoglycemia: A clinical review of 350 cases. Lancet (Minneapolis) 82(7):1962

Chalew S et al. The use of plasma epinephrine response in the diagnosis of idiopathic postprandial syndrome. JAMA 251:612-15, 1984

Clausen J. Chromium induced clinical improvement in symptomatic hypoglycemia. Biol Trace Elem Res 17:229-36, 1988

Conn JW, Newburgh LH. The advantage of a high protein diet in the treatment of spontaneous hypoglycemia. J Clin Invest 15:673-8, 1936

Crapo PA et al. The effects of oral fructose, sucrose, and glucose in subjects with reactive hypoglycemia. Diabetes Care 595):512-17, 1982

Curry DL et al. Magnesium modulation of glucose-induced insulin secretion by the perfused rat pancreas. Endocrinology 101:203, 1977

Davies S, Stewart A. Nutritional Medicine. London, Pan Books, 1987

Freinkel N, Getzger BE. Oral glucose tolerance curve and hypoglycemias in the fed state. N Engl J Med 280:820-8, 1969

Halmos VT et al. [Alcohol-induced hypoglycemia.] Dtsch Z Verdau Stoffwechselkr 39(5):219-26, 1979) (in German

Hopman WPM et al. Glucomannan prevents postprandial hypoglycemia in patients with previous gastric surgery. Gut 29(7):930-4, 1988

Hudspeth WJ et al. Neurobiology of the hypoglycemia syndrome. J Holistic Med 3(1):60-71, 1981

Karlan SC, Cohn C. Hypoglycemic fatigue. JAMA 130:553-5, 1946

Kerr D et al. Effect of caffeine on the recognition of and responses to hypoglycemia in humans. Ann Intern Med 119:799-804, 1993

Langseth L, Dowd J. Glucose tolerance and hyperkinesis. Food Cosmet Toxicol 16(2):129-33, 1978

Nikkila EA, Taskinen MR. Ethanol-induced alterations of glucose tolerance, postglucose hypoglycemia, and insulin secretion in normal, obese, and diabetic subjects. Diabetes 24(10):933-43, 1975

Oettle GJ et al. Glucose and insulin responses to manufactured and whole-food snacks. Am J Clin Nutr 45:86-91, 1987

Rabin D. Hypoglycemia: Physiologic and diagnostic considerations, in GE Abraham, Ed. Radioassay Systems in Clinical Endocrinology. New York, Marcel Dekker, 1981:609-24

Salzer HM. Relative hypoglycemia as a cause of neuropsychiatric illness. J Natl Med Assoc 58(1):12-17, 1966

Sanders LR et al. Refined carbohydrate as a contributing factor in reactive hypoglycemia. South Med J 75:1072, 1982

Schwarz J-M et al. Thermogenesis in men and women induced by fructose vs glucose added to a meal. Am J Clin Nutr 49:667-74, 1989

Shansky A. Vitamin B_3 in the alleviation of hypoglycemia. Drug Cosmetic Industry 129(4):68-9, 104-5, 1981

Snorgaard O. [Functional hypoglycemia. Fancy or fact?] Ugeskr Laeger 154(36):2406-9, 1992) (in Danish)

Sporer KA et al. The incidence of ethanol-induced hypoglycemia. Am J Emerg Med 10(5):403-5, 1992

Stebbing JB et al. Reactive hypoglycemia and magnesium. Magnesium Bull 4(2):131-4, 1982

Sucov A, Woolard RH. Ethanol-associated hypoglycemia is uncommon. Acad Emerg Med 2(3):185-9, 1995

Watson J, Royal Bournemouth Hospital, Bournemouth, England - presented at the annual mtg. of the American Diabetes Association and reported in Medical Tribune August, 1997

Weiss M et al. [Metabolic studies in reactive hypoglycemia.] Harefuah 118(12):691-2, 1990 (in Hebrew)

Wolever TM, Miller JB. Sugars and blood glucose control. Am J Clin Nutr 62(1 Suppl):212S-221S; discussion 221S-227S, 1995

IMMUNODEPRESSION

See Also: **ACQUIRED IMMUNO DEFICIENCY SYNDROME (AIDS)**
CANCER
CANDIDIASIS
INFECTION

NUTRITIONAL TREATMENT GUIDE

✓ = Efficacy generally accepted.
* = Efficacy *demonstrated* by controlled human trials.
[+] = Efficacy *suspected* from uncontrolled human trials.
[-] = Efficacy *suspected* from indirect data.
? = Efficacy *challenged* in a study of similar design.

DIETARY FACTORS

[+] consume adequate **Protein** *(to maintain both cell-mediated and humoral immunity)*
[+] avoid **Coffee** *(to maintain both cell-mediated and humoral immunity)*
[+] avoid **Sugar** *(to maintain both cell-mediated and humoral immunity)*
[+] reduce **Fat** intake to below 30% of calories *(to increase natural killer cell activity)*

NUTRITIONAL FACTORS

✓ **Vitamin A deficiency:** 50,000 IU daily for 6 weeks (10,000 IU during pregnancy)

- -

* **Arginine:** 25 to 30 g daily
* **Dimethylglycine:** 120 mg daily
* **Glutamine deficiency:** 5 to 30 g daily
* **Iron deficiency:** 30 mg twice daily until repletion; then minimal possible dosage (high dosages may be immunosuppressive)
* **Selenium:** 50 to 200 μg daily (high dosages may be immunosuppressive)
* **Vitamin A:** dosage uncertain (high dosages may be immunosuppressive)
* **Vitamin B_6:** ? 50 mg daily
* **Vitamin E:** 200 mg daily
* **Zinc deficiency:** zinc sulfate 220 mg twice daily (high dosages may be immunosuppressive) *AND* **Copper** 2 mg daily
* ? **Beta carotene:** 30 to 60 mg daily
* ? **Vitamin C:** 500 mg to 5 g daily

- -

[+] **Coenzyme Q_{10}:** 60 to 200 mg daily
[+] **Copper deficiency:** 2 mg twice daily for up to 6 weeks (high dosages may be immunosuppressive) *AND* **Zinc** 50 mg daily
[+] **Folic acid deficiency:** 800 μg daily
[+] **Iodine deficiency:** 90 to 300 μg daily
[+] **Magnesium deficiency:** ≈ 400 mg daily
[+] **Pantothenic acid deficiency:** 100 to 200 mg daily
[+] **Vitamin B_{12} deficiency:** 1,000 μg intramuscularly weekly initially and monthly afterwards
[+] **Vitamin C deficiency:** 500 mg twice daily
[+] ? **Omega-3 fatty acids:** *example:* MaxEPA 1 g caps [180 mg EPA; 120 mg DHA] 10 to 20 daily (high dosages may be immunosuppressive)

- -

[-] **Riboflavin deficiency:** 5 to 10 mg daily
[-] **Thiamine deficiency:** 50 mg daily
[-] **Vitamin D deficiency:** 50,000 to 100,000 IU 2 or 3 times during the first week; then, if needed, either 100,000 of ergo- or cholecalciferol every 3 to 6 months *OR* 800 to 1,600 IU daily

OTHER RELATED FACTORS

[+] rule out **Aluminum** toxicity
[+] rule out **Cadmium** toxicity
[+] rule out **Lead** toxicity
[+] rule out **Mercury** toxicity

DIETARY FACTORS

Protein

A deficiency of protein is well known to be immunosuppressive *(Levy)*. Severe protein or calorie malnutrition results in marked impairment of both humoral and cell-mediated immune functions. Usually it is complicated by multiple nutrient deficiencies *(Myrik)*. The major defects in severe protein-calorie malnutrition seem to involve T-lymphocytes and the complement system *(Torún)*.

Fat

Dietary fat intake appears to affect the activity of natural killer cells, a factor of potential importance in early tumor surveillance.

Excessive lipid intake (particularly of cholesterol and of polyunsaturated fatty acids) is associated with immunodepression *(Chandra, 1986)*. Even short-term infusions of lipid emulsions in both healthy volunteers and seriously ill post-operative patients impair monocyte and leukocyte phagocytosis and chemotaxis. Impairment of lymphocyte responses and the generation of anti-tumor natural killer cells have also been observed *(Guillou)*.

A reduced intake of dietary fat appears to stimulate the activity of natural killer cells. Even a modest reduction of the usual fat intake to less than 30% percent of calories in a group of healthy, normal-weight young males may result in a marked increase in natural killer-cell activity *(Barone)*.

Sugar

Sugar has been shown to decrease immunity in several ways. When, for example, healthy adults ingested glucose, lymphocyte transformation was significantly depressed, apparently by increasing serum insulin, which competes with mitogens for binding sites on lymphocytes *(Bernstein)*. Various simple sugars (carbohydrates from glucose, fructose, sucrose, honey or orange juice) were shown to decrease the phagocytic index (the capacity of neutrophils to engulf bacteria) - while starch did not have this effect *(Sanchez)*.

Results of an animal study suggest that sugar may also depress humoral immunity when it is substituted for other dietary nutrients on an equal calorie basis. As the nutritional quality of the diet was reduced by progressively diluting the diet with sucrose in 10% increments, the production of antibodies was decreased proportionately. Even when the diet contained as little as 10% sucrose, antibody production was reduced by one-half *(Nalder)*.

Coffee

While more research is needed, it appears that coffee may depress both cellular and humoral immunity. Results of a crossover study suggest that coffee consumption may suppress the lymphocyte response to mitogens while increasing both suppressor T-cells and natural killer cells and the chemotactic activity of mononuclear cells *(Melamed)*.

Early evidence that coffee may lower immunoglobulin levels comes from a comparison of non-smokers to smokers - a group that may be more sensitive to the effects of immunodepressants due to the adverse effects of tobacco. Among the smokers, the half that consumed 4 or more cups of coffee daily had significantly lower levels of immunoglobulin M than those of the other smokers, while their other immunoglobulin levels also trended lower *(Kraal)*.

NUTRITIONAL FACTORS

VITAMINS

Vitamin A

Deficiency

Vitamin A deficiency has been called an immunodeficiency disorder characterized by widespread alterations in immunity *(Semba,1994)*. The deficiency has been shown to reduce the response of both T and B cells to mitogens and antigens *(Semba,1993)*, impair phagocytosis *(Ongsakul)*, impair antibody responses *(Chavance)*, and impair secretory IgA production *(Dreizen)*. Severe deficiency may also lead to atrophy of the thymus and spleen and a marked decrease in circulating leukocytes and lymphocytes *(Levy)*.

Vitamin A supplementation may reverse post-operative immunosuppression *(Cohen)*. It may boost immune responses in the elderly, persons with parasitic infections and persons with a high exposure to ultraviolet light *(Rumore)*. Moreover, animal work suggests that it may enhance responses to weak immunogens and reverse immunosuppression *(Nuwayri-Salti)*.

Toxicity

An excess of vitamin A may depress the very immune responses that are stimulated by modest increases of the vitamin *(Levy)*. Furthermore, in a recent double-blind study of institutionalized elderly, only 800 micrograms daily (about 2,700 IU) reduced the number of both $CD3^+$ and $CD4^+$ T-lymphocytes *(Fortes)*, suggesting that vitamin A supplements should be used cautiously in this population.

Vitamin B Complex Deficiencies

Deficiencies of various B-complex vitamins are associated with decreased antibody responses and impaired cellular immunity *(Anderson,1983)*. Also, in controlled studies, supplementation of a combination of vitamins B_1, B_6 and B_{12} has been shown to reduce postoperative immunosuppression *(Kurashige;Lettko)*. Whether these supplements were repleting a pre-existing deficiency or exerting a pharmacologic effect is unclear, although the former hypothesis appears more likely.

Folic Acid Deficiency

Human studies have shown that a deficiency of folic acid is associated with impaired responses to mitogens *in vitro* and delayed hypersensitivity responses *(Levy)*.

Pantothenic Acid Deficiency

Pantothenic acid deficiency is known to depress humoral antibody responses to various antigens in humans *(Beisel,1982)*.

Riboflavin Deficiency

In animals, a riboflavin deficiency has been found to be associated with a diminished ability to generate humoral antibodies in response to test antigens *(Beisel,1982)*.

Thiamine Deficiency

Animals made thiamine-deficient demonstrate markedly decreased complement activity, phagocytic activity of peripheral blood leukocytes, and serum bactericidal activity, as well as decreased antibody production in response to sheep red blood cells *(Pletsityi)*.

Vitamin B_6

Since vitamin B_6 is required for normal nucleic acid and protein synthesis and for cellular multiplication, isolated B_6 deficiencies cause more profound effects on immune system functions than deficiencies of any other B-group vitamin. Also, unlike any other B vitamin, deficiencies appear to inhibit cell-mediated immune functions as well as humoral responsiveness to a variety of test antigens *(Axelrod)*.

Specifically, vitamin B_6 deficiency is associated with a reduction in number and function of both T- and B-lymphocytes, reduced delayed hypersensitivity responses, greatly diminished response to antigenic challenge, decreased secretion of immunoglobulins, greatly diminished response to antigenic challenge, decreased secretion of immunoglobulins, reduced thymic epithelial cell function and reduced phagocytic activity of neutrophils *(Levy;Rall)*. Deficiency also impairs interleukin 2 production and lymphocyte proliferation in the elderly, an effect which is reversible with repletion *(Meydani,1991)*.

In several experiments, supplementation of vitamin B_6 has been shown to improve lymphocyte responses. Perhaps the most careful study was of a group of elderly people, some of whom had low baseline levels of pyrioxal-5-phosphate, who received either pyridoxine hydrochloride or placebo. After one to two months, treated subjects showed significant increases in lymphocyte responses to mitogens and antigens, and percentages of T3+ and T4+ (but not of T8+ cells) increased significantly *(Talbott)*.

Vitamin B_{12} Deficiency

Deficiency of vitamin B_{12} associated with impaired lymphocyte response to mitogens and a modest reduction in the phagocytic and bacteriocidal capacity of polymorphonuclear leukocytes *(Levy)*. In untreated pernicious anemia, there is impairment of both lymphocyte *(Das)* and neutrophil *(Kaplan)* functioning.

A recent controlled study found that even a subtle deficiency is detrimental. Elderly patients with low serum B_{12} levels were immunized with pneumococcal vaccine. Compared to age-matched controls, they were found to have impaired antibody responses *(Fata)*.

Vitamin C

Deficiency of vitamin C impairs phagocyte function and cellular immunity *(Chandra,1986)*. This includes inhibition of neutrophil mobility - which, in turn, inhibits the formation of inflammatory reactions *(Beisel,1987)* - and decreased natural killer cell activity *(Dowd)*.

Generally, studies of vitamin C supplementation have been of healthy individuals given megadoses of the vitamin. Based on these studies, supplementation has wide-ranging benefits, bolstering both cellular and humoral immunity. The vitamin may, for example, enhance neutrophil motility and chemotaxis *(Johnston)*, increase neutrophil phagocytosis *(Patrone)*, increase immunoglobulin levels *(Prinz)*, increase complement concentrations *(Prinz)*, increase lymphocyte blastogenesis in response to mitogens *(Kennes)*, and improve delayed hypersensitivity skin reactions *(Kennes)*.

Results of an animal suggest caution in supplementing patients who are highly stressed with megadoses of ascorbic acid. In this study mice that were stressed and then supplemented with the vitamin developed severe lymphopenia. The authors theorize that, since stress abruptly increases adrenal corticosteroids in plasma following the release of vitamin C by the adrenals, large doses of the vitamin may maintain high levels of plasma corticosteroids which, in turn, may reduce the organism's immune response when stressed *(Richardson)*. However, evidence of lymphopenia due to megadose ascorbate has not been reported in humans.

A brother and sister with chronic granulomatous disease (CGD) of the autosomal recessive type, and with markedly defective neutrophil motility and elevated serum IgE levels, were treated with a single oral daily dose of 1 g ascorbate for 6 months. Both children also received prophylactic antibiotics which were always stopped 1 week prior to testing of immune function.

Ascorbate treatment was accompanied by significantly increased neutrophil motility and post-phagocytic metabolic activity, and a reduction in serum IgE levels. Enhanced neutrophil function correlated with clinical improvement. Both children have remained free of infection since ascorbate was added to their regimen and have gained weight (Anderson,1979).

Vitamin D Deficiency

In its active form (1,25-dihydroxyvitamin D_3), vitamin D is an autoregulatory hormone which has been shown *in vitro* to modulate lymphocyte and macrophage functions. While it has no apparent effect on B-lymphocytes, it causes T-cell suppression which indirectly inhibits antibody production by B-cells *(Muller)*.

Vitamin E Deficiency

A deficiency of vitamin E depresses immunoglobulin response to antigens, lymphocytic proliferative responses to mitogens and antigens, delayed dermal hypersensitivity reactions, and general host resistance *(Beisel,1981)*.

Supplementation may enhance immune responses by increasing the number of antibody-forming cells and cell-mediated responses *(Levy)*. Recently, to determine whether long-term supplementation enhances clinically relevant measures of immunity in the healthy elderly, subjects received 60 mg, 200 mg or 800 mg vitamin E for 235 days in a double-blind study published in the *Journal of the American Medical Association*.

While immunoglobulin levels and levels of T- and B-cells were unaffected, certain clinically relevant indices of cell-mediated immunity improved at the 200 mg dosage level, suggesting that the elderly may benefit from higher levels of vitamin E intake than those usually recommended *(Meydani,1997)*. Similar findings have been noted with healthy young subjects *(Meydani,1993)*.

And Vitamin C

A single-blind study published in the *American Journal of Clinical Nutrition* found that the combination of vitamins C and E increased cytokine production significantly more than either vitamin alone, suggesting that supplementation with the combination of the two vitamins may be more effective *(Kee-Ching)*. In a subsequent open trial, combined supplementation of the two vitamins significantly increased lymphoproliferative capacity and the phagocytic functions of polymorphonuclear neutrophils in aged women, whether or not they were healthy *(la Fuente)*.

MINERALS

Copper

Deficiency

A deficiency of copper is associated with an increased incidence of infection and impairment of cell-mediated immunity. The function of the reticuloendothelial system is depressed and the microbicidal activity of granulocytes is reduced. Impaired antibody response to heterologous red blood cells and low levels of thymic hormone activity have been reported *(Chandra,1986)*.

When healthy men were fed a low-copper diet, there was a decrease in proliferation of peripheral blood mononuclear cells when cultured with mitogens and an increase in the percentage of circulating B-cells *(Kelley,1995)*, apparently because T-cells are more sensitive to copper deprivation than B-cells *(Tong)*.

Toxicity

Copper nutriture has an ideal range, as excess copper also suppresses immune responses *(Pocino)*.

Iodine Deficiency

Deficiency of iodine is associated with reduced microbicidal activity of polymorphonuclear leukocytes *(Chandra,1986)*.

Iron

Deficiency

Iron deficiency causes impaired cell-mediated immunity. There may be, for example, impairment of bacteriocidal capacity of neutrophils and impairment of the lymphocyte proliferation response *(Chandra,1986)*. The mean number of total lymphocytes, CD3 and CD4 subsets, and B lymphocytes may be decreased, as well as killer cell activity *(Santos,1990)*. Cellular effector functions involving cytokines and nitric oxide may be impaired *(Weiss)*. As little as a 10% decrease in dietary iron can cause immunodepression *(Levy)*.

Supplementation in cases of deficiency has been demonstrated to improve some of the lymphocyte-related factors mentioned above *(Santos,1990)* although, even after two months, immune functions may not be fully normalized *(Thibault)*.

Toxicity

Iron overload is also associated with significant abnormalities of immune function with impairment of antigen-specific immune responses, a reduction in the number of functional helper precursor cells, impaired generation of cytotoxic T-cells, enhanced suppressor T-cell activity, and reduced proliferative capacity of helper T-cells *(Good)*.

Magnesium Deficiency

Magnesium deficiency produces subtle immunologic sequelae and may be affected by genetic control of blood cell magnesium concentration. Abnormal complement activation, excess antibody production, and susceptibility to allergy and fungal infections have been reported *(Galland)*.

Research has shown that the ability to adapt to a marginal intake of magnesium is limited. In fact, a low intake of the mineral for an extended period of time may be a factor in the pathogenesis of disorders of immune function even though physical signs of magnesium deficiency may be absent *(Kubena)*.

Selenium

Selenium deficiency impairs cell-mediated immunity *(Chandra,1985)*. Phagocytosis is decreased, T-cells appear to be coated by factors that suppress their response to mitogens and antigens *(Levy)*, and helper T-cell numbers are diminished *(Shils)*. Natural killer cell-mediated cytotoxicity is also reduced *(Nair)*.

Supplementation of healthy volunteers *(Kiremidjian-Schumacher;Roy)* and of the institutionalized elderly *(Peretz)* has been demonstrated to enhance lymphocyte responses under double-blind conditions.

Excessive intake may be immunosuppressive, however *(Diplock)*. While the results of *in vitro* studies suggest that immune function in people who already have optimal selenium nutriture is unlikely to improve but could be impaired by additional intake *(LaBue;Nair)*, the results of subsequent experiments using healthy humans suggest instead that selenium has immunoenhancing effects at supplemental levels above those achieved by normal dietary intake *(Kiremidjian-Schumacher;Roy)*. Since it is quite possible that even healthy subjects may be marginally selenium-deficient *(Oster)*, an intracellular selenium assay would be preferable prior to starting high dosage supplementation for the purpose of immunoaugmentation *(LaBue)*.

Zinc Deficiency

Zinc deficiency is associated with impaired immune responses including impaired lymphocyte proliferation, differentiation and maturation and abnormalities in T-lymphocyte subpopulations *(Beck)*. Granulocytes *(Prasad,1995)* and platelets *(Bogden,1987)* have also been shown to be depressed. In addition, zinc deficiency has been correlated with a decrease in natural killer cell and interleukin-2 activity *(Rabbani)* as well as with impairment of leukocyte chemotaxis *(Baer)*.

Supplementation may increase suppressor T-cells *(Mathe)*, restore serum thymulin activity *(Ripa)*, increase interleukin-1 production *(Prasad,1993)*, and enhance natural killer cell activity *(Bogden,1990)*. However, like some of the other micronutrients mentioned above, excessive intake of zinc (300 mg daily) may impair lymphocyte and neutrophil responses *(Bogden,1987; Chandra,1984)*.

A patient with isolated zinc deficiency was found to have lymphopenia, a depressed T-cell mitogen response, increased numbers of circulating T-suppressor cells and decreased circulating T-helper cells. Activity of the patient's natural killer (NK) cells was very depressed, and monocyte cytotoxicity (MC) was 4 times that of normal controls.

Zinc repletion improved the peripheral lymphocyte count, corrected the abnormal helper/suppressor ratio, normalized T-cell response to mitogen, improved NK function, and lowered MC to control values (Allen).

OTHER NUTRITIONAL FACTORS

Amino Acids

Deficiencies or imbalances of essential amino acids interfere with protein synthesis, and thus with production of immunoglobulins, interferons, and all other proteins necessary for host defenses *(Beisel,1982)*.

Arginine

Arginine may become deficient during illness, when a strong immune response is needed *(Visek)*. It is important in immunity because it augments T-lymphocyte activation in response to mitogens. Arginine also appears to mediate a direct effect on components of the immune system which results in enhanced production or use of lymphokines *(Reynolds)*.

Supplementation may increase natural killer cell and lymphokine-activated-killer cell activity *(Park)* and the mean T-lymphocyte response to mitogens *(Daly)*. Although its primary application is to enhance cellular immunity during illness *(Daly)*, it appears to be a safe nutritional stimulator of lymphocyte immune reactivity in healthy people *(Barbul)*.

Glutamine

Deficiency of glutamine is immunosuppressive and falls in glutamine concentration affect T lymphocyte proliferation and macrophage function. Glutamine is depressed in many conditions such as sepsis, surgery, trauma, and burns, where immunity is often compromised, resulting in prolonged illness and an increase in late mortality *(Newsholme)*.

Supplementation

The efficacy of glutamine supplementation has been demonstrated under controlled conditions for patients with multiple organ failure requiring parenteral feeding. These patients demonstrated a significant improvement in six-month survival *(Griffiths)*. Another controlled trial, this time of patients undergoing colorectal resection, showed that, for a group of patients on total parenteral nutrition undergoing colorectal surgery, glutamine increased the T-cell mitogenic response *(O'Riordain)*.

The use of stable dipeptides of glutamine has solved prior problems concerning its bioavailability in supplemental form *(O'Riordain)*.

Beta-Carotene

Modest doses of beta carotene may stimulate immune responses *(Chandra,1986)*. For example, in healthy people, supplementation has been shown under controlled conditions to enhance the response to mitogens *(Moriguchi)*, enhance the CD4-CD8 (helper/suppressor) ratio *(Murata)*, enhance natural killer cell activity *(Santos,1996)*, increase tumor necrosis factor-alpha secretion and improve monocyte functions *(Hughes)*.

However, a recent double-blind study of the healthy elderly failed to find evidence that either short- or long-term beta-carotene supplementation enhanced T-cell-mediated immunity *(Santos,1997)*. The reasons for these conflicting results remain unclear, although it has been suggested that the efficacy of beta-carotene in stimulating immune responses may be largely confined to people with inadequate vitamin A intake or with a previously stressed immune response *(Daudu)*.

Coenzyme Q_{10} (Ubiquinone)

Coenzyme Q_{10} appears to be important for optimal functioning of the immune system *(Blizanov)*.

Results of an open trial suggest that supplementation may increase T-helper cell numbers and the T-helper to T-suppressor ratio, and increase IgG antibody levels in healthy people *(Folkers,1993)*. Chronically ill patients have also shown significant increases of immunoglobulin G following supplementation *(Folkers,1982)*. The results of animal studies also suggest that supplementation may activate macrophages *(Saiki)*.

Dimethylglycine

Under double-blind conditions, supplementation with dimethylglycine has been shown to enhance both humoral and cell-mediated immune responses in both healthy volunteers and in patients with diabetes or sickle cell disease *(Graber)*. Moreover, similar results have been found in animal studies *(Reap)*.

Essential Fatty Acids

A deficiency of essential fatty acids may result in lymphoid atrophy and depressed immune responses. However, an excess of polyunsaturates in the diet may be immunosuppressive *(Chandra,1986)*, especially if there is an imbalance in the ratio between the omega-3 and omega-6 families *(Grimm)*.

Omega-3 Fatty Acids

There are a number of immunoenhancing effects of omega-3 fatty acids *(Calder)*. Supplementation may prevent immunosuppression after trauma *(Ayala)*. Fish oil, a rich source, may combat the immunosuppression caused by the oxygenation of arachidonic acid *(Blackburn)*. Moreover eicosapentaenoic acid may increase the responses of T-cells to mitogens, increase the generation of leukotriene B5, and decrease leukocyte arachidonic acid *(Payan)*.

However, fish oil, especially at high dosages, may have a mild immunodepressant effect and may decrease several indices of cell-mediated immunity *(Payan; Virella)*. Docosahexaenoic acid does not seem to be responsible for these immunosuppressive effects *(Kelley, 1998)*; whether they are due to eicosapentaenoic acid is not known. Unless they are accompanied by adequate antioxidants, omega-3 fatty acids could cause increased free radical formation and lipid peroxidation, leading to a reduction in T cell-mediated function, natural killer cell activity, and macrophage cytotoxicity *(Meydani, 1996)*.

Until more is known about the immunoregulating effects of the omega-3 fatty acids, they should be used cautiously and the immune parameters of concern should be followed.

Omega-6 Fatty Acids

Since either a deficiency or an excess of prostaglandin E_1 can have a deleterious effect in the regulation of T lymphocyte function, precursors from the omega-6 family of essential fatty acids could theoretically promote T-cell activation *(Horrobin)*.

Studies have suggested, however, that omega-6 fatty acids supplementation may have an adverse effect on immune function. For example, total omega-6 fatty acids and linoleic acid correlated inversely with natural killer cell activity in healthy elderly subjects *(Rasmussen)*. Under controlled conditions, a high intake of alpha-linolenic acid (from flaxseed oil), suppressed mononuclear cell responses to mitogens and the delayed hypersensitivity response to recall antigens *(Kelley, 1991)*.

Also, an animal study found that mice on diets enriched with linoleic acid, when compared to mice on diets enriched with oleic, palmitic or eicosapentaenoic acid, were predisposed to suppression of T-cell-mediated cutaneous responses *(Bennett)*.

While other studies have found that high levels of dietary linoleate do not always cause immunosuppression *(Clevel)*, the evidence to date does not suggest employing omega-6 supplementation in order to improve immune responses.

OTHER RELATED FACTORS

Heavy Metal Toxicity

Excess levels of heavy metals such as aluminum *(Nordal)*, cadmium *(Nath; Stacey)*, lead *(Bendich)*, and mercury *(Perlingeiro)* have all been shown to depress various aspects of immune function.

BIBLIOGRAPHY

Allen JI et al. Alterations in human natural killer cell activity and monocyte cytotoxicity induced by zinc deficiency. J Lab Clin Med 102(4):577-89, 1983

Anderson R, Dittrich OC. Effects of ascorbate on leucocytes: Part IV. Increased neutrophil function and clinical improvement after oral ascorbate in 2 patients with chronic granulomatous disease. S Afr Med J 56(12):476-80, 1979

Anderson R, Theron A. Effects of B-complex vitamins on cellular and humoral immune functions in vitro and in vivo. Int J Vitam Nutr Res 24:7-84, 1983

Axelrod AE, Traketellis AC. Relationship of pyridoxine to immunological phenomena. Vitam Horm 22:591-607, 1964

Ayala A, Chaudry IH. Dietary n-3 polyunsaturated fatty acid modulation of immune cell function before and after trauma. Nutrition 11(1):1-11, 1995

Baer MT et al. Nitrogen utilization, enzyme activity, glucose intolerance and leukocyte chemotaxis in human experimental zinc depletion. Am J Clin Nutr 41(6):1220-35, 1985

Barbul A et al. Arginine stimulates lymphocyte immune response in healthy human beings. Surgery 90(2):244-51, 1981

Barone J et al. Dietary fat and natural-killer-cell activity. Am J Clin Nutr 50:861-7, 1989

Beck FW et al. Changes in cytokine production and T cell subpopulations in experimentally induced zinc-deficient humans. Am J Physiol 272(6 Pt 1):E1002-7, 1997

Beisel WR et al. Single-nutrient effects on immunologic functions. JAMA 245(1):53-8, 1981

Beisel WR. Single nutrients and immunity. Am J Clin Nutr 35:417-68 [Suppl], 1982

Beisel WR. Role of nutrition in immune system diseases. Compr Ther 13(1):13-19, 1987

Bendich A et al. Immune response of rats chronically fed subclinical doses of lead. Clin Exp Immunol 43:189-94, 1981

Bennett M et al. Dietary fatty acid effects on T-cell-mediated immunity in mice infected with mycoplasma pulmonis or given carcinogens by injection. Am J Pathol 126(1):103-13, 1987

Bernstein J et al. Depression of lymphocyte transformation following oral glucose ingestion. Am J Clin Nutr 30:613, 1977

Blizanov EG. Coenzyme Q, the immune system and aging, in K Folkers, Y Yamamura, Eds. Biomed & Clin Aspects of Coenzyme Q Vol. 3. Elsevier/North Holland Biomed Press, 1981:311-23, 1981

Blackburn GL. Nutrition and inflammatory events. Abstract. J Am Coll Nutr 149(5):528, 1995

Bogden JD et al. Zinc and immunocompetence in the elderly: Baseline data on zinc nutriture and immunity in unsupplemented subjects. Am J Clin Nutr 46:101-9, 1987

Bogden JD et al. Effects of one year of supplementation with zinc and other micronutrients on cellular immunity in the elderly. J Am Coll Nutr 9(3):214-25, 1990

Calder PC. N-3 polyunsaturated fatty acids and immune cell function. Adv Enzyme Regul 37:197-237, 1997

Chandra RK. Excessive intake of zinc impairs immune responses. JAMA 252:1443-6, 1984

Chandra RK. Trace element regulation of immunity and infection. J Am Coll Nutr 4(1):5-16, 1985

Chandra RK. Nutrition and immunity - Basic considerations. Part I. Contemp Nutr 11(11), 1986

Chavance M et al. Nutritional support improves antibody response to influenza virus in the elderly. Letter. Br Med J [Clin Res] November 9, 1985:1348-9

Cohen B et al. Reversal of postoperative immunosuppression in man by vitamin A. Surg Gynecol Obstet 149:658-62, 1979

Crevel RWR, Saul JAT. Review - Linoleic acid and the immune response. Eur J Clin Nutr 46:847-55, 1992

Daly JM et al. Immune and metabolic effects of arginine in the surgical patient. Ann Surg 208(4):512, 1988

Das KC, Herbert V. The lymphocyte as a marker of past nutritional status: Persistence of abnormal lymphocyte deoxyuridine (uD) suppression test and chromosomes in patients with past deficiency of folate and vitamin B12. Br J Haematol 38:219-33, 1978

Daudu PA et al. Effect of a low b-carotene diet on the immune functions of adult women. Am J Clin Nutr 60:969-72, 1994

Diplock AT. Trace elements in human health with special reference to selenium. Am J Clin Nutr 45:1313-22, 1987

Dowd PS et al. Nutrition and cellular immunity in hospital patients. Br J Nutr 55(3):515-27, 1986

Dreizen S. Nutrition and the immune response - A review. Int J Vit Nutr Res 49:220-8, 1978

Fata FT et al. Impaired antibody responses to pneumococcal polysaccharide in elderly patients with low serum vitamin B12 levels. Ann Intern Med 124(3):299-304, 1996

Folkers K et al. Increase in levels of IgG in serum of patients treated with coenzyme Q10. Res Commun Chem Pathol Pharmacol 38:335-8, 1982

Folkers K et al. The activities of coenzyme Q10 and vitamin B6 for immune response. Biochem Biophys Res Commun 193:88-92, 1993

Fortes C et al. The effect of zinc and vitamin A supplementation on immune response in an older population. J Am Geriatr Soc 46(1):19-26, 1998

Galland L. Magnesium and immune function - an overview. Magnesium 7(5-6):290-9, 1988

Good MF et al. Iron status and cellular immune competence. Blood Rev 2(1);43-9, 1988

Graber CD et al. Immunomodulating properties of dimethylglycine in humans. J Infect Dis 143(1):101-5, 1981

Griffiths RD. Outcome of critically ill patients after supplementation with glutamine. Nutrition 13(7-8):752-4, 1997

Grimm H, Tibell A, Norrlind B, et al. Immunoregulation by parenteral lipids: impact of the n-3 to n-6 fatty acid ratio. JPEN J Parenter Enteral Nutr 18(5):417-21, 1994

Guillou PJ. The effects of lipids on some aspects of the cellular immune response. Proc Nutr Soc 52:91-100, 1993

Horrobin DF et al. The nutritional regulation of T lymphocyte function. Med Hypotheses 5:969-85, 1979

Hughes DA et al. The effect of b-carotene supplementation on the immune function of blood monocytes from healthy male nonsmokers. J Lab and Clin Med 129:309-17, 1997

Johnston CS et al. Antihistamine effect of supplemental ascorbic acid and neutrophil chemotaxis. J Am Coll Nutr 11(2):172-6, 1992

Kaplan SS, Basford RE. Effect of vitamin B12 and folic acid deficiencies on neutrophil function. Blood 47:801-5, 1976

Kee-Ching GJ et al. Supplementation with vitamins C and E enhances cytokine production by peripheral blood mononuclear cells in healthy adults. Am J Clin Nutr 64:960-5, 1996

Kelley DS, Branch LB, Love JE, et al. Dietary alpha-linolenic acid and immunocompetence in humans. Am J Clin Nutr 53(1):40-6, 1991

Kelley DS et al. Effects of low-copper diets on human immune responses. Am J Clin Nutr 62:412-16, 1995

Kelley DS et al. Dietary docosahexaenoic acid and immunocompetence in young healthy men. Lipids 33(6):559-66, 1998

Kennes B et al. Effect of vitamin C supplements on cell-mediated immunity in old people. Gerontology 29:305-10, 1983

Kiremidjian-Schumacher L et al. Supplementation with selenium and human immune cell functions. II. Effect on cytotoxic lymphocytes and natural killer cells. Biol Trace Elem Res 41:115-27, 1994

Kraal JH. Immunoglobulin levels in relation to smoking and coffee consumption. Am J Clin Nutr 31(2):198-200, 1972

Kubena KS, Durlach J. Historical review of the effects of marginal intake of magnesium in chronic experimental magnesium deficiency. Magnes Res 3(3):219-26, 1990

Kurashige S et al. Effect of vitamin B complex on the immunodeficiency produced by surgery of gastric cancer patients. Jpn J Exp Med 58(4):197-202, 1988

LaBue M et al. Dosage window of selenium on phagocytic and natural killer cytotoxic responses. Int Clin Nutr Rev 8(4):198-203, 1988

la Fuente MD et al. Immune function in aged women is improved by ingestion of vitamins C and E. Can J Physiol Pharmacol 76(4):373-80, 1998

Lettko M, Meuer S. Vitamin B-induced prevention of stress-related immunosuppression: results of a double-blind clinical study. Ann NY Acad Sci 585:513-15, 1990

Levy JA. Nutrition and the immune system, in DP Stites et al, Eds. Basic and Clinical Immunology. 4th Edition. Los Altos, CA. Lange Medical Publications, 1982:297-305

Mathe G et al. A phase II trial of immunorestoration with zinc gluconate in immunodepressed cancer patients. Biomed Pharmacother 40(10):383-5, 1986

Melamed I et al. Coffee and the immune system. Int J Immunol 12:129-34, 1990

Meydani SN et al. Vitamin B-6 deficiency impairs interleukin 2 production and lymphocyte proliferation in elderly adults. Am J Clin Nutr 53:1275-80, 1991

Meydani M et al. Effect of long-term vitamin E supplementation on lipid peroxidation and immune responses of young and old subjects. Abstract. FASEB J:A415, 1993

Meydani SN. Effect of (n-3) polyunsaturated fatty acids on cytokine production and their biologic function. Nutrition 12(1 Suppl):S8-14, 1996

Meydani SN et al. Vitamin E supplementation and in vivo immune response in healthy elderly subjects. JAMA 277(17):1380-6, 1997

Moriguchi S et al. Beta-carotene supplementation enhances lymphocyte proliferation with mitogens in human peripheral blood lymphocytes. Nutr Res 16:211-18, 1996

Muller K, Bendtzen K. 1,25-Dihydroxyvitamin D3 as a natural regulator of human immune functions. J Investig Dermatol Symp Proc 1(1):68-71, 1996

Murata T et al. Effect of long-term administration of β-carotene on lymphocyte subsets in humans. Am J Clin Nutr 60:597-602, 1994

Myrik QN. Nutrition and immunology, in ME Shils, VR Young. Modern Nutrition in Health and Disease. Seventh Edition. Philadelphia, Lea & Febiger, 1988, p. 605

Nair MP, Schwartz SA. Immunoregulation of natural and lymphokine-activated killer cells by selenium. Immunopharmacology 19(3):177-83, 1990

Nalder BN et al. Sensitivity of the immunological response to the nutritional status of rats. J Nutr 102(4):535-42, 1972

Nath R et al. Molecular basis of cadmium toxicity. Prog Food Nutr Sci 8(1-2):109-63, 1984

Newsholme EA, Calder PC. The proposed role of glutamine in some cells of the immune system and speculative consequences for the whole animal. Nutrition 13(7-8), 728-30, 1997

Nordal KP et al. Aluminum accumulation and immunosuppressive effect in recipients of kidney transplants. BMJ 297:1581-2, 1988

Nuwayri-Salti N, Murad T. Immunologic and anti-immunosuppressive effects of vitamin A. Pharmacology 30(4):181-7, 1985

Ongsakul M et al. Impaired blood clearance of bacteria and phagocytic activity in vitamin A deficient rats. Proc Soc Exp Biol Med 178(2):204-8, 1985

O'Riordain MG et al. Effect of glutamine on immune function in the surgical patient. Nutrition 12(11-12 Suppl):S82-4, 1996

Oster O. Selenium - an essential supplement. Medwelt 47:12-22, 1996

Park KGM et al. Stimulation of lymphocyte natural cytotoxicity by L-arginine. Lancet 337:645-6, 1991

Patrone F, Dallegri F. Vitamin C and the phagocytic system. Acta Vitaminol Enzymol 1:5-10, 1979

Payan DG et al. Alterations in human leukocyte function induced by ingestion of eicosapentaenoic acid. J Clin Chem 6(5):402-10, 1986

Peretz A et al. Lymphocyte response is enhanced by supplementation of elderly subjects with selenium-enriched yeast. Am J Clin Nutr 53:1323-8, 1991

Perlingeiro RCR, Queiroz MLS. Measurement of the respiratory burst and chemotaxis in polymorphonuclear leukocytes from mercury-exposed workers. Hum Exp Toxicol 14:281-6, 1995

Pletsityi AD. [Change in the activity of specific and nonspecific immunity mechanisms in vitamin B1 deficiency]. Biull Eksp Biol Med 88(7):60-2, 1979) (in Russian)

Pocino M et al. Influence of the oral administration of excess copper on the immune response. Fund Appl Toxicol 16:249-56, 1991

Prasad AS et al. Zinc deficiency in elderly patients. Nutrition 9(3):218-24, 1993

Prasad AS. Zinc: an overview. Nutrition 11(1 Suppl):93-9, 1995

Prinz W et al. The effect of ascorbic acid supplementation on some parameters of the human immunological defense system. Int J Vitam Nutr Res 47(3):248-57, 1977

Rabbani P et al. Dietary model for production of experimental zinc deficiency in man. Am J Clin Nutr 45:1514-25, 1987

Rall LC, Meydani SN. Vitamin B6 and immune competence. Nutr Rev 51(8):217-25, 1993

Rasmussen LB et al. Effect of diet and plasma fatty acid composition on immune status in elderly men. Am J Clin Nutr 39:572-7, 1994

Reap EA, Lawson JW. Stimulation of the immune response by dimethylglycine, a nontoxic metabolite. J Lab Clin Med 115(4):481-6, 1990

Reynolds JV et al. Immunomodulary mechanisms of arginine. Surgery 104(2):142-51, 1988

Richardson J. Vitamin C and immunosuppression. Med Hypotheses 21(4):383-5, 1986

Ripa S, Ripa R. Zinc and immune function. Minerva Med 86(7-8):315-18, 1995

Roy M et al. Supplementation with selenium and human immune cell functions. Biol Trace Elem Res 41:103-14, 1994

Rumore MM. Vitamin A as an immunomodulating agent. Clin Pharm 12(7):506-14, 1993

Saiki I et al. Macrophage activation with ubiquinones and their related compounds in mice. Int J Vitam Nutr Res 53:312-20, 1983

Sanchez A et al. Role of sugars in human neutrophilic phagocytosis. Am J Clin Nutr 26:1180-4, 1973

Santos PC, Falcado RP. Decreased lymphocyte subsets and K-cell activity in iron-deficiency anemia. Acta Haematol 84:118-21, 1990

Santos MS et al. Natural killer cell activity in elderly men in enhanced by β-carotene supplementation. Am J Clin Nutr 64:772-7, 1996

Santos MS et al. Short- and long-term beta-carotene supplementation do not influence T cell-mediated immunity in healthy elderly persons. Am J Clin Nutr 66(4):917-24, 1997

Semba RD et al. Abnormal T-cell subset proportions in vitamin-A-deficient children. Lancet 341:5-8, 1993

Semba RD. Vitamin A, immunity, and infection. Clin Infect Dis 19(3):489-99, 1994

Shils M et al. Selenium deficiency and immune function in home TPN patients. Presentation at the American Society of Clinical Nutrition, 1983

Stacey NH et al. Effects of cadmium on natural killer and killer cell functions in vivo. Environ Res 45:71-7, 1988

Talbott MC et al. Pyridoxine supplementation: Effect on lymphocyte responses in elderly persons. Am J Clin Nutr 46(4):659-64, 1987

Thibault H et al. The immune response in iron-deficient young children: effect of iron supplementation on cell mediated immunity. Eur J Pediatr 152:120-4, 1993

Tong KK et al. The effects of copper deficiency on human lymphoid and myeloid cells: an in vitro model. Br J Nutr 75(1):97-108, 1996

Torún B, Viteri FE. Protein-energy malnutrition, in ME Shils, VR Young. Modern Nutrition in Health and Disease. Seventh Edition. Philadelphia, Lea & Febiger, 1988, p. 752

Virella G et al. Immunosuppressive effects of fish oil in normal human volunteers: correlation with the in vitro effects of eicosapentaenoic acid on human lymphocytes. Clin Immunol Immunopathol 61(2 Pt 1):161-76, 1991

Visek WJ. Arginine needs, physiological state and usual diets. A reevaluation. J Nutr 116(1):36-46, 1986

Weiss G et al. Linkage of cell-mediated immunity to iron metabolism. Immunol Today 16(10):495-500, 1995

INFECTION

See Also: ACQUIRED IMMUNODEFICIENCY SYNDROME (AIDS)
CANDIDIASIS
HERPES SIMPLEX
HERPES ZOSTER
IMMUNODEPRESSION

NUTRITIONAL TREATMENT GUIDE

✓ = Efficacy generally accepted.
* = Efficacy *demonstrated* by controlled human trials.
[+] = Efficacy *suspected* from uncontrolled human trials.
[-] = Efficacy *suspected* from indirect data.
? = Efficacy *challenged* in a study of similar design.

DIETARY FACTORS

✓ rule out **Protein-Calorie Malnutrition**

- -

[+] **low Fat, low Cholesterol diet**
[+] minimize **Glucose, Sucrose** and **Fructose** intakes, especially during infections

NUTRITIONAL FACTORS

* **L-Arginine:** 8 to 20 g daily
* **N-acetyl cysteine:** *for chronic bronchitis or influenza or septic shock:* 200 to 600 mg twice daily
for septic shock: 150 mg/kg bolus, following by a continuous infusion of 50 mg/kg over 4 hours
* **Citrate:** *for urinary tract infections:* sodium citrate 4 g every 8 hours
* **Glutamine:** 5 to 30 g daily
* **Omega-3 fatty acids:** *example:* MaxEPA 1 g caps [180 mg EPA; 120 mg DHA] 10 to 20 daily
* **Selenium:** *for the treatment of sepsis:* 500 μg, 250 μg and 125 μg, each for 3 days
* **Xylitol:** *for acute otitis media:* 8 to 10 g daily
* **Zinc:** *for rhinovirus infections:* zinc gluconate lozenges 180 mg (23 mg elemental Zn) every 2 hours while awake
* ? **Vitamin A:** *especially if deficient:* ? 20,000 IU daily for prophylaxis; 200,000 IU daily for treatment of acute infections (limited to a few days)
* ? **Vitamin C:** ? 500 mg 4 times daily

[+] **Folic acid deficiency:** 800 µg daily
[+] **Iron deficiency:** 30 mg twice daily until repletion; then minimal possible dosage
[+] **Mannose:** *for E. Coli urinary tract infections:* 1 tsp mixed with water 4 times daily
[+] **Pantothenic acid deficiency:** 100 to 200 mg daily
[+] **Vitamin B_{12}:** *for 'post-flu syndrome':* 1 mg intramuscularly
[+] **Vitamin E:** ? 400 to 800 IU daily
[+] **Zinc:** *for vaginal trichomoniasis:* 1% zinc sulfate douche *AND* metronidazole

[-] **Beta-carotene:** ? 30 to 60 mg daily
[-] **L-Carnitine:** acetyl-L-carnitine 2 g daily
[-] **Copper deficiency:** 2 mg twice daily for up to 6 weeks *AND* zinc 50 mg daily

OTHER RELATED FACTORS

* ***Lactobacillus acidophilus*** *for bacterial vaginosis and female urinary tract infections:* oral or vaginal administration

[+] rule out **Food Sensitivities**

[-] rule out **Cadmium** toxicity
[-] rule out **Hydrochloric Acid** deficiency
[-] rule out **Lead** toxicity

DIETARY FACTORS

Protein-calorie Malnutrition

Protein-calorie malnutrition, which is usually associated with concomitant micronutrient deficiencies, increases susceptibility to infection *(Chandra, 1985)*. It is one of the 4 most important deficiency diseases in developing countries *(Latham)*. The elderly are particularly susceptible, as many have poor cell-mediated immune responses due to changes inherent in the aging process *(Lesourd)*.

Low Fat Diet

A diet which is high in fat increases susceptibility to infection. Neutrophil chemotaxis may be slowed, neutrophil phagocytic and bactericidal activity may be depressed, and reticuloendothelial system clearance may be slowed *(Beisel)*. In humans, high fat diets have been shown to increase surgical wound infections *(Edelman)*. The primary danger of a high fat diet appears to be excessive intake of omega-6 fatty acids (see below) which encourage infection via prolonged inflammation, enhanced Gram negative survival, reticuloendothelial blockage, immunosuppression, and monokine depression *(Wan)*.

Low Cholesterol Diet

A diet which is high in cholesterol is believed to increase susceptibility to infection, possibly by suppressing antibody production *(Beisel)*. However, while cholesterol is a potent modulator of T lymphocyte and phagocyte functions in laboratory animals and in leukocyte cultures, its effect in humans in regard to infectious processes is still unclear *(Edelman)*.

Sugars

Glucose, sucrose and fructose all impair resistance to infection by reducing the capacity of neutrophils to engulf bacteria *(Cheraskin)*. When subjects ingested 100 grams of carbohydrate from glucose, fructose, sucrose, honey or orange juice, the phagocytic index (as measured by the capacity of neutrophils to engulf bacteria) was significantly decreased and remained below baseline when reassessed 5 hours later. Starch, by contrast, did not have this effect *(Sanchez)*.

There is recent evidence from controlled studies, however, that *xylitol*, a polyol sugar alcohol that occurs naturally in plums, strawberries and raspberries, may reduce the risk of acute otitis media. This sugar may be administered as a syrup or as a chewing gum. An effective dosage is roughly 8 to 10 grams daily *(Uhari,1996,1998)*. There is also preliminary evidence that *mannose*, an aldohexose, may reduce renal infections caused *by E. Coli (Michaels)* as it coats the lectin projections on the bacteria. This interferes with their ability to attach to the walls of the bladder and urethra, and is said to generally end a kidney infection within 48 hours *(Wright,1996)*.

A 4-year-old girl had chronic kidney infections. She had been seen by numerous doctors. As she had become allergic to nearly every antibiotic she had been prescribed, her mother was advised that she would probably need a kidney transplant in a few years.

Since most urinary tract infections involving the kidneys are caused by Escherichia coli, mannose was prescribed at a dosage of 1/4 teaspoon mixed with water 4 times daily.

Within 3 days, her kidney infection cleared up. She was also prescribed vitamin C and zinc to build up her immune system. More than 2 years later, she had not had a recurrence (Wright,1996).

NUTRITIONAL FACTORS

VITAMINS

Folic Acid Deficiency

Folic acid is necessary for the synthesis of DNA, RNA and proteins in all tissues. Demand for the nutrient increases during infection, particularly due to the bimodal response of lymphocytes, cellular multiplication, and synthesis of specific immunoglobulins.

Folate deficiency is commonly associated with infection. For example, when 260 patients with a variety of viral and mycoplasmal infections were studied, low serum folate concentrations were found in about 60%, and decreased folate levels were associated with evidence of both acute and prolonged infection *(Jacobson)*.

Following a complicated laparoscopic cholecystectomy accompanied by fever and malaise, a 51-year-old obese woman was found to have a liver abscess. On postoperative day 52 the patient's tongue was magenta and sore and she had altered taste, pallor, severe weight loss, diarrhea, and poor appetite and mood. A hematologic blood smear was suggestive of folate deficiency. Premorbidly, the patient had consumed a diet chronically low in folate and had received estrogen therapy for 15 years. Throughout the patient's hospitalization, she had bouts of fever and received numerous antibiotics.

Within a month of initiating nutrition support and vitamin/mineral supplements, her nutritional status improved dramatically (Stolzenberg).

Pantothenic Acid Deficiency

When volunteers were given a formula diet adequate nutritionally except for pantothenic acid, they developed continuous upper respiratory infections, especially acute pharyngitis, as well as a variety of other signs and symptoms. Urine analyses showed a decrease in adrenal hormones which fell progressively as the experiment continued. Digestive enzymes and gastric acid were markedly reduced, and both gastric and intestinal motility decreased *(Thornton)*.

How often a marginal pantothenic acid deficiency contributes to susceptibility to infections is not known. A marginal deficiency appears to be uncommon, however, as pantothenic acid is readily available from diverse dietary sources *(Tahiliani)*.

Vitamin A

Vitamin A status is strongly associated with the severity of infection *(Dudley)*. Even a mild vitamin A deficiency (as manifested by xerophthalmia) may increase the susceptibility to infection *(Sommer)*. Conversely, due to increased urinary retinol excretion, vitamin A requirements are substantially greater during serious infections *(Stephensen,1995)*. For whatever reason, plasma levels of vitamin A have been found to be decreased in both viral hepatitis and chronic bronchitis *(Singh RB)*.

There is substantial evidence, much of it from controlled trials, that supplementation with the vitamin may diminish susceptibility to infection *(Beisel)*. For example, when 147 children with a history of frequent *respiratory infections* randomly received either vitamin A 1,500 IU daily or placebo for 11 months, supplemented children subsequently experienced significantly less frequent episodes of respiratory infections compared to controls - even though their plasma retinol levels were unchanged *(Pinnock)*.

Pharmacologic levels of vitamin A supplementation have also been found to be helpful shorten the duration and complications of *chicken pox* in the absence of clinical evidence of vitamin A deficiency *(Ozsoylu)*. Similar results have been seen with *measles* in presumably well-nourished children (half of which were found to be vitamin A-deficient) *(Arrieta)*. In fact, both WHO and UNICEF have recommended that, in countries where the fatality rate of measles is 1% or higher, vitamin A supplements be provided to all infected children *(Anonymous)*.

The results of treating children with *respiratory syncytial virus* are less clear *(Neuzil;Quinlan)*. There is also evidence of a lack of efficacy of the vitamin by itself in treating acute lower respiratory infections in poorly nourished populations *(Bhandari)*.

In fact, in the absence of clinical evidence of vitamin A deficiency or concurrent measles infection, high-dose vitamin A supplements may cause modest adverse effects in children recovering from pneumonia *(Stephensen,1998)*. There is even evidence that children with probable subclinical deficiency may have an *increased* 2-week prevalence of acute respiratory infections and diarrhea following megadose supplementation *(Stansfield)*.

Vitamin B_{12} Deficiency

A deficiency of vitamin B_{12} may be associated with impaired antibody responses to bacterial antigens *(Fata)*. There is little evidence that supplementation is effective. However, a clinician has reported that one milligram of the vitamin delivered intramuscularly seems to resolve the *'post-flu' syndrome* of lassitude, lethargy, hypersomnia, muscle pains and headaches (which usually lasts for 3 to 4 weeks) within hours *(Engel)*.

Vitamin C

A deficiency of ascorbic acid is associated with impairment of phagocytic cell functions *(Beisel;Patrone)*. Evidence from a study of elderly subjects suggests that acute infections may reduce vitamin C nutriture. Compared to both malnourished subjects and controls, patients with acute infections had poorer vitamin C status *(Pfitzenmeyer)*.

In mammals, infection is followed by a rapid and often sustained fall in the tissue and urine levels of vitamin C *(Stacpoole)*, a transfer from plasma to leukocytes to attempt to keep these levels from becoming depressed *(Tanzer)*, and by localization of the vitamin at the infected site *(Stacpoole)*.

Supplementation may combat infections by stimulating neutrophil motility and enhancing phagocyte antimicrobial activity *(Anderson)*. In fact, ascorbate supplementation may be specific therapy for primary defects of phagocytic function in patients with recurrent infections *(Patrone)*. Moreover, in viral infections, the vitamin may increase serum interferon levels *(Geber)*.

In *chronic bronchitis*, vitamin C intake may be decreased *(Singh RB)*. Furthermore, the risk of the illness appears to be inversely correlated with plasma *(Singh RB)* and serum *(Schwartz)* levels.

Ascorbic acid appears to inhibit the growth of viruses both directly and indirectly. Its antiviral activity may be due, in part, to enhanced interferon production *(Leibovitz)*. The vitamin has also been shown to combat bacterial infections *(Rawal)*.

Numerous studies have investigated the efficacy of vitamin C in treating the *common cold*. While the evidence is that vitamin C supplementation, in doses ranging from 80 to 2,000 mg daily, fails to reduce the frequency of colds, it may reduce both their severity and their duration *(Beisel;Hemilä,1996,1997)*. Anecdotal reports suggest that still higher doses of vitamin C have greater efficacy, but scientific confirmation is lacking.

There is also evidence that supplementation may improve recovery in *severe, acute respiratory infections (Hunt)*, recurrent *furunculosis (Levy)*, and gastric infection with *Helicobacter pylori (Goodman;Rokkas)*.

The effects of vitamin C treatment were studied in a patient with a history of recurrent furunculosis who showed altered neutrophil functions. Chemotaxis, phagocytosis, and superoxide generation of the patient's neutrophils were significantly lower than those of the matched controls.

Treatment with vitamin C 500 mg daily for 30 days caused a dramatic clinical response as well as a significant improvement of all 3 neutrophil functions to values similar to those of the controls (Levy).

Vitamin E

A deficiency of vitamin E is associated with increased infections due to diminished membrane-related chemotaxis and ingestion *(Baehner)*. In a survey of 100 healthy people over age 60, there was an inverse correlation between the plasma alpha tocopherol levels and the number of infections in the previous 3 years *(Chavance)*.

Supplementation enhances both humoral and cellular immune responses. It increases phagocytic defenses to stimulate body defenses against infectious agents *(Tengerdy)*. A variety of animals supplemented with vitamin E have shown increased immune responses and resistance to a number of infectious agents *(Nockels)*.

Six months after children with *chronic respiratory tract infections* began treatment with the vitamin, their clinical status was improved. Moreover, there was normalization of their helper T lymphocytes and the ratio of helper to suppressor cells in their peripheral blood *(Skodinska-Rozewska)*.

MINERALS

Calcium: A Warning

Evidence from a retrospective case-control study *(Pelig)* and from an *in vitro* study *(Apicella)* suggests that calcium supplementation may increase the risk of *urinary tract infections*, perhaps because it enhances the ability of microorganisms to adhere to the lining of the urinary tract *(Apicella)*.

Copper

Copper deficiency is associated with increased susceptibility to infection due to impairment of cell-mediated immunity *(Chandra, 1985)*. However, since excess copper may also increase susceptibility to infection *(Beisel)*, copper supplements are not indicated unless there is a reason to be concerned about copper deficiency.

During infections, copper is removed from tissue storage in order to help fight the infections. Since, as a consequence, serum copper rises *(Watts)*, serum copper in the presence of infection is a poor indicator of copper nutriture.

Iron

Iron deficiency is associated with increased susceptibility to infection due to impairment of cell-mediated immunity *(Beisel)*. However, in contrast to the rise in serum copper during infection, iron is transferred out of the serum into the tissues *(Hershko)*. In bacterial cultures, iron deprivation inhibits bacterial growth; thus hypoferremia may be an important host defense *(Jurado; Hershko)*.

Excessive iron supplementation can increase bacterial growth and replication, as well as increase the release of certain exotoxins *(Beisel)*. The risk of hyperferremia is heightened when the patient receives blood transfusions *(Sobeleva)*.

Selenium

An extensive body of evidence links selenium deficiency with increased susceptibility to viral infections *(Taylor)*. It has been shown to protect against a number of human viruses, including hepatitis B, coxsackie virus, and viruses involved with Keshan disease and viral hemorrhagic fever *(Taylor)*. Moreover, plasma levels decrease during infections, independent of the causative agent *(Srinivas)*.

In a recent controlled study, the clinical outcome of critically ill sepsis patients who received high-dose selenium was significantly improved and the incidence of acute renal failure was reduced *(Gartner)*.

Further studies are needed to ascertain the efficacy of selenium supplementation in the treatment of infectious diseases.

Zinc

Serum zinc levels decrease sharply in many infections *(Srinivas)*; as with iron, this may be a host defense designed to inhibit microbial growth, as levels slightly below normal are associated with optimal phagocytic function, and low concentrations may decrease microbial virulence *(Sugarman)*. Zinc deficiency, however, is associated with impaired immune function and increased susceptibility to infection *(Baer;Shankar;Sugarman)*.

Findings from animal studies suggest that, even when zinc nutriture is normal, supplementation with zinc may improve resistance to infection *(Singh KP)*. Several double-blind studies have investigated the efficacy of zinc supplementation, given in the form of lozenges, in treating the *common (rhinovirus) cold*. While not all studies found the lozenges to be effective, the findings suggest that supplementation - when formulated so as to properly release zinc ions - may lessen the severity and duration of the common cold *(Eby;Garland;Marshall)*. Supplementation (via either the oral or vaginal route) may also be effective in treating *trichomonas* even when metronidazole, the standard treatment, is ineffective alone (*Houang*). While prostatic zinc levels decrease in *bacterial prostatitis*, supplementation appears to be unable to raise prostatic zinc levels and seems ineffective in treating this condition *(Fair)*. (Also see Zinc in the chapter on Inflammation).

However, high levels of zinc supplementation may increase susceptibility to infection. When healthy men ingested 150 mg of zinc twice daily for 6 weeks, there was a reduction in chemotaxis and phagocytosis of bacteria by polymorphonuclear leukocytes as well as a reduction in lymphocytic stimulation response to phytohemagglutinin *(Chandra,1984)*.

A woman with vaginal trichomoniasis failed to respond to metronidazole. She was found to have a low plasma zinc and was placed on zinc supplementation.

After her plasma zinc level achieved the normal range, her infection responded to metronidazole (Willmott).

OTHER NUTRITIONAL FACTORS

Arginine

A growing body of evidence suggests that supplemental arginine upregulates immune function and reduces the risk of infection *(Evoy)*. It appears to protect, for example, against *postoperative infections (Evoy)* and *recurrent respiratory infections (Baligan)*, and animal work suggests that it may improve survival following *sepsis (Adjei)*.

Beta-Carotene

In *chronic bronchitis*, both the intake and plasma levels of beta-carotene may be reduced *(Singh RB)*. Also, the risk of *viral hepatitis* may be inversely correlated with plasma levels of the nutrient *(Singh RB)*.

Beta-carotene supplementation may increase natural killer cell numbers and/or stimulate natural killer cell function *(Cunha)*, and the evidence is increasing that natural killer cells are mediators of natural resistance against viruses, fungi, protozoa and bacteria *(Cavallo)*. The efficacy of supplementation in preventing and treating infections remains to be determined, however, with the possible exception of *AIDS* (see Acquired Immunodeficiency Syndrome).

L-Carnitine

Carnitine metabolism is profoundly impaired in Gram-negative sepsis, usually due to increased urinary excretion causing reduced concentrations in serum and tissues *(Famularo)*.

There is early evidence suggesting that supplementation with L-carnitine or its congeners may be beneficial in treating infections. When acetyl-L-carnitine was administered orally to patients with active *pulmonary tuberculosis* for 30 days in a double-blind study, lymphocyte antibacterial activity either increased or was unchanged in the treatment group, while it decreased in the placebo group *(Jirillo)*.

It also appears that carnitine supplementation may interfere with the pathogenetic cascade that leads to *toxic shock syndrome*. In an animal model, treatment with L-carnitine reduced the severity of the syndrome and accelerated recovery. These effects were mirrored by a reduction in serum levels of TNF-α, interleukin-1 and interleukin-6 *(Famularo)*.

Citrate

In treating *urinary tract infections*, alkalizing the urine appears to be more effective than acidifying it, especially in women without a positive urine culture. Citrate salts are ideal for this purpose as they are rapidly absorbed and metabolized without affecting gastric pH or producing a laxative effect. They raise the urinary pH because they are excreted partly as carbonate *(Pizzorno)*.

For example, in an open trial, 80% of women with urinary tract infections had symptom relief following treatment with sodium citrate while 12% reported aggravation of their symptoms *(Munday)*. Under controlled conditions, 18 hospitalized patients with an indwelling catheter who had developed candiduria were treated with oral potassium-sodium-hydrogen citrate and the dosage was adjusted to achieved a pH of 7 to 7.5. In 16 patients (89%), the treatment raised pH and resulted in the disappearance of candiduria. In 4 patients, the urine became completely sterile while, 12 of the patients developed significant bacteriuria sometime during the treatment. The authors concluded that alkalinization is a simple and effective treatment for this patient population *(Strassner)*.

Findings from another open trial were similar. In cystitis patients with pre-treatment bacteriuria whose symptoms improved following supplementation with sodium citrate, the bacteriuria was cleared, while symptoms were relieved in about 80% of patients who were initially abacteriuric. The investigators concluded that "sodium citrate provides good symptomatic relief for most women with cystitis for whom there is no definite clinical evidence of a bacterial infection, and that failure to respond adequately is very suggestive of persisting bacteriuria for which antibacterial therapy is indicated" *(Spooner)*.

Cysteine

The results of double-blind studies suggest that supplementation of L-cysteine in the form of N-acetyl cysteine (NAC) may reduce the exacerbation rate of *chronic bronchitis (Rasmussen JB)*. It appears that it may do so by normalizing the intrabronchial microbial flora *(Riise)*.

Supplementation has also been shown to reduce *influenza*-like episodes and symptomatology under double-blind conditions *(De Flora)*. Also under double-blind conditions, a short-term intravenous infusion of NAC was effective in treating early *septic shock (Spapen)*.

Essential Fatty Acids

Omega-3 Fatty Acids

Arachidonic-acid-derived eicosanoids modulate the production of pro-inflammatory and immunoregulatory cytokines, overproduction of which is associated with both septic shock and chronic inflammatory diseases. Eicosapentaenoic acid (EPA) and docosahexaenoic acid, omega-3 polyunsaturates which are found in fish oils, suppress the production of arachidonic-acid-derived eicosanoids. Furthermore, EPA is a substrate for the synthesis of an alternative family of eicosanoids. Thus, dietary fats which are rich in omega-3 PUFAs have the potential to alter cytokine production *(Calder)*.

Several human studies have shown that supplementation of the diet of healthy volunteers, or of patients with rheumatoid arthritis or multiple sclerosis, results in reduced production of pro-inflammatory cytokines by peripheral blood mononuclear cells. Results of animal studies indicate that dietary fish oil reduces the response to endotoxin and to pro-inflammatory cytokines, resulting in increased survival; such diets have been beneficial in some models of bacterial challenge, chronic inflammation and auto-immunity *(Calder)*.

When a group of healthy subjects were injected with an endotoxin, those who had consumed fish oil for the previous 6 weeks had less fever and other symptoms such as nausea and shivering *(Endres)*.

Omega-6 Fatty Acids

Eicosanoids formed from the omega-6 fatty acids are generally much more potent in causing biological responses than those formed from the omega-3 fatty acids, including stimulation of cytokine production and inflammatory responses *(Alexander)*. Moreover, a high intake of omega-6 fatty acids may reduce natural killer cell activity and T-cell responsiveness, thus possibly increasing susceptibility to viral infections *(Rasmussen LB)*.

Glutamine

Laboratory and clinical data suggest that glutamine, usually considered to be a nonessential amino acid, may become essential during infections, during which consumption may outstrip endogenous production, resulting in a relative glutamine deficiency *(Wilmore)*.

Results of double-blind studies suggest that glutamine-enriched parenteral or enteral feedings are generally safe and effective in catabolic patients. Intravenous glutamine (either as the L-amino acid or as glutamine-dipeptides) increase plasma levels, exert protein anabolic effects, improve gut structure and/or function and reduce important indices of morbidity, including infection rates and length of hospital stay in selected patient subgroups *(Ziegler)*.

Glutamine supplementation may also be protective against infections for a very different population. A decrease in the plasma glutamine level in athletes after endurance exercise may be partly responsible for the apparent immunosuppression which is known to occur.

In one study, athletes participating in different types of exercise consumed a drink that either contained glutamine or placebo immediately after and 2 hours after exercise. One week later, they completed questionnaires about the incidence of infections during the past week. The percentage of athletes reporting infections was considerably higher in the placebo group, suggesting that glutamine supplementation was protective *(Castell)*.

OTHER RELATED FACTORS

Food Sensitivities

Food reactions cause eustachian tube swelling, blocking fluid outflow from the middle ear and thereby facilitating the development of *otitis media with effusion*.

The *Annals of Allergy* has reported the results of a study of 104 children between the ages of 18 months and 9 years with recurrent serous otitis media. Eighty-one of the children (78%) tested positive for food sensitivities. Cow's milk was the offending agent in 38%, wheat in 33%, egg white in 25%, peanut in 20%, soy in 17%, corn in 15%, orange in 10%, tomato in 5%, chicken in 5% and apple in 4%.

Excluding the offending foods from the diet for 11 weeks led to significant improvement in 70 of the 81 children (86%). Subsequent challenges with suspected foods caused a flare-up of otitis in 66/70 (94%) *(Nsouli)*.

Heavy Metal Toxicity

The results of animal studies suggest that both cadmium and lead toxicity can adversely affect host resistance to bacterial and viral infections *(Cook JA;Gainer)*.

Hydrochloric Acid Deficiency

By compromising the defense mechanisms of the upper gastrointestinal tract, hypochlorhydria predisposes to intestinal bacterial and parasitic infections. Sometimes the infections themselves cause hypochlorhydria *(Cook GC)*.

Lactobacillus acidophilus

Some lactobacilli produce hydrogen peroxide which can be toxic to organisms that produce little or no hydrogen-peroxide-scavenging enzymes such as catalase. Hydrogen-peroxide-producing lactobacillus species were found in the vaginas of 96% of normal women compared to only 6% of women with *bacterial vaginosis (Eschenbach)*. *In vitro*, acidophyllin, the antibacterial component of *L. acidophilus*, caused a 50% inhibition in growth in numerous types of bacteria in lactic-acid-free preparations. Ten of these types were common pathogens *(Shahani)*.

In a crossover study, when women with recurrent *bacterial vaginosis* or *vaginal candidiasis* received a daily intake of 5 ounces (150 ml) of yogurt containing live *L. acidophilus*, they had a greater than 50% reduction in recurrences, while women who consumed pasteurized yogurt that did not contain the bacteria had only a slight reduction *(Shalev)*.

Intravaginal instillation *of L. acidophilus* has been found to be effective in *candidal vaginitis (Hilton)*, *non-specific vaginal discharge and/or vaginitis (Gerstner)* and *trichomoniasis vaginitis (Karkut)*. It has also shown efficacy in treating recurrent *urinary tract infections* in a placebo-controlled study *(Reid)*.

COMBINED NUTRITIONAL INTERVENTIONS

An 8 year-old boy with frequent episodes of influenza as well as respiratory infections presented with earaches, tonsillitis, bronchitis, and pneumonitis. Cervical lymph nodes were chronically swollen and tonsils were enlarged. Physical examination also suggested deficiencies of vitamin A, vitamin D, and zinc, and inadequate functioning of the thymus.

Sugar (except honey), white flour and all refined foods were removed from his diet and he was supplemented with vitamin C 500 mg with meals, vitamin B complex including 10-20 mg of each B vitamin with meals, vitamin A 30,000 IU daily, vitamin D, 1,200 IU daily, chelated zinc 25 µg daily and thymus tablets 3 times daily.

Three weeks later, he returned with another cold, but without complications. Nine months later, the clinical signs of deficiencies were gone, his tonsils were no longer enlarged, and his cervical nodes were normal. His mother reported that he had had no further respiratory infections. One year later, she reported that he had had only "a few sniffles once or twice" which seemed to respond to increased vitamins A and D (Wright, 1979).

BIBLIOGRAPHY

Adjei AA et al. Dietary arginine and glutamine combination improves survival in septic mice. Nutr Res 14:1591-9, 1994

Alexander JW. Immunonutrition: the role of omega-3 fatty acids. Nutrition 14(7-8):627-33, 1998

Anderson R et al. The effects of increasing weekly doses of ascorbate on certain cellular and humeral immune functions in normal volunteers. Am J Clin Nutr 33(1):71-6, 1980

Anonymous. Editorial. Vitamin A for measles. Lancet i:1067-8, 1987

Apicella LL, Sobota AE. Increased risk of urinary tract infection associated with the use of calcium supplements. Urol Res 18:213-17, 1990

Arrieta A et al. Vitamin A levels in children with measles in Long Beach, California. J Pediatr 121(1):75-8, 1992

Baehner RL, Boxer LA. Role of membrane vitamin E and cytoplasmic glutathione in the regulation of phagocytic functions of neutrophils and monocytes. Am J Pediatr Hematol Oncol 191):71-6, 1979

Baer MT et al. Nitrogen utilization, enzyme activity, glucose intolerance and leukocyte chemotaxis in human experimental zinc depletion. Am J Clin Nutr 41(6):1220-35, 1985

Baligan M et al. [L-arginine and immunity. Study of pediatric subjects]. Minerva Pediatr 49(11):537-42, 1997) (in Italian)

Beisel WR. Single nutrients and immunity. Am J Clin Nutr 35:417-68 (Suppl), 1982

Bhandari N et al. Impact of massive dose of vitamin A given to preschool children with acute diarrhoea on subsequent respiratory and diarrhoeal morbidity. BMJ 309:1404-7, 1994

Calder PC. n-3 polyunsaturated fatty acids and cytokine production in health and disease. Ann Nutr Metab 41(4):203-34, 1997

Castell LM et al. Does glutamine have a role in reducing infections in athletes? Eur J Appl Physiol 73(5):488-90, 1996

Cavallo R. [Antimicrobial activity of NK cells.] G Batteriol Virol Immunol 85(1-12):35-46, 1992 Jan-1993 Dec) (in Italian)

Chandra RK. Excessive intake of zinc impairs immune responses. JAMA 252(11):1443-6, 1984

Chandra RK. Trace element regulation of immunity and infection. J Am Coll Nutr 4(1):5-16, 1985

Chavance M et al. Nutritional support improves antibody response to influenza virus in the elderly. Letter to the Editor. Br Med J November 9, 1985, pp. 1348-49

Cheraskin E. Sucrose, neutrophilic phagocytosis and resistance to disease. Dental Survey 52(12):46-8, 1976

Cook GC. Infective gastroenteritis and its relationship to reduced gastric acidity. Scand J Gastroenterol Suppl 111:17-23, 1985

Cook JA et al. Influence of lead and cadmium on the susceptibility of rats to bacterial challenge. Proc Soc Exp Biol Med 150:741-7, 1973

Cunha BA. Beta-carotene stimulation of natural killer cell activity in adult patients with chronic fatigue syndrome. The CFIDS Chronicle Physicians' Forum Fall, 1993, pp. 18-19

De Flora S et al. Attenuation of influenza-like symptomatology and improvement of cell-mediated immunity with long-term N-acetylcysteine treatment. Eur Respir J 10(7):1535-41, 1997

Dudley L et al. Vitamin A status, other risk factors and acute respiratory infection morbidity in children. S Afr Med J 87(1):65-70, 1997

Eby GA. Zinc ion availability--the determinant of efficacy in zinc lozenge treatment of common colds. J Antimicrob Chemther 40(4):483-93, 1997

Edelman R. Obesity: does it modulate infectious disease and immunity? Prog Clin Biol Res 67:327-37, 1981

Endres S et al. Effects of dietary omega-3 fatty acids on the acute phase response during endotoxin fever in humans. J Leuk Biol 42:591, 1987

Engel HG. Validating B12 for postflu use. Cortlandt Forum April, 1995

Eschenbach DA et al. Prevalence of hydrogen peroxide-producingLactobacillus species in normal women and women with bacterial vaginosis. J Clin Microbiol 27(2):251-6, 1989

Evoy D et al. Immunonutrition: the role of arginine. Nutrition 14(7-8):611-17, 1998

Fair WR, Weston WDW, in GJ Brewer, AS Prasad, Eds. Zinc Metabolism: Current Aspects in Health and Disease. New York, Alan R. Liss, 1977:129-40

Famularo G, De Simone C. A new era for carnitine? Immunol Today 16(5):211-13, 1995

Fata FT et al. Impaired antibody responses to pneumococcal polysaccharide in elderly patients with low serum vitamin B12 levels. Ann Intern Med 124(3):299-304, 1996

Gainer JH. Effects of heavy metals and of deficiency of zinc on mortality rates in mice infected with encephalomyocarditis virus. Am J Vet Res 38:869-72, 1977

Garland ML, Hagmeyer KO. The role of zinc lozenges in treatment of the common cold. Ann Pharmacother 32(1):63-9, 1998

Gartner R et al. [Selenium administration in sepsis patients]. Med Klin 92 Suppl 3:12-14, 1997) (in German)

Geber WF et al. Effect of ascorbic acid, sodium salicylate, and caffeine on the serum interferon level in response to viral infection. Pharmacology 13(3):228-33, 1975

Gerstner GJ, Muller G. Intravaginale lyophilisierte Laktobazillen zur therapie des unspezifischen fluor vaginalis. Gynak Rdsch 27:71-78, 1987 (in German)

Goodman KJ et al. Nutritional factors and Helicobacter pylori infection in Colombian children. J Pediatr Gastroenterol Nutr 25(5):507-15, 1997

Hemilä H. Vitamin C and common cold incidence: a review of studies with subjects under heavy physical stress. Int J Sports Med 17(5):370-83, 1996

Hemilä H. Vitamin C intake and susceptibility to the common cold. Br J Nutr 77:1-14, 1997

Hershko C et al. Iron and infection. Br Med J 296:660-4, 1988

Hilton E et al. Ingestion of yogurt containing Lactobacillus acidophilus as prophylaxis for candidal vaginitis. Ann Intern Med 116(5):353-7, 1992

Houang ET et al. Successful treatment of four patients with recalcitrant vaginal trichomoniasis with a combination of zinc sulfate douche and metronidazole therapy. Sex Transm Dis 24(2):116-9, 1997

Hunt C et al. The clinical effects of vitamin C supplementation in elderly hospitalized patients with acute respiratory infection. Int J Vitam Nutr Res 64:212-19, 1994

Jacobson W et al. Serum folate in viral and mycoplasmal infections. J Infect 14:103-11, 1987

Jirillo E et al. Effects of acetyl-L-carnitine oral administration on lymphocyte antibacterial activity and TNF-alpha levels in patients with active pulmonary tuberculosis. A randomized double blind versus placebo study. Immunopharmacol Immunotoxicol 13(1-2):135-46, 1991

Jurado RL. Iron, infections, and anemia of inflammation. Clin Infect Dis 25(4):888-95, 1997

Karkut G. [Effect of lactobacillus immunotherapy on genital infections in women (SolcoTrichovac/Gynatren).] Geburtshilfe Fraunheilkd 44(5):311-14, 1984) (in German)

Latham MC. Protein-energy malnutrition--its epidemiology and control. J Environ Pathol Toxicol Oncol 10(4-5):168-80, 1990

Leibovitz B, Siegel BV. Ascorbic acid and the immune response. Adv Exp Med Biol 135:1-25, 1981

Lesourd BM. Nutrition and immunity in the elderly: modification of immune responses with nutritional treatments. Am J Clin Nutr 66(2):478S-484S, 1997

Levy R, Schlaeffer F. Successful treatment of a patient with recurrent furunculosis by vitamin C: improvement of clinical course and of impaired neutrophil functions. Int J Dermatol 32(11):832-4, 1993

Marshall S. Zinc gluconate and the common cold. Review of randomized controlled trials. Can Fam Physician 44:1037-42, 1998

Michaels EK et al. Effect of D-mannose and D-glucose on Escherichia coli bacteriuria in rats. Urol Res 11(2):97-102, 1983

Munday PE, Savage S. Cymalon in the management of urinary tract symptoms. Letter. Genitourin Med 66(6):461, 1990

Neuzil KM et al. Safety and pharmacokinetics of vitamin A therapy for infants with respiratory syncytial virus infections. Antimicrob Agents Chemother 39:1191-3, 1995

Nockels CF. Protective effects of supplemental vitamin E against infection. Fed Proc 38:2134-8, 1979

Nsouli TM et al. Role of food allergy in serous otitis media. Ann Allergy 73:215-19, 1994

Ozsoylu S et al. Vitamin A for varicella. Letter. J Pediatr 125(6 Pt 1):1017-18, 1994

Patrone F, Dallegri F. [Vitamin C and phagocytic system: present status and perspectives]. Acta Vitaminol Enzymol 1(1-6):5-10, 1979) (in Italian)

Pelig I et al. Dietary calcium supplementation increases the risk of urinary tract infection. Clin Res 40:A562, 1992

Pfitzenmeyer P et al. Vitamin B6 and vitamin C status in elderly patients with infections during hospitalization. Ann Nutr Metab 41(6):344-52, 1997

Pinnock CB et al. Vitamin A status in children who are prone to respiratory tract infection. Aust Paediatr J 22(2):95-99, 1986

Pizzorno JE. Natural medicine approach to the treatment of cystitis. Alternative & Complementary Therapies, October, 1994:32-4

Quinlan KP, Hayani KC. Vitamin A and respiratory syncytial virus infection. Serum levels and supplementation trial. Arch Pediatr Adolesc Med 150(1):25-30, 1996

Rasmussen JB, Glennow C. Reduction in days of illness after long-term treatment with N-acetylcysteine controlled release tablets in patients with chronic bronchitis. Eur Respir J 1:351-3, 1988

Rasmussen LB et al. Effect of diet and plasma fatty acid composition on immune status in elderly men. Am J Clin Nutr 59 (3):572-7, 1994

Rawal BD et al. Inhibition of Pseudomonas aeruginosa by ascorbic acid acting singly and in combination with antimicrobials: in-vitro and in-vivo studies. Med J Aust 1(6):169-74, 1974

Reid G et al. Influence of three-day antimicrobial therapy and lactobacillus vaginal suppositories on recurrence of urinary tract infections. Clin Ther 14:11-16, 1992

Riise GC et al. The intrabronchial microbial flora in chronic bronchitis patients: a target for N-acetylcysteine therapy? Eur Respir J 7:94-101, 1994

Rokkas T et al. Helicobacter pylori infection and gastric juice vitamin C levels. Impact of eradication. Dig Dis Sci 40(3):615-21, 1995

Sanchez A. Role of sugars in human neutrophilic phagocytosis. Am J Clin Nutr 26:180, 1973

Schwartz J, Weiss ST. Dietary factors and their relation to respiratory symptoms. The Second National Health and Nutrition Examination Survey. Am J Epidemiol 132(1):67-76, 1990

Shahani KM et al. Cultured Dairy Prod J 12:8-11, 1977

Shalev E et al. Ingestion of yogurt containing Lactobacillus acidophilus compared with pasteurized yogurt as prophylaxis for recurrent candidal vaginitis and bacterial vaginosis. Arch Fam Med 5(10):593-6, 1996

Shankar AH, Prasad AS. Zinc and immune function: the biological basis of altered resistance to infection. Am J Clin Nutr 68(2 Suppl):447S-463S, 1998

Singh KP et al. Effect of zinc on immune functions and host resistance against infection and tumor challenge. Immunopharmacol Immunotoxicol 14(4):813-20, 1992

Singh RB et al. Dietary intake and plasma levels of antioxidant vitamins in health and disease: a hospital-based case-control study. J Nutr Environ Med 5:235-42, 1995

Skodinska-Rozewska E et al. The effect of vitamin E treatment on the incidence of OKT4+ lymphocytes in the peripheral blood of children with chronic respiratory tract infections. Arch Immunol Ther Exp (Warsz) 35(2):207-10, 1987

Sobeleva MK, Gavalov SM. [The iron overload syndrome in patients with severe bacterial inflammatory diseases and convalescents]. Gematol Transfuziol 38(3):21-4, 1993) (in Russian)

Sommer A et al. Increased risk of respiratory disease and diarrhoea in children with pre-existing mild vitamin A deficiency. Am J Clin Nutr 40:1090-5, 1984

Spapen H et al. Does N-acetyl-L-cysteine influence cytokine response during early human septic shock? Chest 113(6):1616-24, 1998

Spooner JB. Alkalinisation in the management of cystitis. J Int Med Res 12(1):30-4, 1984

Srinivas U et al. Trace element alterations in infectious diseases. Scand J Clin Lab Invest 48(6):495-500, 1988

Stacpoole PW. The role of vitamin C in infectious disease and allergic reactions. Med Hypotheses 1:42-6, 1975

Stansfield SK et al. Vitamin A supplementation and increased prevalence of childhood diarrhoea and acute respiratory infections. Lancet 342:578-82, 1993

Stephensen CB et al. Vitamin A is excreted in the urine during acute infection. Am J Clin Nutr 60:388-92, 1994

Stephensen CB et al. Adverse effects of high-dose vitamin A supplements in children hospitalized with pneumonia. Pediatrics 101(5):E3, 1998

Stolzenberg R. Possible folate deficiency with postsurgical infection. Nutr Clin Pract 9(6):247-50, 1994

Strassner C, Friesen A. [Therapy of candiduria by alkalinization of urine. Oral treatment with potassium-sodium-hydrogen citrate]. Fortschr Med 113(25):359-62, 1995) (in German)

Sugarman B. Zinc and infection. Rev Infect Dis 5(1):137-47, 1983

Tahiliani AG, Beinlich CJ. Pantothenic acid in health and disease. Vitam Horm 46:165-228, 1991

Tanzer F, Ozalp I. Leucocyte ascorbic acid concentration and plasma ascorbic acid levels in children with various infections. Mater Med Pol 25(1):5-8, 1993

Taylor EW et al. Genomic structures of vial agents in relation to the biosynthesis of selenoproteins. Biol Trace Elem Res 56(1):63-91, 1997

Tengerdy RP. Vitamin E, immune response, and disease resistance. Ann N Y Acad Sci 570:335-44, 1989

Thornton GHM et al. J Clin Invest 34:1073, 1955

Uhari M et al. Xylitol chewing gum in prevention of acute otitis media: a double-blind randomized trial. Br Med J 313:1180-4, 1996

Uhari M et al. A novel use of xylitol sugar in preventing acute otitis media. Pediatrics 102(4 Pt 1):879-84, 1998

Wan JM et al. Invited comment: lipids and the development of immune dysfunction and infection. JPEN J Parenter Enteral Nutr 12(6 Suppl):43S-52S, 1988

Watts DL. The nutritional relationships of copper. J Orthomol Med 4(2):99-108, 1989

Willmott F et al. Zinc and recalcitrant trichomoniasis. Letter. Lancet i:1053, 1983

Wilmore DW, Shabert JK. Role of glutamine in immunologic responses. Nutrition 14(7-8):618-26, 1998

Wright JV. Dr. Wright's Book of Nutritional Medicine. Emmaus, Penn, Rodale Press, 1979

Wright JV - interviewed by Richard Leviton in Alternative Medicine Digest, Issue 13, 1996

Ziegler TR et al. Glutamine: from basic science to clinical applications. Nutrition 12(11-12 Suppl):S68-70, 1996

INFERTILITY

NUTRITIONAL TREATMENT GUIDE

✓ = Efficacy generally accepted.
* = Efficacy *demonstrated* by controlled human trials.
[+] = Efficacy *suspected* from uncontrolled human trials.
[-] = Efficacy *suspected* from indirect data.
? = Efficacy *challenged* in a study of similar design.

I. MALES

DIETARY FACTORS

[-] avoid **Alcohol**
[-] avoid **Caffeine**
[-] avoid **Tea**

NUTRITIONAL FACTORS

* **Glutathione**: 600 mg intramuscularly daily (2 month trial)
* **Vitamin B_{12}**: methylcobalamin 1,500 μg daily (12 week trial)
* **Vitamin C**: 200 mg daily (60 day trial)

- -

[+] **L-Arginine deficiency:** 4 g daily (3 to 6 month trial)
[+] **L-Carnitine:** 1 g 3 times daily (3 month trial)
[+] **Coenzyme Q_{10}:** ? 60 mg daily
[+] **Folic acid:** folinic acid 15 mg daily (3 month trial)
[+] **Vitamin B_{12} deficiency:** 1000 μg IM weekly initially; then monthly
[+] **Vitamin E:** 400 mg daily *AND* **Selenium** 100 μg daily
[+] **Zinc deficiency:** zinc sulfate 220 mg twice daily *AND* **Copper** 2 mg daily

OTHER RELATED FACTORS

[+] rule out **Cadmium toxicity**
[+] rule out **Lead toxicity**

II. FEMALES

DIETARY FACTORS

[-] avoid **Caffeinated Soft Drinks**
[-] avoid **Coffee**
[-] avoid **Milk and Dairy Products** (only if galactosemic)
[-] avoid **Tea**
[-] ? avoid **Alcohol**
[-] ? avoid **Caffeine**

NUTRITIONAL FACTORS

[+] **Folic acid deficiency:** 5 mg 3 times daily
[+] **Iron deficiency:** 35 mg daily *AND* **Vitamin C** 200 mg daily
[+] **Vitamin B_{12} deficiency:** 1000 µg IM weekly initially; then monthly
[+] **Vitamin C** *AND* **clomiphene:** *enhances efficacy of clomiphene in inducing ovulation*
[+] **Zinc deficiency:** zinc sulfate 220 mg twice daily *AND* **Copper** 2 mg daily
[+] ? **Vitamin B_6:** pyridoxal-5-phosphate ? 50 mg daily

OTHER RELATED FACTORS

[+] rule out **Gluten intolerance**
[+] rule out **Lead toxicity**

DIETARY FACTORS

About 12% of primary infertility due to ovulatory dysfunction is related to abnormal weight. Perhaps half of all infertile women become amenorrheic following a period of weight loss *(Wynn)*. In one study, a body weight of 85% of less than ideal was associated with a 4.7-fold increase in the risk of ovulatory infertility, while a body weight of 120% or more was associated more than double the relative risk *(Green)*.

Coffee and Tea

Females

The results of several observational studies have been consistent with the hypothesis that caffeine reduces fertility *(Bolumar;Stanton)*. In regard to women, caffeine reduces the serum concentration of prolactin, and low serum prolactin is known to be associated with female infertility *(Casas)*.

In a prospective study of 104 healthy women who had been attempting to get pregnant for 3 months, women who consumed more than the equivalent of one cup of coffee daily were half as likely to become pregnant, per cycle, as women who drank less, and a dose-response effect was present *(Wilcox,1988)*.

Questions remain concerning whether caffeine is the substance responsible for impairing fertility in caffeinated beverages. A recent study of 2,607 planned pregnancies over the previous 30 years found no difference in fecundability between women who ingested 100 mg or less of caffeine daily and those who ingested more than 100 mg daily. However, women who were coffee drinkers, and men who were tea drinkers, had significantly decreased fecundability scores *(Curtis)*.

Another study failed to find an relationship between tea intake and female fertility, while one caffeinated soft drink per day was associated with a 50% reduction in fecundability after controlling for coffee consumption, frequency of intercourse, and age. The strength of this association exceeded the prediction from the study's data on coffee consumption if caffeine were the responsible agent *(Wilcox,1991)*.

Whether caffeine or some other substance associated with caffeinated beverages is responsible for impairing fertility will remain uncertain until these beverages are eliminated in controlled clinical trials.

Males

There is little evidence implicating caffeine in male infertility. One small study found weak evidence for an association between sperm nuclear morphometric parameters and caffeine intake *(Vine)*. However, when men who consumed up to 100 mg of caffeine daily were compared to those who consumed more than 100 mg daily, the fecundability (monthly probability of conception) of their mates was similar *(Curtis)*.

Alcohol

Females

Excessive alcohol ingestion may provoke hyperprolactinemia in women *(Mendleson)*, a cause of menstrual cycle dysfunction and infertility. When a group of infertile women were compared to women who recently gave birth, alcohol use was found to be associated with an increased risk of infertility due to an ovulatory factor or to endometriosis. These findings suggest that even moderate alcohol consumption may contribute to some types of infertility *(Grodstein)*.

Males

Ethanol has a toxic effect on the Leydig cells *(van Thiel)*, with the degree of impairment depending upon the amount of ethanol ingested and the duration of ethanol exposure *(Anderson)*. Animal studies suggest that, following moderate periods of abstinence, male alcoholics with reproductive disorders could have at least a partial recovery *(Anderson)*.

Milk and Dairy Products

Relatively high intestinal lactase activity, or low activity of an enzyme involved in galactose catabolism, reduces fertility in women in the presence of galactosemia *(Herrinton)*. Moreover, in populations with higher *per capita* milk consumption and a greater ability to digest its lactose component into glucose and galactose, fertility at older ages was lower, and the decline in fertility rates was steeper *(Cramer,1994)*.

However, results of a recent study suggest that the biologic variation in galactose metabolism that exists in the general population has no influence on fertility *(Herrinton)*. The need to avoid the intake of galactose from milk and dairy products (and to substitute other foods or supplements to provide an adequate calcium intake) thus appears to be limited to women with galactosemia *(Cramer,1989)*.

NUTRITIONAL FACTORS

VITAMINS

Folic Acid Deficiency

Females

Folate deficiency may cause women to become infertile *(Dawson DW)*. In addition to dietary inadequacy, deficiency may be caused by diseases affecting the jejunal mucosa, such as celiac disease and tropical sprue, and certain drugs, such as antacids, diphenylhydantoin and ethanol.

Three women, all close to 30 years old, who had been infertile for several years, and who were found to show evidence of folate deficiency secondary to celiac disease, were treated with folate supplementation. Hematologic indices returned to normal and all became pregnant during the following 3 to 15 months *(Dawson DW)*.

Males

There is evidence from an open trial that folic acid supplementation may improve the number of sperm and their motility in infertile men. Moreover, in this study, the most remarkable improvements in sperm were seen in men whose partners later became pregnant *(Bentivoglio)*.

Vitamin B_6

While the results of open trials are mixed, some report that supplementation with vitamin B_6 seemed to successfully treat female infertility *(Abraham)*. Even amenorrhea with galactorrhea and hyperprolactinemia sometimes responded *(Kidd;McIntosh)*.

The mechanism is unclear although, in one study, 5 out of 7 infertile women had significant increases in progesterone levels following supplementation *(Abraham)*. This finding may be relevant as inadequate progesterone may fail to maintain the endometrium sufficiently to support the fertilized ovum.

Vitamin B_{12}

Pernicious anemia, although rare during childbearing ages, usually leads to infertility in both sexes *(Marty)*. As with folate deficiency, fertility is restored following vitamin B_{12} supplementation *(Gulden)*.

In addition, under double-blind conditions, vitamin B_{12} supplementation has seemed effective in treating oligospermia (sperm counts of 20 million per milliliter or less) in perhaps one-half of patients *(Kumamoto)*.

Vitamin C

Males

Since ascorbic acid is a powerful antioxidant, it is not surprising that a marginal deficiency of the vitamin in the seminal plasma has been shown to cause oxidative damage to sperm DNA *(Fraga)*. Asthenospermia (reduced sperm motility) may be associated with both increased free radical activity and marginal ascorbate deficiency, suggesting that the latter may be causative *(Lewis, 1997)*. Moreover, oxidative damage to semen is believed to be responsible for many cases of idiopathic oligospermia *(Aitken)*; thus oligospermia could also result from inadequate ascorbate in the seminal plasma *(Luck)*.

The benefit of vitamin C supplementation to infertile males can be dramatic. One week after 30 infertile males received either zero, 200 mg or 1000 mg of ascorbic acid daily, the placebo group showed few changes, while the 1,000 mg group showed a 140% increase in sperm count as well as improvements in sperm viability, motility, and reductions in abnormalities, immaturity and agglutination. The 200 mg group also improved, although the improvement was not as dramatic.

After 3 weeks, both treatment groups showed further improvement, and the 200 mg group caught up to the 1,000 mg group. After 60 days, *all* of the men who received ascorbic acid had impregnated their wives, compared to *none* of the men in the placebo group. The investigators concluded that vitamin C supplementation is effective for male infertility characterized by sperm agglutination in excess of 25% *(Dawson EB)*.

When compared to treatment with mesterolone *(Hargreave)* or clomiphene citrate *(Abel)*, vitamin C supplementation appears to be equally effective.

Females

The ovary is a site of ascorbate accumulation and turnover; in fact, the mid-cycle change in its retention and excretion has been proposed as a definitive marker of ovulation. Moreover, preliminary data suggest that the supply of ascorbic acid to the ovary might be a limiting factor in the ability of the preovulatory follicle to grow in response to gonadotropin stimulation *(Luck)*.

While the efficacy of vitamin C alone in treating anovulatory women has not been reported, when ascorbic acid was added to clomiphene, ovulation and menses were induced in 17 out of 42 women (41%) who were not responsive to clomiphene alone *(Igarashi)*.

Vitamin E

Based on early rat studies, it appears that a deficiency of vitamin E destroys testicular function *(Mason)*. There is recent evidence that the percentage of motile spermatozoa may be related to sperm alpha-tocopherol content *(Therond)*.

In a placebo-controlled study of 52 asthenospermic males, supplementation improved sperm motility. Eleven of the treated men impregnated their spouses versus none of the 35 men given placebo *(Suleiman)*. Moreover, in open trials, vitamin E supplementation has been reported to be effective in treating oligospermia *(Shute; Warren)*, abnormal sperm *(Shute)*, and even low *in vitro* fertilization rates despite normal sperm counts and sperm function *(Geva)*.

Evidence that the vitamin may be functioning as an antioxidant comes from studies showing that vitamin E supplementation reduces the level of malondialdehyde, a measure of lipid peroxidation, in the sperm *(Geva; Suleiman)*.

MINERALS

Iron Deficiency

Depleted iron stores, as evidenced by reduced serum ferritin, may be associated with infertility despite the lack of an iron-deficiency anemia.

When a group of 113 women with hair loss and reduced serum ferritin were given iron supplementation along with vitamin C to increase its absorption, 7 of the women became pregnant within 28 weeks. All of these 7 women previously had a long history of infertility *(Rushton)*.

Controlled trials are needed to confirm these findings.

Selenium Deficiency

Males

Selenium is important to male fertility. Two selenium-containing proteins found in sperm are structurally important *(Schrauzer)* and selenium deficiency has been linked to decreased testosterone secretion, decreased spermatozoa motility, and increased abnormal spermatozoa (*Bedwal)*. Also, there is some evidence that infertility may be associated with a metabolic defect concerning the incorporation of selenium into sperm cells *(Hansen)*.

The question of whether infertile men benefit from selenium supplementation remains to be answered. Both low and high sperm selenium concentrations appear to have a negative influence on the number and motility of spermatozoa, but the optimal sperm selenium concentration is not yet defined *(Hansen)*. When a group of subfertile men took selenium supplements for 12 weeks, those supplemented with selenium-rich yeast showed increased selenium and glutathione peroxidase activity in both blood components and seminal fluid, yet sperm count, motility and morphology failed to improve *(Iwanier)*.

However, when selenium was combined with vitamin E in an open trial, the combination appeared to be effective in increasing sperm motility, percent live sperm, and percent normal spermatozoa in oligo-astheno-terato-zoospermic infertile men *(Vezina)*. As selenium and vitamin E were not given to separate control groups, it is possible that these effects were solely due to the vitamin E.

Females

In women, selenium deficiency appears to result in infertility and abortions *(Bedwal)*. In fact, one study noted that mean glutathione peroxidase activity (which is selenium-dependent) in follicles yielding oocytes which were subsequently fertilized was greater than that of the follicles with non-fertilized oocytes *(Paszkowski)*. Whether selenium supplementation is effective for treating infertility in women remains to be studied.

Zinc Deficiency

Males

Zinc has an important influence on male reproductive function. Serum and semen zinc levels are lower in infertile males than in normals *(Mohan)*. Both the number *(Abbasi)* and motility *(Skandhan)* of sperm appear to correlate with semen zinc levels. Blood zinc as measured in granulocytes and platelets may correlate with serum testosterone and dihydrotestosterone levels *(Prasad,1988,1996)*. Moreover, during zinc restriction, serum testosterone and dihydrotestosterone levels decrease along with the sperm count *(Abbasi)*.

Zinc supplementation has been shown in open trials to increase both sperm count and sperm motility in oligospermic men, as well as acid phosphatase activity *(Tikkiwal)*. Among oligospermic men, those with low plasma testosterone may be the best candidates, as their plasma testosterone increases and they are more likely to become fertile *(Netter;Prasad,1996)*.

Females

Animal studies have shown that zinc deficiency interferes with ovulation or leads to a very high number of degenerated ovocytes *(Favier,1992)*. In randomized studies, zinc supplementation has been shown to exert a beneficial effect on fertility in women. However, too high a supplemental dosage may be as harmful as a deficiency *(Favier,1993)*.

OTHER NUTRITIONAL FACTORS

L-Arginine Deficiency

Arginine is the dietary precursor to nitric oxide, and within spermatozoa, nitric oxide appears to be necessary for adequate sperm motility *(Lewis,1996)*. It is also precursor in the synthesis of putrescine, spermidine, and spermine, polyamines which may have an important role as initiators in spermatic motility processes *(Mendez)*. Moreover, pathospermia (abnormal sperm) is sometimes marked by abnormal arginine metabolism *(Papp)*.

When free and bound arginine was measured in the semen of normal and infertile men, there was a positive correlation between sperm motility and free arginine content, as well as a positive correlation between sperm count and bound arginine *(Tanimura)*. Confirmation of the causative role of arginine in affecting sperm count comes from a study in which normal men received an arginine-deficient diet for 9 days. Their sperm count was decreased and did not return to normal for several weeks after arginine was restored to the diet *(Holt)*.

Several open trials have found that arginine supplementation often seems effective for treating male infertility. In a typical study, arginine supplementation resulted in improvement in three-quarters of a group of 178 men with decreased sperm count and sperm motility *(Schachter)*. Men with severe oligospermia (less than 10 million sperm per ejaculate) are unlikely to benefit, however *(Pryor)*.

A man who had been unable to impregnate his wife for 6 years had only 25 million sperm per milliliter in his ejaculate, less than 50% of which were motile.

He was treated with L-arginine 4 grams daily. Six weeks later, his sperm count was "100% improved" and, shortly afterwards, his wife was found to be pregnant (Wright).

L-Carnitine

Both extracellular and intracellular acetylcarnitine play an important role in sperm energy metabolism, providing the primary fuel for sperm motility *(Bruns)*. In fact, the increase of carnitine and acetylcarnitine content in spermatozoa during epididymal passage is coincident with the acquisition of progressive motility *(Jeulin)*. Also, seminal-free carnitine content correlates with sperm count and motility *(Bornman)*.

In open trials, L-carnitine supplementation has appeared to be effective in increasing sperm counts and improving sperm motility. Three months after 47 infertile men with idiopathic asthenospermia but with sperm counts of at least 10 million per milliliter started L-carnitine supplementation, 79% responded with greatly increased sperm counts, a doubling of the percentage of motile sperms, and an increase in progressive-rapid-motility (a measure of sperm function) from 21% to 32% *(Vitale)*. Improvements following supplementation are greatest in men whose pretreatment sperm motility is most impaired *(Costa)*.

Coenzyme Q_{10}

In sperm cells, coenzyme Q_{10} (CoQ_{10}) is concentrated in the mitochondria of the midpiece. The energy for movement and all other energy-dependent processes in the sperm cell also depend on the availability of CoQ_{10}. As ubiquinol, its reduced form, it also acts as an antioxidant, preventing lipid peroxidation in sperm membranes *(Lewin)*.

Seminal fluid Co Q_{10} may be reduced in men with low sperm count or motility *(Mancini)*. Moreover, in infertile men, ubiquinol content in seminal plasma correlates with sperm count *(Alleva)*.

As expected, the results of open trials suggest that supplementation with CoQ_{10} may be beneficial for men with low sperm counts or low sperm motility *(Lewin; Tanimura)*. The effect on sperm motility has also been studied *in vitro* using samples of asthenospermic and normal motility sperm. While, after incubation with CoQ_{10}, there was no change in motility in normal sperm, motility significantly increased in the sperm from asthenospermic men *(Lewin)*.

Glutathione

One of the few known mechanisms for male infertility is the excessive generation of reactive oxygen species by abnormal spermatozoa and by contaminating leukocytes. Glutathione is important to the antioxidant defense of the spermatogenic epithelium, the epididymis, and perhaps in ejaculated spermatozoa *(Irvine)*. Men with oligozoospermia (reduced live sperm count in the ejaculated semen) may have reduced sperm concentrations of glutathione *(Ochsendorf)*.

When men who may be infertile due to excessive oxidative stress receive glutathione, it appears to act at the epididymis and during spermatogenesis to improve the function of ejaculated spermatozoa *(Irvine)*. Both sperm morphology and motility improve *(Lenzi,1992,1993)*.

While, because of the limited absorption of oral glutathione, the substance was administered intramuscularly in these studies, larger oral doses may possibly be effective. Alternatively, *N-acetylcysteine* (NAC), a glutathione precursor, may be administered as a means of increasing intracellular glutathione levels. Since NAC appears to chelate zinc and copper, it is suggested that these minerals be supplemented during long-term NAC administration *(Gaby)*.

When his wife failed to become pregnant after 8 months of trying, a 31-year-old male had his sperm tested and was told that his sperm count was much lower than normal and that sperm motility was more than slightly reduced. For several months he tried to time intercourse to ovulation, but his efforts were unsuccessful.

He then saw his doctor who placed him on a nutrient formula which included copper (for the prostate), iron and various antioxidants (to reduce damage to sperm due to free radical production) along with L-arginine (for sperm motility) to take between meals and at bedtime. He was also placed on zinc (for the prostate) with breakfast and dinner.

Two months later, his wife missed her period and was found to be pregnant. Laboratory testing showed that his sperm count had reached near normal levels and that sperm motility was now normal (Chrein).

OTHER RELATED FACTORS

Toxic Minerals

Heavy metal accumulation can adversely affect fertility, especially when the heavy metals interact with deficiencies of nutrient minerals *(Gerhard)*.

Cadmium

Males with excessive cadmium exposure, especially if zinc nutriture is low, may be particularly liable to develop infertility. Several observational studies have found a correlation between exposure to toxic levels of cadmium and low sperm counts and semen volume *(Xu)*.

In men with asthenozoospermia, higher cadmium concentrations have been found in both blood *(Chia)* and semen *(Omu)*. Also, in the seminal plasma of men with varicocele-associated infertility, cadmium was elevated and zinc was decreased, suggesting that excessive cadmium exposure, or a defect in transition metal regulation, is involved in its development *(Benoff)*.

Lead

In males, exposure to even low levels of lead can lead to reduced libido, reduced sperm motility, abnormal sperm morphology, chromosomal damage, infertility, abnormal prostatic function and changes in serum testosterone.

In females, effects include infertility, miscarriage, premature membrane rupture, pre-eclampsia, pregnancy hypertension and premature delivery *(Winder)*.

Gluten Intolerance

Women with intolerance to gluten may be unable to conceive until they are placed on a gluten-free diet. Resumption of fertility may take as long as one year *(Fielding)*.

Judith, a 36 year-old housewife, complained of increasing pain and stiffness in her back and knees which corresponded to evidence of osteoarthritis on x-rays. She also complained of tiredness, mild eczema and premenstrual symptoms. Though she had delivered two children over 10 years earlier, she had been unable to conceive since then. Laboratory testing showed her to have deficiencies of chromium, iron, magnesium, selenium and zinc, as well as evidence of a mild diabetic tendency. Treatment with nutritional supplements corrected all of her deficiencies except for iron and her arthritic symptoms improved considerably.

As it was suspected that her deficiencies were based on malabsorption due to food sensitivities, she was asked to avoid dairy produce and all gluten-containing grains (wheat, oats, barley and rye). There was a considerable improvement in her energy level, further reduction in her arthritic pains and she became pregnant. However, on reintroducing wheat into her diet, her symptoms strongly recurred, and she was advised to have a full evaluation for celiac disease (Davies).

BIBLIOGRAPHY

Abbasi AA et al. Experimental zinc deficiency in man: Effect on testicular function. J Lab Clin Med 96(3):544-50, 1980

Abel BJ et al. Randomized trial of clomiphene citrate treatment and vitamin C for male infertility. Br J Urol 54(6):780-84, 1982

Abraham GE, Hargrove JT - reported in Med World News March 19, 1979

Alleva R et al. The protective role of ubiquinol-10 against formation of lipid hydroperoxides in human seminal fluid. Mol Aspects Med 18 Suppl:S221-S228, 1997

Anderson RA Jr et al. Spontaneous recovery from ethanol-induced male infertility. Alcohol 2(3):479-84, 1985

Aitken RJ. The role of free oxygen radicals and sperm function. Int J Androl 12:95-7, 1989

Bedwal R, Bahuguana A. Zinc, copper and selenium in reproduction. Experientia 50:626-40, 1994

Benoff S et al. A potential role for cadmium in the etiology of varicocele-associated infertility. Fertil Steril 67(2):336-47, 1997

Bentivoglio G et al. Folinic acid in the treatment of human male infertility. Fertil Steril 60(4):698-701, 1993

Bolumar F. Caffeine intake and delayed conception: a European multicenter study on infertility and subfecundity. European Study Group on Infertility Subfecundity. Am J Epidemiol 145(4):324-34, 1997

Bornman MS et al. Seminal carnitine, epididymal function and spermatozoal motility. S Afr Med J 75:20-1, 1989

Bruns KA, Casillas ER. Partial purification and characterization of an acetylcarnitine hydrolase from bovine epididymal spermatozoa. Arch Biochem Biophys 277:1-7, 1990

Casas M et al. Dopaminergic mechanism for caffeine induced decrease in fertility? Letter. Lancet i:731, 1989

Chia SE. Blood concentrations of lead, cadmium, mercury, zinc, and copper and human semen parameters. Arch Androl 29(2):177-83, 1992

Chrein L. Supplements delivered us a baby. Natural Health Jan.-Feb. 1995:66-8

Costa M et al. L-carnitine in idiopathic asthenozoospermia: a multicenter study. Andrologia 26(3):155-9, 1994

Cramer DW. Galactose-1-phosphate uridyl transferase activity associated with age at menopause and reproductive history. Fertil Steril 51(4):609-15, 1989

Cramer DW et al. Adult hypolactasia, milk consumption, and age-specific fertility. Am J Epidemiol 139(3):282-9, 1994

Curtis KM et al. Effects of cigarette smoking, caffeine consumption, and alcohol intake on fecundability. Am J Epidemiol 146(1):32-41, 1997

Davies S, Stewart A. Nutritional Medicine. London, Pan Books, 1987

Dawson DW, Sawers AH. Infertility and folate deficiency. Case reports. Br J Obstet Gynaecol 89:678-80, 1982

Dawson EB et al. Effect of ascorbic acid on male fertility. Ann N Y Acad Sci 498:312-23, 1987

Favier A. The role of zinc in reproduction: Hormonal mechanisms. Biol Trace Elem Res 32:363-82, 1992

Favier A. [Current aspects about the role of zinc in nutrition]. Rev Prat 43(2):146-51, 1993) (in French)

Fielding JF. Pregnancy and coeliac disease. J Ir Med Assoc 67(15):422, 1974

Fraga CG et al. Ascorbic acid protects against endogenous oxidative DNA damage in human sperm. Proc Natl Acad Sci 88:11003-6, 1991

Gaby AR. Literature review and commentary: Glutathione therapy for male infertility. Townsend Letter for Doctors, April 1993

Gerhard I, Runnebaum B. [Environmental pollutants and fertility disorders. Heavy metals and minerals.] Geburtshilfe Frauenheilkd 52(7):383-96, 1992) (in German)

Geva E et al. The effect of antioxidant treatment on human spermatozoa and fertilization rate in an in vitro fertilization program. Fertil Steril 66:430-4, 1996

Green BB et al. Risk of ovulatory infertility in relation to body weight. Fertil Steril 50(9):621-6, 1988

Grodstein F et al. Infertility in women and moderate alcohol use. Am J Public Health 84(9):1429-32, 1994

Gulden KD. Pernicious anemia, vitiligo, and infertility. J Am Board Fam Pract 3(3):217-20, 1990

Hansen JC, Deguchi Y. Selenium and fertility in animals and man--a review. Acta Vet Scand 37(1):19-30, 1996

Hargreave TB et al. Randomised trial of mesterolone versus vitamin C for male infertility. Br J Urol 56(6):740-44, 1984

Herrinton LJ et al. Lactose metabolism and time to pregnancy. Fertil Steril 66(3):384-8, 1996

Holt et al cited in Tanimura J. Studies on arginine supplementation in human semen. Part I: the arginine contents of normal and sterile human semen. Bull Osaka Med Sch 13:76-83, 1967

Igarashi M. Augmentative effect of ascorbic acid upon induction of human ovulation in clomiphene-ineffective anovulatory women. Int J Fertility 22:168-73, 1977

Irvine DS. Glutathione as a treatment for male infertility. Rev Reprod 1(1):6-12, 1996

Iwanier K et al. Selenium supplementation enhances the element concentration in blood and seminal fluid but does not change the spermatozoal quality characteristics in subfertile men. J Androl 16(5):441-7, 1995

Jeulin C et al. Acetylcarnitine and spermatozoa: relationship with epididymal maturation and motility in the boar and men. Reprod Nutr Dev 28:1317-27, 1988

Kidd GS et al. The effects of pyridoxine on pituitary hormone secretion in amenorrhea-galactorrhea syndromes. J Clin Endocrinol Metab 54(4):872-5, 1982

Kumamoto Y et al. Clinical efficacy of mecobalamin in treatment of oligozoospermia: Results of double-blind comparative clinical study. Acta Urol Jpn 34:1109-32, 1988

Lenzi A et al. Glutathione therapy for male infertility. Arch Androl 29(1):65-8, 1992

Lenzi A et al. Placebo-controlled, double-blind, cross-over trial of glutathione therapy in male infertility. Hum Reprod 8(10):1657-62, 1993

Lewin A, Lavon H. The effect of coenzyme Q10 on sperm motility and function. Mol Aspects Med 18 Suppl:S213-S219, 1997

Lewis SE et al. Nitric oxide synthase and nitrite production in human spermatozoa: evidence that endogenous nitric oxide is beneficial to sperm motility. Mol Hum Reprod 2(11):873-8, 1996

Lewis SE. Comparison of individual antioxidants of sperm and seminal plasma in fertile and infertile men. Fertil Steril 1997 Jan;67(1):142-7, 1997

Luck MR et al. Ascorbic acid and fertility. Biol Reprod 52:262-6, 1995

Mancini A et al. Coenzyme Q10 concentrations in normal and pathological human seminal fluid. J Androl 15(6):591-4, 1994

Marty H. [Pernicious anemia as cause of secondary sterility.] Schweiz Med Wochenschr 114(5):178-9, 1984 (in German)

Mason KE. A histological study of sterility in the albino rat due to a dietary deficiency. Proc Natl Acad Sci 11:377-82, 1925

McIntosh EN. Treatment of women with the galactorrhea-amenorrhea syndrome with pyridoxine (vitamin B6). J Clin Endocrinol Metab 42(6):1192-5, 1976

Mendez JD, Hernandez MP. [Effect of L-arginine and polyamines on sperm quality. Ginecol Obstet Mex 61:229-34, 1993 (in Spanish)

Mendleson JH. Alcohol effects on reproductive function in women. Psychiatry Letter 4(7):35-8, 1986

Mohan H et al. Inter-relationship of zinc levels in serum and semen in oligospermic infertile patients and fertile males. Indian J Pathol Microbiol 40(4):451-5, 1997

Netter A et al. Effect of zinc administration on plasma testosterone, dehydrotestosterone and sperm count. Arch Androl 7(1):69-73, 1981

Ochsendorf FR. Glutathione in spermatozoa and seminal plasma of infertile men. Hum Reprod 13(2):353-9, 1998

Omu AE. Significance of trace elements in seminal plasma of infertile men. Nutrition 11(5 Suppl):502-5, 1995

Papp G et al. The role of basic amino acids of the seminal plasma in fertility. Int Urol Nephrol 15(2):195-203, 1983

Paszkowski T et al. Selenium dependent glutathione peroxidase activity in human follicular fluid. Clin Chim Acta 236:173-80, 1995

Prasad AS. Zinc in growth and development and spectrum of human zinc deficiency. J Am Coll Nutr 7(5):377-84, 1988

Prasad A et al. Zinc status and serum testosterone levels of healthy subjects. Nutrition 12(5):344-8, 1996

Pryor JP et al. Controlled clinical trial of arginine for infertile men with oligospermia. Br J Urol 50:47-50, 1978

Rushton DH et al. Ferritin and fertility. Letter. Lancet 337:1554, 1991

Schachter A et al. Treatment of oligospermia with the amino acid arginine. J Urol 110(3):311-13, 1973

Schrauzer GN. Benefits of natural selenium. Anabolism 7(4):5, 1988

Shute E. Effect of vitamin E on sperm. Urol Cutaneous Rev 48:423-6, 1944

Skandhan KP et al. Semen electrolytes in normal and infertile subjects. II. Zinc. Experientia 34(11):1476-7, 1978

Stanton CK, Gray RH. Effects of caffeine consumption on delayed conception. Am J Epidemiol 142(12):1322-9, 1995

Suleiman SA et al. Lipid peroxidation and human sperm motility: protective role of vitamin E. J Androl 17(5):530-7, 1996

Tanimura J. Studies on arginine supplementation in human semen. Part I: the arginine contents of normal and sterile human semen. Bull Osaka Med Sch 13(2):76-83, 1967a

Therond P et al. alpha-Tocopherol in human spermatozoa and seminal plasma: relationships with motility, antioxidant enzymes and leukocytes. Mol Hum Reprod 2(10):739-44, 1996

Tikkiwal M et al. Effect of zinc administration on seminal zinc and fertility of oligospermic males. Indian J Physiol Pharmacol 31(1):30-34, 1987

Van Thiel DH et al. Ethanol, a Leydig cell toxin: evidence obtained in vivo and in vitro. Pharmacol Biochem Behav 18 Suppl 1:317-23, 1983

Vezina D et al. Selenium-vitamin E supplementation in infertile men: Effects on semen parameters and micronutrient levels and distribution. Biol Trace Elem Res 53:65-83, 1996

Vine MF et al. Human sperm morphometry and smoking, caffeine, and alcohol consumption. Reprod Toxicol 11(2/3):179-84, 1997

Vitale G et al. Carnitine supplementation in human idiopathic asthenospermia: clinical results. Drugs Exp Clin Res 21(4):157-9, 1995

Warren N. Summary of a presentation to the Family Planning Association's Conference on infertility. Lancet ii:542-4, 1948

Wilcox A et al. Caffeinated beverages and decreased fertility. Lancet ii:1473-76, 1988

Wilcox AJ, Weinberg CR. Tea and fertility. Letter. Lancet 337:1159-60, 1991

Winder C. Lead, reproduction and development. Neurotoxicology 14(2-3):303-17, 1993

Wright JV. A case of low sperm count. Prevention August 1983, pp. 66-69

Wynn A, Wynn M. The need for nutritional assessment in the treatment of the infertile patient. J Nutr Med 1:315-24, 1990

Xu B et al. Trace elements in blood and seminal plasma and their relationship to sperm quality. Reprod Toxicol 7:613-18, 1993

INFLAMMATION

See Also: ALLERGY

NUTRITIONAL TREATMENT GUIDE

✓ = Efficacy generally accepted.
* = Efficacy *demonstrated* by controlled human trials.
[+] = Efficacy *suspected* from uncontrolled human trials.
[-] = Efficacy *suspected* from indirect data.
? = Efficacy *challenged* in a study of similar design.

NUTRITIONAL FACTORS

* **Copper salicylate**: *for anti-inflammatory and analgesic effects:* 60 mg twice daily
* **Omega-6 fatty acids (gamma linolenic acid)**: 1.5 to 6 g daily

- -

[+] **Omega-3 fatty acids (eicosapentaenoic acid)**: 3.2 g daily
[+] **Vitamin B_{12}**: *for bursitis:* 1000 µg IM daily for 7-10 days, then 3 times weekly for 2-3 weeks, then 1-2 times weekly for 2-3 weeks, depending on rate of improvement
[+] **Vitamin C**: at least 500 mg daily (maximum effective dosage is uncertain)
[+] **Vitamin E**: ? 400 IU daily
[+] **Zinc deficiency**: zinc sulfate 220 mg twice daily *AND* **Copper** 2 mg daily

- -

[-] **Copper deficiency**: 2 mg twice daily for up to 6 weeks *AND* **Zinc** 50 mg daily
[-] **L-Glutamine**: 5 to 30 g daily
[-] **Hydrolytic enzymes**: *example:* Wobenzyme® 10 tablets twice daily
[-] **Quercetin**

OTHER RELATED FACTORS

[+] rule out **Gluten** sensitivity

NUTRITIONAL FACTORS

VITAMINS

Vitamin B_{12}

In open trials, vitamin B_{12} injections have been found to helpful in rapidly reducing the pain and subjective symptoms found in both acute and chronic *bursitis (Gaby;Klemes)*. (Most of the experience has been with *subdeltoid* bursitis.) An anti-inflammatory effect of the vitamin has been confirmed in an animal study *(Hanck)*.

Vitamin C

The inflammatory process enhances the degradation and excretion of ascorbic acid *(Hemila;Roberts)*; thus patients with inflammatory conditions may require higher than normal intakes of the vitamin to prevent depletion.

In both animal and *in vitro* studies, vitamin C has been found to have an anti-inflammatory effect *(Williams,1986)*. Supplementation inhibits the activity of myeloperoxidase in polymorphonuclear leukocytes, thus preventing potential tissue damage by the enzyme when it is released during leukocyte degranulation in inflammation *(Nowak;Williams,1984).*

In a recent study of patients with *cystic fibrosis*, all indices of inflammation of those with low plasma ascorbate levels were relatively high, while clearly lower values were noted in those with high plasma ascorbate. This finding is consistent with the hypothesis that, by scavenging oxygen free radicals, vitamin C interacts with an inflammation-amplifying cycle of activation of alveolar macrophages and neutrophils, release of proinflammatory cytokines and oxygen free radicals, and inactivation of antiproteases *(Winklhofer-Roob).*

Ascorbate status has also been found to influence the early stages of *gingival inflammation*. Young men received varying amounts of the vitamin. The propensity of the gingiva to become inflamed or bleed on probing was reduced after normal intakes (65 mg/day) as compared to deficient intakes (5 mg/day), and upon supplementary intakes (605 mg/day) as compared to normal intakes *(Jacob).*

Vitamin C supplementation is often combined with flavonoids as they may enhance its bioavailability *(Vinson)*:

A 38-year-old male presented with severe subpatellar bursitis with extensive local swelling and heat, extreme tenderness, severe pain and limitation of motion.

He was treated with vitamin C along with citrus bioflavonoids 200 mg 3 times daily. Within 24 hours there was noticeable diminution in swelling and pain, and in 72 hours the lesion had subsided almost completely, leaving only slight local tenderness (Biskind).

Vitamin E

In activated neutrophilic granulocytes, vitamin E was found to inhibit both chemotaxis and chemiluminescence *(Blankenhorn).* Moreover, based on animal studies, its anti-inflammatory effect has been theorized to be due to its strong action to protect lysosome and other membranes which may inhibit histamine liberation from granules of mast cells, and serotonin liberation from inside the tissue cells. Supporting this theory is that fact that vitamin E acts slowly, protects enlargement of inflammation, shortens its prognosis, and has lesser effects in suppressing inflammation that is already existing *(Kamimura,1972).*

Little has been done to investigate the anti-inflammatory action of vitamin E in humans. Supplementation appeared effective in treating various *inflammatory skin diseases* in open trials *(Kamimura,1956;Yasuda).* However, for patients with active *ulcerative colitis*, it was ineffective in modulating arachidonate metabolism or in affecting disease activity *(Lauritsen).*

MINERALS

Copper

Inflammation increases the dietary copper requirement. In an animal study, for example, an acute phase response in rats increased the amount of dietary copper required to maintain hepatic Cu,Zn superoxide dismutase activity at levels equal to those of nonstressed, copper-adequate rats *(DiSilvestro).* If dietary copper were not increased, accumulation of the superoxide radical due to reduced activity of Cu,Zn superoxide dismutase could further the inflammatory process *(Sorenson,1989).*

Moreover, inflammation produces an acute phase response that includes elevated levels of copper *(Beshgetoor;Milanino)* and of ceruloplasmin, the main copper component of plasma *(DiSilvestro).* Maintaining adequate copper nutriture is therefore an important goal.

Copper supplementation also has an anti-inflammatory and analgesic effect related to its ability to form complexes which serve as selective antioxidants *(Sorenson,1980).* Copper salicylate appears to be one of the most effective of these complexes *(Jacka; Sorensen,1977)*, and its ulcerogenic effect appears to be low *(Korolkiewicz).* For patients with rheumatoid arthritis, it was more effective than either copper acetate or salicylic acid *(Hangarter).*

Zinc

As with copper, adequate zinc is needed during inflammation for healing *(Denko).* Zinc in physiological concentrations can cause approximately a 40% inhibition of immunologically induced histamine and leukotriene release from both basophils and mast cells. In addition, zinc modulates serotonin release from platelets, macrophage and neutrophil phagocytosis, lymphocyte proliferation, and immune hemolysis *(Marone)*. Zinc supplementation may also have inflammatory effects because of its ability to inhibit polymorphonuclear leukocyte chemotaxis *(Dreno)*.

Animal work suggest that zinc is an effective anti-inflammatory by itself, and it has an additive effect when given with non-steroidal anti-inflammatory drugs *(Abou-Mohamed)*. Zinc also has an analgesic action during early inflammation and this may be the consequence of reducing levels of the inflammatory cytokine IL-beta and nerve growth factor *(Safieh-Garabedian*

The most common form of prostatitis is abacterial *inflammatory prostatitis*. In this condition, despite normal serum zinc levels, semen and prostatic zinc levels may be depressed. In an informal clinical setting, when more than 200 patients with chronic abacterial prostatitis received zinc for between 2 and 16 weeks, over 70% reported symptom relief. Semen zinc levels, which were initially depressed, usually increased *(Bush)*. However, results of a controlled study failed to find evidence that zinc supplementation was beneficial to patients with chronic *inflammatory rheumatic diseases (Peretz)*.

Clearly, more studies are needed to clarify the role of zinc supplementation in treating inflammatory disorders.

OTHER NUTRITIONAL FACTORS

Essential Fatty Acids

Omega-3 Fatty Acids

alpha-linolenic acid → EPA → 3 series prostaglandins
└→ DHA

Arachidonic acid, precursor to the pro-inflammatory eicosanoids, is released from membrane phospholipids in the course of inflammatory activation and is metabolized to prostaglandins and leukotrienes. Encouraging results have been obtained by dietary supplementation with long chain omega-3 fatty acids like eicosapentaenoic acid (EPA). In states of inflammation, EPA is released to compete with arachidonic acid for enzymatic metabolism inducing the production of less inflammatory and chemotactic derivatives *(Heller)*.

For example, in a study published in the *New England Journal of Medicine*, normal subjects were supplemented with EPA for 6 weeks. EPA in neutrophils was increased 7-fold without any increase in arachidonic acid. When the neutrophils were activated, there was a 37% reduction in the release of arachidonic acid and a 48% reduction in the inflammatory products of this pathway. In addition, the adherence of neutrophils to bovine epithelial cells as monolayers treated with leukotriene B4 was completely inhibited.

These results suggest that diets enriched with fish oil-derived fatty acids have anti-inflammatory effects by inhibiting the 5-lipoxygenase pathway, thus causing a reduction in the release of leukotrienes along with a reduction in the release of superoxide from neutrophils *(Lee)*.

Omega-6 Fatty Acids

linoleic acid → GLA → DGLA → prostaglandin E_1

While, in general, eicosanoids formed from the omega-3 fatty acids are much less potent in causing biological responses than those formed from the omega-6 fatty acids, including stimulation of cytokine production and inflammatory responses *(Alexander)*, sources of gamma-linolenic acid (GLA) have also demonstrated significant anti-inflammatory effects even though GLA is a precursor to pro-inflammatory arachidonic acid (AA).

Following GLA supplementation, dihomogammalinolenic acid (DGLA), but not arachidonic acid, accumulates in neutrophil glycerolipids. This increase in DGLA relative to AA within inflammatory cells such as the neutrophil may attenuate the biosynthesis of AA metabolites and represent a mechanism by which dietary GLA exerts an anti-inflammatory effect *(Johnson)*. GLA supplementation has also been shown to decrease the capacity of polymorphonuclear cells to generate pro-inflammatory leukotriene B4 in parallel to the increase in DGLA *(Ziboh)*.

Flavonoids

In animal studies, various flavonoids have shown potent anti-inflammatory activity *(Pelzer)*. They may inhibit arachidonic acid metabolism *(Baumann;Ferràndiz)*, inhibit histamine release from basophils and mast cells *(Amella;Middleton)*, and decrease neutrophil lysosomal enzyme secretion to stabilize cell membranes and decrease lipid peroxidation, leukotriene release, and collagen breakdown by hyaluronidase *(Busse)*.

Quercetin is one of the most promising of the flavonoids. *In vitro*, it protected human skin fibroblasts, keratinocytes and endothelial cells from oxidative damage due to depletion of glutathione. Moreover, while ascorbic acid is not cryoprotective by itself, it had a synergistic cryoprotective effect when supplied with quercetin *(Skaper)*.

The efficacy of quercetin treating inflammation *in vivo* remains to be shown, however.

L-Glutamine

Glutamine has traditionally been thought of as a nonessential amino acid. However, laboratory and clinical data suggest that it may be essential during certain inflammatory conditions during which glutamine consumption may outstrip endogenous production and a relative glutamine deficiency state may exist. The results of animal and clinical studies suggest that improved outcome may be possible by providing the appropriate dose of glutamine by the appropriate route to achieve adequate tissue concentrations *(Wilmore)*.

While its mechanism of action is not well understood, a recent *in vitro* study found that L-glutamine inhibits the generation of nitric oxide from L-arginine in endothelial cells, thus providing regulation of this important pathway *(Meininger)*.

In animal work, L-glutamine supplementation has been shown to have marked anti-inflammatory activity and moderate analgesic activity. It was effective orally in suppressing various experimentally-induced inflammatory reactions and did not show any gastric irritation in anti-inflammatory doses. Its anti-inflammatory activity was comparable to that of phenylbutazone *(Jain)*.

OTHER RELATED FACTORS

Hydrolytic Enzymes

Wobenzyme® is an enteric-coated tablet consisting of a mixture of pancreatin (beef) 100 mg, bromelain 45 mg, papain 60 mg, lipase 10 mg, amylase 10 mg, trypsin 24 mg and alpha-chymotrypsin 1 mg combined with rutin 50 mg. Under double-blind conditions, patients received Wobenzyme® prior to dental surgery and postoperatively for several days. By postoperative day 3, the levels of C-reactive protein (a measure of inflammation) were 3-fold higher in the controls *(Vizenz)*.

Individual enzymes have also shown promise. For example, in a study of 538 patients with acute inflammation published in *JAMA*, there was a dramatic subsidence of all signs and symptoms of acute inflammation in 94.3% when they received trypsin intravenously *(Innerfield)*. Trypsin would also be expected to have an anti-inflammatory effect when given orally as, in a double-blind crossover study, plasma levels rose in a dose-dependent manner *(Donath)*.

More studies are needed to better ascertain the anti-inflammatory effects of the various hydrolytic enzymes.

Food Sensitivities

Celiac disease (gluten sensitivity) is associated with various inflammatory conditions. These include recurrent *pericarditis (Dawes)* and *inflammatory rheumatic disorders (Carli)*.

BIBLIOGRAPHY

Abou-Mohamed G et al. Effect of zinc on the anti-inflammatory and ulcerogenic activities of indomethacin and diclofenac. Pharmacology 50(4):266-72, 1995

Alexander JW. Immunonutrition: the role of omega-3 fatty acids. Nutrition 14(7-8):627-33, 1998

Amella M et al. Inhibition of mast cell histamine release by flavonoids and bioflavonoids. Planta Medica 51:16-20, 1985

Baumann J et al. Flavonoids and related compounds as inhibition of arachidonic acid peroxidation. Prostaglandins 20(4):627-39, 1980

Beshgetoor D, Hambidge M. Clinical conditions altering copper metabolism in humans. Am J Clin Nutr 67(5 Suppl):1017S-1021S, 1998

Biskind MS, Martin WC. The use of citrus flavonoids in infection. II. Am J Digest Dis 22:41-45, 1955

Blankenhorn G. Vitamin E: Clinical research from Europe. Nutr Dietary Consult, June, 1988

Bush IM, Chairman, Dept. of Urology, Chicago Medical School, and associates. Zinc: a key urological element. Presented at the Am. Medical Assoc. annual meeting, Chicago, 1974

Busse WW et al. Flavonoid modulation of human neutrophil function. J Allergy Clin Immunol 73:801-9, 1984

Carli P et al. [Inflammatory rheumatism and celiac disease in adults. Coincidence or pathogenic relationship]? Presse Med 24(13):606-10, 1995) (in French)

Dawes PT, Atherton ST. Coeliac disease presenting as recurrent pericarditis. Lancet i:1021-2, 1981

Denko CW et al. Inflammation in relation to dietary intake of zinc and copper. Int J Tissue React 3(2):73-6, 1981

DiSilvestro RA, Marten JT. Effects of inflammation and copper intake on rat liver and erythrocyte Cu-Zn superoxide dismutase activity levels. J Nutr 120(10):1223-7, 1990

Donath F et al. Dose-related bioavailability of bromelain and trypsin after repeated oral administration. Clin Pharmacol Ther 61:157, 1997

Dreno B et al. Zinc salts effects on granulocyte zinc concentration and chemotaxis in acne patients. Acta Derm Venereol 72(4):250-2, 1992

Ferràndiz ML, Alcaraz MJ. Anti-inflammatory activity and inhibition of arachidonic metabolism by flavonoids. Agents Actions 32(3-4):283-8, 1991

Gaby AR. Vitamin B12, Part II. More benefits of this versatile vitamin. Nutrition & Healing 2(7), August, 1995

Hanck A, Weiser H. Analgesic and anti-inflammatory properties of vitamins. Int J Vitam Nutr Res (suppl)27:189-206, 1985

Hangarter W. [Copper salicylate in rheumatoid arthritis and rheumatism--like degenerative diseases]. Med Welt 31(45):1625-8, 1980) (in German)

Heller A et al. Lipid mediators in inflammatory disorders. Drugs 55(4):487-96, 1998

Hemila H, Roberts P, Wikstrom M. Activated polymorphonuclear leucocytes consume vitamin C. FEBS Lett 178(1):25-30, 1984

Innerfield I, et al. Parenteral administration of trypsin: Clinical effect of 538 patients. JAMA 152:597-9, 1953

Jacka T et al. Copper salicylate as an anti-inflammatory and analgesic agent in arthritic rats. Life Sci 32(9):1023-30, 1983

Jacob RA et al. Experimental vitamin C depletion and supplementation in young men. Nutrient interactions and dental health effects. Ann N Y Acad Sci 498:333-46, 1987

Jain P, Khanna NK. Evaluation of anti-inflammatory and analgesic properties of L-glutamine. Agents Actions 11(3):243-9, 1981

Johnson MM et al. Dietary supplementation with gamma-linolenic acid alters fatty acid content and eicosanoid production in healthy humans. J Nutr 127(8):1435-44, 1997

Kamimura M. Shinyaku to Rinsho 5:363, 1956 (in Japanese)

Kamimura M. Antiinflammatory effect of vitamin E. J Vitaminol 18:204-09, 1972

Klemes IS. Vitamin B12 in acute subdeltoid bursitis. Indust Med Surg 26:290-2, 1957

Korolkiewicz Z, et al. The pharmacologic activity of complexes and mixtures with copper and salicylates or aminopyrine following oral dosing in rats. Agents Actions 26(3-4):355-9, 1989

Lauritsen K et al. Does vitamin E supplementation modulate in vivo arachidonate metabolism in human inflammation? Pharmacol Toxicol 61(4):246-9, 1987

Lee TH et al. Effect of dietary enrichment with eicosapentaenoic acid and docosahexaenoic acids on in vitro neutrophil and monocyte leukotriene generation and neutrophil function. N Engl J Med 312:1217-23, 1985

Marone G et al. Physiological concentrations of zinc inhibit the release of histamine from human basophils and lung mast cells. Agents Actions 18:103-6, 1986

Meininger CJ, Wu G. L-glutamine inhibits nitric oxide synthesis in bovine venular endothelial cells. J Pharmacol Exp Ther 281(1):448-53, 1997

Middleton E, Drzewieki G. Naturally occurring flavonoids and human basophil histamine release. Arch Allergy Appl Immunol 77:155-57, 1985

Milanino R et al. Copper and zinc body levels in inflammation: an overview of the data obtained from animal and human studies. Agents Actions 39(3-4):195-209, 1993

Nowak D et al. Ascorbic acid enhances the decrease in peroxidase activity in inflamed tissues of mice. Arch Immunol Ther Exp (Warsz) 41(5-6):321-6, 1993

Pelzer LE et al. Acute and chronic antiinflammatory effects of plant flavonoids. Farmaco 53(6):421-4, 1998

Peretz A et al. Zinc distribution in blood components, inflammatory status, and clinical indexes of disease activity during zinc supplementation in inflammatory rheumatic diseases. Am J Clin Nutr 57(5):690-4, 1993

Roberts P et al. Vitamin C and inflammation. Med Biol 62:88, 1984

Safieh-Garabedian B et al. Zinc reduces the hyperalgesia and upregulation of NGF and IL-1 beta produced by peripheral inflammation in the rat. Neuropharmacology 35(5):599-603, 1996

Skaper SD et al. Quercetin protects cutaneous tissue-associated cell types including sensory neurons from oxidative stress induced by glutathione depletion: cooperative effects of ascorbic acid. Free Radic Biol Med 22(4):669-78, 1997

Sorenson JR, Hangarter W. Treatment of rheumatoid and degenerative diseases with copper complexes: a review with emphasis on copper-salicylate. Inflammation 2(3):217-38, 1977

Sorenson J. Copper aspirinate: A more potent anti-inflammatory and anti-ulcer agent. J Int Acad Prev Med 1980, pp. 7-21

Sorenson JRJ. Copper complexes offer a physiological approach to treatment of chronic diseases. Progress in Medical Chemistry Vol. 26, 1989

Vinson JA, Bose P. Comparative bioavailability of synthetic and natural vitamin C in guinea pigs. Nutr Rep Int 27:875-80, 1983

Vinzenz K. [Edema therapy in dental interventions with hydrolytic enzymes]. Quintessenz 42(7):1053-64, 1991) (in German)

Williams RN et al. Ascorbic acid inhibits the activity of polymorphonuclear leukocytes in inflamed ocular tissues. Exp Eye Res 39(3):261-5, 1984

Williams RN, Paterson CA. A protective role for ascorbic acid during inflammatory episodes in the eye. Exp Eye Res 42(3):211-8, 1986

Wilmore DW, Shabert JK. Role of glutamine in immunologic responses. Nutrition 14(7-8):618-26, 1998

Winklhofer-Roob BM et al. Plasma vitamin C concentrations in patients with cystic fibrosis: evidence of associations with lung inflammation. Am J Clin Nutr 65(6):1858-66, 1997

Yasuda T et al. Theor Dermatol Urol (Japan) 19:69, 1957 (in Japanese)

Ziboh VA, Fletcher MP. Dose-response effects of dietary g-linolenic acid-enriched oils on human polymorphonuclear-neutrophil biosynthesis of leukotriene B4. Am J Clin Nutr 55:39-45, 1992

INNER EAR DISORDERS

(including HEARING LOSS, MENIERE'S SYNDROME, TINNITUS and VERTIGO)

See Also: ATHEROSCLEROSIS
'HYPOGLYCEMIA' (FUNCTIONAL)

NUTRITIONAL TREATMENT GUIDE

✓ = Efficacy generally accepted.
* = Efficacy *demonstrated* by controlled human trials.
[+] = Efficacy *suspected* from uncontrolled human trials.
[-] = Efficacy *suspected* from indirect data.
? = Efficacy *challenged* in a study of similar design.

DIETARY FACTORS

* **Low Fat, low Cholesterol diet** *(to reduce the risk of hearing loss)*

- - - - - - - - - - - - - - - - - - - -

[+] **Diabetic diet** *(for hyperglycemia/hyperinsulinemia)*
[+] **Hypoglycemic diet** *(for 'reactive hypoglycemia')*
[+] **moderate Alcohol consumption**
[+] low **Sodium diet** *(for Meniere's syndrome)*

- - - - - - - - - - - - - - - - - - - -

[-] increase dietary **Sodium** *(for sensorineural hearing loss IF accompanied by hypoglycemia)*

NUTRITIONAL FACTORS

* **Fluoride:** *for otosclerosis*: sodium fluoride 6 to 16 mg daily (Beware of side effects.)
* **Hydroxyethylrutosides:** *for Meniere's syndrome*: 2 g daily

- - - - - - - - - - - - - - - - - - - -

[+] **Coenzyme Q_{10}:** ? 30 mg daily
[+] **Hydroxyethylrutosides:** *for acute deafness of vascular origin:* 2 g daily
[+] **Iron deficiency:** 30 mg twice daily until repletion; then minimal possible dosage
[+] **Magnesium deficiency:** *to protect against noise-induced hearing loss:* ≈ 400 mg daily
[+] **Vitamin A deficiency:** 50,000 IU daily for 6 weeks (10,000 IU daily during pregnancy) (Has been combined with **vitamin E** to increase efficacy.)
[+] **Vitamin B_6:** ? 50 mg daily
[+] **Vitamin B_{12} deficiency:** 1,000 μg intramuscularly weekly initially and monthly afterwards
[+] **Vitamin D deficiency:** repletion (? 500-1000 IU daily) combined with calcium (? 500 mg daily)
[+] **Zinc deficiency:** *for tinnitus and sensorineural hearing loss:* ? 100 mg daily

OTHER RELATED FACTORS

[+] rule out **Food Sensitivities**
[+] rule out **Impaired Carbohydrate Metabolism**

DIETARY FACTORS

Low Fat, Low Cholesterol Diet

Hyperlipidemia may reduce the flow of oxygen and nutrients to the inner ear by increasing erythrocyte aggregation *(Spencer,1975)* and rigidity *(Browning)*. Chinchillas made hyperlipidemic by being fed a high cholesterol diet developed a high-frequency hearing loss and were more susceptible to noise-induced hearing loss *(Sikora)*. Similarly, when spontaneously hypertensive rats received a diet that promoted hyperlipoproteinemia, they had greater hearing losses when noise-exposed than rats fed a normal diet, and exhibited significantly decreased cochlear blood flow *(Pillsbury)*.

In humans, sensorineural hearing loss is frequently associated with hyperlipidemia *(Yanick,1975)*, and interventions to normalize serum lipid levels may be effective. When 120 patients with inner ear disease and hypolipoproteinemia were treated with vasodilators and a 500-calorie, high-protein, low-carbohydrate diet, 83% noted reduced symptoms within 5 months *(Pulec)*. In a crossover study, a low saturated fat diet not only protected against hearing loss (usually of the sensorineural type), but partly restored hearing *(Rosen)*. Moreover, these relationships extend to children with bilateral fluctuating sensorineural hearing loss and hyperlipidemia. For a group of these children, hearing correlated with lipid levels, and a low fat diet was followed by improvement *(Strome)*.

Hypercholesterolemia also appears to increase the risk of sudden hearing loss in humans. In a group of these patients, both cholesterol and fibrinogen levels were significantly higher than those of controls, leading to significantly elevated values of erythrocyte aggregation and plasma viscosity. Furthermore, drastic lowering of plasma cholesterol and fibrinogen by a selective extracorporal apheresis resulted in an immediate improvement in hearing for 6 out of 7 patients *(Suckfull)*.

Impaired Carbohydrate Metabolism

Impaired carbohydrate metabolism, sometimes with hyperinsulinemia, has been associated with a variety of inner ear disturbances, including Meniere's syndrome *(Proctor B)*, fluctuant hearing loss *(Goldman; Spencer,1975)*, sudden deafness *(Currier)*, and sensorineural hearing loss *(Gosselin)*.

Within one group of 42 patients with sensorineural hearing loss who displayed a rising, progressively improving audiometric pattern, 68% had impaired carbohydrate metabolism. This included 9 patients with abnormally low readings on glucose, 7 who were diabetic, 5 with impaired glucose tolerance and 9 with nondiagnostic glucose intolerance *(Carmen)*. This figure agrees with that of an early study of 90 patients with sensorineural hearing loss in which 58% were found to have abnormal 5-hour glucose tolerance curves *(Gosselin)*.

When a group of 59 patients with audio-vestibular disturbances received a prolonged glucose tolerance test, 17% had glucose intolerance while 51% had reactive hypoglycemia. The latter finding was statistically significant as compared to normal controls *(Carrillo)*.

Nearly 75% of 50 patients with Meniere's disease had either an abnormal glucose tolerance test or high insulin levels *(Proctor B)*. However, in a series of 100 patients with vertigo, insulin resistance (predominantly in overweight patients) appeared to be the basic abnormality; only 4 patients had hypoglycemia *(Lehrer)*.

Many of these patients should respond to diets designed to improve carbohydrate metabolism. (See Diabetes Mellitus and 'Hypoglycemia'.)

Alcohol

In a study of 3,751 patients with an average age of 66 years, hearing loss prevalence was inversely related to alcohol consumption. This relationship is theorized to be due to the protective effect of alcohol on atherosclerosis, a process that causes hearing loss due to its effects on the cochlear blood supply *(Popelka)*.

Dietary Sodium

Since the endolymph is higher in potassium, while the perilymph is higher in sodium, electrolyte imbalances may affect the function of the inner ear *(Yanick,1983)*.

A low sodium diet appears to have some efficacy in treating Meniere's syndrome. When, in an open trial, patients received this diet along with diuretics, the number of attacks of vertigo decreased in more than 70% and hearing improved in 46%. Moreover, patients remaining on the program for an average of 6 years of follow-up reported sustained improvement *(Anonymous,1991b)*.

The rationale for treating Meniere's syndrome with a low sodium diet is based on the hypothesis that individual susceptibility to the syndrome occurs due to inflammatory changes in the endolymphatic sac or cochlear aqueduct secondary to viral infections. As these changes predispose the affected tissues to fluid retention, sodium restriction is needed to combat it *(Proctor C)*.

The opposite dietary intervention may be indicated for patients with sensorineural hearing loss who also have hypoglycemia. On the basis of a 24-hour urinary electrolyte clearance test, a group of such patients were found to have higher levels of potassium than of sodium as well as a negative nitrogen balance. After dietary sodium was increased, not only did their sodium-potassium balance improve, but their nitrogen balance also showed improvement *(Goldman)*.

COMBINED DIETARY INTERVENTIONS

Preliminary findings suggest that combining that a diet that is *low in saturated fat* (with increased polyunsaturates), *low in cholesterol*, *low in carbohydrates* and *sugar-free* may benefit patients with a variety of inner ear disorders. One clinician reported that "most" of a total of more than 1,400 patients with inner ear symptoms and hyperlipoproteinemia responded to this diet. Not only did hearing improve and stabilize (as demonstrated in the pure tone audiogram and in speech discrimination scores), but dizziness cleared promptly, the sensation of pressure in the ears and associated headache was quickly relieved, and tinnitus often lessened in severity and sometimes disappeared *(Spencer,1981)*.

Headaches, pressure in the head, and fullness in the ears were among the first symptoms relieved. In some, the improvement was dramatic within 4 to 8 weeks on the diet, the first lasting symptomatic improvement in all the years of their disease. Phenomenal gain in hearing resulted with as much as a 30 decibel improvement in the affected ear. Fluctuating hearing loss fluctuated less and often became stabilized at an improved level. Recruitment disappeared along with the fullness and discomfort in the ears. Acute vertiginous attacks ceased or became much less frequent and severe *(Spencer,1975)*.

Another clinician reports that symptoms of half of the patients with Meniere's disease were completely controlled by combining a *low fat, low carbohydrate diet* with the treatment of *food sensitivities* (see Food Sensitivities below) *(Powers)*.

NUTRITIONAL FACTORS

VITAMINS

Vitamin A Deficiency

The cochlea has a high concentration of vitamin A and all special sensory receptor cells contain, or are functionally dependent upon, the vitamin *(Chole)*. Low serum vitamin A levels are associated with decreased auditory function *(Lohle)*. Feeding young rats a vitamin-A deficient diet causes changes in the cochlea which are visible on electron microscopy *(Lohle)*. A study utilizing guinea pigs found evidence that vitamin A deficiency increases the sensitivity of the inner ear to noise, and that this increased sensitivity increases the probability of noise-induced hearing loss *(Biesalski)*.

Early work suggests that vitamin A supplementation may improve hearing and reduce tinnitus, presumably by repleting a marginal deficiency. In an open trial reported in the *Archives of Otolaryngology*, 300 patients with hearing loss received a series of intramuscular injections of vitamin A; 83% reported an average hearing gain of roughly 18% in each ear with very definite gains in hearing of conversational tones. Tinnitus was reduced or ceased in a similar percentage of patients *(Lobel)*.

AND **Vitamin E**

Vitamin E protects vitamin A from oxidation *(Tappel)*, and it has been combined with vitamin A in the treatment of sensorineural hearing loss. Particularly when the auditory symptoms are due to presbyacusis, results of a number of studies suggest that the combination may result in a 5 to 15 decibel improvement of the pure-tone threshold *(Romeo)*. It remains unclear, however, if the addition of vitamin E contributes to the efficacy of vitamin A.

Vitamin B_6

In an open trial, 47 patients with Meniere's disease who had failed to respond to previous treatments received pyridoxine supplementation. Fifteen of them improved, presumably due to the supplement. Three patients failed to improve, and others gradually improved, but it was uncertain whether pyridoxine supplementation was responsible in their case.

Also, in the same study, 23 patients with vertigo due to unknown causes received pyridoxine, and many of them improved. Intravenous administration relieved symptoms more rapidly than oral administration. While oral administration was effective, intravenous administration relieved symptoms more rapidly *(Lewy)*.

These promising results have yet to be confirmed by a controlled clinical trial. Moreover, presuming that pyridoxine was responsible for the improvements noted, it is not known whether the supplement was repleting a pre-existing deficiency.

Vitamin B_{12} Deficiency

A study of army personnel who were exposed to military noise during their service found that reduced serum levels of vitamin B_{12} may be associated with susceptibility to noise-induced chronic tinnitus and hearing loss *(Shemesh)*.

Twelve of these patients who had low serum cobalamin levels received cobalamin by injection until serum levels were normalized. A slight improvement was noted in almost all symptoms. Improvement was significant for measures of the loudness of sounds, disturbance in a noisy environment, and "general feeling" *(Shemesh)*. Controlled trials will better ascertain the efficacy of vitamin B_{12} in treating inner ear disorders.

Vitamin D Deficiency (Also see Calcium below.)

A deficiency of vitamin D appears to cause hearing loss by depressing the concentration of ionized calcium in the perilymph *(Ikeda,1987)*. Reduced serum vitamin D levels may be surprisingly common among, for example, patients with bilateral sensorineural hearing loss. In one study, 23 out of 28 patients had depressed levels of 1,25-dihydroxyvitamin D3, the activated form of the vitamin. *(Ikeda,1989)*. While, in this study, the levels of 25-hydroxyvitamin D3 were normal, a study of 47 patients with otosclerosis (mean age 45 years) found depressed levels of 25-hydroxyvitamin D in 10 and borderline low levels in 2. Moreover, raised serum alkaline phosphatase levels were found in 32.6%, calcium in 6.5% and inorganic phosphate in 4.3%.

The 16 patients with either an abnormally low 25-hydroxyvitamin D level and/or a raised alkaline phosphatase level were placed on vitamin D and calcium therapy. Hearing significantly improved in 3 of them (19%) *(Brookes,1985)*. Similarly, 2 out of 4 patients with bilateral cochlear deafness and abnormally low 25-hydroxyvitamin D levels showed unilateral hearing improvement following supplementation with these 2 nutrients *(Brookes,1983)*. Further studies are needed for confirmation.

Yet another study involved 56 patients with senile deafness. Their serum calcium levels were significantly depressed, and there was a significant correlation between hearing levels and serum alkaline phosphatase levels. The 12 patients in the group who the investigators judged to have abnormal bone metabolism were treated with an active vitamin D preparation (1-alpha-hydroxyvitamin D3 for 6 to 10 months, and hearing improvement was noted for 6 ears (4 patients) *(Yamazaki,1988)*.

MINERALS

Calcium (Also see Vitamin D above.)

The results of animal studies suggest that both Meniere's syndrome *(Meyer zum Gottesberge)* and sensorineural hearing loss *(Ikeda,1987)* may be due to shift in the homeostasis of ionized calcium towards a higher concentration of free ionized calcium in the fluid compartments and the adjacent intracellular spaces. For Meniere's syndrome, further animal work suggests that ionized calcium becomes raised in the endolymph, but not in the perilymph *(Wang)*.

There is no evidence that calcium supplementation will correct this abnormality or reduce symptoms.

Fluoride

Confirming the results of open trials, double-blind studies have found that sodium fluoride administration may slow the progression of otosclerosis *(Bretlau;Colletti)*. However, there may be damage to the gastric mucosa *(Spak)*, interference with the assimilation of other minerals *(Yanick,1985)* and, possibly, an increased risk of osteosarcoma *(Anonymous,1991a)*.

Iron Deficiency

Growing rats raised on an iron-deficient diet show raised auditory thresholds which are unrelated to the hypoxia of anemia *(Sun,1987)*. Evidence that iron deficiency is an etiology of sensorineural deafness comes from a study of patients with both sensorineural deafness and reduced serum iron levels. Following iron supplementation, hearing improved in some of the patients; only these patients showed increases in serum iron *(Sun,1982)*. Red cell basic ferritin appears to be a particularly sensitive assay for assessing iron nutriture in these cases, as patients with most kinds of sensorineural hearing loss have reduced levels compared to normal controls *(Sun,1991)*.

Idiopathic sudden hearing loss was studied in 426 patients. They showed low concentrations of hemoglobin, serum iron, serum ferritin, and red cell basic ferritin as well as abnormal circadian variations in the serum iron level.

Treatment consisted of iron therapy, medication to combat disturbances in iron metabolism, vitamins, or a combined regimen. Of the different treatments, the results were significantly better in the patients who received iron therapy. There was improvement in over half of the patients who started treatment more than 3 months after the onset of the disease *(Sun,1992)*.

Magnesium

Animal studies have shown that noise-induced hearing loss is facilitated by magnesium deficiency *(Gunther)*. A placebo-controlled study of healthy young male military recruits has explored the protective effect of magnesium supplementation. Following 2 months of basic training during which the recruits were repeatedly exposed to high levels of impulse noises, permanent hearing loss was significantly more frequent and more severe in the placebo group as compared to the magnesium group *(Attias)*.

Zinc Deficiency

The soft tissues of the cochlea and vestibule have the highest zinc level of any part of the body *(Shambaugh,1989)*. Zinc deficiency appears to be associated with sensorineural hearing loss, tinnitus - which tends to be continuous rather than intermittent *(Gersdorff,1987a)* - or both. Evidence for the association with tinnitus comes from a study of 74 patients who had not received any drug and were free of known diseases. When compared to age-matched normal controls, their serum zinc levels were significantly lower *(Ochi)*.

Their tinnitus was rated on a numerical scale and they were started on zinc supplementation. Two weeks later, blood zinc levels had risen significantly while ratings on the tinnitus scale were significantly decreased *(Ochi)*. Other open trials of zinc for tinnitus patients with reduced zinc nutriture have also reported improvement in some patients following zinc supplementation *(Gersdorff,1987b;Shambaugh,1989)*, while a trial of zinc for tinnitus patients with normal zinc nutriture found the supplement to be ineffective *(Paaske)*.

For elderly, hypozincemic patients with progressive hearing deterioration, one study found that 35% had at least a 10% improvement in discrimination and at least a 5 dB improvement in pure-tone hearing. Moreover, imbalance occasionally improved *(Shambaugh,1986)*. The same investigator has reported that it often takes between 3 months and 1 year to bring serum zinc levels up to normal in these patients *(Shambaugh,1984)*.

Confirmation of these therapeutic benefits awaits controlled studies.

OTHER NUTRITIONAL FACTORS

Coenzyme Q_{10} (ubiquinone)

One animal study found that coenzyme Q_{10} (CoQ_{10}) may promote recovery from acute sensorineural hearing loss due to hypoxia *(Sato)*, while another found that pretreatment with CoQ_{10} prevented hearing loss due to intermittent intense sound stimuli *(Morimitsu)*.

Two open trials have reported good results with CoQ_{10} in the treatment of patients with paroxysmal deafness. One of these studies noted that 38 out of 42 patients (who also suffered from dizziness) responded to some degree *(Yamazaki)*. The other study, which involved 154 patients who received CoQ_{10} within 2 weeks of the onset of symptoms, reported that the patients responded whether or not they received concurrent treatment with steroids *(Shitara)*.

Controlled clinical trials are needed to confirm these results.

Hydroxyethylrutosides

This standardized mixture of semisynthetic flavonoids act primarily on the microvascular endothelium to reduce hyperpermeability and edema and may also have a protective effect on the vascular epithelium *(Wadworth)*. In addition, they may improve microcapillary blood flow by reducing red cell aggregation and whole blood viscosity, and by increasing erythrocyte deformability *(Schmidt-Schönbein;van Haeringen)*.

Hydroxyethylrutosides were found to be effective in treating Meniere's syndrome in a double-blind crossover study. Despite a marked tendency to a carryover effect when hydroxyethylrutosides were given prior to placebo, there was a clear trend to greater symptomatic improvement as compared to placebo, and audiometric findings showed a uniform, significant superiority for both air and bone conduction in the treated group. Side effects in both groups were similar *(Moser)*.

Sudden deafness of vascular origin may also be responsive. Four patients have been described whose tinnitus disappeared and hearing improved following administration of the flavonoid mixture *(Madej)*.

Controlled studies are needed to confirm these results.

OTHER RELATED FACTORS

Food Sensitivities

Food sensitivities have repeatedly been implicated in inner ear dysfunction, with symptoms sometimes remitting following food eliminations *(Shambaugh,1981)*.

In Meniere's syndrome, for example, the symptoms are thought to be produced by a sudden influx of fluid into the endolymphatic sac, and this sac is known to be capable of trapping antigen and generating an immune response *(Derebery,1996)*. While the majority of patients have been found to have only a low sensitivity to inhalent antigens, they have reactions to very common "hidden" foods (such as corn) in the diet.

In addition to history, reasons to suspect food sensitivities or allergies in these patients include bilaterality and refractoriness to the usual medical and surgical treatments *(Derebery,1992)*. Other suspicious symptoms include fluid retention, nuchal myalgia, postprandial fatigue, early morning insomnia, periodic mental depression or amnesia, or specific food cravings *(Wilson)*.

One study reports on 23 patients who presented with incapacitating vertigo plus one or more of the other Meniere's disease symptoms (e.g. tinnitus, low frequency hearing loss, fullness of the ears) without evidence of metabolic, infective, or tumor-related etiologies, and who had failed to respond to anti-vertiginous drugs. They received RAST food and inhalent testing. Positive foods according to RAST results were then tested with intradermal provocation. Foods that produced any ear symptoms were completely eliminated and immunotherapy started.

All 23 patients were better within 2 weeks. Audiograms at 3 months showed improvement in sensorineural hearing losses, especially in the low frequencies *(Hoover)*.

Two patients with Meniere's syndrome had symptoms that were so severe that they would fall helpless to the ground. Both obtained relief by avoiding specific foods. Ingestion of the offending food, or injection of the food extract, reproduced their symptoms (Duke).

Besides Meniere's syndrome, other inner ear disorders, and especially the complaint of tinnitus, have been reported to respond to food eliminations in informal clinical settings *(DeBartolo;Shambaugh,1981)*. However, despite the numerous anecdotal reports which have appeared at least since 1923, placebo-controlled clinical trials have yet to be published to confirm the efficacy of this approach.

A 49 year-old Chinese female complained of a buzzing in the left ear associated with decreased hearing. She also had recurrent attacks of mild vertigo, recurrent headaches, and gastrointestinal complaints. Lobsters, and occasionally fish, caused diarrhea. She drank 8 to 9 cups of coffee daily.

The ENT exam was essentially negative. A pure tone audiogram revealed a mild low tone sensorineural hearing loss in the left ear. There was a Type II tracing by the Bekesy audiometry.

On provocative food testing, she was quite allergic to coffee. With coffee avoidance, her hearing became normal, the Bekesy tracing was Type I, and her buzzing ceased (Pang).

BIBLIOGRAPHY

Anonymous. FDA Consumer May, 1991a, p.4

Anonymous. Unpublished study reported in Am Fam Pract 44:1786, 1991b

Attias J et al. Oral magnesium intake reduces permanent hearing loss induced by noise exposure. Am J Otolaryngol 15:26-32, 1994

Biesalski HK et al. Vitamin A deficiency increases noise susceptibility in guinea pigs. J Nutr 120(7):726-37, 1990

Bretlau P et al. Otospongiosis and sodium fluoride. A clinical double-blind, placebo-controlled study on sodium fluoride treatment in otospongiosis. Am J Otol 10(1):20-2, 1989

Brookes GB. Vitamin D deficiency - a new cause of cochlear deafness. J Laruyngol Otol 97(5):405-20, 1983

Brookes GB. Vitamin D deficiency and otosclerosis. Otolaryngol Head Neck Surg 93(3):313-21, 1985

Browning GG et al. Blood viscosity as a factor in sensorineural hearing impairment. Lancet i:121-3, 1986

Carmen RE et al. Audiometric configuration as a reflection of low plasma glucose and diabetes. Am J Otol 10(5):372-9, 1989

Carrillo V et al. [Disorders of glucose tolerance and pathology of the labyrinth.] Acta Otorhinolaryngol Belg 38(5):474-84, 1984) (in French)

Chole Q. Vitamin A in the cochlea. Arch Otorhinolaryngol 124:379-82, 1978

Colletti V, Fiorino FG. Effect of sodium fluoride on early stages of otosclerosis. Am J Otol 12(3):195-8, 1991

Currier WD. Metabolic errors and sudden deafness. Otolaryngol Clin North Am 8:501-6, 1975

Derebery MJ, Valenzuela S. Meniere's syndrome and allergy. Otolaryngol Clin North Am 25(1):213-24, 1992

Derebery MJ. Allergic and immunologic aspects of Meniere's disease. Otolaryngol Head Neck Surg 114(3):360-5, 1996

DeBartolo HM Jr. Zinc and diet for tinnitus. Am J Otol 10(3):256, 1989

Duke WW. Meniere's syndrome caused by allergy. JAMA 81:2179, 1923

Gersdorff M et al. A clinical correlation between hypozincemia and tinnitus. Arch Otorhinolaryngol 244(3):190-3, 1987a

Gersdorff M et al. [The zinc sulfate overload test in patients suffering from tinnitus associated with low serum zinc. Preliminary report.] Acta Otorhinolaryngol Belg 41(3):498-505, 1987b

Goldman H. Metabolic causes of fluctuant hearing loss. Otolaryngol Clin North Am 8:369-73, 1975

Gosselin EJ, Yanick P Jr. Audiologic and metabolic findings in 90 patients with fluctuant hearing loss. J Am Audiol Soc 2:15-18, 1976

Gunther T et al. Biochemical mechanisms affecting susceptibility to noise-induced hearing loss. Am J Otol 10(1):36-41, 1989

Hoover SN. Food allergy and Meniere's disease. Annual Meeting Abstracts AAOA News 5(4):10, 1987

Ikeda K et al. The effect of vitamin D deficiency on the cochlear potentials and the perilymphatic ionized calcium concentration of rats. Acta Ocolaryngol Suppl (Stockh) 435:64-72, 1987

Ikeda K et al. Evaluation of vitamin D metabolism in patients with bilateral sensorineural hearing loss. Am J Otol 10(1):11-3, 1989

Lehrer JF et al. Identification and treatment of metabolic abnormalities in patients with vertigo. Arch Intern Med 146(8):1497-500, 1986

Lewy A, Fox N. Clinical notes; New instruments and technics: pyridoxine (B6) used in the treatment of vertigo. Arch Otolaryngol November, 1947, pp.681-3

Lobel MJ. Arch Otolaryngol May, 1951

Lohle E. The influence of chronic vitamin A deficiency on human and animal ears. Arch Otorhinolaryngol 234:167-73, 1982

Madej S. [Treatment of sudden deafness of vascular etiology with venoruton.] Otolyngol Pol 43(3):214-17, 1989 (in Polish)

Meyer zum Gottesberge AM. Imbalanced calcium homeostasis and endolymphatic hydrops. Acta Otolaryngol Suppl (Stockh) 460:18-27, 1988

Morimitsu T et al. Effect of intermittent sound stimulation on cochlear microphonics and the possible preventive effect of coenzyme Q10. Hear Res 3(2):155-66, 1980

Moser M et al. A double-blind clinical trial of hydroxyethylrutosides in Meniere's disease. J Laryngol Otol 98(3):265-72, 1984

Ochi K et al. [The serum zinc level in patients with tinnitus and the effect of zinc treatment]. Nippon Jibiinkoka Gakkai Kaiho 100(9):915-9, 1997) (in Japanese)

Paaske PB et al. Zinc in the management of tinnitus. Ann Otol Rhinol Laryngol 100:647-9, 1991

Pang LQ. The importance of allergy in otolaryngology, in LD Dickey, Ed. Clinical Ecology. Springfield, Illinois, Charles C. Thomas, 1976

Pillsbury HC. Hypertension, hyperlipoproteinemia, chronic noise exposure: Is there synergism in cochlear pathology? Laryngoscope 96(10): 1112-38, 1986

Popelka MM et al. Moderate alcohol consumption and hearing loss: a protective effect. Am J Epidemiol 145(11):SER Abstracts 241, 1997

Powers WH. Allergic factors in Meniere's disease. Trans Am Acad Ophthalmol Otolaryngol 77:22-9, 1973

Proctor B, Proctor C. Metabolic management in Meniere's disease. Ann Otol Rhinol Laryngol 90(6 Pt 1):615-18, 1981

Proctor CA et al. Etiology and treatment of fluid retention (hydrops) in Meniere's syndrome. Ear Nose Throat J 71(12):631-5, 1992

Pulec JL et al. Progressive sensorineural hearing loss, subjective tinnitus and vertigo caused by elevated blood lipids. Ear Nose Throat J 76(10):716-20,725-6,728 passim, 1997

Romeo G. The therapeutic effect of vitamins A and E in neurosensory hearing loss. Acta Vitaminol Enzymol 7 Suppl:85-92, 1985

Rosen S et al. Dietary prevention of hearing loss. Acta Otolaryngol (Stockh) 70(4):242-7, 1970

Sato K. Pharmacoklinetics of coenzyme Q10 in recovery of acute sensorineural hearing loss due to hypoxia. Acta Otolaryngol Suppl (Stockh) 458:95-102, 1988

Schimdt-Schönbein H et al. Vasa 4:263, 1975

Shambaugh G. Allergy and the inner ear. Ear Clin Int 1:166-7, 1981

Shambaugh GE Jr. Zinc: An essential trace element. Clin Ecology 2(4):203-06, 1984

Shambaugh GE Jr. Zinc for tinnitus, imbalance, and hearing loss in the elderly. Am J Otol 7(6):476-7, 1986

Shambaugh GE Jr. Zinc: the neglected nutrient. Am J Otol 10(2):156-60, 1989

Shemesh Z et al. Vitamin B12 deficiency in patients with chronic tinnitus and noise-induced hearing loss. Am J Otolaryngol 14(2):94-9, 1993

Shitara T et al. Otal Fukuoka Vol. 24, 1978 (in Japanese)

Sikora MA et al. Diet-induced hyperlipidemia and auditory dysfunction. Acta Otolaryngol (Stockh) 102(5-6):372-81, 1986

Spak C-J et al. Tissue response of gastric mucosa after ingestion of fluoride. Br Med J 298:1686-7, 1989

Spencer JT Jr. Hyperlipoproteinemia and inner ear disease. J Int Acad Metabology 4:38-42, 1975

Spencer JT Jr. Hyperlipoproteinemia, hyperinsulinism and Meniere's disease. South Med J 74:1194-7, 1981

Strome M et al. Hyperlipidemia in association with childhood sensorineural hearing loss. Laryngoscope 98(2):165-9, 1988

Suckfull M et al. [Hypercholesteremia and hyperfibrinogenemia in sudden deafness]. Laryngorhinootologie 76(8):453-7, 1997) (in German)

Sun AH. A preliminary report on combined traditional Chinese and Western medicine in semsorineural hearing loss. An analysis of 108 cases. J Tradit Chin Med 2:215-22, 1982

Sun AH et al. Iron deficiency and hearing loss. ORL 49:118-22, 1987

Sun AH et al. Red cell basic ferritin concentration in sensorineural hearing loss. ORL J Otorhinolaryngol Relat Spec 53(5):270-2, 1991

Sun AH et al. Idiopathic sudden hearing loss and disturbance of iron metabolism. A clinical survey of 426 cases. ORL J Otorhinolaryngol Relat Spec 54(2):66-70, 1992

Tappel AL. Nutrition Today July-August 1973

van Haeringen NJ et al. Bibl Anat 12:459, 1973

Wadworth AN, Faulds D. Hydroxyethylrutosides. A review of its pharmacology, and therapeutic efficacy in venous insufficiency and related disorders. Drugs 44(6):1013-32, 1992

Wang Q, Zhang L. [The changes of Ca++ concentrations of endolymph and perilymph of the experimental endolymphatic hydrops]. Chung Hua Erh Pi Yen Hou Ko Tsa Chih 29(5):263-5, 1994) (in Chinese)

Wilson WH. Antigenic excitement in Meniere's disease. Laryngoscope 82:1726-35, 1972

Yamazaki T et al. Jibi Rinsyo 70(suppl 5):1799-1813, 1977 (in Japanese)

Yamazaki T, Ogawa K, Imoto T, et al. Senile deafness and metabolic bone disease. Am J Otol 9(5):376-82, 1988

Yanick P, Gosselin EJ. Audiologic and metabolic findings in 90 patients with fluctuant hearing loss. J Am Audiol Soc 2:15-18, 1975

Yanick P. Holistic applications to ear disorders. J Int Acad Prev Med 1983, pp. 24-7

Yanick P. Solving problematic tinnitus. A clinical scientific approach. Townsend Letter for Doctors. February - March , 1985, p.31

INSOMNIA

See Also: ANXIETY
DEPRESSION

NUTRITIONAL TREATMENT GUIDE

✓ = Efficacy generally accepted.
* = Efficacy *demonstrated* by controlled human trials.
[+] = Efficacy *suspected* from uncontrolled human trials.
[-] = Efficacy *suspected* from indirect data.
? = Efficacy *challenged* in a study of similar design.

DIETARY FACTORS

[+] avoid **Alcohol**
[+] avoid **Caffeine**
[+] avoid **Very-Low-Calorie diets**

NUTRITIONAL FACTORS

✓ **L-Tryptophan** 1 to 4 g one hour before bedtime

- -

* avoid **Chromium** supplementation
* **Potassium deficiency:** potassium chloride 96 mEq daily for one week)
* **Thiamine deficiency:** 10 mg daily

- -

[+] **L-5-Hydroxytryptophan:** 100 to 300 mg one half hour before retiring
[+] **Magnesium deficiency:** ≈ 400 mg daily
[+] **Niacinamide:** 1 g one half hour before bedtime
[+] **Vitamin B_{12}:** *to treat sleep-wake rhythm disorders:* 1.5 mg daily to 3 times daily

OTHER FACTORS

* rule out **Food Sensitivities**

- -

[+] rule out **Reactive Hypoglycemia**

DIETARY FACTORS

Very-low-calorie diets may interfere with sleep. When overweight premenopausal women were placed on an 800 kcal/day diet, sleep onset latency was lengthened and slow-wave sleep decreased *(Karklin)*.

Alcohol

Alcohol, although it produces initial sedation, interferes with REM and slow wave sleep *(Stone)*. There is sympathetic activation which does not return to baseline levels until blood alcohol levels have returned to zero *(Onen)*. Moreover, among people who consume 2 or more alcoholic drinks per day, there is a 3-fold risk of having a 20 or more periodic leg movements per hour during sleep *(Aldrich)*. Whether these movements cause the alcohol-induced sleep disturbance is not known.

Caffeine

Caffeine has been repeatedly shown to adversely affect sleep *(Brown)*. Among normals, the equivalent of one cup of coffee ½ hour before retiring has no effect, two cups primarily affects sleep latency and the other parameters related to the early part of the night, and four cups adversely affects all sleep parameters *(Karacan)*.

Plasma caffeine clearance is slowed in people with caffeine-induced wakefulness *(Levy)*. In a large cross-sectional study, the proportion of subjects reporting insomnia increased significantly with mean caffeine intake even after controlling for age, adiposity, smoking, alcohol intake and occupation *(Shirlow)*.

In one study, 16 patients complaining of psychological distress and sleep disturbances were placed on a caffeine- and sucrose-free diet for up to 2 weeks. Those who improved were challenged double-blind with caffeine and sucrose. Symptoms returned for 7 of the 16 patients when they were challenged with caffeine or sucrose, but not when they were challenged with placebos *(Christensen)*.

NUTRITIONAL FACTORS

VITAMINS

Niacinamide

Animal studies suggest that niacinamide has effects similar to that of the benzodiazepines. These include hypnotic and muscle relaxant qualities *(Möhler)*.

Thiamine Deficiency

In a double-blind study of healthy elderly who were likely to be marginally thiamine-deficient, supplementation improved sleep patterns and general well-being, while it reduced daytime sleep time and fatigue *(Smidt)*. More studies are needed to better assess this vitamin's efficacy.

Vitamin B_{12}

Disturbances in the usual sleep-wake rhythm are a cause of insomnia, especially as patients with this disturbances are often only able to sleep at inappropriate times. Some of these patients have been reported to respond to oral supplementation with vitamin B_{12} with normalization of sleeping patterns and of hormonal circadian rhythms *(Okawa;Ohta;Tomoda)*.

A 55 year-old man suffering from delayed sleep phase syndrome since age 18 was treated with vitamin B_{12} 1.5 mg daily. His sleep-wake rhythm was improved and the improvement lasted more than 6 months while he remained on the supplement (Okawa).

MINERALS

Chromium: A Warning

Following anecdotal and self-supplementation trials which suggested that chromium supplements may interfere with sleep, a research group provided 16 healthy volunteers (average age of 40 years) with either a commercial chromium yeast containing 50 μg chromium or a brewer's yeast placebo at 7:30 PM nightly for 6 nights. They were asked to discontinue any vitamin or mineral supplements for one week prior to the study.

While, with 2 exceptions, no effects were attributed to the placebo, 100% of chromium-supplemented volunteers noted increased and more vivid dreams, 75% noted

increased sleep interruption, and 50% noted difficulty falling asleep. Additional comments in that group included complaints of unrefreshing sleep and fatigue *(Schrauzer)*.
The results of this study suggest that patients with insomnia who are taking a chromium supplement should discontinue the supplement on a trial basis to see if it adversely affects their sleep patterns.

Magnesium Deficiency

Insomnia is one of the central or neurotic, symptoms of chronic magnesium deficiency *(Durlach)*. A number of parasomnias (night terrors; nocturnal verbal and motor automatisms; restless legs syndrome) may be related to magnesium deficiency *(Popoviciu,1990,1993)*.

Sleep is usually agitated with frequent nocturnal awakenings. Nocturnal instrument monitoring reveals major disorders of sleep organization. The deficiency may be severe enough to be diagnosed on the basis of hypomagnesemia *(Papoviciu,1993)*.

Conversely, a high magnesium, low aluminum diet has been found to be associated with high-quality sleep time and few nighttime awakenings *(Penland)*, and magnesium supplementation has been reported to reduce sleep latency and result in uninterrupted sleep *(Davis)*.

Potassium Deficiency

Evidence that a marginal potassium deficiency interferes with sleep comes from a double-blind crossover study of normal young men. While on a low-potassium diet, they randomly received either oral potassium chloride or placebo. Potassium supplements were found to improve sleep consolidation *(Drennan)*.

OTHER NUTRITIONAL FACTORS

L-Tryptophan

The nutritional precursor to serotonin, L-tryptophan has been extensively studied and has been found to be an effective hypnotic. For younger insomniacs suffering purely from extended sleep latency, it is effective starting the first night of supplementation. For more chronic and severe insomniacs with both extended sleep latencies and problems in sleep maintenance, it may take several days or longer before improvement occurs. Sometimes, in these cases, improvement occurs only after supplementation is discontinued; for such patients, intermittent treatment may be most effective *(Schneider-Helmert)*.

Supplementation with L-tryptophan does not impair visuomotor performance, cognition or memory, does not elevate the threshold for arousal from sleep, and does not distort sleep stages. Tolerance does not develop and there is a negligible to low incidence of side effects *(Hartmann; Schneider-Helmert)*. It is unavailable in many countries, however, ever since a contaminant introduced by one manufacturer resulted in an epidemic of eosinophilia myalgia syndrome several years ago.

L-5-Hydroxytryptophan

While much less studied than L-tryptophan for treating insomnia, L-5-hydroxytryptophan, the immediate precursor to serotonin, also appears to be effective in promoting sleep. Moreover, there is reason to believe that L-5-hydroxytryptophan may be more effective than L-tryptophan in improving sleep. L-tryptophan, while increasing the time spent in non-REM sleep, may decrease the time spent in REM sleep *(Wyatt,1972)*. L-5-hydroxytryptophan, by contrast, has been shown to *increase* the amount of time spent in REM sleep *(Wyatt,1971)*.

Susan, a lively 75-year-old woman, reported increasing problems with sleep. After thrashing around for an hour after bedtime, she would get up and do some quiet activity until she became sleepy enough to doze off. Although she awoke feeling rested, by midmorning she was sleepy again and complained that her sleep patterns were interfering with her normal quality of life.

She initially was placed on melatonin 3 mg one-half hour before bedtime. While she did well at first, after a few weeks her insomnia returned. She was switched to 5-hydroxytryptophan 300 mg at bedtime and reported a few weeks later that she no longer had a sleeping problem (Murray).

OTHER RELATED FACTORS

Food Sensitivities

Insomnia has been attributed at times to food sensitivities. While most of the literature is anecdotal, a reaction to cow's milk was shown in a double-blind crossover study to cause insomnia for a group of children below 5 years of age *(Kahn)*.

'Reactive Hypoglycemia'

There appears to be a relationship between insomnia and low blood sugar levels (which, presumably, serve as a marker for low brain sugar levels). In 1966, insomnia was found to be a symptom of half of a group of 300 patients who demonstrated a drop of 20 mg% or more below the fasting blood sugar level during a 6-hour glucose tolerance test *(Salzer)*.

Also, 30 years later, responses of a group of 2,415 female workers were analyzed. Insomnia was found to be one of the risk factors for hypoglycemia (a blood glucose reading of less than 60 mg/dl); other risk factors were histories of hypotension and glycosuria, eating snacks and desserts, and a history of occupation as a nurse *(Mogi)*.

(See 'Hypoglycemia' for further information.)

BIBLIOGRAPHY

Aldrich MS, Shipley JE. Alcohol use and periodic limb movements of sleep. Alcohol Clin Exp Res 17(1):192-6, 1993

Brown SL et al. Occult caffeine as a source of sleep problems in an older population. J Am Geriatr Soc 43(8):860-4, 1995

Christensen L. Psychological distress and diet - effects of sucrose and caffeine. J Appl Nutr 40(1):44-50, 1988

Davis W, Ziady F. U. of Pretoria, S. Africa - presented at the Second International Symposium on Magnesium, Montreal, 1976

Drennan MD et al. Potassium affects actigraph-identified sleep. Sleep 14(4):357-60, 1991

Durlach J et al. Magnesium and therapeutics. Magnes Res 7(3/4):313-28, 1994

Hartmann EL - presented at a symposium sponsored by the Am. Med. Assoc. and quoted in Clin Psychiatry News, March, 1985

Kahn A et al.. Milk intolerance in children with persistent sleeplessness: a prospective double-blind crossover evaluation. Pediatrics 84(4):595-603, 1989

Karacan I et al. Dose-related sleep disturbances induced by coffee and caffeine. Clin Pharmacol Ther 20:682-89, 1976

Karklin A et al. Restricted energy intake affects nocturnal body temperature and sleep patterns. Am J Clin Nutr 59:346-9, 1994

Levy M, Zylber-Katy E. Caffeine metabolism and coffee-attributed sleep disturbances. Clin Pharmacol Ther 33(6):770-75, 1983

Mogi T et al. Epidemiological study on hypoglycemia endemic to female nurses and other workers. Ind Health 34(4):335-46, 1996

Möhler H et al. Nicotinamide is a brain constituent with benzodiazepine-like actions. Nature 278:563-65, 1979

Murray MT. 5-HTP: The Natural Way to Overcome Depression, Obesity, and Insomnia. New York, Bantam Books, 1998

Okawa M et al. Vitamin B12 treatment for sleep-wake rhythm disorders. Sleep 31(1):15-23, 1990

Ohta T et al. Treatment of persistent sleep-wake schedule disorders in adolescents with methylcobalamin (vitamin B12). Sleep 14(5):414-8, 1991

Onen SH et al. [Prevention and treatment of sleep disorders through regulation] of sleeping habits]. Presse Med 23(10):485-9, 1994 (in French)

Penland J. Effects of trace element nutrition on sleep patterns in adult women. Fed Am Soc Exp Biol J 2:A434, 1988

Popoviciu L et al. Parasomnias (non-specific nocturnal episodic manifestations) in patients with magnesium deficiency. Rom J Neurol Psychiatry 28(1):19-24, 1990

Popoviciu L et al. Clinical, EEG, electromyographic and polysomnographic studies in restless legs syndrome caused by magnesium deficiency. Rom J Neurol Psychiatry 31(1):55-61, 1993

Salzer HM. Relative hypoglycemia as a cause of neuropsychiatric illness. J Natl Med Assoc 58(1):12-17, 1966

Schneider-Helmert D, Spinweber CL. Evaluation of L-tryptophan for treatment of insomnia: a review. Psychopharmacology (Berlin) 89(1):1-7, 1986

Schrauzer G et al. Somatopsychological effects of chromium supplementation. J Nutr Med 3:43-8, 1992

Shirlow MJ, Mathers CD. A study of caffeine consumption and symptoms: Indigestion, palpitations, tremor, headache and insomnia. Int J Epidemiol 14(2):239-48, 1985

Smidt LJ et al. Influence of thiamin supplementation on the health and general well-being of an elderly Irish population with marginal thiamin deficiency. J Gerontol 46(1):M16-M22, 1991

Stone BM. Sleep and low doses of alcohol. Electroencephalogr Clin Neurophysiol 48(6):706-09, 1980

Tomoda A et al. Circadian rhythm abnormalities in adrenoleukodystrophy and methyl B12 treatment. Brain Dev 17:428-31, 1995

Wyatt RJ et al. Effects of 5-hydroxytryptophan on the sleep of normal human subjects. Electroencephalogr Clin Neurophysiol 30(6):505-9, 1971

Wyatt RJ. The serotonin-catecholamine-dream bicycle: A clinical study. Biol Psychiatry 5:33-64, 1972

IRRITABLE BOWEL SYNDROME

NUTRITIONAL TREATMENT GUIDE

✓ = Efficacy generally accepted.
* = Efficacy *demonstrated* by controlled human trials.
[+] = Efficacy *suspected* from uncontrolled human trials.
[-] = Efficacy *suspected* from indirect data.
? = Efficacy *challenged* in a study of similar design.

DIETARY FACTORS

* **low Fat diet**
* ? **high Fiber diet** *OR* add dietary fiber supplements such as **Psyllium** 1 tsp twice daily or unprocessed **Wheat Bran** 4 to 5 tsp twice daily, along with generous amounts of fluid

- - - - - - - - - - - - - - - - - - - -

[+] avoid **Sugar** (except in infantile colic)

- - - - - - - - - - - - - - - - - - - -

[-] avoid **Refined Carbohydrates**

OTHER RELATED FACTORS

* ? rule out **Food Sensitivities**

- - - - - - - - - - - - - - - - - - - -

[+] ***Lactobacillus acidophilus*:** dosage varies with preparation (minimum 6 week trial)

DIETARY FACTORS

High Fiber Diet

A high intake of dietary fiber is commonly recommended. Moreover, gastric emptying and small bowel motility are slowed by soluble fiber, while both soluble and insoluble fiber reduce sigmoidal intraluminal pressures and overcome spastic constipation when given in progressive graded doses *(Friedman)*.

A high fiber diet has proved to be effective for constipation, a common complaint in this disorder. Moreover, several studies found that the addition of wheat bran increases stool weight and decreases transit time in IBS patients *(Müller-Lissner)*. Nevertheless, several double-blind studies failed to find evidence that the addition of bran to the diet reduced symptoms *(Cann;Cook;Lucei)*.

Since the experimental subjects may have already had sufficient dietary fiber in their baseline diets to obtain its full benefits, it may be that increased dietary fiber is only beneficial to patients whose diet is too low in fiber. For example, a controlled study that did find bran to be effective compared supplemented patients with patients who had excluded wholegrain cereal products from their diet *(Manning)*.

Another explanation for the negative findings is that some patients react adversely to certain dietary fibers. In a survey of 100 patients, 55% stated that wholemeal wheat and bran products made them worse, while only 10% found them helpful. Of the other sources of fiber, citrus fruits, especially oranges, were most likely to be offenders, while proprietary fiber products such as psyllium (ispaghula) showed some benefit, with 39% of patients indicating that it reduced symptoms and 22% indicating that it aggravated symptoms *(Francis)*.

A double-blind study has confirmed the efficacy of psyllium. Both constipation and intestinal transit times were significantly improved following its addition to the diet as compared to placebo. Abdominal pain and bloating also lessened, although the improvement was similar to that obtained with placebo *(Prior)*.

Because patients vary in their response to dietary fiber, its use needs to be individualized. If the patient is not eating whole grains, switching to them should be tried first. If indicated, a trial of psyllium, or of unprocessed bran, can be performed separately.

A 14 year-old female had a history for several years of increasingly severe abdominal cramps in varying locations throughout her abdomen largely relieved by antispasmodics. Stools were normal and defecation was once every 2 to 3 days. Dietary analysis revealed a lack of dietary bulk and fiber.

She was told to add raw, bulky, fibrous vegetables, honey-sweetened granola for breakfast, and 2 tablespoons of unprocessed bran daily. On follow-up one month later, she reported no further spasms (Wright J).

Refined Carbohydrates

In a low fiber, "junk food" diet, dietary carbohydrates are largely refined. Results of a survey of the diets of 18 women with functional bowel disorder as compared to the diets 37 normal controls were consistent with the hypothesis that a high intake of refined carbohydrates may contribute to the syndrome. Calorie, fat, fiber and protein intakes were found to be similar in the two groups. However, the symptomatic women were found to consume more refined carbohydrate *(Jarrett)*.

One theory is that a diet high in refined carbohydrate provokes spasm of the smooth muscle. A diet high in refined carbohydrate allows the intense muscle spasm to occur because the physical buffering effect of fecal bulk is considerably reduced due to lack of dietary fiber *(Grimes)*.

Sugar

Dietary sugars, including lactose, fructose, sucrose and sorbitol, may contribute to the illness. When a group of patients was assessed for sugar malabsorption by a breath hydrogen test, 96% malabsorbed at least one sugar, and ingestion of a malabsorbed sugar provoked symptoms *(Fernandez-Banares)*.

Sucrose, for example, increases fecal bile acid concentrations and bacterial fermentation activity, and decreases intestinal transit time. These alterations are associated with an elevated risk of developing irritable bowel syndrome *(Kruis)*. By contrast, in *infantile colic*, feeding a sucrose solution found to *reduce* symptoms in a double-blind crossover study *(Markestad)*.

An infant developed diarrhea and colic during the first year of her life. She was found to have isolated fructose malabsorption and responded to a fructose-free diet (Wales).

Dietary Fat

Fat is the major dietary stimulant of the gastrocolonic response *(Wright S)* which is believed to be initiated by the secretion of cholecystokinin. Compared to normals, IBS patients were found to have an exaggerated and prolonged release of cholecystokinin following ingestion of a fatty meal *(Sjolund)*.

Furthermore, as compared to normals, a small intestinal infusion of a fatty meal provokes excessive intestinal dysmotility in IBS patients, and the dysmotility is often accompanied by abdominal symptoms, suggesting that small bowel dysfunction contributes to the symptoms of irritable bowel syndrome. Patients with diarrhea tend to be more sensitive than those with constipation *(Kellow)*.

OTHER RELATED FACTORS

Food Sensitivities

Food sensitivities provoke symptoms in perhaps half of the patient population *(Parker;Stefanini)*. This relationship has been observed, not only in adults, but also in infants who are experiencing colic *(Hill)*. Some of the research has consisted of controlled studies; however, all had major limitations in their trial designs *(Niec)*. Patients with an allergic history or an elevated total IgE level may be more likely to respond to a food elimination diet, although the results of IgE RAST testing may not correlate with those of provocative testing *(Petitpierre)*.

Dairy products are frequently found to be offenders due to fact that lactose intolerance is a common problem *(Bohmer;Griffith)*. While most milk products tend to cause symptoms in lactose-intolerant patients, some may be able to tolerate butter and certain aged cheeses (because they are low in lactose) and yogurt (due to the lactase activity of the bacterial culture).

Additional research has found wheat, corn, coffee, tea, and citrus fruits to be some of the other more common offending agents *(Gallo)*.

A 42 year-old woman with a diagnosis of irritable bowel syndrome had an 8-year history of almost daily bloating, loose stools, abdominal pain and gas. Fourteen days after stopping all dairy products, she was symptom-free. The following day she drank 3 glasses of milk and ate a bowl of ice cream, and discovered that her symptoms returned worse than before. She tried avoidance and provocation twice more, each time with the same result (Manahan).

Lactobacillus acidophilus

Lactobacillus acidophilus is a beneficial bacterium. Successful implantation has been reported to produce symptom relief, although it may require weeks or months before improvement is noted *(Rettger)*. Its efficacy has recently been confirmed in a small double-blind crossover study *(Halpern)*. While its mechanism of action is uncertain, the benefits of *L acidophilus* could be due to its antimicrobial activity when symptoms are due to undiagnosed chronic intestinal infections.

BIBLIOGRAPHY

Bohmer CJ, Tuynman HA. The clinical relevance of lactose malabsorption in irritable bowel syndrome. Eur J Gastroenterol Hepatol 8(10):1013-16, 1996

Cann P et al. What is the benefit of coarse wheat bran in patients with irritable bowel syndrome? Gut 25:168-73, 1984

Cook IJ et al. Effect of dietary fiber on symptoms and rectosigmoid motility in patients with irritable bowel syndrome. A controlled, crossover study. Gastroenterology 98(1):66-72, 1990

Fernandez-Banares F et al. Sugar malabsorption in functional bowel disease: clinical implications. Am J Gastroenterol 88:2044-50, 1993

Francis CY, Whorwell PJ. Bran and irritable bowel syndrome: time for reappraisal. Lancet 344:39-40, 1994

Friedman G. Diet and the irritable bowel syndrome. Gastroenterol Clin North Am 20(2):313-24, 1991

Gallo C et al. Irritable bowel: A food allergy? Hightlights in Food Allergy 32:198-203, 1996

Griffith CJ. Lactose Intolerance. Phys Asst 56-62, Nov. 1997

Grimes DS. Refined carbohydrate, smooth-muscle spasm and disease of the colon. Lancet i:395-7, 1976

Halpern GM et al. Treatment of irritable bowel syndrome with lacteol fort: a randomized, double-blind, cross-over trial. Am J Gastroenterol 91(8):1579-85, 1996

Hill DJ et al. A low allergen diet is a significant intervention in infantile colic: results of a community-based study. Part I. J Allergy Clin Immunol 96(6):886-92, 1995

Jarrett M et al. Comparison of diet composition in women with and without functional bowel disorder. Gastroenterol Nurs 16(6):253-8, 1994

Kellow JF et al. Dysmotility of the small intestine in irritable bowel syndrome. Gut 29(9):1236-43, 1988

Kruis W et al. Influence of diets high and low in refined sugar on stool qualities, gastrointestinal transit time and fecal bile acid excretion. Gastroenterology 92:1483, 1987

Lucei MR et al. Is bran efficacious in irritable bowel syndrome? A double-blind, placebo controlled, cross-over study. Gut 28:221, 1990

Manahan B. Eat for Health. Tiburon, CA, HJ Kramer, Inc., 1988

Manning AP et al. Wheat fibre and irritable bowel syndrome: A controlled study. Lancet ii:417, 1977

Markestad T. Use of sucrose as a treatment for infant colic. Arch Dis Child 76:356-8, 1997

Müller-Lissner SA. Effect of wheat bran on weight of stool and gastrointestinal transit time: A meta analysis. Br Med J 296:615-17, 1988

Niec AM et al. Are adverse food reactions linked to irritable bowel syndrome? Am J Gastroenterol 93(11):2184-90, 1998

Parker TJ et al. Management of patients with food intolerance in irritable bowel syndrome: the development and use of an exclusion diet. J Hum Nutr Diet 8:159-66, 1995

Petitpierre M et al. Irritable bowel syndrome and hypersensitivity to food. Ann Allergy 54:538-40, 1985

Prior A, Whorwell PJ. Double blind study of ispaghula in irritable bowel syndrome. Gut 28(11):1510-13, 1987

Rettger LF et al. Lactobacillus Acidophilus. Its Therapeutic Application. New Haven, Yale U. Press, 1935

Sjolund K et al. Disturbed motilin and cholecystokinin release in the irritable bowel syndrome. Scand J Gastroenterol 31(11):1110-4, 1996

Stefanini GF et al. Oral cromolyn sodium in comparison with elimination diet in the irritable bowel syndrome, diarrheic type. Multicenter study of 428 patients. Scand J Gastroenterol 30(6):535-41, 1995

Wales JK et al. Isolated fructose malabsorption. Arch Dis Child 65(2):227-9, 1990

Wright JV. Dr. Wright's Book of Nutritional Therapy. Emmaus, PA, Rodale Press, 1979

Wright SH et al. Effect of dietary components on the gastrocolonic response. Am J Physiol 238(3):G228-32, 1980

KIDNEY STONES (CALCIUM OXALATE)

NUTRITIONAL TREATMENT GUIDE

✓ = Efficacy generally accepted.
* = Efficacy *demonstrated* by controlled human trials.
[+] = Efficacy *suspected* from uncontrolled human trials.
[-] = Efficacy *suspected* from indirect data.
? = Efficacy *challenged* in a study of similar design.

DIETARY FACTORS

✓ drink plenty of **Fluids**

- -

* avoid **Sugar** *(especially in nondietary hypercalciuria)*

- -

[+] drink **Hard Water**
[+] **low Sodium, high Potassium diet** *(in hypercalciuria)*
[+] **high Fiber diet**
[+] **low Fat diet**
[+] restrict **Oxalate** intake *(in hyperoxaluria)*

NUTRITIONAL FACTORS

* **Essential Fatty Acids:** evening primrose & fish oil mixture to provide a 1 to 4 ratio of EPA to GLA
* **Magnesium:** 200 mg twice daily with meals

- -

[+] **Calcium:** Consider a trial of mild calcium restriction in selected patients.
[+] **Citrate:** *in hypocitraturia:* potassium citrate 30 to 80 mEq daily (or 2 liters lemonade daily)
[+] **Glycosaminoglycans:** *to reduce oxalate excretion:* 30 mg twice daily of a mixture (15 day trial)
[+] **Phosphorus:** *in hyperphosphaturia:* orthophosphate 1 to 1.5 g daily
[+] **Vitamin B_6:** *in hyperoxaluria:* pyridoxine 150 mg daily

- -

[-] **Vitamin A deficiency:** 50,000 IU daily for 6 weeks (10,000 IU daily during pregnancy)

OTHER RELATED FACTORS

[-] avoid **Cadmium** exposure

DIETARY FACTORS

Fluids

Inadequate body fluid due either to insufficient intake or fluid loss encourages stone formation by reducing urinary output and increasing the concentration of stone-forming minerals in the urine *(Robertson,1980).* Fluid intake is inversely related to the risk of kidney stones *(Curhan,1993).* In fact, there is evidence that a low protein, high fiber, high fluid diet has no advantage over merely increasing fluid intake *(Hiatt).* Unless they have a tendency to retain fluid, stone formers should have a daily intake of 2 to 2.5 liters of fluid spread evenly throughout the day *(Vahlensieck).*

As to drinking water, hard water is preferable. Water hardness has been shown to negatively correlate with the incidence of kidney stones *(Sierakowski).* The higher calcium content of hard water is one reason for its superiority; dietary calcium precipitates oxalate to form calcium oxalate which is not absorbed from the intestines, thus reducing the risk of calcium oxalate precipitating in the urine.

When, for a group of calcium oxalate stone-formers, 24-hour urines following the ingestion of calcium- and magnesium-rich mineral water was compared to tap water, several risk factors were favorably altered by both water regimens, but more so by the mineral water. In addition, the mineral water produced some unique favorable changes *(Rodgers).*

Other minerals besides calcium may also be important as, when tap water from a soft water, high kidney stone area was compared to that from a hard water, low stone area, the calcium content of the water was not significantly different *(Shuster,1982).*

Animal Protein

Vegetarians have about half the risk of urinary stones of omnivores *(Robertson,1982.* Moreover, the intake of animal protein is directly related to the risk of kidney stones *(Curhan,1993).* Recurrent stone formers have higher intakes of animal protein than do single stone formers, while non-stone formers consume less animal protein than single stone formers *(Robertson,1979).*

In addition to increasing urinary excretion of both calcium and oxalate, animal protein increases urinary excretion of uric acid *(Blacklock,1983).* Uric acid excretion promotes calcium oxalate stone formation by interfering with the action of naturally occurring inhibitors in the urine *(Rao)*, and by serving as seeds for stone formation and growth *(Noda).*

Despite these considerations, a recent randomized, controlled trial of 99 first-time calcium oxalate stone formers found unexpectedly that, 2 ½ years after half of the patients received a low-animal protein, high fiber diet, 13 of the patients on the "therapeutic" diet developed recurrent stones compared to only 2 patients on the control diet *(Hiatt).*

This finding suggests that lowering animal protein consumption could actually *increase* the risk of recurrent kidney stones, and thus the efficacy of restricting animal protein must be considered to be uncertain until further controlled trials are completed.

One possible explanation is that only *hypercalciuric* calcium oxalate stone formers should restrict animal (or all) protein intake, as there is evidence that they are particularly sensitive to the hypercalciuric effect of a high protein intake *(Jungers).* In any event, a vegetarian diet is not recommended for patients with *absorptive hyperoxaluria* as it may increase oxalic acid excretion *(Siener).*

Dietary Fat

If fat is not fully absorbed from the gut, it binds to intraluminal calcium, thus reducing its ability to bind oxalate and increasing urinary oxalate excretion *(Smith).* In renal stone formers, fat intake is positively correlated with urinary oxalate excretion *(Masai).* Moreover, compared to healthy controls, urinary stone formers tend to consume more fat *(Griffith).*

Dietary Fiber

Patients with renal stones have a lower dietary fiber intake than normals *(Fellström)*, and renal stones are rare in Third World countries where the fiber intake is still high *(Modlin).* When stone formers are supplemented with fiber, urinary calcium excretion is substantially reduced *(Jahnen)*, sometimes normalizing excretion for patients with hypercalciuria *(Shah).*

In a study of stone formers with hypercalciuria, the addition of rice bran to the diet resulted in an 84% decrease in kidney stone formation in the following year and less than 10% of the patients developed new stones *(Ohkawa).* However, dietary fiber increases urinary oxalate excretion *(Holmes)*, so its efficacy in reducing calcium oxalate stones in patients with hyperoxaluria is questionable.

Low Sodium, High Potassium Diet

Hypercalciuria, which is a pivotal risk factor for stone formation and growth *(Unwin)*, may be sodium-dependent. As a low salt diet may correct hypercalciuria *(Silver)*, it should therefore be tried when patients are hypercalciuric *(Massey,1995;Burtis)*.

Potassium intake has been inversely related to the risk of kidney stones *(Curhan,1993)*. While table salt (sodium chloride) increases urinary calcium loss, potassium chloride does not *(Bell)*. In fact, during potassium administration, urinary calcium declines *(Lemann)*. Moreover, a high potassium intake reverses the hypercalciuria caused by a diet high in meat *(Kaneko)*.

Potassium has natriuretic effects. It also inhibits renal calcitriol synthesis, thus promoting phosphate retention which, in turn, reduces urinary calcium excretion (see Phosphorus below) *(Green;Lemann)*.

Oxalate

Stone formers often have an increased tendency to absorb oxalate and excrete it in the urine *(Zarembski)*. In patients with hyperoxaluria, since dietary oxalate contributes to urinary oxalate excretion, it may be beneficial to limit the intake of high oxalate foods. (Urinary oxalate also comes from glycine and ascorbic acid.)

However, most stone formers do not have hyperoxaluria *(Rao)*, and it is possible to have hyperoxaluria without developing kidney stones *(Butz)*.

Foods with the Highest Oxalate Concentration (25 mg/100 gm)
Beans
Cocoa
Instant Coffee
Parsley
Rhubarb
Spinach
Tea

Other Relatively High Oxalate Foods
Beet Tops
Carrot
Celery
Chocolate
Cucumber
Grapefruit
Kale
Peanut
Pepper
Sweet Potato

Sugar

Sugar ingestion may foster stone formation, as a positive correlation has been found between sugar intake and the incidence of idiopathic renal stones *(Yoshida)*. Furthermore, over 70% of idiopathic stone formers respond to sucrose ingestion by an exaggerated increase in the excretion of calcium, oxalate and uric acid. There is also evidence that sugar promotes oversaturation of the urine with calcium oxalate, and induces calcific lesions within the kidney on which crystal aggregation may take place as a preliminary step to stone formation *(Blacklock,1987)*.

Alcohol

Alcohol consumption among stone formers is almost double that of healthy controls *(Fellström)*. In fact, the correlation between alcohol consumption and the levels of urinary calcium and uric acid is almost linear *(Goldfarb)*.

However, a large prospective study of the risk of symptomatic kidney stones found, after 6 years of follow-up, a 21% *decrease* in risk of stone formation for each 240 ml (8 oz) serving of beer consumed daily, and a 39% decrease in risk for each daily serving of wine *(Curhan,1996a)*. This surprising finding makes the efficacy of avoiding alcohol questionable for the purpose of reducing kidney stone risk and suggests that controlled clinical trials are needed to ascertain the role of alcohol in kidney stone formation.

Coffee and Caffeine

The same prospective study whose findings suggested that beer and wine intake may reduce kidney stone risk also found that coffee (whether or not it contained caffeine) and tea reduced risk *(Curhan,1996a)*. This finding contrasts with findings from experimental

(Massey,1985;Morgan) and observational *(Heaney)* studies which found that caffeine and decaffeinated coffee cause hypercalciuria and suggests that controlled clinical trials may be needed to ascertain whether caffeine and/or decaffeinated coffee should be avoided by stone formers.

Soft Drinks

In a study of more than 1,000 men with a history of kidney stones, soft drink consumption was eliminated for 3 years. After that time, significantly fewer new stones developed in the no-soft-drink group compared to controls.

However, the improvement only occurred in men whose usual soft drinks contained *phosphoric acid* (primarily *cola* beverages); for these men the risk of recurrence of kidney stones was reduced by as much as 36%. Among those who consumed soft drinks other than colas, discontinuing them failed to reduce the risk of stones *(Shuster,1992)*. This finding is consistent with experimental evidence that patients with idiopathic hypercalciuria have an inappropriately high phosphate excretion which promotes increased activation of 1,25-dihydroxyvitamin D leading to increased stone formation *(Williams)*.

However, there is also evidence that phosphate supplementation may be beneficial (see Phosphorus below), suggesting that further studies are needed to clarify the relationship between phosphoric acid intake and kidney stones before dietary recommendations can be made.

NUTRITIONAL FACTORS

VITAMINS

Vitamin A Deficiency

Even with a normal dietary intake, patients may have reduced serum vitamin A levels *(Khanam)*. However, a study of 20 living patients and 78 autopsy cases failed to find objective evidence of vitamin A deficiency *(Jewett)*.

The results of animal studies have suggested that, if vitamin A should be deficient, hypercalciuria would be found and calcium oxalate stone formation would be enhanced *(Bichler;Gershoff,1981)*. While human trials of vitamin A supplementation are lacking, an animal study in which oxalate lithiasis was induced found evidence that vitamin A supplements have an inhibitory effect on lithogenesis - but probably no litholytic action *(Sakly)*.

Vitamin B_6 Deficiency

The results of tryptophan loading studies suggest that patients may be vitamin B_6-deficient *(Gershoff,1960; Grimm)*. This deficiency appears to be associated with a metabolic block in the degradation of oxalic acid resulting in hyperoxaluria and stone precipitation.

Several open trials have shown that this block can be at least partially corrected with pyridoxine supplementation *(Mitwalli)*, resulting in a reduction in the rate of recurrence of urolithiasis *(Revusova)*. Even hyperoxaluric patients without evidence of vitamin B_6 deficiency may benefit *(Gibbs;Ruml)*.

Also, in *primary oxalosis*, a rare genetic disorder associated with severe, recurrent calcium oxalate stone formation, supplementation with massive doses may be beneficial *(Will)*.

Vitamin C: Should Supplementation be Avoided?

Since ascorbate can be metabolized to oxalate, concern has been raised that vitamin C supplementation may increase urinary oxalate levels and thus contribute to stone formation in predisposed individuals. However, when more than 45,000 males with no history of kidney stones were followed by 6 years, men who had been consuming 1,500 mg or more of vitamin C daily had 22% *fewer* kidney stones than those who consumed less than 250 mg daily *(Curhan,1996b)*. Several other studies have also found no evidence that vitamin C supplementation increases the risk of kidney stone formation *(Bendich)*.

Urinary oxalate excretion does not increase significantly following supplementation with the vitamin *(Diplock)*. In fact, findings from one study suggested that oxalate found in urine after vitamin C ingestion may be due to an artifact in laboratory methodology *(Wandzilak)*. Thus, when urinary oxalate is being measured in ascorbate-supplemented patients, the urine should be collected in disodium EDTA. This will prevent erroneous results due to the conversion of ascorbate to oxalate after collection *(Chalmers)*.

Vitamin D

Recent research has suggested that excessive phosphate excretion may induce increased activation of 1,25-dihydroxy-vitamin D *(Williams)*. The result is not only absorptive hypercalciuria *(Breslau)*, but greater oxalate absorption and hyperoxaluria with subsequent stone formation *(Giannini)*.

MINERALS

Calcium

About 30 to 50% of patients have idiopathic hypercalciuria. Calcium restriction is usually not indicated, however, as:

1. Chronic high calcium intake (up to 2 grams daily) in patients with normal vitamin D levels does not significantly increase urinary calcium, presumably because of a parathormone-mediated decrease in 1,25-dihydroxyvitamin D levels which, in turn, decreases the fraction of calcium absorbed *(Pacifici)*.

2. Some hypercalciuric patients will continue to have high urinary calcium excretion rates despite a low calcium diet due to overproduction of 1,25-dihydroxyvitamin D which stimulates bone resorption along with intestinal calcium absorption *(Coe)*.

3. Urinary oxalate increases as dietary calcium is reduced *(Brockis)* - perhaps because dietary calcium precipitates oxalate in the intestines to form calcium oxalate which is not absorbed *(Liebman)*.

4. Hypercalciuria in perimenopausal women with renal calculi and osteoporosis may be due to excessive bone resorption consequent to estrogen deficiency. In that case, estrogen replacement, rather than calcium restriction, is the indicated treatment *(Wasserstein)*.

In fact, there is evidence that dietary calcium intake may be *inversely* associated with the risk of kidney stone formation *(Curhan,1997;Leonetti)* - although it is possible that this association is due to the presence of some other protective factor besides the calcium content in dairy products (the major source of dietary calcium). For example, dairy products are a major source of phosphorus, which may reduce urinary calcium excretion and calcium oxalate supersaturation *(Curhan,1997)*.

Increased calcium intake in the form of supplements taken with meals may effectively reduce oxalate absorption in patients with malabsorption, yet supplemental calcium, in contrast to dietary calcium, has been found to be associated with a slightly increased risk for kidney stones. This contradiction may be because supplemental calcium is often taken away from meals. Because of this possibility, when calcium supplements are prescribed, they should be taken with meals to coincide with the time of oxalate ingestion *(Curhan,1997)*.

In the event that calcium supplementation is indicated to prevent bone resorption in a patient with recurrent kidney stones, it should be given in the form of carbonate, citrate, gluconate or lactate, all of which tend to alkalinize the urine which decreases urinary calcium excretion *(Wasserstein)*.

Despite the above arguments, a minority of patients with recurrent renal stones and idiopathic hypercalciuria will benefit from calcium restriction. If calcium restriction were to be tried, proof of its efficacy should be sought. Specifically, calciuria would need be significantly reduced while both oxaluria and serum 1,25-dihydroxyvitamin D levels remain low.

A man with frequently recurrent kidney stones was found to have 7 mg/kg/d urinary calcium excretion when drinking tap water. When, however, he began to boil his water for 10 minutes (to lower the calcium content by precipitating calcium carbonate), urinary calcium excretion decreased to 3 mg/kg/d.

He subsequently remained free of symptoms during 3 years of follow-up (Popovtzer).

Magnesium

Kidney stones have repeatedly been produced in magnesium-deficient animals *(Hodgkinson)*. Total serum magnesium and erythrocyte magnesium levels may be low in recurrent stone formers *(Schmiedl)*. Perhaps 5% of stone formers have hypomagnesiuria *(Preminger,1990)*, and the urine of over 25% of stone formers has a lowered magnesium to calcium ratio *(Labeeuw)*. The hypomagnesiuria appears to be due to inadequate magnesium intake, as magnesium absorption following supplementation appears to be normal *(Johansson,1980)*.

Supplementation with magnesium salts may inhibit stone formation, even in patients without magnesium deficiency *(Johannson,1982)*. Magnesium decreases the urinary saturation of calcium oxalate by combining with urinary oxalate to form soluble magnesium oxalate *(Goldwasser)* so long as it is administered with meals *(Lindberg)*. In some studies, magnesium was combined with vitamin B_6 with good results *(Rattan)*.

Phosphorus

In stone formers, urinary phosphorus may be elevated, thus creating the risk of phosphate deficiency *(Schwille)*. Hyperphosphaturia appears to correlate with urinary calcium levels *(Kitamura)*; in fact, there is evidence that patients with idiopathic hypercalciuria excrete excessive phosphate for any given serum calcium concentration *(Williams)*.

Loss of phosphate may increase the activation of 1,25-dihydroxyvitamin D (see Vitamin D above) *(Williams)*. There also appears to be a failure of the kidneys to convert orthophosphate to pyrophosphate *(Conte,1989a)*.

Supplementation with orthophosphate reduces urinary calcium *(Palmqvist)* with reduction in calcium oxalate supersaturation and stone formation. However, unless baseline phosphate levels are low *(Alvarez-Arroyo)*, the reduction in stone formation appears to be limited *(Palmqvist)*, especially as compared to other treatments such as alkali citrate or magnesium *(Tiselius)*.

A 29-year-old insulin-dependent diabetic woman developed phosphate depletion, nephrolithiasis and bilateral ureteric obstruction due to antacid abuse. There were no musculoskeletal symptoms. Laboratory testing revealed hypophosphatemia, hypercalciuria, hypophosphaturia, elevated plasma, 1,25-dihydroxyvitamin D and low plasma intact parathyroid hormone.

These abnormalities were corrected when antacid ingestion was reduced and phosphate intake supplemented (Harmelin).

OTHER NUTRITIONAL FACTORS

Citrate

Hypocitraturia, which is found in roughly 15 to 30 percent of stone formers *(François;Menon)*, correlates with hypercalciuria in these patients *(Conte,1989b)*. In fact, people with recurrent stones are more likely to have hypocitraturia than those with first-time stones *(Yagisawa)*.

In open trials, potassium citrate supplementation in hypocitraturic stone formers has been shown to successfully reduce stone formation *(Pak,1986a; Whalley)*. Citrate augments inhibitor activity against calcium oxalate crystallization *(Harvey)* and reduces calcium excretion *(Khanniazi)*. Hyperuricosuric patients may also benefit *(Pak,1986b)*, as may patients with distal renal tubular acidosis *(Preminger,1985)*.

It appears possible to achieve at least some of these benefits of citrate supplementation with lemon juice. One of the richest food sources of citrate, lemon juice has been shown to decrease hypocitraturia and decrease urinary calcium excretion *(Seltzer)*.

Essential Fatty Acids

Patients with idiopathic calcium oxalate stones have a lower concentration of linoleic acid and a higher concentration of arachidonic acid in both plasma and erythrocyte membrane phospholipids *(Baggio,1996)*.

The administration of *fish oils* was found to reduce urinary calcium and oxalate excretion in these patients *(Baggio,1996;Buck,1991)*. This confirms the results of an animal study in which nephrocalcinosis following intraperitoneal injections of calcium gluconate was prevented by pre-treatment with fish oil *(Buck,1991)*.

The administration of *evening primrose oil*, a rich source of the omega-6 fatty acid gamma-linolenic acid, may also be beneficial. When rats were made hypercalciuric and diabetic, urine calcium excretion was significantly less in the animals that received the oil than in controls *(Tulloch)*.

Animal work has shown a synergism between the omega-3 fatty acid eicosapentaenoic acid (EPA) and the omega-6 fatty acid gamma-linolenic acid (GLA) in reducing renal parenchymal calcification *(Burgess)*. This combination was tested in a double-blind study in which recurrent stone formers received a mixture of fish and evening primrose oils with a EPA to GLA ratio of 1 to 4. Kidney stone formation was successfully reduced as well as hypercalciuria *(Buck,1993).*

Glycosaminoglycans

In vitro evidence suggests that glucosaminoglycans (GAGs) may be potent inhibitors of growth and aggregation of calcium oxalate crystals *in vitro* *(Michelacci).* Furthermore, stone formers may excrete less GAGs than normals *(Michelacci).*

In an open trial of patients with idiopathic calcium oxalate nephrolithiasis, supplementation of GAGs reduced renal clearance of oxalates *(Baggio,1991)*, suggesting that they may be beneficial in reducing stone formation.

COMBINED NUTRITIONAL INTERVENTIONS

A man who passed 15 calcium oxalate stones over 9 years had an increased 24-hour urinary oxalate excretion, a low normal calcium excretion, a high normal phosphate excretion, a low magnesium excretion, and a normal uric acid excretion. Serum calcium, phosphorus and uric acid were normal, but magnesium was slightly low. Hair calcium and phosphorus were high normal and hair magnesium was quite elevated, suggesting magnesium deficiency.

He was placed on chelated magnesium 100 mg twice daily and pyridoxine 50 mg twice daily. In addition, he was told to limit vitamin C to a maximum of 2 to 3 gm daily, to eliminate high-oxalate foods, and to limit calcium for the first few weeks.

Three months later, his tests for magnesium and oxalate were normal; after 6 months, his elevated hair magnesium had reduced to nearly normal. On follow-up 3 years later, he had not passed any stones (Wright).

OTHER RELATED FACTORS

Cadmium Toxicity

Cadmium exposure is associated with an increased prevalence of urolithiasis *(Scott).* Cadmium both damages the renal tubules which can lead to calcific foci in the kidneys *(Axellson)* and encourages oxalate crystallization *(Eusebio).*

Cadmium toxicity may be fairly widespread among stone formers. In one study, calcium oxalate stone formers were found to excrete significantly more cadmium than normals *(Elliot).*

BIBLIOGRAPHY

Alvarez-Arroyo MV et al. Correlation between 1.25 dihydroxyvitamin D serum levels and fractional rate of intestinal calcium absorption in hypercalciuric nephrolithiasis. Role of phosphate. Urol Res 20(1):96-7, 1992

Axellson B, Piscator M. Renal change after prolonged exposure to cadmium. Arch Environ Health 12:360-72, 1969

Baggio B et al. Correction of erythrocyte abnormalities in idiopathic calcium-oxalate nephrolithiasis and the reduction of urinary oxalate by oral glycosaminoglycans. Lancet 338:403-5, 1991

Baggio B et al. Anomalous phospholipid n-6 polyunsaturated fatty acid composition in idiopathic calcium nephrolithiasis. J Am Soc Nephrol 7(4):613-20, 1996

Bell R et al. The influence of NaCl and KCl on urinary calcium excretion in healthy young women. Nutr Res 12:17-26, 1992

Bendich A, Langseth L. The health effects of vitamin C supplementation: a review. J Am Coll Nutr 14(2):124-36, 1995

Bichler KH et al. Influence of vitamin A deficiency on the excretion of uromucoid and other substances in the urine of rats. Clin Nephrol 20:32-39, 1983

Blacklock NJ. Influence of diet on the formation of bladder and kidney stones. Nutr Health 2:89-99, 1983

Blacklock NJ. Sucrose and idiopathic renal stone. Nutr Health 5(1/2):9-17, 1987

Breslau NA. Pathogenesis and management of hypercalciuric nephrolithiasis. Miner Electrolyte Metab 2096):328-39, 1994

Brokis JG et al. The effects of vegetable and animal protein diets on calcium, urate and oxalate excretion. Br J Urol 54(6):590-3, 1982

Buck AC et al. The protective role of eicosapentaenoic acid [EPA] in the pathogenesis of nephrolithiasis. J Urol 146(1):188-94, 1991

Buck AC et al. The treatment of idiopathic recurrent urolithiasis with fish oil and evening primrose oil: a double blind study. Abstract. J Urol 149:253A, 1993

Burgess NA et al. Evaluation of four animal models of intrarenal calcium deposition and assessment of the influence of dietary supplementation with essential fatty acids on calcification. Urol Res 23(4):239-42, 1995

Burtis WJ et al. Dietary hypercalciuria in patients with calcium oxalate kidney stones. Am J Clin Nutr 60:424-9, 1994

Butz M et al. Dietary influence on serum and urinary oxalate in healthy subjects and oxalate stone formers. Urol Int 35:309-15, 1980

Chalmers AH et al. Stability of ascorbate in urine: relevance to analyses for ascorbate and oxalate. Clin Chem 31:1703, 1985

Coe FL et al. Effects of low-calcium diet on urine calcium excretion, parathyroid function and serum 1,25 (OH)2D3 levels in patients with idiopathic hypercalciuria and normal patients. Am J Med 72:25-32, 1982

Conte A et al. The relation between orthophosphate and pyrophosphate in normal subjects and in patients with urolithiasis. Urol Res 17(3):173-5, 1989a

Conte A et al. On the relation between citrate and calcium in normal and stone-former subjects. Int J Nephrol 21(4):369-73, 1989b

Curhan GC et al. A prospective study of dietary calcium and other nutrients and the risk of symptomatic kidney stones. N Engl J Med 328(12):833-8, 1993

Curhan GC et al. Prospective study of beverage use and the risk of kidney stones. Am J Epidemiol 143(3):240-7, 1996a

Curhan GC et al. A prospective study of the intake of vitamins C and B6, and the risk of kidney stones in men. J Urol 155:(6)1847-51, 1996b

Curhan GC et al. Comparison of dietary calcium with supplemental calcium and other nutrients as factors affecting the risk for kidney stones in women. Ann Intern Med 126:497-504, 1997

Diplock AT. Safety of antioxidant vitamins and β-carotene. Am J Clin Nutr 62(suppl):10S-16S, 1995

Elliot JS, Ribeiro ME. The urinary excretion of trace metals in patients with calcium oxalate urinary stone. Invest Urol 10:253-5, 1973

Eusebio E, Elliot JS. Effect of trace metals on crystallisation of calcium oxalate. Invest Urol 4:431, 1967

Fellström B et al. Dietary history and dietary records in renal stone patients and controls. Urol Res 12:58, 1984

François B et al. Inhibitors of urinary stone formation in 40 recurrent stone formers. Br J Urol 58(5):479-83, 1986

Gershoff SN, Prien EL. Excretion of urinary metabolites in calcium oxalate urolithiasis: Effect of tryptophan and vitamin B6 administration. Am J Clin Nutr 8:812, 1960

Gershoff SN, McGandy RB. The effects of vitamin A-deficient diets containing lactose in producing bladder calculi and tumors in rats. Am J Clin Nutr 34:483, 1981

Giannini L et al. Possible link between vitamin D and hyperoxaluria in patients with renal stone disease. Clin Sci 84:51-4, 1993

Gibbs DA, Watts RWE. The action of pyridoxine in primary hyperoxaluria. Clin Sci 38:277-86, 1970

Goldfarb S. Dietary factors in the pathogenesis and prophylaxis of calcium nephrolithiasis. Kidney Int 34:544-55, 1988

Goldwasser B et al. Calcium stone disease: An overview. J Urol 135:1, 1986

Green TJ, Whiting SJ. Potassium bicarbonate reduces high protein-induced hypercalciuria in adult men. Nutr Res 14:991-1002, 1994

Griffith HM et al. A control study of dietary factors in renal stone formation. Br J Urol 53:416-20, 1981

Grimm U et al. [Studies on tryptophan metabolism in calcium oxalate urolithiasis.] Z Urol Nephrol 81(5):299-303, 1988 (in German)

Harmelin DL et al. Antacid-induced phosphate depletion syndrome presenting as nephrolithiasis. Aust N Z J Med 20(6):803-5, 1990

Harvey JA et al. Calcium citrate: Reduced propensity for the crystallization of calcium oxalate in urine resulting from induced hypercalciuria of calcium supplementation. J Clin Endocrinol Metabol 61(6):1223-25, 1985

Heaney RP, Recker RR. Effects of nitrogen, phosphorus, and caffeine on calcium balance in women. J Lab Clin Med 99:46-55, 1982

Hiatt RA et al. Randomized controlled trial of a low animal protein, high fiber diet in the prevention of recurrent calcium oxalate kidney stones. Am J Epidemiol 144(1):25-33, 1996

Hodkinson A. Proc Roy Soc Med 51:970, 1958

Holmes RP et al. Dietary oxalate and its intestinal absorption. Scanning Microscopy 9(4):1109-20, 1995

Jahnen A et al. Dietary fibre: the effectiveness of a high bran intake in reducing renal calcium excretion. Urol Res 20(1):3-6, 1992

Jewett HJ et al. Does vitamin A deficiency exist in clinical urolithiasis? JAMA 121:566-69, 1943

Johansson G et al. Biochemical and clinical effects of the prophylactic treatment of renal calcium stones with magnesium hydroxide. J Urol 124:770-4, 1980

Johansson G et al. Effects of magnesium hydroxide in renal stone disease. J Am Coll Nutr 1(2):179-85, 1982

Jungers P et al. [Correlation between protein and sodium intake and calciuria in calcium lithiasis]. Nephrologie 14(6):287-90, 1993) (in French)

Kaneko K et al. Urinary calcium and calcium balance in young women affected by high protein diet of soy protein isolate and adding sulfur-containing amino acids and/or potassium. J Nutr Sci Vitaminol (Tokyo) 36(2):105-16, 1990

Khanam A et al. Role of vitamins in urolithiasis. Biomed Pharmacother 42(9):609-13, 1988

Khanniazi MK et al. Study of potassium citrate treatment of crystalluric nephrolithiasis. Biomed Pharmacother 47:25-8, 1993

Kitamura T et al. [Urinary calcium and phosphorus excretion and their relationship in calcium-containing urinary stone formers.] Nippon Hinyokika Gakkai Zasshi 80(2):197-203, 1989

Labeeuw et al. Magnesium in the physiopathology and treatment of renal calcium stones. Press Med 16:25-7, 1987

Lemann J et al. Potassium causes calcium retention in healthy adults. J Nutr 123:1623-6, 1993

Leonetti F et al. Dietary and urinary risk factors for stones in idiopathic calcium stone formers compared with healthy subjects. Nephrol Dial Transplant 13(3):617-22, 1998

Liebman M, Chai W. Effect of dietary calcium on urinary oxalate excretion after oxalate loads. Am J Clin Nutr 65:1453-9, 1997

Lindberg J et al. Effect of magnesium citrate and magnesium oxide on the crystallization of calcium salts in urine: changes produced by food-magnesium interaction. J Urol 143(2):248-51, 1990

Masai M et al. Effect of dietary intake on urinary oxalate excretion in calcium renal stone formers. Br J Urol 76(6):692-6, 1995

Massey LK, Berg TA. The effect of dietary caffeine on urinary excretion of calcium, magnesium, phosphorus, sodium, potassium, chloride and zinc in healthy males. Nutr Res 5:1281-4, 1985

Massey LK, Whiting SJ. Dietary salt, urinary calcium and kidney stone risk. Nutr Rev 53(5):131-9, 1995

Menon M, Mahle CJ. Urinary citrate excretion in patients with renal calculi. J Urol 129(6):1158-60, 1983

Michelacci YM et al. Urinary excretion of glycosaminoglycans in normal and stone forming subjects. Kidney Int 36(6):1022-8, 1989

Mitwalli A et al. Control of hyperoxaluria with large doses of pyridoxine in patients with kidney stones. Int J Nephrol 20(4):353-59, 1988

Modlin M. Urinary phosphorylated inositols and renal stone. Lancet ii:1113-14, 1980

Morgan LJ et al. Caffeine-induced hypercalciuria and renal prostaglandins: effect of aspirin and n-3 polyunsaturated fatty acids. Am J Clin Nutr 60:362-8, 1994

Noda S et al. Oxalate crystallization in the kidney in the presence of hyperuricemia. Scanning Microsc 3(3):829-35, 1989

Ohkawa T et al. Rice bran treatment for patients with hypercalciuric stones: experimental and clinical studies. J Urol 132(6):1140-5, 1984

Pacifici R et al. Effect of Ca and vitamin D supplementation on urinary calcium excretion in the adult female population. Abstract. J Am Coll Nutr 6(5):430, 1987

Pak CY, Fuller C. Idiopathic hypocitraturic calcium-oxalate nephrolithiasis successfully treated with potassium citrate. Ann Intern Med 104:33-37, 1986a

Pak CY, Peterson R. Successful treatment of hyperuricosuric calcium oxalate nephrolithiasis with potassium citrate. Arch Intern Med 146(5):863-7, 1986b

Palmqvist E, Tiselius HG. Phosphate treatment of patients with renal calcium stone disease. Urol Int 43(1):24-28, 1988

Popovtzer MM et al. Letter. N Engl J Med 310(11):721, 1984

Preminger GM et al. Prevention of recurrent calcium stone formation with potassium citrate therapy in patients with renal tubular acidosis. J Urol 134(1):20-3, 1985

Preminger G et al. Hypomagnesiuric hypocitraturia. An apparent new entity for calcium nephrolithiasis. J Lithotripsy Stone Dis, 1990

Rao PN. Dietary habit and urolithiasis, in DLJ Freed, Ed. Health Hazards of Milk. London, Balliere Tindall, 1984

Rattan VF et al. Effect of combined supplementation of magnesium oxide and pyridoxine in calcium-oxalate stone formers. Urol Res 22(3):161-5, 1994

Revusova V et al. The significance of oxaluria reduction by pyridoxine in prevention of calcium oxalate nephrolithiasis. Cas Lek Ces 121(6):163-6, 1982

Robertson WG et al. Should recurrent calcium oxalate stone formers become vegetarian? Br J Urol 51:427-31, 1979

Robertson WG et al. Epidemiological risk factors in calcium stone disease. Scand J Urol Nephrol 53(suppl):15-30, 1980

Robertson WG et al. The prevalence of urinary stone disease in vegetarians. Eur Urol 8:334, 1982

Rodgers AL. Effect of mineral water containing calcium and magnesium on calcium oxalate urolithiasis risk factors. Urol Int 58(2):93-9, 1997

Rao RN et al. Dietary management of urinary risk factors in renal stone formers. Br J Urol 54:578-83, 1982

Ruml LA et al. Medical therapy: calcium oxalate urolithiasis. Urolithiasis 24(1):117-33, 1997

Sakly R et al. [Antilithogenic and litholytic action of vitamin A vis-a-vis experimental calculi in rats]. Ann Urol (Paris) 28(3):128-31, 1994) (in French)

Schmiedl A, Schwille P. Magnesium status in idiopathic calcium urolithiasis - An orientational study in younger males. Eur J Clin Chem Clin Biochem 34:393-40, 1996

Schwille PO et al. Urinary phosphate excretion in the pathophysiology of idiopathic recurrent calcium urolithiasis: hormonal interactions and lipid metabolism. Urol Res 25(6):417-26, 1997

Scott R et al. The importance of cadmium as a factor in calcified upper urinary stone disease - A prospective 7-year study. Br J Urol 54:584, 1982

Seltzer MA et al. Dietary manipulation with lemonade to treat hypocitraturic calcium nephrolithiasis. J Urol 156(3):907-9, 1996

Shah PJ et al. Idiopathic hypercalciuria: its control with unprocessed bran. Br J Urol 52(6):426-29, 1980

Shuster J et al. Water hardness and urinary stone disease. J Urol 128:422-5, 1982

Shuster J et al. Soft-drink consumption and urinary-stone recurrence: a randomized prevention trial. J Clin Epidemiol 45:911-16, 1992

Siener R, Hesse A. [The effect of different food forms on the urine composition and the risk of calcium oxalate stone formation]. Z Ernahrungswiss 32(1):46-55, 1993) (in German)

Sierakowski R et al. Stone incidence as related to water hardness in different geographical regions in the United States. Urol Res 7:157-60, 1979

Silver J et al. Sodium-dependent idiopathic hypercalciuria in renal-stone formers. Lancet ii:484-6, 1983

Smith IH et al. Nutrition and urolithiasis. N Engl J Med 298:87-89, 1978

Tiselius HG, Sandvall K. How are urine composition and stone disease affected by therapeutic measures at an outpatient stone clinic? Eur Urol 17(3):206-12, 1990

Tulloch I et al. Evening primrose oil reduces urinary calcium excretion in both normal and hypercalciuric rats. Urol Res 22(4):227-30, 1994

Unwin R et al. Grand round: unraveling the molecular mechanisms of kidney stones. Lancet 348:1561-5, 1996

Vahlensieck W. Review: The importance of diet in urinary stones. Urol Res 14(6):283-8, 1986

Wandzilak TR et al. Effect of high dose vitamin C on urinary oxalate levels. J Urol 151:834-7, 1994

Wasserstein A. The calcium stone former with osteoporosis. JAMA 257(16):2215, 1987

Whalley NA et al. Long-term effects of potassium citrate therapy on the formation of new stones in groups of recurrent stone formers with hypocitraturia. Br J Urol 78:10-14, 1996

Will EJ, Bijvoet OL. Primary oxalosis: Clinical and biochemical response to high-dose pyridoxine therapy. Metabolism 28(5):542-8, 1979

Williams CP et al. Inappropriate phosphate excretion in idiopathic hypercalciuria: the key to a common cause and future treatment? J Clin Pathol 49(11):881-8, 1996

Wright JV. Dr. Wright's Book of Nutritional Therapy. Emmaus, Penn., Rodale Press, 1979

Yagisawa T et al. Metabolic risk factors in patients with first-time and recurrent stone formations as determined by comprehensive metabolic evaluation. Urology 52(5):750-5, 1998

Yoshida O. Epidemiology of urolithiasis in Japan. Jap U Urol 70:975-83, 1979

Zarembski PM, Hodgkinson. Some factors increasing the urinary excretion of oxalate in man. Clin Chim Acta 25:1-10, 1969

LEARNING DISORDERS

See Also: ATTENTION-DEFICIT HYPERACTIVITY DISORDER

NUTRITIONAL TREATMENT GUIDE

✓ = Efficacy generally accepted.
* = Efficacy *demonstrated* by controlled human trials.
[+] = Efficacy *suspected* from uncontrolled human trials.
[-] = Efficacy *suspected* from indirect data.
? = Efficacy *challenged* in a study of similar design.

DIETARY FACTORS

✓ avoid **Malnutrition**

- -

* ? avoid **Sugar** (especially when consumed away from meals)

- -

[+] eat a **Diet Balanced in Protein, Fat, Complex Carbohydrate and Fiber**

- -

[-] avoid **Refined Carbohydrates**
[-] avoid chronic, high **Caffeine** intake

NUTRITIONAL FACTORS

✓ **Iron deficiency:** 30 mg twice daily until repletion (adult dosage); then minimal possible dosage

- -

* **Docosahexaenoic acid (DHA):** 420 mg daily (adult dosage)
* **Choline:** phosphatidylcholine ? 25 g 3 times daily (25 g supplies 3.75 g choline)
* **Thiamine deficiency:** 50 mg daily

- -

[+] **Magnesium deficiency:** ≈ 400 mg daily (adult dosage)
[+] **Vitamin C deficiency:** 50 mg daily (for children and adolescents)
[+] **Zinc deficiency:** adult dosage: zinc sulfate 220 mg twice daily *AND* **Copper** 2 mg daily

- -

[-] **Iodine deficiency:** 90 to 300 μg daily
[-] avoid **Manganese** toxicity

OTHER RELATED FACTORS

[+] rule out **Food Sensitivities**

- -

[-] rule out **Aluminum** toxicity
[-] rule out **Cadmium** toxicity
[-] rule out **Lead** toxicity

DIETARY FACTORS

The diet must be nutritionally adequate, as malnutrition is a known cause of learning failure *(Galler)*. Eating breakfast primarily appears to improve learning in children who are poorly nourished *(Hill)*.

While it has been well documented that adequate caloric intake is important, equally as important is proper balance of the macronutrients. A balanced diet should minimize the danger of a neuroglycopenic ('hypoglycemic') response to sugar ingestion which could interfere with learning *(Jones)*. (See 'Hypoglycemia'.)

Sugar

Findings from the numerous research studies investigating the effects of sugar ingestion on learning have been highly conflicting. There is evidence that sugar ingestion may adversely affect learning. For example, consumption of the amount of glucose in two 12-ounce cans of cola was followed by a fall in plasma glucose concentration which was sufficient to induce hormonal, symptomatic, and neurophysiologic changes in healthy children *(Jones)*.

In a double-blind study, when normal preschool children received 6 ounces of juice sweetened with sucrose, they showed a performance decrement in a structured testing situation and demonstrated more inappropriate behavior during free play; these changes did not occur when the juice was sweetened with an artificial sweetener *(Goldman)*. Also, children, but not adults, exhibit a dramatic rise in blood adrenalin levels after the equivalent of 2 frosted cupcakes for breakfast, suggesting that they may be particularly prone to anxiety, irritability and difficulty concentrating following a sugary meal *(Tamborlane)*.

Most of the research, however, suggests that acute sucrose ingestion is not a common cause of learning problems in children *(Wolraich)*. This is probably because any adverse effects of sugar, such as the neuroglycopenic response referred to earlier, are usually mitigated by the presence of other macronutrients in the diet when the sugar is consumed as part of a balanced meal *(Conners)*.

Refined Carbohydrates

In a study of 184 children aged 5 to 16 years published in the *Annals of the New York Academy of Sciences*, of all the dietary measures, only the proportion of refined foods in the diet was significantly related to reading performance. It accounted for 2.59% of the reading score variance *(Thatcher, 1984)*.

While the findings of this study fail to prove that refined carbohydrates adversely affect learning, there is a plausible rationale for this finding: Zinc is more concentrated in the germ and bran of grains, while cadmium is more concentrated in the endosperm; thus refined carbohydrates have a much lower zinc to cadmium ratio than whole grains *(Schoeder)*.

Evidence for the relevance of this ratio comes from a study of 150 children aged 5 to 16 years. The proportion of refined carbohydrates in the diet was positively related to hair cadmium concentrations and negatively correlated with intelligence and school achievement scores, suggesting that the consumption of refined low-nutrient foods increases the body cadmium burden. (Also see Cadmium Toxicity below.)

Furthermore, the relationship between diet and cognitive functioning remained even after the effects of cadmium, age, sex, socioeconomic status, and race were regressed out *(Lester, 1982)*. These findings add to the evidence cited above which suggests that the consumption of foods both high in sucrose and low in nutrient density may contribute to childhood learning disorders.

Caffeine

Since caffeinism is characterized by heightened anxiety, depression and various psychophysiological reactions, investigators have begun to explore the relationship between caffeine consumption and learning. Evidence suggesting a relationship comes from a survey of college students which found that heavy caffeine consumers reported poorer academic performance than abstainers *(Gilliland)*.

Moreover, the apparently beneficial effects of caffeine on psychomotor performance may actually be due to the cessation of caffeine withdrawal symptoms *(James)*. The well-known stimulant effect of caffeine which is utilized by students to maintain alertness in learning situations may thus also be partly due to the same mechanism.

However, controlled clinical trials are needed before any conclusions can be drawn.

NUTRITIONAL FACTORS

VITAMINS

In addition to the known adverse effects of classical vitamin deficiency diseases on learning, there are a few studies whose results suggest that marginal vitamin deficiencies (which are far more common in industrialized societies) may adversely affect learning.

Thiamine Deficiency

Overt thiamine deficiency is well known to produce Wernicke-Korsakoff syndrome, a memory disorder. Evidence that a marginal thiamine deficiency may impair learning comes from a 1946 study of children living at an orphanage whose diets were supplemented with thiamine. Compared to their baselines, their performances on a battery of tests of intellectual function significantly improved *(Harrel)*.

More recently, 31% of a group of epileptics taking phenytoin were found to have reduced blood levels of thiamine and received supplementation of the vitamin under placebo-controlled conditions. After 6 months, thiamine-supplemented patients showed significant improvements in both the verbal and nonverbal scales of the Weschler IQ scale. Specific improvements suggested that thiamine improved such neuropsychological functions as visuospatial analysis, visuomotor speed and verbal abstracting ability *(Botez)*.

Vitamin C Deficiency

While little has been done to investigate the effects of marginal vitamin C nutriture on learning, there is an intriguing study in which 72 pairs of students (kindergarten to college) were matched on the basis of socioeconomic levels and then divided into higher and lower plasma ascorbic acid groups.

The average IQ of the higher ascorbic acid group was found to be significantly greater than that of the lower ascorbic acid group. Both groups then received supplementary orange juice for 6 months. Afterwards, the average IQ of the lower ascorbic acid group increased significantly more than did that of the higher ascorbic acid group.

The average IQ of students in the lower ascorbic acid group was raised by 3.6 units when plasma ascorbic acid was increased by 50%. This is the same as increasing dietary vitamin C for the average adult from 100 mg to 150 mg daily.

The study was subsequently continued with 32 pairs of students for a second school year. The results were similar. *(Kubala)*.

MINERALS

Copper Toxicity

Several studies have found hair copper to be higher in learning disabled *(Rimland)* and dyslexic *(Capel)* children than in normal controls, and one study found both hair and sweat copper concentrations to be higher in dyslexic children than in matched controls *(Grant)*.

The explanation for this finding is unknown, but could well be related to reduced zinc nutriture (see Zinc below), since copper reduces zinc absorption *(Castillo-Durán)*, while zinc decreases copper absorption *(Bremmer)*.

Iodine Deficiency

In studies from India *(Tiwari)*, Sicily *(Vermiglio)*, and China *(Boyages)*, iodine deficiency in childhood has been shown to be associated with cognitive impairment, poor motivation to achieve, and defective visual perceptual integrative motor ability.

Iron Deficiency

Infants with iron deficiency anemia have lower mental and motor developmental scores *(Lozoff)*. Among older children, iron deficiency appears to interfere with specific neurophysiological processes supporting attention *(Tucker)*.

Double-blind studies have shown that iron-deficient adolescent girls, including those with non-anemic iron deficiency, may improve on measures of verbal learning and memory with supplementation *(Ballin;Bruner)*. Moreover, 4 months after starting iron supplementation, non-anemic iron-deficient preschool children, who at baseline had poorer learning ability and long-term memory retention, no longer showed differences from normal controls *(Pollitt)*.

However, the cognitive defects found in children with iron-deficiency anemia during infancy may persist *(Walter)*, and some iron-deficient children may continue to have lower developmental IQ and achievement test scores after iron repletion *(Lozoff)*.

Magnesium Deficiency

Chronically magnesium-deficient children often have normal IQ scores, yet may present with learning problems. They display excess fidgeting, anxious restlessness and psychomotor instability *(Durlach)*.

Manganese Toxicity

Manganese toxicity particularly affects the central nervous system *(Donaldson)*. Observational studies have found that learning disabled children tend to have higher hair manganese levels than normals *(Pihl)*. It has been postulated that infant formulas, which may contain 3 to 100 times the manganese content of breast milk, may contribute to a manganese overload *(Collipp)*.

Due to its inhibitory effect on iron absorption, elevated manganese may promote the development of iron deficiency. More studies are needed to confirm a relationship between manganese toxicity and learning disorders.

Selenium Toxicity

Hair selenium is a useful measure of selenium intake *(Gallagher)*, and at least two studies have found evidence suggesting that elevated hair selenium levels may be associated with learning problems. The first study, which investigated 400 public school children, found that learning disabled children had significantly higher hair selenium than normal controls, and learning disabled children who were in special classes had significantly higher hair selenium than those who remained in the regular classroom *(Ely)*.

The second study, which investigated 120 public school children, found a significant direct correlation between hair selenium and scores on the Walker Problem Behavior Identification Checklist scales measuring acting out, withdrawal, and total scale score *(Marlowe,1986)*.

Consistent with these findings, selenium toxicity has been associated with both irritability and lassitude, and these behavioral changes could cause learning disabilities. However, further studies are needed before it can be concluded that excessive selenium intake is a cause of learning problems.

Zinc Deficiency

Although hair zinc levels in 26 dyslexic children were not significantly different from those of normal controls, their sweat zinc was only 66% that of controls, a significant difference *(Grant)*. Since sweat zinc is a reliable measure of zinc status, while hair zinc may fail to reflect zinc deficiency, these findings suggest that at least some dyslexic children may have reduced zinc nutriture.

Zinc-deficient children are irritable, tearful and sullen, and would therefore be prone to developing learning disabilities. Moreover, adequate zinc nutriture may protect against the neurotoxic effects of cadmium which interferes with biochemical processes catalyzed by zinc by displacing it. Consistent with this hypothesis, the results of a study of school-aged children suggested that the degree of negative correlation between cadmium and cognitive performance depended upon hair zinc concentrations *(Lester,1985)*.

OTHER NUTRITIONAL FACTORS

Choline

The cholinergic system is implicated in normal learning and memory function *(Durkin)*. In animal models, cholinergic agents have been shown to stimulate consciousness and the reticular activating system *(Yasuhara)*.

Results of human and animal studies suggest that

supplementation with cholinergic agents may be temporarily helpful in improving serial learning, especially for slow learners *(Gillin;Ladd)*, as well as for improving memory function in children with developmental *(Woodbury)* problems.

Studies are needed to assess whether these effects improve learning over the long term.

Two 4-year-old children with multiple developmental problems received choline starting at 500 mg/d and titrated up to 3 g daily. The fish-like odor was used as a signal that the maximum dose had been passed; then the dose was decreased until no odor was secreted.

After several months, both showed improvements as documented by the Denver Developmental Screening Test, the abbreviated version of the Conner's Scale, and psychiatric follow-up (Woodbury).

Omega-3 Fatty Acids

There is evidence that the occurrence of learning problems is correlated with reduced total plasma omega-3 fatty acid concentrations as well as with symptoms of essential fatty acid deficiency including thirst, frequent urination and dry skin *(Stevens)*.

Research interest specifically in regard to dyslexia has focused on docosahexaenoic acid (DHA), an omega-3 fatty acid which is a key fatty acid in both the brain and the retina and is present in large quantities in these tissues *(Stordy)*. In dyslexia, there is evidence for reduced incorporation of DHA into cell membranes *(Horrobin)*. Moreover, in addition to their obvious central processing defects, dyslexics have retinal processing defects *(Galaburda;Grosser)*; for example, they have poorer dark adaptation than normals *(Stordy)*.

One month after 5 dyslexics and 5 normal controls started supplementation with DHA, the dyslexics with poor scotopic vision had consistent and significant improvements in dark adaptation, while only one of the controls, a vegan, clearly improved *(Stordy)*.

Studies are badly needed to ascertain whether DHA supplementation also enhances learning, at least in this specific population.

COMBINED NUTRITIONAL INTERVENTIONS:

Many controlled studies have investigated the effects of dietary changes, sometimes along with nutritional supplementation, upon intelligence and academic performance. Long-term improvements have been found in several studies *(Benton)*. Other studies, however, have failed to find evidence of efficacy *(Nelson)*, possibly because the populations studied were not limited to children preselected on the basis of screening criteria that are appropriate for the specific experimental intervention. For example, dietary changes designed to improve nutritional status would most likely benefit children with a poor nutritional status, while elimination diets would most likely benefit children who have been found to be sensitive to foods or food additives.

Perhaps the largest and most intriguing study involved 803 New York City public schools. Over 4 years, these schools introduced a diet policy which lowered sucrose and synthetic food additives. While, on a standardized test, there had usually been less than a 1% annual change in mean academic percentile ranking as compared to the rest of the nation's schools, there was a 15.7% increase following the dietary change. In addition, each school's academic performance ranking was negatively correlated with the percent of children who ate school food prior to the dietary change and, after the change, the percent of children who ate school meals within each school became positively correlated with that school's rate of gain in mean academic percentile ranking *(Schoenthaler)*.

OTHER RELATED FACTORS

Food Sensitivities

Experimental studies proving a relationship between food sensitivities and learning disorders are lacking. This lack of evidence is striking when one considers that a large number of studies have found a relationship between food sensitivities and attention-deficit hyperactivity disorder (ADHD), since ADHD is believed to be a contributor to the development of learning disabilities.

Despite the lack of an experimental literature, clinicians have encountered patients for whom food sensitivities appeared to play an important etiologic role:

> *Two days after delivery, a white male infant developed a severe rash. The rash became chronic; later it was diagnosed as eczema. He also developed difficulty pronouncing words, spoke in incomplete sentences and appeared forgetful and confused. His symptoms were so severe that he was unable to sit quietly in class and failed to learn at a normal rate.*
>
> *In the second grade, his mother tried a Feingold salicylate and food additive elimination diet as well as nutritional supplements with uncertain results. He was seen at the Learning Disabilities Unit of the Massachusetts General Hospital in Boston where he was diagnosed as having a Learning Disorder with Developmental Dyslexia. Individualized teaching was unsuccessful due to "hyperactivity, distractibility, moodiness and unpredictable behavior."*
>
> *When examined at age 9 ½, his face was stark white, while his eyes were edematous and black. He had constant pruritus with scabs and scars from scratching, and over-reacted to loud noises.*
>
> *All dairy products were removed from his diet. Four days later, he had an episode of violent behavior; afterwards he became relatively calm and his school behavior markedly improved. The presence of multiple sensitivities was confirmed by placing solutions of various substances under his tongue. Numerous foods and chemicals provoked reactions, including changes in behavior and penmanship, fluid retention, nasal discharge and sneezing (Challem).*

Aluminum Toxicity

There is evidence that aluminum toxicity may play a role in learning problems. For example, compared to controls, serum aluminum levels were elevated in a group of 28 children with learning disorders or hyperactivity *(Howard)*. Similarly, hair aluminum has been found to be elevated in some of the studies of dyslexic or learning disabled children *(Capel;Marlowe,1984)*.

Lead Toxicity

The evidence of an adverse effect upon learning is strongest for lead *(Dudek;Tong)*. A meta-analysis of 24 studies found that the hypothesis that low-level lead exposure impairs children's IQ was strongly supported *(Needleman)*.

This is a serious public health problem. It is estimated, for example, that between 10 and 50 percent of American children harbor unsafe lead levels *(Preuss)*. In fact, the American Academy of Pediatrics recommends that, as part of their routine health care, all children undergo blood lead screening when they are 9 to 12 months old and again at age 2.

While prevention is obviously preferable, chelation therapy can improve the cognitive performance of children with moderate lead poisoning *(Ruff)*.

***AND/OR* Cadmium Toxicity**

When 26 dyslexic children aged 6 to 14 were compared to controls, they tended to have higher lead and cadmium concentrations in both sweat and hair *(Grant)*. Similarly, when 150 unselected school children were evaluated, polynomial regression analysis of either hair lead or cadmium concentrations as the independent variables and WISC-R verbal and performance IQ scores as the dependent variables showed a continuous negative relationship between intelligence measures and both dependent variables.

Further analysis suggested that lead independently accounted for a significant amount of the performance but not verbal IQ variance, while the reverse was true for cadmium *(Thatcher,1985)*.

COMBINED TREATMENT REGIMEN

In the sixth grade, even though intelligence tests showed Michael to be in the high-average range, he had difficulty in understanding the meaning of printed words. Neurological examination revealed only slight clumsiness of gross motor activity and he was diagnosed as dyslexic.

On examination, he had very dry, patchy, dull skin, and both his skin and his hair failed to reflect light with a normal luster. His hair was easily tousled and, when pulled between the fingers, it had a straw-like texture. He had dandruff and "chicken skin" (follicular hyperkeratosis) on the back of his arms, and his fingernails were soft and frayed at the ends. As these findings suggested an essential fatty acid imbalance, his blood was tested for essential fatty acids. Results suggested a need for larger amounts of polyunsaturated fats and less saturated fats in his diet. Also, laboratory studies revealed evidence of vitamin B_6, iron and zinc deficiencies.

He was placed on linseed and evening primrose oils, told to reduce saturated fats in his diet, and supplemented with vitamins and minerals as well as with additional vitamin B_6 in the form of pyridoxal phosphate. A marked symptomatic improvement ensued which coincided with the return of normal luster and texture to his skin and hair.

Also, his history had revealed milk intolerance in infancy, so he was asked to avoid all dairy products for 5 days and then to challenge himself with them. His stuffy nose cleared noticeably by the fifth day; when he returned to dairy products he became congested, cranky and "spacey." He therefore agreed to avoid them.

Less than one year after starting treatment, he was doing well in school and catching up in reading (Baker).

BIBLIOGRAPHY

Ballin A et al. Iron state in female adolescents. Am J Dis Child 146(7):803-5, 1992

Baker S McD. A biochemical approach to the problem of dyslexia. J Learn Disabil 18(10):581-4, 1985

Benton D. Vitamin and mineral intake and cognitive function, in A Bendich, CE Butterworth, Eds. Micronutrients in Health and in Disease. New York, Marcel Dekker, 1991

Botez MI et al. Thiamine and folate treatment of chronic epileptic patients: a controlled study with the Wechsler IQ scale. Epilepsy Res 16:157-63, 1993

Boyages SC et al. Iodine deficiency impairs intellectual and neuromotor development in apparently-normal persons. A study of rural inhabitants of north-central China. Med J Aust 150(12):676-82, 1989

Bremner I, Beattie JH. Copper and zinc metabolism in health and disease: speciation and interactions. Proc Nutr Soc 54:489-99, 1995

Bruner AB et al. Randomized study of cognitive effects of iron supplementation in non-anaemic iron-deficient adolescent girls. Lancet 348:992-6, 1996

Capel ID et al. Comparison of concentrations of some trace, bulk, and toxic metals in the hair of normal and dyslexic children. Clin Chem 27(6):879-81, 1981

Castillo-Durán C et al. Oral copper supplementation: effect on copper and zinc balance during acute gastroenteritis in infants. Am J Clin Nutr 51:1088-92, 1990

Challem JJ, Lewin R. The miracle of little Andy Alexander. Lets Live May, 1983, pp. 32-9

Collipp PJ. Manganese in infant formulas and learning disability. Ann Nutr Metab 27:488-94, 1983

Conners CK - reported in Medical Tribune January 9, 1985

Donaldson J. The physiopathologic significance of manganese in brain: its relation to schizophrenia and neurodegenerative disorders. Neurotoxicology 8(3):451-62, 1987

Dudek B, Merecz D. Impairment of psychological functions in children environmentally exposed to lead. Int J Occup Med Environ Health 10(1):37-46, 1997

Durkin T. Central cholinergic pathways and learning and memory processes: presynaptic aspects. Comp Biochem Physiol 93:273-80, 1989

Durlach J. Clinical aspects of chronic magnesium deficiency, in MS Seelig, Ed. Magnesium in Health and Disease. New York Spectrum Publications, 1980

Ely DL et al. Aerometric and hair trace metal content in learning disabled. Environ Res 25:325-39, 1981

Galaburda A, Livingstone M. Evidence for a magnocellular defect in developmental dyslexia. Ann N Y Acad Sci 682:71-81, 1993

Gallagher ML et al. Selenium levels in new growth hair and in whole blood during injection of a selenium supplement for six weeks. Nutr Res 4:577-82, 1984

Galler JR. Malnutrition - a neglected cause of learning failure. Postgrad Med 80:225-30, 1986

Gilliland K, Andress D. Ad lib caffeine consumption, symptoms of caffeinism, and academic performance. Am J Psychiatry 138(4):512-14, 1981

Gillin JC et al. Effects of lecithin on memory and plasma choline levels: a study in normal volunteers, in G Pepeu, H Ladinsky, Eds. Cholinergic Mechanisms. New York, Plenum Press:937-45, 1981

Goldman JA et al. Behavioral effects of sucrose on preschool children. J Abnorm Child Psychol 14(4):656-77, 1986

Grant ECG et al. Zinc deficiency in children with dyslexia: Concentrations of zinc and other minerals in sweat and hair. Br Med J 296:607-9, 1988

Grosser GS, Spafford CS. Light sensitivity in peripheral retinal fields of dyslexic and proficient readers. Perceptual Motor Skills 71:467-77, 1990

Harrel RF. Mental response to added thiamine. J Nutr 31:283, 1946

Hill GM. The impact of breakfast especially ready-to-eat cereals on nutrient intake and health of children. Nutr Res 15(4):595-613, 1995

Horrobin DF et al. Possible relevance of phospholipid abnormalities and genetic interactions in psychiatric disorders: the relationship between dyslexia and schizophrenia. Med Hypotheses 45(6):605-13, 1995

Howard JMH. Clinical import of small increases in serum aluminum. Clin Chem 30(10):1722-3, 1984

James JE. Caffeine and psychomotor performance. Neuropsychobiology 31:202-3, 1995

Jones TW et al. Enhanced adrenomedullary response and increased susceptibility to neuroglycopenia: mechanisms underlying the adverse effects of sugar ingestion in healthy children. Pediatrics 126(2):171-7, 1995

Kubala AL, Katz MM. Nutritional factors in psychological test behavior. J Genet Psychol 96:343-52, 1960

Ladd SL et al. Effect of phosphatidylcholine on explicit memory. Clin Neuropharmacol 16(6):540-9, 1993

Lester ML et al. Refined carbohydrate intake, hair cadmium levels and cognitive functioning in children. Nutr Behav 1:3-13, 1982

Lester ML et al. Protective effects of calcium and zinc against heavy metal impairment of cognitive function - summarized in Thatcher RW, Lester ML. Nutrition, environmental toxins and computerized EEG: A mini-max approach to learning disabilities. J Learn Disabil 18(5):287-97, 1985

Lozoff B. Iron and learning potential in childhood. Bull N Y Acad Med 65(10):1050-66, 1989

Marlowe M et al. Hair selenium levels and children's classroom behavior. J Orthomol Med 1(2):91-6, 1986

Marlowe M et al. Hair mineral content as a predictor of learning disabilities. J Learn Disabil 17(7):418-21, 1984

Needleman HL, Gatsonis CA. Los-level lead exposure and the IQ of children. A meta-analysis of modern studies. JAMA 263(5):673-8, 1990

Nelson M. Workshop on 'nutrition and the school child' - food, vitamins and IQ. Proc Nutr Soc 50:29-35, 1991

Pihl RO, Parkes M. Hair element content in learning disabled children. Science 198:204-6, 1977

Pollitt E. Cognitive effects of iron deficiency anaemia. Letter. Lancet i:158, 1985

Preuss HG. A review of persistent, low-grade lead challenge: neurological and cardiovascular consequences. J Am Coll Nutr 12(3):246-54, 1993

Rimland B, Larson GE. Hair mineral analysis and behavior: an analysis of 51 studies. J Learn Disabil 16(5):279-85, 1983

Ruff HA et al. Declining blood lead levels and cognitive changes in moderately lead-poisoned children. JAMA 269(13):1679-81, 1993

Schoeder HA. Losses of vitamins and trace minerals resulting from processing and preservation of foods. Am J Clin Nutr 24:562-73, 1971

Schoenthaler SJ. The impact of a low food additive and sucrose diet on academic performance in 803 New York City public schools. Int J Biosoc Res 8(2):185-95, 1986

Stevens LJ et al. Omega-3 fatty acids in boys with behavior, learning and health problems. Physiol Behav 59(4-5):915-20, 1996

Stordy BJ. Benefit of docosahexaenoic acid supplements to dark adaptation in dyslexics. Letter. Lancet 346:385:1995

Tamborlane WV, professor of pediatrics, Yale School of Medicine, and Jones, TM, visiting scientist from Australia - reported in The New York Times, 1990

Thatcher RW et al. Comparisons among EEG, hair minerals and diet predictions of reading performance in children. Ann NY Acad Sci 433:87-96, 1984

Thatcher RW, Lester ML. Nutrition, environmental toxins and computerized EEG: A mini-max approach to learning disabilities. J Learn Disabil 18(5):287-97, 1985

Tiwari BD et al. Learning disabilities and poor motivation to achieve due to prolonged iodine deficiency. Am J Clin Nutr 63:782-6, 1996

Tong S et al. Lifetime exposure to environmental lead and children's intelligence at 11-13 years: The Port Pirie Cohort Study. BMJ 312:1569-75, 1996

Tucker DM et al. Iron status and brain function: Serum ferritin levels associated with asymmetries of cortical electrophysiology and cognitive performance. Am J Clin Nutr 39(1):105-13, 1984

Vermiglio F et al. Defective neuromotor and cognitive ability in iodine-deficient schoolchildren of an endemic goiter region in Sicily. J Clin Endocrinol Metab 70(2):379-84, 1990

Walter T. Impact of iron deficiency on cognition in infancy and childhood. Eur J Clin Nutr 47:307-16, 1993

Wolraich ML et al. The effect of sugar on behavior or cognition in children. JAMA 274:1617-21, 1995

Woodbury MM, Woodbury MA. Neuropsychiatric development: two case reports about the use of dietary fish oils and/or choline supplementation in children. J Am Coll Nutr 12(3):239-45, 1993

Yasuhara M, Naito H. Characteristic actions of CDP choline on the central nervous system. Curr Ther Res 16:346-74, 1974

LUPUS

NUTRITIONAL TREATMENT GUIDE

✓ = Efficacy generally accepted.
* = Efficacy *demonstrated* by controlled human trials.
[+] = Efficacy *suspected* from uncontrolled human trials.
[-] = Efficacy *suspected* from indirect data.
? = Efficacy *challenged* in a study of similar design.

DIETARY FACTORS

[+] **low Phenylalanine, low Tyrosine diet** *(for chronic discoid lupus)* (A **Vegan diet** qualifies.)

- -

[-] **low Calorie, low Fat diet**

NUTRITIONAL FACTORS

* **Omega-3 fatty acids:** *example:* MaxEPA 20 g daily (180 mg EPA & 120 mg DHA per gram)

- -

[+] **Beta-carotene:** *for sun sensitivity in discoid lupus:* 50 mg 3 times daily
[+] **Magnesium deficiency:** ≈ 400 mg daily (Consider IM or IV administration, especially in hypomagnesemia.)
[+] **Niacin:** ? 200 mg niacin (or niacinamide) daily
[+] **Selenium:** 200 μg daily *AND*
Vitamin E (tocopheryl succinate)10 mg daily
[+] **Vitamin B_{12}:** ? 1,000 μg intramuscularly daily
[+] ? **Pantothenic acid:** ? 10 g daily
[+] ? **Vitamin E:** ? 1,200-1,600 IU daily

- -

[-] avoid **Tryptophan** supplementation

OTHER RELATED FACTORS

[+] rule out **Food Sensitivities**

DIETARY FACTORS

Low Calorie, Low Fat Diet

The results of studies using an animal model of systemic lupus erythematosus (SLE) have suggested that diets high in fat may affect the onset and severity of the disease by weakening immune responses *(Morrow)*. A low calorie, low fat diet appears to be beneficial *(Corman)*.

Low Phenylalanine, Low Tyrosine Diet

There is evidence suggesting that patients should avoid both dietary and supplemental sources of phenylalanine and its metabolite, tyrosine. L-tyrosine supplementation aggravated the clinical symptoms of 4 out of 5 patients with diffuse collagen diseases. One of these patients, for example, was a woman with subacute disseminated lupus erythematosus. When she received 1 gram of L-tyrosine daily, her lesion became reddish.

This effect appears to be due to a specific intermediary block in phenylalanine and tyrosine metabolism which was confirmed in all of a group of 18 patients with various forms of lupus *(Nishimura,1958)*.

The results of treating 3 hospitalized women with chronic discoid lupus with a diet that minimized phenylalanine (1.1 g daily) and tyrosine were reported in the *Archives of Dermatology* in 1959. Steroids and ACTH were avoided. All had excellent recoveries even though one of the patients (who also had acute exacerbations) had failed to respond to previous treatments. In her case, despite a history of repeated episodes of pyrexia, her temperature normalized after 5 days and an ulcerative lesion gradually cleared over a one-month period.
The diet produced no notable side effects. However, discontinuation of the diet often led to an exacerbation *(Nishimura,1959)*.

Subsequent studies using a mouse model of SLE have confirmed the beneficial effects of limiting proteins with a high content of phenylalanine and tyrosine *(Corman)*.

As beef and dairy products are rich in phenylalanine and tyrosine, a *vegan* diet may be effective because of its low content of these amino acids. In a 1934 report, a woman with SLE and typical skin lesions started on the diet of a "well-known food faddist" which consisted entirely of fruit and vegetables. Within one week, the authors were surprised to discover that 95% of her facial lesions had disappeared and, at the end of 2 weeks, her face was entirely clear. They then tried the diet on a few of their SLE patients. Most showed considerable resolution of skin lesions within 2 weeks *(Anderson N)*.

A 16-year-old girl with SLE presented with proteinuria, hypocomplementemia and positive antinuclear and anti-DNA titers despite treatment with prednisolone 60 mg daily.

She was tapered off the steroids and started on a vegan diet in which protein and calorie intake was much reduced, but with little reduction in fat. Her antibody titers fell to normal, proteinuria decreased and serum albumin rose (Shigemasa).

NUTRITIONAL FACTORS

VITAMINS

Niacin

Back in 1944, daily injections of nicotinamide were reported to rapidly improve skin lesions in SLE. Lesions were less intense even the first day after the injections were started, and the improvement was very marked after several days. With continuing treatment, the lesions remained stationery *(Daïnow)*.

There is also a recent report of a woman with SLE whose condition only worsened with ACTH and steroids. However, a few months after starting injections of nicotinic acid, her symptoms disappeared and even her poor kidney function improved. Over the next several years, she continued on nicotinic acid and remained in full remission *(Hoffer)*.

Pantothenic Acid

Two reports a half a century ago by the same investigator noted that patients with subacute or chronic discoid lupus improved following "massive" therapy with calcium pantothenate or panthenol (pantothenyl alcohol) *(Goldman1948,1950)*.

These positive findings were not confirmed by a subsequent trial performed by different investigators. Similar patients were supplemented with between 200 and 600 mg daily of calcium pantothenate for 2 to 14 weeks or with panthenol 1 to 4 mg daily for 4 to 16 weeks. All patients were either unchanged or worse *(Cochrane)*.

Other investigators that have used pantothenic acid in conjunction with vitamin C *(Swartz)* or vitamin E *(Welsh)* have used much higher dosages (7 to 15 g daily), suggesting that the negative findings could have been due to the use of too low a dosage.

A woman with acute disseminated lupus erythematosus recovered coincidentally with the administration of 7 to 12 grams daily of calcium pantothenate. Each time the supplement was stopped, she relapsed.

During her last relapse, she was tried on cortisone, but developed a psychic disturbance so it had to be stopped. Since calcium pantothenate was restarted, she has been in remission (Swartz).

Vitamin A

While one animal study using a murine model of SLE suggested that vitamin A deficiency may hasten and worsen disease development *(Gershwin)*, a similar study found evidence that the deficiency may slow the disease process *(Liao)*.

Very limited data from human studies display a similar dichotomy. Treating SLE patients with a high dosage of vitamin A (100,000 IU daily) enhanced antibody-dependent cell-mediated cytotoxicity, natural killer cell activity and blastogenic response to plant mitogens and interleukin-2 *(Vien)*. However, several lines of indirect evidence suggest that systemic lupus erythematosus (SLE) could reflect a toxicity reaction to excessive tissue levels of the vitamin. For example, the remission often associated with long-term hemodialysis in patients with end-stage renal disease may be due to a gradual reduction in vitamin A levels at the sites of SLE activity *(Mawson)*.

Until the safety and efficacy of vitamin A supplementation is clarified, it is probably best to avoid it in SLE.

Vitamin B_{12}

Serum cobalamin levels may be reduced in SLE. In one group of 43 female patients, 8 of them had levels which were 180 pg/mL or less *(Molad)*. Moreover, SLE patients may have increased levels of the vitamin B_{12}-binding protein transcobalamin II due to increased production or stimulation of its secretion *(Lasser)*. This increase is directly correlated with disease activity *(Lasser;Molad)*.

The efficacy of vitamin B_{12} supplementation has been poorly investigated. One study from 1953 did report on 3 SLE patients who had previously failed to respond to oral and intramuscular vitamin E supplementation. Six weeks after staring intramuscular vitamin B_{12} injections, all 3 patients had complete clearing of their skin lesions *(Block)*.

Vitamin E

There have been several open trials of vitamin E supplementation. In one study, 4 patients with discoid lupus received between 900 and 1,600 IU daily and showed complete and almost complete clearing, while 2 similar patients who received only 300 IU daily failed to benefit *(Ayres,1978)*. A more recent study of 7 similar patients provided them with 400 mg of vitamin E 3 times daily for 12 weeks during the summer when the disease is likely to be most active. The lesions remained stable in all patients, neither improving nor worsening *(Yell)*.

When 12 patients with SLE received 100 to 150 mg of vitamin E orally 3 times daily after meals plus 150 mg intramuscularly (in an aqueous solution) 2 to 3 times weekly, 8 had excellent results, 1 had good results and 3 had poor results in regard to their skin lesions *(Block)*.

***AND* Pantothenic Acid**

In an open trial, 67 patients with biopsy-confirmed SLE were treated with the combination of vitamin E 1,000 to 2,000 mg daily and pantothenic acid 10 to 15 grams daily as calcium pantothenate. Patients with chronic discoid lupus began to show objective improvement in 4 to 6 months. Patients with disseminated discoid lupus improved in 2 months, while patients in the subacute disseminated group improved in 1 month.

The 3 patients in the acute disseminated group also received steroid hormones initially; however, they were later maintained on the supplements alone without relapse for 7 to 19 months. The only side effects were transient nausea and gastric distress *(Welsh)*.

MINERALS

Magnesium Deficiency

While plasma magnesium levels may be normal, erythrocyte magnesium has been found to be low for SLE patients *(Romano)*. The following case report suggests that, as with other patients with magnesium deficiency, repletion may relieve the deficiency symptoms:

A 35-year-old white female with a 9-year history of SLE presented with a 3-month history of gradually increasing myalgias. Her SLE was well controlled with prednisone and azathioprine, and she needed occasional non-steroidal anti-inflammatory drugs.

On examination, there was some diffuse tenderness on muscle palpation. Only 4 of 19 fibromyalgia tender points were noted, and she did not fulfill the ACR criteria for fibromyalgia syndrome. Plasma magnesium level was 1.7 mg/dl (reference mean 2.05 mg/dl). Erythrocyte magnesium level was 3.8 mg/dl (reference mean 5.5 mg/dl).

She was treated with 6 weekly intramuscular injections of magnesium sulfate 1 gram. Afterwards, her erythrocyte magnesium level increased to 4.3 mg/dl and her myalgias improved significantly. After a second course of 6 magnesium injections, her erythrocyte magnesium level increased to 5.4 mg/dl and myalgias almost disappeared. She was then treated continuously with magnesium chloride (Slow-Mag) 64 mg 3 times daily with food.

Six months later, her erythrocyte magnesium level was 5.2 mg/dl. Subsequently, she remains free of myalgias (Romano).

Selenium

In a murine model, selenium supplementation as sodium selenite significantly improved survival and increased natural killer cell activity *(O'Dell)*.

AND Vitamin E

Supplementation of selenium along with vitamin E was reported to be beneficial for a patient with SLE and low glutathione peroxidase levels. These levels increased slowly over 6 to 8 weeks *(Juhlin)*.

OTHER NUTRITIONAL FACTORS

Beta-carotene

Case reports suggest that, in discoid lupus, the administration of beta-carotene may reduce sun sensitivity, even in treatment-resistant patients *(Haeger-Aronsen;Newhold)*.

Essential Fatty Acids

In SLE, both linoleic acid (omega-6 series) and alpha-linolenic acid (omega-3 series) metabolites are significantly reduced in the plasma phospholipid fraction, suggesting that essential fatty acid metabolism is altered *(Suryaprabha)*.

Supplementation of the omega-3 fatty acids EPA and DHA, often in fish oil, has been shown to be beneficial with SLE patients in both animal and human studies. For example, in a double-blind crossover study, 17 patients with active SLE randomly received MaxEPA (a proprietary fish oil preparation) 20 g daily or 20 g olive oil daily in matching capsules, in either order, added to a standardized isoenergetic low-fat diet.

When individual outcome measures were considered following the completion of the 34-week study, 14 patients achieved useful or ideal status while they were receiving MaxEPA, while 13 patients were rated as worse or unchanged while receiving olive oil placebo. The difference between the two types of capsules was statistically significant *(Walton)*. These findings are consistent with those of open trials *(Das;Mohan)*.

Tryptophan: A Warning

SLE is characterized by abnormal tryptophan metabolism with excretion of metabolites *(Cardin de'Stefani)*. There is concern that some of these metabolites could promote auto-antibody production *(McCormick)*. Indeed, SLE patients demonstrate autoantibodies against tryptophanyl-tRNA synthetases - just as they demonstrate autoantibodies against tyrosyl- and phenylalanyl-tRNA synthetases (see Low Phenylalanine, Low Tyrosine Diet above) *(Vartanian)*. Moreover, SLE patients with neuropsychiatric dysfunction have elevate cerebrospinal levels of quinolinic acid, a neuroactive metabolite *(Vogelgesang)*.

Supplementation with tryptophan, or with 5-hydroxytryptophan, should thus be avoided unless it is first shown to be safe for this population.

OTHER RELATED FACTORS

Food Sensitivities

An increased prevalence of food reactions have been noted in SLE patients *(Diumenjo)*. Furthermore, elimination of offending foods has appeared to produce remissions *(Cooke)*.

There is a case report of an infant with symptoms and lab tests suggestive of lupus who was found to have antibodies to milk. Milk was eliminated from his diet and his symptoms resolved; however, symptoms returned on 2 occasions when he drank milk *(Anderson J)*. Similarly, when 15 lupus-prone (NZB/W) mice were raised without casein in their diets, 12 were still alive at 10 months of age, while only 1 of 12 similar mice eating the normal diet was still alive *(Carr)*.

A 36-year-old female developed episodic vomiting at age 5 and migraine at age 11. At age 16 she developed a polyarthritis and a diagnosis of SLE was made. Her disease progressed over the years with further involvement of the gastrointestinal, genitourinary, and respiratory tracts as well as progressive vascular symptoms. Spontaneous bruising and petechiae occurred, together with peripheral edema. Antinuclear antibodies and LE preparations were positive repeatedly and she was placed on cortisone and cytotoxic drugs.

Following admission to an environmental control unit, all medications were stopped. Joint stiffness and swelling gradually disappeared and her erythrocyte sedimentation rate fell from 63 to 15 mm in 1 week, the lowest value in years. Food and chemical challenges precipitated a return of her symptoms (Rea).

COMBINED NUTRITIONAL TREATMENT

A 34-year-old female had recently gone through the third of 3 hospitalizations and was taking prednisone and non-steroidal anti-inflammatory drugs. On her own, she went on a diet of whole foods, organically grown without artificial flavors, colors or preservatives, sugar, artificial sweeteners, hydrogenated oils, and practically no canned foods, and worked her way up to 6 grams vitamin C 4 times daily (bowel tolerance). She found that she was then able to taper her prednisone dosage faster than after her previous 2 hospitalizations.

After evaluation, she was told to eliminate grains containing gluten and gliadin (all grains except corn and rice) as well as cow milk and dairy products, and to take hydrochloric acid, pepsin and pancreatic enzymes. She was also tested for other food sensitivities and placed on vitamin B_6 500 mg 3 times daily (since almost all drugs that cause lupus and related symptoms inhibit B_6-dependent enzymes) along with vitamin B complex, one tablespoonful of flax oil daily, 240 mg of gamma-linolenic acid from primrose, black current or borage oils, 800 IU vitamin E, 30 mg zinc picolinate, DHEA and testosterone (usually below normal in lupus patients), along with vitamin and mineral injections.

It took over one and one-half years of following the program and making further adjustments before she became symptom-free. When seen after another 5 years, she was still in a full remission (Wright,1995).

BIBLIOGRAPHY

Anderson JA et al. Hyperreactivity to cow-s milk in an infant with LE and tart cell phenomenon. J Pediatr 84:59-67, 1974

Anderson NP, Ayres S Jr. Light sensitive dermatoses. JAMA 103(17):1279-85, 1934

Ayres S, Mihan R. Is vitamin E involved in the autoimmune mechanism? Cutis 21:321-5, 1978

Block MT. Vitamin E in the treatment of diseases of the skin. Clin Med January 1953, pp. 31-4

Cardin de'Stefani E, Costa C. [Changes in the metabolism of tryptophan in erythematosus.] Boll Soc Ital Bio Sper 60(8):1535-40, 1984 (in Italian)

Carr R et al. Abnormal responses to ingested substances in murine systemic lupus erythematosus: apparent effect of a casein-free diet on the development of systemic lupus erythematosus in NZB/W mice. J Rheumatol 14 Suppl 13:158-65, 1987

Cochrane T, Leslie G. The treatment of lupus erythematosus with calcium pantothenate and panthenol. J Invest Dermatol 18:365-7, 1952

Cooke HM, Reading CM. Dietary intervention in systemic lupus erythematosus: 4 cases of clinical remission and reversal of abnormal pathology. Int Clin Nutr Rev 5(4):166-76, 1985

Corman LC. The role of diet in animal models of systemic lupus erythematosus: Possible implications for human lupus. Semin Arthritis Rheum 15(1):61-9, 1985

Daïnow I. Recherches cliniques sur certaines proprietes anti-allergiques de la nicotinamide. Z Vitaminforsch 15:245-50, 1944 (in French)

Das UN. Beneficial effect of eicosapentaenoic and docosahexaenoic acids in the management of systemic lupus erythematosus and its relationship to the cytokine network. Prostaglandins Leukot Essent Fatty Acids 51:207-13, 1994

Diumenjo MS et al. [Allergic manifestations of systemic lupus erythematosus.] Allergol Immunopathol (Madr) 13(4):323-6. 1985 (in Spanish)

Gershwin ME et al. Nutritional factors and autoimmunity. IV. Dietary vitamin A deprivation induces a selective increase in IgM autoantibodies and hypergammaglobulinemia in New Zealand Black mice. J Immunology 133(1):222-6, 1984

Goldman L. Treatment of subacute and chronic discoid lupus erythematosus with intensive calcium pantothenate therapy. J Invest Dermatol 11:95, 1948

Goldman L. Preliminary and short report: Intensive panthenol therapy for lupus erythematosus. J Invest Dermatol 15:291, 1950

Haeger-Aronsen B et al. Oral carotenoids for photohypersensitivity in patients with erythrohepatic protoporphyria, polymorphous light eruptions and lupus erythematodes discoides. Int J Dermatol 18(1):73-82, 1979

Hoffer A. Lupus erythematosus. Townsend Letter for Doctors & Patients October, 1997:74-5

Juhlin L et al. Blood glutathione-peroxidase levels in skin diseases: Effect of selenium and vitamin E treatment. Acta Derm Venereal (Stockh) 62(3):211-4, 1982

Lasser U et al. Transcobalamin II, a serum protein reflecting autoimmune disease activity, its plasma dynamics, and the relationship to established serum parameters in systemic lupus erythematosus. Clin Immunol Immunopathol 36(3):345-57, 1985

Liao CH et al. Dietary vitamin A deficiency and the immune system in a murine model of systemic lupus erythematosus. Nutr Res 16:279-92, 1996

Mawson AR. Systemic lupus erythematosus, renal disease, hemodialysis and vitamin A. Med Hypotheses 18(4):387-98, 1985

McCormick JP et al. Characterization of a cell-lethal product from the photooxidation of tryptophan: Hydrogen peroxide. Science 191:468-9, 1976

Mohan IK Das UN. Oxidant stress, anti-oxidants and essential fatty acids in systemic lupus erythematosus. Prostaglandins Leukot Essent Fatty Acids 56(3):193-8, 1997

Molad Y et al. Serum cobalamin and transcobalamin levels in systemic lupus erythematosus. Am J Med 88(2):141-4, 1990

Morrow J et al. Dietary fat and immune function. J Immunol 135(6):3857, 1985

Newbold PCH. Beta-carotene in the treatment of discoid lupus erythematosus. Br J Dermatol 95:100-1, 1976

Nishimura N et al. Intermediary metabolism of phenylalanine and tyrosine in diffuse collagen diseases. Arch Dermatol 77:255-62, 1958

Nishimura N et al. Intermediary metabolism of phenylalanine and tyrosine in diffuse collagen diseases. Arch Dermatol 80:466-77, 1959

O'Dell JR et al. Improved survival in murine lupus as the result of selenium supplementation. Clin Exp Immunol 73(2):322-7, 1988

Rea WJ, Brown OD. Mechanisms of environmental vascular triggering. Clin Ecology 3(3):122-8, 1985

Romano TJ. Magnesium deficiency in systemic lupus erythematosus. J Nutr Environ Med 7:107-11, 1997

Shigemasa C et al. Effect of vegetarian diet on systemic lupus erythematosus. Letter. Lancet 339:1177, 1992

Suryaprabha P et al. Reactive oxygen species, lipid peroxides and essential fatty acids in patients with rheumatoid arthritis and systemic lupus erythematosus. Prostaglandins Leukot Essent Fatty Acids 43(4):251-5, 1991

Swartz JH - verbal report in discussion of the paper by Welsh AL (Lupus erythematosus: Treatment by combined use of massive amounts of pantothenic acid and vitamin E.) Arch Dermatol Syphilol 70:181-98, 1954

Vartanian OA. [Detection of autoantibodies against phenylalanyl-, tyrosyl-, and tryptophanyl-tRNA-synthetase and anti-idiotypic antibodies to it in serum from patients with autoimmune diseases]. Mol Biol (Mosk) 25(4):1033-9, 1991) (in Russian)

Vien CV et al. Effect of vitamin A treatment on the immune reactivity of patients with systemic lupus erythematosus. J Clin Lab Immunol 26(1):33-5, 1988

Vogelgesang SA et al. Quinolinic acid in patients with systemic lupus erythematosus and neuropsychiatric manifestations. J Rheumatol 23(5):850-5, 1996

Walton AJ et al. Dietary fish oil and the severity of symptoms in patients with systemic lupus erythematosus. Ann Rheum Dis 50(7):463-6, 1991

Welsh AL. Lupus erythematosus: Treatment by combined use of massive amounts of pantothenic acid and vitamin E. Arch Dermatol Syphilol 70:181-98, 1954

Wright JV. Treatment of lupus. Nutrition & Healing 2(12), December, 1995

Yell JA et al. Vitamin E and discoid lupus erythematosus. Lupus 1(5):303-5, 1992

MACULAR DEGENERATION

NUTRITIONAL TREATMENT GUIDE

✓ = Efficacy generally accepted.
* = Efficacy *demonstrated* by controlled human trials.
[+] = Efficacy *suspected* from uncontrolled human trials.
[-] = Efficacy *suspected* from indirect data.
? = Efficacy *challenged* in a study of similar design.

DIETARY FACTORS

[-] eat plenty of **Fruits** and **Vegetables**
[-] ? moderate **Wine** consumption

NUTRITIONAL FACTORS

* ? **Zinc:** ? 100 mg daily (taken away from meals)

- -

[+] **Carotenoids:** *to increase macular pigment density:* lutein esters equivalent to 30 mg free lutein daily
[+] **Vitamin E:** ? 800 IU daily (Supplement concurrently with **Vitamin A**.)

- -

[-] **Selenium:** ? 400 to 800 μg daily
[-] **Taurine deficiency:** ? 500 mg to 5 g daily
[-] **Vitamin A deficiency:** 50,000 IU daily (10,000 IU daily during pregnancy)
[-] **Vitamin C:** ? 500 mg twice daily

OTHER RELATED FACTORS

[+] rule out **Gluten** sensitivity

DIETARY FACTORS

Fruits and Vegetables

When the diets of patients who were diagnosed with the advanced stage of age-related macular degeneration (AMD) within the previous year were compared to those of normals, the consumption of carotenoid-rich, dark green, leafy vegetables (especially spinach and collard greens) was most strongly associated with a reduced risk of developing the disease *(Seddon)*.

Moreover, a similar study found that the consumption of fruits and vegetables rich in vitamin A was inversely correlated with AMD risk *(Goldberg)*.

Wine

In a group of more than 3,000 adults 45 to 75 year of age with macular changes indicative of AMD, fundoscopy revealed that 6% did in fact have AMD. There was a statistically significant negative association between the risk of AMD and the consumption of alcohol which varied according to the type of alcohol consumed. The effect of wine consumption dominated this negative association, with a 19% reduction in risk after adjustments for confounding variables *(Obesesan)*.

However, this finding was not confirmed in a similar study which failed to find the lesions of age-related maculopathy to be associated with wine consumption *(Moss)*.

NUTRITIONAL FACTORS

VITAMINS

Vitamin A Deficiency

In a logistic regression analysis, after adjusting for demographic and medical factors, only the frequency of consumption of fruits and vegetables rich in vitamin A was negatively correlated with AMD on the basis of data from the first American National Health and Nutrition Examination Survey *(Goldberg)*. Moreover, when monkeys were made vitamin A-deficient, they developed retinal degeneration *(Hayes)*.

However, serum vitamin A levels appear to be normal in AMD *(Ishihara)*, and so far there is no evidence that supplementation is beneficial.

Vitamin C

The dietary intake of vitamin C has been inversely correlated with the risk of age-related maculopathy *(Mares-Perlman,1996;Seddon)*, although serum ascorbate levels appear to be normal in the disease *(Ishihara)*.

Experimental studies have demonstrated that bright light preferentially damages precisely the region that degenerates in age-related macular degeneration *(Young)*. When rats received ascorbate supplementation prior to photic exposure, their retinas were protected from damage due to the oxidative insult *(Organisciak)*. Furthermore, in a large retrospective study, vitamin C supplementation was associated with a decreased incidence of early AMD *(Mares-Perlman,1993)*.

Vitamin E

Animal studies have found that vitamin E deficiency results in a significant loss of photoreceptor cells *(Hayes:Robison)*. Some, but not all, human epidemiological studies have found evidence for an inverse relationship between vitamin E nutriture and macular degeneration.

When, for example, the incidence of specific lesions of larger drusen and pigmentary abnormalities, as well as the incidence of age-related maculopathy were assessed in more than 1,700 people 5 years after baseline, there was a modest, but significant, inverse relationship between dietary vitamin E intake and the incidence of large drusen *(VandenLangenberg)*. Another study found the odds of age-related maculopathy were lower in people with the highest versus lowest quintile of vitamin E intake *(Mares-Perlman,1996)*, although a study of patients with advanced AMD failed to confirm such a relationship *(Sedden)*.

Similarly mixed findings have been noted in studies of plasma/serum vitamin A levels. In a group of well-nourished patients, those with plasma vitamin E levels in the lowest quartile had double the risk of AMD of patients in the medium and highest quartiles. However, there was no association between AMD and the use of vitamin supplements *(West)*, and two studies failed to find a significant association between serum vitamin E levels and the presence of AMD *(Mares-Perlman,1995;Smith)*.

Supplementation

While controlled trials are lacking, the frequent response of patients to vitamin E supplementation in open trials appears promising. In one study, 28 of a group of 39 patients (72%) with dystrophy of the macula lutea showed evidence of improved vision following supplementation *(Adayeva)*.

Furthermore, in an informal clinical setting, when 20 patients were treated with vitamin E along with the replacement of table salt with mineral-rich sea salt, 19 improved while only 1 deteriorated. Four patients whose vision had deteriorated to mere hand movements improved sufficiently to read a newspaper (20/50). A few patients deteriorated after stopping the supplement, only to improve again when vitamin E was reinstituted. Improvement was sometimes very slow, taking up to 12 months *(Todd).*

Results of studies done on rats suggest that vitamin E may act as an inhibitor of vitamin A uptake and/or storage *(Katz)*. Moreover, vitamin A deficiency increases the extent of retinal damage induced by vitamin E deficiency *(Robison)*. Thus, vitamin E supplementation should always be accompanied by supplementation with vitamin A.

MINERALS

Copper

Elevations of both serum copper *(Silverstone)* and ceruloplasmin, a copper-binding alpha-globulin, *(Newsome,1986)* have been noted. Furthermore, a rabbit study found that chronic copper toxicity may cause retinal pathology *(Gahlot)*. Whether copper toxicity is a cause of macular degeneration is not known.

Selenium Deficiency

Since selenium is an important antioxidant, and photo-oxidation is believed to be an important factor in promoting macular degeneration, selenium nutriture may be important. Two studies have examined blood selenium levels in this disorder. One looked at whole blood selenium levels in 10 patients with exudative age-related maculopathy and found that the selenium concentration was significantly lower in patients than in normal controls *(Mayer)*.

The other study examined fasting serum selenium levels in patients with AMD. Compared to normal controls, there was a borderline association between AMD and serum selenium levels *(Tsang)*.

The efficacy of selenium supplementation is not known.

Zinc

The concentration of zinc is higher in the retina than in any other organ *(Underwood)* and decreases with age *(Wyszynski)*.

Several studies have examined the relationship between zinc nutriture and macular degeneration. Population-based studies have found an inverse relationship between dietary zinc intake and abnormalities of the retinal pigment *(Mares-Perlman,1996;VandenLangenberg)*. One of these studies found the relationship to be strongest for some types of early age-related maculopathy, but late age-related maculopathy was unrelated to zinc intake *(Mares-Perlman,1996)*.

Studies concerning serum zinc levels have had conflicting results. Some have found reduced levels *(Ishihara)*, while others have found elevated levels *(Silverstone)*.

In eyes from 57 donors, soluble macular zinc was 45% less in eyes over 70 years of age, and there was a greater reduction in the soluble fraction of macular retinal pigment epithelium in eyes with signs of macular disease *(Newsome,1995)*. This reduction in zinc may cause the disease as, when rats were fed a zinc-deficient diet, they developed impaired retinal function and loss of visual acuity *(Mobarhan)*.

Furthermore, when lack of dietary zinc caused rats to develop a reduced concentration of retinal zinc, the utilization of vitamin A was impaired *(Huber)*. Since, as noted above, monkeys made vitamin A-deficient develop retinal degeneration, this may be a mechanism by which retinal zinc deficiency fosters the disorder.

Also, retinal zinc deficiency may reduce the activity of catalase, an antioxidant metalloenzyme found in the macular human retinal pigment epithelium *(Newsome,1991)*. This finding is significant because macular degeneration is associated with reduced catalase activity *(Newsome,1991)*.

Supplementation

In an double-blind study, 151 patients with drusen or macular degeneration randomly received either 100 mg of zinc supplementation or placebo with meals. One to two years later, although some eyes in the zinc-treated group lost vision, this group had significantly less loss of visual acuity than the placebo group. In vision testing, 33% of the placebo-treated patients lost at least 10 letters of vision compared to only 10% of patients in the zinc-treated group. Moreover, 66% of the placebo group and 86% of the zinc group lost 9 or fewer letters of vision *(Newsome,1988)*.

These findings are consistent with those of a retrospective study of 2,152 subjects between the ages of 43 and 86 years for whom zinc supplementation was associated with a reduced risk of retinal pigment degeneration *(Mares-Perlman,1993)*. However, when, in another double-blind study, 112 patients with macular degeneration including exudative lesions in a single eye were supplemented with only 46 mg elemental zinc daily, no effect of zinc supplementation could be found 2 years later *(Stur)*, suggesting that a larger dosage may be needed.

OTHER NUTRITIONAL FACTORS

Carotenoids

Two of the roughly 600 naturally-occurring carotenoids, lutein and zeaxanthin, the major carotenoids of maize and melon respectively, are the constituents of the macula lutea, the yellow spot in the macula (the central part of the retina). Their concentration in the macula may possibly prevent or limit damage due to their physicochemical properties and their capability to quench oxygen free radicals and singlet oxygen which are generated in the retina as a consequence of the simultaneous presence of light and oxygen *(Schalch)*.

When patients with advanced AMD were questioned about diet, those in the highest quintile of carotenoid intake had a 43% lower risk than those in the lowest quintile. Lutein and zeaxanthin were the carotenoids most strongly associated with reduced risk *(Seddon)*.

Another survey found significant, but modest inverse associations between the intakes of pro-vitamin A carotenoids and the incidence of large drusen *(Vanden Langenberg)*, and yet another found that the risk of developing AMD was significantly reduced in populations whose diets were high in fruits and vegetables rich in beta-carotene *(Goldberg)*. However, two other surveys failed to confirm a relationship between carotenoid intake and macular degeneration *(Mares-Perlman; Smith)*.

Further evidence suggesting a relationship between carotenoids and macular degeneration comes from a study of 22 eyes with AMD which found that 77% of the affected eyes had total amounts of lutein and zeaxanthin in the central retina which were below the mean for the control group *(Landrum,1997a)*. Moreover, there is evidence that serum levels of total carotenoids appear to be inversely associated with risk *(Mares-Perlman,1995)*.

Supplementation

Increased serum lutein levels correspond to increases in the concentration of lutein in the macula of the human eye. Serum levels of lutein can be increased significantly with lutein supplementation. Thus, when levels of macular pigmentation are low, long-term lutein supplementation could result in significant increases in the level of pigmentation within the macula *(Landrum,1997a)*.

While it is not yet known whether carotenoid supplementation can retard or even reverse macular degeneration, the findings of 2 recent studies appear hopeful. Twenty to 40 days after 2 subjects began lutein supplementation, their macular pigment density began to increase. The optical density curve eventually leveled off 40 to 50 days after the subjects discontinued the supplement, and little or no decrease in optical density was observed subsequently. The mean increases in macular pigment optical density were 39% and 21%, respectively. This means there was a substantial reduction in blue light reaching tissues vulnerable to being affected by AMD *(Landrum,1997b)*.

Another study of 11 subjects and 2 controls increased the dietary intake of lutein and zeaxanthin from foods for up to 15 weeks. Eight of the experimental subjects were responders, with increases in macular pigment density. As in the previous study, these increases remained for at least several months after subjects returned to their former diets *(Hammond)*.

Taurine Deficiency

Taurine, which is necessary for normal vision, is released from the retina following light exposure and is actively transported from retina to choroid by the retinal pigment epithelium *(Scharschmidt)*.

In animal studies, taurine deficiency has been found to be associated with retinal degeneration *(Imaki)*. Whether taurine supplementation is beneficial is not yet known.

COMBINED NUTRIENT TREATMENT

There are numerous studies in the literature in which combinations of supplementary nutrients were tested. In perhaps the best study to date, patients with advanced AMD received a daily multivitamin-mineral-antioxidant supplement containing vitamin C, vitamin E, selenium and beta-carotene, or placebo.

Distance visual acuity stabilized over 18 months in the supplemented group but declined in the placebo group.

However, compared to the placebo group, the supplemented group had increased cortical opacification of the right lens *(Age-related Macular Degeneration Study Group)*.

OTHER RELATED FACTORS

Gluten Sensitivity

The following case report illustrates the possible relationship between sensitivity to gluten and progressive loss of vision:

A 32-year-old woman first presented with diarrhea and a 7 kg weight loss. No symptoms were identified and eventually the symptoms settled. She had a premature menopause at age 34, and at age 38 she complained of some visual deterioration which seemed to stabilize.

At age 43, she presented with blurring of vision in the right eye and reported progressive visual loss over several years. attributable to macular degeneration. While her left eye was normal, 2 years later vision began to deteriorate in that eye. Visual loss was progressive and, at age 50, her vision was barely 6/60 in both eyes and she was registered as blind.

At age 52, she was seen due to weight loss, lethargy, and burning feet. Work-up revealed anemia, positive IgA antigliadin antibody, and high fecal fat excretion. A jejunal biopsy showed total villous atrophy.

She was placed on a gluten-free diet, with a good symptomatic response and reduction of antigliadin antibody to normal. Moreover, her progressive visual loss seemed to stabilize, suggesting that a nutrient deficiency rather than neurotoxicity due to antibodies was the responsible etiologic agent (Mitchell).

BIBLIOGRAPHY

Adayeva Y et al. Vitamin E treatment in dystrophy of the macula lutea. Abstract. Am J Ophthalmol 56:498, 1963

Age-related Macular Degeneration Study Group. Multicenter ophthalmic and nutritional age-related macular degeneration study - Part 2: antioxidant intervention and conclusions. J Am Optom Assoc 67:30-49, 1996

Gahlot DK, Ratnakar KS. Effect of experimentally induced chronic copper toxicity on retina. Indian J Ophthalmol 29(4):351-3, 1981

Goldberg J et al. Factors associated with age-related macular degeneration. An analysis of data from the first National Health and Nutrition Examination Survey. Am J Epidemiol 128(4):700-10, 1988

Hammond BR Jr et al. Dietary modification of human macular pigment density. Invest Ophthalmol Vis Sci 38(9):1795-801, 1997

Hayes KC. Retinal degeneration in monkeys induced by deficiencies of vitamin E or A. Invest Ophthalmol Vis Sci 13(7):499-510, 1974

Huber AM, Gershoff SN. Effects of zinc deficiency on the oxidation of retinol and ethanol in rats. J Nutr 105(11):1486-90, 1975

Imaki H et al. Retinal degeneration in 3-month-old rhesus monkey infants fed a taurine-free human infant formula. J Neurosci Res 18(4):602-14, 1987

Ishihara N et al. [Antioxidants and angiogenetic factor associated with age-related macular degeneration]. Nippon Ganka Gakkai Zasshi 101(3):248-51, 1997 (in Japanese)

Katz ML et al. Dietary vitamins A and E influence retinyl ester composition and content of the retinal pigment epithelium. Biochim Biophys Acta 924(3):432-41, 1987

Landrum JT et al. The macular pigment: a possible role in protection from age-related macular degeneration. Adv Pharmacol 38:537-55, 1997a

Landrum JT et al. A one year study of the macular pigment: the effect of 140 days of a lutein supplement. Exp Eye Res 65(1):57-62, 1997b

Mares-Perlman J et al. Relationship between age-related maculopathy and intake of vitamin and mineral supplements. Abstract. Invest Ophthalmol Vis Sci 34:1133, 1993

Mares-Perlman JA et al. Serum antioxidants and age-related macular degeneration in a population-based case-control study. Arch Ophthalmol 113:1518-23, 1995

Mares-Perlman JA et al. Association of zinc and antioxidant nutrients with age-related maculopathy. Arch Ophthalmol 114:991-7, 1996

Mayer MJ et al. Whole blood selenium in exudative age-related maculopathy. Acta Ophthanlmol Scand 76(1):62-7, 1998

Mitchell M, Robinson TJ. Gluten sensitivity and neurological dysfunction. Letter. Lancet 347:903-4, 1996

Mobarhan S et al. Dietary zinc deficiency produces electroretinogram (ERG) abnormalities without depleting total ocular zinc. Fed Proc 43:685, 1984

Moss SE, et al. Alcohol consumption and the 5-year incidence of age-related maculopathy: the Beaver Dam eye study. Ophthalmology 105(5):789-94, 1998

Newsome DA et al. Macular degeneration and elevated serum ceruloplasmin. Invest Ophthalmol Vis Sci 27(12):1675-80, 1986

Newsome DA et al. Oral zinc in macular degeneration. Arch Ophthalmol 106(2):192-8, 1988

Newsome D et al. The trace element and antioxidant economy of the human macula: can dietary supplementation influence the course of macular degeneration? Abstract. J Am Coll Nutr 10(5):536, 1991

Newsome DA et al. Zinc content of human retinal pigment epithelium decreases with age and macular degeneration but superoxide dismutase activity increases. J Trace Elem Exp Med 8:193-9, 1995

Obisesan TO et al. Moderate wine consumption is associated with decreased odds of developing age-related macular degeneration in NHANES-1. J Am Geriatr Soc 46(1):1-7, 1998

Organisciak DT et al. The protective effect of ascorbate in retinal light damage of rats. Invest Ophthalmol Vis Sci 26(11):1580-8, 1985

Robison WG Jr et al. Vitamin E deficiency and the retina: photoreceptor and pigment epithelial changes. Invest Ophthalmol Vis Sci 18(7):683-90, 1979

Schalch W. Carotenoids in the retina--a review of their possible role in preventing or limiting damage caused by light and oxygen. EXS 62:280-98, 1992

Scharschmidt BF et al. Effect of taurine on the isolated retinal pigment epithelium of the frog: electrophysiologic evidence for stimulation of an apical, electrogenic Na^{+}-K^{+} pump. J Membr Biol 106(1):71-81, 1988

Seddon JM et al. Dietary carotenoids, vitamins A, C, and E, and advanced age-related macular degeneration. JAMA 272:1413-20, 1994

Silverstone BZ et al. A metabolic analysis of high myopia and senile macular degeneration. Metab Pediatr Syst Ophthalmol 11(3):122-5, 1988

Smith W et al. Serum beta carotene, alpha tocopherol, and age-related maculopathy: the Blue Mountains Eye Study. Am J Ophthalmol 124(6):838-40, 1997

Stur M et al. Oral zinc and the second eye in age-related macular degeneration. Invest Ophthalmol Visual Sci 37(7):1225-35, 1996

Todd GP. Nutrition, Health & Disease. Norfolk, Virginia, The Donning Company, 1988

Tsang NC et al. Serum levels of antioxidants and age-related macular degeneration. Doc Ophthalmol 81(4):387-400, 1992

Underwood EJ. Trace Elements in Human and Animal Nutrition, 4th Edition. London, Academic press, 1977:198

VandenLangenberg GM et al. Associations between antioxidant and zinc intake and the 5-year incidence of early age-related maculopathy in the Beaver Dam Eye Study. Am J Epidemiol 148(2):204-14, 1998

West S, et al. Are antioxidants or supplements protective for age-related macular degeneration? Arch Ophthalmol 112:222-7, 1994

Wyszynski RE et al. A donor-age-dependent change in the activity of alpha-mannosidase in human cultured RPE cells. Invest Ophthalmol Vis Sci 30:2341-7, 1989

Young RW. Solar radiation and age-related macular degeneration. Surv Ophthalmol 32(4):252-69, 1988

MENOPAUSAL SYMPTOMS

NUTRITIONAL TREATMENT GUIDE

✓ = Efficacy generally accepted.
* = Efficacy *demonstrated* by controlled human trials.
[+] = Efficacy *suspected* from uncontrolled human trials.
[-] = Efficacy *suspected* from indirect data.
? = Efficacy *challenged* in a study of similar design.

DIETARY FACTORS

* eat **Plants rich in Phytoestrogens**

- -

[+] moderate **Alcohol** consumption

NUTRITIONAL FACTORS

* ? **Vitamin E:** *for hot flashes and senile vulvovaginitis:* ? 800 IU daily (6 week trial)

- -

[+] **Boron deficiency:** *to increase estrogen levels:* 3 mg daily
[+] **Essential Fatty Acids:** *for mastalgia:* evening primrose oil 1 g 4 times daily
[+] **Flavonoids:** *for hot flashes, nocturnal leg cramps, easy bruising or nosebleeds:* hesperidin 200 mg after meals and at bedtime for 2 weeks; then reduce dosage to half for 4 weeks; then further reduce dosage as tolerated.
(Combine with **Vitamin C** 250 mg 3 times daily.)
[+] **Gamma-Oryzanol:** 100 mg 3 times daily (results in 2 to 8 weeks)

- -

[-] **L-Tryptophan:** 1 to 6 g daily

DIETARY FACTORS

Phytoestrogen-rich Plants

PLANTS RICH IN PHYTOESTROGENS

soy
fennel, celery, and parsley
clover sprouts
high-lignan flaxseed oil
nuts and seeds

Phytoestrogens (usually isoflavones, phytosterols, saponins, or lignans) are compounds in plants that are capable of exerting mild estrogenic effects.

The high intake of dietary phytoestrogens is thought to explain why hot flashes and other menopausal symptoms rarely occur in cultures consuming predominantly a plant-based diet *(Adlercreutz, 1997; Kaldas)*.

Dietary phytoestrogens and phytoestrogen-containing herbs may offer significant advantages over the use of estrogens in the treatment of menopausal symptoms. While both synthetic and natural estrogens pose significant health risks, including increasing the risk of cancer, gallbladder disease, and thromboembolic disease, phytoestrogens have not been associated with these risks *(Rose)*.

Several commonly eaten plants contain clinically meaningful amounts of phytoestrogens. For example, one cup of soybeans provides approximately 300 mg of isoflavones, the equivalent of about 0.45 mg of conjugated estrogens or one tablet of Premarin *(Messina)*.

Hot flashes and other menopausal symptoms are rare in Japanese women as compared to American and European women. In one study, the consumption of soy products and boiled beans resulted in 100 to 1,000-fold higher amounts of urinary isoflavonoid phytoestrogens than those of endogenous estrogens in normal omnivorous women consuming either a Western or Asian diet. These high amounts are adequate to have biological effects, especially in postmenopausal women with low estrogen levels *(Adlercreutz,1992)*.

The efficacy of consuming phytoestrogen-rich plant foods in reducing hot flashes has been investigated in 2 double-blind studies. The first of these studies compared soy flour, which contains the potent phytoestrogen daidzin, with wheat flour, which contains the less potent enterolactones. Post-menopausal women with at least 14 hot flashes per week randomly received dietary supplementation with either of the two flours. After 12 weeks, both groups had significant reductions of hot flashes, and both had significantly reduced menopausal symptom scores *(Murkies)*.

Evidence that this improvement was not due to a placebo effect comes from the second study. Post-menopausal women received either isolated soy protein or casein placebo for 12 weeks. Soy was significantly superior to placebo. Women taking soy had a 26% reduction in the mean number of hot flashes by week 3, and a 33% reduction by week 4. By the end of the twelfth week, they had a 45% reduction as compared to a 30% reduction for the women taking placebo *(Albertazzi)*.

Further evidence of the efficacy of phytoestrogenic plants comes from a study in which postmenopausal women received one of these plants, namely soybean flour, red clover sprouts or linseed, at levels which approximated 10% of their energy intake. After 6 weeks there were significant increases in vaginal cell maturation and reductions in follicle stimulating hormone *(Wilcox)*. Similarly, postmenopausal women consuming enough soyfoods to provide about 200 mg of isoflavones demonstrated signs of estrogenic activity - such as an increased number of superficial cells which line the vaginal wall, a change which would combat vaginal dryness and irritation *(Messina)*.

Alcohol

Moderate alcohol consumption is a newly recognized determinant of endogenous estrogen levels in postmenopausal women. Phytoestrogens have now been isolated and identified in both *beer* and *bourbon*. (See Phytoestrogens below.) Bourbon is made from corn, and corn oil possesses estrogenic activity, while beer contains hops, which have also been shown to have estrogenic activity *(Gavaler)*.

There is preliminary evidence that regular alcohol consumption may delay menopause. When 2,240 women between the ages of 45 and 49 years were surveyed, those who consumed the least amount of alcohol were more likely to be postmenopausal *(Torgerson)*.

However, specifically for postmenopausal women receiving oral estrogen and progestin replacement therapy, alcohol ingestion has been shown to cause a 3-fold increase in circulating estradiol. These elevated levels may remain above baseline for 5 hours. The health implications of this elevation are unknown *(Ginsburg)*.

NUTRITIONAL FACTORS

VITAMINS

Vitamin E

In several preliminary studies of menopausal women, all performed between 1942 and 1952, vitamin E supplementation was associated with improvement in vasomotor symptoms, depression and anxiety as well as in a number of physical complaints of uncertain cause such as dizziness, palpitations, dyspnea and fatigue. These results were confirmed in two placebo-controlled studies *(Finkler;Rubenstein)*, although vitamin E proved no better than placebo in a third *(Blatt)*.

Vitamin E has also been reported to produce clinical improvement in senile vulvovaginitis associated with what appears to be the proliferation of new blood vessels on biopsy after 4 weeks of treatment *(Shute)*. In a study reported in the *British Medical Journal*, half of the patients eventually responded *(McLaren)*.

In a survey of hundreds of menopausal women, many reported relief from hot flashes 2 days after starting supplementation with vitamin E. According to the clinician who took the survey, hot flashes may disappear completely, usually within one week, when vitamin C and calcium are added to the vitamin E *(Reitz)*; this impression remains to be confirmed by controlled trials.

> *A 57 year-old postmenopausal woman who was not on estrogen replacement had a 12-year history of episodic hot flashes, palpitations and shortness of breath. The hot flashes came in waves, lasted about 90 seconds, and were associated with a feeling of malaise. The palpitations were sometimes associated with the hot flashes, but could also occur alone. Two years earlier her doctor found that, during an episode of palpitations, her pulse rate was 220 beats per minute. She described her breathing problem as a constant need to yawn, sigh or to try to take a deep breath, and noted that it seemed worse when she was nervous or in a rush.*
>
> *She was given a trial of vitamin E 200 IU daily. When next seen 3 months later, she reported that she had also begun to take a "megavitamin." Her hot flashes were better, although not entirely gone. She was generally much calmer, her pulse rate was slower and she stated that her shortness of breath was 75% improved. In addition, she felt more energetic and was able to do more physical work before tiring.*

MINERALS

Boron

Supplemental boron may both enhance and mimic some of the effects of estrogen in postmenopausal women *(Nielsen,1992)*. Two open trials have found that supplementation may increase serum 17-β-estradiol concentrations. The first study placed postmenopausal women who were not on estrogen therapy on a low boron diet for 119 days. When they the women were then supplemented with boron, serum 17-β-estradiol increased. *(Nielsen,1987)*.

The other study found that, for a group of postmenopausal women, boron supplementation only increased 17-β-estradiol concentrations in those receiving estrogen therapy *(Nielsen,1992)*. Taken together, these findings suggest that supplementary boron may have estrogenic effects for postmenopausal women who are either boron-depleted or receiving estrogen replacement therapy.

OTHER NUTRITIONAL FACTORS

Essential Fatty Acids

While one-third of a group of perimenopausal women complained of mastalgia at baseline, 3 months after they started hormone replacement therapy two-thirds of the group had developed this complaint. In a open trial, 10 women with hormone replacement therapy-induced mastalgia received *evening primrose oil*, a rich source of the omega-6 essential fatty acid gamma-linolenic acid. Seven of these women noted a reduction in breast pain *(Harding)*. These findings have yet to be confirmed in a controlled study.

Evening primrose oil supplementation has been tested under double-blind conditions in a group of post-menopausal women complaining of vasomotor flushing. After 6 months, when compared to women who received placebo, the only significant improvement with evening primrose oil administration was a reduction in the maximum number of flushes occurring during the night. This was not a clinically meaningful improvement, suggesting that evening primrose oil is ineffective for this symptom *(Chenoy)*.

Flavonoids

Flavonoids in the capillary wall may maintain the integrity of the capillary endothelium with an additional contribution from estrogen *(Clemetson)*.

Hesperidin, the predominant flavonoid in oranges and lemons, has been combined with vitamin C to treat menopausal symptoms. In a placebo-controlled study, hesperidin complex, hesperidin methyl chalcone and ascorbic acid were given to 94 menopausal women complaining of hot flashes. The supplements were found to be markedly more effective than any of the 3 placebo control substances. Symptoms were relieved in 53% and moderated in 34%. The only adverse effect was a slightly offensive perspiration odor with a tendency for perspiration to discolor the clothing *(Smith)*.

Also, in an open trial, menopausal women with nocturnal leg cramps, easy bruising or spontaneous nosebleeds - all of which worsened during the time of month when menses formerly occurred - received hesperidin and vitamin C. When symptoms remitted, the dosage was reduced and, later, an attempt was made to discontinue supplementation.

Of 14 women with nocturnal leg cramps, 4 achieved symptom relief within 2 weeks, and the rest within an average of 7 weeks. Eleven out of 15 women with easy bruising improved after 8 weeks, while the other 4 responded by 16 weeks. Nosebleeds stopped in 6 to 11 weeks in the 8 moderate cases and the dosage was successfully reduced. Of the remaining 3 cases, one was under control after 3 months and was then able to successfully reduce the dosage. The other 2 patients improved; however, their nosebleeds were never completely controlled until they stopped spontaneously in the fourth year *(Horoschak)*.

Gamma-Oryzanol

An antioxidant extracted from rice bran oil, gamma-oryzanol has been reported to relieve a wide range of menopausal symptoms in several open trials. Using the Kupperman index of menopausal symptoms, up to 85% of patients report improvement *(Ishihara)*.

Phytoestrogens

See 'Phytoestrogen-containing Plants' above.

L-Tryptophan

Low blood tryptophan levels may be correlated with estrogen levels in depressed women who have recently gone through menopause *(Anonymous)*. Moreover, for 3 perimenopausal women with climacteric symptoms including hot flashes, insomnia and depression, there was a significant positive correlation between total plasma estrogen concentration and the concentration of *free* plasma tryptophan (but not with *total* plasma tryptophan) during the night.

The majority of tryptophan is bound to albumin, and plasma estrogens can bind to albumin. It thus seems likely that this relationship is due to a direct action of estrogen on the tryptophan binding site of albumin. Since the metabolism of brain serotonin depends partly on the concentration of free plasma tryptophan, these results suggest a possible means by which estrogens might influence cerebral serotonin metabolism, and perhaps mood, in perimenopausal women *(Thomson)*.

There is already evidence that tryptophan supplementation has anti-depressant effects (see Depression). Controlled trials of tryptophan in the treatment of perimenopausal depression are needed to ascertain its efficacy in this specific patient group.

BIBLIOGRAPHY

Adlercreutz H et al. Dietary phyto-oestrogens and the menopause in Japan. Letter. Lancet 339:1233, 1992

Adlercreutz H, Mazur W. Phyto-oestrogens and Western diseases. Ann Med 29(2):95-120, 1997

Albertazzi P et al. The effect of dietary soy supplementation on hot flushes. Obstet Gynecol 91(1):6-11, 1998

Anonymous. Editorial: Tryptophan and depression. Br Med J 1:242-3, 1976

Blatt MHG et al. Vitamin E and climacteric syndrome: Failure of effective control as measured by menopausal index. Arch Intern Med 91:792-9, 1953

Chenoy R et al. Effect of oral gammalinolenic acid from evening primrose oil on menopausal flushing. BMJ 308:501-3, 1994

Clemetson CAB et al. Capillary strength and the menstrual cycle. Ann N Y Acad Sci 93:277-300, 1962

Finkler RS. The effect of vitamin E in the menopause. J Clin Endocrinol Metab 9:89-94, 1949

Gavaler JS. Alcohol and nutrition in postmenopausal women. J Am Coll Nutr 12(4):349-56, 1993

Ginsburg ES et al. Effects of alcohol ingestion on estrogens in postmenopausal women. JAMA 276(21):1747-51, 1996

Harding C et al. Hormone replacement therapy-induced mastalgia responds to evening primrose oil. Br J Surg 83(Suppl 1):24, 1996

Horoschak A. Nocturnal leg cramps, easy bruisability and epistaxis in menopausal patients: Treated with hesperidin and ascorbic acid. Del State Med J, January, 1959:19-22

Ishihara M. Effect of gamma oryzanol on serum peroxide level and climacteric disturbances. Asia-Oceania J Obstet Gynaecol 10(3):317, 1984

Kaldas RS, Hughes CL. Reproductive and general metabolic effects of phytoestrogens in mammals. Reprod Toxicol 3:81-9, 1989

McLaren HC. Vitamin E in the menopause. Br Med J 2:1378, 1949

Messina M, Barnes S. The roles of soy products in reducing risk of cancer. J Natl Cancer Inst 83:541-6, 1991

Murkies A et al. Dietary flour supplementation decreases post-menopausal hot flashes: Effect of soy and wheat. Maturitas 21(3):189-95, 1995

Nielsen FH et al. Effect of dietary boron on mineral, estrogen, and testosterone metabolism in postmenopausal women. FASEB J 1:394-7, 1987

Nielsen FH et al. Boron enhances and mimics some effects of estrogen therapy in postmenopausal women. J Trace Elem Exp Med 5:237-46, 1992

Reitz R. Menopause: A Positive Approach. New York, Penguin Books, 1979

Rose DP. Dietary fiber, phytoestrogens, and breast cancer. Nutrition 8:47-51, 1992

Rubenstein BB. Vitamin E diminishes the vasomotor symptoms of menopause. Abstract. Fed Proc 7:106, 1948

Shute E. J Obstet Gynecol Br Emp 49:482, 1942

Smith CJ. Non-hormonal control of vaso-motor flushing in menopausal patients. Chic Med March 7, 1964

Thomson J et al. Relationship between nocturnal plasma oestrogen concentration and free plasma tryptophan in perimenopausal women. J Endocrinol 72(3):395-6, 1977

Torgerson DJ et al. Alcohol consumption may influence onset of the menopause. BMJ 315:188, 1997

Wilcox G et al. Oestrogenic effects of plant foods in postmenopausal women. Br Med J 301:905-6, 1990

MENORRHAGIA

NUTRITIONAL TREATMENT GUIDE

✓ = Efficacy generally accepted.
* = Efficacy *demonstrated* by controlled human trials.
[+] = Efficacy *suspected* from uncontrolled human trials.
[-] = Efficacy *suspected* from indirect data.
? = Efficacy *challenged* in a study of similar design.

NUTRITIONAL FACTORS

* **Iron deficiency:** 30 mg twice daily until repletion; then minimal maintenance dosage

- -

[+] **Manganese deficiency:** 3 to 5 mg daily
[+] **Vitamin A deficiency:** 25,000 IU twice daily for 15 days
[+] **Vitamin B complex:** B "50" daily

OTHER RELATED FACTORS

* **Flavonoids** *AND* **Vitamin C**: 200 mg of each 3 times daily

NUTRITIONAL FACTORS

VITAMINS

Vitamin A Deficiency

Patients may have reduced serum levels of vitamin A *(Lithgow*). In an open trial, women with menorrhagia whose vitamin A levels were low received vitamin A supplementation for 15 days. Menstruation returned to normal in 57.5% and diminished in an additional 35%. Moreover, 17-β-estradiol production was increased more than 100% *(Lithgow)*.

Vitamin B Complex Deficiencies

Results on an animal study suggest that deficiency of one or more components of the vitamin B complex could promote menorrhagia. Estrone pellets were implanted in the spleens of adult castrate female rats so that the absorbed estrogen passed through the liver before reaching the systemic circulation. On a normal diet the animals remained anestrous but, when they were placed on a vitamin B complex-free diet, protracted estrus occurred.

Studies performed in the early 1940s provided preliminary evidence suggesting the relevance of B complex deficiencies to menorrhagia. The addition of brewer's yeast as a source of vitamin B complex caused rats to become anestrous, while subsequent dietary depletion again led to estrus, suggesting that the liver may have an important role in maintaining the body's estrogen level within the normal range, and that a vitamin B deficiency may impair the hepatic estrogen-inactivating function *(Biskind, 1942)*.

These findings were consistent with those of a subsequent human study. Upon evaluation, *all* of a group of 52 women who presented with menorrhagia, metrorrhagia, cystic mastitis and/or premenstrual tension had signs or symptoms of vitamin B complex deficiency, while all but 2 of a group of 39 women who presented with signs and symptoms of nutritional deficiency were found to have conditions suggestive of estrogen excess. Both groups were treated with vitamin B complex with good results *(Biskind, 1943, 1944)*. Unfortunately, this promising early research failed to lead to controlled clinical trials of members of the B complex.

MINERALS

Iron Deficiency

Women who lose more than 60 to 80 ml of blood per menses tend to become progressively iron-deficient *(Fraser)*. Many such women, even though they may suffer from iron-deficiency anemia, are unaware of their excessive menstrual blood loss *(McKenna)*.

Even despite the absence of iron-deficiency anemia, menorrhagic patients may still be iron-deficient *(Lewis)*. In fact, one study found that menorrhagia correlated with depleted bone marrow iron stores irrespective of serum iron level *(Taymor)*.

Chronic iron deficiency is not only a result of menorrhagia; it is also a cause, as iron repletion is an effective treatment. For example, under double-blind conditions, menorrhagia improved in 75% of a group of chronically iron-deficient patients placed on iron supplementation as compared to only 33% of placebo-treated controls, a statistically significant difference *(Taymor)*.

The iron-deficient patients who fail to respond to supplementation frequently have organic pathology such as fibroids, polyps or adenomyosis *(Taymor)*.

Manganese Deficiency

Manganese deficiency has been associated with menorrhagia. Five and one-half months after healthy young women were placed on a diet that contained one-half of the average American intake of manganese, their menstrual fluid had increased about 50% in volume. Furthermore, they were now losing between 50 and 100% more manganese, as well as iron, copper and zinc, in the menstrual fluid *(Johnson)*.

OTHER NUTRITIONAL FACTORS

Flavonoids

Certain flavonoids have structural formulae that resemble that of estradiol *(Clemetson, 1962b)*. With help from estrogen, flavonoids in the capillary wall are important to maintaining the integrity of the capillary endothelium *(Clemetson, 1962b)*.

AND Vitamin C

Citrus-derived flavonoids have been combined with vitamin C to treat menorrhagia. In an open trial, menorrhagia was reduced in 14 out of 16 patients who received the combined supplement. Of the 2 women who failed to respond, one had endometriosis, while the other had metrorrhagia *(Cohen)*.

These findings were confirmed in a placebo-controlled trial. After 2 months, 32 of the 37 supplemented women had decreased menstrual blood loss compared to only one of the 13 women who received placebo. Two months were often required before improvement was noted, and menorrhagia tended to return with one to two months after supplementation was discontinued *(Clemetson, 1962a)*.

BIBLIOGRAPHY

Biskind MS, Biskind GR. Effect of vitamin B complex deficiency on inactivation of estrone in the liver. Endocrinology 31:109-14, 1942

Biskind MS. Nutritional deficiency in the etiology of menorrhagia, cystic mastitis and premenstrual tension, treatment with vitamin B complex. J Clin Endocrinol Metabol 3:227-34, 1943

Biskind MS et al. Nutritional deficiency in the etiology of menorrhagia, cystic mastitis and premenstrual tension, treatment with vitamin B complex. II. Further observations of treatment with the vitamin B complex. Surg Gynecol Obstet 78:49-57, 1944

Clemetson CAB, Blair LM. Capillary strength of women with menorrhagia. Am J Obstet Gynecol 83(10):1269-79, 1962a

Clemetson CAB et al. Capillary strength and the menstrual cycle. Ann N Y Acad Sci 93:277-300, 1962b

Cohen JD, Rubin HW. Functional menorrhagia: Treatment with bioflavonoids and vitamin C. Curr Ther Res 2:539, 1960

Fraser IS. Menorrhagia--a pragmatic approach to the understanding of causes and the need for investigations. Br J Obstet Gynaecol 101 Suppl 11:3-7, 1994

Johnson P, Human Nutrition Center, US Dept of Agriculture, Grand Forks, N. Dakota - reported in the Townsend Letter for Doctors, May, 1991

Lewis GJ. Do women with menorrhagia need iron? Br Med J 284:1158, 1982

Lithgow DM, Politzer WM. Vitamin A in the treatment of menorrhagia. S Afr Med J 51:191-3, 1977

McKenna DM et al. Iron deficiency in pre-menopausal females. Ir Med J 82(2):69-70, 1989

Taymor ML et al. The etiological role of chronic iron deficiency in production of menorrhagia. JAMA 187:323-7, 1964

MITRAL VALVE PROLAPSE

NUTRITIONAL TREATMENT GUIDE

✓ = Efficacy generally accepted.
* = Efficacy *demonstrated* by controlled human trials.
[+] = Efficacy *suspected* from uncontrolled human trials.
[-] = Efficacy *suspected* from indirect data.
? = Efficacy *challenged* in a study of similar design.

DIETARY FACTORS

* avoid **Caffeine**

NUTRITIONAL FACTORS

* **Coenzyme Q_{10}:** 3.0 to 3.4 mg/kg daily initially. Once improvement occurs, gradually reduce to a maintenance dosage.
* **Magnesium deficiency:** ≈ 400 mg daily (1 year trial)

- -

[+] **L-Carnitine:** 1 g 3 times daily (4 month trial)

- -

[-] **Vitamin C deficiency:** 500 mg twice daily

DIETARY FACTORS

Caffeine

In a controlled study, 12 cardiac patients who usually drank 3 to 5 cups of coffee a day first underwent 2 days of caffeine withdrawal. They then received a dose of caffeine orally or intravenously equivalent of 2 cups of coffee. Both before and after the caffeine dose, they received programmed cardiac stimulation, a procedure which produces arrhythmias in people who are already prone to them.

All but one of the 5 patients who had a history of rhythm disturbances associated with caffeine ingestion had mitral valve prolapse (MVP), and all 5 of these patients had arrhythmias produced with programmed cardiac stimulation following the caffeine administration, a finding which suggests that patients with MVP may be especially caffeine-sensitive *(Dobmeyer)*.

Caffeine sensitivity in MVP patients may be due to autonomic nervous system abnormalities and increased catecholamine levels *(Dobmeyer)*. Also, heavy caffeine use can cause a magnesium deficit which, in turn, could provoke the symptoms of MVP (see Magnesium below) *(Zeana)*.

NUTRITIONAL FACTORS

VITAMINS

Vitamin C Deficiency

A deficiency of ascorbic acid may contribute to the valvular changes seen in mitral valve prolapse by altering collagen metabolism *(Zeana)*. Whether repletion has any effect on the resulting lesions is not known.

MINERALS

Magnesium Deficiency

Magnesium deficiency hinders the mechanism by which fibroblasts degrade defective collagen, increases circulating catecholamines, and predisposes to dysregulation of the autonomic nervous system *(Galland,1986)*. It is therefore not unexpected that it promotes the development of mitral valve prolapse.

Signs and symptoms of the disorder, most commonly palpitations and precordial pain, may be a late complication of latent tetany (spasmophilia) due to a magnesium deficit *(Zeana)*. For example, in a group of 75 patients, 85% showed EMG changes suggestive of latent tetany, and 73% had a positive Chvostek sign *(Gerard)*. Conversely, out of a group of 170 patients with neuromuscular hyperexcitability, 26% of the 143 patients with evidence of latent tetany (positive Chvostek sign, EEG or EMG findings) were found to have mitral valve prolapse compared to none of the other 27 patients without latent tetany *(Durlach,1985)*.

In this population, erythrocyte *(Durlach,1994)* and lymphocyte *(Cohen)* magnesium levels are often reduced. Serum magnesium levels, which are far less sensitive to reductions in magnesium nutriture, are usually normal *(Galland,1985)*, but may be reduced in heavily symptomatic patients *(Lichodziejewska)*.

Supplementation

If the diagnosis of latent tetany due to a magnesium deficit is made early enough, mitral valve prolapse is preventable with magnesium supplementation. Once prolapse has developed, magnesium supplementation may take months or longer to be fully effective in reversing the process and is not always curative; therefore medications may still be required for symptomatic patients. After one year of magnesium treatment, the symptoms may be partially or totally reversed in about one-third of cases *(Durlach,1985)*.

There have been several studies of magnesium supplementation, some of which were placebo-controlled. *All* of these studies found the supplement to be effective. For example, a recent double-blind crossover study investigated magnesium supplementation for 84 heavily symptomatic patients with primary mitral valve prolapse and reduced serum magnesium levels. After 5 weeks, the mean number of symptoms was reduced by half, and there was a significant reduction in weakness, chest pain, dyspnea, palpitations, and anxiety. Moreover, while 63% of the patients had increased noradrenaline excretion at baseline, only 17% now had this finding (*Lichodziejewska*).

In a placebo-controlled study of patients with symptomatic mitral valve prolapse and latent tetany, only magnesium-treated patients responded; of the 24 who received magnesium lactate for 16 weeks, 29% became asymptomatic after 4 to 12 weeks, 46% became asymptomatic except for emotional symptoms, and the rest had a less marked improvement *(Simoes Fernandes)*.

OTHER NUTRITIONAL FACTORS

L-Carnitine

Carnitine is a naturally occurring compound found in the diet that is involved in mammalian energy metabolism. One of its functions is to facilitate mitochondrial long-chain fatty acid oxidation, which provides the major energy source for the myocardium.

Since essential fatty acid metabolism may be impaired in latent tetany *(Galland,1985b)*, and a similar impairment may occur when young rats or puppies are made magnesium-deficient *(Rayssiguier)*, the availability of carnitine to the myocardium (which is unable to manufacture it) may influence the development of the syndrome.

After a group of investigators found a treatment-resistant patient who responded dramatically to supplementation with L-carnitine, they randomly sampled carnitine levels of 4 other patients; all were found to be below the normal range for both free plasma and urinary carnitine *(Trivellato)*. Since 1984, when their paper was published, no further studies on carnitine for mitral valve prolapse have been reported, although carnitine continues to be investigated for its possible benefits in other cardiac conditions.

A 44 year-old male presented with a 5-year history of mitral valve prolapse and numerous associated symptoms that were resistant to drug therapy. He was found to have below normal values for free plasma and urinary carnitine.

After treatment with L-carnitine 1 gram 3 times daily for 4 months, symptoms resolved and his heart rate decreased from 115 bpm to 70 bpm (Trivellato).

Coenzyme Q_{10} (ubiquinone)

Like carnitine, coenzyme Q_{10} (CoQ_{10}), which is found primarily in the myocardium, plays an important role in energy metabolism. The efficacy of supplementation with CoQ_{10} has been investigated in several studies, all with positive findings.

In a study of 400 children between the ages of 8 and 16 with symptomatic mitral valve prolapse, CoQ_{10} supplementation was "definitely effective" and there were no side effects. With adequate doses, rapid normalization of symptomatic, stress-induced cardiac dysfunction could be achieved in one week. When the supplement was withdrawn, symptoms returned; however, it was possible to gradually decrease the dosage to a maintenance level *(Oda,1985)*.

Similarly, for adult patients who received CoQ_{10}, often with the goal of producing a whole blood levels of ≥ 2.1 µg/dl, there was significant improvement based on the New York Heart Association functional scale as well as significant objective improvement in myocardial function *(Langsjoen)*.

While these trials were uncontrolled, there is a report of a controlled study of children with symptomatic mitral valve prolapse, all of whom initially showed an abnormal response to a standard isometric hand grip test as a measure of cardiac performance. Eight of these children received CoQ_{10} while another 8 of them received placebo.

After 8 weeks, hand grip testing had normalized in all but one of the treated children compared to none of the placebo controls. The researchers note that relapse to their former condition was frequently noted if the children discontinued CoQ_{10} within 1 year to 17 months, but rarely occurred in those who continued to take the supplement for 18 months or longer *(Oda,1984)*.

BIBLIOGRAPHY

Cohen L et al. Idiopathic magnesium deficiency in mitral valve prolapse. Am J Cardiol 57(6):486-7, 1986

Dobmeyer DJ et al. The arrhythmogenic effects of caffeine in human beings. N Engl J Med 308(14):814-16, 1983

Durlach J et al. Latent tetany and mitral valve prolapse due to chronic primary magnesium deficit, in Halpern and Durlach, Eds. Magnesium Deficiency. First European Congress on Magnesium. Karger, Basel, 1985

Durlach J. Primary mitral valve prolapse: a clinical form of primary magnesium deficit. Magnes Res 7:3/4:339-40, 1994

Galland L. Magnesium deficiency in mitral valve prolapse, in Halpern and Durlach, Eds. Magnesium Deficiency. First European Congress on Magnesium. Karger, Basel, 1985

Galland L. Impaired essential fatty acid metabolism in latent tetany. Magnesium 4:333-8, 1985b

Galland LD et al. Magnesium deficiency in the pathogenesis of mitral valve prolapse. Magnesium 5(3-4):165-74, 1986

Gerard R et al. [Mitral valve prolapse and spasmophilia in the adult.] Arch Mal Coeur 72(7):715-20, 1979

Langsjoen H et al. Usefulness of coenzyme Q10 in clinical cardiology: a long-term study. Mol Aspects Med 15(suppl ps):S165-S175, 1994

Lichodziejewska B et al. Clinical symptoms of mitral valve prolapse are related to hypomagnesemia and attenuated by magnesium supplementation. Am J Cardiol 79(6):768-72, 1997

Oda T, Hamamoto K. Effect of coenzyme Q10 on the stress-induced decrease of cardiac performance in pediatric patients with mitral valve prolapse. Jpn Circ J 48(12):1387, 1984

Oda T. Effect of coenzyme Q10 on stress-induced cardiac dysfunction in paediatric patients with mitral valve prolapse: A study by stress echocardiography. Drugs Exp Clin Res 11(8):557-76, 1985

Rayssiguier Y, Genex E. New data on magnesium and lipids inter-relationship in the pathogenesis of vascular diseases, in Halpern, Durlach. Magnesium Deficiency. 1st European Congress on Magnesium. Karger, Basel, 1985

Simoes Fernandes J et al. Therapeutic effect of a magnesium salt in patients suffering from mitral valvular prolapse and latent tetany. Magnesium 4(5-6):283-90, 1985

Trivellato M et al. Carnitine deficiency as the possible etiology of idiopathic mitral valve prolapse: Case study with speculative annotation. Texas Heart Inst J 11(4):370, 1984

Zeana CD. Recent data on mitral valve prolapse and magnesium deficit. Magnesium Res 1(3-4):203-11, 1988

MULTIPLE SCLEROSIS

See Also: NEUROMUSCULAR DISORDERS (GENERAL)

NUTRITIONAL TREATMENT GUIDE

✓ = Efficacy generally accepted.
* = Efficacy *demonstrated* by controlled human trials.
[+] = Efficacy *suspected* from uncontrolled human trials.
[-] = Efficacy *suspected* from indirect data.
? = Efficacy *challenged* in a study of similar design.

DIETARY FACTORS

* **Fat** to come mainly from **Polyunsaturates**

- -

[+] avoid **Cow's Milk**, especially as a substitute for breast milk in infancy
[+] consume **Fish** rather than land-based animal products
[+] **low Fat diet**
[+] **low Sugar, low Pectin, high Leafy, Green Vegetable** diet

- -

[-] minimize **Coffee** and **Tea**

NUTRITIONAL FACTORS

* **Omega-3 fatty acids (fish oil):** 25 ml daily
* **Omega-6 fatty acids (evening primrose oil):** 4 g daily
* **L-Threonine:** 6 to 7.5 g daily

- -

[+] **L-5-Hydroxytryptophan:** *for cerebellar ataxia:* 16 mg/kg daily (1 year trial)
[+] **Folic acid:** 200 to 300 μg daily
[+] **Thiamine:** thiamine hydrochloride 150 mg IV *AND* **Liver extract** 20 μg IM every 7-10 days for a trial of 10 treatments
[+] **Vitamin B_6 deficiency:** 50 to 100 mg daily
[+] **Vitamin B_{12} deficiency:** 1,000 μg intramuscularly weekly initially and monthly afterwards
[+] ? **Vitamin B_{12}:** ? 20,000 μg IM weekly (1 year trial)

- -

[-] **Calcium deficiency:** ≈ 1 g daily
[-] **Magnesium deficiency:** ≈ 400 mg daily (Consider IM or IV administration, especially in hypomagnesemia.)
[-] **Selenium deficiency:** 200 μg daily
[-] **Vitamin D deficiency:** 50,000 to 100,000 IU 2 or 3 times during the first week; then, if needed, either 100,000 IU or ergo- or cholecalciferol every 3 to 6 months *OR* 800 to 1,600 IU daily

OTHER RELATED FACTORS

[+] **Proteolytic Enzymes:** Dosage depends upon preparation.
[+] rule out **Food Sensitivities**
[+] rule out **Mercury Amalgam** toxicity

DIETARY FACTORS

Dietary Fat

Epidemiological studies have repeatedly found a direct relationship between the risk of multiple sclerosis (MS) and dietary fat intake *(Ben-Shlomo)* and, more specifically, between MS risk and *animal* fat intake *(Sepcic;Tola)*. The intakes of meat *(Gusev)* and of unskimmed dairy products *(Sepcic)* have also been repeatedly associated with the risk of the disease.

By contrast, the intake of polyunsaturated fats has been *inversely* correlated with MS risk *(Alter)*. In MS patients, moreover, polyunsaturates may be deficient in the brain, cerebrospinal fluid, serum and erythrocytes *(Gul;Manley; Neu)*.

These findings have led to suggestions to reduce the intakes of total and saturated fats, and to increase the intake of polyunsaturates, particularly the intake of essential fatty acids *(Di Biase;Hutter)*. There is some evidence that such a diet may be beneficial:

Swank and his associates conducted a 34-year study on 150 patients who were placed on a diet that was low in saturated animal fats. At each level of severity of disability, patients who adhered to the diet showed significantly less deterioration and much lower death rates than did those who consumed more fat than prescribed (more than 20g/d). The greatest benefit was seen in those with minimal disability at the start of the trial. In this group, when those who died from non-MS diseases were excluded, 95% survived and remained physically active.

Defaulting from the diet even after 5 to 10 years was, in almost all cases, followed by reactivation of the disease. Patients consuming 10 to 15 grams daily or less had even better improvement in energy and fatigue levels *(Swank)*.

Another research group has reported their findings from a 3-year study. Eighty-three patients increased the polyunsaturate to saturate ratio of the diet. Initially the ratio was 0.8; after 6 months it was 1.5 and, at 36 months, it was 1.3. While matched controls continued to deteriorate, treated patients who were compliant showed a reduction in the exacerbation rate and improvement in neurological status *(Fitzgerald)*.

While such results are promising, patients who are well are more likely to continue on treatment than those who deteriorate. Thus "good compliers" are likely to be self-selected from those who do well, giving the predictable "positive" result *(Anonymous,1990)*.

Carbohydrates

There appears to be a relationship between MS and carbohydrate intake, although the nature of this relationship remains unclear. One small study has noted a correlation between the risk of MS and a high intake of complex carbohydrates (bread and pasta) between infancy and adolescence *(Tola)*, and there is a report of clinical improvement following the removal of carbohydrates from the diet *(Eckel)*.

Even if we were to assume that carbohydrate intake promotes MS, there are many possible mechanisms to explain the relationship - and most explanations would not suggest the necessity of such an extreme diet as one that is devoid of carbohydrates. One theory is that the removal of certain carbohydrates (such as wheat and rye proteins) to which patients are sensitive is the underlying mechanism (see Food Sensitivities below) *(Shatin)*.

Schwyzer has suggested a different approach to dietary carbohydrates, noting that the presentation of MS resembles that of methanol poisoning and suggesting that methanol overload can occur due to diet:

> If methanol, which is abundant in fruit pectin, is incompletely metabolized due to inadequate activity of alcohol dehydrogenase in the liver, it could leave free formaldehyde in the circulation which could eventually trigger an autoimmune reaction in sensitive individuals.
>
> Since alcohol dehydrogenase preferentially metabolizes fructose, sucrose or fructose ingestion

may further reduce the enzyme's ability to metabolize methanol. As little as 2 to 3 oz of fructose can temporarily overload hepatic capacity to produce adequate alcohol dehydrogenase.

Folic acid, which is abundant in leafy green vegetables, offers an alternative pathway for methanol metabolism and may explain why pregnant women, who are commonly given folate supplements, sometimes experience a temporary remission of MS (see Folic Acid below).

Schwyzer suggests a diet which is low in sugar and pectin, and high in leafy, green vegetables and notes that, within 9 to 12 months of starting this diet, chronic fatigue may disappear. Subsequently, so long as the diet continues to be followed, the patient may gradually go into permanent remission *(Schwyzer)*.

The efficacy of this diet has yet to be confirmed in controlled clinical trials.

Coffee and Tea

One study as found an association between MS and the frequent consumption of coffee and tea between infancy and adolescence *(Tola)*. Whether this finding has etiologic relevance is unknown.

NUTRITIONAL FACTORS

VITAMINS

Folic Acid

Folate nutriture does *not* appear to be reduced *(Nijst)* unless patients have been treated with high dosages of corticosteroids *(Frequin)*.

In addition to Schwyzer's work (see Carbohydrates above), there has been an open trial of folic acid supplementation as part of the treatment program for a group of MS patients with chronic gastritis. The supplement appeared to produce a "pronounced therapeutic effect" on the patients' neurological status which caused improvement in their general condition. Moreover, the reparative process in the gastric mucosa was improved *(Kanevskaia)*.

Thiamine

Thiamine is an essential component of myelin *(Anonymous,1970)*. Several case reports appeared many years ago suggesting that it may be effective when delivered by injection. Dramatic, although transient, improvements were noted after intraspinal injections *(Stern)*. Also, the combination of thiamine with niacin has been reported to be beneficial when injected intravenously *(Moore)*.

The most recent report concerns 14 patients with a history of neurologic deficits suggestive of MS which had been confirmed by neurologic investigation. They were treated with intravenous thiamine hydrochloride along with intramuscular injections of liver extract every 7 to 10 days for a series of 10 treatments. Following neurologic re-evaluation, further treatment was provided if there was evidence of a positive response.

Patients were treated for periods ranging from several months to 29 years. None had progression of the disease while on treatment. When symptoms recurred on cessation of treatment, they were controlled by resumption of therapy. Patients treated early in the disease responded best, while those with more advanced disease responded more slowly. Thiamine hydrochloride 100 mg daily by mouth combined with regular liver extract therapy was tried with one patient, but symptoms soon returned; the symptoms remitted again when intravenous thiamine was resumed *(Mount)*.

These findings have yet to be confirmed in controlled clinical trials.

Vitamin B_6 Deficiency

It has been suggested, but not demonstrated, that a vitamin B_6 deficiency may cause MS in susceptible persons. Pigs on a B_6-deficient diet develop a syndrome that has features resembling MS, namely demyelinization of peripheral nerves and spinal cord and sensory neuronal degeneration along with epileptiform convulsions, fatty degeneration of the liver and microcytic anemia *(Wintrobe)*.

Also, exposure to carbon monoxide increases the need for vitamin B_6, and there are data suggesting a relationship between carbon monoxide exposure and demyelinating disease. For example, humans poisoned by carbon monoxide sometimes develop a demyelinating condition, while animals exposed to carbon monoxide develop central nervous system degeneration. Moreover, carbon monoxide air pollution is the one environmental factor present only in the localities where MS is common *(Mitchell)*.

Vitamin B_{12}

Like thiamine, vitamin B_{12} is an essential component of myelin *(Norman)*. Also, demyelination of long nerve axons is characteristic of severe vitamin B_{12} deficiency while, in combined system disease, supplementation arrests demyelination *(Mount)*.

A significant association between cobalamin metabolism and MS has been postulated based on the observations that patients with MS have lower serum cobalamin levels, higher unsaturated cobalamin binding capacities, and a higher prevalence of macrocytosis than do normal controls *(Goodkin)*. Moreover, serum vitamin B_{12} levels in MS patients are lower in those who experienced the onset of neurological symptoms prior to 18 years of age *(Sandyk, 1993)*.

One explanation is that vitamin B_{12} deficiency leads to a vulnerability to the viral or immunologic mechanism that is reputed to cause multiple sclerosis. Alternatively, vitamin B_{12} deficiency may aggravate an existing immune system impairment. There also are speculations that multiple sclerosis may increase the need for vitamin B_{12}, leading to a deficiency state *(Gruener)*.

The presence of cobalamin deficiency should routinely be considered as it may aggravate the disorder or impair recovery *(Reynolds)*. Case reports and the results of early trials suggest that vitamin B_{12} supplementation, usually delivered parenterally, is occasionally beneficial, especially for patients with cobalamin deficiency.

In a controlled study, 62 patients randomly received intramuscular hydroxocobalamin injections or placebo weekly for 15 months. While there were no significant differences between the 2 experimental groups, the only patient who initially had a low serum cobalamin level and received hydroxocobalamin injections showed a moderate improvement *(Simpson)*.

Furthermore, when 6 patients with chronic progressive disease received methylcobalamin for 6 months, abnormalities in both the visual and brainstem auditory evoked potentials improved more frequently during therapy than in the pretreatment period, although the motor disability failed to improve *(Kira)*.

A 46-year-old woman had painful paresthesias associated with progressive right leg weakness. Multiple sclerosis was diagnosed. During the following 15 years she was admitted about every 18 months for symptom exacerbation and responded each time to ACTH infusions. In June, 1987, a brain MRI showed bilateral high-signal-intensity, white matter abnormalities. About 2 months later, a mean corpuscular volume of 100.8 fl suggesting erythrocyte macrocytosis was recorded.

When evaluated the next year, she had severe spastic monoparesis of the right leg associated with distal wasting. Vibration appreciation was bilaterally absent in the feet, with decreased pinprick appreciation in the right mid-thigh. Reflexes were symmetrically depressed with bilateral plantar extensor responses. Hemoglobin was 14.4 g/dL, MCV was 98.3 fl. The blood smear contained rare hypersegmented polymorphonuclear leukocytes. Serum B_{12} was less than 100 pg/ml and folic acid was 8.2 ng/ml. Plasma concentrations of vitamin B_{12}-dependent metabolites were normal (total serum homocystine and serum methylmalonic acid). Rheumatoid factor was raised with an antinuclear factor titer of 20. Serum intrinsic factor antibodies were present.

She was treated with vitamin B_{12} injections 1000 µg daily for 1 week followed by weekly injections. Initial improvement was such that she could climb stairs without circumduction of the right leg. After 6 months, she showed evidence of increased right leg strength. Blood count was normal with a decreased in MCV to 92.7 fl and no hypersegmented polymorphonuclear cells. Serum B_{12} was 210 pg/ml.

Since pernicious anemia has an autoimmune basis, both ACTH and steroids produce amelioration of the disease with hematological remission. It is suggested that ACTH produced temporary remissions, giving rise to the mistaken impression that she had a classic clinical course for multiple sclerosis (Ransohoff).

Vitamin D Deficiency

Activated (1,25-dihydroxy) vitamin D can completely prevent experimental autoimmune encephalomyelitis, a widely accepted mouse model of human multiple sclerosis. It has been suggested that the environmental factor in MS is the degree of sunlight exposure catalyzing the production of vitamin D3 in the skin, and that the hormonal form of vitamin D3 is a selective immune system regulator inhibiting the autoimmune disease.

This theory can explain the striking geographic distribution of multiple sclerosis and also explains the high incidence of multiple sclerosis in Switzerland at low altitudes and the low rates at high altitudes, as well as the high incidence in inland areas of Norway and lower prevalence along the coast. Ultraviolet light intensity is higher at high altitudes, resulting in a greater vitamin D3 synthetic rate, accounting for the low multiple sclerosis rates at higher altitudes. Moreover, on the Norwegian coast, fish are consumed at high rates and fish oils are rich in vitamin D3 *(Hayes)*.

Also, this theory would explain the epidemiological relationship between MS and dental caries. MS and dental caries may share certain etiological factors, two of which may be dietary excess of certain fats (see Dietary Fat above), and vitamin D deficiency. In the United States, a strong positive correlation exists between MS death rates and dental caries indices *(Craelius)*.

The prevalence of MS in 45 countries or areas correlates well with the frequencies of decayed, missing or filled teeth among children of school age. The prevalence of MS also correlates well with the percentage of edentulous individuals in certain countries. Furthermore, a review of the literature shows that the risk for dental caries is higher among the same groups for which the risk of MS is higher *(Craelius)*.

Whether vitamin D supplementation can benefit MS patients remains to be determined.

MINERALS

Calcium Deficiency

In the white matter of the brains of MS patients, the calcium content is depressed *(Yasui,1992)*. Based on epidemiologic, biochemical and genetic evidence, it has been theorized that a deficiency of calcium and vitamin D during adolescence may interfere with myelination in predisposed people *(Goldberg)*. Epidemiologic studies also suggest a link between MS in young adults and a specific history of high milk intake during childhood followed by a large or sudden reduction during the adolescent growth spurt *(Butcher,1986)*. Consistent with this hypothesis, electrophoresis of solubilized proteins from mouse brain tissue has shown that a dietary reduction in calcium carbonate in early life can cause a change in the electrophoretic pattern which is similar to the abnormality seen in multiple sclerosis plaque *(Butcher,1992)*.

Calcium supplementation has not been shown to either prevent or treat multiple sclerosis.

Copper

In animal studies, copper deficiency causes defective myelination *(Underwood)*. Multiple sclerosis appears to be associated with abnormal copper metabolism. Erythrocyte *(Smith)* and serum *(Kapaki)* copper levels may be reduced, while ceruloplasmin, a copper-binding protein, tends to be increased *(Smith)*, especially during acute exacerbations *(Becus)*.

The clinical importance of these changes is not known, and there is no evidence that copper supplementation is beneficial.

Magnesium

Magnesium nutriture may affect the maintenance and function of nerve cells as well as the proliferation and synthesis of lymphocytes. Thus, a deficit may induce dysfunction of nerve cells or lymphocytes directly and/or indirectly *(Yasui,1992)*.

The few studies of magnesium in MS patients have consistently found evidence of reduced magnesium nutriture *(Yasui,1997)*. The average magnesium content in central nervous system tissues is reduced, especially in the white matter including demyelinated plaque. Moreover, the magnesium content of the visceral organs, except for the spleen, is also reduced *(Yasui,1990)*. While plasma levels may be normal, erythrocyte magnesium levels are significantly depressed *(Stelmaskiak)*.

Magnesium supplementation has not been shown to either prevent or treat multiple sclerosis.

Selenium

The geographical distribution of MS suggests that selenium may be involved in its etiology *(Foster)*. For example, MS prevalence is high in Ostrobothnia, a low selenium district in Finland, while in Lapland, a high selenium district, the prevalence is low *(Wikstrom)*. In one group of 20 patients, their dietary selenium was evaluated and was found to be below the minimum values recommended by the US Food and Nutrition Board *(Mazzella)*.

Studies of selenium nutriture have found mixed results. One study of 40 patients found hair selenium levels to be significantly lower than those of controls *(Ryan)*. However, most studies of erythrocyte and plasma selenium levels have failed to find significant decreases from those of normal controls *(Smith)*.

Some of the studies of the activity of glutathione peroxidase, a selenium-dependent enzyme, have found reductions *(Jensen)*, while others have found normal activity *(Szeinberg)*.

Supplementation

It appears that, for patients with reduced glutathione peroxidase activity, selenium supplementation may be beneficial. Among a group of patients who demonstrated significantly lowered selenium values and lowered glutathione peroxidase activities of major types of hematogenous cells (which showed an increased peroxidation rate), increasing the daily intake of selenium along with vitamins C and E resulted in normalization of all these abnormalities *(Clausen)*. Similarly, among a group of patients with reduced glutathione peroxidase activity, supplementation with selenium along with vitamins C and E resulted in a 5-fold increase in enzyme activity *(Mai)*.

Controlled clinical trials are needed to ascertain whether selenium supplementation results in clinical benefits for MS patients who are selenium-deficient.

Zinc

A study of the demyelinated area in the central nervous system of a patients revealed a decreased zinc level *(Yasui,1991)*. While the evidence is conflicting, there appear to be abnormalities in the compartmentalization of zinc *(Dore-Duffy; Wong)*. In one study, plasma and erythrocyte zinc levels were higher than those of controls, but decreased dramatically during relapses *(Ho)*, suggesting that patients in remission should be studied separately from those who are relapsing.

The clinical efficacy of zinc supplementation in MS has yet to be investigated.

OTHER NUTRITIONAL FACTORS

Essential Fatty Acids

Multiple sclerosis appears to share with many other neurological diseases a lipid imbalance arising from faulty lipid metabolism and involving the essential fatty acids linoleic and linolenic acids as well as trace fatty acids *(Marshall)*. More specifically, reductions in levels of docosahexaenoic acid (DHA) *(Wilson)*, eicosapentaenoic acid (EPA) *(Nightingale)*, linoleic acid *(Cunnane)*, and arachidonic acid have been noted in nervous tissue and/or erythrocytes of MS patients.

Many studies have investigated the efficacy of essential fatty acids in the treatment of multiple sclerosis. While these trials have had different lengths, electrophoretic mobility studies of red cells from MS patients indicate that treatment with unsaturated fatty acids must continue for at least 2 years before normal reactivity is restored. Assuming this also applies to myelin, clinical trials need to last longer than 2 years if treatment is to be effective *(Field)*.

Omega-3 Fatty Acid Supplementation

In a 6-month trial, the immunologic effects of omega-3 fatty acid supplementation were studied in 20 patients with relapsing-remitting MS and healthy controls. In both groups, supplementation reduced the production of proinflammatory eicosanoids, and the decreased some cytokines with an immunoenhancing effect. These changes could modulate some immune functions which have been demonstrated to be altered in the disease *(Gallai)*.

When 12 patients received MaxEPA, a proprietary fish oil preparation, for just 1 to 4 months, the 5 patients with acute remitting MS showed a slight but significant reduction in total neurologic scores, while the 7 patients with slowly progressive MS continued to deteriorate *(Cendrowski)*.

This study was followed by a randomized double-blind study of 312 patients with acute remitting MS. Both groups received dietary advice to increase their intake of omega-6 fatty acids, while just the treatment group was supplemented with omega-3 fatty acids. Although, after 2 years, there were no significant differences between the two groups in regard to the duration, frequency and severity of relapses and the number of patients who had improved or remained unchanged, there was a trend in favor of the treatment group in all of these parameters *(Bates)*.

Omega-6 Fatty Acid Supplementation

Three double-blind trials of patients with a remitting-relapsing course were reanalyzed together due to inconsistency in the findings. The combined data consisted of neurologic assessments over two and one-half years of trials for 87 treated patients and 85 control patients.

Treated patients with minimal or no disability at entry had a significantly smaller increase in disability than did controls. In addition, treatment reduced the severity and duration of relapses at all levels of disability and duration of illness at entry to the trials. The authors suggest that the study design may have failed to reveal the full extent of potential benefits as oleic acid, the placebo used, may itself ameliorate MS-like illnesses *(Dworkin)*. Moreover, Horrobin has suggested that the results were suboptimal due to inadequate dosages and the use of dyes in the supplements which block the conversion of essential fatty acids to prostaglandins *(Horrobin)*.

L-5-Hydroxytryptophan

There is early evidence from an open trial that supplementation with L-5-hydroxytryptophan, the immediate precursor to serotonin, may reduce cerebellar ataxia in MS. Twenty-one patients with hereditary ataxias as well as patients with multiple sclerosis and surgical lesions of the anterior lobe vermis were treated for one year. There was a significant regression of symptoms, primarily in the static (versus the kinetic) form of ataxia and in the speed of speech, suggesting that the treatment was effective in treating the cerebellar syndrome, no matter what the cause *(Trouillas)*.

No further trials of L-5-hydroxytryptophan in multiple sclerosis have been published. However, in subsequent trials involving patients with cerebellar ataxia due to other causes, the results have been mixed.

L-Threonine

Threonine is a precursor to glycine, an inhibitory neurotransmitter that readily passes the blood-brain barrier and serves as the major inhibitory neurotransmitter of the spinal cord, affecting specific inhibitory receptors on spinal interneurons and motoneurons *(Davidoff)*.

In 2 double-blind crossover studies, oral L-threonine supplementation exerted a modest but definite antispastic effect *(Hauser;Lee)*.

L-Tryptophan

While brain tissue tryptophan levels appear to be normal *(Langemann)*, levels in the cerebrospinal fluid and blood plasma may be reduced *(Sandyk,1996)*.

A subgroup of MS patients experiences symptom exacerbations following periods of mental stress. Psychological stress may also contribute to the onset and long term clinical deterioration of the disease. Mental stress is associated with activation of the hypothalamic-pituitary-adrenal axis resulting in increased release of ACTH and cortisol secretion. Stress-induced activation of this axis is associated with an increased metabolism of cerebral serotonin, the synthesis of which is dependent upon the availability of its precursor tryptophan. This suggests that tryptophan supplementation could theoretically diminish these patients' exacerbations and even halt progression of the disease *(Sandyk,1996)*.

While this hypothesis has yet to be fully tested, 12 patients received L-tryptophan as well as placebo for 30 days each under double-blind conditions. After the 30 days on tryptophan, there was a slight alleviation of changeable symptoms, especially in motility and bladder disturbances as well as in mood *(Hyyppä)*.

COMBINED NUTRITIONAL THERAPY

In an open trial, 16 patients aged 22 to 37 years who exhibited unambiguous exacerbations within the previous one to two years received calcium (16 mg/kg) and magnesium (10 mg/kg) supplementation in the form of dolomite along with cod liver oil (20 g/d) to furnish vitamin D (5000 IU) as well as omega-3 fatty acids.

After one or two years, the number of exacerbations was less than half of the number expected from their case histories *(Goldberg)*.

OTHER RELATED FACTORS

Proteolytic Enzymes

Immune complexes are associated with multiple sclerosis *(Glenk)* and particularly with clinical exacerbations *(Neuhofer,1990)*, while reduction of disease activity is associated with a reduction in immune complexes *(Dasgupta)*.

Immune complexes can be reduced by the administration of proteolytic enzymes *(Glenk;Steffen)*. In an open trial, patients received oral and/or injectable enzyme mixtures and they were placed on a whole food diet containing a very high level of raw foods and polyunsaturated fatty acids.

Results were tabulated for patients who had been treated for at least 2 years. Forty-five out of 83 patients with chronic progressive MS were appreciably improved and progression in another 26 patients was at least diminished, while the condition of 12 patients, all of whom had previously been treated with azathioprine (an immunotoxic drug), deteriorated.

Moreover, 35 out of 43 patients with step-wise, episodic progression (intervals of at least 4 weeks between acute episodes) exhibited appreciable improvement. In some, paralysis disappeared. The condition of the other 8 patients stabilized.

Enzyme injections needed to be initiated at the first signs of an exacerbation to be effective. There were no serious side effects from the treatment *(Neuhofer,1986)*.

Controlled clinical trials of enzyme therapy are needed to validate these interesting findings.

Food Sensitivities

Numerous studies have reported an association between food reactions and symptoms in multiple sclerosis. Foods that are particularly suspicious in regard to inciting exacerbations fall into 3 groups:

Chocolate

Epidemiological studies have documented a correlation between high cocoa consumption and high MS incidence. When cocoa is introduced to an area, MS incidence rises sharply. Some dogs develop muscle weakness, twitching, loss of sphincter function and myocardial damage when fed chocolate. Moreover, cases have been reported in which chocolate ingestion by MS patients was followed by exacerbations *(Maas)*.

Dairy Products

There is a striking correlation between the incidence of multiple sclerosis and the world distribution of dairy production and consumption *(Butcher,1976)*. This correlation appears to be primarily due to the consumption of cow's milk as it is lower for cream and butter consumption and absent for the consumption of cheese *(Malosse)* - which also suggests that it is not due to the milk fat. In a small study of 46 patients and 92 controls living in a high-risk area, a high consumption of full-fat, unskimmed milk increased the risk of MS by 22-fold *(Sepcic)*.

Whether the avoidance of dairy products is beneficial to a sub-group of patients is not known.

Gluten

Epidemiological evidence is consistent with the hypothesis that the ingestion of high-gluten grains by genetically predisposed individuals may cause MS *(Shatin)*. Compared to controls, MS patients have a statistically higher rate of positive responses to rye and wheat during provocative ophthalmic testing *(Ehrentheil)*. Gluten avoidance has been used occasionally as a treatment, and there are informal reports suggesting that patients with especially difficult food sensitivities improve on a cereal-free diet *(Jonez)*.

However, celiac disease appears to be uncommon in this patient population. Studies of the jejunal mucosa of MS patients have failed to find evidence of celiac-like changes *(Bateson;Jones)*, and most MS patients fail to respond to gluten withdrawal *(Hewson)*.

One study of 36 patients only found gluten antibodies in one of the patients, and the level of antibodies in this patient was not even elevated enough to justify a trial of a gluten-free diet *(Hunter)*. Although anti-gliadin antibodies may be rarer among MS patients than among patients with neurological dysfunction of unknown cause *(Hadjivassiliou)*, an occasional patient could theoretically respond to a gluten-free diet.

A 44 year-old woman with a 20-year history of multiple sclerosis went into remission as soon as foods she was found to be sensitive to were removed from her diet.

After 8 months, these foods were reintroduced. Within 4 days, symptoms of weakness and ataxia returned (Mandell).

Mercury Amalgam Toxicity

The role of mercury from dental amalgams in promoting MS is controversial. There is epidemiological evidence suggesting that dental caries may be a precursor of one form of MS *(Craelius)*. Although this data can be interpreted many ways (see Vitamin D above), one possibility is that the association is due to the placement of mercury-containing amalgams.

It has been theorized that, when amalgam fillings are exposed to gingival action and oxidation, inorganic mercury in the fillings (especially class V fillings and root canals) may be converted to an organic form which may act as a neurotoxin *(Ingalls)*. Although brain mercury concentrations are not abnormally elevated *(Fung)*, when MS patients were compared to controls who had the same number of mercury amalgam fillings, the patients had, on average, 7.5 times higher cerebrospinal fluid (CSF) mercury levels than the controls *(Ahlot-Westerlund)*. This finding suggests either that they were more likely to absorb mercury leached from the amalgams into the CSF, or that their higher mercury levels came from other sources than dental amalgams. Moreover, *all* the patients had above normal CSF mercury levels *(Ahlot-Westerlund)*.

Two preliminary studies have investigated objective changes following amalgam removal. In one study, 4 patients had CSF samples taken by lumbar puncture before and after the removal of all dental amalgams and their replacement with biocompatible materials. (They also received megadoses of vitamin C each visit, were placed on special diets based on nutritional blood chemistries, and advised to limit sugar, alcohol and caffeine.) Although the baseline gels of all 4 patients showed abnormal heavy photolabeling of multiple proteins, the follow-up gels showed a near absence of such labeling *(Huggins)*.

In the other study, 7 patients had their amalgams removed. Six months later, the visual evoked response, a measure of nerve conduction velocity, showed significantly decreased latencies, indicating improvement in nerve conduction *(Siblerud)*.

Controlled studies are needed to confirm and extend these initial findings before the controversy concerning the role of dental amalgams can be resolved.

BIBLIOGRAPHY

Ahlrot-Westerlund B. Mercury in cerebrospinal fluid in multiple sclerosis. Swed J Biol Med 1:6, 1989

Alter M et al. Multiple sclerosis and nutrition. Arch Neurol (Chicago) 31(4):267-72, 1974

Anonymous. "Cures" for multiple sclerosis. Br Med J i:59-60, 1970

Anonymous. Editorial: Lipids and multiple sclerosis. Lancet 336:25-6, 1990

Bates D et al. A double-blind controlled trial of long chain n-3 polyunsaturated fatty acids in the treatment of multiple sclerosis. J Neurol Neurosurg Psychiatry 52(1):18-22, 1989

Bateson MC et al. Jejunal morphology in multiple sclerosis. Lancet i:1108-10, 1979

Becus T et al. Study of serum and cerebrospinal fluid ceruloplasmin in multiple sclerosis and other neurologic diseases. Rev Roum Neurol 8:3-12, 1971

Ben-Shlomo Y et al. Dietary fat in the epidemiology of multiple sclerosis: has the situation been adequately addressed? Neuroepidemiology 11(4-6):214-25, 1992

Butcher J. The distribution of multiple sclerosis in relation to the dairy industry and milk consumption. N Z Med J 83:427-30, 1976

Butcher PJ. Milk consumption and multiple sclerosis - an etiological hypothesis. Med Hypotheses 19(2):169-78, 1986

Butcher PJ. Calcium intake and the protein composition of mouse brain: relevance to multiple sclerosis. Med Hypotheses 39(3):275-80, 1992

Cendrowski W. Multiple sclerosis and MaxEPA. Br J Clin Pract 40:365-7, 1986

Clausen J et al. Selenium in chronic neurologic diseases. Multiple sclerosis and Batten's disease. Biol Trace Elem Res 15:179-203, 1988

Craelius W. Comparative epidemiology of multiple sclerosis and dental caries. J Epidemiol Community Health 32(3):155-65, 1978

Cunnane SC et al. Essential fatty acid and lipid profiles in plasma and erythrocytes in patients with multiple sclerosis. Am J Clin Nutr 50:801-6, 1989

Dasgupta MK et al. Circulating immune complexes in multiple sclerosis. Relation with disease activity. Neurology 32:1000-4, 1982

Davidoff RA. Antispasticity drugs: mechanisms of action. Ann Neurol 17(2):107-16, 1985

Di Biase A, Salvati S. Exogenous lipids in myelination and myelination. Kao Hsiung I Hsueh Ko Hsueh Tsa Chih 13(1):19-29, 1997

Dore-Duffy P et al. Zinc in multiple sclerosis. Ann Neurol 14(4):450-4, 1983

Dworkin RH et al. Linoleic acid and multiple sclerosis: A reanalysis of three double-blind trials. Neurology 34:1441-5, 1984

Eckel K, Lutz W. [The treatment of multiple sclerosis by the removal of carbohydrates.] Wien klin Wschr 73:493, 1961 (in German)

Ehrentheil OF et al. Role of food allergy in multiple sclerosis. Neurology 2:412, 1952

Field EJ, Joyce G. Multiple sclerosis: effect of gamma linolenate administration upon membranes and the need for extended clinical trials of unsaturated fatty acids. Eur Neurol 22(1):78-83, 1983

Fitzgerald G et al. The effect of nutritional counseling on diet and plasma EFA status in multiple sclerosis patients over 3 years. Hum Nutr Appl Nutr 41(5):297-310, 1987

Foster HD. The iodine-selenium connection: its possible roles in intelligence, cretinism, sudden infant death syndrome, breast cancer and multiple sclerosis. Med Hypotheses 40(1):61-5, 1993

Frequin ST et al. Decreased vitamin B12 and folate levels in cerebrospinal fluid and serum of multiple sclerosis patients after high-dose intravenous methylprednisolone. J Neurol 240(5):305-8, 1993

Fung YK et al. Brain mercury in neurodegenerative disorders. J Toxicol Clin Toxicol 35(1):49-54, 1997

Gallai V et al. Cytokine secretion and eicosanoid production in the peripheral blood mononuclear cells of MS patients undergoing dietary supplementation with n-3 polyunsaturated fatty acids. J Neuroimmunol 56(2):143-53, 1995

Glenk W, Neu S. Enzyme Die Bausteine des Lebens Wie sie wirken, helfen und heilen. Munich, Wilhelm Heyne Verlag, 1990 (in German)

Goldberg P et al. Multiple sclerosis: decrease relapse rate through dietary supplementation with calcium, magnesium, and vitamin D. Med Hypotheses 21(2):193-20, 1986

Goodkin DE et al. Serum cobalamin deficiency is uncommon in multiple sclerosis. Arch Neurol 51(11):1110-4, 1994

Gruener DM et al. Dietary vitamin B12 deficiency in a patient with multiple sclerosis. Gen Hosp Psychiatry 16(3):224-8, 1994

Gul S et al Fatty acid composition of phospholipids from platelets and erythrocytes in multiple sclerosis. J Neurol Neurosurg Psychiatry 33(4):506-10, 1970

Gusev E et al. Environmental risk factors in MS: a case-control study in Moscow. Acta Neurol Scand 94(6):386-94, 1996

Hadjivassiliou M et al. Does cryptic gluten sensitivity play a part in neurological illness? Lancet 347:369-71, 1996

Hauser SL et al. An antispasticity effect of threonine in multiple sclerosis. Arch Neurol 49(9):923-6, 1992

Hayes CE et al. Vitamin D and multiple sclerosis. Proceed Society Exp Biol Med 216:21-7, 1997

Hewson DC. Is there a role for gluten-free diets in multiple sclerosis? Human Nutr 38:417-20, 1984

Ho S-Y et al. Zinc in multiple sclerosis. II. Correlation with disease activity and elevated plasma membrane-bound zinc in erythrocytes from patients with multiple sclerosis. Ann Neurol 20:712-15, 1986

Horrobin D. Multiple sclerosis: the rational basis for treatment with colchicine and evening primrose oil. Med Hypotheses 5:365-78, 1979

Huggins HA, Levy TE. Cerebrospinal fluid protein changes in multiple sclerosis after dental amalgam removal. Altern Med Rev 3(4):295-300, 1998

Hunter AL et al. Gluten antibodies in patients with multiple sclerosis. Hum Nutr Appl Nutr 38(2):142-3, 1984

Hutter C. On the causes of multiple sclerosis. Med Hypotheses 41(2):93-6, 1993

Hyyppä MT et al. Effect of L-tryptophan treatment on central indoleamine metabolism and short-lasting neurologic disturbances in multiple sclerosis. J Neural Trans 37(4):297-304, 1975

Ingalls TH. Epidemiology, etiology and prevention of multiple sclerosis. Am J Forensic Med Pathol 4:55-61, 1983

Jensen GE et al. Leucocyte glutathione peroxidase activity and selenium level in multiple sclerosis. J Neurol Sci 48(1):61-7, 1980

Jones PE et al. Morphological and biochemical findings in jejunal biopsies from patients with multiple sclerosis. J Neurol Neurosurg Psychiatry 42(5):402-6, 1979

Jonez HD. Management of multiple sclerosis. Postgrad Med 11(5):415-22, 1952

Kanevskaia SA et al. [Folic acid in the combined treatment of patients with disseminated sclerosis and chronic gastritis]. Vrach Delo (4):96-7, 1990) (in Russian)

Kapaki E et al. Zinc, copper and magnesium concentration in serum and CSF of patients with neurological disorders. Acta Neurol Scand 79(5):373-8, 1989

Kira J et al. Vitamin B12 metabolism and massive-dose methyl vitamin B12 therapy in Japanese patients with multiple sclerosis. Intern Med 33(2):82-6, 1994

Langemann H et al. Measurement of low-molecular-weight antioxidants, uric acid, tyrosine and tryptophan in plaques and white matter from patients with multiple sclerosis. Eur Neurol 32(5):248-52, 1992

Lee A, Patterson V. A double-blind study of L-threonine in patients with spinal spasticity. Acta Neurol Scand 88(5):334-8, 1993

Maas AG, Hogenhuis LA. Multiple sclerosis and possible relationship to cocoa: A hypothesis. Ann Allergy 59(1):76-9, 1987

Mai J et al. High dose antioxidant supplementation to MS patients. Biol Trace Element Res 24(2):109-17, 1990

Malosse D et al. Correlation between milk and dairy product consumption and multiple sclerosis prevalence: a worldwide study. Neuroepidemiology 11(4-6):304-12, 1992

Mandell, Marshall - reported in Let's Live January, 1984, pp. 26-31

Manley P. Diet in multiple sclerosis. Practitioner 238:358-63, 1994

Marshall BH. Lipids and neurological diseases. Med Hypotheses 34(3):272-4, 1991

Mazzella GL et al. Blood cells glutathione peroxidase activity and selenium in multiple sclerosis. Eur Neurol 22(6):442-6, 1983

Mitchell DA, Schandl EK. Carbon monoxide, vitamin B6, and multiple sclerosis: a theory of interrelationship. Am J Clin Nutr 26(8):890-6, 1973

Moore MT. Treatment of multiple sclerosis with nicotinic acid and vitamin B1. Arch Intern Med 65:18, 1940

Mount HTR. Multiple sclerosis and other demyelinating diseases. Letter. Can Med Assoc J 108:1356-7, 1973

Neu IS. [Metabolic aspects of multiple sclerosis.] Wien Med Wochenschr 135(1-2):20-2, 1985) (in German)

Neuhofer C. Enzymtherapie bei Multipler Sklerose. Hufeland Journal Biologisch-medizinisches Zentralorgan, 1986

Neuhofer C. Multiple sclerosis: treatment with enzyme preparations. Lecture. First Int. Conf. on Systemic Enzyme Therapy, September 12, 1990

Nightingale S et al. Red blood cell and adipose tissue fatty acids in mild inactive multiple sclerosis. Acta Neurol Scand 82(1):43-50, 1990

Nijst TQ et al. Vitamin B12 and folate concentrations in serum and cerebrospinal fluid of neurological patients with special reference to multiple sclerosis and dementia. J Neurol Neurosurg Psychiatry 53(11):951-4, 1990

Norman CS. Vitamin B12 plasma clearance in multiple sclerosis. Ir J Med Sci 6:333, 1966

Ransohoff RM et al. Vitamin B12 deficiency and multiple sclerosis. Letter. Lancet 335:1285-6, 1990

Reynolds EH. Multiple sclerosis and vitamin B12 metabolism. J Neuroimmunol 40(2-3):225-30, 1992

Ryan DE et al. Trace elements in the scalp-hair of persons with multiple sclerosis and normal individuals. Clin Chem 24(11):1996-2000, 1978

Sandyk R, Awerbuch GI. Vitamin B12 and its relationship to age of onset of multiple sclerosis. Int J Neurosci 71(1-4):93-9, 1993

Sandyk R. Tryptophan availability and the susceptibility to stress in multiple sclerosis: a hypothesis. Int J Neurosci 86(1-2):47-53, 1996

Schwyzer RU. Multiple sclerosis: prevention of serious illness: vision of a desired future for newly ascertained patients. Med Hypotheses 37(2):115-18, 1992

Sepcic J. Nutritional factors and multiple sclerosis in Gorski Kotar, Croatia. Neuroepidemiology 12:234-40, 1993

Shatin R. Multiple sclerosis and geography: new interpretations of epidemiological observations. Neurology 14(1-6):338-44, 1964

Siblerud RL, Kienholz E. Evidence that mercury from silver dental fillings may be an etiological factor in reduced nerve conduction velocity in multiple sclerosis patients. J Orthomol Med 12(3):169-72, 1997

Simpson CA et al. The treatment of multiple sclerosis with massive doses of hydroxocobalamin. Neurology 15(7):599-603, 1965

Smith DK et al. Trace element status in multiple sclerosis. Am J Clin Nutr 50:136-40, 1989

Steffen C, Menzel J. Enzymbbau von Immunkomplexen. Z Rheumatol 42(5):249-55, 1983 (in German)

Stelmasiak Z et al. Magnesium concentration in plasma and erythrocytes in MS. Acta Neurol Scand 92(1):109-11, 1995

Stern EI. The intraspinal injection of vitamin B1 for the relief of intractable pain, and for inflammatory and degenerative diseases of the central nervous system. Am J Surg 34:495, 1938

Swank RL, Dugan BB. Effect of low saturated fat diet in early and late cases of multiple sclerosis. Lancet 336:37-9, 1990

Szeinberg A et al. Glutathione peroxidase activity in various types of blood cells in multiple sclerosis. Acta Neurol Scand 63(1):67-75, 1981

Tola MR et al. Dietary habits and multiple sclerosis. A retrospective study in Ferrara, Italy. Acta Neurol (Napoli) 16(4):189-97, 1994

Trouillas P. Regression of cerebellar syndrome with long-term administration of 5-HTP or the combination 5-HTP-benserazide. Ital J Neurol Sci 5(3):253-66, 1984

Underwood EJ. Trace Elements in Human and Animal Nutrition, 4th Ed. New York, Academic Press, 1971

Wikstrom J et al. Selenium, vitamin E and copper in multiple sclerosis. Acta Neurol Scand 54(3):287-90, 1976

Wilson R, Tocher DR. Lipid and fatty acid composition is altered in plaque tissue from multiple sclerosis brain compared with normal white brain matter. Lipids 26:9-12, 1991

Wintrobe MM et al. Pyridoxine deficiency in swine, with particular reference to anemia, epileptiform convulsions and fatty liver. Bull Johns Hopkins Hosp 72:1-25, 1943

Wong EK et al. [A hypothesis: multiple sclerosis a systemic disease.] J Fr Ophtalmol 6(3):243-9, 1983 (in French)

Yasui M et al. Magnesium concentration in brains from multiple sclerosis patients. Acta Neurol Scand 81(3):197-200, 1990

Yasui M et al. [Zinc concentration in the central nervous system in a case of multiple sclerosis--comparison with other neurological diseases]. No To Shinkei 43(10):951-5, 1991 (in Japanese)

Yasui M, Ota K. Experimental and clinical studies on dysregulation of magnesium metabolism and the aetiopathogenesis of multiple sclerosis. Magnes Res 5(4):295-302, 1992

Yasui M et al. Magnesium-related neurological disorders, in Mineral and Metal Neurotoxicology. CRC Press, 1997:219-26

MUSCLE CRAMPS (FUNCTIONAL)

See Also: 'HYPOGLYCEMIA' (FUNCTIONAL)
PAIN
PREGNANCY-RELATED ILLNESS

NUTRITIONAL TREATMENT GUIDE

✓ = Efficacy generally accepted.
* = Efficacy *demonstrated* by controlled human trials.
[+] = Efficacy *suspected* from uncontrolled human trials.
[-] = Efficacy *suspected* from indirect data.
? = Efficacy *challenged* in a study of similar design.

NUTRITIONAL FACTORS

* **L-Carnitine:** *for muscle pain from over-exercise:* 3 g daily
* ? **Vitamin E:** ? 500 IU daily (1 month trial)

- -

[+] **Calcium:** *for night cramps:* calcium gluconate 4.8 g at bedtime
[+] **Magnesium deficiency:** ≈ 400 mg daily (Consider IM or IV supplementation, especially in hypomagnesemia.)
[+] **Potassium deficiency:** ? 80 to 100 mEq daily total intake, preferably from potassium-rich foods
[+] **Riboflavin:** 10 mg daily
[+] **Sodium deficiency:** *for exercise-related heat cramps:* repletion
[+] **Taurine:** *for muscle cramps from cirrhosis of the liver:* 6 g 3 times daily (1 month trial)
[+] **Vitamin B_6:** 50 mg daily (3 month trial)
[+] **Vitamin B_{12}:** *for night cramps:* 500 μg intramuscularly every 4 to 6 weeks as needed

OTHER RELATED FACTORS

[+] rule out **Reactive Hypoglycemia**

NUTRITIONAL FACTORS

VITAMINS

Riboflavin

Supplementation with megadose riboflavin moderately reduces neuromuscular irritability *(Haralambie).* Although there is no recent literature, a 1946 French study found riboflavin supplementation to be effective in treating muscle cramps secondary to other medical disorders, specifically diabetes mellitus, cardiovascular diseases, infections and toxicities *(Perrault).*

Vitamin B_6

John Ellis has proposed that carpal tunnel syndrome can often be successfully treated with vitamin B_6, and his observation has been confirmed by a number of studies (see Carpal Tunnel Syndrome). He has also noted that some patients with carpal tunnel syndrome complain of nocturnal muscle spasms in the extremities. According to Ellis, these muscle spasms will also respond to supplementation with the vitamin *(Ellis,1966)*.

A 69 year-old tractor driver presented with stiffness in both hands. They were swollen, and flexion was very limited. He also complained of frequent cramps in his thighs during the day, and nocturnal leg cramps about twice a week.

Four weeks after starting on pyridoxine 50 mg daily, hand stiffness was dramatically relieved, and he reported that, after one week on pyridoxine, his leg cramps vanished (Ellis,1973).

Vitamin B_{12}

Sixteen consecutive middle-aged and elderly patients with night cramps all had dramatic relief for 4 to 6 weeks or even longer following an injection of vitamin B_{12}. By far the great majority spontaneously requested another injection within the 6-week period *(Aitchison)*.

This interesting report has yet to be followed-up with a controlled clinical trial.

Vitamin E

Vitamin E supplementation has been reported to be highly effective in providing relief for recurrent muscle cramps in several studies, including one of two double-blind studies *(Connolly;Roca)*. The largest group studied consisted of 125 patients with nocturnal leg and foot cramps, over half of whom had suffered for over 5 years.

Following supplementation, 82% reported complete or nearly complete relief, usually within one week, while another 16% had a moderate to good response. Many had to continue vitamin E to prevent cramps from recurring.

The authors noted similar success treating nocturnal rectal cramps, abdominal muscle cramps, and cramps following heavy exercise *(Ayres)*.

A woman suffered from severe leg cramps every night after going to bed. By trial and error, she found that if she took vitamin E at precisely 5 PM each day, the cramps would not occur (Anonymous).

MINERALS

Calcium

Calcium deficiency causes neuromuscular irritability *(Tonner)*. While calcium supplementation is a popular remedy for muscle cramps, the literature on its use in the absence of calcium deficiency is largely limited to reports of its efficacy in relieving leg cramps of pregnancy, which are believed to be due to alterations in the endocrine regulation of calcium homeostasis (see Pregnancy-related Illness). One clinician found that calcium supplementation was more effective than quinine in preventing nocturnal leg cramps, but had better results when the two treatments were combined *(Knowles)*.

In primary hypoparathyroidism, the serum calcium concentration is elevated and about 50% of patients present with muscle cramps and paresthesias, the most common neuromuscular complaints seen in this disorder *(Turken)*. This suggests that a serum calcium level should be part of the work-up of patients presenting with idiopathic recurrent muscle cramps.

At age 75, a man had been suffering for many years from cramps in the soles of the feet at night when turning or stretching. Within one or two days of starting supplementation with calcium lactate, the cramps disappeared. Previously, he wore arch supporters and stayed away from walking on the beach barefoot due to the pains occurring after each walk. Now a daily beach walk of 4 to 5 miles never causes cramps (Bricklin).

Magnesium Deficiency

Magnesium deficiency causes spasmophilia (latent tetany). Even though the serum magnesium level is not a sensitive measure of magnesium deficiency, hypomagnesemia is commonly associated with muscle cramps *(Khokhlov;Moorkens)*.

The important role of magnesium in determining muscle contractility has been objectively demonstrated in an animal study. When rat phrenic nerve-diaphragm preparations were placed in magnesium solutions, significantly lower stimulation frequencies were needed to produce tetanic contractions when intra- and extracellular magnesium levels were low than when they were plentiful *(Schindler)*.

In one of the few published human studies not concerning pregnancy-associated muscle cramps, 68 patients with varicose veins of the lower limbs received magnesium preparations. Circulation in the involved limb was improved, and muscular spasms were completely relieved *(Khokhlov)*.

A 17-year-old soldier exercised too strenuously and developed muscle spasms so severe that he was immobilized and required hospitalization. Upon evaluation, the only abnormality found was a low serum magnesium concentration.

He received two intravenous infusions of magnesium sulfate in saline. Within 48 hours, his pain lessened significantly, and it was gone after 4 days (Bilbey).

Potassium Deficiency

Muscle cramps may be associated with hypokalemia. These cramps will usually respond to potassium supplementation *(Portier)*. However, when there is a concurrent magnesium deficiency, magnesium repletion is also necessary, since the potassium deficiency may otherwise prove to be refractory *(Whang)*.

Exercise-related muscle cramps are not usually associated with hypokalemia *(Maughan)*. Therefore, potassium supplementation does not appear to be indicated in their treatment.

A woman who had foot cramps for months realized that they always occurred 10 days before her menstrual period. She began to increase her dietary potassium intake at that time of her monthly cycle, and her foot cramps ceased. When, however, she forgot to change her diet, the cramps would return (Anonymous).

Sodium

Heat cramps occurring during heavy exercise may be due to sodium and fluid depletion from profuse sweating. These can be prevented by increasing the daily dietary sodium intake *(Bergeron)*.

There is also a clinical report suggesting that increasing sodium intake may be effective in treating nocturnal calf cramps *(Glatzel)*. This observation has yet to be confirmed by a controlled clinical trial.

OTHER NUTRITIONAL FACTORS

L-Carnitine

In a placebo-controlled study, 6 untrained males received a placebo for 3 weeks. Then, after a week's interval, they received L-carnitine for another 3 weeks.

On the first day of the third and seventh weeks of the study, the quadriceps muscle was exercised in an eccentric manner for 20 minutes. L-carnitine reduced the pain and tenderness after exertion significantly more than did placebo *(Giamberardino)*.

Taurine

Muscle cramps are common in patients with liver cirrhosis *(Matsuzaki)*. Compared to similar patients who do not experience muscle cramps, plasma taurine appears to be reduced *(Yamamoto,1994a)*.

Supplementation with taurine usually relieves the cramps *(Matsuzaki;Yamamoto,1994b)*, and there is a good correlation between rising plasma taurine levels and decreasing muscle cramps *(Yamamoto,1994a)*.

COMBINED NUTRITIONAL INTERVENTIONS

A 57 year-old woman had a 3-year history of muscle spasms of her hands and wrists about twice monthly. Sometimes the muscle of her toes, feet and ankles or knees would also spasm. The severe cramping pains lasted about 30 minutes, with residual discomfort for days afterward. A rheumatologist was unable to make a diagnosis, and only Butazolidin provided partial relief.

She had a strong craving for sweets and recognized that sugar could trigger a attack. A glucose tolerance test was performed; the nadir was 45 mg% and was associated with syncope. Also, her sedimentation rate was moderately elevated.

She was asked to avoid refined sugar, caffeine and alcohol, and to eat small, frequent meals. A multiple vitamin and mineral formula was prescribed along with additional calcium, magnesium, vitamin B complex, and vitamins C and E.

She returned one week later with early symptoms of an attack. A slow intravenous injection of pyridoxine 150 mg and magnesium 600 mg was begun, and the spasm ceased before the injection was completed. Subsequently she has followed the treatment program and her muscle cramping has subsided. On several occasions, when hand spasms returned, a pyridoxine and magnesium injection relieved the symptoms within seconds (Gaby).

OTHER RELATED FACTORS

Bone Meal

A study reported in the *Canadian Medical Association Journal* back in 1944 described the treatment of 112 children with "growing pains" or who kicked and screamed at night. All were given vitamins A and D. In addition, half were given dicalcium phosphate while the other half were given bone meal. Over a 2-year period, all 57 children on bone meal were completely relieved, while only 22 of the 56 children on dicalcium phosphate were relieved. When these 22 children were switched to bone meal, *all* were completely relieved *(Martin)*.

Among other things, these intriguing findings suggest that bone meal (perhaps along with vitamins A and D) may be effective for children with "growing pains" - and possibly for reasons other than its calcium and phosphorus content. Unfortunately, further studies to confirm and clarify these results have not been reported. Also, bone meal, especially for growing children, is only recommended if a laboratory analysis has failed to find a significant amount of lead or other toxic substances in the specific product.

A 6-year-old girl was awakened every night by terrible leg cramps. She was evaluated medically, and was found to be entirely normal.

Three weeks after taking 6 tablets a day of bone meal, she started sleeping through the night. When the bone meal was stopped, after about a week the cramps returned until it was restarted (Bricklin).

Reactive Hypoglycemia

While systematic research has not been done, Roberts has treated over 350 patients with severe symptoms of either spontaneous leg cramps or restless legs. With few exceptions, they also experienced typical features of functional hypoglycemia which was confirmed by afternoon glucose tolerance testing. Occasionally, in fact, a muscle cramp would occur concurrent with the development of hypoglycemia during testing.

A sugar-free, high protein diet with snacking was effective for the "vast majority" of patients. Moreover, when cramps recurred, they were usually related to a dietary indiscretion within the preceding 24 hours *(Roberts)*. (Also see 'Hypoglycemia' - Functional.)

BIBLIOGRAPHY

Aitchison WR. Nocturnal cramps. Letter. N Z Med J 80:137, 1974

Anonymous. Home Remedies for Everyday Health Problems. Emmaus, Penn., Rodale Press, 1987

Ayres S Jr, Mihan R. Leg cramps (systremma) and "restless legs" syndrome. A progress report on response to vitamin E (tocopherol). South Med J 67(11):1308-12, 1974

Bergeron MF. Heat cramps during tennis: a case report. Int J Sport Nutr 6(1):62-8, 1996

Bilbey DJ, Prabhakaran VM. Muscle cramps and magnesium deficiency: case reports. Can Fam Physician 42:1348-51, 1996

Bricklin M., Ed. Rodale's Encyclopedia of Natural Home Remedies. Emmaus, Penn., Rodale Press, 1982

Connolly PS et al. Treatment of nocturnal leg cramps. A crossover trial of quinine vs vitamin E. Arch Intern Med 152(9):1877-80, 1992

Ellis JM. The Doctor who Looked at Hands. New York, Vantage Press, 1966, pp. 266-67

Ellis JM, Presley J. Vitamin B6: The Doctor's Report. New York, Harper & Row, 1973

Gaby A. The Doctor's Guide to Vitamin B6. Emmaus, PA, Rodale, 1984

Giamberardino MA et al. Effects of prolonged L-carnitine administration on delayed muscle pain and CK release after eccentric effort. Int J Sports Med 17(5):320-4, 1996

Glatzel H. [Nocturnal calf cramps.] Letter. Dtsch Med Wochenschr 105(20):736, 1980 (in German)

Haralambie G. Vitamin B2 status in athletes and the influence of riboflavin administration on neuromuscular irritability. Nutr Metab 20(1):1-8, 1976

Khokhlov AM et al. [Role of electrolytes in the pathogenesis of arterial spasm and muscle cramps in varicose veins of the lower limbs.] Khirurgiia (Mosk) (9):88-92, 1989 (in Russian)

Knowles FW. Fluoride and leg cramps. Letter. N Z Med J 93:60, 1981

Martin EM. Report on the clinical use of bone meal. Can Med Assoc J 50:562, 1944

Matsuzaki Y et al. Is taurine effective for treatment of painful muscle cramps in liver cirrhosis? Am J Gastroenterol 88:1466-7, 1993

Maughan RJ. Exercise-induced muscle cramp: a prospective biochemical study in marathon runners. J Sports Sci 4(1):31-4, 1986

Moorkens G et al. Magnesium deficit in a sample of the Belgian population presenting with chronic fatigue. Magnes Res 10(4):329-37, 1997

Perrault M et al. Paris médicale 36:549-54, 1946 (in French)

Portier C. [Muscle cramps and hypokalemia.] Letter. Nouv Presse Med 2(25):1717, 1973) (in French)

Roberts HJ. Spontaneous leg cramps and "restless legs" due to diabetogenic (functional) hypoinsulinism: A basis for rational therapy. J Fla Med Assoc 60(5):29-31, 1973

Roca AO et al. Dialysis leg cramps. Efficacy of quinine versus vitamin E. ASAIO J 38(3):M481-5, 1992

Schindler R et al. The role of magnesium in the generation and therapy of benign muscle cramps. Combined in-vivo/in-vitro studies on rat phrenic nerve-diaphragm preparations. Arzneimittelforschung 48(2):161-6, 1998

Tonner DR, Schlechte JA. Neurologic complications of thyroid and parathyroid disease. Med Clin North Am 77(1):251-63, 1993

Turken SA et al. Neuromuscular involvement in mild, asymptomatic primary hyperparathyroidism. Am J Med 87(5):553-7, 1989

Whang R et al. Refractory potassium repletion: a consequence of magnesium deficiency. Arch Intern Med 152:40-5, 1992

Yamamoto S et al. [Painful muscle cramps in liver cirrhosis and effects of oral taurine administration]. Nippon Shokakibyo Gakkai Zasshi 91(7):1205-9, 1994a (in Japanese)

Yamamoto S. Oral taurine therapy for painful muscle cramp in liver cirrhosis. Am J Gastroenterol 89(3):457-8, 1994b

MYOPIA

(NEARSIGHTEDNESS)

NUTRITIONAL TREATMENT GUIDE
✓ = Efficacy generally accepted. * = Efficacy *demonstrated* by controlled human trials. [+] = Efficacy *suspected* from uncontrolled human trials. [-] = Efficacy *suspected* from indirect data. ? = Efficacy *challenged* in a study of similar design.
DIETARY FACTORS * consume adequate **Animal Protein**, especially **Milk Protein** - [-] avoid **Undernutrition** [-] consume **Unrefined Carbohydrates** and other sources of **Dietary Fiber** [-] minimize **Refined Carbohydrates** including **Refined Sugar**
NUTRITIONAL FACTORS [+] **Calcium deficiency:** ≈ 1 g daily - [-] **Chromium deficiency:** 200 µg daily [-] **Folic acid:** High dietary intake may increase the chance of myopia reversal. [-] **Vitamin D deficiency:** 50,000 to 100,000 IU 2 or 3 times during the first week; then, if needed, either 100,000 IU of ergo- or cholecalciferol every 3 to 6 months *OR* 800 IU daily

DIETARY FACTORS

Undernutrition

Several studies have investigated the relationship between body stature as an index of nutritional status and myopia. While the findings are conflicting, by far the largest study reviewed the data of over 100,000 consecutive male miliary recruits aged 17 to 19 years. It found that persons with severe myopia were slightly shorter and weighed less than those with mild myopia, while the non-myopes were taller and heavier than the myopes. Similarly, the mean body-mass index among the myopes was slightly smaller than among the non-myopes *(Rosner)*.

In contrast to studies of people who had already become myopic, one small study compared 24 children who subsequently became myopic between the ages of 7 to 10 years to 68 children who still were not myopic at the age of 10 years. While there were no significant differences in high and weight between the two groups at age 7 years, the children who were to develop myopia had a generally lower intake of many food components, including total calories, protein and fat as well as several micronutrients *(Edwards)*, suggesting that they could have nutritional insufficiencies that were too subtle to affect growth.

Protein

Compared with normally sighted children, myopic children were found to refuse *animal protein* (from fish, milk, cheese and eggs) more often - although they did eat meat. Moreover, myopia in children who refused to eat animal protein from those sources was found to be both more common and more severe. While 5% of normal children refused 2 protein sources, 7% of stationary myopes and 11% of active myopes did so. The most striking difference between the 2 groups was in milk consumption, with over 3 times as many advancing myopes refusing milk as compared to stationary myopes (16% vs. 5%) *(Gardiner,1956).*

In a controlled clinical trial, 91 myopic school children were placed on a diet in which 10% of caloric intake was animal protein without any change in total calories. Calcium caseinate was used as a supplement for the 72 children who refused animal protein as ordinary food due to taste or lack of appetite.

After 1 to 2 years, compared to untreated controls, treated children showed a substantially lower average annual increase in myopia. In the younger children, the deterioration was greater in the controls by a mean of 0.5 diopter per annum while, in the older children, the progress of myopia was all but arrested in the treated group. The more severe the myopia at the start of treatment, the bigger the difference between treated and untreated groups. In general, the treated group deteriorated at about one-third the rate of the untreated group.

After 6 months, in the 16 children who consumed the amount of calcium caseinate advised, the mean change in refraction was an improvement of 0.02 diopters; in the 42 who took some calcium caseinate, the mean change was a deterioration of 0.16 diopters; and in the 14 who refused any calcium caseinate, there was a deterioration of 0.22 diopters, suggesting that milk plays an important role in the control of myopia *(Gardiner,1958).*

Dietary Fiber

There is preliminary data suggesting a relationship between the intake of dietary fiber and myopia. In a retrospective study of 120 consecutive binocular non-strabismic optometric patients aged 7 to 38 years, dietary fiber intake was significantly related to refractive strata, with myopes consuming a median of only 39% as much fiber in grams as hyperopes (farsighted people) (5.3 g vs. 13.55 g).

The author suggests that this finding may be because hyperopes with higher fiber status were eating more unrefined foods with better trace mineral availability, that the higher fiber intakes may result in more thorough admixture with saliva resulting in improved nutrient absorption, or because dietary fiber is often correlated with dietary folate, and the intake of dietary folate is highly correlated with myopia prevention/reversal *(Lane,1982a).*

Refined Carbohydrates

Consistent with the hypothesis that a high intake of dietary fiber may be protective, there is evidence that a high intake of refined carbohydrates may promote myopia. When rats received a high sucrose diet upon weaning, the normal hypermetropia was significantly reduced (that is, a relative myopia developed) compared to controls. Then, when the sucrose and control group were reversed, myopia developed in the rats that were now receiving the high-sucrose diet. This myopia failed to reverse, however, when they were switched to a sucrose-free diet *(Bardiger).*

There is also preliminary data in humans suggesting that the consumption of refined carbohydrates may be associated with the development of myopia. When the diets of optometric patients between the ages of 7 and 38 years were studied, myopes were found to have a significantly higher ratio of consumption of refined carbohydrates to total carbohydrates than hyperopes. Moreover, hyperopes had a lower ratio of consumption of refined to total carbohydrates than emmetropes (people who are neither near- or farsighted) *(Lane,1982a).*

NUTRITIONAL FACTORS

VITAMINS

Folic Acid

When, in a group of 110 optometric patients, the intake of various nutrients was examined, the strongest association with myopia reduction over 12 months for patients aged 6 to 38 years appeared to be with food-derived folic acid in proportion to body weight, and there was a strong association of food-folate intake with diopters of reversal of myopia.

Habitual food folate ingestion, while correlated with intraocular pressure reduction, was far more strongly correlated with myopia reduction, suggesting that the efficacy of folate in reducing myopia was not simply due to an effect on intraocular pressure.

If we assume that that this correlation is due to a therapeutic effect of folic acid, folate's efficacy could be partly due to enhanced absorption of dietary calcium and chromium, nutrients which are also implicated in myopia reduction. Supplemental folic acid, in the form of pteroylglutamic acid, did not show the same correlation with myopia reduction, and thus appears to be less effective *(Lane,1994)*.

MINERALS

Calcium, the Calcium to Phosphorus Ratio, and Vitamin D

Calcium

The normal sclera is rich in calcium *(Strebel)*. It has been suggested that blood calcium concentrations may be directly related to the distensibility of the globe *(Law)* as, in progressive myopia, low blood calcium concentrations are often found *(Fleming; Wood)*.

Calcium to Phosphorus Ratio

Myopia incidence is also correlated with a low dietary ratio of calcium to phosphorus, and a low calcium to phosphorus ratio has also been noted in the serum and urine of myopic patients *(Kolosov)*. The low dietary ratio appears to promote the development of nutritionally-induced secondary hyperparathyroidism in the body's attempt to correct for the imbalance *(Lane,1985)*.

In one study of 13 patients aged 6 to 16 years with early myopia, the 7 patients who ingested less than 800 mg of calcium daily *all* showed evidence of increasing myopia, while *none* of the 6 patients who ingested at least 800 mg daily showed evidence of increasing myopia, a highly significant difference, and their ratio of dietary calcium to phosphorus was significantly negatively correlated with increasing myopia. Similarly, *none* of 6 young adult control subjects who ingested less than 500 mg daily of calcium from milk and egg products showed evidence of decreasing myopia, while *all* 3 controls who ingested at least 500 mg daily showed evidence of decreasing myopia, again a highly significant difference *(Lane,1985)*.

These findings are in agreement with those of a Russian study which found a highly significant decrease in the calcium to phosphorus ratio in both the serum and urine of patients with progressive myopia compared to those with stable myopia. Moreover, the patients with progressive myopia showed a highly significant increase in alkaline phosphatase activity *(Kolosov)*.

Further evidence suggesting that myopia may be associated with secondary hyperparathyroidism comes from a study of 120 optometric patients aged 7 to 38 years. High hair calcium is believed to occur primarily when calcium is being mobilized from bone into blood and urine as a result of secondary hyperparathyroidism to prevent hyperphosphatemia with loss of bone calcium through excessive excretion. In this study, hair calcium concentrations were found to be significantly higher in myopes than in emmetropes. When the groups were sub-divided based on age, the significant differences were found to be due to the younger age group (ages 7 to 17 years) *(Lane,1982a)*.

Also, among myopes ages 18 to 38 years, high hair calcium was found to be highly correlated with an increased ratio of flesh-protein (animal meat) ingestion to total protein intake. Flesh protein would also be expected to promote secondary hyperparathyroidism due to its low calcium to phosphorus ratio *(Lane,1982b)*.

There is also a retrospective analysis of children who were very-low-birthweight infants found that, among those given both calcium and phosphorus supplements to prevent postnatal bone mineral deficiency, 6 out of 55 (11%) subsequently developed myopia compared to 5 out of 14 (61%) who were unsupplemented *(Pohlandt)*.

Vitamin D

Calcium has important interactions with vitamin D. Vitamin D promotes calcium absorption and mobilizes it from bone *(Passmore)*, while diets deficient in calcium stimulate parathyroid hormone secretion which increases the degradation of 25-hydroxy vitamin D leading to a secondary vitamin D deficiency *(Siu-Caldera)*.

In an avian model of experimental myopia, deficiencies of both calcium and vitamin D were found to affect eye growth *(Hodos)*. Moreover, in an earlier study, *all* experimental animals fed a low-calcium, vitamin D-deficient diet developed prominence of the eyes, wide palpebral fissures, and deep anterior chambers, findings that are very frequently associated with myopia in humans *(Knapp)*.

Laboratory data and controlled clinical trials of calcium supplementation are badly needed to test the hypothesis that nutritionally-induced secondary hyperparathyroidism promotes the development and progression of myopia.

Meanwhile, we do have the findings from an informal open clinical trial reported in 1939. Fifty-three patients aged 3 to 20 years with progressive myopia received vitamin D. Also, depending upon milk intake, they received a calcium-containing mineral tablet that also contained smaller amounts of copper, iron, magnesium phosphorus, potassium and sodium.

After a 5 to 28 month observation period, the majority of patients noted increased near and distant visual acuity and were not as dependent upon their glasses as formerly. For distinct near vision without lenses, they found that reading matter could be held at a greater distance from the eyes.

Six of the 12 patients who took their medications regularly showed a reduction in their myopia, 2 remained stationary, while 4 progressed. Sixteen of the 46 patients (35%) on whom there was sufficient data had a reduction in their myopia; 7 of them (15%) remained stationary, and 2 (4%) displayed decreased myopia in the left eye despite progression in the right. Moreover, objective testing showed that the cornea and sclera may shrink following treatment (*Knapp*).

Chromium Deficiency

In a study of 120 optometric patients, mean hair chromium concentrations were significantly lower for myopia patients than for patients with normal refractions. When followed for 2 years, median hair chromium concentrations for patients with increasing refractive power relative to the retina (increasing myopia or decreasing hyperopia) or no change, was less than one-third of the value for patients showing decreasing refractive power *(Lane, 1982a)*.

There is also evidence that chromium deficiency, as measured by erythrocyte concentration, is an important risk factor for the development of high (severe) myopia *(Lane, 1995)*.

The efficacy of chromium supplementation remains to be tested.

Copper and Zinc Metabolism

Copper

Copper metabolism in myopia may be abnormal. In children with progressive myopia, the lacrimal fluid has been found to contain a reduced concentration of copper *(Vinetskaia)*. Similarly, eyes of cadavers with myopia show a significant reduction of scleral copper and abnormal distribution of copper in the scleral tissue *(Avetisov)*.

Among Caucasian (but not African) groups with high myopia, many patients show low serum copper levels *(Silverstone, 1990)*. By contrast, *high* serum copper levels were found in high myopes who had developed retinal detachment *(Silverstone, 1990)*. This group was also found to exhibit a high level of urinary copper excretion and an inverse ratio between the subretinal fluid levels and serum concentrations *(Silverstone, 1986)*.

Zinc

The metabolism of zinc also appears to be abnormal. In Caucasian, but not African, patients with high myopia, many show high serum zinc levels. When highly myopic Caucasian patients were studied, both serum zinc and urine zinc levels were significantly elevated *(Silverstone, 1986, 1990)*.

Zinc to Copper Ratio

A Chinese study of children aged 9 to 14 years performed a logistic regression analysis. One finding was a close relationship between the hair zinc to copper ratio and juvenile myopia *(Qiang)*.

Until copper and zinc metabolism in myopia is better understood, and until experimental studies find benefits from attempts to correct their abnormalities, attempts to intervene nutritionally are inappropriate.

COMBINED NUTRITIONAL SUPPLEMENTATION

In an open trial, 193 patients with high, progressive myopia were placed on a nutritional treatment program that included increased fruits and vegetables, increased folate from food, an increase in the dietary ratio of calcium to phosphorus, and supplementation with chromium.

Over time, these patients were found to have enhanced resistance to the common complication of myopic degeneration *(Lane, 1995)*.

BIBLIOGRAPHY

Avetisov ES et al. [Copper metabolism in scleral tissue and possibilities of its correction in myopia]. Vestn Oftalmol 107(5):31-4, 1991) (in Russian)

Bardiger M, Stock AL. The effects of sucrose-containing diets low in protein on ocular refraction in the rat. Proc Nutr Soc 31(1):4A-5A, 1972

Edwards MH. Do variations in normal nutrition play a role in the development of myopia? Optom Vis Sci 73(10):638-43, 1996

Fleming N. Discussion of the paper by F. W. Law: Calcium and parathyroid therapy in progressive myopia. Trans Ophthalmol Soc U K 44:281-90, 1934

Gardiner PA. Observations on the food habits of myopic children. Br Med J ii:699-700, 1956

Gardiner PA. Dietary treatment of myopia in children. Lancet i:1152-5, 1958

Hodos W. Avian models of experimental myopia: environmental factors in the regulation of eye growth. Ciba Found Symp 155:149-59, 1990

Knapp AA. Vitamin-D complex in progressive myopia. Am J Ophthalmol 22:1329-37, 1939

Kolosov VI et al. [Further studies of the role of changes in phosphorocalcium metabolism in the mechanism of progression of myopia in children.] Oftalmol Zh 36(1):25-9, 1981 (in Russian)

Lane BC. Myopia prevention and reversal: new data confirms the interaction of accommodative stress and deficit-inducing nutrition. J Int Acad Prev Med November, 1982a:17-30

Lane BC. Milk, sugar and myopia prevention and reversal. Abstract. Proceedings 148th Natl. Mtg., Am. Assn. For the Advancement of Science. Wash., DC, 1982b:149

Lane BC. Nutrition and Vision, in J Bland, Ed. 1984-85 Yearbook of Nutritional Medicine. New Caanan, CT, Keats Pub., 1985

Lane BC. Food folate vs. supplemental folate in eye disorders. Abstract. J Am Coll Nutr 13(5):534, 1994

Lane BC et al. Dietary intervention enhances resistance to myopic degenerations. Abstract. J Am Coll Nutr 14(5):545, 1995

Law FW. Calcium and parathyroid therapy in progressive myopia. Trans Ophthalmol Soc U K 54:281-90, 1934

Passmore R, Eastwood MA. Davidson and Passmore: Human Nutrition and Dietetics. Eighth Edition. London, Churchill Livingstone, 1986:139

Pohlandt F. Hypothesis: myopia of prematurity is caused by postnatal bone mineral deficiency. Eur J Pediatr 153(4):234-6, 1994

Qiang M, Zhao R. [A logistic regression analysis of relations between juvenile myopia and TV-watching, trace elements, and psychological characteristics]. Chung Hua Yu Fang I Hsueh Tsa Chih 25(4):222-4, 1991 (in Chinese)

Rosner M et al. Myopia and stature: findings in a population of 106,926 males. Eur J Ophthalmol 5(1):1-6, 1995

Silverstone BZ et al. Copper and zinc metabolism in high myopic patients with retinal detachment evaluation of the Cu/Zn ratio. Metab Pediatr Syst Ophthalmol 9(1):581-3, 1986

Silverstone BZ. Effects of zinc and copper metabolism in highly myopic patients. Ciba Found Symp 155:210-7, discussion 217-21, 1990

Siu-Caldera ML et al. Diets deficient in calcium increase the degradation of 25(OH) vitamin D. Abstract. J Am Coll Nutr 12:618, 1993

Strebel J. [Qualitative inorganic analysis of the sclera in normal human eyes.] Schweiz Med Woch 61:1102, 1931 (in German)

Vinetskaia MI, Iomdina EN. [Study of lacrimal fluid trace elements in several eye diseases]. Vestn Oftalmol 110(4):24-6, 1994 (in Russian)

Wood DJ. Calcium deficiency in the blood with reference to spring catarrh and malignant myopia. Br J Ophthalmol 11:224-30, 1927

NEURALGIA AND NEUROPATHY

See Also: CARPAL TUNNEL SYNDROME
DIABETES MELLITUS
HERPES ZOSTER
PAIN

NUTRITIONAL TREATMENT GUIDE

✓ = Efficacy generally accepted.
* = Efficacy *demonstrated* by controlled human trials.
[+] = Efficacy *suspected* from uncontrolled human experiments
[-] = Efficacy *suspected* from indirect data
? = Efficacy *challenged* in at least one study of similar design

DIETARY FACTORS

[+] avoid **Caffeine**

NUTRITIONAL FACTORS

* **Vitamin B_{12}:** 1,000 µg IM as needed
* **Zinc Deficiency:** *for optic neuropathy:* zinc sulfate 400 mg daily for 1 month

- -

[+] **Essential fatty acids:** *for Guillian-Barré Syndrome*
[+] **Folic acid deficiency:** 800 µg daily
[+] **Magnesium:** *for chronic neuropathic pain:* magnesium sulfate (0.5mol.1-1) 5 ml IV over 5 min. followed by the same dose by continuous infusion for 1 hr. once weekly (3 mo. trial)
[+] **Niacin:** 100 to 300 mg daily
[+] **Thiamine deficiency:** 50 mg daily
[+] **Vitamin B_6 deficiency:** 50 to 100 mg daily
[+] **Vitamin E deficiency:** D,L-alpha-tocopheryl acetate 200 to 2,000 mg or IU daily for 6 weeks; then maintenance levels as needed

OTHER RELATED FACTORS
[+] rule out **Cadmium** toxicity
[+] rule out **Lead** toxicity
[+] rule out **Gluten** sensitivity

DIETARY FACTORS

Caffeine

A case report suggests that caffeine ingestion may provoke pain for some patients with neurogenic pain. This possibility remains to be investigated, however, with controlled clinical trials, although caffeine has been shown to reduce the efficacy of transcutaneous electrical nerve stimulation (TENS) in reducing pain *(Marchand)*.

A 55 year-old woman with a 5-year history of trigeminal neuralgia drank 3 to 4 cups of coffee daily. When she switched to decaffeinated coffee, her severe facial pain disappeared for a full year. She then began to drink hot cocoa (which contains caffeine-like compounds) and the pain returned. She stopped the cocoa and, within 3 weeks, the pain subsided again. Later, she drank a single cup of regular coffee and her pain returned for an entire week.

In the 2 years following, she has avoided all caffeine and remains free of pain (Glore).

NUTRITIONAL FACTORS

VITAMINS

Vitamin B Complex Deficiencies

Since deficiencies of any of several of the B complex vitamins may promote neuralgias and neuropathies, and since members of the complex work closely together, there is an argument for using the B complex in combination, even to rule out the possibility of a nutritional neuropathy due to a B vitamin deficiency *(Weber)*.

In a German study, 1,149 patients with polyneuropathy, neuralgia, radiculopathy or neuritis under treatment with 234 different doctors received various dosages of a vitamin B complex preparation. Most had clear improvements in pain, muscle weakness and paresthesias. About 3 weeks after starting treatment, 69% of patients noted a reduction in pain, and improvements in the other target symptoms were similar *(Eckert)*.

Folic Acid Deficiency

Folate deficiency can cause a peripheral neuropathy. For example, 21% of a group of 34 patients with severe folate deficiency and megaloblastosis due to poor diet or gastrointestinal disease were found to have a peripheral neuropathy. This neuropathy, which was diagnosed either clinically or electrophysiologically, was usually mild and predominantly sensory *(Shorvon, 1979)*.

Patients receiving carbamazepine are particularly susceptible to folate deficiency, as the drug impairs folate absorption *(Hendal)*. For example, the dietary folate intake of a group of trigeminal neuralgia patients receiving carbamazepine treatment was similar to that of matched controls, while their red cell folate levels were significantly lower *(al-Musaed)*.

Folic acid supplementation has been shown to be beneficial in treating neuropathies when it repletes a folate deficiency *(Parry, 1994)*. This includes otherwise unexplained optic neuropathies *(Golnik)*.

A 26-year-old male complaining of left wrist and hand weakness and paresthesias in the forearm and dorsum of the hand due to a polyneuropathy was found to have a folate deficiency (in the absence of other vitamin deficiencies) and celiac disease.

The discrete clinical signs and the relatively pronounced electrophysiologic signs did not improve after therapy with vitamin B complex, but improved after treatment with folic acid 2.5 mg daily, suggesting that the polyneuropathy was due to the folate deficiency (Fehling).

Niacin

Niacin deficiency does not appear to promote neuralgia or neuropathy. In fact, in treating pellagra, the classic niacin deficiency disease, neuropathies may worsen if patients received niacin supplementation without the rest of the vitamin B complex *(Wadia)*.

However, in older open trials, megadosage niacin supplementation has been reported to be effective in the treatment of both Bell's palsy *(Kime)* and trigeminal neuralgia *(Adams;Anonymous,1943)*, suggesting that its efficacy is due to a pharmacological effect.

Thiamine Deficiency

Thiamine deficiency is known to cause a polyneuropathy (the essential feature of dry beriberi) in addition to other neurologic disorders. Typical complaints are of weakness and burning feet *(Skelton)*. Based on erythrocyte transketolase activation, perhaps one-third of patients with neurologic disorders are thiamine -deficient *(Langohr)*.

When thiamine is deficient, the results of open trials suggest that supplementation may be helpful for treating acute neuropathies *(Skelton)*, idiopathic facial neuralgia and some cervicobrachial neuralgias *(Ropert)*.

Vitamin B_6

A deficiency of vitamin B_6 may cause a peripheral neuropathy *(Byers;Heller;Snider)*. While data are sparse, it appears that this neuropathy responds to vitamin repletion *(Byers)*.

Conversely, long-term ingestion of pyridoxine (2 to 3 years or more) in massive dosages of 1 to 5 grams daily can *cause* a sensory neuropathy. There have even been occasional reports of neuropathies occurring at supplemental dosages as low as 200 mg when ingested over an extended period of time *(Berger;Dalton; Parry,1985)*.

Vitamin B_{12}

Deficiency of vitamin B_{12} may cause peripheral neuropathy *(Shorvon,1980)*. This neuropathy is now believed to be related to interference with methylation reactions in the central nervous system *(Weir)*. The classic findings of pernicious anemia may be absent. In fact, hematologic indices are normal in up to 30% of patients with deficiency, and the results of the Schilling test may also be normal *(Fine)*.

Supplementation with vitamin B_{12} has been found to be beneficial for neuropathies *(Dettori;Fine)*, including Bell's palsy *(Jalaludin)* and trigeminal neuralgia *(Surtees)*. It is uncertain if supplementation is of any value except in cases of deficiency.

A 56-year-old woman had a 14-month history of sciatica that was unresponsive to conservative care. X-rays and a CT myelogram were negative; an MRI showed a mild bulge at L5-S1. She failed to respond to oral anti-inflammatory medications and epidural steroid injections. Further tests included a CBC, blood chemistries, bone scan, EMG, and MRIs of her brain and thoracic spine, all of which were negative.

Later, however, a second EMG showed a left sciatic neuropathy with mild polyneuropathy. She began to suffer from paresthesias in both arms and her right leg. Additional blood tests were done, and a mildly low serum cobalamin level was noted.

She was then treated successfully with vitamin B_{12} injections (Anonymous,1996a).

Vitamin E Deficiency

Vitamin E is essential for normal neurological structure and function, with severe deficiency resulting in a characteristic neurological syndrome. A deficiency results in a 'distal or dying back' axonal neuropathy which predominantly involves the centrally directed fibers of sensory neurons, with the large caliber myelinated fibers being particularly affected *(Muller)*. Patients with, for example, lipid malabsorption syndromes, are liable to develop the neuropathy *(Traber)*.

If the vitamin is deficient, supplementation may improve neurologic functioning, or at least prevent further neurologic deterioration *(Traber)*. Supplementation has also been found to be beneficial for disorders such as leprous nerve involvement *(Floch)* and, in combination with vitamin B complex, tic douloureux *(Hoffer)*.

A middle-aged woman with a biliary-colonic fistula presented with chronic polyneuropathy due to vitamin E deficiency caused by malabsorption. Once plasma tocopherol levels were normalized by parenteral administration, there was substantial clinical improvement (Ayuso Blanco).

MINERALS

Magnesium

Following a nerve block, intravenous administration of magnesium, a N-methyl-D-aspartate (NMDA) receptor antagonist, once weekly relieved chronic neuropathic pain in 4 out of 8 patients after 3 to 11 weeks *(Tanaka)*. There is no evidence than oral administration would be effective and this study has yet to be replicated under controlled conditions.

Zinc Deficiency

Guinea pigs fed a zinc-deficient diet showed decreased motor nerve conduction velocity which correlated with the degree of deficiency and was associated with abnormal posture and locomotion, and with hypersensitivity to touch. The neuropathy was reversible by increasing zinc intake *(O'Dell)*.

While little has been done to explore the efficacy of zinc repletion, a randomized, placebo-controlled trial provided zinc supplementation to a group of patients, mainly males in their forties, with bilateral, retrobulbar, axial, optic neuropathy related to smoking and drinking. Treatment, which normalized low plasma zinc levels, significantly improved visual capacity of the central scotoma area *(Bechetoille)*.

OTHER RELATED FACTORS

Heavy Metal Toxicity

Cadmium

Cadmium toxicity is known to cause a peripheral neuropathy *(Blum)*.

Lead

Lead exposure has repeatedly been shown to result in a reduction in nerve conduction velocity *(Cordeiro; Yeh)*. In fact, the simple finger tapping test is one way of easily screening for an incipient lead neuropathy, since decreased finger tapping ability directly correlates with blood lead levels *(Matsumoto)*.

Gluten Sensitivity

Gluten sensitivity may be common in patients with neurological disease of unknown cause and may have etiological significance *(Anonymous, 1996b)*. Moreover, peripheral neuropathy is one of the neurologic manifestations of celiac disease *(Cooke)*.

A 65-year old woman with a right peroneal nerve palsy superimposed on a diffuse peripheral neuropathy was found to have folic acid deficiency. Further evaluation led to the diagnosis of adult celiac disease. Electrophysiological and histological studies demonstrated a predominantly demyelinating peripheral neuropathy which responded first to parenteral folic acid supplementation and second to a gluten-free diet (Viader).

COMBINED NUTRITIONAL TREATMENT

A man who had been unable to work for 3 weeks due to sciatica had improved only slightly with chiropractic manipulation. He had a history of a back injury resulting in a severe sprain several years earlier, and prior orthopedic and neurological evaluations had resulted in non-surgical treatments. One year earlier, an orthopedist noted early disc degeneration.

Examination revealed tenderness in an area 3 inches to the left of the lumbar spine extending along the course of the sciatic nerve into the posterior thigh. He was started on daily intramuscular injections of vitamin B_{12} 1000 µg and thiamine 50 mg. The first injection resulted in 50% relief and each subsequent injection provided slight additional relief.

After 1 week, his limp was considerably less as was his local tenderness. After another week, the limp and the pain had disappeared, although he continued to have mild, aching low back pain. Vitamin C 3 gms daily was added. Two weeks later the back pain ceased.

On follow-up several months later, he reported that, with the aid of occasional chiropractic manipulation, he had had no significant pain in his low back or leg (Wright).

BIBLIOGRAPHY

Adams WE, Robinson W. Trigeminal neuralgia. Lancet ii:555-6, 1941

al-Musaed AA et al. Carbamazepine and folic acid in trigeminal neuralgia patients. J R Soc Med 85(1):19-22, 1992

Anonymous. Trigeminal neuralgia treated with nicotinic acid. Lancet ii:295-6, 1943

Anonymous. Back Letter 11(7):77, 1996a

Anonymous. Does cryptic gluten sensitivity play a part in neurological illness? Lancet 347:369-71, 1996b

Ayuso Blanco T et al. [Chronic polyneuropathy due to vitamin E deficiency.] Neurologia 9(7):300-2, 1994 (in Spanish)

Bechetoille A et al. [Therapeutic affect of zinc sulfate on central scotoma due to optic neuropathy of alcohol and tobacco abuse]. J Fr Ophtalmol 6(3):237-42, 1983 (in French)

Berger A et al. Dose response, coasting, and differential fiber vulnerability in human toxic neuropathy. Neurology 42:1367-70, 1992

Blum LW et al. Peripheral neuropathy and cadmium toxicity. Pa Med 92(4):54-6, 1989

Byers CM et al. Pyridoxine metabolism in carpal tunnel syndrome with and without peripheral neuropathy. Arch Phys Med Rehabil 65(11):712-16, 1984

Cooke WT. Neurologic manifestations of malabsorption, in Handbook of Clinical Neurology, Volume 28, Metabolic and Deficiency Diseases of the Nervous System, Part II. Amsterdam: North-Holland Publishing Co. 1976:225-41

Cordeiro R et al. [Neurological disorders in workers with low levels of lead in the blood. I: Peripheral neuropathy]. Rev Saude Publica 30(3):248-55, 1996 (in Portuguese)

Dalton K, Dalton MJT. Characteristics of pyridoxine overdose neuropathy syndrome. Acta Neurol Scand 76:8-11, 1987

Dettori AG, Ponari O. Effetto antalgico della cobamamide in corso di neuropatie periferiche di diversa etiopatogenesi. Minerva Med 64:1077-82, 1973

Eckert M, Schejbal P. [Therapy of neuropathies with a vitamin B combination. Symptomatic treatment of painful diseases of the peripheral nervous system with a combination preparation of thiamine, pyridoxine and cyanocobalamin]. Fortschr Med 110(29):544-8, 1992 (in German)

Fehling C et al. Folate deficiency and neurological disease: One case with a close association. Arch Neurol 30:263-5, 1974

Fine EJ, Soria ED. Myths about vitamin B12 deficiency. South Med J 84(12):1475-81, 1991

Floch H, Horth R. La vitaminotherapie E dans la lepre: Nevrites et troubles trophiques. Bull Soc Pathol Exot 45:157-60, 1952 (in French)

Glore S, Ricker A. Trigeminal neuralgia: case study of pain cessation with a low-caffeine diet. J Am Diet Assoc 91:1120-1, 1991

Golnik KC, Schaible ER. Folate-responsive optic neuropathy. J Neuroophthalmol 14(3):163-9, 1994

Heller CA, Friedman PA. Pyridoxine deficiency and peripheral neuropathy associated with long-term phenelzine therapy. Am J Med 75(5):887-8, 1983

Hendal J et al. The effects of carbamazepine and valproate on folate metabolism. Acta Neurol Scand 69(4):226-31, 1984

Hoffer A. An alternative treatment for tic douloureux. Letter. J Orthomol Psychiatry 9(4):245-6, 1994

Jalaludin MA. Methylcobalamin treatment of Bell's palsy. Methods Find Exp Clin Pharmacol 17:539-44, 1995

Kime CE. Bell's palsy: A new syndrome associated with treatment by nicotinic acid. Arch Otolaryngol 68:28-32, 1958

Langohr HD et al. Vitamin B-1, B-2 and B-6 deficiency in neurological disorders. J Neurol 225:95-108, 1981

Marchand S et al. Effects of caffeine on analgesia from transcutaneous electrical nerve stimulation. Letter. N Engl J Med 333(5):325-6, 1995

Matsumoto T et al. Relations between lead exposure and peripheral neuromuscular functions of lead-exposed workers--results of tapping test. Environ Res 61(2):299-307, 1993

Muller DP, Goss-Sampson MA. Neurochemical, neurophysiological, and neuropathological studies in vitamin E deficiency. Crit Rev Neurobiol 5(3):239-63, 1990

O'Dell B et al. Zinc status and peripheral nerve function in guinea pigs. FASEBJ 4:2919-22, 1990

Parry GJ. Sensory neuropathy with low-dose pyridoxine. Neurology 35:1466-8, 1985

Parry TE. Folate responsive neuropathy. Presse Med 23(3):131-7, 1994

Ropert R. Utilisation de la vitamine B_1 fortes doses dans le traitement de divers syndromes douloureux facio-cephaliques. Sem Hop 34:508-9, 1958 (in French)

Shorvon SD, Reynolds EH. Folate deficiency and peripheral neuropathy, in MI Botez, EH Reynolds, Eds. Folic Acid in Neurology, Psychiatry, and Internal Medicine. New York, Raven Press, 1979

Shorvon SD et al. The neuropsychiatry of megaloblastic anaemia. Br Med J 281:1036-43, 1980

Skelton WP 3rd, Skelton NK. Thiamine deficiency neuropathy. It's still common today. Postgrad Med 85(8):301-6, 1989

Snider DE Jr. Pyridoxine supplementation during isoniazid therapy. Tubercle 61(4):191-6, 1980

Surtees SJ, Hughes RR. Treatment of trigeminal neuralgia with vitamin B12. Lancet i:439-41, 1954

Tanaka M et al. [Relief of neuropathic pain with intravenous magnesium.] Masui 47(9):1109-13, 1998 (in Japanese)

Traber MG et al. Lack of tocopherol in peripheral nerves of vitamin E-deficient patients with peripheral neuropathy. N Engl J Med 317:262-5, 1987

Viader F et al. [Celiac disease in adults revealed by sensory-motor neuropathy]. Presse Med 24(4):222-4, 1995 (in French)

Wadia NH, Swami RK. Pattern of nutritional deficiency disorders of nervous system in Bombay. Neurology India 18:207, 1970

Weber GA et al. Nutritionally induced peripheral neuropathies. Clin Podiatr Med Surg 7(1):107-28, 1990

Weir DG, Scott JM. The biochemical basis of the neuropathy in cobalamin deficiency. Baillieres Clin Haematol 8(3):479-97, 1995

Wright JV. Dr. Wright's Book of Nutritional Therapy. Emmaus, PA, Rodale Press, 1979

Yeh JH et al. Combined electroneurographic and electromyographic studies in lead workers. Occup Environ Med 52(6):415-9, 1995

OBESITY

NUTRITIONAL TREATMENT GUIDE

✓ = Efficacy generally accepted.
* = Efficacy *demonstrated* by controlled human trials.
[+] = Efficacy *suspected* from uncontrolled human experiments
[-] = Efficacy *suspected* from indirect data
? = Efficacy *challenged* in at least one study of similar design

DIETARY FACTORS

✓ **Balanced Hypocaloric diet**

- -

* eat a daily **Breakfast**
* substitute **Fructose** for Glucose or Sucrose
* **Low-Insulin-Response diet** (especially for hyperinsulinemic patients)
* **Low-Fat Hypocaloric diet**
* increase **dietary Fiber**

- -

[+] **Very-Low-Calorie diet**
[+] **High Carbohydrate Hypocaloric diet**
[+] **Low Carbohydrate Hypocaloric diet**
[+] **High Protein Hypocaloric diet**
[+] increase intake of **Raw Foods**
[+] drink **Caffeine**-containing beverages, especially before exercise

- -

[-] ? minimize **Sugar** intake

NUTRITIONAL FACTORS

* **Omega-6 Essential Fatty Acids:** evening primrose oil 4 to 8 g daily in divided doses
* **5-Hydroxytryptophan:** ? 100 to 300 mg 3 times daily (6 week trial)
* **Vitamin C:** 1 g 3 times daily (6 week trial)
* ? **Chromium:** chromium picolinate 200 to 400 μg daily *OR* niacin-bound chromium 200 μg 3 times daily

- -

[+] **Coenzyme Q_{10} deficiency:** 50 mg twice daily
[+] **Pantothenic acid:** 2.5 g 4 times daily (1 to 3 g daily for maintenance)

OTHER RELATED FACTORS

[+] rule out **Food Sensitivities**

DIETARY FACTORS

In order for the average person to lose one pound per week, caloric intake must be reduced by 500 calories per day. Most people will begin to lose weight if they reduce their daily calorie intake to below 1,500 calories; some may require an intake of less than 1,000 calories to lose weight *(Friedman)*. For optimal results, an exercise program and a psychological and/or behavioral program should be combined with the diet plan.

Obesity-related health risks do not start until a patient is 20% or more above ideal body weight, or if there is an existing condition, such as hypertension *(Pi-Sunyer)*. Despite the many health benefits of dieting, numerous studies suggest that dieting may increase a person's relative mortality risk about 1.5 to 2.5 times. These data also demonstrate a strong relationship between weight loss and cardiovascular mortality, perhaps due to the loss of lean muscle tissue *(Williamson)*.

Breakfast

Obese or overweight people have less satisfactory breakfast habits than people who are normal in weight *(Ortega)*. In a controlled study, moderately obese women who ate breakfast were more successful at losing weight than those who did not. Analysis of behavioral data suggested that eating breakfast helped reduce dietary fat and minimized impulsive snacking *(Schlundt)*.

WEIGHT REDUCTION DIETS

Balanced Diets

Balanced diets, such as Weight Watchers, the Setpoint Diet and the Prudent Diet, are considered to be the safest for weight loss. They generally provide for 800 to 1,500 calories daily using a wide variety of foods *(Morgan)*.

Insulin-control Diets

A variation of the balanced diet is the insulin-control diet based on the hypothesis that weight gain is promoted overconsumption of carbohydrates *(Heller;Sears)*. Instead of formally restricting calories, it focuses on a balance of carbohydrate, protein, and fat intake, generally in a 40:30:30 ratio, which is designed to minimize insulin response without reaching a ketotic state. The Zone Diet and the Healthy for Life Diet are examples.

A crossover study of obese hyperinsulinemic females has demonstrated that a low-insulin-response hypocaloric diet may be preferable to a standard hypocaloric diet for this patient group *(Slabber)*. However, there is no evidence that an elevated blood insulin level, by itself, causes weight gain, or that eating equal amounts of protein and carbohydrate at every meal lowers insulin levels *(Reaven)*.

High Carbohydrate (Low Protein) Diets

High carbohydrate (low protein) diets, such as the Pritikin Diet, are believed to induce weight loss by limiting food choices *(Morgan)*. One study compared a low calorie diet to a low-fat, complex carbohydrate diet without calorie restriction. While both resulted in weight loss (3.8 kg versus 4.4 kg, respectively), the high carbohydrate diet was preferred by the subjects as it was more palatable and the quality of life was superior while following it *(Shah)*.

Several versions of this diet, such as the Beverly Hills Diet *(Mirkin)* and certain Macrobiotic diets *(Anonymous,1971)*, are nutritionally unbalanced. Furthermore, there have been concerns that, compared to balanced diets, these diets may promote loss of body protein *(Blackburn)* and dysinsulinism *(Heller;Sears)*.

Low Fat Diets

The rationale for the low fat diet, such as the diet advocated by Dean Ornish in Eat More, Weigh Less, is that dietary fat induces overconsumption and weight gain through its low satiety properties and high caloric density *(Golay,1997)*. Other studies have also noted that a reduction in fat and caloric intake without a reduction in proteins and carbohydrates can lead to successful weight loss *(Roust;Sheppard)*.

However, there is evidence that its successful, long term applicability may be limited. It appears to work best with individuals genetically predisposed to obesity *(Heitmann; Lissner)*. Also, the evidence is that a low fat diet must be complemented by a reduction in carbohydrate intake in order to be successful *(Flatt,1995)*.

Ketogenic Low Carbohydrate Diets

Ketogenic low carbohydrate diets satisfy hunger because of their high protein and fat contents. Ketosis soon develops leading to a diuresis causing a rapid initial weight loss. Plasma insulin levels are lowered, causing increased release of fatty acids from adipose tissue and, thereby, enhanced fat mobilization *(Flatt,1974)*.

These diets have many potential adverse effects. These include hyperuricemia, sodium and potassium loss, diarrhea, glucose intolerance, hyperlipidemia, constipation, postural hypotension, fatigue, and nutritional inadequacy *(Friedman)*, as well as adverse effects on cognition *(Wing)* and mood *(Stenson)*.

High Protein Diets

Closely related to ketogenic low carbohydrate diets are non-ketogenic high protein diets such as the Healthy for Life and Zone diets. These tend to severely limit food choices and, if the protein comes mainly from animal sources, are high in cholesterol. They are often deficient in vitamins and minerals *(Friedman)*.

Assuming that total calorie intake is equal, two studies found greater weight loss may on a low, rather than on a high, carbohydrate diet *(Rabast;Young)*, while another had opposite findings and noted that patients had fewer cravings and better overall moods on the high carbohydrate diet *(Stenson)*. Still another study found weight loss to be similar, but found the low carbohydrate diet superior as it uniquely lowered fasting plasma glucose, insulin, cholesterol, and triacylglycerol concentrations *(Golay,1996)*.

With such conflicting findings, it seems that diets should be individualized; if patients have difficulty with one type of diet, they may do better with another.

High Fat Diets

High fat diets such as Dr. Atkins' New Diet Revolution, while they taste good and satisfy hunger well for their low calorie content, suffer from the combined dangers of a high fat intake and inadequate nutrition *(Anonymous,1973)*.

Very-low-calorie Diets

Very-low-calorie diets generally contain 300 to 400 calories per day, although there does not appear to be any advantage in reducing energy intake to below 800 calories daily *(Foster)*. Compared to balanced diets of equal calorie content, the greater weight loss frequently noted from liquid protein diets, a popular form of this type of diet, is solely due to a larger amount of fluid loss *(Yang)*. Adding fiber to these diets may reduce hunger and improve bowel function *(Astrup)*.

Very-low-calorie diets should be limited to persons who are at least 30 percent and 18 kg overweight, have received a recent physical examination and EKG, are free of cancer, type I diabetes, significant psychiatric disturbances, a cardiac conduction disorder, a recent myocardial infarction or a history of cerebrovascular, renal or hepatic disease *(Wadden)*. Potential adverse effects of these diets include hypoglycemia *(Marsoobian)*, cold intolerance *(Prasad)*, headaches, muscle cramps, halitosis, abdominal cramps *(Atkinson)*, anemia *(Fisler)*, and gallstone formation *(Klawansky)*. Other potential negative sequelae include negative nitrogen balance, brittle nails, and dry skin *(Morgan)*.

Furthermore, long-term maintenance of weight loss with very-low-calorie diets is not very satisfactory and is no better than other forms of obesity treatment *(National)*. On the positive side, a very-low calorie diet in diabetics may reduce serum and fasting blood glucose levels plus serum lipid levels *(Bistrian)*.

Fasting

Over the long term, the results of temporary or intermittent fasting are variable *(Fisler)*. About one-third of the weight lost during a 24-day fast is fluid and lean body mass *(Apfelbaum)*. Possible adverse effects include severe ketosis, electrolyte imbalance, hyperuricemia, gouty arthritis, abdominal cramps, orthostatic hypotension, muscle wasting, hepatic and renal impairment, and a negative nitrogen balance *(Blackburn)*.

DIETARY CONSTITUENTS

Dietary Fiber

Increasing dietary fiber adds non-calorie bulk; the result is that satiety develops after less food intake, leading to weight loss *(Smith)*. Increasing the intake of raw foods in the diet can be an effective intervention for promoting weight loss *(Douglass)*. This may be due to the high fiber content of these foods or to the reduction in energy intake resulting from substituting raw foods for other foods of higher caloric value. Several specific sources of dietary fiber appear to be effective in promoting weight loss, including bean husk *(Lecomte)*, glucomannan *(Walsh)*, guar gum *(Pasman)*, sugar beet fiber *(Burley)*, and xanthum gum *(Cairella)*.

While insoluble fiber (such as wheat bran) may reduce appetite at mid-morning more effectively than soluble fiber (such as psyllium gum), soluble fiber may have a greater effect on satiety later in the day, suggesting that a combination of soluble and insoluble fibers may be most effective in reducing food intake throughout the day *(Delargy)*.

A Warning

There is evidence from a controlled study that high fiber weight reduction may significantly increase annual bone loss from the lumbar spine in postmenopausal women. Moreover, this loss may not be reversed if the weight is regained; thus repeated cycles of high fiber weight loss and gain may increase the risk of spinal osteoporosis *(Avenell)*.

Sugars

Animal studies have found that sucrose consumption stimulates increased calorie consumption *(Marks-Kaufman)* and fat accumulation accompanied by insulin resistance *(Toida)*. Similar effects appear to occur in humans *(Geiselman;Vasselli)*; moreover, it appears that sugar may act as a vehicle for fat intake by making fat more palatable *(Emmett)*. However, a recent large cross-sectional survey failed to find evidence that either sugary fatty foods, or diets high in sugars, are associated with obesity *(Gibson)*.

Compared to both sucrose and glucose, fructose may be preferable as there is preliminary data suggesting that it may reduce subsequent fat consumption *(Moyer;Rodin)*. Since a thermogenic defect may contribute to the development of obesity *(Donnelly;Dulloo,1987)*, the finding that it causes greater thermogenesis *(Schwarz)* could be relevant.

Caffeine

Caffeine is another promoter of thermogenesis whose intake may contribute to weight loss *(Dulloo,1989)*. In obese mice, caffeine decreased body fat content without affecting food intake *(Chen,1994)*.

Moreover, a low dose of caffeine prior to low-intensity exercise increases post-exercise energy expenditure and thus may help to prevent or treat mild obesity *(Donnelly)*. However, because of caffeine's other effects, high levels of caffeine consumption cannot be recommended on a long-term basis.

Reduced-Fat and Reduced-Sugar Foods

In recent years a variety of reduced-fat and reduced-sugar foods have become available. In order to discover if their substitution results in weight loss, or if people eating these foods simply eat larger quantities, a group of non-obese, free-living females, all initially non-users of reduced-fat and reduced-sugar products, were placed on reduced-fat or reduced-sugar foods, or served as controls. After 10 weeks, both experimental dietary changes failed to produce changes in total energy intake or body weight status *(Gatenby)*.

NUTRITIONAL FACTORS

VITAMINS

Pantothenic Acid

An open trial found that 100 patients on weight-loss diets who were supplemented with massive dosages of pantothenic acid were not hungry despite an average of 1.2 kg (2.7 lb) weight loss per week. After the desired weight was achieved, there were able to maintain it with a maintenance diet and continued pantothenic acid supplementation.

The author of the study notes that individuals who are deficient in pantothenic acid lose their capacity to utilize fat effectively, while body fat burns more effectively when pantothenic acid is plentiful during dieting, delaying the onset of ketosis and allowing weight loss without hunger and weakness *(Leung)*.

These preliminary findings have yet to be confirmed with controlled clinical trials.

Vitamin C

Both plasma *(Singh)* and serum *(Moor de Burbos)* levels of ascorbic acid may be inversely related to the risk of obesity. In fact, in one of these studies, the group with extreme obesity had the lowest serum levels *(Moor de Burbos)*.

This finding by itself would mean little if it were not for the results of two double-blind studies of obese patients supplemented with vitamin C. In the first, large doses of ascorbic acid led to weight loss. The greatest response was in patients who were more than one-third above their ideal body weight *(Naylor,1982)*.

The other study of ascorbate supplementation was of women who were about 50% above ideal weight and who had failed to lose weight on various reducing programs. The difference in weight loss between the experimental and control groups became significant after only 2 weeks. After 6 weeks of supplementation, mean weight loss in the experimental group was 2.53 kg compared to only 0.95 kg in the controls, a significant difference *(Naylor,1985)*.

While the mechanism by which vitamin C may promote weight loss is unknown, it may theoretically reduce obesity by increasing cellular energy consumption through increasing sodium pump activity *(Naylor,1985)*.

MINERALS

Chromium

Several double-blind studies have found that chromium supplementation fostered the loss of body fat in obese individuals while preserving lean muscle mass. For example, 90 days after moderately overweight patients randomly received either chromium picolinate or placebo, patients in the chromium group lost significantly more weight (7.79 vs. 1.81 kg, respectively) and fat mass (7.71 kg vs. 1.53 kg, respectively), and had a greater reduction in percent body fat (6.3% vs. 1.2%, respectively) without any loss of fat-free mass *(Kaats)*.

While these results are impressive, two double-blind studies failed to find efficacy from chromium supplementation. The body composition of football players (who would be expected to have a high muscle mass and relatively little body fat) was unaffected by chromium picolinate *(Clancy)*. Also, active duty Navy personnel (men's body fat ≥ 22% of body composition; women's body fat ≥ 30%) failed to lose weight on the supplement *(Trent)*.

Zinc

Most epidemiologic studies have found an inverse correlation between either plasma/serum *(Singh)* or hair *(Ming-Der Chen)* zinc levels and obesity, although a few studies have had the opposite finding *(Taneja;Yakinci)*.

In a controlled study, obese patients received zinc sulfate and/or 0.1 mg thyroxine for 8 weeks. Only the patients receiving zinc had significant weight loss, whether or not they were on thyroxine. Moreover, serum zinc levels were inversely related to body weight reduction *(Chen,1991a)*.

A Warning

Despite these promising findings, dietary zinc treatment *increased* body fat deposition in mice that were obese, whether due to genetic or dietary factors *(Chen,1991b; Chen,1996)*. Moreover, at baseline these mice had higher amounts of zinc in their liver and adipose tissues than lean mice - even though zinc levels were markedly low in most of the peripheral tissues *(Chen,1991b)*.

Until more is known concerning zinc metabolism in obesity, supplementation cannot be recommended as a treatment.

OTHER NUTRITIONAL FACTORS

Coenzyme Q_{10} (ubiquinone)

About half of a group of 27 morbidly obese patients were found to have reduced levels of coenzyme Q_{10} (CoQ_{10}) *(van Gaal)*.

In an open trial, 9 morbidly obese patients, 5 of whom were deficient in CoQ_{10}, were placed on a very-low-calorie diet (650 kcal) and supplemented with the coenzyme. After 8 to 9 weeks, the mean weight loss of the 5 patients with reduced CoQ_{10} levels at baseline was more than twice that of the 4 patients with normal levels (13.5 kg vs. 5.8 kg) *(van Gaal)*.

These impressive early findings suggest that supplementation with coenzyme Q_{10} may substantially increase weight loss in morbidly obese patients who have low levels of the coenzyme. However, they require confirmation from controlled clinical trials.

5-Hydroxytryptophan

In double-blind studies, obese patients supplemented with 5-hydroxytryptophan had significant weight loss within 6 weeks, even without any dietary changes. They reduced their carbohydrate intake and noted early satiety. Mood was unchanged *(Cangiano;Ceci)*.

Omega-6 Essential Fatty Acids

The preponderance of early data suggests that *evening primrose oil*, a source of omega-6 fatty acids, may promote weight loss in obese patients who have failed to lose weight despite following an appropriate diet. Very obese patients may have reduced brown fat activity which the oil, when effective, appears to normalize. Moreover, these patients have a poor response to ephedrine which dramatically increases following treatment *(Lowndes)*.

Following the encouraging results of open trials *(Lowndes;Vaddadi)*, 2 double-blind studies have been performed. When a group of women with "substantial" obesity was studied, evening primrose oil was no more effective than placebo *(Haslett)*. However, when another study restricted treatment to patients with a family history of obesity, only the supplemented group had significant weight loss *(Garcia)*, suggesting that candidates for evening primrose oil administration should have a family history of obesity.

The results of one of the open trials suggest that, the greater the excess weight, the more effective the supplement will be; evening primrose oil was ineffective for people within 10 percent of ideal body weight. Furthermore, its efficacy appears to be dose-related *(Vaddadi)*.

OTHER RELATED FACTORS

Food Sensitivities

On the basis of clinical observations, Randolph has hypothesized that obesity may result from cravings for certain frequently eaten foods to which people have become sensitized, as avoidance of those foods precipitates a variety of mental and physical symptoms. In that situation, a weight reduction diet may be exceedingly difficult until the masked food allergens have first been avoided for several days, during which a diuresis will often occur. Corn, wheat and milk appear to be the most frequent offenders *(Randolph)*.

While others have reported similar observations *(Mandell;McDowell)*, this hypothesis has yet to be explored under controlled conditions.

A 33-year-old chronically obese woman also had a history of depression, migraine headaches, irritability, perceptual and learning problems, periodic motor problems, and childhood hyperactivity. Upon repeated testing, several foods were found to produce consistent irregular behavioral and physiological states. Although calorie intake remained constant during her evaluative period, she gained weight during 6-day phases when sensitive foods were eaten and lost weight during phases when nonsensitive foods were eaten.

She was instructed to avoid the substances to which she reacted, and found that she was more effective in controlling her weight and was also greatly improved in other problem areas (O'Banion).

BIBLIOGRAPHY

Anonymous. Council on Foods and Nutrition. Zen macrobiotic diets. JAMA 218:397, 1971

Anonymous. A critique of low-carbohydrate ketogenic weight reduction regimens: A review of Dr. Atkins' Diet Revolution. JAMA 224:1415-9, 1973

Apfelbaum M et al. [The composition of weight loss during the water diet. Effects of protein supplementation.] Gastroenterologia 108(3):121-34, 1967

Astrup A et al. Dietary fibre added to very low calorie diet reduces hunger and alleviates constipation. Int J Obes 14:105-12, 1990

Atkinson RL. Low and very low calorie diets. Med Clin North Am 73(1):203-15, 1989

Avenell A et al. Bone loss associated with a high fibre weight reduction diet in postmenopausal women. Eur J Clin Nutr 48(8):561-6, 1994

Bistrian BR et al. Nitrogen metabolism and insulin requirements in obese diabetic adults on a protein sparing modified diet. Diabetes 25:494-504, 1976

Blackburn GL. Fad reducing diets: Separating fads from facts. Contemp Nutr 8(7), 1983

Burley VJ et al. Sustained post-ingestive action of dietary fibre: effects of a sugar-beet-fibre-supplemented breakfast on satiety. J Hum Nutr Diet 6:253-60, 1993

Cairella M, Godi R. Clinical observations on the use of xanthum gum in obesity. Clin Dietol 13(1):37-40, 1986

Cangiano C et al. Eating behavior and adherence to dietary prescriptions in obese adult subjects treated with 5-hydroxytryptophan. Am J Clin Nutr 56:863-7, 1992

Ceci F et al. The effects of oral 5-hydroxy-tryptophan administration on feeding behaviour in obese adult female subjects. J Neural Transm 76(2):109-17, 1989

Chen MD et al. [Zinc sulfate and thyroxine treatment on the obese patients]. Chung Hua I Hsueh Tsa Chih (Taipei) 48(3):210-6, 1991a (in Chinese)

Chen MD et al. [Investigation of the relationships between zinc and obesity]. Kao Hsiung I Hsueh Ko Hsueh Tsa Chih 7(12):628-34, 1991b (in Chinese).

Chen MD et al. Effect of caffeine on the levels of brain serotonin and catecholamine in the genetically obese mice. Chung Hua I Hsueh Tsa chih (Taipei) 53(5):257-61, 1994

Chen MD et al. Zinc supplementation aggravates body fat accumulation in genetically obese mice and dietary-obese mice. Biol Trace Elem Res 52(2):125-32, 1996

Clancy SP et al. Effects of chromium picolinate supplementation on by composition, strength, and urinary chromium loss in football players. Int J Sports Nutr 4(2):142-53, 1994

Delargy HJ et al. Effects of amount and type of dietary fiber (soluble and insoluble) on short-term control of appetite. Int J Food Sci Nutr 48:67-77, 1997

Donnelly K, McNaughton L. The effects of two levels of caffeine ingestion on excess postexercise oxygen consumption in untrained women. Eur J Appl Physiol 65:459-63, 1992

Douglass J et al. Effects of a raw food diet on hypertension and obesity. South Med J 78(7):841, 1985

Dulloo AG et al. Normal caffeine consumption: influence on thermogenesis and daily energy expenditure in lean and postobese human volunteers. Am J Clin Nutr 49:44-50, 1989

Dulloo AG, Miller DS. Obesity: A disorder of the sympathetic nervous system. World Rev Nutr Diet 50:1-56, 1987

Emmett PM, Heaton KW. Is extrinsic sugar a vehicle for dietary fat? Lancet 345:1537-40, 1995

Fisler JS, Drenick EJ. Starvation and semistarvation diets in the management of obesity. Ann Rev Nutr 7:465-84, 1987

Flatt JP, Blackburn GL. The metabolic fuel regulatory system: Implications for protein-sparing therapies during caloric deprivation and disease. Am J Clin Nutr 27:175-87, 1974

Flatt JP. McCollum Award Lecture, 1995: Diet, Lifestyle and weight maintenance. Am J Clin Nutr 62:820-36, 1995

Foster GD et al. A controlled comparison of three very-low-calorie diets: effects on weight, body composition, and symptoms. Am J Clin Nutr 55:811-17, 1992

Friedman RB. Fad diets: Evaluation of five common types. Postgrad Med 89(1):249-58, 1986

Geiselman PJ. Sugar-induced hyperphagia: is hyperinsulinemia, hypoglycemia, or any other factor a 'necessary' condition? Appetite 11 Suppl 1:26-34, 1988

Garcia CM et al. Gamma linolenic acid causes weight loss and lower blood pressure in overweight patients with family history of obesity. Swed J Biol Med 4:8-11, 1986

Gatenby SJ et al. Extended use of foods modified in fat and sugar content: nutritional implications in a free-living female population. Am J Clin Nutr 65:1867-73, 1997

Gibson SA. Are high-fat, high-sugar foods and diets conducive to obesity? Int J Food Sci Nutr 47(5):405-15, 1996

Golay A et al. Similar weight loss with low- or high-carbohydrate diets. Am J Clin Nutr 63:174-8, 1996

Golay A, Bobbioni E. The role of dietary fat in obesity. Int J Obesity 21(Suppl 3):S2-S11, 1997

Haslett C et al. A double-blind evaluation of evening primrose oil as an antiobesity agent. Int J Obes 7(6):549-53, 1983

Heitmann BL et al. High dietary fat intake may have an obesity-promoting effect in women with a genetic predisposition. Am J Clin Nutr 61:1213-17, 1995

Heller RF, Heller RF. Hyperinsulinemic obesity and carbohydrate addiction: the missing link is the carbohydrate frequency factor. Med Hypotheses 42:307-12, 1994

Kaats GR et al. A randomized, double-masked, placebo-controlled study of the effects of chromium picolinate supplementation on body composition: a replication and extension of a previous study. Curr Therapeut Res 59(6):379-88, 1998

Klawansky S, Chalmers TC. Fat content of very-low-calorie diets and gallstone formation. Letter. JAMA 268(7):873, 1992

Lecomte A. A double-blind study confirms the effects of weight of bean husk Arkocaps. Revue de L'association Mondiale de Phytotherapie 1:41-4, 1985

Leung L. Pantothenic acid as a weight-reduction agent: fasting without hunger, weakness and ketosis. Med Hypotheses 44(5):403-5, 1995

Lissner L, Heitmann BL. Review of dietary fat and obesity: evidence from epidemiology. Eur J Clin Nutr 49:79-90, 1995

Lowndes RH, Mansel RE. The effects of evening primrose oil (Efamol) on serum lipid levels of normal and obese subjects, in DF Horrobin, Ed. Clinical Uses of Essential Fatty Acids. Montreal, Eden Press, 1982:37-52

Mandell M, Mandell FG. The Mandells' Its Not Your Fault You're Fat Diet. New York, Harper & Row, 1983

Marks-Kaufman R et al. The effects of dietary sucrose on opiate receptor binding in genetically obese (ob/ob) and lean mice. J Am Coll Nutr 8(1):9-14, 1989

Marsoobian V et al. Very-low-energy diets alter the counterregulatory response to falling plasma glucose concentrations. Am J Clin Nutr 61:373-8, 1995

McDowell M. Appetite control: An addiction-like component in overeating and its cure. Obesity/Bariatric Med 9(5):138-43, 1980

Ming-Der Chen, MA et al. Zinc in hair and serum of obese individuals in Taiwan. Am J Clin Nutr 48:1307-9, 1988

Mirkin GB, Shore RN. The Beverly Hills diet: Dangers of the newest weight loss fad. JAMA 246(19):2235-7, 1981

Moor De Burbos A. et al. Blood vitamin and lipid levels in overweight and obese women. Eur J Clin Nutr 46:803-8, 1992

Morgan SL. Rational weight loss programs: A clinician's guide. J Am Coll Nutr 8(3):186-94, 1989

Moyer AE, Rodin J. Fructose and behavior: does fructose influence food intake and macronutrient selection? Am J Clin Nutr 58(suppl):810S-4S, 1993

National Task Force on the Prevention and Treatment of Obesity. Very low-calorie diets. JAMA 270(8):967-74, 1993

Naylor GJ et al. A double blind placebo controlled trial of ascorbic acid in obesity. IRCS Med Sci 10:848, 1982

Naylor GJ et al. A double blind placebo controlled trial of ascorbic acid in obesity. Nutr Health 1985, p. 425

O'Banion D, Greenberg M. Behavioral effects of food sensitivity, in DR O'Banion, Ed. An Ecological and Nutritional Approach to Behavioral Medicine. Springfield, IL, Charles C. Thomas, 1981

Ortega RM et al. Difference in the breakfast habits of overweight/obese and normal weight schoolchildren. Int J Vitam Nutr Res 68(2):125-32, 1998

Pasman WJ et al. Effect of one week of fibre supplementation on hunger and satiety ratings and energy intake. Appetite 29(1):77-87, 1997

Pi-Sunyer FX, co-director of the Center for Research in Clinical Nutrition, St. Luke's/Roosevelt Hospital Center, New York City - reported in The diet dilemma. Med World News May, 1992

Prasad N. Very-low-calorie diets. Postgrad Med 88(3):179-88, 1990

Rabast U et al. Comparative studies in obese subjects fed carbohydrate-restricted and high carbohydrate 1,000-calorie formula diets. Nutr Metab 22(5):269-77, 1978

Randolph TG. Masked food allergy as a factor in the development and persistence of obesity. J Lab Clin Med 32:1547, 1947

Reaven, Gerald, emeritus professor of medicine, Stanford University - interviewed by Leibman B in Cardo-phobia. Zoning out on the new diet books. Nutrition Action Newsletter, July-August, 1996

Rodin J. Comparative effects of fructose, aspartame, glucose and water preloads on calorie and macronutrient intake. Am J Clin Nutr 51:428-35, 1990

Roust LR et al. Effects of isoenergetic low-fat diets on energy metabolism in lean and obese women. Am J Clin Nutr 60:470-5, 1994

Schlundt DG et al. The role of breakfast in the treatment of obesity: a randomized clinical trial. Am J Clin Nutr 55:645-51, 1992

Schwarz J-M et al. Thermogenesis in men and women induced by fructose vs. glucose added to a meal. Am J Clin Nutr 49:667-74, 1989

Sears B. Enter the Zone. New York, Harper Collins, 1995

Shah M et al. Comparison of a low-fat, ad libitum complex-carbohydrate diet with a low-energy diet in moderately obese women. Am J Clin Nutr 59:980-4, 1994

Sheppard L et al. Weight loss in women participating in a randomized trial of low-fat diets. Am J Clin Nutr 54:821-8, 1991

Singh RB et al. Association of low plasma concentrations of antioxidant vitamins, magnesium and zinc with high body fat per cent measured by bioelectrical impedance analysis in Indian men. Magnes Res 11(1):3-10, 1998

Slabber M et al. Effects of low-insulin-response, energy-restricted diet on weight loss and plasma insulin concentrations in hyperinsulinemic obese females. Am J Clin Nutr 60:48-53, 1994

Smith U. Dietary fibre, diabetes and obesity. Int J Obes 11 Suppl 1:27-31, 1987

Stenson J. High-protein diets may defeat their purpose. Obesity April 4, 1996:8

Taneja S et al. Excess bioavailability of zinc may cause obesity in humans. Experientia 52(1):31-3, 1996

Toida S et al. Effect of high sucrose feeding on fat accumulation in the male Wistar rat. Obes Res 4(6):561-8, 1996

Trent L, Thieding-Cancel D. Effects of chromium picolinate on body composition. J Sports Med Phys Fitness 35:273-80, 1995

Vaddadi KS, Horrobin DF. Weight loss produced by evening primrose oil administration in normal and schizophrenic individuals. IRCS J Med Sci 7:52, 1979

van Gaal L et al. Exploratory study of coenzyme Q10 in obesity, in K Folkers, Y Yamamura, Eds. Biomedical and Clinical Aspects of Coenzyme Q. Volume 4. Amsterdam, Elsevier Science Publishers, 1984, pp. 369-73

Vasselli JR. Carbohydrate ingestion, hypoglycemia and obesity. Appetite 6:53-9, 1985

Wadden TA et al. Responsible and irresponsible use of very-low-calorie diets in the treatment of obesity. JAMA 263(1):83-5, 1990

Walsh DE et al. Effect of glucomannan on obese patients: A clinical study. Int J Obes 8(4):289-93, 1984

Williamson DF., epidemiologist, Centers for Disease Control, Atlanta, USA - reported in The diet dilemma. Med World News May, 1992

Wing RR et al. Cognitive effects of ketogenic weight-reducing diets. Int J Obesity 19:811-16, 1995

Yakinci C et al. Serum zinc, copper, and magnesium levels in obese children. Acta Paediatr Jpn 39(3):339-41, 1997

Yang MU, Van Itallie TB. A composition of weight loss during short-term weight reduction. J Clin Invest 58:722-30, 1976

Young CM et al. Effect of body composition and other parameters in obese young men of carbohydrate level of reduction diet. Am J Clin Nutr 24(3):290-6, 1971

ORGANIC MENTAL DISORDERS

See Also: ALCOHOLISM
ANXIETY
BIPOLAR DISORDER
DEMENTIA
DEPRESSION

NUTRITIONAL TREATMENT GUIDE

✓ = Efficacy generally accepted.
* = Efficacy *demonstrated* by controlled human trials.
[+] = Efficacy *suspected* from uncontrolled human experiments
[-] = Efficacy *suspected* from indirect data
? = Efficacy *challenged* in at least one study of similar design

NUTRITIONAL FACTORS

* **Lithium deficiency:** 400 μg daily from lithium-rich brewer's yeast (4 week trial)
* ? **Folic acid deficiency:** 0.5 mg daily

- -

[+] rule out **Copper** toxicity
[+] **Magnesium deficiency:** ≈ 400 mg daily
[+] **Niacin deficiency:** 50 mg to 100 mg daily
[+] **Potassium deficiency:** ? 80 to 100 mEq daily total intake, preferably from potassium-rich foods
[+] **Sodium deficiency:** repletion
[+] **Thiamine deficiency:** 50 mg daily
[+] **Vitamin B_{12} deficiency:** 1000 μg IM weekly for 3 weeks, then 1000 μg IM monthly
[+] **Zinc deficiency:** zinc sulfate 220 mg twice daily *AND* **Copper** 2 mg daily

OTHER RELATED FACTORS

✓ ? rule out **Food Sensitivities**

- -

[-] rule out **Aluminum** toxicity
[-] rule out **Lead** toxicity
[-] rule out **Mercury** toxicity

NUTRITIONAL FACTORS

VITAMINS

Vitamin B Complex Deficiencies

Deficiencies of multiple B complex vitamins often coexist among populations of hospitalized psychiatric patients *(Carney)*. While individual B complex vitamins known to cause organic mental syndromes will be discussed, supplementation with the entire B complex should be considered whenever there is suspicion that nutriture of any member of the complex is inadequate.

Folic Acid

Folic acid deficiency, which is found in about one-quarter of psychiatric patients hospitalized in public facilities, is associated with a wide variety of psychiatric symptoms including psychosis, depression, confusion, disorientation, and dementia. One clue to the deficiency is that the psychiatric symptoms are often accompanied by neurologic symptoms of weakness, numbness, stiffness and spasticity, both with and without muscular atrophy *(Howard)*.

The vulnerability of the brain to adverse effects from folate deficiency is due to the important role of folates in the synthesis of neurotransmitters and elements of the neuronal structure. Folates are involved in the synthesis of S-adenosylmethionine (the main contributor of methyl groups in the nervous system), in the synthesis of glutamate (an excitatory neurotransmitter), and in the formation of purine and pyrimidine bases. Moreover, tetrahydrobiopterin is an essential cofactor for hydroxylation processes within the brain *(Ortega)*.

Whether a folate deficiency is primary or secondary to the psychiatric disorder, there is growing evidence that folate replacement may improve mental function *(Crellin)*. In addition to many open trials, two placebo-controlled studies have demonstrated beneficial effects from folic acid supplementation, one in patients with a syndrome of psychiatric and neuropsychological changes associated with folate deficiency and the other in patients on long-term lithium therapy. However, several placebo-controlled studies have not demonstrated therapeutic effects, possibly because the high dosages used in those studies (15-20 mg daily) are known to be potentially toxic and to cause mental symptoms *(Young)*.

A patient presented with an organic brain syndrome associated with subacute combined degeneration of the cord. As the cause of the illness was suspected to be a dietary folate deficiency, the patient was treated with methyl tetrahydrofolate (the form in which folic acid is transported into the CNS). There was a striking psychiatric, neurological and hematological response (Lever).

Niacin

A deficiency of niacin may cause delirium, dementia or psychosis *(Peterman)* which responds, often within days, to supplementation *(Sydenstricker)*.

Thiamine

Deficiency of thiamine has been associated with forgetfulness, difficulty in orderly thinking, and ideas of persecution *(Peterman)*. It is also related to postoperative mental confusion *(Older)* and risk of delirium in the elderly *(O'Keffe)*.

Vitamin B_{12}

Vitamin B_{12} deficiency may cause an organic psychosis *(Phillips)*. Paranoia, violence and depression are common *(Zucker)*. Psychiatric changes often predate the development of anemia and spinal cord disease *(Evans)*, although paresthesias, sensory loss, and ataxia may be noted *(Lindenbaum)* and the EEG may show abnormalities *(Evans)*.

Among hospitalized psychiatric patients, vitamin B_{12} deficiency is not uncommon. When every patient over 30 years old admitted to a Norwegian mental hospital during a one-year period was evaluated, 5.8% of the 396 patients were deficient (<75 pmol/L), while another 9.6% were subnormal (75-110 pmol/L) *(Edwin)*.

Especially for elderly patients, vitamin B_{12} supplementation should be started when serum cobalamin concentrations are below 200 pmol/L *(Nilsson)*. In an open trial reported in the *New England Journal of Medicine*, all of 39 patients with neuropsychiatric abnormalities and cobalamin deficiency improved following cobalamin supplementation *(Lindenbaum)*.

A young adult was evaluated following the acute onset of neuropsychiatric symptoms consistent with vitamin B_{12} deficiency. The lab findings were atypical in that, despite a normal hematocrit, a normal MCV, a normal peripheral blood smear, a normal bone marrow biopsy, and a normal Schilling test, he had abnormally low serum vitamin B_{12} levels.

He responded quickly to parenteral vitamin B_{12} therapy but, at the time of his last clinic visit, still had mild residual symptoms (Shanoudy).

MINERALS

Calcium

Hypocalcemia is usually due to hypoparathyroidism *(Joborn)*, and over half the patients with hypoparathyroidism develop psychiatric symptoms. Cognitive impairment is most frequent, while irritability, agitation, hyperactivity and delusions may also be noted (*Webb*), or an organic anxiety syndrome may develop *(Carlson)*.

Affective and organic symptoms are overwhelmingly dominant in *hypercalcemic* patients, the majority of whom are women 50 years or older who have been vaguely ill for a prolonged time before the actual endocrinopathy appears. The severity of the psychiatric symptoms seems unrelated to the degree of hypercalcemia *(Alarcon)*. Personality changes characterized by irritability and a lack of initiative and spontaneity are most frequently seen. Depression may be prominent, manifested by a loss of interest, social withdrawal, anorexia, anhedonia, and memory impairment *(Webb)*.

In both cases, treatment should be directed at correcting the underlying condition.

Copper Toxicity

Copper toxicity can cause brain dysfunction. When 30 patients with unusually elevated hair copper levels were evaluated, mental symptoms included profound mental fatigue, poor memory, lack of concentration, insomnia, severe depression, apprehension, and irritability along with somatic complaints. Serum and urine copper levels were normal.

Chelation therapy with D-penicillamine often elicited a prompt reduction of symptoms, and 24-hour urine output of copper during chelation therapy was generally proportional to the hair copper level *(Nolan)*.

Lithium Deficiency

Low levels of tap water and/or urine lithium have been correlated with higher mental hospital admissions due to diagnoses of psychosis, neurosis, schizophrenia, personality disorders and homicides *(Dawson)*. Moreover, lithium-deficient male rats demonstrated decreased aggression both in response to handling and in social interactions, and wheel-running activity was inhibited *(Klemfuss)*.

While little research has been conducted on the efficacy of nutritional levels of lithium supplementation, in a placebo-controlled study of 24 former drug users, some of whom had a history of violence, subjects received nutritional levels of lithium or placebo for 4 weeks. In the lithium group, total mood test scores increased steadily and significantly, suggesting that nutritional lithium had mood-improving and mood-stabilizing effects *(Schrauzer)*.

Magnesium

One of the first symptoms of magnesium deficiency is the development of an organic mental disorder *(Webb)*. Confusional states, depression, and neuromuscular irritability may be noted *(Gatewood)*.

Interestingly, within the psychiatric hospital population, plasma magnesium levels may be either higher and lower than normal in the more disturbed, excitable patients, suggesting that an abnormality of magnesium metabolism may contribute to their disorder *(Kirow)*.

Potassium

Hypokalemia (low serum potassium) is associated with dysphoric mood, tearfulness, weakness, and fatigue, and an overt organic mental syndrome is not uncommon *(Webb)*.

As part of the toxicity syndrome, *hyperkalemia* frequently results in the development of an organic mental syndrome *(Webb).*

In both cases, treatment should be directed primarily at correcting the underlying disorder. Also, in hypokalemia, potassium repletion should be considered.

Sodium

Hyponatremia (low serum sodium) is often associated with apathy, impaired concentration, emotional lability, lethargy, memory impairment, social withdrawal, and anorexia as part of the deficiency syndrome. When severe, disorientation, somnolence, illusions and hallucinations may occur *(Webb).*

Hypernatremia causes neuropsychiatric signs such as irritability and hyperactivity in about one out of four patients. Irritability and hyperactivity appear early, with a frank organic brain syndrome appearing in more severe cases *(Webb).*

As with abnormal serum potassium levels, therapy should be directly at correcting the underlying cause, although low serum levels may require repletion.

Zinc Deficiency

Zinc deficiency is associated with apathy, lethargy, amnesia, and mental retardation, often with considerable irritability, depression and paranoia *(Prasad).* Acute zinc deficiency, which is rare, produces a syndrome of mental apathy and depression along with diarrhea and a moist eczematoid dermatitis *(Kay).*

OTHER RELATED FACTORS

Food Sensitivities

In susceptible individuals, foods may cause a wide variety of mental and behavioral symptoms *(Rippere).* When 30 patients with psychological symptoms and abnormal scores on the Minnesota Multiphasic Personality Inventory were tested under double-blind conditions following an elimination diet, there were significantly greater cognitive-emotional symptoms when they were tested with foods than when they were tested with placebo *(King).*

However, when 19 patients who believed their neurotic symptoms were due to food sensitivities were investigated with elimination diets, open food reintroductions, and double-blind provocation testing for the foods reported to cause reactions during the reintroductions, there was no evidence that any of the patients was food sensitive *(Pearson).* This finding suggests that blind food challenges after several days of following a diet eliminating all suspicious foods (most often the common foods) may be necessary to establish whether true food sensitivities exist.

Heavy Metal Toxicity

When 37 emotionally disturbed children were compared to controls, the disturbed children had significantly higher hair lead and mercury levels. Using discriminant function analysis, subjects could be correctly classified as disturbed or normal by using aluminum, arsenic, lead and mercury with 77.8% accuracy.

Stepwise discriminant analysis showed that lead was the most significant metal in separating the two groups, followed by mercury, arsenic and aluminum. There was also a significant positive correlation between aluminum, lead and mercury levels and ratings on the Walker Problem Behavior Identification checklist *(Marlowe).*

Aluminum

Memory loss and depression are characteristic of aluminum toxicity. Incoordination is the most common physical finding *(White).*

Lead

Excessive lead exposure produces a variety of nonspecific symptoms, including depression, fatigue, irritability *(Schottenfeld)*, restlessness, talkativeness, illusions, mania, anxiety, aggression, and even some forms of schizophrenia *(Hunter).* Neuropsychological testing usually reveals multiple deficits *(Schottenfeld).*

Mercury

Mental symptoms from exposure to elemental or organic mercury include fatigue, irritability, nervousness, shyness, memory loss, lack of concentration, apathy, intellectual decline, depression, anxiety, drowsiness and insomnia *(Kupsinel).*

BIBLIOGRAPHY

Alarcon RD, Franceschini JA. Hyperparathyroidism and paranoid psychosis: Case report and review of the literature. Br J Psychiatry 145:477, 1984

Carlson RJ. Longitudinal observations of two cases of organic anxiety syndrome. Psychosomatics 27(7):529-31, 1986

Carney MW. Thiamine, riboflavin and pyridoxine deficiency in psychiatric in-patients. Br J Psychiatry 141:271-2, 1982

Crellin R et al. Folates and psychiatric disorders. Clinical potential. Drugs 45(5):623-36, 1993

Dawson EB. The relationship of tap water and physiological levels of lithium to mental hospital admission and homicide in Texas, in Schrauzer & Klippel, Eds. Lithium in Biology and Medicine. Cambridge VCH, 1991:169-88

Edwin E et al. Vitamin B12 hypovitaminosis in mental diseases. Acta Med Scand 177:689-99, 1965

Evans DL et al. Organic psychosis without anemia or spinal cord symptoms in patients with vitamin B12 deficiency. Am J Psychiatry 140(2):218-21, 1983

Gatewood JW et al. Mental changes associated with hyperparathyroidism. Am J Psychiatry 132(2):129-32, 1975

Howard JS III. Folate deficiency in psychiatric practice. Psychosomatics 16:112-15, 1975

Hunter D. The Disease of Occupation. 4th Edition. London, English University Press, 1969:283

Joburn C et al. Psychiatric symptomatology in patients with primary hyperthyroidism. Ups J Med Sci 91(1):77-87, 1986

Kay RG, Tasman-Jones C. Acute zinc deficiency in man during intravenous alimentation. Aust N Z J Surg 45(4):325-30, 1975

King DS. Can allergic exposure provoke psychological symptoms? a double-blind test. Biol Psychiatry 16(1):3-19, 1981

Kirow GK et al. Plasma magnesium levels in a population of psychiatric patients: correlation with symptoms. Neuropsychobiology 30(2-3):73-8, 1994

Klemfuss H, Schrauzer GN. Effects of nutritional lithium deficiency on behavior in rats. Biol Trace Elem Res 48(2):131-9, 1995

Kupsinel R. Mercury amalgam toxicity: A major common denominator of degenerative disease. J Orthomol Psychiatry 13(4):240-57, 1984

Lever EG et al. Subacute combined degeneration of the cord due to folate deficiency: response to methyl folate treatment. J Neurol Neurosurg Psychiatry 49(10):1203-7, 1986

Lindenbaum J et al. Neuropsychiatric disorders caused by cobalamin deficiency in the absence of anemia or macrocytosis. N Engl J Med 318(26):1720-8, 1988

Marlowe M et al. J Orthomol Psychiatry 12:260-7, 1983

Nilsson K et al. Plasma homocysteine in relation to serum cobalamin and blood folate in a psychogeriatric population. Europ J Clin Invest 24:600-6, 1994

Nolan KR. Copper toxicity syndrome. J Orthomol Psychiatry 12:270-82, 1983

O'Keffe ST et al. Thiamine deficiency in hospitalized elderly patients. Gerontology 40:18-24, 1994

Older J. Thiamine deficiency: Cause of postoperative mental confusion. Geriatr Med Today 5(4):103-6, 1986

Ortega TM et al. [The role of folates in the diverse biochemical processes that control mental function]. Nutr Hosp 9(4):251-6, 1994) (in Spanish)

Pearson DJ et al. Food allergy: How much in the mind? An objective clinical and psychiatric study of suspected food hypersensitivity. Lancet i:1259-61, 1983

Peterman RA, Goodhart RS. Current status of vitamin therapy in nervous and mental disease. J Clin Nutr 2(1):11-21, 1954

Phillips SL, Kahaner KP. An unusual presentation of vitamin B12 deficiency. Letter. Am J Psychiatry 145(4):529, 1988

Prasad AS et al. Experimental zinc deficiency in humans. Ann Intern Med 89:483, 1978

Rippere V. Some varieties of food intolerance to psychiatric patients: An overview. Nutr Health 3(3):125-36, 1984

Schottenfeld RS, Cullen MR. Organic affective illness associated with lead intoxication. Am J Psychiatry 141(11):1423-6, 1984

Schrauzer G et al. Effects of nutritional lithium supplementation on mood: A placebo-controlled study with former drug users. Biol Trace Elem Res 40(1):89-101, 1994

Shanoudy H, Salem AG. Neuropsychiatric manifestations of vitamin B12 deficiency in the absence of anemia or macrocytosis: a case report. S D J Med 45(5):129-31, 1992

Sydenstricker VP, Cleckley HM. The effect of nicotinic acid in stupor, lethargy and various other psychiatric disorders. Am J Psychiatry 98:83-92, 1941

Webb WL, Gehi M. Electrolyte and fluid imbalance: Neuro-psychiatric manifestations. Psychosomatics 22(3):199-203, 1981

White DM et al. Neurologic syndrome in 25 workers from an aluminum smelting plant. Arch Intern Med 152(7):1443-8, 1992

Young SN, Ghadirian AM. Folic acid and psychopathology. Prog Neuropsychopharmacol Biol Psychiatry 13(6):841-63, 1989

Zucker DK et al. B12 deficiency and psychiatric disorders: case report and literature review. Biol Psychiatry 16(2):197-205, 1981

OSTEOARTHRITIS

See Also: PAIN

NUTRITIONAL TREATMENT GUIDE

✓ = Efficacy generally accepted.
* = Efficacy *demonstrated* by controlled human trials.
[+] = Efficacy *suspected* from uncontrolled human experiments
[-] = Efficacy *suspected* from indirect data
? = Efficacy *challenged* in at least one study of similar design

NUTRITIONAL FACTORS

* **Boron:** 6 mg daily as borax 50 mg (preferably derived from fruits, vegetables and nuts)
* **Glucosamine Sulfate:** 500 mg 3 times daily
(May be preceded with 400 mg IM or IV daily for 7 days.)
* **Chondroitin Sulfate:** *example:* Condrosulf (IBSA, Lugano) 400 mg 2 to 3 times daily
* **Folic acid:** 6,400 μg daily
AND **Vitamin B_{12}**: cobalamin 20 μg daily (2 month trial)
* **Glycosaminoglycans:** dosage depends upon biological source and manufacturing procedures
* **Molybdenum:** 500 μg as amino acid chelate daily. Start with 1 cap with meals and at bedtime. Increase to maximum of 5 caps daily, or decrease to 2 to 3 caps daily, depending upon response. (1 month trial)
* **Niacinamide:** 1. Start with 500 mg twice daily
2. Gradually increase dosage as indicated to a maximum of 1 g 3 times daily.
3. Taper to a maintenance dosage after efficacy is established.
* **S-Adenosyl-L-Methionine:** 400 mg 3 times daily (1 month trial)
* **Selenium:** sodium selenite 140 μg daily
AND **Vitamin E:** 100 mg daily
* **Vitamin E:** D-alpha tocopherol acetate 400 mg daily (3 week trial)

- -

[+] **D-Phenylalanine:** 375 mg daily
[+] **Sulfur:** Dosage and routes of administration are poorly explored.
[+] **Zinc deficiency:** zinc sulfate 220 mg twice daily *AND* **Copper** 2 mg daily

- -

[-] **Vitamin C:** 500 mg twice daily
[-] **Vitamin D deficiency:** 800 IU daily

OTHER RELATED FACTORS

* **Cartilage extract:** dry powder 1 g per 3-5 lbs body weight *OR* Cartilade™ four 740 mg capsules. Take 3 times daily 15 to 30 minutes before meals. Reduce dosage if effective. (1 month trial)
* **Superoxide Dismutase:** Orgotein 16 mg intra-articularly weekly for 2 weeks, and then as needed.

- -

[+] rule out **Food Sensitivities**

- -

[-] avoid **Obesity**

NUTRITIONAL FACTORS

VITAMINS

Niacinamide

Kaufman has written for four decades about his extensive clinical experience with treating joint dysfunction with megadoses of niacinamide, which he found particularly effective for degenerative arthritis of the knee. Using an index of joint range of motion as the outcome measure, several hundred patients receiving niacinamide had superior scores to those of untreated age-matched control patients *(Kaufman,1955)*. He reports that, while niacinamide is not an analgesic, pain may decrease as joint mobility increases.

More recently, a double-blind study has provided substantiation for Kaufman's findings. Three months after starting niacinamide, compared to patients who received placebo, treated patients had significant improvement in joint mobility and in overall severity of arthritis. Moreover, they showed a reduction in their erythrocyte sedimentation rate and were able to reduce the anti-inflammatory medication by 13%. Beneficial effects started after 1 to 3 months and maximal benefits were reached in 1 to 3 years. The only side effects were gastrointestinal, and these were mild *(Jonas)*.

While the exact mechanisms of action are unknown, it has been suggested that niacinamide may provide energy and nucleic acids to cartilage through nonoxidative mechanisms to increase cartilage repair rates *(Jonas)*. Also, it may enhance the secretion of glucocorticoids *(Shneider)* or act in a similar manner *(Kosogorova; Rosenberg;Yamada)*.

A 61 year-old married housewife reported a history of joint discomfort for many years, and moderate deformities of the fingers for at least 10 years. Six to seven years earlier, she first noted severe pain in her hip joints. Her knees were very stiff. She had a lifelong curvature of the spine, and had a good deal of back pain. Recently she noted increased fatigability and insomnia.

On examination she had tenderness on digital pressure over the sternum, medial epicondyles, iliac crest, trochanter, styloid process of the radius, and sacroiliac joints. Marked kyphoscoliosis was noted and her tongue showed evidence of infiltration and atrophy of papillae. The liver edge was one finger's breath below the rib margin on deep inspiration and was tender to palpation. Bony prominences of the lower extremities were hyperpallesthetic to the tuning fork. Tickle sense was absent and plantar dysesthesia was present. Her low Joint Range Index of 68.2 indicated severe joint dysfunction.

She was started on niacinamide 100 mg every 30 minutes. One month later, she noted marked improvement in her Joint Range Index, and considerable subjective relief from joint discomfort. Plantar dysesthesia was no longer present and hyperpallesthesia of the lower extremities was replaced by normal vibratory sensation. Her tongue showed improvement and liver enlargement had diminished markedly. Fatigability and insomnia were no longer a problem.

Niacinamide dosage was adjusted according to her response and eventually stabilized at 2,000 mg daily. After 2 years, her Joint Range Index had risen to 92.8 (slight joint dysfunction) (Kaufman,1949).

Pantothenic Acid

For a group of 77 patients, the dietary intake of pantothenic acid was found to be below 80% of the recommended dietary allowance *(White-O'Connor)*. Moreover, rats made acutely deficient in pantothenic acid developed pathologic joint changes which closely resembled those of osteoarthrosis - including osteoporosis, calcification of cartilage, and the formation of osteophytes and lipping *(Nelson)*.

In an open trial, patients supplemented with pantothenic acid along with vitamin B complex demonstrated a limited, variable improvement which ended upon discontinuation of supplementation *(Annand)*. However, a randomized double-blind study of pantothenic acid supplementation failed to confirm these findings *(Anonymous)*.

It is possible that only patients with marginal nutriture of the vitamin will benefit due to repletion of the vitamin, but this hypothesis remains to be tested.

Vitamin B_{12} *AND* Folic Acid

A double-blind crossover study of patients receiving non-steroidal anti-inflammatory drugs (NSAIDs) compared cobalamin and folate, folate alone, and placebo with NSAIDs for 2 months each following a 10-day drug and supplement washout period. Acetaminophen was taken as needed during the study.

For all subjects, mean right and left hand grip values were higher with combined cobalamin-folate ingestion than with folate alone or with placebo and were equivalent to those obtained during NSAID use. Moreover, the number of tender hand joints were reduced with the use of the combination of cobalamin and folate compared to the use of NSAIDs *(Flynn)*.

Further controlled trials are needed, especially a trial employing a larger dosage of cobalamin.

Vitamin C

When patients were re-evaluated 7 to 10 years after baseline, while *incident* osteoarthritis was unaffected by vitamin C intake, there was a 3-fold reduction in the risk of osteoarthritis *progression* for both the middle and highest tertile of vitamin C intake. This related mainly to a reduced risk of cartilage loss, but also included a reduced risk of developing knee pain *(McAlindon, 1996a)*.

Consistent with this finding, cartilage taken from guinea pigs with experimental osteoarthritis fed 2 to 4 mg of vitamin C daily showed classic signs of advanced osteoarthritis while cartilage from animals fed 150 mg daily showed only minor arthritic changes *(Schwartz)*.

Unfortunately, controlled clinical trials of ascorbate supplementation have yet to be performed.

Vitamin D Deficiency

For a group of 77 patients, the dietary intake of vitamin D was found to be below 80% of the recommended dietary allowance *(White-O'Connor)*.

There is evidence that inadequate vitamin D nutriture may be associated with the risk of osteoarthritis progression. In a study of osteoarthritis of the knee in 556 subjects, incident osteoarthritis was found in 75 knees, and progressive osteoarthritis was found in 62 knees. The risk for progression increased 3-fold in subjects who were in the middle and lower tertile for both the intake and serum levels of vitamin D compared with those who were in the upper tertile. Low serum levels also predicted loss of cartilage and osteophyte growth *(McAlindon, 1996b)*.

The efficacy of repleting a vitamin D deficiency is not known.

Vitamin E

Much like the NSAIDs, vitamin E appears to be a prostaglandin inhibitor *(Partkhomets; White)*. Moreover, *in vitro* studies have suggested that this vitamin may modulate osteoarthritic development by enhancing the stability of sulfated proteoglycans in articular cartilage *(Schwartz)*.

In two double-blind studies, one with a crossover design, vitamin E was significantly more effective than placebo in providing pain relief *(Blankenhorn; Machtey)*. It has also been found to be as effective as Diclofenac, a NSAID, under double-blind conditions. Both treatments were equally effective in significantly reducing the circumference of the knee joints, increasing walking time, and increasing joint mobility *(Scherak)*.

MINERALS

Boron

Epidemiologic studies from a number of countries have shown an inverse relationship between soil boron levels and the prevalence of osteoarthritis *(de Fabio).* In areas of the world where boron intake is routinely 1 mg per day or less, the estimated incidence of arthritis is 20 to 70%, while in areas of the world where boron intake is 3 to 10 mg per day, the estimated incidence of arthritis is zero to 10% *(Newnham,1994a).* Moreover, the boron concentration in femur heads, bones, and synovial fluid is lower in arthritics than in normals *(Newnman,1994b).* In a small double-blind study, 5 out of 7 boron-supplemented patients subjectively improved compared to only 1 out of 8 placebo-treated controls after 8 weeks. There was a significantly greater improvement in the condition of all joints on boron than on placebo, as well as significantly less pain on passive movement *(Travers).* These findings are consistent with those in animals which noted that arthritic symptoms disappeared within a month following the start of supplementation as evidenced by the resumption of normal activity *(Newnham,1994c).*

Newnham has reported that, in his experience, boron supplementation is effective for about 90% of patients, and that most have complete symptom remission *(Newnham,1979).* Adults under age 70 often require 2 months to improve, while those of more advanced age may require 4 months to detect benefits *(Newnham,1994c).*

While the human requirement for boron is not yet known, it has been estimated to be near 1 to 2 mg daily *(Nielsen).* Until the results of long-term toxicity studies are reported, it is preferable to increase boron intake by increasing its quantity in the diet. Excellent sources are fruits, vegetables and nuts.

Molybdenum

Molybdenum is required for the synthesis of 4 detoxifying enzymes *(Rajagopalan).*

In a single-blind crossover study, 14 people with chronic aches and pains due to "arthritis" including osteo- or rheumatoid arthritis, frozen shoulder or undiagnosed low back pain graded their pain level and general health for 28 days. They then took either molybdenum or placebo capsules for the next 28 days; then the groups were crossed over for a third 28-day period.

Within one week of starting molybdenum, aches and pains significantly improved, as did their rating of their general health. When discontinued after 28 days, the effects of the supplement wore off within one week *(Moss).*

Selenium

Patients may have reduced blood levels of glutathione peroxidase, an important selenium-containing enzyme *(Jameson).*

While the effects of selenium supplementation alone have yet to be reported, selenium has been combined with vitamin E in two studies. This is because, due to their closely-related mechanisms of action, deficiency syndromes of the two nutrients overlap and most can be treated successfully with either nutrient *(Combs)*; therefore it makes sense to combine them.

The first study was an open trial involving patients with either osteo- or rheumatoid arthritis. Following supplementation, pain relief was found to be correlated with increased levels of glutathione peroxidase *(Bruce).*

In the other study, which was double-blind, 81 patients with chronic, disabling muscular pain, stiffness and aching, many of whom had osteoarthrosis, received selenium and vitamin E or placebo. Glutathione peroxidase levels increased in 75% of the patients. Similar to the open trial, mean pain score reduction was significantly more frequent and more marked among patients whose glutathione peroxidase levels increased than among those whose levels decreased. However, while pain score reduction was more pronounced among the total group of treated patients, pain reduction as compared to patients on placebo was not significant *(Jameson).*

A non-significant trend towards improvement in certain clinical parameters was also found in a double-blind study of a formulation which combined selenium with vitamins A, C and E ("selenium-ACE"). At both 3 and 6 months, investigators failed to find significant evidence for the compound over placebo *(Hill).*

Perhaps selenium supplementation is specifically indicated specifically to replete a selenium deficiency as marked, for example, by reduced blood levels of glutathione peroxidase. This hypothesis has remains to be tested in a controlled clinical trial.

Sulfur

Early in the development of osteoarthritis, there is a loss of sulfated proteoglycans from the involved hyaline cartilage. The value of sulfur supplementation has been poorly investigated, even though sulfur baths and injections are old-fashioned arthritis treatments which are still popular in many countries.

Some support for sulfur administration is provided by studies from the 1920s and 1930s. Sulfur baths were shown to increase blood sulfur levels *(Osterberg)*. The cystine (a sulfur-containing amino acid) content of fingernails in "arthritics" was found to be 8.9% compared to 12% in normals, suggesting that sulfur levels may be depressed *(Sullivan)*. Moreover, in an open trial, "arthritics" received colloidal sulfur intravenously. Pain and effusions disappeared, and the cystine fingernail test normalized *(Woldenberg)*.

Half a century later, these intriguing studies have failed to stimulate further research. One exception is a recent study of osteoarthritic cartilage in horses in which the sulfur concentration was found to be only one-third that of normal tissue *(Rizzo)*. (Sulfur, by the way, is often provided in glycosaminoglycan preparations.)

OTHER NUTRITIONAL FACTORS

Glycosaminoglycans (mucopolysaccharides)

The matrix of hyaline cartilage consists of a framework of collagen within which hydrophilic, aggregated proteoglycans are entrapped. These proteoglycan molecules consist of a backbone of long chain, random-coil hyaluronic acid with alternating side chains of glycosaminoglycans. The glycosaminoglycans are long-chain carbohydrate polymers of repeating disaccharide units (glucosamine or galactosamine), glucuronic acid and a protein core, regions of which are enriched in chondroitin sulfate or keratan sulfate.

Compared to normals, the urinary sugar components of glycosaminoglycans appear to be increased in osteoarthritis. Patients were found to excrete significantly more galactosamine, glucosamine and mannose and their total uronic acid excretion was higher *(Krajickova)*.

Chondroitin Sulfate

Chondroitin sulfate is a glycosaminoglycan composed of repeating units of N-acetylchondrosine with one sulfate group per disaccharide unit. In the early stages of joint disease, both in animal models and in man, there are changes in chondroitin sulfate that affect the chain length and the pattern of sulfation. These changes appear to reflect part of the cellular response by the chondrocytes to damage to the articular cartilage matrix *(Hardingham)*.

The oral administration of chondroitin sulfate has been shown to be effective in several double-blind studies. *(Bourgeois;Bucsi;Verbruggen)*. While it takes longer than NSAIDs to become effective, the therapeutic effect lasts up to 3 months following termination of treatment *(Morreale)*.

Glucosamine Sulfate

Glucosamine is the building block of the proteoglycans, the ground substance of articular cartilage. Sulfate, another important component, appears to potentiate its therapeutic effect *(D'Ambrosio)*.

Administration has been shown in double-blind studies to reduce pain, joint tenderness and swelling, and to increase range of motion *(Noack;Tapadinhas)*. In one double-blind study, electron microscopy of articular cartilage was used to compare cartilage from placebo-treated patients with that of patients treated with glucosamine sulfate. The results were intriguing: cartilage taken from the controls showed typical findings of established osteoarthritis, while cartilage taken from experimental patients appeared more similar to healthy cartilage, suggesting that the damaged cartilage was healing *(Drovanti)*.

While NSAIDs are believed to inhibit proteoglycan synthesis, glucosamine sulfate inhibits proteoglycan degradation *(Vidal y Plana)*. Pain relief following glucosamine sulfate administration is slower but, by 8 weeks, it may be significantly greater than that obtained from NSAIDs *(Lopes Vaz)*. Compared to NSAIDs, glucosamine sulfate has repeatedly been shown to yield similar or even superior benefits with less adverse effects under double-blind conditions *(Muller-Fassbender;Qiu; Rovati)*.

When compared to Arteparon^{R} (glycosaminoglycan polysulfate) (see Animal Tissue Extracts below), glucosamine was superior, particularly in mild arthritis for which 90% of pts. had pain reduction, while glycosaminoglycan polysulfate was successful in advanced cases *(Hehne)*.

However, despite its promise, there are serious limitations in the studies to date. Further research is thus needed before the appropriate place in the therapeutic armamentarium is established for this substance *(Barclay;da Camara)*.

D-Phenylalanine

The analgesic effect of D-phenylalanine is well known *(Dove)*. In open trials, supplementation with D-phenylalanine appeared to be effective for the treatment of a variety of arthritic conditions. In fact, in one study, over 75% of patients experienced good to complete pain relief within one week to one month *(Balagot; Ehrenpreis).*

S-Adenosylmethionine

S-adenosyl-L-methionine, produced from the sulfur amino acid L-methionine and adenosine triphosphate by the action of methionine-adenosyl-transferase, is another beneficial sulfur-containing physiologic compound. It has been shown to be analgesic and anti-inflammatory and to stimulate proteoglycan synthesis by articular chondrocytes *(diPadova).*

On the basis of clinical trials on over 22,000 patients and a number of double-blind studies, investigators have concluded that SAMe is as effective as the NSAIDs, but without their adverse side-effects *(diPadova).* As with glucosamine sulfate, pain relief takes longer when compared to NSAIDs. In one double-blind study, even after 5 days of intravenous loading prior to starting oral administration, it took 2 weeks before the earliest effects were seen *(Bradley).*

COMBINED NUTRIENT SUPPLEMENTATION

A 71 year-old man presented with osteoarthritis confirmed by x-rays which was worst in the knees, but also present in the hands and spine. he also complained of low energy and slight memory problems. Blood tests for rheumatoid factor were negative. Physical exam revealed slight swelling of knees and swelling and slight tenderness in several finger joints. His skin was slightly dry and he appeared to have a slight excess of gas in the abdomen.

He was placed on niacinamide 1000 mg 3 times daily, glucosamine 500 mg 3 times daily, cod-liver oil 1 tbs. daily, vitamin E 600-800 IU daily and selenium 300 μg daily along with a multiple vitamin/mineral supplement.

By the fourth week, he noted a definite lessening of arthritis symptoms, especially in the knees. By 4 months, he was walking well without his cane as the pain and swelling were gone. As testing revealed evidence of digestive problems, he also received hydrochloric acid-pepsin capsules, pancreatic enzymes and B vitamin injections. Two months later, he reported improvement in his energy level and memory (Wright,1994).

OTHER RELATED FACTORS

Obesity

Using Hartley albino guinea pigs which develop spontaneous osteoarthritis of the knee joint, a study was done to determine the importance of body weight in the pathogenesis of the disease. Body mass was found to be an important predisposing factor *(Bendele).*

Similarly, in a study of osteoarthritis patients, obesity was positively to pain from osteoarthritis and was more prevalent among these osteoarthritis patients than it is among the general geriatric population *(White-O'Connor).*

Animal Tissue Extracts

There has been some success in treating osteoarthritis with various preparations derived from animal tissues which are rich in glycosaminoglycans.

In osteoarthritis, neovascularization is involved in the reinitiation of cartilage growth and mineralization *(Brown),* while animal cartilage contains a protein that may inhibit angiogenesis *(Folkman;Langer;Moses).* This could be why animal cartilage preparations appear to reduce symptoms and disease activity.

For example, in a double-blind study, 147 patients received one of two cartilage extracts or placebo. The placebo group was encouraged to use various NSAIDs during active episodes. After 5 years, average pain scores dropped 85% in the cartilage-treated groups compared to only a 5% decrease in the controls. Moreover, joint deterioration was significantly less in the cartilage-treated groups (37% that of the control group) and the treated groups lost significantly less time from work *(Rejholec).*

Cartilade™ is a standardized shark cartilage preparation. In an unpublished study, 70% of a group of 16 dogs with severe secondary osteoarthritis due to hip dysplasia demonstrated remarkable improvement following the administration of the supplement for 21 days. Fifteen days after the preparation was discontinued, their condition regressed, with about half the improvement remaining *(Rauis)*.

Similar results were found when 6 elderly patients who had failed to benefit from standard agents stopped all prescriptions for pain and inflammation and received Cartilade™ in another unpublished study. Improvement began to be noted by the end of the third week. The 3 patients who completed the study required lower doses of NSAIDs and achieved greater pain relief from them *(Orcasita)*.

Clinicians report that about 60 to 70 percent of patients note pain reduction starting about 2 to 3 weeks after starting shark cartilage. When taken as a dry powder, it can be mixed in a blender with nonacidic fruit juice or water *(Sculti)*.

Standardized preparations derived from bovine cartilage and bone marrow (Rumalon®), and from bovine lung and tracheal tissue (Arteparon®), are other products whose efficacy may be primarily due to their glycosaminoglycan content.

Rumalon®, which is given intramuscularly, has been found effective in controlled studies *(Rejholec)*, but has caused nephrotic syndrome and hepatotoxicity as well as other untoward reactions *(Berg)*. Arteparon® is prepared by extraction from bovine lung and tracheal tissues followed by sulfate esterification of certain sugar hydroxy groups resulting in glycosaminoglycan polysulfuric esters. It is given intra-articularly or intramuscularly, and was effective in several double-blind studies *(Ishikawa)*.

Superoxide Dismutase

The activity of superoxide dismutase (SOD), an important and well-recognized antioxidant, is increased in osteoarthritic joints, suggesting that it is a marker of articular destruction and repair *(Sumii)*.

In double-blind studies, bovine copper-zinc SOD (Orgotein) has been shown to be an effective treatment when injected directly into an involved joint *(Flohë)*. A series of 2 weekly treatments gave relief for up to 3 months *(McIlwain)*.

The oral absorption of SOD is controversial. Animal studies have shown that administration of oral, non-enteric-coated SOD fails to increase tissue levels *(Giri)*; however, under double-blind conditions, an enteric-coated, wheat-sprout-derived product rich in SOD and catalase (SOD/CAT, Biomed, Honolulu) raised serum SOD levels in human subjects in an unpublished study *(Ordonez)*. Furthermore, in a recent pilot study on humans, orally-administered SOD significantly raised erythrocyte SOD levels for 4 hours *(Introna)*.

In an unpublished study, osteoarthritic dogs responded to oral administration of the enteric-coated wheat-sprout-derived product *(Randall)*. Moreover, 90% of a group of patients responded to the product in a large, but again unpublished, open trial *(Rothschild)*.

Controlled clinical trials are needed to determine the efficacy of oral SOD products in the treatment of osteoarthritis.

Food Sensitivities

Non-steroidal anti-inflammatory drugs (NSAIDs), which are commonly used in the treatment of osteoarthritis, have been shown to increase intestinal permeability to food antigens in osteoarthritis patients *(Bjarnason)*. This implies that patients receiving NSAIDs may be especially liable to food-mediated reactions.

Childers has hypothesized that a buildup of cholinesterase-inhibiting glycoalkaloids and steroids from consumption of substances in the nightshade (Solanaceae) family may cause inflammation, muscle spasms, pain, and stiffness, and eventually result in osteoarthritis. He believes that osteoarthritis is a result of long-term consumption and/or use of these substances as they contain vitamin D_3, which in excess eventually causes crippling disability.

According to Childers, rigid omission of the nightshades, (which include tomato, potato, tobacco, and black pepper) will, over several months, gradually result in improvement *(Childers)*. He has collected numerous anecdotal reports of improvement of both osteo- and rheumatoid arthritis on a nightshade-free diet; however, neither epidemiological studies nor controlled clinical trials have been undertaken to validate his hypothesis.

In addition to Childers' hypothesis, a few case reports have appeared which involve foods other than the nightshades. These reports suggest that the elimination of certain foods that are specific to the individual may sometimes result in dramatic symptomatic improvement *(Chao; Wright, 1979)*.

A 50-year-old housewife had a 16-year history of osteoarthritis. Medications consisted of 3 grains of Thyrolar, buffered aspirin for pain, and Premarin. She had a strong craving for bread and developed leg cramps if she drank more than a glass of milk daily. White wine caused hiccups and sneezing, while red wine and chocolate caused a headache. She developed hives when she ate cherries. Her total IgE was 22.5 units (normal values are less than 20, while probable atopy is above 100).

She agreed to follow an elimination diet, which restricted her to eating foods which were usually not in her diet more often than once weekly, and to discontinue her Thyrolar. Three weeks later she reported that her arthritic symptoms were clearly better. Although she had experienced some sudden pains, she no longer was having constant aching. While previously she complained of constant coughing and choking, these symptoms had entirely ceased at least 10 days earlier and her voice, which had been hoarse, was now normal.

On two occasions she had ingested a small amount of a dairy product and soon developed a cramp in her toes. She also noted that her energy level was quite low off of thyroid. A free thyroxine index confirmed that she was hypothyroid, so she was started on a small dose of Synthroid and told to add a new food to her diet every 3 days. After one 50 microgram Synthroid she noted throat congestion; after two she became so ill that she couldn't function for a few hours. She tried to return to Thyrolar but found that her throat congestion returned when she restarted it. She was switched her to a hypoallergenic thyroid supplement and her throat returned to normal.

Currently she is on a four-day rotary diet (i.e. she eats foods from a particular food group one out of four days). Her energy level is excellent on 2 grains of thyroid, her voice is entirely normal, and her joint pains are minimal.

BIBLIOGRAPHY

Anonymous. Calcium pantothenate in arthritic conditions. A report from the General Practitioner Research Group. Practitioner 224:208-11, 1980

Annand JC. Pantothenic acid and osteoarthritis. Letter to the Editor. Lancet ii:1168, 1963

Balagot RC et al. Analgesia in mice and humans by D-phenylalanine: Relation to inhibition of enkephalin degradation and enkephalin levels. Adv Pain Res Ther 5:289-92, 1983

Barclay TS et al. Glucosamine. Ann Pharmacother 32(5):547-9, 1998

Bendele AM, Hulman JF. Effects of body weight restriction on the development and progression of spontaneous osteoarthritis in guinea pigs. Arthritis Rheum 34(9):1180-4, 1991

Berg PA et al. Bovine cartilage and marrow extract. Letter. Lancet i:1275, 1989

Bjarnason I et al. Intestinal permeability and inflammation in rheumatoid arthritis: Effects of non-steroidal anti-inflammatory drugs. Lancet ii:1171-74, 1984

Blankenhorn G. [Clinical effectiveness of Spondyvit (vitamin E) in activated arthroses. A multicenter placebo-controlled double-blind study.] Z Orthop 124(3):340-3, 1986 (in German)

Bourgeois P et al. Efficacy and tolerability of chondroitin sulfate 1200 mg/day vs chondroitin sulfate 3 x 400 mg/day vs placebo. Osteoarthritis Cartilage 6 Suppl A:25-30, 1998

Bradley JD et al. A randomized, double blind, placebo controlled trial of intravenous loading with S-adenosylmethionine (SAM) followed by oral SAM therapy in patients with knee osteoarthritis. J Rheumatol 21(5):905-11, 1994

Brown RA, Weiss JB. Neovascularisation and its role in the osteoarthritic process. Ann Rheum Dis 47(11):881-5, 1988

Bruce A et al. The effect of selenium and vitamin E on glutathione peroxidase levels and subjective symptoms in patients with arthrosis and rheumatoid arthritis, in Proceedings New Zealand Workshop on Trace Elements in New Zealand. Dunedin, U. of Otago, 1981:92

Bucsi L, Poor G. Efficacy and tolerability of oral chondroitin sulfate as a symptomatic slow-acting drug for osteoarthritis (SYSADOA) in the treatment of knee osteoarthritis. Osteoarthritis Cartilage 6 Suppl A:31-6, 1998

Chao IT. Food incompatibility as a major cause of chronic arthritis of different forms. Ann Allergy 47:128, 1981

Childers NF, Margoles MS. An apparent relation of nightshades (Solanaceae) to arthritis. J Neurol Orthop Med Surg 14:227-31, 1993

Combs GF. Assessment of vitamin E status in animals and man. Proc Nutr Soc 40:187-94, 1981

D'Ambrosio E et al. glucosamine sulphate: A controlled clinical investigation in arthrosis. Pharmatherapeutica 2(8):504-8, 1981

da Camara CC, Dowless GV. Glucosamine sulfate for osteoarthritis. Ann Pharmacother 32(5):580-7, 1998

deFabio A. Treatment & prevention of osteoarthritis. Townsend Letter for Doctors, Feb.-March, 1990:143-8 diPadova C. S-adenosylmethionine in the treatment of osteoarthritis. Review of the clinical studies. Am J Med 83(5A):60-65, 1987

Dove B et al. [The analgesic action of d-phenylalanine in combination with morphine or methadone]. Pharmazie 46(12):875-7, 1991 (in German).

Drovanti A et al. Therapeutic activity of oral glucosamine sulfate in osteoarthritis: A placebo-controlled double-blind investigation. Clin Ther 3(4):260-72, 1980

Ehrenpreis S et al. Further studies on the analgesic activity of D-phenylalanine in mice and humans. EL Way, Ed. Proceedings of the International Narcotic Research Club Convention 1979:379-82

Flohë L. Superoxide dismutase for therapeutic use: clinical experience, dead ends and hopes. Mol Cell Biochem 84(2):123-31, 1988

Flynn MA et al. The effect of folate and cobalamin on osteoarthritic hands. J Am Coll Nutr 13(4):351-6, 1994

Folkman J et al. Induction of angiogenesis during the transition from hyperplasia to neoplasia. Nature 339:58-61, 1989

Giri SN, Misra HP. Fate of superoxide dismutase in mice following oral route of administration. Med Biol 62(5):285-9, 1984

Hardingham T. Chondroitin sulfate and joint disease. Osteoarthritis Cartilage 6 Suppl A:3-5, 1998

Hehne HJ et al. Treatment of gonarthritis with chondroprotective substances: A prospective comparative study of glucosamine sulphate and glycosaminoglycan polysulphate. Fortschr Med 102(24):676-82, 1984

Hill J, Bird HA. Failure of selenium-ACE to improve osteoarthritis. Br J Rheumatol 29(3):211-3, 1990

Introna M et al. The effect of oral supplementation with legume derived superoxide dismutase on erythrocyte superoxide dismutase in healthy volunteers. J Appl Nutr 49(1-2):12-17, 1997

Ishikawa K et al. Clinical evaluation of the intraarticular injection of glycosaminoglycan polysulfate for osteoarthritis of the knee joint. A multi-centric double-blind controlled study. Zschr Orthop 120:708-16, 1982

Jameson S et al. Pain relief and selenium balance in patients with connective tissue disease and osteoarthritis: A double-blind selenium tocopherol supplementation study. Nutr Res Suppl:391-7, 1985

Jonas WB et al. The effect of niacinamide on osteoarthritis: a pilot study. Inflamm Res 45:330-4, 1996

Kaufman W. The Common Form of Joint Dysfunction: Its Incidence and Treatment. Brattleboro, Vt., E.L. Hildreth & Co., 1949

Kaufman W. The use of vitamin therapy to reverse certain concomitants of aging. J Am Geriatr Soc 3:927, 1955

Kosogorova LS et al. [Recovery of immunological responsiveness in patients with bronchial asthma during nicotinamide treatment]. Probl Tuberk (5):41-4, 1996 (in Russian)

Krajickova J, Macek J. Urinary proteoglycan degradation product excretion in patients with rheumatoid arthritis and osteoarthritis. Ann Rheum Dis 47(6):468-71, 1988

Langer R et al. Isolations of a cartilage factor that inhibits tumor neovascularization. Science 193:70-2, 1976

Lopes Vaz A. Double-blind clinical evaluation of the relative efficacy of ibuprofen and glucosamine sulphate in the management of osteoarthrosis of the knee in out-patients. Curr Med Res Opin 8:145-59, 1982

Machtey I, Ouaknine, L. Tocopherol in osteoarthritis: A controlled pilot study. J Am Geriatr Soc 26:328-30, 1978

McAlindon TE et al. Do antioxidant micronutrients protect against the development and progression of knee osteoarthritis? Arthritis Rheum 39(4):648-56, 1996a

McAlindon T et al. Relation of dietary intake and serum levels of vitamin D to progression of osteoarthritis of the knee among participants in the Framingham study. Ann Intern Med 125(5):353-9, 1996b

McIlwain H et al. Intra-articular orgotein in osteoarthritis of the knee: a placebo-controlled efficacy, safety, and dosage comparison. Am J Med 87(3):295-300, 1989

Morreale P et al. Comparison of the antiinflammatory efficacy of chondroitin sulfate and diclofenac sodium in patients with knee osteoarthritis. J Rheumatol 23(8):1385-91, 1996

Moses MA et al. Identification of an inhibitor of neovascularization from cartilage. Science 248:1408-10, 1990

Moss M. Effects of molybdenum on pain and general health: a pilot study. J Nutr Environ Med 5:55-61, 1995

Muller-Fassbender H et al. Glucosamine sulfate compared to ibuprofen in osteoarthritis of the knee. Osteoarthritis Cartilage 2:61-9, 1994

Nelson MN et al. Proc Soc Exp Biol 73:31, 1950

Newnham RE. Boron beats arthritis. Proc ANZAAS, Australian Academy of Science, Canberra, 1979

Newnham RE. Agricultural practices affect arthritis. Nutr Health 7:49-53, 1994a

Newnham RE. Essentiality of boron for healthy bones and joints. Environ Health Perspect 102 Suppl 7:83-5, 1994b

Newnham RE. The role of boron in human nutrition. J Appl Nutr 46(3):81-5, 1994c

Nielsen FH. Boron - An overlooked element of potential nutritional importance. Nutr Today 23(1):4-7, 1988

Noack W et al. Glucosamine sulfate in osteoarthritis of the knee. Osteoarthritis Cartilage 2:51-9, 1994

Orcasita JA - reported in Walker M. Therapeutic effects of shark cartilage. Townsend Letter for Doctors June, 1989:288-91

Ordonez L, Rothschild PR. Absorption study with SOD/CAT[R] whole food antioxidant enzyme complex. Biotec Food Corporation, 1215 Center St., Honolulu, HI 96816-3226, 1989

Osterberg AE et al. Absorption of sulphur compounds during treatment by sulphur baths. Arch Derm Syph 20:156-66, 1929

Parkhomets VP, Donchenko GV. [Arachidonic acid metabolism and vitamin E]. Ukr Biokhim Zh 64(6):3-11, 1992 (in Russian)

Qiu GX et al. Efficacy and safety of glucosamine sulfate versus ibuprofen in patients with knee osteoarthritis. Arzneimittelforschung 48(5):469-74, 1998

Rajagopalan KV. Molybdenum: an essential trace element in human nutrition. Ann Rev Nutr 8:401-27, 1988

Randall D et al. Effect of oral Dismutase[R] enzyme supplementation upon musculo-skeletal inflammation. Biotec Food Corporation, 1215 Center St., Honolulu, HI 96816-3226, 1989

Rauis J - reported in Walker M. Therapeutic effects of shark cartilage. Townsend Letter for Doctors June, 1989:288-91

Rejholec V. Long-term studies of antiosteoarthritic drugs: an assessment. Semin Arthritis Rheum 17(Suppl 1):35-53, 1987

Rizzo R et al. Calcium, sulfur, and zinc distribution in normal and arthritic articular equine cartilage: a synchrotron radiation-induced X-ray emission (SRIXE) study. J Exp Zool 273(1):82-6, 1995

Rosenberg MR et al. Effect of hydrocortisone and nicotinamide on gamma glutamyltransferase in primary cultures of rat hepatocytes. In Vitro 18(9):775-82, 1982

Rothschild PR et al. Effect of oral antioxidant enzyme supplementation upon musculo-skeletal inflammation. Biotec Food Corporation, 1215 Center St., Honolulu, HI 96816-3226, 1989

Rovati LC et al. A large, randomized, placebo-controlled, double-blind study of glucosamine sulfate vs. piroxicam and vs. their association, on the kinetics of the symptomatic effect in knee osteoarthritis. Osteoarthritis Cartilage 2(Suppl 1):56, 1994

Scherak O et al. [High dosage vitamin E therapy in patients with activated arthrosis]. Z Rheumatol 49(6):369-73, 1990 (in German).

Schwartz ER. The modulation of osteoarthritic development by vitamins C and E. Int J Vit Nutr Res Suppl 26:141-46, 1984

Sculti L. Arthritis benefits from shark cartilage therapy. Alt Comp Therap, Oct. 1994:35-7

Shneider AB. [Stereometric evaluation of the myocardial cardiomyocyte-capillary ratio of thiamine and nicotinamide.] Kardiologiia 29(4):97-9, 1989 (in Russian)

Sullivan MX, Hess WC. Cystine content of fingernails in arthritis. J Bone Joint Surg 16:185, 1935

Sumii H et al. Superoxide dismutase activity in arthropathy: its role and measurement in the joints. Hiroshima J Med Sci 45(2):51-5, 1996

Tapadinhas MJ et al. Oral glucosamine sulphate in the management of arthrosis: report on a multi-centre open investgation in Portugal. Pharmatherapeutica 3(3):157-68, 1982

Travers RL et al. Boron and arthritis: the results of a double-blind pilot study. J Nutr Med 1:127-32, 1990

Verbruggen G et al. Chondroitin sulfate: S/DMOAD (structure/disease modifying anti-osteoarthritis drug) in the treatment of finger joint OA. Osteoarthritis Cartilage 6 Suppl A:37-8, 1998

Vidal y Plana RR et al. Articular cartilage pharmacology: I. In vitro studies on glucosamine and non-steroidal anti-inflammatory drugs. Pharmacol Res Commun 10(6):557-69, 1978

White G. Vitamin E inhibition of platelet prostaglandin biosynthesis. Fed Proc 36:350, 1977

White-O'Connor B, Sobal J. Nutrient intake and obesity in a multidisciplinary assessment of osteoarthritis. Clin Ther 9 Suppl B:30-42, 1986

Woldenberg SC. The treatment of arthritis with colloidal sulfur. J South Med Assoc 28:875-81, 1935

Wright JV. A case of food-induced arthritis. Prevention October, 1979, pp. 55-9

Wright JV. Degenerative arthritis. Nutrition & Healing 1(2), September, 1994

Yamada K et al. Endogenous tumor necrosis factor-alpha production by a pancreatic beta-cell line: inhibitory effects of hydrocortisone and nicotinamide. Life Sci 59(17):1423-9, 1996

OSTEOPOROSIS
(including OSTEOMALACIA)

See Also: KIDNEY STONES

NUTRITIONAL TREATMENT GUIDE

✓ = Efficacy generally accepted.
* = Efficacy *demonstrated* by controlled human trials.
[+] = Efficacy *suspected* from uncontrolled human experiments
[-] = Efficacy *suspected* from indirect data
? = Efficacy *challenged* in at least one study of similar design

---

DIETARY FACTORS

* drink **Milk** regularly (or consume adequate calcium from other sources)
* avoid excessive **Phosphorus**
* avoid excessive **Protein**
* consume **Soybeans**

- -

[+] moderate (*NOT* excessive) **Alcohol** consumption
[+] ? avoid **Caffeine** (especially if calcium consumption is low)
[+] ? minimize **Salt** intake

- -

[-] **Alkaline Ash diet**
[-] consume **Olive Oil**
[-] **High Potassium diet**
[-] restrict **Saturated Fat**
[-] minimize **Sugar** intake
[-] **Vegetarian diet**
[-] consume **Fruit**

NUTRIENTS

I. *To Prevent or Reverse Osteoporosis*

* **Copper deficiency:** 2 mg twice daily for up to 6 weeks *AND* **Zinc** 50 mg daily
* **Magnesium deficiency:** ≈ 400 mg daily
* **Omega-3 fatty acids:** *example:* MaxEPA 1 g caps [180 mg EPA; 120 mg DHA] 10 to 20 daily *AND* **Omega-6 fatty acids:** *example:* evening primrose oil 500 mg caps [7-10% GLA] 6 to 8 daily
* **Vitamin D deficiency:** 800 IU daily including dietary sources
* **Vitamin K deficiency:** phylloquinone 5 mg daily *OR* phytonadione 10 mg IM as needed
* ? **Calcium deficiency:** ≈ 1 g daily (may be more effective when combined with vitamin D)
* ? **Fluoride:** sodium fluoride 25 to 40 mg twice daily (in selected cases)

- -

- -

[-] **Boron deficiency:** 3 mg daily *OR* a diet rich in fruits and vegetables
[-] **Manganese deficiency**: 3 to 5 mg daily
[-] **Vitamin B_6 deficiency:** 50 to 100 mg daily
[-] **Vitamin B_{12} deficiency:** 1,000 μg intramuscularly weekly initially and monthly afterwards
[-] **Vitamin C deficiency:** 500 mg twice daily
[-] **Zinc deficiency:** zinc sulfate 220 mg twice daily *AND* **Copper** 2 mg daily

II. *To Reduce Fracture Risk*

* **Vitamin D deficiency:** 800 IU daily including dietary sources
* **Vitamin K deficiency:** phylloquinone 5 mg daily *OR* phytonadione 10 mg IM as needed
* ? **Calcium deficiency:** ≈ 1 g daily (may be more effective when combined with vitamin D)

- -

[+] **Coenzyme Q_{10}:** 30 to 90 mg daily

- -

[-] **Vitamin B_6 deficiency:** 50 to 100 mg daily
[-] avoid **Vitamin C** supplements in the form of ascorbic acid

III. *To Reduce Calcium Loss*

* **Boron deficiency:** 3 mg daily *OR* a diet rich in fruits and vegetables
* **Potassium bicarbonate:** 60 to 120 mmol daily

- -

[+] **L-Lysine deficiency:** 400 mg daily
[+] **Vitamin D deficiency:** 800 IU daily including dietary sources
[+] **Vitamin K deficiency:** phylloquinone 5 mg daily *OR* phytonadione 10 mg IM as needed

OTHER RELATED FACTORS

[+] rule out **Aluminum toxicity** (inhibits bone mineralization)
[+] rule out **Lactose Intolerance** (may cause patients to fail to ingest adequate calcium)
[+] ? rule out **Hydrochloric Acid deficiency** (decreases calcium absorption)

DIETARY FACTORS

Alkaline Ash Diet

The acidity of the ash resulting from the diet has a substantial affect on bone density. High in animal protein and low in fruits and vegetables, the average Western diet generates a large amount of acid, mainly as sulfates and phosphates. The kidney responds to this acid challenge with a net excretion of acid, as well as by excretion of ammonium and titratable acid, while the skeleton supplies buffer by actively resorbing bone which increases calcium excretion *(Barzel;Hu)*.

Different food proteins differ greatly in their potential acid load, and therefore in their acidogenic effect. Meat and other high-protein animal foods, as well as most cereal grains and other starches, produce an acid ash. Fruits (except for cranberries and plums), vegetables (except for corn and lentils) and dairy products (except for cheese) produce an alkaline ash. Generally, vegetarian diets are more alkaline than omnivore diets, and vegan diets are more alkaline than lacto-ovo-vegetarian diets *(Dwyer)*.

ALKALINE ASH-FORMING FOODS

Milk
certain Nuts (almonds, chestnuts, coconut)
Vegetables (except corn and lentils)
Fruits (except cranberries and plums)
Molasses

ACID ASH-FORMING FOODS

Meat (including fish, poultry, shellfish and eggs)
Grains (including wheat, corn, rye, barley, rice)
Buckwheat
Lentils
Cranberries
Plums (and prunes)
Sugar (refined)
Cheese

The addition of exogenous alkali buffers (whether as chemical salts or as high-potassium fruits and vegetables) to a diet rich in animal protein results in a less acid urine, a reduction in net acid excretion, reduced ammonium and titratable acid excretion, and decreased calciuria. Bone resorption may be halted, and bone accretion may actually occur. *(Barzel).*

Potassium bicarbonate is a specific salt which neutralizes endogenous acid. At a dosage sufficient to do so, it not only improves calcium and phosphorus balance, but reduces bone resorption and increases the rate of bone formation *(Green;Sebastian).*

Protein

Protein intake should be moderate. Dietary protein appears to be a determinate of peak bone mass in women *(Cooper).* Moreover, following a bone fracture, a controlled study found that protein supplementation significantly improved the clinical course *(Tkatch).*

Excessive protein intake, however, tends to promote osteoporosis. Dietary protein intake is directly correlated with calcium loss *(Blank)* as well as with the risk of bone fracture *(Meyer).*

Saturated Fats

Saturated fatty acids, by forming calcium soaps *(Weiser),* may decrease calcium absorption *(Wohl).* The adverse effects of a high saturated fat diet on adult cancellous (but not cortical) bone has been confirmed in an animal study *(Wohl),* and growing animals have shown similar findings *(Wohl).*

However, when bone mineral density (BMD) of healthy children and adolescents was related to diet, BMD in the distal (but not ultradistal) forearm was *positively* related to saturated fat intake, suggesting that restriction of saturated fat intake in children and adolescents for the purpose of protecting against osteoporosis may not be warranted *(Gunnes).*

Further studies are needed to confirm or repudiate this isolated finding before any conclusions can be reached.

Sugar

Sucrose ingestion has been shown to induce hypercalciuria in experimental subjects, probably due to the effects of insulin secretion *(Holl).* Moreover, a high sucrose diet has been shown to decrease the mechanical strength of bones in growing rats *(Tjaderhane).*

The finding that, for a group of young women, trabecular bone density was inversely related to dietary carbohydrate independently of sex steroid hormones *(Leuenberger)* could well be due to dietary sugar. In fact, when healthy men and women between the ages of 25 and 69 were interviewed, carbohydrate intake was also inversely related to bone mineral density - however, upon further analysis, the association was significant only with respect to the intake of mono- and disaccharides *(Trichopoulou).*

AND Fat

Animal studies have found that short-term exposure to a diet high in both sucrose and fat can induce hyperinsulinemia, affect calcium and magnesium metabolism, and adversely alter bone mineralization and mechanical properties *(Li;Zernicke).* More recently, rats were randomly assigned to a long-term high-fat, high-sucrose diet or to a low-fat, complex-carbohydrate diet. After 2 years, bone morphology, bone mineral content, and the mechanical properties of bone were all altered adversely *(Zernicke).*

Meat

Animal, but not vegetable, protein intake appears to be associated with an increased risk of bone fractures *(Abelow;Feskanich).* A similar relationship may exist for the intake of red meat *(Feskanich).*

Although some studies have found that older lacto-ovo-vegetarian women have greater bone mineral density than omnivorous women *(Marsh;Sanchez)*, others have failed to find such an association *(Lloyd;Tesar)*. Moreover, a recent study of Chinese women found *lower* hip bone mineral density in elderly vegetarians than in omnivores *(Lau)*; thus the effect of meat-eating on bone mineral density is uncertain.

One of the possible advantages to avoiding meat is due to its high phosphorus content. (See Calcium to Phosphorus Ratio below.) In a study of men on a high meat diet, long-term calcium and phosphorus balances were 4 mg and 184 mg, respectively, while for men on a control diet, balances were -15 mg and 12 mg. The difference was not significant for calcium, but was for phosphorus *(Spencer,1983)*.

Olive Oil

In contrast to the effects of saturated fatty acids, the intake of olive oil, which is a major source of the monounsaturate oleic acid, appears to be positively associated with bone mineral density *(Trichopoulou)*. More studies are needed to confirm this relationship and to establish whether olive oil intake affects bone mineral density and susceptibility to osteoporosis.

Dietary Fiber

The relationship between dietary fiber intake and bone mineral density is uncertain. A positive association has been found between fiber intake and bone mineral density in the lumbar spine in premenopausal women *(New)*, and between fiber intake and bone mineral density in the ultradistal forearm in children and adolescents *(Gunnes)*.

However, in a group of young women, trabecular bone density was *inversely* related to dietary fiber intake *(Leuenberger)*. There is also evidence that, in women, fiber intake is inversely associated with both the blood level of 17-beta-estradiol *(Feng)* and the serum level of androgens *(Leuenberger)*. These hormonal changes would be expected to decrease bone mineral density and thus increase the risk of osteoporosis. Thus, it is premature to make any recommendations concerning dietary fiber in regard to preventing or treatment osteoporosis.

Salt (sodium chloride)

Increased dietary sodium increases urinary calcium and decreases serum calcium, causing an increase in parathyroid hormone. Parathyroid hormone, in turn, increases calcium absorption and renal calcium resorption, and bone resorption *(Evans)*. In fact, salt is believed to be a more important determinant of urinary calcium excretion than calcium intake within the usual ranges of salt and calcium intake *(Antonios)*. For each 100 mmol of sodium excreted, there is approximately 1 mmol loss of urinary calcium; thus those individuals consuming 2,000 mg sodium chloride daily need to replace 1,000 mg of excreted calcium *(Massey)*.

Patients with hypertension are especially sensitive to the deleterious effect of sodium on bone. They have a higher urinary calcium excretion for a given urinary sodium excretion, as well as a tendency for lower ionized calcium and higher parathyroid hormone and 1,25-dihydroxy-vitamin D concentrations *(MacGregor)*.

High Potassium Diet

(Also see Potassium below.)

While dietary sodium increases urinary calcium excretion, dietary potassium reduces it *(Siani)*. Moreover, in a study of 994 healthy premenopausal women, higher potassium intakes were associated with higher lumbar spine bone mineral densities *(New)*.

Alcohol

Ethanol contains a meaningful amount of phytoestrogens (*Rosenblum)* and can aromatize androgens, converting them into estrogens (*Gavaler)*; thus moderate alcohol consumption (3-6 drinks per week) has been theorized to reduce the risk of postmenopausal osteoporosis by increasing serum estradiol levels *(Gavaler)*. Support for this hypothesis can be found in two recent epidemiologic studies *(Felson;Holbrook)*.

Alcohol abuse, however, is believed to be an important risk factor for fractures and osteoporosis, and has been shown to be associated with decreased bone mineral density *(Laitinen)*. Ethanol-associated osteopenia seems to be a direct effect of alcohol on bone cells and an indirect or modulating effect through mineral regulating hormones such as vitamin D metabolites, parathyroid hormone, and calcitonin *(Sampson)*.

Caffeine

Caffeine consumption increases urinary and fecal calcium loss *(Heaney,1982;Massey,1994)*. It is inversely correlated with bone density *(Hernandez-Avila)* and bone mineral content *(Harris)*, and may adversely affect calcium metabolism and the mobilization of bone calcium

(Massay,1994). Moreover, caffeine intake has been directly correlated with the risk of hip fractures *(Meyer;Tavani)*. These adverse effects are mainly relevant to low calcium consumers (*Barger-Lux;Massey,1994*).

Milk

Frequent milk consumption before age 25 has been associated with higher hip bone mineral density in middle-aged and elderly women, suggesting that it should be encouraged among children and young adults *(Murphy S)*. Moreover, in both men and women aged 30 to 69, those who drank at least one glass of milk daily had lower serum alkaline phosphatase activity, suggesting that milk has osteostatic effects in adults via a mechanism different from that of estrogens *(Yoshida)*.

However, a recent 12-year prospective study of 77,761 women who were initially between 34 and 59 years old, and who had never taken calcium supplements, found no evidence that a higher intake of milk or calcium from food reduced the risk of forearm or hip fractures. Even their history of milk consumption as teenagers was unrelated to the risk of adult fractures.

While these findings suggest that calcium from milk or other foods is less effective than calcium supplements, a 2-year placebo-controlled study of postmenopausal women which compared milk power and calcium tablets found that either form of calcium supplementation was equally effective in stopping bone loss *(Prince)*. Therefore, based on current knowledge, milk consumption should probably be encouraged.

Soybeans

Soybeans are essentially the unique dietary source of isoflavones. These substances have chemical structures similar to estrogen but with 1/1,000-1/10,000th of the estrogenic activity. They are also a rich source of potassium *(Siani)*.

Under double-blind conditions, they have been shown to increase bone mineral content and density in the lumbar spine *(Potter)*. This confirms the findings from animal studies which found that soy protein isoflavones prevent ovariectomy-induced bone loss *(Arjmandi)*.

Fruit

In a study of almost 1,000 premenopausal women, lumbar spine and femoral trochanter bone mineral densities were lower in women reporting a low intake of fruit in early adulthood than in women with a medium or high intake *(New)*.

HOMOCYSTEINE

In homocystinuria, the toxic amino acid homocysteine is believed to interfere with collagen cross-linking, leading to a defective bone matrix and osteoporosis *(Lubec)*. Osteoporosis is a common finding in homocystinuria, even among children *(Kaur)*.

However, among homocystinurics, the reduction in cross-links may fail to correlate with serum homocysteine levels. If this finding extends to the general population with mildly elevated serum homocysteine levels, it suggests that reduction of homocysteine in the latter group may fail to affect osteoporosis. (See Atherosclerosis for information on lowering serum homocysteine levels with nutrients.)

NUTRITIONAL FACTORS

VITAMINS

Vitamin B_6 Deficiency

Vitamin B_6 is co-factor in the production of intracellular putrescine which is a metabolic regulator of the vitamin K cycle. Vitamin K, in turn, is a primary factor involved in the binding of hydroxyapatite to bone matrix (see Vitamin K below) *(Reynolds)*.

In rats, vitamin B_6 deficiency has been shown to cause both osteoporosis *(Benke)* and abnormalities in the healing of bone fractures *(Dodds)*. When 30 elderly women with hip fractures following minimal trauma were compared to 21 control women admitted for elective arthroplasty, half of the women with fractures had below normal levels of serum pyridoxal-5'-phosphate compared to only 3 of the controls *(Reynolds)*.

Controlled clinical trials are needed to ascertain the efficacy of vitamin B_6 repletion.

Vitamin B_{12} Deficiency

Pernicious anemia, a manifestation of vitamin B_{12} deficiency, is well-recognized as a risk factor for osteoporosis and fractures *(Melton)*. Patients who are B_{12}-deficient tend to have reduced levels of blood skeletal alkaline phosphatase and osteocalcin, and the degree of megaloblastic anemia correlates with the reduction in skeletal alkaline phosphatase, suggesting that osteoblast activity depends upon cobalamin, and that bone metabolism is affected by cobalamin deficiency *(Carmel)*. Moreover, findings from an *in vitro* study suggest that a vitamin B_{12} deficiency may promote osteoporosis *(Kim)*.

As with vitamin B_6, controlled clinical trials are needed to ascertain the efficacy of vitamin B_{12} repletion.

Vitamin C Deficiency

Adequate amounts of vitamin C are necessary for the activity of lysine and proline hydroxylases, enzymes needed for collagen synthesis. While its role in bone cell differentiation and formation is less well characterized, there is evidence of a positive association of vitamin C intake with bone mineral density in postmenopausal women with dietary calcium intakes of at least 500 mg *(Hall)*.

A study of premenopausal women found a significant difference in lumbar spine bone mineral density between the lowest and higher quartiles for vitamin C intake *(New)*. While this finding was not confirmed in a study of postmenopausal women, the study did find evidence of a positive association between dietary vitamin C intake and femoral neck bone mineral density *(Wang)*. There is also evidence that, in adolescents (but not in children), bone mineral density in both the distal and ultradistal forearm may be predicted by vitamin C intake *(Gunnes)*.

Despite these positive correlations, ascorbic acid depletion does not appear to be closely associated with osteoporosis *(Banerjee;Bhammhani)*, although animal work does suggest that ascorbate deficiency, extending both during the period of rapid growth and the slower phases of skeletal maturation, may result in bone abnormalities *(Kipp)*.

A Warning

From an initial cohort of 65,000 women aged 40 to 75, there were 272 subsequent cases of hip fractures. A comparison with matched controls revealed an increased risk of fracture with high dietary intakes of vitamin C which was non-significant when calcium intake was low and more pronounced when calcium intake was high *(Michaelsson)*.

This worrisome finding confirms the results of an animal study in which young guinea pigs that were fed high dosages of vitamin C developed decreases in bone density *(Bray)*. The same study found, however, that non-acidic forms of vitamin C failed to have the same effect, suggesting that neutral forms of ascorbate may be safe.

Vitamin D Deficiency

Vitamin D is essential for the maintenance of a healthy skeleton. Without vitamin D, children develop rickets and adults exacerbate their osteoporosis and develop osteomalacia. 1,25-dihydroxyvitamin D3, the activated form, stimulates intestinal calcium absorption and mobilizes stem cells to mobilize calcium stores from bone *(Holick)*.

Patients with recent hip fractures usually have lower vitamin D and higher parathyroid hormone levels. Vitamin D deficiency in elderly subjects, through a secondary hyperparathyroidism, plays a significant role in decreasing bone density and increasing bone fragility and fracture risk *(Quesada-Gomez)*. Moreover, osteoporotic patients may have a deficit in converting vitamin D into its active form *(Rudman;Tsai)*, possibly due to hepatic or renal disease, or to hypoparathyroidism, leading to depressed fractional calcium absorption, especially at low calcium intakes, causing a negative calcium balance *(Pak)*.

Supplementation

Vitamin D supplementation in the elderly has been shown to rapidly improve vitamin D status, increase serum calcitriol levels *(Quesada-Gomez)*. It also normalizes calcium absorption *(Riggs,1985)* and prevents secondary hyperparathyroidism and bone loss *(Lips)*. Moreover, regular exposure to sunlight, or the use of full spectrum lighting, will safely promote vitamin D synthesis. Supplementation specifically with active vitamin D is indicated for patients who are unable to convert the vitamin sufficiently into its active form *(Kawakami)*.

However, vitamin D intoxication from over-supplementation is not uncommon. Intoxication is marked by hypercalciuria and encourages bone resorption *(Adams)*. As the optimal supplemental dosage that promotes calcium absorption without causing bone resorption has yet to be established *(Eufemio,1990)*, pharmacologic doses are not generally recommended.

Vitamin K Deficiency

Vitamin K plays a substantial role in calcification *(Hauschka)* and its intake influences bone mineral density and calcium excretion *(Binkley)*. Compared to normals, osteoporosis patients may have reduced plasma vitamin K levels *(Hart)*. A deficiency of the vitamin is associated with increased urinary calcium losses *(Robert)* and bone fractures *(Hodges)*.

When supplemented with vitamin K, urinary calcium losses can be reduced in patients by up to 50% *(Jie;Tomita)* and bone density may increase *(Orimo)*. In a controlled study, vitamin K_2 was effective in reducing further vertebral fractures in a group of osteoporotic patients *(Shiraki)*. Moreover, fractures in rabbits healed faster when rabbits were supplemented with vitamin K even though they were an a diet which was considered to contain adequate levels of the vitamin *(Bouckaert)*.

MINERALS

Boron Deficiency

Boron is a trace element whose potential importance in osteoporosis is just becoming recognized. While meat and fish are poor sources, foods of plant origin, especially fruits, vegetables and nuts, are rich sources of the mineral.

The role of boron in bone metabolism is most likely to be due to its interactions with other nutrients such as calcium, magnesium, phosphorus and vitamin D *(McCoy;Meacham;Volpe)* as well as its effects on sex hormones. For example, in a group of postmenopausal women, compared to a low-boron baseline diet, the addition of a boron supplement reduced total plasma calcium concentrations and the urinary excretions of calcium and magnesium. Moreover, it elevated the serum concentrations of 17-beta-estradiol and testosterone *(Nielsen,1994)*. Since estrogen administration has been shown to be effective in slowing calcium loss from bone in postmenopausal women, and estradiol-17-beta is the most biologically active form of estrogen, this finding may be of particular importance.

Because boron deprivation (much like magnesium deprivation) causes changes similar to those seen in women with postmenopausal osteoporosis, this element is apparently needed for optimal calcium metabolism and to prevent the excessive bone loss which often occurs in postmenopausal women and older men *(Nielsen,1990)*. Long-term controlled clinical trials are needed to ascertain when boron supplementation may be indicated.

Calcium Deficiency

Since 99% of the body's calcium is in the bones, the relationship between calcium metabolism and bone density has been extensively studied. Calcium deficiency is a primary contributor to the high incidence of osteoporosis *(Heaney,1992;Nordin)*.

A high calcium intake during childhood and adolescence clearly helps to maximize peak bone mineral density and thus reduces osteoporosis risk *(Cadogan;Kerstetter)*, although there is some controversy over the efficacy of calcium supplementation following menopause. One reason may be that calcium supplementation appears more effective in preventing loss of *cortical* bone (as measured, for example, in a phalanx) than in preventing loss of *trabecular* bone (for example, in the vertebrae) where most osteoporotic fractures occur *(Trachtenbarg)*. Also, calcium supplements are not always well absorbed, particularly by older people who are more likely to be hypochlorhydric

However, there is a growing body of controlled trials showing a benefit from calcium with or without vitamin D which strongly suggests that some of the age-related bone loss in elderly women could be prevented by higher intake of both nutrients *(Heaney,1993)*. Furthermore, numerous trials have found that substantially greater increases in bone mass occur when osteoporotic women add calcium to estrogen or calcitonin as part of their antiresorptive regimen *(Kilgore)*. This may because patients, under conditions of calcium deficiency, are unable to adequately increase calcitriol production in order to enhance calcium absorption *(Prince)*.

By contrast, the results of double-blind studies suggest that calcium supplementation fails to prevent bone loss during lactation and only slightly enhances the gain in bone density after weaning *(Prentice)*.

The question of whether older men should ingest calcium supplements is yet another area of controversy. In normal older men, calcium administration suppresses biological markers of bone resorption for at least 6 hours *(Horowitz)*. However, a recent study failed to find a relation between calcium intake in older men and the incidence of forearm or hip fractures *(Owusu)*.

Osteoporosis is a well-recognized complication of the prolonged use of corticosteroid medications. In an open trial, patients on a median dosage of 15 mg prednisone daily took a nightly calcium supplement. When measured 2 months later, the urinary hydroxyproline to creatinine ratio, an index of bone resorption, had significantly decreased, suggesting the supplement may help to prevent steroid-associated osteoporosis *(Reid)*.

Copper Deficiency

Several enzymes involved in collagen synthesis require copper, a trace element that is necessary in bone metabolism *(Saltman)*. The results of animal studies suggest that a mild dietary copper deficiency may enhance bone resorption and lead to reduced bone mineral density and bone strength *(Andon;Smith)*.

In human studies, copper levels of osteoporotic patients were lower in serum *(Conlan)*, bone and hair *(Okono)*. Furthermore, in postmenopausal women, serum copper levels have been found to be directly associated with bone mass density *(Strause)*.

While there has been relatively little research exploring the efficacy of copper supplementation, one study provided 73 healthy women between the ages of 45 and 56 with a copper supplement or a placebo. Two years later, the 32 women who took the placebo had a significantly lower vertebral bone mineral density of the lumbar spine (L2-4), while the vertebral bone mineral density for the 24 women who took the copper supplement was not significantly different *(Eaton-Evans)*.

Fluoride

The concentration of fluoride in drinking water has been found to be inversely related to bone mineral density *(Phipps)* and the risk of osteoporotic hip fractures *(Lehmann)*. However, some studies have found evidence of a weak *positive* correlation between fluoridated drinking water and hip fracture risk *(Hillier)*, while high levels of fluoride in drinking water have been found to be associated with reduced radial bone mass *(Raheb)*.

Similarly, the results of clinical studies of fluoride supplementation have been mixed. Sodium fluoride appears to be one of the most potent agents for increasing trabecular bone density *(Eufemio,1989)*. Supplementation increases the rate of bone formation, the number of osteoblasts, and the level of skeletal alkaline phosphatase *(Anonymous)*. However, it decreases cortical bone, increases skeletal fragility *(Riggs,1990)*, and impairs osteoblast activity *(Balena)*. It also used to frequently produce worrisome gastrointestinal side effects including damage to the gastric mucosa *(Spak)*, although the availability of enteric-coated sodium fluoride has eliminated this problem *(Murray TM)*.

Because of the complexity of its effects, the advisability of sodium fluoride treatment remains uncertain and its use should be limited to selected cases. A recent review makes the following suggestions:

1. Do not prescribe sodium fluoride without calcium supplementation in order to avoid bone loss at the appendicular skeleton.
2. For the same reason, do not prescribe a supra-physiological dosage of vitamin D concurrently.
3. To avoid a calcium shift from cortical to trabecular bone and osteomalacia, keep the dosages small.
4. Avoid sodium fluoride in renal insufficiency *(Devogelaer)*.

Magnesium Deficiency

Magnesium, whose intake correlates with bone mineral density *(Argus)*, has a number of functions which may explain this relationship. It is required for the activation of alkaline phosphatase, an enzyme involved in forming calcium crystals in bone and in converting vitamin D into its active form. It also promotes and regulates parathormone which, in turn, stimulates osteoclasts to resorb calcified bone.

Magnesium intake has been repeatedly correlated with bone mineral density *(New;Tranquilli)*. In fact, in a study of women aged 23 to 75, magnesium intake was a significant predictor of forearm bone mineral content *(Angus)*. Among patients with osteoporosis, magnesium deficiency is common and bone magnesium content may be below normal *(Cohen;Seelig)*.

Supplementation

While bone density normally decreases about one percent a year after menopause, almost three-quarters of 31 women who took 250 to 750 mg daily of magnesium for 2 years showed bone density increases of 1 to 8 percent. Bone density remained unchanged in most of the rest of the subjects, and 17 women who refused supplements experienced bone density losses of between 1 and 3 percent *(Stendig-Lindberg)*.

For patients prone to osteoporosis due to gluten-sensitive enteropathy, magnesium supplementation has been shown to significantly increase bone mineral density *(Rude)*. Furthermore, magnesium supplements may reduce the adverse side effects of sodium fluoride treatment *(Muenzenberg)*.

Manganese Deficiency

Manganese, necessary for bone metabolism *(Saltman)*, is another mineral whose nutriture is decreased in osteoporosis. Serum manganese levels may be greatly reduced in osteoporotic women *(Reginster)*. Moreover, when young men were fed manganese-deficient diets, serum calcium, phosphate, and alkaline phosphatase concentrations increased significantly, consistent with the hypothesis that manganese deficiency may affect bone remodeling *(Friedman)*.

Animal studies have provided further evidence that manganese deficiency may contribute to osteoporosis. Rats fed a manganese-deficient diet had smaller, less dense bones with less resistance to fractures than controls *(Amdur)*. Moreover, bone mineral density in the femoral shaft was significantly lower than that of the controls *(Andon)*.

The effects of repleting a manganese deficiency have yet to be reported.

Phosphorus and the Calcium to Phosphorus Ratio: A Warning

Although high phosphorus intakes, by reducing urinary calcium excretion, may increase calcium retention *(Hegsted;Spencer,1978)*, epidemiologic data suggests that women at high risk of developing osteoporosis typically follow a high phosphorus, low calcium diet - especially with the growing use of phosphorus-containing food additives. Such a diet appears to cause a mild secondary hyperparathyroidism and may eventually impair the usual homeostatic mechanisms that operate when dietary calcium intake is marginal in order to protect bone *(Calvo)*.

In animal models, a high phosphorus, low calcium diet produces a significant reduction in vertebral bone mass *(Calvo)*. Moreover, when 7 patients were supplemented with phosphorus, examination of bone biopsies showed a decrease in bone-forming surface and an increase in bone surface involved in resorption *(Goldsmith)*.

The ideal dietary ratio of calcium to phosphorus is estimated to be 1 to 1, while the typical Western diet yields a ratio of between 1 to 2 and 1 to 4. In fact, data from animal studies suggest that calcium to phosphorus ratios of less than 1 to 2 enhance bone resorption regardless of calcium intake *(Worthington-Roberts)*, while the results of a controlled study of women aged 43 to 65 suggest that the treatment of osteoporosis may be fruitless so long as dietary calcium to phosphorus ratios are less than 1 to 1.25 *(Albanese)*.

Potassium

(Also see Alkaline Ash Diet above.)

Compared to a baseline diet, while supplementation with sodium chloride increases urinary calcium excretion, supplementing with potassium chloride does not do so *(Bell)*. Moreover, dietary potassium promotes calcium retention, and thus may protect bone from osteoporotic changes *(Lemann)*.

Sodium

See Salt above.

Strontium

In an animal study, low doses of strontium increased the number of bone forming sites and vertebral bone volume, but did not have detectable adverse effects on the mineral profile, bone mineral chemistry or bone matrix mineralization *(Grynpas)*. This confirmed the results of an earlier study which found that small doses of oral strontium stimulated bone formation without altering bone resorption *(Marie)*.

In a long-term human trial, following 3 months to 3 years of supplementation, 84% of 32 patients (10 of whom also received estrogen and testosterone) experienced marked reduction of bone pain. X-rays showed possible improvement in 78% *(McCaslin)*.

However, because of the interaction between strontium and vitamin D, high doses of the vitamin are needed during strontium supplementation in order to avoid a reduction in calcium absorption *(Rousselet)*. Controlled clinical trials are needed to ascertain whether strontium supplementation should be part of osteoporosis treatment.

A 34-year-old woman had experienced aching in the lower back since delivery of a child 5 years earlier. The diagnosis of osteoporosis was made, and for 3 years prior to admission she had been treated with hormones and wore a back brace, but without improvement. Examination showed stiffness of the spinal column with limitation of movement, grade 4; and x-rays revealed generalized osteoporosis with compression of the second lumbar vertebrae.

She was started on treatment with strontium lactate and showed steady improvement. Three years later she was free of pain. X-rays of the vertebrae made before and after treatment provided objective confirmation of her dramatic improvement (McCaslin).

Zinc

Zinc is essential for normal bone formation *(Saltman)*, and its intake has been directly correlated with bone mineral density, at least in premenopausal women *(New)*.

Both serum and bone zinc levels may be depressed in elderly osteoporotic patients *(Atik)*. In addition, urinary zinc excretion may be elevated, but probably due to bone resorption rather than inadequate intake or zinc depletion *(Relea)*. In fact, urinary zinc excretion has been proposed as a simple marker of bone resorption *(Szathmari)*.

Results of a study on weanling rats suggest that the effect of vitamin D3 on bone metabolism is enhanced by orally administered zinc sulfate *(Yamaguchi)*. However, clinical studies of efficacy of zinc supplementation have yet to be reported.

OTHER NUTRITIONAL FACTORS

Coenzyme Q_{10} (ubiquinone)

While little research has been conducted on the efficacy of coenzyme Q_{10} in osteoporosis, a preliminary study of 5 patients reported such excellent results that the authors proposed that it may be an effective treatment option *(Neri Stagnaro)*.

Essential Fatty Acids

Animals made deficient in the essential fatty acids develop severe osteoporosis coupled with increased renal and arterial calcification. This is similar to osteoporosis in elderly patients, where the loss of bone calcium is associated with ectopic calcification of other tissues.

Essential fatty acids increase calcium absorption from the gut (in part by enhancing the effects of vitamin D), reduce urinary excretion of calcium, increase calcium deposition in bone, and improve bone strength and enhance the synthesis of bone collagen, while reducing ectopic calcification *(Kruger,1997)*.

When rats were supplemented with diets containing 8% of either fish oil (high in the omega-3 fatty acids DHA & EPA), evening primrose oil (high in omega-6 fatty acids, especially GLA), or sunflower oil (high in omega-6 fatty acids), only those fed fish oil had increased calcium absorption which resulted in an improvement in calcium balance *(Kruger,1995)*. This findings suggests that the omega-3 fatty acids are superior to the fatty acids of the omega-6 family.

Two double-blind studies, both of elderly osteoporotic women, have explored supplementation with both families of essential fatty acids. In one, patients received fish oil, evening primrose oil, both oils together, or olive oil placebo. After 16 weeks, alkaline phosphatase decreased in the fish oil and combination groups, suggesting an increase in bone mineral density, while osteocalcin, an indicator of bone formation activity, rose in the fish oil group and more significantly in the combination group. These findings confirm the superior efficacy of the omega-3 fatty acids and further suggest that the omega-6 fatty acids potentiate their effect *(van Papendorp)*.

In the other double-blind study, all patients were supplemented with calcium and randomly received either a combination of EPA (omega-3 family), GLA (omega-6 family) or placebo. After 18 months, bone density of the lumbar spine declined and that of the hip was unchanged in the placebo group while, in the supplemented group, bone density increased at both sites. Moreover, the calculated risk of hip fracture was significantly lower in the supplemented group than in the placebo group *(Kruger,1996)*.

L-Lysine Deficiency

Bone matrix, necessary for bone development, contains hydroxylysine which is apparently essential for bone mineralization. This amino acid must be synthesized *de novo* in the body from dietary lysine *(Heather)*.

As supplementation with L-lysine can both enhance intestinal calcium absorption and improve renal conservation of absorbed calcium, it may be of value in preventing and treating osteoporosis *(Civitelli)*. However, if dietary intake is adequate, it is possible that supplementation will provide no extra benefit *(Flodin;Spencer,1963)*. Controlled clinical trials would help to clarify its efficacy.

OTHER RELATED FACTORS

Hydrochloric Acid Deficiency

A deficiency of hydrochloric acid impairs calcium absorption *(Recker)* and should thus be repleted with proper supplementation.

Lactose Intolerance

Several studies have found an increased frequency of lactose maldigestion in patients with osteoporosis. However, a connection between lactose maldigestion and decreased absorption of calcium has not been shown. Instead, the increased tendency toward osteoporosis appears to be caused by a lower calcium intake because of milk intolerance *(Corazza;Gudmand-Hoyer;Larouche)*.

Aluminum Toxicity

Aluminum inhibits bone mineralization; the greater the aluminum exposure, the higher the risk of an early fracture *(Mjoberg)*. Even small amounts, such as in aluminum-containing antacids, bind inorganic phosphorus in the intestines resulting in phosphorus depletion which, in turn, increases fecal calcium excretion, causing a negative calcium balance. Fecal fluoride is also significantly increased, thus decreasing the intestinal absorption of fluoride *(Spencer,1985)*.

Calcium supplementation may be highly effective in reversing the effects of aluminum-induced metabolic bone disease:

A man received long-term home parenteral nutrition following extensive small bowel resection after mesenteric vein thrombosis. He developed bone disease caused by aluminum intoxication which had components of osteomalacia and low-turnover osteoporosis. Aluminum was detected at the surface of mineralized bone and was elevated in the serum, resulting in a positive deferoxamine infusion test.

One year of treatment with high doses of calcium (up to 24 mEq per day) significantly diminished his bone pain, increased the serum levels of calcium, abolished aluminum deposits in the mineralized trabecula, improved bone formation, and increased trabecular bone volume (Lidor).

BIBLIOGRAPHY

Abelow BJ et al. Cross-cultural association between dietary animal protein and hip fracture: a hypothesis. Calcif Tissue Int 50(1):14-8, 1992

Adams JS, Lee G. Gains in bone mineral density with resolution of vitamin D intoxication. Ann Intern Med 127(3):203-6, 1997

Albanese AA et al. Effects of dietary calcium:phosphorus ratios on utilization of dietary calcium for bone synthesis in women 20-75 years of age. Nutr Rep Int 33(6):879-91, 1986

Amdur MO et al. The need for manganese in bone development by the rat. Proc Soc Exp Biol Med 59:254-5, 1945

Andon M et al. Effects of dietary copper and manganese restriction on serum mineral concentrations and femoral shaft bone density in rats. J Am Coll Nutr 11:600, 1992

Angus RM et al. Dietary intake and bone mineral density. Bone Mineral 4(3):265-78, 1988

Anonymous. Editorial: Fluoride and the treatment of osteoporosis. Lancet i:547, 1984

Antonios TFT, MacGregor GA. Salt - more adverse effects. Essay. Lancet 348:250-1, 1996

Arjmandi BH et al. Bone-sparing effect of soy protein in ovarian hormone-deficient rats is related to its isoflavone content. Am J Clin Nutr 68(6 Suppl):1364S-1368S, 1998

Atik OS. Zinc and senile osteoporosis. J Am Geriatr Soc 31:790-1, 1983

Balena R et al. Effects of different regimens of sodium fluoride treatment for osteoporosis on the structure, remodeling and mineralization of bone. Osteoporosis Int 8(5):428-35, 1998

Banerjee AK et al. Vitamin C and osteoporosis in old age. Age Ageing 7(1):16-18, 1978

Barger-Lux MJ et al. Effects of moderate caffeine intake on the calcium economy of premenopausal women. Am J Clin Nutr 52:722-5, 1990

Barzel US, Massey LK. Excess dietary protein can adversely affect bone. J Nutr 128(6):1051-3, 1998

Bell R et al. The influence of NaCL and KCl on urinary calcium excretion in healthy young women. Nutr Res 12:17-26, 1992

Benke PH et al. Osteoporotic bone disease in the pyridoxine-deficient rat. Biochem Med 6:526-35, 1972

Bhammhani MM et al. Plasma ascorbic acid concentrations in osteoporotic outpatients. Br J Rheumatol 31(2):142-3, 1992

Binkley N, Suttie J. Vitamin K nutrition and osteoporosis. J Nutr 125:1812-21, 1995

Blank RP et al. Calcium metabolism and osteoporotic ridge absorption: A protein connection. J Prostet Dent 58(5):590-5, 1987

Bouckaert JH, Said AH. Fracture healing by vitamin K. Nature 185:849, 1960

Bray DL, Briggs GM. Decrease in bone density in young male guinea pigs fed high levels of ascorbic acid. J Nutr 114(5):920-8, 1984

Cadogan J et al. Milk intake and bone mineral acquisition in adolescent girls: Randomized, controlled intervention trial. Br Med J 315:1255-60, 1997

Calvo MS, Park YK. Changing phosphorus content of the U.S. diet: potential for adverse effects on bone. J Nutr 126:1168S-1180S, 1996

Carmel R et al. Cobalamin and osteoblast-specific proteins. N Engl J Med 319(2):70-5, 1988

Civitelli R et al. Dietary L-lysine and calcium metabolism in humans. Nutrition 8(6):400-5,

Cohen L, Kitzes R. Infrared spectroscopy and magnesium content of bone mineral in osteoporotic women. Israel J Med Sci 17:1123-25, 1981

Conlan D et al. Serum copper levels in elderly patients with femoral-neck fractures. Age Aging 19:212-14, 1990

Cooper C et al. Dietary protein intake and bone mass in women. Calcif Tissue Int 58:320-5, 1996

Corazza GR et al. Lactose intolerance and bone mass in postmenopausal Italian women. Br J Nutr 73(3):479-87, 1995

Devogelaer JP et al. Fluoride therapy of type I osteoporosis. Clin Rheumatol 14 Suppl 3:26-31, 1995

Dodds RA et al. Abnormalities in fracture healing induced by vitamin B6-deficiency in rats. Bone 7(6):489-95, 1986

Dwyer J et al. Acid/alkaline ash diets: time for assessment and change. J Am Diet Assoc 85(7):841-5, 1985

Eaton-Evans J et al. Copper supplementation and bone mineral density in middle-aged women. Proc Nutr Sci 54:191A, 1995

Eufemio MA. Fluoride therapy: Advances in the therapy of osteoporosis, part III. Geriatr Med Today 8(9):79-88, 1989

Eufemio MA. Vitamin D: Advances in the therapy of osteoporosis - Part VIII. Geriatr Med Today 9(11):37-49, 1990

Evans C, Eastell R. Adaptation to high dietary sodium intake. Challenges in Modern Medicine 7:413-18, 1995

Felson DT et al. Alcohol intake and bone mineral density in elderly men and women: The Framingham Study. Am J Epidemiol 142:485-92, 1995

Feng W et al. Low follicular oestrogen levels in New Zealand women consuming high fibre diets: a risk factor for osteopenia? N Z Med J 106(985):419-22, 1993

Feskanich D et al. Protein consumption and bone fractures in women. Am J Epidemiol 143(5):472-9, 1996

Flodin NW. The metabolic roles, pharmacology, and toxicology of lysine. J Am Coll Nutr 16(1):7-21, 1997

Friedman BJ et al. Manganese balance and clinical observations in young men fed Mn-deficient diets. J Nutr 117:133-43, 1987

Gavaler JS, Van Thiel DH. The association between moderate alcoholic beverage consumption and serum estradiol and testosterone levels in normal postmenopausal women: relationship to the literature. Alcohol Clin Exp Res 16(1):87-92, 1992

Goldsmith RS et al. Effects of phosphorus supplementation on serum parathyroid hormone and bone morphology in osteoporosis. J Clin Endocrinol Metab 43:523-32, 1976

Green TJ, Whiting SJ. Potassium bicarbonate reduces high protein-induced hypercalciuria in adult men. Nutr Res 14:991-1002, 1994

Grynpas MD et al. Strontium increases vertebral bone volume in rats at a low dose that does not induce detectable mineralization defect. Bone 18(3):253-9, 1996

Gudmand-Hoyer E. The clinical significance of disaccharide maldigestion. Am J Clin Nutr 59(3 Suppl):735S-741S, 1994

Gunnes M, Lehmann E. Dietary calcium, saturated fat, fiber, and vitamin C as predictors of forearm cortical and trabecular bone mineral density in healthy children and adolescents. Acta Paediatr 84:388-92, 1995

Hall SL, Greendale GA. The relation of dietary vitamin C intake to bone mineral density: results from the PEPI study. Calcif Tissue Int 63(3):183-9, 1998

Harris SS, Dawson-Hughes B. Caffeine and bone loss in healthy postmenopausal women. Am J Clin Nutr 60:573-8, 1994

Hart JP et al. Electrochemical detection of depressed circulating levels of vitamin K1 in osteoporosis. J Clin Endocrinol Metab 60(6):1268-9, 1985

Hauschka PV et al. Vitamin K and mineralization. Trends Biochem Sci 3:75, 1978

Heaney RP, Recker RR. Effects of nitrogen, phosphorus, and caffeine on calcium balance in women. J Lab Clin Med 99:46-55, 1982

Heaney R. Calcium in the prevention and treatment of osteoporosis. J Intern Med 231:169-80, 1992

Heaney RP. Thinking straight about calcium. Editorial. N Engl J Med 328(7):503-5, 1993

Heather AJ. Osteoporosis: role of lysine. Med Trial Tech Q , pp. 167-71, 1966

Hegsted M et al. Urinary calcium and calcium balance in young men as affected by level of protein and phosphorus intake. J Nutr 111:553-62, 1981

Hernandez-Avila M et al. Caffeine and other predictors of bone density among pre- and perimenopausal women. Epidemiology 4(2):128-33, 1993

Hillier S et al. Water fluoridation and osteoporotic fracture. Community Dent Health 13 Suppl 2:63-8, 1996

Hodges SJ et al. Depressed levels of circulating menaquinones in patients with osteoporotic fractures of the spine and femoral neck. Bone 12:387-9, 1991

Holbrook TL, Barrett-Conner E. A prospective study of alcohol consumption and bone mineral density. Br Med J 306:1506-8, 1993

Holick MF. Noncalcemic actions of 1,25-dihydroxyvitamin D3 and clinical applications. Bone 17(2 Suppl):107S-111S, 1995

Holl M, Allen L. Sucrose ingestion, insulin response and mineral metabolism. J Nutr 117:1229-33, 1987

Horowitz M et al. Oral calcium suppresses biochemical markers of bone resorption in normal men. Am J Clin Nutr 60(6):965-8, 1994

Hu J-F et al. Dietary intakes and urinary excretion of calcium and acids: a cross-sectional study of women in China. Am J Clin Nutr 58:398-406, 1993

Jie K-SG et al. Effects of vitamin K and oral anticoagulants on urinary calcium excretion. Br J Haematol 83:100-4, 1993

Kaur M et al. Clinical and biochemical studies in hypocystinuria. Indian Pediatr 32(10):1067-75, 1995

Kawakami H, Morii H. [Treatment of osteoporosis by active vitamin D.] Nippon Rinsho 56(6):1505-10, 1998 (in Japanese)

Kerstetter JE. Do dairy products improve bone density in adolescent girls? Nutr Rev 53(11):328-32, 1995

Kilgore C. Calcium enhances antiresorptive drugs' effectiveness: bone mass increases threefold, on average, when calcium is added to an HRT regimen. Family Practice News 27(14):1-2, 1997

Kim GS et al. Effects of vitamin B12 on cell proliferation and cellular alkaline phosphatase activity in human bone marrow stromal osteoprogenitor cells and UMR106 osteoblastic cells. Metabolism 45(12):1443-6, 1996

Kipp DE et al. Long-term low ascorbic acid intake reduces bone mass in guinea pigs. J Nutr 126(8):2044-9, 1996

Kruger MC et al. Eicosapentaenoic acid and docosahexaenoic acid supplementation increases calcium balance. Nutr Res 15:211-19, 1995

Kruger MC et al. Calcium, gamma-linolenic acid (GLA) and eicosapentaenoic acid (EPA) supplementation in osteoporosis. Osteoporosis Int 6(suppl):250, 1996

Kruger MC, Horrobin DF. Calcium metabolism, osteoporosis and essential fatty acids: a review. Prog Lipid Res 36(2-3):131-51, 1997

Laitinen K, Valimaki M. Alcohol and bone. Calcif Tissue Int 49 Suppl:S70-3, 1991

Laroche M et al. Lactose intolerance and osteoporosis in men. Rev Rhum Engl Ed 62(11):766-9, 1995

Lau EM et al. Bone mineral density in Chinese elderly female vegetarians, vegans, lacto-vegetarians and omnivores. Eur J Clin Nutr 52(1):60-4, 1998

Lehmann R et al. Drinking water fluoridation: bone mineral density and hip fracture incidence. Bone 22(3):273-8, 1998

Lemann J et al. Potassium causes calcium retention in healthy adults. J Nutr 123:1623-6, 1993

Leuenberger PK et al. Determination of peak trabecular bone density: Interplay of dietary fiber, carbohydrate, and androgens. Am J Clin Nutr 50:955-61, 1989

Li KC et al. Effect of a high fat-sucrose diet on cortical bone morphology and biomechanics. Calif Tissue Int 47(5):308-13, 1990

Lidor C et al. Successful high-dose calcium treatment of aluminum-induced metabolic bone disease in long-term home parenteral nutrition. JPEN J Parenter Enteral Nutr 15(2):202-6, 1991

Lips P. Vitamin D deficiency and osteoporosis: The role of vitamin D deficiency and treatment with vitamin D analogues in the prevention of osteoporosis-related fractures. Eur J Clin Invest 26:436-42, 1996

Lloyd T et al. Urinary hormonal concentrations and spinal bone densities of premenopausal vegetarian and nonvegetarian women. Am J Clin Nutr 54:1005-10, 1991

Lubec B et al. Evidence for McKusick's hypothesis of deficient collagen cross-linking in patients with homocystinuria. Biochim Biophys Acta 1315(3):159-62, 1996

Leuenberger PK et al. Determination of peak trabecular bone density: Interplay of dietary fiber, carbohydrate, and androgens. Am J Clin Nutr 50:955-61, 1989

MacGregor GA, Cappuccio FP. The kidney and essential hypertension: a link to osteoporosis? J Hypertens 11:781-5, 1993

Marie PJ et al. Effect of low doses of stable strontium on bone metabolism in rats. Miner Electrolyte Metab 11(1):5-13, 1985

Marsh AG. Cortical bone density of adult lacto-ovo-vegetarian and omnivorous women. J Am Diet Assoc February, 1980, pp. 148-51

Massey LK et al. Interactions between dietary caffeine and calcium on calcium and bone metabolism in older women. J Am Coll Nutr 13(6):592-6, 1994

Massey LK, Whiting SJ. Dietary salt, urinary calcium, and bone loss. J Bone Miner Res 11(6):731-6, 1996

McCaslin FE Jr., Janes JM. The effect of strontium lactate in the treatment of osteoporosis. Proc Staff Mtgs Mayo Clin 34:329-34, 1983

McCoy H et al. Relation of boron to the composition and mechanical properties of bone. Environ Health Perspect 102 Suppl 7:49-53, 1994

Meacham SL et al. Effect of boron supplementation on blood and urinary calcium, magnesium, and phosphorus, and urinary boron in athletic and sedentary women. Am J Clin Nutr 61:341-5, 1995

Melton ME, Kochman ML. Reversal of severe osteoporosis with vitamin B12 and etidronate therapy in a patient with pernicious anemia. Metabolism 43(4):468-9, 1994

Meyer HE et al. Dietary factors and the incidence of hip fracture in middle-aged Norwegians: a prospective study. Am J Epidemiol 145:117-23, 1997

Mjoberg B et al. Aluminum, Alzheimer's disease and bone fragility. Acta Orthop Scand 68(6):511-4, 1997

Muenzenberg KJ, Koch W. Mineralogic aspects in the treatment of osteoporosis with magnesium. Abstract. J Am Coll Nutr 8(5):461, 1989

Murphy S et al. Milk consumption and bone mineral density in middle aged and elderly women. BMJ 308:939-41, 1994

Murray TM, Ste-Marie LG. Prevention and management of osteoporosis: consensus statements from the Scientific Advisory Board of the Osteoporosis Society of Canada. 7. Fluoride therapy for osteoporosis. CMAJ 155(7):949-54, 1996

Neri Stagnaro M, Stagnaro S. [CoQ10 in the prevention and treatment of primary osteoporosis. Preliminary data.] Clin Ter 146(3):215-19, 1995 (in Italian)

New SA et al. Nutritional influences on bone mineral density: a cross-sectional study in premenopausal women. Am J Clin Nutr 65:1831-9, 1997

Nielsen FH. Studies on the relationship between boron and magnesium which possibly affects the formation and maintenance of bones. Magnes Trace Elem 9(2):61-9, 1990

Nielsen FH. Biochemical and physiologic consequences of boron deprivation in humans. Environ Health Perspect 102 Suppl 7:59-63, 1994

Nordin BE. Calcium and osteoporosis. Nutrition 13(7-8):664-86, 1997

Okano T. [Effects of essential trace elements on bone turnover--in relation to the osteoporosis]. Nippon Rinsho 54(1):148-54, 1996 (in Japanese)

Orimo H et al. Clinical evaluation of menatetrenone in the treatment of involutional osteoporosis - a double-blind multicenter comparative study with 1 α hydroxy vitamin D3. J Bone Miner Res (suppl 1)7:S122, 1992

Owusu W et al. Calcium intake and the incidence of forearm and hip fractures among men. J Nutr 127:1782-7, 1997

Pak CYC. Calcium metabolism. J Am Coll Nutr 8(S):46S-53S, 1989

Phipps KR et al. The association between water-borne fluoride and bone mineral density in older adults. J Dent Res 77(9):1739-48, 1998

Potter SM et al. Soy protein and isoflavones: their effects on blood lipids and bone density in postmenopausal women. Am J Clin Nutr 68(6 Suppl):1375S-1379S, 1998

Prentice A. Editorial. Calcium supplementation during breast feeding. N Engl J Med 337(8):558-9, 1997

Prince RL et al. The pathogenesis of age-related osteoporotic fracture: Effects of dietary calcium deprivation. J Clin Endocrinol Metab 82(1):260-4, 1997

Quesada-Gomez JM et al. Vitamin D insufficiency as a determinant of hip fractures. Osteoporosis Int Suppl 3:S42-S47, 1996

Raheb J. Water fluoridation, bone density and hip fractures: a review of recent literature. Community Dental Oral Epidemiol 23:309-16, 1995

Recker RR. Calcium absorption and achlorhydria. N Engl J Med 313(2):70-3, 1985

Reginster JY et al. Trace elements and postmenopausal osteoporosis: a preliminary study of decreased serum manganese. Med Sci Res 16:337-8, 1988

Reid IR, Ibbertson HK. Calcium supplements in the prevention of steroid-induced osteoporosis. Am J Clin Nutr 44:287-90, 1986

Relea P et al. Zinc, biochemical markers of nutrition, and type-I osteoporosis. Age Aging 24(4):303-7, 1995

Reynolds TM et al. Hip fracture patients may be vitamin B6 deficient. Acta Orthop Scand 63(6):635-8, 1992

Riggs BL Nelson KI. Effect of long term treatment with calcitriol on calcium absorption and mineral metabolism in postmenopausal osteoporosis. J Clin Endocrinol Metab 61(3):457-61, 1985

Riggs BL et al. Effect of fluoride treatment on the fracture rate in postmenopausal women with osteoporosis. N Engl J Med 322:802-9, 1990

Robert D et al. Hypercalciuria during experimental vitamin K deficiency in the rat. Calcif Tissue Int 37:143-7, 1985

Rosenblum ER et al. Isolation and identification of phytoestrogens from beer. Alcohol Clin Exp Res 16(5):843-5, 1992

Rousselet F et al. [Strontium and calcium metabolism. Interaction of strontium and vitamin D.] C R Soc Biol (Paris) 169(2):322-9, 1975 (in French)

Rude RK, Olerich MI. Magnesium deficiency: possible role in osteoporosis associated with gluten-sensitive enteropathy. Osteoporosis Int 6(6):453-61, 1996

Rudman D et al. Fractures in the men of a Veterans Administration nursing home: Relation to 1,25-dihydroxyvitamin D. J Am Coll Nutr 8(4):324-34, 1989

Saltman PD, Strause LG. The role of trace minerals in osteoporosis. J Am Coll Nutr 12(4):384-9, 1993

Sampson HW. Alcohol, osteoporosis, and bone regulating hormones. Alcohol Clin Exp Res 21(3):400-3, 1997

Sanchez TV et al. Bone mineral mass in elderly vegetarian females. Am J Roentgenol 131:542, 1978

Sebastian A et al. Improved mineral balance and skeletal metabolism in postmenopausal women treated with potassium bicarbonate. N Eng J Med 333:1776-81, 1994

Seelig MS. Interrelationship of magnesium and estrogen in cardiovascular and bone disorders, eclampsia, migraine and premenstrual syndrome. J Am Coll Nutr 12(4):442-58, 1993

Shiraki M. [Vitamin K2.] Nippon rinsho 56(6):1525-30, 1998 (in Japanese)

Siani A, Strazzullo P. Why and how to increase dietary potassium intake. Nutr Metab Cardiovasc Dis 6:245-54, 1996

Smith RT et al. Mechanical properties of bone from copper deficient rats fed starch or fructose. Fed Proc 44:541, 1985

Spak C-J et al. Tissue response of the gastric mucosa after ingestion of fluoride. Br Med J 298:1686-7, 1989

Spencer H, Samachson J. Effect of lysine on calcium metabolism in man. J Nutr 81:301-6, 1963

Spencer H et al. Effect of phosphorus on the absorption of calcium and on the calcium balance in man. J Nutr 108:447-57, 1978

Spencer H et al. Further studies of the effect of a high protein diet as meat on calcium metabolism. Am J Clin Nutr 37:924-9, 1983

Spencer H, Kramer L. Osteoporosis: Calcium, fluoride, and aluminum interactions. J Am Coll Nutr 4(1):121-8, 1985

Stendig-Lindberg G et al. Trabecular bone density in a two year controlled trial of peroral magnesium in osteoporosis. Magnes Res 6(2):155-63, 1993

Strause L et al. Dietary calcium intake, serum copper concentration and bone density in postmenopausal women. Abstract. FASEB J 5:A576, 1991

Szathmari M et al. [Zinc excretion in osteoporotic women]. Orv Hetil 134(17):911-4, 1993 (in Hungarian)

Tavini A et al. Coffee intake and risk of hip fracture in women in northern Italy. Prev Med 24:396-400, 1995

Tesar R et al. Axial and peripheral bone density and nutrient intakes of postmenopausal vegetarian and omnivorous women. Am J Clin Nutr 56:699-704, 1992

Tjaderhane L, Larmas M. A high sucrose diet decreases the mechanical strength of bones in growing rats. J Nutr 128(10):1807-10, 1998

Tkatch L et al. Benefits of oral protein supplementation in elderly patients with fracture of the proximal femur. J Am Coll Nutr 11(5):519-25, 1992

Tomita A. Post menopausal osteoporosis 47Ca study with vitamin K2. Clin Endocrinol (Jpn) 19:731-6, 1971

Tractenbarg DE. Treatment of osteoporosis: What is the role of calcium? Postgrad Med 87(4):263-70, 1990

Tranquilli AL et al. Calcium, phosphorus and magnesium intakes correlate with bone mineral content in postmenopausal women. Gynecol Endocrinol 8(1):55-8, 1994

Trichopoulou A et al. Energy intake and monounsaturated fat in relation to bone mineral density among women and men in Greece. Prev Med 26(3):395-400, 1997

Tsai KS et al. Impaired vitamin D metabolism in women: Possible role in pathogenesis of senile osteoporosis. J Clin Invest 73:1668-72, 1984

van Papendorp DH et al. Biochemical profile of osteoporotic patients on essential fatty acid supplementation. Nutr Res 15(3):325-34, 1995

Volpe SL et al. The relationship between boron and magnesium status and bone mineral density in the human: a review. Magnes Res 6(3):291-6, 1993

Wang MC et al. Associations of vitamin C, calcium and protein with bone mass in postmenopausal Mexican American women. Osteoporos Int 7(6):533-8, 1997

Weisner NM, in NW Solomons, IH Rosenberg, Eds. Absorption and Malabsorption of Mineral Nutrients. New York, Alan R. Liss, 1984:15

Wohl GR et al. Effects of high-Fat diet on mature bone mineral content, structure, and mechanical properties. Calcif Tissue Int 63(1):74-9, 1998

Worthington-Roberts B. Contemporary Developments in Nutrition. St. Lewis, Mo., C.V. Mosby Co., 1981:240-53

Yamaguchi M, Sakashita T. Enhancement of vitamin D3 effect on bone metabolism in weanling rats orally administered zinc sulphate. Acta Endocrinol 111:285-8, 1986

Yoshida H et al. Milk consumption decreases activity of human serum alkaline phosphatase: a cross-sectional study. Metabolism 44(9):1190-3, 1995

Zernicke RF et al. Long-term, high-fat-sucrose diet alters rat femoral neck and vertebral morphology, bone mineral content, and mechanical properties. Bone 16(1):25-31, 1995

PAIN

See Also: **DYSMENORRHEA**
FIBROMYALGIA
HEADACHE
MUSCLE CRAMPS (FUNCTIONAL)
NEURALGIA AND NEUROPATHY
PREMENSTRUAL SYNDROME

NUTRITIONAL TREATMENT GUIDE

✓ = Efficacy generally accepted.
* = Efficacy *demonstrated* by controlled human trials.
[+] = Efficacy *suspected* from uncontrolled human experiments
[-] = Efficacy *suspected* from indirect data
? = Efficacy *challenged* in at least one study of similar design

DIETARY FACTORS

* **high Fiber diet** *(for non-pathological, recurrent abdominal pain in childhood)*
* add **Caffeine** *(to increase the strength of peripherally-acting analgesics)*

- -

[+] **low Oxalate diet** *(for vulvar pain)*, preferably *WITH* calcium citrate tabs (200 mg calcium; 750 mg citrate) 2 to 3 tabs with each meal (1 year trial)

NUTRITIONAL FACTORS

* **L-Carnitine:** *to protect against damage and pain in deconditioned muscles due to exercise:* 3 g daily starting 2 weeks before resuming the activity and continuing for 1 week.
* **Magnesium:** *to reduce intra- and postoperative analgesia requirements:* intravenous infusion
* **Molybdenum:** 500 μg as amino acid chelate daily. Start with 1 cap with meals and at bedtime. Increase to maximum of 5 caps daily, or decrease to 2 to 3 caps daily, depending upon response. (1 month trial)
* **Selenium deficiency:** 200 μg daily
* **Vitamin C:** *for moderate to severe pain:* calcium, potassium and/or magnesium ascorbates: 10 to 50 g daily as needed (under medical supervision)
for delayed-onset muscle soreness following strenuous exercise: 1 g 3 times daily
* ? **D-Phenylalanine:** 250 mg 15 to 30 minutes before meals.
May take up to 3 weeks for results.
If ineffective, double the dosage.
* ? **Thiamine** ? 100 mg daily,
AND **Vitamin B_6** ? 50 mg daily
AND **Vitamin B_{12}** ? 0.25 mg daily (*for chronic pain*) (6 month trial)

- -

[+] **Magnesium deficiency:** ≈ 400 mg daily
[+] **Thiamine:** thiamine hydrochloride ? 1 to 4 g daily

[+] **Vitamin B_6:** ? 50 mg daily
[+] **Vitamin B_{12}:** ? 5000 µg IM daily (2 week trial)
[+] **Vitamin E:** Titrate dosage upwards until effective. (Use high doses under medical supervision.)

- -

[-] **Copper deficiency:** 2 mg twice daily for up to 6 weeks *AND* **Zinc** 50 mg daily

OTHER RELATED FACTORS

[+] ? rule out **Food Sensitivities**

DIETARY FACTORS

High Fiber Diet

Recurrent, non-pathological, abdominal pain is the most common chronic complaint of school-aged children. The diets of a group of children and adolescents with this complaint was found to contain only 10 grams of dietary fiber daily as contrasted to the RDA of 20 to 35 grams daily *(Rosenberg)*.

In a double-blind study, either high- or low-fiber cookies were randomly added to the diets of children with this complaint. Half of the children who received the high-fiber cookies, but not of those who received the low-fiber cookies, improved *(Christensen)*. It appears that their positive response to increased dietary fiber may be because the majority of patients with this presentation fulfill standardized criteria for the diagnosis of irritable bowel syndrome in adults *(Hyams)*, and the symptoms of irritable bowel syndrome may respond to dietary fiber supplementation (see Irritable Bowel Syndrome).

Low Oxalate Diet

As a group, women with vulvodynia have a normal 24-hour urinary oxalate excretion, although about half have elevated 24-hour urinary oxalate concentrations (greater than 1 mg per 40 dl) *(Baggish)*. When women with this complaint and elevated urinary oxalate were placed on an anti-oxalate dietary regimen, 24% demonstrated objective improvement, and 10% became able to have pain-free sexual intercourse *(Baggish)*.

When women were *not* selected for a low-oxalate diet based on their urinary oxalate excretion, only 3 to 4% responded to the diet. However, when calcium citrate was added, three-quarters of the patients responded within one year. The improved response is probably because calcium binds to oxalate in the bowel, while citrate inhibits the formation of oxalate crystals in the urine *(Melmed)*.

A woman suffered for 4 years from vulvar vestibulitis which affected her ability to work, her home life and sexual functioning. She had multiple treatments and operations with no relief. Her urine showed excess oxalate.

She was placed on a nutritionally balanced, low-oxalate diet and calcium citrate 6 tablets daily in divided doses, and her fluid intake and urine output were significantly increased.

After 3 months, her symptoms were significantly reduced; after one year, she was pain-free and able to resume normal activities. Withdrawing the calcium citrate resulted in a return of the symptoms and reinstitution alleviated them. She also noted marked exacerbation of her symptoms after an intake of high-oxalate containing foods such as rhubarb, peanuts, spinach and celery (Solomons).

Caffeine

In vitro, instant coffee powders were shown to compete with naloxone for binding to opiate receptors *(Boublik)*. These finding were not confirmed *in vivo*, however, as an animal study found that high doses of coffee, whether or not they contained caffeine, failed to show opiate-antagonizing activity *(Stubelt)*. Recent animal work has provided evidence suggesting that the antinociceptive effect of caffeine is mediated by central amplification of cholinergic transmission *(Ghelardini).*

When data on 131 patients with chronic back pain were reviewed, there were no significant differences between low, moderate and high caffeine users on subjective measures of pain severity or affective distress, suggesting that chronic caffeine intake fails to alter chronic pain *(Currie).*

The primary application of caffeine supplementation in pain control has been as an analgesic adjuvant when combined with certain analgesic drugs. In a review of 30 clinical trials involving over 10,000 patients, it was found that 40% higher dosages of aspirin, acetaminophen or salicylamide would be needed if they were not given in combination with caffeine *(Laska).* A similar adjuvant effect was found when caffeine was added to propyphenazone *(Kraetsch)*, or to ibuprofen, a non-steroidal anti-inflammatory drug *(Forbes).*

A double-blind study found that the potentializing action of caffeine on acetaminophen-induced pain relief enables a degree of pain relief equivalent to that of a combination using an analgesic with a peripheral action (such as acetaminophen) and another with a central action, in this case dextroproxyphen. The fact that combining a peripheral analgesic drug with caffeine does not have a central action avoids the secondary effects induced by central analgesics (drowsiness, constipation) in pain patients *(Kuntz).* However, meta-analyses of randomized controlled trials have questioned the efficacy of caffeine as an adjuvant as they found that caffeine added little to the analgesic effect of acetaminophen *(Zhang,1996)*, and was ineffective in enhancing the analgesic effect of aspirin *(Zhang,1997).*

A Warning

Caffeine can also have negative effects on pain. Distress due to somatic dysfunction may be caused by acute caffeine withdrawal. Subjects in one study normally consumed 300 mg or more of caffeine a day and abstained from caffeine for 4 days. The number of somatic dysfunctions increased significantly during caffeine withdrawal. By day 4, most of the individuals had not fully returned to baseline *(Reeves).* Also, a double-blind crossover study found that caffeine ingestion may reduce the effectiveness of transcutaneous electrical nerve stimulation *(Marchand).*

NUTRITIONAL FACTORS

VITAMINS

Vitamin B Complex

Supplementation with 3 members of the vitamin B complex, namely thiamine, vitamin B_6 and/or vitamin B_{12}, may reduce pain. Besides their individual effect (which we discuss shortly), their combination appears to suppress nociceptive transmission at the spinal level *(Fu).* Using the writhing test in the mouse, oral administration of these vitamins either alone or in combination resulted in dose-related antinociceptive properties *(Leuschner).*

This finding is consistent with the results of a study of 376 patients with acute pain of the lumbar vertebrae which investigated supplementation with these 3 vitamins as an adjunct to treatment with diclofenac, a non-steroidal anti-inflammatory drug. Under double-blind conditions, the combination of the vitamins with the drug was found to be significantly superior for patients with severe pain *(Brüggemann).*

Similarly, a double-blind study of patients with chronic back pain found that, after 6 months, supplemented patients had a significantly better psychosomatic state, a tendency toward greater range of motion, and half the relapse rate. Of the non-relapsing patients, the clinical condition tended to improve over time in the B vitamin group, whereas it tended to deteriorate in the placebo group *(Schwieger).* However, a subsequent double-blind crossover study failed to confirm this finding using normal subjects in a noninflammatory experimental pain model *(Bromm).*

The mechanism by which this B vitamin combination exerts its antinociceptive effect was explored with single neurons in the spinal cord dorsal horn in anesthetized cats. Findings suggested that these vitamins may suppress nociceptive transmission at the spinal level *(Fu).*

Thiamine

Massive intravenous doses of thiamine suppress the transmission of neural stimuli to skeletal muscles by producing ganglionic blockade *(Mazzoni).* In an open trial, 1 to 2 grams of thiamine hydrochloride was given once or twice daily to 133 pain patients who had failed to benefit from analgesics or physical therapy. Seventy-eight percent of the 69 headache patients improved compared to 71% of the 56 patients with pain in the spine and joints, and 63% of the 8 patients with neuralgia. Five of the 8 headache patients complained of nausea; otherwise there were no side effects *(Quirin)*.

Vitamin B_6

Vitamin B_6 is required in the conversion of dietary tryptophan to serotonin, a neurotransmitter which modulates pain perception, making it a serotonin-stimulating agent. Since chronic pain patients have decreased serotonin levels, the vitamin may be particularly beneficial for patients being withdrawn from analgesics as well as those with pain due to temporomandibular joint dysfunction *(Bernstein)*.

Vitamin B_{12}

Oral administration of vitamin B_{12} to rats has been shown to have a dose-dependent analgesic effect *(Hanck)*. In an open trial, daily injections of 5,000 μg of hydroxocobalamin appeared to reduce pain in all but 10 of a group of 400 patients with vertebral pain accompanied by sensory disturbances *(Hieber)*, while a smaller trial reported pain relief in 60% of cancer patients following 2 weeks of daily injections of 10,000 μg of cobamamide *(Dettori)*.

Although numerous similar trials attest to the efficacy of the vitamin, none meets current methodological requirements to prove its analgesic effect *(Dordain)*. Moreover, animal studies have failed to confirm its efficacy *(Eschalier)*. Scientific proof of the efficacy of vitamin B_{12} in treating pain is therefore still awaiting further investigations.

Vitamin C

Supplementation with megadoses of vitamin C has repeatedly been shown to reduce pain, although the mechanism of action remains to be elucidated. Some of these studies were done under controlled conditions *(Creagan;Gupta)*. In rats, an analgesic effect was found at a dosage of 500 mg/kg *(Hanck)*.

Pain reduction following megadose ascorbate supplementation has been reported in cases of advanced cancer *(Creagan;Hanck)*, Paget's disease *(Basu)*, and osteogenesis imperfecta *(Kurz)*, in patients with dental *(Lytle)* or lumbar disc *(Greenwood)* pains, and in patients with post-suxamethonium pain following procedures such as esophagoscopy, bronchoscopy and direct laryngoscopy *(Gupta)*. Moreover, in a double-blind crossover study, supplementation was shown to reduce muscle soreness after strenuous exercise *(Kaminski)*.

Vitamin E

Blood vitamin E levels decrease in rats when they are subjected to emotionally painful stress *(Tverdokhlib)*.

In open trials, vitamin E supplementation appeared to be effective in the treatment of dysmenorrhea *(Kryzhanovskii;Luzina)*. As this effect was reversed following naloxone administration, the endogenous opioid system appear to be involved.

Controlled clinical trials are needed to elucidate its clinical efficacy in treating pain.

MINERALS

Copper

Copper deficiency has been shown under experimental conditions to lower enkephalin levels, thus affecting the endogenous control of pain perception *(Bhathena)*. Conversely, intracerebral injection of cupric ion caused naloxone-reversible analgesia in mice and showed potency close to that of morphine *(Marzullo)*, and intracerebral injection of copper sulfate in mice potentiated morphine analgesia. *(Bhargava)*.

For a group of children and adolescents with recurrent abdominal pain, copper intake was only 0.82 mg daily compared to the RDA of 1 to 2.5 mg daily *(Rosenberg)*. However, studies have yet to be performed to evaluate whether copper supplementation is of any value in treating pain.

Magnesium

A deficiency of magnesium may be associated with cramping of both striated and smooth muscle, causing a wide variety of pain syndromes including headache, muscle cramps, angina pectoris, and epigastric cramps *(Durlach)*. In addition, the pain threshold decreases *(Clauw;Webb)*. Recent evidence from animal work suggests that magnesium deficiency may cause hyperalgesia through its effect on the NMDA (N-methyl-D-aspartate) receptors *(Dubray)*.

When symptoms are due to a magnesium deficiency, they can be expected to respond to magnesium repletion *(Bilbey)*. Magnesium has also been given intravenously as a pharmacotherapeutic nutrient. When given as an infusion perioperatively, it has been shown to reduce both intra- and postoperative analgesic requirements under double-blind conditions *(Koinig)*. Also, in an open trial, weekly magnesium injections successfully treated neuropathic pain syndromes after a nerve block was performed initially *(Tanaka).*

Molybdenum

Molybdenum is required for the synthesis of 4 detoxifying enzymes *(Rajagopalan).* It has been theorized that, by interfering with the activity of the detoxifying enzyme sulfite oxidase (which requires molybdenum), a deficiency may increase the risk of developing non-specific symptoms due to toxicity from sulfur dioxide and dietary sulfites *(Calabrese).*

Also, in a single-blind crossover study, 14 people with chronic aches and pains due to "arthritis" including osteo- or rheumatoid arthritis, frozen shoulder or undiagnosed low back pain graded their pain level and general health for 28 days. They then took either molybdenum or placebo capsules for the next 28 days; then the groups were crossed over for a third 28-day period.

Within one week of starting molybdenum, aches and pains significantly improved, as did the ratings of general health. When discontinued after being taken for 28 days, the effects of the supplement wore off within 1 week *(Moss).* This intriguing study awaits replication.

Selenium

Selenium deficiency may be associated with muscular pain *(van Rij).*

Results of the few clinical studies which have been published suggest that selenium supplementation may reduce pain, perhaps because the pain was secondary to a marginal selenium deficiency. For example, in a Swedish study, middle-aged women with chronic back and shoulder pains were found to have low serum selenium levels as compared to healthy controls. They were treated with selenium along with vitamin E (due to its closely-related mechanism of action) or placebo under double-blind conditions along with physiotherapy. The women with relatively higher initial selenium levels, or those whose serum selenium increased with supplementation, also responded better to physiotherapy, suggesting that a marginal selenium deficiency may have contributed to their complaints *(Jameson,1985a).*

When patients with chronically disabling muscular pain and stiffness received selenium and vitamin E, serum glutathione peroxidase (which requires selenium) increased in three-quarters of the supplemented patients, and mean pain score reduction was significantly more frequent and marked among those patients than among the rest of the group *(Jameson,1985b).* There is also some evidence that "growing pains" in children may respond to selenium supplementation *(Brahme-Istren).*

OTHER NUTRITIONAL FACTORS

L-Carnitine

Supplementation with L-carnitine has been found in a single-blind study to reduce delayed muscle pain after eccentric effort *(Giamberardino,1996).* The investigator suggests that the supplement may be appropriate for deconditioned people who are resuming their physical activity or sport in order to protect them against muscle damage and pain *(Giamberardino,1997).*

D-Phenylalanine

Supplementation with D-phenylalanine reduces pain by inhibiting enkephalin degradation *(Ehrenpreis).* When healthy volunteers took the submaximal effort tourniquet test, D-phenylalanine attenuated the increase in the intensity of both ischemic and pressure pain as the duration of the ischemia lengthened *(Nurmikko).*

D-phenylalanine was found to be effective for chronic pain in a double-blind crossover study *(Budd)*, but was ineffective in another study with a similar design *(Walsh)*, leaving its efficacy for chronic pain in question.

There is evidence from both placebo-controlled studies *(Kitade)* and an animal study *(Takeshirge)* that D-phenylalanine potentiates acupuncture analgesia, presumably by the same mechanism. Moreover, the results of animal studies suggest that it may potentiate morphine analgesia and antagonize morphine tolerance and dependence *(Dove;Hachisu)*, perhaps because chronic morphine administration increases enkephalinase activity leading to reduced endorphin levels *(Malfroy).*

A 70 year-old man was suffering from severe bone pain due to metastatic prostate cancer. Both analgesics and DES (diethylstilbestrol) failed to give him pain relief. However, D-phenylalanine 1.5 g twice daily completely controlled the pain (Budd).

L-Tryptophan

Tryptophan is the dietary precursor of 5-hydroxytryptamine (serotonin), an important neurotransmitter in the modulation of pain. It has been shown under double-blind conditions to raise the pain tolerance threshold *(Seltzer,1982)*. In open trials, tryptophan has reversed opiate tolerance *(Hosobuchi)* and restored the initial post-operative analgesia experienced by patients who had undergone dorsal rhizotomies or cordotomies for intractable pain *(King)*.

There are also reports of tryptophan reducing complaints of both acute *(Shpeen)* and chronic *(Selzer,1981)* pain, although it has not always been found to be effective *(Stockstill)*.

OTHER RELATED FACTORS

Food Sensitivities

Food sensitivities may be a cause of pain. Dental pain *(Lytle)*, muscle and joint pain *(Borok)*, and vulvar pain *(Melmed)* have all remitted following food elimination diets. Lactose intolerance has long been suspected as a cause of recurrent abdominal pain, and findings from several open trials suggest that a lactose-free diet may benefit patients with evidence of lactose malabsorption *(Gold)*.

However, *Pediatrics* has published the results of a double-blind study suggesting that lactose elimination may not be beneficial. Lactase deficiency was found to be as common in normals as it was in patients with recurrent abdominal pain. Moreover, after one year, lactase-deficient patients on a lactose-free diet, lactase-sufficient patients on a lactose-free diet, and lactase-sufficient patients on a regular diet all had about the same rates of remission *(Lebenthal)*.

Controlled clinical trials remain to be done to establish the etiologic role of foods.

A 42 year-old woman had pain between the shoulders, in the hands, wrists, and elbows and left hip for 20 years which gradually worsened and eventually forced her to discontinue work as a waitress. In addition, fatigue was constant. Frequent and, at times, prolonged bed rest was ineffectual. Sick headaches had occurred all of her life; 3 to 4 had occurred during the previous year. She also developed hives at various intervals.

Physical examination revealed pain and soreness with motion in various joints. Allergy skin testing was negative.

She was placed on a fruit- and cereal-free elimination diet, and her pains disappeared in 10 days. After 3 months she had no distress or discomfort even when doing physical work. During 8 years of follow-up, her relief continued so long as she eliminated fruits, fish and condiments from her diet, and restricted wheat, milk and eggs (Rowe).

BIBLIOGRAPHY

Baggish MS et al. Urinary oxalate excretion and its role in vulvar pain syndrome. Am J Obstet Gynecol 177(3):507-11, 1997

Basu TK et al. Ascorbic acid therapy for the relief of bone pain in Paget's disease. Acta Vitaminol Enzymol (Milano) 32:45-9, 1978

Bernstein AL. Vitamin B6 in neurology. Ann N Y Acad Sci 585:250-60, 1990

Bhargava HN. The effects of divalent ions on morphine analgesia and abstinence syndrome in morphine-tolerant and -dependent mice. Psychopharmacology (Berl) 57(2):223-5, 1978

Bhathena S et al. Decreased plasma enkephalins in copper deficiency in man. Am J Clin Nutr 43:42-6, 1986

Bilbey DL, Prabhakaran VM. Muscle cramps and magnesium deficiency: case reports. Can Fam Physician 42:1348-51, 1996

Borok G et al. Atopy: The Incidence of Chronic Recurrent Maladies. XVI European Congress of Allergology and Clinical Immunology. June 24-25, 1995

Boublik JH et al. Coffee contains potent receptor binding activity. Nature 301:246-8, 1983

Brahme-Istren M et al. [Oral selenium therapy against growing pain in children.] Lakartidningen 92(38):3450-2, 1995 (in Swedish)

Bromm K et al. Do the B-vitamins exhibit antinociceptive efficacy in men? Results of a placebo-controlled repeated-measures double-blind study. Neuropsychobiology 31(3):156-65, 1995

Brüggemann G et al. [Results of a double-blind study of diclofenac & vitamin B1, B6, B12 versus declofenac in patients with acute pain of the lumbar vertebrae. A multicenter study.] Klin Wochenschr 68(2):116-20, 1990 (in German)

Budd K. Use of D-phenylalanine, an enkephalinase inhibitor, in the treatment of intractable pain. Adv Pain Res Ther 5:305-8, 1983

Calabrese E et al. Sulfite oxidase deficiency: a high risk factor in SO2, sulfite, and bisulfite toxicity? Med Hypotheses 7(2):133-45, 1981

Christensen MF. Recurrent abdominal pain and dietary fiber. Letter. Am J Dis Child 140(8):738-9, 1986

Clauw DJ et al. Muscle intracellular magnesium levels with pain tolerance in fibromyalgia (FM). Abstract. Arthritis Rheumatol S213:324, 1994

Creagan ET et al. Failure of high-dose vitamin C (ascorbic acid) to benefit patients with advanced cancer. N Engl J Med 301:687-90, 1979

Currie SR et al. Caffeine and chronic low back pain. Clin J Pain 11(3):214-19, 1995

Dettori AG, Ponari O. Effectto antalgico della cobamide in corso di neuropatie periferiche di diversa etiopatogenesi. Minerva Med 64:1077-82, 1973 (in Italian)

Dordain G et al. [Vitamin B12, an analgesic vitamin? Critical examination of the literature]. Acta Neurol Belg 84(1):5-11, 1984 (in French)

Dove B et al. [The analgesic action of d-phenylalanine in combination with morphine or methadone]. Pharmazie 46(12):875-7, 1991 (in German)

Dubray C et al. Magnesium deficiency induces an hyperalgesia reversed by the NMDA receptor antagonist MK801. Neuroreport 8(6):1383-6, 1997

Durlach J. Clinical aspects of chronic magnesium deficiency, in MS Seelig, M Cantin, Eds. Magnesium in Health and Disease. New York, Spectrum Books, 1980

Ehrenpreis S et al. D-phenylalanine and other enkephalinase inhibitors as pharmacological agents: Implications for some important therapeutic applications. Acupunct Electrother Res 7(2-3):157-72, 1982

Eschalier A et al. A comparison of the effects of vitamin B12 and aspirin in three experimental pain models in rats and mice. Psychopharmacology (Berl) 81(3):228-31, 1983

Forbes JA et al. Effect of caffeine on ibuprofen analgesia in postoperative oral surgery pain. Clin Pharmacol Ther 49(6):674-84, 1991

Fu QG et al. B vitamins suppress spinal dorsal horn nociceptive neurons in the cat. Neurosci Lett 95(1-3):192-7, 1988

Ghelardini C et al. Caffeine induces central cholinergic analgesia. Naunyn Schmiedebergs Arch Pharmacol 356(5):590-5, 1997

Giamberardino MA et al. Effects of prolonged L-carnitine administration on delayed muscle pain and CK release after eccentric effort. Int J Sport Med 17:320-4, 1996

Giamberardino MA - interviewed in Clinical Pearls News 7(5):1997

Gold DM et al. Empiric dairy restriction in recurrent abdominal pain (RAP) of childhood. Abstract. J Am Coll Nutr 14(5):549, 1995

Greenwood JR. Optimum vitamin C intake as a factor in the preservation of disc integrity. Med Ann DC 33:274, 1964

Gupta SR, Savant NS. Post suxamethonium pains and vitamin C. Anasethesia 26:436-40, 1971

Hachisu M et al. Relationship between enhancement of morphine analgesia and inhibition of enkephalinase by 2S, 3R 3-amino-2-hydroxy-4-phenylbuanoic acid derivatives. Life Sci 30:1739-46, 1982

Hanck A, Weiser H. Analgesic and anti-inflammatory properties of vitamins. Int J Vitam Nutr Res (suppl)27:189-206, 1985

Hieber H. . [Treatment of vertebragenous pain and sensitivity disorders using high doses of hydroxocobalamin]. Med Monatsschr 28:545-8, 1974 (in German)

Hosobuchi Y et al. Tryptophan loading may reverse tolerance to opiate analgesics in humans: A preliminary report. Pain 9:161-9, 1980

Hyams JS et al. Characterization of symptoms in children with recurrent abdominal pain: resemblance to irritable bowel syndrome. J Pediatr Gastroenterol Nutr 20(2):209-14, 1995

Jameson S et al. Effekter av selenvitamin E-behandling till kvinnor med lång variga arbetsrelaterade nack-och skuldersmärtor. En dubbelblindstudie. Läkaresällskapets Riksstämma, 1985a (in Swedish)

Jameson S et al. Pain relief and selenium balance in patients with connective tissue disease and osteoarthrosis: A double-blind selenium tocopherol supplementation study. Nutr Res Suppl 1:391-7, 1985b

Kaminski M, Boal R. An effect of ascorbic acid on delayed-onset muscle soreness. Pain 50(3):317-21, 1992

King RB. Pain and tryptophan. J Neurosurg 53(1):44-52, 1980

Kitade T et al. Studies on the enhanced effect of acupuncture analgesia and acupuncture anesthesia by D-phenylalanine (2nd report) - schedule of administration and clinical effects in low back pain and tooth extraction. Acupunct Electrother Res 15(2):121-35, 1990

Koinig H et al. Magnesium sulfate reduces intra- and postoperative analgesic requirements. Anesth Analg 87(1):206-10, 1998

Kraetsch HG et al. Analgesic effects of propyphenazone in comparison to its combination with caffeine. Eur J Clin Pharmacol 49(5):377-82, 1996

Kryzhanovskii GN et al. [Endogenous opioid system in the realization of the analgesic effect of alpha-tocopherol.] Biull Eksp Biol Med 105(2):148-50, 1988 (in Russian)

Kuntz D, Brossel R. [Analgesic effect and clinical tolerability of the combination of paracetamol 500 mg and caffeine 50 mg versus paracetamol 400 mg and dextropropoxyphene 30 mg in back pain]. Presse Med 25(25):1171-4, 1996 (in French)

Kurz D, Eyring EJ. Effect of vitamin C on osteogenesis imperfecta. Pediatrics 54:56-61, 1974

Laska EM et al. Caffeine as an analgesic adjuvant. JAMA 251(13):1711-18, 1984

Lebenthal E et al. Recurrent abdominal pain and lactose absorption in children. Pediatrics 67(6):828-32, 1981

Leuschner J. Antinociceptive properties of thiamine, pyridoxine and cyanocobalamin following repeated oral administration to mice. Arzneimittelforschung 42(2):114-5, 1992

Luzina NL, Vakuleva LP. [Use of an antioxidant, alpha-tocopherol acetate, in the complex treatment of algomenorrhea.] Akush Ginekol (Mosk) (5):67-9, 1987 (in Russian)

Lytle RL. Chronic dental pain: Possible benefits of food restriction and sodium ascorbate. J Appl Nutr 40(2):95-8, 1988

Malfroy B et al. High-affinity enkephalin-degrading peptidase in brain is increased after morphine. Nature 276:523-6, 1978

Marchand S et al. Effects of caffeine on analgesia from transcutaneous electrical nerve stimulation. Letter. N Engl J Med 333(5):325-6, 1995

Marzullo G, Hine B. Opiate receptor function may be modulated through an oxidation-reduction mechanism. Science 208(4448):1171-3, 1980

Mazzoni P, Valenti F. Un nuovo anestetico generale per via endovenosa - la tiamina. Acta Anesh (Padova) 15:815-28, 1964 (in Italian)

Melmed MH. A low oxalate diet and calcium citrate administration are effective treatment for vulvar pain syndrome (vestibulitis). J Gynecol Surg 217, 1996

Moss M. Effects of molybdenum on pain and general health: a pilot study. J Nutr Environ Med 5:55-61, 1995

Nurmikko T et al. Attenuation of tourniquet-induced pain in man by D-phenylalanine, a putative inhibitor of enkephalin degradation. Acupunct Electrother Res 12(3-4):185-91, 1987

Quirin H. Pain and vitamin B1 therapy. Biblthca Nutr Dieta (38):110-11, 1986

Rajagopalan KV. Molybdenum: an essential trace element in human nutrition. Ann Rev Nutr 8:401-27, 1988

Reeves RR et al. Somatic dysfunction increase during caffeine withdrawal. J Am Osteopath Assoc 97(8):454-6, 1997

Rosenberg AJ et al. Dietary deficiency in children with recurrent abdominal pain. J Am Coll Nutr 14(5):548, 1995

Rowe AH. Allergic fatigue and toxemia. Ann Allergy 17:9-18, 1959

Schwieger G et al. Relapse prevention of painful vertebral syndromes in follow-up treatment with a combination of vitamins B1, B6, and B12. Ann N Y Acad Sci 585:540-2, 1990

Seltzer S et al. Perspectives in the control of chronic pain by nutritional manipulation. Pain 11(2):141-8, 1981

Seltzer S et al. Alteration of human pain thresholds by nutritional manipulation and L-tryptophan supplementation. Pain 13(4):385-93, 1982

Shpeen SE et al. The effect of tryptophan on postoperative endodontic pain. Oral Surg Oral Med Oral Pathol 58(4):446-9, 1984

Solomons CC et al. Calcium citrate for vulvar vestibulitis: a case report. J Reprod Med 36(12):879-82, 1991

Stockstill JW et al. The effect of L-tryptophan supplementation and dietary instruction on chronic myofascial pain. J Am Dent Assoc 118(4):457-60, 1989

Strubelt O et al. Failure of coffee to inhibit the pharmacodynamic activity of morphine in vivo. Experientia 42(1):35-7, 1986

Takeshirge M et al. Parallel individual variations in effectiveness of acupuncture, morphine analgesia, and dorsal PAG-SPA and their abolition by D-phenylalanine. Adv Pain Res Ther 5:563-8, 1983

Tanaka M et al. [Relief of neuropathic pain with intravenous magnesium.] Masui 47(9):1109-13, 1998 (in Japanese)

Tverdokhlib VP et al. [Effect of emotional and pain stress on the level of antioxidant vitamins in the blood serum of rats]. Vopr Pitan 6:52-4, 1987 (in Russian)

van Rij AM et al. Selenium deficiency in total parenteral nutrition. Am J Clin Nutr 32:2076-85, 1979

Walsh NE et al. Analgesic effectiveness of D-phenylalanine in chronic pain patients. Arch Phys Med Rehabil 6797):436-9, 1986

Webb WL, Gehi M. Electrolyte and fluid imbalance: neuropsychiatric manifestations. Psychosomatics 22:199-203, 1981

Zhang WY, Li Wan Po A. Analgesic efficacy of paracetamol and its combination with codeine and caffeine in surgical pain--a meta-analysis. J Clin Pharm Ther 21(4):261-82, 1996

Zhang WY, Po AL. Do codeine and caffeine enhance the analgesic effect of aspirin?--A systematic overview. J Clin Pharm Ther 22(2):79-97, 1997

PARKINSON'S DISEASE

NUTRITIONAL TREATMENT GUIDE

✓ = Efficacy generally accepted.
* = Efficacy *demonstrated* by controlled human trials.
[+] = Efficacy *suspected* from uncontrolled human experiments
[-] = Efficacy *suspected* from indirect data
? = Efficacy *challenged* in at least one study of similar design

DIETARY FACTORS

✓ restrict **dietary Protein** to 0.8 mg/kg body weight. (Also, consume 90% of the daily protein intake at the evening meal.)

- -

[-] minimize **Fat**, especially **Animal Fat**

NUTRITIONAL FACTORS

✓ **L-Dopa:** 0.5 to 1 g daily initially. Increase gradually as tolerated by 100-500 mg every 2 days (or more slowly) until maximal benefits or the appearance of adverse reactions. Give with food. Optimal dosage is generally reached in 6 to 8 weeks and usually ranges from 4 to 8 g daily.

- -

* **Choline:** citicoline (CDP-choline) 500 mg to 1,200 mg daily (one month trial)
* **Octacosanol:** Viobin 5 mg 3 times daily
* **Vitamin C:** *to improve functional performance in patients on L-dopa:* ? 1 g daily

- -

[+] **Coenzyme Q_{10}:** 300 mg to 600 mg daily
[+] **L-5-Hydroxytryptophan:** *to improve depression:* 200 to 900 mg daily in divided doses
[+] **Glutathione (reduced):** 600 mg intravenously twice daily for 30 days
[+] **L-Methionine:** Start with 1 g daily and increase gradually to 5 g daily. (2 month trial)
[+] **Octacosanol:** 1 to 2 mg daily (6 week trial)
[+] **Omega-6 fatty acids:** *to reduce tremor:* evening primrose oil 1 g 3 times daily
[+] **D-Phenylalanine:** *to improve rigidity, speech and depression:* 100 to 250 mg twice daily (4 week trial)
[+] **L-Tryptophan:** *to improve levodopa-induced "on-off" symptoms:* 2 to 8 g daily *WITH* niacin 25 mg daily *AND* pyridoxine 50 mg daily
[+] **L-Tyrosine:** ? 100 mg/kg daily (instead of L-dopa)
[+] **Vitamin B_6:** pyridoxal-5-phosphate ? 50 mg daily
[+] **Vitamin C:** 3 g daily
AND **Vitamin E:** 3,200 IU daily: *to delay progression to drug treatment*

- -

[-] **Beta-carotene deficiency:** 30 to 120 mg daily
[-] avoid **Copper** toxicity
[-] avoid **Iron** toxicity
[-] **Magnesium deficiency:** ≈ 400 mg daily

[-] avoid **Manganese** toxicity
[-] **N-Acetylcysteine:** ? 4 to 6 g daily
[-] **Niacin deficiency:** 50 to 100 mg daily
[-] **Vitamin E:** *to slow functional decline:* 400 IU to 3,200 IU daily

OTHER RELATED FACTORS

[-] rule out **Aluminum** toxicity
[-] rule out **Food Sensitivities**
[-] rule out **Mercury** toxicity

While a single, primary etiology of Parkinson's disease has not been identified, the disease is known to result from degeneration of neurons in the substantia nigra and locus ceruleus which produce dopamine.

DIETARY FACTORS

Dietary Protein

L-dopa, which is commonly given for the treatment of Parkinsonian symptoms, is one of several large, neutral amino acids which must compete with one another for passage across the blood-brain barrier. Restricting dietary protein to 0.8 g/kg (the US RDA), and serving 90% of it with the evening meal, increases its efficacy. The most striking result of the diet is a reduction in the daily fluctuations in L-dopa's efficacy (the "on-off" phenomenon) *(Tsui;Vilming)*. The introduction of a low protein diet may also permit a reduction in the dosage of L-dopa *(Paré)*.

A low protein diet, however, may foster the development of nutrient deficiencies when the usual diet is only marginally adequate in those nutrients *(Paré)*. Moreover, in the elderly, protein restrictions may lead to a negative nitrogen balance *(Vilming)*. This diet must thus be used with caution.

Animal Fat

When the fat intake of 110 patients was compared to that of matched controls, animal fat intake was strongly related to Parkinson's disease *(Logroscino,1996)*. It has been suggested that fatty diets impair essential fatty acid metabolism, causing changes in the membrane structure resulting in increased electron spillage and superoxide radical formation. Chronic oxidative stress generated by faulty mitochondria could eventually affect the neuromelanin-containing dopaminergic midbrain neurons, known to be susceptible to oxidation, and could also cause the mitochondrial DNA mutations seen in Parkinson's disease *(Peers)*.

Low fat diets could, theoretically, not only prevent the disease, but also arrest its progression in established cases by improving mitochondrial membrane structure in the surviving nigral neurons *(Peers)*.

NUTRITIONAL FACTORS

VITAMINS

Niacin

Compared to normals, a group of 342 patients was found to ingest a markedly lower intake of niacin *(Hellenbrand)*. Even if their dietary niacin intake were in the accepted normal range, the elderly may become niacin-deficient; in fact, oral niacin supplementation may still not protect them from biochemical evidence of niacin deficiency *(Frank)*. Moreover, treatment with L-dopa, particularly when given concurrently with a decarboxylase inhibitor (such as carbidopa or benserazide), further increases the risk of niacin deficiency *(Bender)*.

Supplementation with niacin or with 1-N-methyl-nicotinamide, its metabolite, may increase the efficacy of L-dopa by extending the length of time that L-dopa levels remain elevated in the brain *(Black)*. Also, nicotinamide adenine dinucleotide (NADH), a coenzyme formed from niacin, is required for the synthesis of tetrahydro-biopterin, the cofactor for the enzyme (tyrosine hydroxylase) which catalyzes the conversion of tyrosine to L-dopa *(Vrecko)*.

Several open trials have reported excellent results using reduced NADH. For example, for a group of 15 patients, 7 days of intravenous infusions of 10 mg daily was followed by significant improvement in the Unifed Parkinson's Disease Rating Scale and significantly increased the bioavailability of plasma levodopa *(Kuhn,1996)*.

While these preliminary results are impressive, a double-blind study which provided 25 mg daily intravenously for 4 days, followed by 25 mg intramuscularly after 2 and 4 weeks, failed to find more than a tendency to clinical improvement in both the NADH and placebo groups *(Dizdar)*.

More controlled clinical trials are needed to ascertain whether NADH has notable efficacy in treatment.

Vitamin B_6

Deficiency of vitamin B_6 is common in the elderly, even despite adequate intake and oral supplementation *(Frank)*. In fact, treatment with the combination of L-dopa and a decarboxylase inhibitor, a common therapeutic regimen, may provoke a marginal vitamin B_6 deficiency *(Bender)*. This deficiency may be of particular importance in Parkinson's disease because the enzyme dopa decarboxylase, which catalyzes the conversion of dopa to dopamine, is dependent upon pyridoxal phosphate, the activated form of the vitamin.

There have been several open trials of supplementation with pyridoxine. Most concluded that the supplement appeared to reduce the clinical signs of Parkinsonism, including decreases in tremor, muscle cramps and rigidity, and improvements in bladder control, gait and energy *(Baker;Vaïnshtok)*. It is not known whether responsive patients were initially vitamin B_6-deficient, and we lack controlled studies confirming this finding.

A Warning

If patients are receiving L-dopa without a decarboxylase inhibitor, pyridoxine supplementation may counteract the effects of the drug *(AMA)*.

Vitamin C

Evidence is accumulating that oxidative mechanisms affecting the dopaminergic neurons may contribute to cell death and thus to the progression of PD *(Grimes)*. Ascorbic acid is a highly effective inhibitor of dopamine oxidation *in vitro* and has been shown to be decreased in the amygdaloid nucleus of Parkinsonian brains *(Riederer)*.

Other lines of evidence suggest that vitamin C nutriture may be reduced in Parkinson patients. Studies have repeatedly found an inverse relationship between the dietary intake of vitamin C and risk of the disease *(Cerhan;de Rijk;Singh)*. Plasma/serum levels have sometimes been noted to be low compared to normals *(Singh;Yapa)*, although not in all studies *(Fernandez-Calle)*. Furthermore, patients show classic vitamin C deficiency symptoms much more frequently than similar patients without the disease *(Yapa)*.

The effects of vitamin C supplementation on unmedicated patients have not been reported, and it is not known whether supplementation can help to protect people from developing the disease. *In vitro*, ascorbic acid was one of the most effective inhibitors of dopamine oxidation out of a wide range of compounds *(Florence; Offen)* although, compared to the thiol antioxidants (such as reduced glutathione), it was not terribly effective in rescuing neurons from dopamine-induced apoptosis *(Offen)*.

There is also evidence that vitamin C supplementation may counteract the adverse effects of L-dopa treatment. L-dopa is toxic to dopaminergic neurons; *in vitro*, however, its toxicity is prevented by the addition of ascorbate *(Mena)*.

Under double-blind conditions, it produced a modest improvement in 6 patients with "on-off" effects from L-dopa. However, it failed to change the pattern of "on-off" effects, the severity of parkinsonism/dyskinesia, or self-assessment ratings *(Reilly)*.

Further controlled trials are needed to better ascertain the place of vitamin C supplementation in the treatment of this disorder.

A 62 year-old male had stopped L-dopa because of intolerable nausea and salivation. L-dopa was re-instituted along with ascorbic acid. After 4 weeks, his ability to move his head increased, salivation decreased, and speech and handwriting improved considerably. Hand coordination improved so markedly that he began to play the organ for the first time in several years.

Several times placebo was substituted for vitamin C on a double-blind basis. Each time his condition deteriorated on placebo and improved with vitamin C (Sacks).

Vitamin E

Like vitamin C, vitamin E is an antioxidant. When rats were made vitamin E-deficient, there was nigral dopaminergic neuronal loss due to oxidative damage, suggesting that the same may occur in Parkinson's disease *(Dexter,1994)*.

The development of Parkinson's disease has been found to be associated with a low intake of vitamin E-rich foods in early life *(Golbe,1988,1990)*, suggesting that a higher intake of vitamin E early in life may protect against the eventual development of the disease. This possible prophylactic effect of the vitamin may also extend to later life. The largest epidemiological study to date concerned more than 5,000 non-demented individuals aged 55 to 95 years, including 31 with Parkinson's disease. Not only was the odds ratio for the disease found to be only 0.5 per 10 mg of daily dietary vitamin E intake, but this association was dose-dependent *(de Rijk)*.

Despite the importance of vitamin E as a lipid-soluble antioxidant, experiments in which vitamin E supplementation was provided to patients with established disease have generally failed to find evidence of benefit *(Kieburtz;Parkinson Study Group,1993,1996; Shoulson)*. One hint of possible benefit, however, comes from a retrospective study of 14 patients aged 55 to 76 years who had taken vitamin E for an average of 7 years. When matched for age, the duration of illness and levodopa dosage, these patients had significantly lower mean scores for Parkinson's disease, suggesting that their illness was less severe *(Factor)*.

***AND* Vitamin C**

Vitamin E has been given together with vitamin C in an a small open trial. Compared to unsupplemented patients, 15 patients with early disease receiving the two antioxidants were able to delay starting standard drug treatment for an additional 2 ½ years *(Fahn)*, suggesting that the combination may delay the progression of the disease.

MINERALS

Copper

Excessive copper has pro-oxidant effects, and chronic occupational exposure to copper is associated with an elevated risk of developing the disease *(Gorell)*. Moreover, elevated cerebrospinal fluid copper levels appear to exert a pro-oxidative effect *(Snyder)*, and at least one of the studies of cerebrospinal fluid copper levels in Parkinson patients have found the levels to be elevated *(Pall)*.

Copper deficiency in second generation rats produces low dopamine levels in the corpus striatum and results in clinical signs analogous to those of Parkinson's disease. In this situation, the dopamine concentration correlates with striatal copper, but not with liver copper - which is an index of copper nutriture. Moreover, the dopamine concentration is not readily reversed by copper supplementation *(O'Dell)*.

In patients, there is evidence that copper levels in the substantia nigra may be depressed *(Dexter,1989;Uitti)*.

There is no evidence so far that copper supplementation is an effective treatment intervention to correct the abnormality.

Iron

As with copper, excessive levels exert pro-oxidant effects. In fact, it has been theorized that iron participates in the mechanism of nerve cell death in Parkinson's disease *(Hirsh,1998)* and occupational exposure to iron is associated with an increased risk of the disease *(Zayed)*.

Systemic iron metabolism appears to be altered in Parkinson's disease. The defect seems to be in the systems that regulate the synthesis of the major proteins of iron metabolism in the liver as well as the brain. Over time, it may expedite entry of iron into the brain and decrease iron in the extracellular compartment *(Logroscino,1997)*.

Tyrosine hydroxylase, an enzyme involved in the production of dopa from tyrosine, requires iron as coenzyme. The activity of this enzyme is reduced in Parkinson's disease, and can be stimulated by iron supplementation. In an open trial, oxyferriscarbone, an iron complex, was given intravenously to 10 patients in akinetic crisis who were being treated with L-dopa. All improved remarkably, and there were no side effects. Seven of the patients were able to reduce or discontinue L-dopa. The effects were dose-dependent and lasted one to two days *(Birkmayer,1986)*.

The safety of iron supplementation is questionable, however, since patients have elevated iron levels in the substantia nigra pars compacta *(Jellinger)*. This elevation cannot be solely attributed to neuronal degeneration *(Hirsch)*; it may exert a pro-oxidative effect by participating in the auto-oxidation of dopamine *(Sofic)* and may thereby promote the progress of the disease. Further studies are therefore needed before the safety of iron supplementation is established.

Also, ferrous sulfate, when given with levodopa and carbidopa, may reduce the drugs' efficacies due to the formation of iron complexes *(Campbell)*.

Magnesium Deficiency

Studies have consistently shown evidence of reduced magnesium nutriture *(Yasui,1997)*, and magnesium is reduced in multiple regions of the brain *(Uitti; Yasui,1992)*. There is so far no evidence, however, that magnesium supplementation is effective other than to reverse the usual effects of magnesium deficiency.

Manganese Toxicity

Excessive manganese exposure, which is usually occupational, increases the risk of Parkinsonism *(Gorell)* due to the depletion of dopamine and the production of neurotoxins *(Florence)*.

A woman with symptoms suggestive of early Parkinsonism reported taking 1,500 mg manganese daily as a nutritional supplement for the past 6 months. Hair mineral analysis revealed 30 times the normal manganese level (Kunin).

Zinc

Zinc metabolism is altered. Such changes may be important, not only in Parkinson's disease, but also in other neurological disorders in which oxidative stress is implicated *(Cuajungco)*.

Specifically, zinc levels in the substantia nigra, the caudate nucleus and lateral putamen may be increased *(Dexter)*, while cerebrospinal fluid *(Jimenez-Jimenez,1998)* and plasma *(Abbott)* levels may be reduced.

There is no evidence that zinc supplementation is beneficial.

OTHER NUTRITIONAL FACTORS

Carotenoids

Epidemiological studies have found that beta-carotene intake may be lower in patients than in normals. In one study of more than 5,000 independently living individuals without dementia aged 55 to 95 years, the odds ratio for Parkinson's disease was 0.6 per milligram of beta-carotene intake *(de Rijk)*. Less clear is whether plasma/serum levels of the carotenoids may be reduced *(Jimenez-Jimenez,1993;Singh)*.

The efficacy of carotenoid supplementation has not been studied.

Choline

The rationale for choline supplementation rests on the postulated balance between dopamine and acetylcholine neurotransmission in the striatum, and pathological evidence for atrophy of the cholinergic cells in the nucleus basalis of Meynert *(Growdon,1987)*.

Choline or lecithin supplementation may decrease levodopa-induced dyskinetic movements. Unfortunately, as supplementation may increase rigidity and akinesia, it cannot be recommended *(Barbeau;Papavasiliou)*.

There is, however, another method of providing cholinergic supplementation which is more promising. Cytidine 5'-diphosphocholine, also identified as CDP-choline or citicoline, is an essential intermediate in the biosynthetic pathway of the structural phospholipids of cell membranes, especially that of phosphatidylcholine. Following oral or parenteral administration, CDP-choline releases its two principle components, cytidine and choline. Once absorbed, the cytidine and choline disperse widely throughout the organism, cross the blood-brain barrier, and reach the central nervous system, where they are incorporated into the phospholipid fraction of the membrane and microsomes *(Secades)*.

Considerable accumulated evidence supports the use of citicoline to enhance membrane maintenance, membrane repair, and neuronal function *(Weiss)*. Citicoline has been shown in animal work to increase striatal dopamine content *(Shibuya)*. In humans, it increased plasma dopa and homovanillic acid concentrations and increased lymphocytic dopaminergic receptors *(Cubells)*.

For patients on L-dopa, citicoline has been shown to decrease the incidence of side effects and retard the loss of its efficacy during long-term treatment. Moreover, the dosage of L-dopa can usually be cut in half *(Eberhardt)*.

In a double-blind crossover study, patients receiving levodopa plus a decarboxylase inhibitor showed significant improvements in rigidity and bradykinesia *(Agnoli)*. Furthermore, when one of two groups of patients was treated with citicoline, only the untreated group showed evidence of cortical cognitive impairment *(Garcia-Mas)*.

Toxicological tests have found citicoline to be safe. It has no serious adverse effects on the cholinergic system and is well-tolerated *(Secades)*.

Coenzyme Q_{10}

Deficiency of the mitochondrial transport enzyme complex I (NADH:ubiquinone oxidoreductase) appears to be one of the basic abnormalities responsible for mitochondrial respiratory failure in Parkinson's disease *(Mizuno)*. The defect appears to be genetic, arising from mitochondrial DNA, and may play an important role in the neurodegeneration by fostering reactive oxygen species production and conferring increased neuronal susceptibility to mitochondrial toxins *(Swerdlow)*.

The activities of complex I and complex II/III in platelet mitochondria are reduced in patients with early, untreated Parkinson's disease. Coenzyme Q_{10} (CoQ_{10}) is the electron acceptor for both complex I and complex II. In Parkinson's patients, the levels of CoQ_{10} and the activities of these complexes are correlated. Moreover, the level of mitochondrial coenzyme Q_{10} is significantly lower *(Shults)*.

In a study of aged mice, supplementation with a massive dosage of CoQ_{10} (200 mg/kg/d) attenuated MPTP-induced loss of striatal dopamine and dopaminergic axons, suggesting that CoQ_{10} may be beneficial in Parkinson's disease *(Beal)*. Although two open trials have failed to find improvement on the Unified Parkinson's Disease Rating Scale following supplementation for at least on month with dosages as high as 200 mg 4 times daily *(Shults;Strijks)*, there was a trend toward an increase in complex I activity *(Shults)*.

Despite the lack of scientific evidence supporting the clinical efficacy of CoQ_{10}, two reports of patients who were already being treated with niacin suggest that selected patients may respond:

1. An 84 year-old man with a history of mental illness had been supplemented with niacin 1 g 3 times daily as well as ascorbic acid, vitamin E and selenium for at least 25 years. Parkinson's disease was diagnosed a couple of years prior to evaluation and, one year earlier, he was started on Sinemet®. Although the drug provided slight benefit, he continued to deteriorate. On examination, he had a typical Parkinson gait with leg muscle weakness and tremor. Coenzyme Q_{10} 600 mg daily was added and, within 2 weeks, he was much better. The dosage was subsequently reduced to 300 mg daily. When re-evaluated one year later, he had regained the use of his limbs, had very little tremor, and had been able to return to playing golf.

2. A woman receiving high-dosage niacin as part of a treatment regimen for mental illness had a history of difficulty walking for many years. While her neurologist had not established a diagnosis, her gait resembled that of Parkinson's disease and the diagnosis was being considered. She was started on coenzyme Q_{10} 300 mg daily. Within one month, there was a marked improvement in her gait as well as in her mood (Hoffer).

L-Dopa

Dopa (dihydroxyphenylalanine) is the precursor to the neurotransmitter dopamine, and Parkinsonian brains show a massive deficit of striatal dopamine *(Hornykiewicz)*. L-dopa and levodopa, its synthetic form, have become mainstays in the standard treatment of Parkinson's disease *(AMA)*.

Since dopa is one of several large, neutral amino acids in competition with one another for passage across the blood-brain barrier, L-dopa supplementation should be routinely combined with a low protein diet (see discussion above). It should only be administered under close medical supervision because of its potential for side effects.

Glutathione

Depletion of reduced glutathione (GSH), an important antioxidant, occurs in the substantia nigra in Parkinson's disease. In fact, GSH depletion is found in incidental Lewy body disease, the presymptomatic stage of Parkinson's disease *(Pearce)*.

Recently it has been theorized that GSH depletion, which can enhance oxidative stress and increase the levels of excitotoxic molecules, may initiate the neuronal loss *(Bains)*. *In vitro*, GSH depletion was shown to induce a redux desequilbrium which appeared to trigger apoptosis in neuronal cells *(Nicole)*.

In animal work, the exogenous administration of GSH led to a significant decrease of lipoperoxidation in the brain areas of cortex and hippocampus *(Calabrese)*. *In vitro*, GSH partially protected cells from dopamine-induced apoptosis. N-acetylcysteine, a GSH precursor, was even more effective (see N-acetylcysteine below), while neither vitamin C nor vitamin E offered any protection despite their importance as antioxidants *(Offen)*.

In an open trial, 9 patients with early, untreated Parkinson's disease received GSH by intravenous injection for 30 days; then it was discontinued and patients were followed-up for 2 to 4 months after which they were treated with carbidopa-levodopa. Based on 2 ratings scales and the Webster Step-Second Test, *all* patients improved significantly after GSH therapy with a 42% decline in disability. Once GSH was stopped, the effect lasted 2 to 4 months *(Sechi)*.

Controlled clinical trials of GSH are warranted to see if these interesting preliminary findings can be confirmed.

L-Methionine

Methionine, an essential sulfur amino acid, readily crosses the blood-brain barrier where it is converted to S-adenosylmethionine (SAMe). L-dopa supplementation has been found to reduce brain SAMe levels *(Surtees)*.

In an open trial, supplementation of 11 previously untreated patients with L-methionine was followed in about 3 weeks by improvement in clinical signs, particularly akinesia and rigidity, with a less marked effect on tremor. The authors noted that the efficacy of this essential amino acid seemed similar to that of L-dopa *(Meininger)*.

Other investigators then tested L-methionine supplementation on 15 patients who had shown maximal improvement from standard medications. After 2 months, 10 of the patients (67%) showed further improvement. Improvements were seen in activity level, ease of movement, rigidity and dyskinesia, mood, sleep, attention span, muscular strength, concentration and voice. Tremor and drooling were unimproved, however. Side effects were limited to nausea in two patients, and diarrhea in one *(Smythies)*.

Controlled clinical trials of L-methionine are needed to confirm these early reports. Also, supplementation with SAMe deserves to be evaluated.

N-Acetylcysteine

The importance of reduced glutathione in protected neuronal cells has already been discussed. N-acetylcysteine is a nutritional precursor for glutathione synthesis and appears to be better absorbed orally. Compared to cysteine, the addition of an acetyl group makes it more stable as well as more active biologically *(Issels)*.

While N-acetylcysteine has yet to be studied in controlled clinical trials for its efficacy in Parkinson's disease, the result of early work with another neurodegenerative condition is encouraging *(Hurd)*.

Octacosanol

This long-chain alcohol extracted from wheat germ oil was given to 10 patients with mild to moderate symptoms in a double-blind crossover study. Compared to placebo baselines, the experimental group showed a small but statistically significant improvement in their self-ratings of "activities of daily living" and "mood." Three patients

(30%) were rated as significantly improved on octacosanol, and none worsened *(Snider)*. Additional controlled studies are needed to further clarify its efficacy.

> *A man who had developed hallucinations and disorientation on medication requiring hospitalization received octacosanol 300 µg 3 times daily. Within 6 weeks dramatic improvement began to be noted in strength, mobility and appetite. His neurologist remarked that he had never before seen such a marked improvement in a Parkinsonian patient (England).*

Omega-6 Fatty Acids

Evening primrose oil is a source of omega-6 fatty acids and a particularly rich source of gamma-linolenic acid, a key intermediary in omega-6 fatty acid metabolism.

In a preliminary trial, 11 patients with tremor were given evening primrose oil. In 6 patients (55%), the tremor improved *(Critchley)*. Controlled trials are need to confirm this hopeful finding.

D-Phenylalanine

Patients may have reduced urinary levels of phenylethylamine, a metabolite of phenylalanine *(Heller,1973)*.

D-phenylalanine (but not L-phenylalanine) has been shown to have a therapeutic effect on drug-induced Parkinsonism in animals *(Fernandez Pardel)*. In an open trial, 15 patients received D-phenylalanine starting 10 days after suspending their medications. Four weeks later, repeat neurological examinations revealed highly significant improvements in rigidity, difficulty ambulating, speech difficulty and depression compared to the drug-free baseline. Tremor, however, failed to improve *(Heller,1976)*. Controlled studies are needed to confirm these early results.

As phenylalanine is, like L-dopa, a large, neutral amino acid, supplements should be taken as far away as possible from L-dopa with which it competes for transport across the blood-brain barrier *(Nutt)*.

L-Tryptophan

Tryptophan is the dietary precursor of the neurotransmitter serotonin. In patients unmedicated with L-dopa, cerebrospinal fluid concentrations of L-tryptophan are reduced, while L-dopa supplementation further reduces L-tryptophan concentrations *(Tohgi,1993b)*. Moreover, the more advanced the symptoms, the lower the L-tryptophan concentration in the cerebrospinal fluid *(Tohgi,1993a)*.

There is evidence that the serotonergic deficit in Parkinson patients contributes to the depression often seen in patients with advanced symptoms *(McCance-Katz)*, and depressed patients with Parkinson's disease may have a significant reduction in the cerebrospinal fluid of the serotonin metabolite 5-HIAA *(Mayeux)*.

Furthermore, in an open trial, supplementation with 5-hydroxytryphophan, the metabolite of L-tryptophan and immediate precursor to serotonin, improved depression in a group of Parkinson patients *(Mayeux)*.

Supplementation with L-tryptophan (or, possibly, with 5-hydroxytryptophan) appears to be particularly beneficial for patients receiving L-dopa. Competition between tryptophan and L-dopa for passage across the gut mucosa could result in tryptophan malabsorption leading to depression and other side effects of L-dopa treatment *(Lehmann)*. Moreover, competition between these two large, neutral amino acids for transport across blood-brain barrier could be a cause of the fluctuating ("on-off") response to L-dopa *(Nutt)* as well as further reduction in the availability of tryptophan in the brain for conversion to serotonin.

Studies investigating the efficacy of L-tryptophan supplementation have had mixed results. One study compared the combination of levodopa and L-tryptophan with levodopa and placebo. Only the group that received both agents showed significant improvements in tests of functional ability to perform certain tasks as well as a small but significant improvement in mood and drive *(Coppen)*. When, however, L-tryptophan was given to patients with levodopa-induced psychiatric symptoms under double-blind conditions, the psychiatric disturbances were not greatly altered *(Beasley)*.

Two women with levodopa-induced "on-off" symptoms responded dramatically to L-tryptophan along with niacin and pyridoxine (to facilitate conversion to serotonin) *(Sandyk)*. These case reports have yet to be confirmed by controlled clinical trials.

Patients who have had the disease for a relatively short period of time are those most likely to benefit from L-tryptophan supplementation, while those who have had the disease for a long time could have an adverse reaction *(Bryant)*.

Because of their competitive interaction, L-tryptophan should not be taken at the same time in the day as L-dopa *(Nutt)*.

L-Tyrosine

Tyrosine, derived from phenylalanine, is the precursor to dopa. Tyrosine hydroxylase is the enzyme required for the conversion of tyrosine to dopa (which is the rate-limiting step in the biosynthesis of dopamine); thus Parkinson's disease can be considered as a tyrosine hydroxylase deficiency of the striatum *(Haavik)*. In fact, the disease appears to be associated with biopterin, the cofactor for tyrosine hydroxylase *(Yamaguchi)*.

Supplementation with L-tyrosine increases the cerebrospinal fluid level of homovanillic acid, the major dopamine metabolite, suggesting that it may enhance dopaminergic transmission by increasing dopamine turnover *(Growdon,1982)*.

The possibility of substituting L-tyrosine for L-dopa has been explored in a small pilot study. After 3 years of follow-up, the authors concluded that L-tyrosine supplementation was associated with better clinical results and many fewer side effects than L-dopa or dopamine antagonists in some of the patients *(Lemoine)*. As with the other large, neutral amino acids, L-tyrosine supplements should not be taken at the same time as L-dopa *(Nutt)*.

OTHER RELATED FACTORS

Food Sensitivities

People with well defined food reactions are significantly more likely to have difficulty carrying out sulfur oxidation reactions (*Scadding*), and Parkinson's disease patients are more likely than normals to demonstrate a reduced sulfur oxidation capacity *(Steventon)*. Parkinson's disease patients have been reported to have more adverse reactions to foods such as tomatoes, oranges, and wheat compared to controls. Furthermore, they may have a significantly higher prevalence of irritable bowel syndrome, a disorder that may be promoted by food sensitivities *(Bell)*.

Aluminum Toxicity

Aluminum concentrations in the substantia nigra, caudate nucleus and globus pallidus may be elevated in the brains of patients who had Parkinson's disease and even more elevated in the gray matter and the basal ganglia *(Yasui,1992)*. Also, aluminum is present in Lewy bodies in the substantia nigra of Parkinsonian brains, but not in patients with supranuclear palsy, suggesting that its presence is not solely due to neuronal degeneration *(Hirsch)*.

Furthermore, there is evidence that long-term occupational exposure to aluminum may increase the risk of developing Parkinson's disease *(Zayed)*.

Lead Toxicity

Findings from epidemiological studies suggest that long-term exposure to lead may play a role in the development of Parkinson's disease *(Kuhn,1998)*. Moreover, the combination of lead with either iron or copper is even more closely associated with the disease *(Gorell)*.

Mercury Toxicity

Mercury is another heavy metal which may foster the development of Parkinson's disease. In a case-control study, after controlling for age, sex, ethnicity, fish consumption, medication intake, smoking and alcohol consumption, blood and urinary mercury were excellent predictors of the risk of Parkinson's disease, while hair mercury was a poor predictor *(Ngim)*.

BIBLIOGRAPHY

Abbott RA et al. Diet, body size and micronutrient status in Parkinson's disease. Eur J Clin Nutr 46:879-84, 1992

Agnoli A et al. New strategies in the management of Parkinson's disease: a biological approach using a phospholipid precursor (CDP-choline). Neuropsychobiology 8(6):289-96, 1982

AMA Drug Evaluations, Fifth Edition. Chicago, American Medical Association, 1983

Bains JS, Shaw CA. Neurodegenerative disorders in humans: the role of glutathione in oxidative stress-mediated neuronal death. Brain Res Brain Res Rev 25(3):335-58, 1997

Baker AB. Treatment of paralysis agitans with vitamin B6. JAMA 116:2484, 1941

Barbeau A. Lecithin in movement disorders, in A Barbeau, JH Growdon, RJ Wurtman, Eds. Choline and Lecithin in Brain Disorders. Nutrition and the Brain, Volume 5. New York, Raven Press, 1979:263-71

Beal MF et al. Coenzyme Q10 attenuates the 1-methyl-4-phenyl-1,2,3,tetrahydropyridine (MPTP) induced loss of striatal dopamine and dopaminergic axons in aged mice. Brain Res 783(1):109-14, 1998

Beasley BL et al. Treatment with tryptophan of levodopa-associated psychiatric disturbances. Arch Neurol 37(3):155-6, 1980

Bell IR et al. Irritable bowel and specific food intolerances in Parkinson's disease. Abstract. J Am Coll Nutr 12:615, 1993

Bender DA et al. Niacin depletion in Parkinsonian patients treated with L-dopa, benserazide and carbidopa. Clin Sci 56(1):89-93, 1979

Birkmayer W, Birkmayer JGD. Iron, a new aid in the treatment of Parkinson patients. J Neural Trans 67:287-92, 1986

Black MJ, Brandt RB. Nicotinic acid or N-methyl nicotinamide prolongs elevated brain dopa and dopamine in L-dopa treatment. Biochem Med Metab Biol 36(2):244-51, 1986

Bryant RC. Duration of illness and response to tryptophan in Parkinson's disease. Letter. Arch Neurol 37(10):677, 1980

Calabrese V et al. Cysteine-induced enhancement of lipid peroxidation in substantia nigra: comparative effect with exogenous administration of reduced glutathione. Drugs Exp Clin Res 23(1):25-31, 1997

Cambpell NR et al. Sinemet-ferrous sulphate interaction in patients with Parkinson's disease. Br J Clin Pharmacol 30(4):599-605, 1990

Cerhan JR et al. Antioxidant intake and risk of Parkinson's Disease in older women. Am J Epidemiol 139(11):S65, 1994

Coppen A et al. Levodopa and L-tryptophan therapy in parkinsonism. Lancet i:654-7, 1972

Critchley EMR. Evening primrose oil (Efamol) in parkinsonism and other tremors: A preliminary study, in DF Horrobin, Ed. Clinical Uses of Essential Fatty Acids. Montreal, Eden Press, 1982:205-8

Cuajungco MP, Lees GJ. Zinc metabolism in the brain: relevance to human neurodegenerative disorders. Neurobiol Dis 4(3-4):137-69, 1997

Cubells JM, Hernando C. Clinical trial on the use of cytidine diphosphate choline in Parkinson's disease. Clin Ther 10(6):664-71, 1988

de Rijk MC et al. Dietary antioxidants and Parkinson disease: The Rotterdam study. Arch Neurology 54:762-5, 1997

Dexter DT et al. Increased nigral iron content and alterations in other metal ions occurring in brain in Parkinson's disease. J Neurochem 52(6):1830-6, 1989

Dexter DT et al. Nigral dopaminergic cell loss in vitamin E deficient rats. Neuroreport 5(14):1773-6, 1994

Dizdar N et al. Treatment of Parkinson's disease with NADH. Acta Neurol Scand 90(5):345-7, 1994

Eberhardt R et al. Citicoline in the treatment of Parkinson's disease. Clin Ther 12(6):489-95, 1990

England H. Octacosanol helped his Parkinson's disease. Prevention, March, 1983

Factor SA et al. Vitamin E therapy in Parkinson's disease. Adv Neurol 53:457-61, 1990

Fahn S. An open trial of high-dosage antioxidants in early Parkinson's disease. Am J Clin Nutr 53:380S-1S, 1991

Fernandez-Calle P et al. Serum levels of ascorbic acid (vitamin C) in patients with Parkinson's disease. J Neurol Sci 118(1):25-8, 1993

Fernandez Pardal J et al. Ann Psiq Biol 3:234-6, 1974

Florence TM, Stauber JL. Neurotoxicity of manganese. Letter. Lancet i:363, 1988

Frank O et al. Superiority of periodic intramuscular vitamins over daily oral vitamins in maintaining normal vitamin titers in a geriatric population. Am J Clin Nutr 30:630, 1977

Garcia-Mas A et al. Effects of citicholine in subcortical dementia associated with Parkinson's disease assessed by quantified electroencephalography. Clin Ther 14(5):718-29, 1992

Golbe LI et al. Case-control study of early life dietary factors in Parkinson's disease. Arch Neurol 45:1350-3, 1988

Golbe LI et al. Follow-up study of early-life protective and risk factors in Parkinson's disease. Mov Disord 5(1):66-70, 1990

Gorell JM et al. Occupational exposures to metals as risk factors for Parkinson's disease. Neurology 48(3):650-8, 1997

Grimes JD et al. Prevention of progression of Parkinson's disease with antioxidative therapy. Prog Neuropsychopharmacol Biol Psychiatry 12(2-3):165-72, 1988

Growdon JH et al. Effects of oral L-tyrosine and homovanillic acid levels in patients with Parkinson's disease. Life Sci 30(10):827-32, 1982

Growdon JH. An overview of phosphatidylcholine, in I Hanin, GB Ansell, Eds. Lecithin. New York, Plenum Publishing Co., 1987

Haavik J, Toska K. Tyrosine hydroxylase and Parkinson's disease. Mol Neurobiol 16(3):285-309, 1998

Heller B, Fischer E. Diminution of phenylethylamine in the urine of Parkinson patients. Arzneimittelforschung 23(6):884-5, 1973

Heller B et al. Therapeutic action of D-phenylalanine in Parkinson's disease. Arzneimittelforschung 26:577-9, 1976

Hellenbrand W et al. Diet and Parkinson's disease. II: A possible role for the past intake of specific nutrients. Results from a self-administered food-frequency questionnaire in a case-control study. Neurology 47(3):644-50, 1996

Hirsch EC et al. Iron and aluminum increase in the substantia nigra of patients with Parkinson's disease: an X-ray microanalysis. J Neurochem 56(2):446-51, 1991

Hirsch EC, Faucheux BA. Iron metabolism and Parkinson's disease. Mov Disord 13 Suppl 1:39-45, 1998

Hoffer A. How to live longer and feel better - even with cancer. J Orthomol Med 11(3):147-67, 1996

Hornykiewicz O. Parkinson's disease: from brain homogenate to treatment. Fed Proc 32:183-90, 1973

Hurd RW et al. Treatment of four siblings with progressive myoclonus epilepsy of the Unverricht-Lundborg type with N-acetylcysteine. Neurology 47(5):1264-8, 1996

Issels RD et al. Promotion of cystine uptake and its utilization for glutathione biosynthesis induced by cysteamine and N-acetylcysteine. Biochem Pharmacol 37:881, 1988

Jellinger K et al. Brain iron and ferritin in Parkinson's and Alzheimer's diseases. J Neural Transm Park Dis Demt Sect 2(4):327-40, 1990

Jimenez-Jimenez FJ et al. Serum levels of beta-carotene and other carotenoids in Parkinson's disease. Neurosci Lett 157(1):103-6, 1993

Jimenez-Jimenez FJ et al. Cerebrospinal fluid levels of transition metals in patients with Parkinson's disease. J Neural Transm 105(4-5):497-505, 1998

Kieburtz K et al. The effect of deprenyl and tocopherol on cognitive performance in early untreated Parkinson's disease. Parkinson Study Group. Neurology 44(9):1756-9, 1994

Kuhn W et al. Parenteral application of NADH in Parkinson's disease: clinical improvement partially due to stimulation of endogenous levodopa biosynthesis. J Neural Transm 103(10):1187-93, 1996

Kuhn W et al. High prevalence of parkinsonism after occupational exposure to lead-sulfate batteries. Neurology 50(6):1885-6, 1998

Kunin RA. Meganutrition. New York, McGraw-Hill, 1980

Lehmann J. Levodopa and depression in Parkinsonism. Lancet i:140, 1971

Lemoine P et al. [L-tyrosine: a long-term treatment of Parkinson's disease.] C R Acad Sci [III] 309(2):43-7, 1989

Logroscino G et al. Dietary lipids and antioxidants in Parkinson's disease: a population-based, case-control study. Ann Neurol 39:89-94, 1996

Logroscino G et al. Altered systemic iron metabolism in Parkinson's disease. Neurology 49(3):714-7, 1997

Mayeux R et al. The relationship of serotonin to depression in Parkinson's disease. Mov Disord 3(3):237-44, 1988 (in German)

McCance-Katz EF et al. Serotonergic dysfunction in depression associated with Parkinson's disease. Neurology 42(9):1813-4, 1992

Meininger V et al. [L-methionine treatment of Parkinson's disease: preliminary results.] Rev Neurol (Paris) 138(4):297-303, 1982 (in French)

Mena MA et al. Levodopa toxicity is foetal rat midbrain neurones in culture: modulation by ascorbic acid. Neuro Rep 4:438-40, 1993

Mizuno Y et al. Mitochondrial dysfunction in Parkinson's disease. Ann Neurol 44(3 Suppl 1):S99-109, 1998

Ngim CH, Devathasan G. Epidemiologic study on the association between body burden mercury level and idiopathic Parkinson's disease. Neuroepidemiology 8(3):128-41, 1989

Nicole A et al. Direct evidence for glutathione as mediator of apoptosis in neuronal cells. Biomed Pharmacother 52(9):349-55, 1998

Nutt JG et al. The "on-off" phenomenon in Parkinson's disease. Relation to levodopa absorption and transport. N Engl J Med 310 (8):483-8, 1984

O'Dell BL. Roles of zinc and copper in the nervous system. Prog Clin Biol Res 380:147-62, 1993

Offen D et al. Prevention of dopamine-induced cell death by thiol antioxidants: possible implications for treatment of Parkinson's disease. Exp Neurol 141(1):32-9, 1996

Pall HS et al. Raised cerebrospinal-fluid copper concentration in Parkinson's disease. Lancet ii:238-41, 1987

Papavasiliou PS, Rosal V. Effects of choline in patients with levodopa-induced dyskinesia, in A Barbeau, JH Growdon, RJ Wurtman, Eds. Choline and Lecithin in Brain Disorders. Nutrition and the Brain, Volume 5. New York, Raven Press, 1979:335-41

Paré S et al. Effect of daytime protein restriction on nutrient intakes of free-living Parkinson's disease patients. Am J Clin Nutr 55:701-7, 1992

Parkinson Study Group. Effects of tocopherol and deprenyl on the progression of disability in early Parkinson's disease. N Engl J Med 328:176-83, 1993

Parkinson Study Group. Impact of deprenyl and tocopherol treatment on Parkinson's disease in DATATOP patients requiring levodopa. Ann Neurol 39(1):37-45, 1996

Pearce RK et al. Alterations in the distribution of glutathione in the substantia nigra in Parkinson's disease. J Neural Transm 104(6-7):661-77, 1997

Peers R. Fatty diet, mitochondria and Parkinson's disease. Letter. N Z Med J 110(1041):132, 1997

Reilly DK et al. On-off effects in Parkinson's disease: a controlled investigation of ascorbic acid therapy. Adv Neurol 37:51-60, 1983

Riederer P et al. Transition metals, ferritin, glutathione, and ascorbic acid in parkinsonian brains. J Neurochem 52(2):515-20, 1989

Sacks W, Simpson GM. Ascorbic acid in levodopa therapy. Letter. Lancet i:527, 1975

Sandyk R, Fisher H. L-tryptophan supplementation in Parkinson's disease. Int J Neurosci 45(3-4):215-9, 1989

Scadding GK et al. Poor sulphoxidation ability in patients with food sensitivity. Br Med J 297:105-7, 1988

Secades JJ, Frontera G. CDP-choline: pharmacological and clinical review. Methods Find Exp Clin Pharmacol 17 Suppl B:2-54, 1995

Sechi G et al. Reduced intravenous glutathione in the treatment of early Parkinson's disease. Prog Neuropsychopharmacol Biol Psychiatry 20:1159-70, 1996

Shibuya M et al. Effects of CDP-choline on striatal dopamine level and behavior in rats. Jpn J Pharmacol 31(1):47-52, 1981

Shoulson I. DATATOP: a decade of neuroprotective inquiry. Parkinson Study Group. Deprenyl And Tocopherol Antioxidative Therapy Of Parkinsonism. Ann Neurol 44(3 Suppl 1):S160-1, 1998

Shults CW et al. Absorption, tolerability, and effects on mitochondrial activity of oral coenzyme Q10 in parkinsonian patients. Neurology 50(3):793-5, 1998

Singh RB et al. Dietary intake and plasma levels of antioxidant vitamins in health and disease: a hospital-based case-control study. J Nutr Environ Med 5:235-42, 1995

Smythies JR, Halsey JH. Treatment of Parkinson's disease with L-methionine. South Med J 77:1577, 1984

Snider SR. Octacosanol in parkinsonism. Letter. Ann Neurol 16(6):723, 1984

Snyder RD, Friedman MB. Enhancement of cytotoxicity and clastogenicity of L-DOPA and dopamine by manganese and copper. Mutat Res 405(1):1-8, 1998

Sofic E et al. Selective increase of iron in substantia nigra zona compacta of parkinsonian brains. J Neurochem 56(3):978-82, 1991

Steventon GB et al. Xenobiotic metabolism in Parkinson's disease. Neurology 39(7):883-7, 1989

Strijks E et al. Q10 therapy in patients with idiopathic Parkinson's disease. Mol Aspects Med 18 Suppl:S237-40, 1997

Surtees R, Hyland K. L-3,4-dihydroxyphenylalanine (levodopa) lowers central nervous system S-adenosylmethionine concentrations in humans. J Neurol Neurosurg Psychiatry 53(7):569-72, 1990

Swerdlow RH et al. Origin and functional consequences of the complex I defect in Parkinson's disease. Ann Neurol 40(4):663-71, 1996

Tohgi H et al. Concentrations of serotonin and its related substances in the cerebrospinal fluid of parkinsonian patients and their relations to the severity of symptoms. Neurosci Lett 150(1):71-4, 1993a

Tohgi H et al. Alterations in the concentration of serotonergic and dopaminergic substances in the cerebrospinal fluid of patients with Parkinson's disease, and their changes after L-dopa administration. Neurosci Lett 159(1-2):135-8, 1993b

Tsui J et al. The effect of dietary protein on the efficacy of L-dopa: A double-blind study. Neurology 39:549-52, 1989

Uitti RJ et al. Regional metal concentrations in Parkinson's disease, other chronic neurological diseases, and control brains. Can J Neurol Sci 16(3):310-4, 1989

Vaĭnshtok AB. [Treatment of parkinsonism with large doses of vitamin B6.] Sov Med (7):14-9, 1979 (in Russian)

Vilming ST. [Diet therapy in Parkinson disease.] Tidsskr Nor Laegeforen 115(10):1244-7, 1995 (in Norwegian)

Vrecko K et al. Stimulation of dopamine biosynthesis in cultured PC 12 phaeochromocytoma cells by the coenzyme nicotinamide adeninedinucleotide (NADH). J Neurol Transm Park Dis Dement Sect 5(2):147-56, 1993

Weiss GB. Metabolism and actions of CDP-choline as an endogenous compound and administered exogenously as citicoline. Life Sci 56(9):637-60, 1995

Yamaguchi T et al. Effects of tyrosine administration on serum biopterin in normal controls and patients with Parkinson's disease. Science 219:75-7, 1983

Yapa S. Detection of subclinical ascorbate deficiency in early Parkinson's disease. Public Health 106:393-5, 1992

Yasui M et al. Calcium, magnesium and aluminum concentrations in Parkinson's disease. Neurotoxicology 13(3):593-600, 1992

Yasui M et al. Magnesium-related neurological disorders, in Mineral and Metal Neurotoxicology CRC Press, 1997:219-26

Zayed J et al. [Environmental factors in the etiology of Parkinson's disease.] Can J Neurol Sci 17(3):286-91, 1990

PEPTIC ULCERS

NUTRITIONAL TREATMENT GUIDE

✓ = Efficacy generally accepted.
* = Efficacy *demonstrated* by controlled human trials.
[+] = Efficacy *suspected* from uncontrolled human experiments
[-] = Efficacy *suspected* from indirect data
? = Efficacy *challenged* in at least one study of similar design

DIETARY FACTORS

* avoid **Milk**
* ? high **dietary Fiber** intake

- - - - - - - - - - - - - - - - - - - -

[+] avoid **Alcohol**
[+] avoid **Caffeine**
[+] avoid **Coffee**, even if decaffeinated
[+] avoid **Tea** except for **Black Tea (*Camellia sinensis*)**
[+] avoid **refined Sugar**

NUTRITIONAL FACTORS

✓ **Aluminum:** aluminum hydroxide gel 5 to 30 ml daily
✓ **Bismuth:** 120 mg 4 times daily 20 minutes before meals and at bedtime
✓ **Magnesium:** magnesium hydroxide (dosage depends upon the frequency and intensity of the pain and upon bowel function)

- - - - - - - - - - - - - - - - - - - -

* **Calcium:** calcium carbonate ? 1 g one and three hours after meals and at bedtime
* **Cysteine:** *to protect against ulcer recurrence:* D,L-cysteine 200 mg 4 times daily
* **Omega-3 fatty acids:** *to prevent NSAID-induced injury AND to treat peptic ulcers:* ? 2 g of a combination of EPA & DHA 3 times daily
* **S-Methylmethionine:** *to protect against ulcer recurrence:* raw cabbage juice 1 liter daily
* **Vitamin A:** *to improve ulcer healing:* 50,000 IU 3 times daily (short term only)
* **Vitamin C:** *to prevent aspirin-induced gastroduodenal injury:* 1 g twice daily (as mineral ascorbates)
* **Zinc:** *to prevent NSAID-induced gastroduodenal injury AND to treat peptic ulcers:* zinc acexamate 300 mg at bedtime *OR* zinc sulfate 220 mg 3 times daily

- - - - - - - - - - - - - - - - - - - -

[+] **Glutamine:** *to protect against aspirin-induced gastric lesions and to improve healing of peptic ulcers:* L-glutamine 400 mg 4 times daily 1 hour before meals and before retiring
[+] **Iron deficiency:** *to replete low iron stores from hemorrhage:* 30 mg twice daily until repletion
[+] **Omega-6 fatty acids:** *example:* evening primrose oil 3 g daily (6 week trial)
[+] **Vitamin C deficiency:** *to reduce the risk of hemorrhage:* 500 mg twice daily
[+] **Vitamin E:** ? 400 to 800 IU daily

- - - - - - - - - - - - - - - - - - - -

[-] **Selenium deficiency:** 200 μg daily
[-] **Vitamin A:** *to reduce the risk of peptic ulcers from hyperchlorhydria or non-steroidal anti-inflammatory drugs*

OTHER RELATED FACTORS

* rule out **Food Sensitivities**

DIETARY FACTORS

There are various recommendations regarding the timing of meals, although few are based on scientific studies. Small, frequent feedings, while they used to be recommended, have not been shown to be preferable to 3 meals a day. If fact, although some patients find that they have less symptoms with more frequent feedings - especially during exacerbations - authorities now advise against extra feedings because of increased acid secretion, although stomach distension with large quantities of food is generally discouraged *(Marotta)*.

Advice to consume an early dinner is one recommendation that is based on experimental evidence. When healthy volunteers ate standardized meals at 7 am and 12 noon, dinner at either 6 pm or 9 pm in random order, and went to bed at a standardized time, nocturnal pH was significantly higher when they ate the early dinner, suggesting that an early dinner may be beneficial by reducing nocturnal gastric acidity *(Duroux)*.

Bland Diet

Current evidence does not support the tradition of placing ulcer patients on restrictive bland diets. The major goal of diet is to avoid extreme elevations of gastric acid secretion and the direct irritation of gastric mucosa.

Spices, in particular *black pepper*, *red pepper*, and *chilli* powder, may produce dyspepsia *(Marotta)*. However, when duodenal ulcer patients were given red chilli powder with each meal for 4 weeks, their rate of ulcer healing was unchanged *(Kumar, 1984)*.

If fact, recent animal work suggests that *capsaicin*, the pungent principle of hot pepper, actually has a gastroprotective effect *(Abdel-Salam)*. It thus seems unwarranted to restrict spices unless they cause discomfort.

Dietary Fiber

Soluble dietary fiber slows gastric emptying by increasing the viscosity of the stomach contents. A study of 47,000 male health professionals followed for 6 years found a one-third reduction in risk for men who had 7 or more servings of fruit or vegetables per day compared to those who had fewer than 3 servings per day. Moreover, total dietary fiber, and particularly soluble fiber, was inversely related with duodenal ulcer risk *(Aldoori, 1997a)*.

There is also some evidence from experimental studies that a high intake of dietary fiber may be protective against the formation and relapse of duodenal ulcers *(Malhotra; Rydning, 1982)*, perhaps because refined foods move faster from the stomach to the duodenum, resulting in less buffering and greater acidity *(Grimes)*.

Not all experimental studies have found the addition of dietary fiber to be effective, however *(Kang, 1988; Rydning, 1985)*. Because of the many differences between studies, more studies are needed to clarify the picture.

Alcohol

Epidemiological studies have generally failed to find evidence that alcohol intake is associated with the risk of peptic ulcers *(Aldoori, 1997b; Kato)*. Yet, in a study of roughly 1,000 patients, alcohol ingestion precipitated pain in half those with duodenal ulcer compared to none of the patients with biliary disease *(Kang, 1992)*.

Ethanol ingestion may stimulate an increase in gastric acid secretion *(Lenz)* and a superficial injury to gastric mucosa *(Yeomans)*. Even though the injury is usually resurfaced in 1 or 2 hours *(Yeomans)*, this finding suggests that ethanol may cause pain in peptic ulcer disease by irritating the area of injury.

Coffee

Coffee strongly stimulates gastric acid secretion and can induce dyspepsia *(Marotta;McArthur)* and abdominal pain *(Kang,1992)* in patients. In a study of 150 duodenal ulcer patients, they were found to stop drinking coffee or to reduce the intake significantly after symptoms started due to dyspeptic complaints *(Eisig)*. However, coffee intake does not appear to be associated with the risk of duodenal ulcer *(Aldoori,1997b)*.

Tea

Primarily due to a local chemical action on the gastric mucosa, many teas are potent stimulators of gastric acid secretion *(Dubey)*. However, results of an animal study suggest that black tea (*Camellia sinensis*) actually has anti-ulcer activity, probably mediated through prostaglandins. Black tea extract favorably altered the changes in acid and peptic activity of gastric secretion produced by a number of inciting substances and significantly reduced ulcer formation *(Maity)*.

Caffeine

The question of the contribution of caffeine to the effect of coffee and other caffeine-containing beverages has been explored in several studies. A large, recent prospective cohort study found little association between caffeine-containing beverages and the risk of duodenal ulcer *(Aldoori,1997b)*. However, noncoffee caffeine-containing beverages (tea and soft drinks) stimulate acid secretion *(Marotta)*, and there is evidence that caffeine may exacerbate preexisting conditions and increase ulcer symptoms *(Turnberg)*. Therefore, like coffee, it is best avoided by patients, especially if its intake worsens their symptoms.

Decaffeinated Coffee

Since both regular coffee and caffeine stimulate acid secretion, it is possible that decaffeinated coffee may not do so. Unfortunately, decaffeinated coffee also stimulates gastric acid secretion *(Elta;Marotta)*. As with regular coffee and caffeine, it has not been shown to cause peptic ulceration.

Milk

Milk, formerly recommended in the treatment of peptic ulcer *(Farrar)*, has been found to have only a transient neutralizing effect on gastric acidity, after which gastric secretion rises *(McArthur;Ippoliti)*.

In one study, 65 duodenal ulcer patients being treated with cimetidine were randomized to receive either a normal hospital diet or one consisting exclusively of milk, with both groups allowed to add fruit and sugar as desired. After 4 weeks, endoscopic exams showed that, while the ulcers had healed in 78% of patients who consumed the hospital diet, only 53% of the patients on the milk diet had healing of their ulcers, suggesting that milk, at least when not consumed as part of a regular meal, is contraindicated for patients with active ulcers *(Kumar,1986)*.

Sugar

Refined sugar intake appears to be correlated with the risk of duodenal ulcers, even after controlling for smoking, social class and relative weight *(Katschinski)*. The results of experimental work suggest that this association exists because sugar promotes the development of peptic ulcers.

In one study, 41 ulcer patients followed a low-carbohydrate diet (60-70 gm/day) for 3 months followed by a high-carbohydrate diet (the standard "gastric diet") for 3 months. Twenty-eight of the patients felt better on the low-carbohydrate diet, 11 noted no difference and only 2 of the 41 felt better on the high-carbohydrate diet *(Yudkin)*.

In order to ascertain whether the reduction in dietary starch or the reduction in sugar (sucrose) was the cause of symptomatic improvement from the low-carbohydrate diet, healthy young volunteers were placed on a high sugar diet in which dietary starch was reduced by the same amount that sugar was increased. A test meal before breakfast revealed an increase in peak gastric and pepsin activities, suggesting that sugar had a detrimental effect as compared to starch *(Yudkin)*.

NUTRITIONAL FACTORS

VITAMINS

Vitamin A

A recent prospective study of 47,000 males found that vitamin A from all sources (including supplements) was the only nutrient whose intake was inversely related to the risk of duodenal ulcer. Men who had the highest intake had a 45% reduction in ulcer risk *(Aldoori,1997a)*.

Moreover, there is evidence that supplementation may protect against peptic ulceration. In an animal study, supplementation with vitamin A prevented the development of duodenal ulcers due to excessive stomach acid *(Mahmood)*.

Results of another animal study suggest that vitamin A supplementation is effective in preventing the development of peptic ulcers due to the use of aspirin *(Rettura)*. There is also evidence vitamin A supplementation may prevent the development of stress ulcers. In a randomized controlled trial, part of a group of 52 patients who had had severe physiological stresses from burns, organ injuries or post-operative organ disturbances received vitamin A. Sixty-three percent of the controls but only 18% of those receiving vitamin A developed stress ulcers, a significant difference *(Chernow)*.

Vitamin A supplementation appears to aid in ulcer healing. Fours weeks after patients with chronic gastric ulcers received either antacids alone or antacids plus vitamin A in a controlled trial, the addition of vitamin A resulted in a significantly greater number of patients with completely healed ulcers and a significantly greater reduction in ulcer size *(Patty)*.

Vitamin B_6

Patients with active gastric, but not duodenal, peptic ulcers usually have below normal levels of fasting serum pyridoxal *(Sanderson,1975)*. As patients with other forms of gastric pathology have a similar finding *(Sanderson,1976)*, pyridoxal deficiency appears to be a non-specific indicator of gastric pathology.

Unfortunately, only one preliminary trial has been published concerning the efficacy of vitamin B_6 supplementation in preventing or treating peptic ulceration *(Lemeshko)*. There are, however, animal studies which found that pyridoxine supplementation combated the development of stress-induced gastric ulcerations *(Henrotte)*.

Until more is known, the efficacy of the vitamin in preventing or treating peptic ulcers remains uncertain.

Vitamin C

Results of an early study suggest that patients with chronic peptic ulcer commonly have an inadequate intake of vitamin C *(Riggs)*. A more recent study reached a similar conclusion, but also found that, after treatment, ascorbate intake returned to normal *(Cohen)*, suggesting that the low intake may have been due to ulcer symptoms. Laboratory studies have repeatedly found that patients have evidence of reduced vitamin C nutriture *(Dubey; Esposito)*.

Guinea pigs fed a vitamin-C deficient diet develop peptic ulcerations *(Smith)*, suggesting that vitamin C deficiency may contribute to the development of the illness. In addition, vitamin C nutriture is poorer in patients with gastrointestinal hemorrhage (whether or not they have peptic ulcers) as compared to patients with uncomplicated peptic ulcers, suggesting that patients with vitamin C deficiency are more prone to hemorrhage *(Portnoy;Russell)*.

It appears that vitamin C is secreted by the stomach *(O'Connor;Sobala)*, and patients have been found to have reduced gastric vitamin C levels *(O'Connor)*. Infection with *Helicobacter pylori* is now known to be a major contributor to the development of peptic ulcers, and gastric juice vitamin C is lower in *H. pylori*-positive patients than in *H. pylori*-negative patients *(Rokkas)*. Furthermore, eradication of *H. pylori* is associated with a normalization of gastric juice ascorbate levels *(Rokkas)*.

Supplementation

Whether vitamin C supplementation aids in the eradication of *H. Pylori* is unknown, and there are few studies investigating the treatment of peptic ulcers by providing vitamin C supplementation, even with the relatively modest goal of normalizing ascorbate nutriture.

We do know that treatment with intravenous vitamin C (along with atropine) appears to be at least as effective as other intravenous therapies *(Debray)*. When combined with ferrous sulfate, the healing index of gastric, but not of duodenal, ulcers was higher than that of controls *(Miwa)*. Moreover, when combined with antacids, the addition of ascorbic acid was associated with longer remissions and fewer relapses when compared to controls *(Nash)*.

There is another application of vitamin C therapy that has demonstrated its efficacy. In a double-blind crossover study, vitamin C was shown to protect against aspirin-induced duodenal injury *(McAlindon)*.

More studies are needed to better ascertain the therapeutic efficacy of vitamin C in treating peptic ulcerations, although correction of a vitamin C deficiency is certainly warranted. Since ascorbic acid is mildly acidic, and thus could irritate the ulcer, the vitamin should be given as an ascorbate salt.

Vitamin E

Healthy volunteers placed on a vitamin E-deficient diet develop gastric ulcers *(Horwitt)*. Recent Russian work has suggested that peptic ulcer disease may be associated with both an enhancement of lipid peroxidation and a deficit of vitamin E *(Litinskaia)*. Moreover, an animal model of gastric mucosal injury (ischemia-reperfusion) found that both serum and gastric mucosal alpha-tocopherol levels decreased after injury, suggesting that vitamin E is consumed in the process *(Yoshikawa)*.

Animal *(Yoshikawa)* and human *(Litinskaia)* studies have found vitamin E supplementation to protect against gastric ulceration, and early Russian studies have suggested that vitamin E supplementation may aid in the healing of peptic ulcers of both the stomach and the duodenum *(Arutiniunian;Toteva)*. Controlled studies are needed to confirm these findings.

MINERALS

Aluminum

Aluminum hydroxide is well known to enhance the healing of peptic ulcers *(Poynard)*. The use of aluminum salts has been questioned recently, however, because of growing evidence that aluminum exposure may promote the development of Alzheimer's dementia.

There is a highly significant increase in serum aluminum concentrations following the ingestion of aluminum hydroxide *(Berstad)* although, due to its rapid excretion, it appears that there is no danger of aluminum accumulation in the tissues so long as renal function is normal *(Nagy)*. In fact, in a case-control study, the overall adjusted odds ratio for the use of aluminum-containing antacids in regard to the risk of Alzheimer's dementia was only 0.7, and there was no significant dose-response trend *(Graves)*.

A Warning

Although current evidence fails to implicate aluminum hydroxide in Alzheimer's dementia, it has been shown to bind phosphorus and thus interfere with its absorption *(Lotz)*. Therefore, if aluminum hydroxide is taken regularly over a period of time, a phosphorus deficiency could develop leading to osteomalacia and other adverse effects.

Bismuth

Bismuth inhibits the growth of *Helicobacter pylori* both *in vitro* and *in vivo (McNulty)*, and it also appears to have other ulcer-healing properties *(Qvigstad)*. Commercial bismuth compounds have been shown to be as effective as the H2-receptor antagonists but with a lower relapse rate *(Gorbach; Wagstaff)*.

However, due to the suspicion that neurological toxicity could develop with chronic use, a course of bismuth treatment should be limited to a maximum of 6 to 8 weeks with an 8-week interval between a further course of treatment *(Gorbach)*.

Calcium

Calcium carbonate is a potent antacid which is converted in the stomach to calcium chloride. However, its ingestion is followed by increased gastric acid secretion. While magnesium and aluminum hydroxide may do the same, the data are less convincing. The clinical relevance of this acid rebound has yet to be thoroughly investigated, and limited data suggest no obvious clinically significant deleterious effect from the use of calcium carbonate in peptic ulcer *(Hade;McGuigan)*.

A Warning

Regular ingestion of large doses of calcium carbonate over a long period of time may occasionally cause the milk-alkali syndrome marked by hypercalcemia and low parathormone *(Olshewski)*. It should therefore be used with appropriate caution.

Iron Deficiency

The presence of iron deficiency should suggest an evaluation for peptic ulcers and other gastrointestinal pathology. Among patients with chronic iron deficiency anemia, benign duodenal ulceration was found in between 6 and 16 percent of patients in 3 different studies *(Jolobe)*. Moreover, when patients with serum ferritin values of $\leq$ 50 ng/ml were evaluated, 46 out of 143 (about one-third) were found to have acid peptic disease *(Lee)*.

Magnesium

Magnesium hydroxide is a potent and effective antacid when prescribed as a liquid formulation *(McGuigan)*. Compared to aluminum hydroxide, magnesium hydroxide appears to be more effective in treating both gastric and duodenal ulcers *(Grebenev)*.

As magnesium salts may produce loosening of the stools, they are often combined with aluminum hydroxide (which is constipating) *(McGuigan)*. The efficacy of this combination may be at least equal to that of drugs such as ranitidine (an H2-blocker), omeprazole (a gastric acid pump inhibitor) and misoprostol (a prostaglandin E1 analog) *(Caspary;Mach;Schmassmann)*.

Warnings

Like aluminum hydroxide, magnesium supplements may interfere with phosphorus absorption. Thus, with chronic use at high dosages, osteomalacia and other adverse effect could occur *(Lotz)*.

Also, magnesium absorption and urinary excretion causes alkalinization of the urine. Magnesium supplementation could thus cause hypermagnesemia in the presence of renal insufficiency *(Herzog)*.

Selenium

Gastric tissue levels of patients with ulcers are markedly low when compared, not only to healthy subjects, but also when compared to patients with a variety of other gastric pathologies *(Burguera)*.

Conversely, the results of animal studies suggest that selenium possesses important anti-ulcer properties *(al-Moutairy;Parmar)*. Therefore, until more is known about the relationship between selenium nutriture and peptic ulcers, it appears reasonable to replete any evidence of selenium deficiency, especially since marginal selenium nutriture is fairly common.

Zinc

Patients may have reduced plasma and serum zinc levels *(Bandyopadhyay;Erzinkian)*. However, the zinc content of the gastric mucosa may be elevated, suggesting a shift of zinc from the serum to the gastric mucosa *(Bandyopadhyay)*.

Zinc is an important element in the process of wound healing. While, in an animal model, zinc deficiency did not affect the formation of acetic acid-induced gastric ulcers, it reduced cell proliferation and delayed ulcer healing *(Watanabe)*.

Supplementation

When duodenal ulcer patients received zinc supplementation, basal acid secretion was reduced by more than half *(Puscas)*. When zinc acexamate, the first zinc compound developed for use in peptic ulcer therapy, was compared under double-blind conditions to famotidine in the treatment of acute duodenal ulcer, both treatments were equally effective, with a reduction of more than half of the ulcer diameter in about 80% of each of the two patient groups after 4 weeks *(Garcia-Plaza)*. In another double-blind study, zinc acexamate was found effective in the prevention of gastroduodenal damage due to non-steroidal anti-inflammatory drugs, with a 92% reduction in the incidence of gastric and duodenal ulcers *(Rodriguez de la Serna)*.

In a review of 13 randomized studies of zinc acexamate, the salt was found to be superior to placebo and equal to H2 receptor antagonist drugs for patients with either gastric or duodenal peptic ulcers *(Jimenez)*.

Zinc acexamate is not the only zinc salt to have shown evidence of efficacy. Zinc sulfate has been compared to placebo under double-blind conditions. Fifteen patients with gastric ulcers and normal zinc levels randomly received either zinc sulfate or placebo. The 2 patient groups were comparable in all respects, including initial ulcer size.

After 3 weeks the absolute reduction in size of the ulcer crater based on barium-meal x-ray films was 3 times as great in the treated group. Complete healing of ulcers occurred more frequently in the patients taking zinc sulphate than in patients treated with placebo, while the placebo group contained more patients whose ulcers did not heal at all than the group taking zinc sulphate *(Frommer)*.

OTHER NUTRITIONAL FACTORS

Glutamine

L-glutamine has been shown in animal studies to protect against gastric lesions produced by aspirin *(Mitra;Okabe)*. Moreover, 4 weeks after 57 patients received either glutamine or lactose in addition to standard treatment, all but 2 of the 24 patients receiving glutamine showed complete healing on x-ray compared to only half of the lactose group *(Shive)*.

Sulfhydryl-containing Nutrients

Various nutrients which contain a sulfhydryl group have been found to provide protection against early vascular injury in ulcers due to chemical injury without inhibiting acid secretion *(Szabo,1986)*. They have also been shown to be effective in reducing the recurrence rate of duodenal ulceration under double-blind conditions *(Salim)*.

While prostaglandins have a similar effect, only sulfhydryl compounds enter directly into protective reactions such as free radical scavenging, modification of receptor sulfhydryl groups, and oxidation of certain structural and enzyme proteins *(Szabo,1986)*. Moreover, they stimulate the formation of gastrointestinal mucus *(Salim)*.

Glutathione

Important to cellular defense against the damaging effects of free radicals, glutathione is a tripeptide composed of the amino acids cysteine, glutamic acid and glycine. In gastric ulcer, there is a dramatic decrease in stomach glutathione levels *(Giorgi)*.

In vitro, cellular stores of reduced glutathione have been shown to protect against acid-induced gastric mucosal cell damage. Moreover, the addition of L-cysteine successfully increased cellular glutathione and decreased cell lysis by acid *(Mutoh)*. Since the systemic bioavailability of oral glutathione supplements is uncertain *(Smith C; Witchi)*, cysteine supplementation should thus be a method of assuring adequate cellular glutathione levels cells vulnerable to acid damage.

Cysteine

The efficacy of cysteine in protecting against ulcer recurrence was demonstrated in a double-blind study. Two hundred twenty-one smokers with healed duodenal ulcerations received D,L-cysteine, cimetidine, or placebo. The cumulative relapse rate after one year was 64% for placebo, 30% for cimetidine, and only 11% for cysteine *(Salim)*.

S-Methylmethionine ('Vitamin U')

Found in trace amounts in certain raw foods, particularly green vegetables, S-methylmethionine appears to speed the healing of peptic ulcers. In one study, 26 patients received concentrated cabbage juice, a rich source of S-methylmethionine. Ninety-two percent of a group of 26 treated patients showed healing on x-ray after 3 weeks of treatment as compared to 32% of 19 controls *(Cheney)*. (Cabbage juice is also rich in glutamine which may also have contributed to its benefits.) Moreover, S-methylmethionine has been shown to protect dogs against the development of experimental ulcers *(Szabo,1960)*.

A man was informed by his physician that x-rays showed that his old peptic ulcer had returned and a new one had formed. The pain ceased almost as soon as he started drinking 5 glasses of raw cabbage juice daily. After one week, he decreased the cabbage juice to 3 glasses daily.

When, two months later, he was re-examined, both ulcers had healed (Bricklin).

Omega-3 Fatty Acids

Supplementation with fish oil, a rich source of omega-3 fatty acids, may reduce gastric erosions and ulcers caused by the ingestion of ethanol, aspirin, acid or alkali, perhaps by 'stealing' glutathione available for leukotriene synthesis *(Rogers;Szabo,1988)*. Also, *in vitro*, omega-3 fatty acids have been shown to inhibit the growth of *Helicobacter pylori (Thompson)*.

When 21 patients received a fish oil preparation, 85% demonstrated cicatrization of the ulcer compared to 60% of those who did not take fish oil, suggesting that it stimulated the reparative process (*Matushevskaia*). In an animal study, fish oil was shown to inhibit indomethacin-induced gastric ulceration in a dose-dependent manner *(Al-Meshal)*.

Omega-6 Fatty Acids

There is some evidence that patients may have a reduced intake of linoleic acid *(Kearney)*. Moreover, some studies of adipose tissue levels of linoleic acid in patients have found those levels to be decreased *(Grant;Kearney)*.

While, *in vitro*, omega-6 fatty acids have been found to inhibit the growth of *Helicobacter pylori (Thompson)*, their efficacy in preventing and treating peptic ulcers has been poorly studied. In an open trial, patients who received evening primrose oil had healing of their ulcers in 4 to 6 weeks *(Das)*.

FOOD SENSITIVITIES

Food sensitivities, including atopic allergies, are common among patients *(De Lazzari;Budagovskaia;Kaess)* and appear to contribute to the development of peptic ulceration. Back in 1942, Pollard and Stuart demonstrated that reactive foods delayed gastric emptying and caused severe gastric hyperemia and edema *(Pollard).* Siegel found that 98% of patients with x-ray evidence of peptic ulcer had coexisting respiratory tract allergies *(Siegel,1974).*

Biopsies from the edges of gastric and duodenal ulcers demonstrate a marked increase of immunoglobulin E-containing cells at the lesion edges, suggesting a local anaphylactic reaction *(Andre).*

When 30 patients with food allergies confirmed by double-blind challenge studies had food allergens applied to the gastric mucosa, all showed macroscopic reactions such as swelling, erosions and bleeding, although skin and RAST tests were positive for those foods only half of the time *(Reimann).* Avoiding the implicated foods may improve healing and prevent recurrence *(Siegel,1977).*

A 46 year-old woman with x-ray evidence of a gastric ulcer and a history of migraines failed to respond to a high-milk diet. She was placed on a 5-day lamb, pear and bottled spring water diet.

Initially she experienced the worst migraine of her life, requiring injections of pain relievers. When foods were reintroduced, she found that she reacted to cow's milk products; by avoiding these, she experienced a rapid clearing of her ulcer symptoms and subsequently remained asymptomatic (Davies).

BIBLIOGRAPHY

Abdel-Salam OM et al. Capsaicin and the stomach. A review of experimental and clinical data. J Physiol Paris 91(3-5):151-71, 1997

Aldoori WH et al. Prospective study of diet and the risk of duodenal ulcer in men. Am J Epidemiol 145(1):42-50, 1997a

Aldoori WH et al. A prospective study of alcohol, smoking, caffeine, and the risk of duodenal ulcer in men. Epidemiology 8(4):420-4, 1997b

Al-Meshal MA et al. Cod liver oil inhibits indomethacin induced gastropathy without affecting its bioavailability and pharmacological activity. Life Sci 48:1401-9, 1991

al-Moutairy AR, Tariq M. Effect of vitamin E and selenium on hypothermic restraint stress and chemically-induced ulcers. Dig Dis Sci 41(6):1165-71, 1996

Andre C et al. Evidence for anaphylactic reactions in peptic ulcer and varioliform gastritis. Ann Allergy 51:325-7, 1983

Arutiniunian VM et al. [Use of alpha-tocopherol acetate (vitamin E) and sodium nucleinate in the treatment of patients with stomach and duodenal ulcer.] Klin Med (Mosk) 6194):52-4, 1983

Bandyopadhyay B et al. Serum zinc level : a possible index in the pathogenesis of peptic ulcer syndrome. Biochem Mol Biol Int 36(5):965-72, 1995

Berstad A et al. Controlled clinical trial of duodenal ulcer healing with antacid tablets. Scand J Gastroenterol 17(7):953-9, 1982

Bricklin M. Rodale's Encyclopedia of Natural Home Remedies. Emmaus, PA, Rodale Press, 1982

Budagovskaia VN, Voitko, NE. [Allergic reactions in patients with peptic ulcer; incidence of food and drug allergy.] Vopr Pitan (3):30-3, 1984 (in Russian)

Burguera JL et al. Gastric tissue selenium levels in healthy persons, cancer and non-cancer patients with different kinds of mucosal damage. J Trace Elem Med Biol 9(3):160-4, 1995

Caspary WF et al. Low-dose antacid therapy in the treatment of duodenal ulcer--a multicentre double-blind trial vs. misoprostol. Z Gastroenterol 29(9):411-6, 1991

Cheney G. Calif Med, January, 1956

Chernow MS et al. Stress ulcer: A preventable disease. J Trauma 12:831, 1972

Cohen MM, Duncan AM. Ascorbic acid nutrition and gastroduodenal disorders. Br Med J 4:516-18, 1967

Das UN et al. Essential fatty acids and peptic ulcer disease. Letter. Gut 28(7):914-16, 1987

De Lazzari F et al. High IgE serum levels and "peptic" ulcers: clinical and functional approach. Ital J Gastroenterol 26(1):7-11, 1994

Davies S, Stewart A. Nutritional Medicine. London, Pan Books, 1987

Debray C et al. [Treatment of gastro-duodenal ulcers with large doses of ascorbic acid.] Sem Ther 44:393-8, 1968 (in French)

Dubey SS et al. Ascorbic acid, dehydroascorbic acid, glutathione and histamine in peptic ulcer. Indian J Med Res 76:859-62, 1982

Duroux P et al. Early dinner reduces nocturnal gastric acidity. Gut 30(8):1063-7, 1989

Eisig JN et al. Coffee drinking in patients with duodenal ulcer and a control population. Scand J Gastroenterol 24(7):796-8, 1989

Elta GH et al. Comparison of coffee intake and coffee-induced symptoms in patients with duodenal ulcer, nonulcer dyspepsia, and normal controls. Am J Gastroenterol 85(10):1339-42, 1990

Erzinkian KL et al. [Zinc metabolism in duodenal ulcer.] Ross Med Zh (5-12):14-5, 1992 (in Russian

Esposito R, Valentini R. Vitamin C and gastroduodenal disorders. Letter. Br Med J 2(597):118, 1968

Farrar GE Jr. Milestones in clinical pharmacology. Remember the Sippy regimen for peptic ulcer? Clin Ther 11(2):278-9, 1989

Frommer DJ. The healing of gastric ulcers by zinc sulphate. Med J Aust 793-6, 1975

Garcia-Plaza A et al. [A multicenter clinical trial. Zinc acexamate versus famotidine in the treatment of acute duodenal ulcer. Study Group of Zinc acexamate]. Rev Esp Enferm Dig 88(11):757-62, 1996 (in Spanish)

Giorgi G et al. Glutathione (GSH) in human stomach mucosa. Riv Eur Sci Med Farmacol 11(2):163-7, 1989

Gorbach SL. Bismuth therapy in gastrointestinal diseases. Gastroenterology 99(3):863-75, 1990

Grant HW et al. Duodenal ulcer is associated with low dietary linoleic acid intake. Gut 31(9):997-8, 1990

Graves AB et al. The association between aluminum-containing products and Alzheimer's disease. J Clin Epidemiol 43(1):35-44, 1990

Grebenev AL et al. [A comparative evaluation of the antacid properties of the preparations Maalox and Almagel]. Ter Arkh 66(8):44-7, 1994 (in Russian)

Grimes DS, Goddard J. Gastric emptying of wholemeal and white bread. Gut 18:725, 1977

Hade JE, Spiro HM. Calcium and acid rebound: a reappraisal. J Clin Gastroenterol 15(1):37-44, 1992

Henrotte JG et al. Effect of pyridoxine on mice gastric ulcers and brain catecholamines after an immobilization stress. Ann Nutr Metab 36(5-6):313-7, 1992

Herzog P, Holtermuller KH. Antacid therapy—changes in mineral metabolism. Scand J Gastroterol Suppl 75:56-82, 1982

Horwitt MK. Fed Proc 18:530, 1959

Ippoliti AF et al. The effect of various forms of milk on gastric-acid secretion. Ann Intern Med 84:286-9, 1976

Jimenez E et al. Meta-analysis of efficacy of zinc acexamate and peptic ulcer. Digestion 51:18-26, 1992

Jolobe OMP. Iron deficiency in benign duodenal ulcer. Letter. Lancet 349:809-10, 1997

Kaess H et al. Food intolerance in duodenal ulcer patients, non ulcer dyspepsia patients and healthy subjects. A prospective study. Klin Wochenschr 66(5):208-11, 1988

Kang JY et al. Dietary supplementation with pectin in the maintenance treatment of duodenal ulcer: A controlled study. Scand J Gastroenterol 23(1):95-9, 1988

Kang JY et al. Chronic upper abdominal pain: site and radiation in various structural and functional disorders and the effect of various foods. Gut 33(6):743-8, 1992

Kato I et al. A prospective study of gastric and duodenal ulcer and its relation to smoking, alcohol, and diet. Am J Epidemiol 135(5):521-30, 1992

Katschinski BD et al. Duodenal ulcer and refined carbohydrate intake: a case-control study assessing dietary fibre and refined sugar intake. Gut 31(9):993-6, 1990

Kearney J et al. Dietary intakes and adipose tissue levels of linoleic acid in peptic ulcer disease. Br J Nutr 62(3):699-706, 1989

Kumar N et al. Do chillies influence healing of duodenal ulcer? Br Med J 288:1803-4, 1984

Kumar N et al. Effect of milk on patients with duodenal ulcers. Br Med J 293:666, 1986

Lee JG et al. Serious gastrointestinal pathology found in patients with serum ferritin values ≤ 50 ng/ml. Am J Gastroenterol 93(5):772-6, 1998

Lemeshko FP, Grebenshchikova VG. [Experience with treatment of gastric ulcer and duodenal ulcer with pyridoxine.] Sov Med 29(2):31-3, 1966 (in Russian)

Lenz HJ et al. Wine and five percent ethanol are potent stimulators of gastric acid secretion in humans. Gastroenterology 85(5):1082-7, 1983

Litinskaia EV et al. [The vitamin E concentration and lipid peroxidation status of patients with peptic ulcer undergoing laser therapy.] Vrach Delo (8):70-2, 1989 (in Russian)

Lotz M et al. Evidence for a phosphorus-depletion syndrome in man. N Engl J Med 278(8):409-15, 1968

Mach T. [A clinical trial on the effect of aluminum containing antacids on the course of duodenal ulcer healing and morphology of the gastric mucosa]. Folia Med Cracov 36(1-4):3-20, 1995 (in Polish)

Mahmood T et al. Prevention of duodenal ulcer formation in the rat by dietary vitamin A supplementation. JPEN J Parenter Enteral Nutr 10(1):74-7, 1986

Maity S et al. Anti-ulcer effect of the hot water extract of black tea (Camellia sinensis). J Ethnopharmacol 46(3):167-74, 1995

Malhotra SL. A comparison of unrefined wheat and rice diets in the management of duodenal ulcer. Postgrad Med J 54:6-9, 1978

Marotta RB, Floch MH. Diet and nutrition in ulcer disease. Med Clin North Am 75(4):967-9, 1991

Matushevskaia VN et al. [Optimization of dietary fat composition in erosive and ulcerative diseases of the gastroduodenal area]. Vopr Pitan (6):35-7, 1996 (in Russian)

McAlindon ME et al. Effect of allopurinol, sulphasalazine, and vitamin C on aspirin induced gastroduodenal injury in human volunteers. Gut 38(4):518-24, 1996

McArthur K et al. Relative stimulatory effects of commonly ingested beverages on gastric acid secretion in humans. Gastroenterology 83:199-203, 1982

McGuigan JE. Peptic ulcer, in KJ Isselbacher et al, Eds. Harrison's Principles of Internal Medicine, Ninth Edition. New York, McGraw-Hill Book Company, 1980

McNulty CAM et al. Susceptibility of clinical isolates of Campylobacter pyloridis to 11 antimicrobial agents. Antimicrob Agents Chemther 28:837-8, 1985

Mitra R, Pal SP. Inhibition of mast cell population by L-glutamine in aspirin-induced ulceration in rat stomach. Indian J Physiol Pharmacol 21(4):374-8, 1977

Miwa M et al. The therapeutics of peptic ulcers: Clinical evaluation of C-Fe therapy. Tokai J Exp Clin Med 5(1):41-4, 1980

Mutoh H et al. Reduced glutathione protects cultured gastric mucosal cells from suckling rats against acid. Am J Physiol 261(1 Pt 1):G65-70, 1991

Nagy E, Jobst K. The kinetics of aluminium-containing antacid absorption in man. Eur J Chem Clin Biochem 32(3):119-21, 1994

Nash EC. A comparative study of an antacid with and without vitamin C in the treatment of peptic ulcer. Am Pract Digest Treatments 3:117-20, 1952

O'Connor JH et al. Vitamin C in the human stomach: relation to gastric pH, gastroduodenal disease, and possible sources. Gut 30(4):436-42, 1989

Okabe S et al. Effects of acetylsalicylic acid (ASA), ASA plus L-glutamine and L-glutamine on healing of chronic gastric ulcer in the rat. Digestion 14(1):85-8, 1976

Olschewski P et al. [The milk-alkali syndrome--a rare differential diagnosis for hypercalcemia]. Dtsch Med Wochenschr 121(33):1015-8, 1996 (in German)

Parmar NS et al. Gastric anti-ulcer and cytoprotective effect of selenium in rats. Toxicol Appl Pharmacol 92(1):122-30, 1988

Patty I et al. Cytoprotective effect of vitamin A and its clinical importance in the treatment of patients with chronic gastric ulcer. Int J Tissue React 5(3):301-7, 1983

Pollard HM, Stuart GJ. Experimental reproduction of gastric allergy in human beings with controlled observations on the mucosa. J Allergy 13:467-73, 1942

Portnoy B, Wilkinson JP. Vitamin C deficiency in peptic ulceration and hematemesis. Br Med J 554-60, 1938

Poynard T et al. Randomized double-blind clinical trial of aluminum phosphate versus ranitidine in the acute treatment of duodenal ulcer. Digestion 47(2):105-10, 1990

Puscas I et al. Effect of ZnSO4 upon gastric acid secretion and carbonic anhydrase. Int J Clin Pharmacol Ther Toxicol 23(11):609-12, 1985

Qvigstad G, Waldum HL. [Bismuth. An old medicine of current interest]. Tidsskr Nor Laegeforen 115(11):1353-7, 1995 (in Norweigian)

Reimann HJ, Ewin J. Gastric mucosal reactions in patients with food allergy. Am J Gastroenterol 83(11):1212-19, 1988

Rettura G et al. Vitamin A protects against aspirin toxicity. J Am Coll Nutr 3:291-2, 1984

Riggs HE et al. JAMA 124:639, 1944

Rodriguez de la Serna A, Diaz-Rubio M. Multicenter clinical trial of zinc acexamate in the prevention of nonsteroidal antiinflammatory drug induced gastroenteropathy. Spanish Study Group on NSAID Induced Gastroenteropathy Prevention. J Rheumatol 21(5):927-33, 1994

Rogers C et al. Role for leukotrienes in the pathogenesis of hemorrhagic mucosal lesions induced by ethanol or HCl in the rat. Gastroenterology 90:1797, 1986

Rokkas T et al. Helicobacter pylori and gastric juice vitamin C levels. Impact of eradication. Dig Dis Sci 40(3):615-20, 1995

Russell RL et al. Ascorbic acid levels in leucocytes of patients with gastrointestinal hemorrhage. Lancet ii:603-6, 1968

Rydning A et al. Prophylactic effect of dietary fiber in duodenal ulcer disease. Lancet ii:736-9, 1982

Rydning A, Berstad A. Fiber diet and antacids in the short-term treatment of duodenal ulcer. Scand J Gastroenterol 20(9):1078-82, 1985

Salim AS. Sulphydryl-containing agents and the prevention of duodenal ulcer relapse. Pharmacology 46(5):281-8, 1993

Sanderson CR, Davis RE. Serum pyridoxal in patients with active peptic ulceration. Gut 16(3):177-80, 1975

Sanderson CR, Davis RE. Serum pyridoxal in patients with gastric pathology. Gut 17(5):371-4, 1976

Schmassmann A et al. Antacid provides better restoration of glandular structures within the gastric ulcer scar than omeprazole. Gut 35(7):896-904, 1994

Shive W et al. Glutamine in treatment of peptic ulcer. Texas State J Med 53:840-3, 1957

Siegel J. Gastrointestinal ulcer - Arthus reaction! Ann Allergy 32:127-30, 1974

Siegel J. Immunologic approach to the treatment and prevention of gastrointestinal ulcers. Ann Allergy 38:27-41, 1977

Smith CV. Will glutathione become a hot new supplement? Nutr Report 11(11), November, 1993

Smith DT, McConkey M. Peptic ulcers (gastric, pyloric and duodenal) occurrence in guinea-pigs fed on a diet deficient in vitamin C. Arch Intern Med 51:413-26, 1933

Sobala GM et al. Effect of eradication of Helicobacter pylori on gastric juice ascorbic acid concentrations. Gut 34(8):1038-41, 1993

Szabo S, Vargha G. Unhtersuchung de Wirkungswiese des sogenannten "Vitamin U" mit histochemischen Reaktionen. Arzneimittelforsch 10:23-8, 1960 (in German)

Szabo S. Experimental basis for a role for sulfhydryls and dopamine in ulcerogenesis: a primer for cytoprotection--organoprotection. Klin Wochenschr 64 Suppl 7:116-22, 1986

Szabo S, Rogers C. Diet, ulcer disease, and fish oil. Letter. Lancet i:119, 1988

Thompson L et al. Inhibitory effect of polyunsaturated fatty acids on the growth of Helicobacter pylori: a possible explanation of the effect of diet on peptic ulceration. Gut 35(11):1557-61, 1994

Toteva ETs et al. [Use of alpha-tocopherol in the complex treatment of patients with peptic ulcer.] Vrach Delo (2):79-81, 1988 (in Russian)

Turnberg LA. Coffee and the gastrointestinal tract. Editorial. Gastroenterology 75(3):529-30, 1978

Wagstaff AJ et al. Colloidal bismuth subcitrate. A review of its pharmacodynamic and pharmacokinetic properties, and its therapeutic use in peptic ulcer disease. Drugs 36(2):132-57, 1988

Watanabe T et al. Zinc deficiency delays gastric ulcer healing in rats. Dig Dis Sci 40(6):1340-4, 1995

Witschi A et al. The systemic availability of oral glutathione. Eur J Clin Pharmacol 43(6):667-9, 1992

Yeomans ND, Skeljo MV. Repair and healing of established gastric mucosal injury. J Clin Gastroenterol 13 Suppl 1:S37-41, 1991

Yoshikawa T et al. Vitamin E in gastric mucosal injury induced by ischemia-reperfusion. Am J Clin Nutr 53:210S-4S, 1991

Yudkin J. Eating and ulcers. Letter. Br Med J 280:483-4, 1980

PERIPHERAL VASCULAR DISEASE

(including THROMBOPHLEBITIS)

See Also: ATHEROSCLEROSIS

NUTRITIONAL TREATMENT GUIDE

✓ = Efficacy generally accepted.
* = Efficacy *demonstrated* by controlled human trials.
[+] = Efficacy *suspected* from uncontrolled human experiments
[-] = Efficacy *suspected* from indirect data
? = Efficacy *challenged* in at least one study of similar design

DIETARY FACTORS

* **low Fat, low Cholesterol diet**

- -

[-] moderate **Alcohol** intake
[-] high **dietary Fiber** intake
[-] minimize **Meat**
[-] minimize **Sugar**

NUTRITIONAL FACTORS

* **L-Carnitine**: *for arterial insufficiency and vasospasm:* L-carnitine 2 g twice daily *OR* propionyl-L-carnitine 1 to 2 g daily
* **Flavonoids**: *for venous insufficiency:* Hydroxyethylrutosides 1,000 mg daily *OR* Rutin 270 mg daily *OR* Daflon 500 mg
for varicose veins: Pycnogenol® 30 mg 3 times daily
for post-thrombotic syndrome: Hydroxyethylrutosides 1,000 mg daily
* **Inositol hexanicotinate:** *for arterial insufficiency:* 1 to 2 g daily
* **Omega-6 fatty acids:** *for arterial insufficiency:* ? evening primrose oil 4 g daily
* **Vitamin C**: *to prevent deep venous thromboses:* 1 g daily
for arterial insufficiency: 500 mg 3 times daily
* **Vitamin E:** *for arterial insufficiency:* 300 IU to 1600 IU daily (6 month trial)
to prevent postoperative thromboembolism: ? 800 IU to 1600 IU daily

- -

[+] **Flavonoids:** *for arterial insufficiency:* Hydroxyethylrutosides 1,000 mg daily
[+] **Folic acid:** *for arterial insufficiency:* ? 5 to 7.5 mg daily
to reduce elevated homocysteine levels: 1 to 2 mg daily
[+] **Glycosaminoglycans:** *for arterial or venous insufficiency and for varicose veins:* Mesoglycan 50 mg twice daily
[+] **Magnesium deficiency:** examples: magnesium sulfate 4 to 8 mmol IV or IM daily *OR* magnesium hydroxide 250 mg twice daily by mouth
[+] **Vitamin B_6:** *to reduce elevated homocysteine levels:* ? 100 mg daily

- -

[-] **Iron deficiency:** 30 mg twice daily until repletion; then minimal possible dosage

[-] **Omega-3 fatty acids (fish oil)**

OTHER RELATED FACTORS

* rule out **Food Sensitivities** *(recurrent intractable thrombophlebitis)*

- -

[+] rule out **Arsenic** toxicity
[+] **Hydrolytic Enzymes:** Wobenzyme N® 3 to 10 tablets 3 times daily

DIETARY FACTORS

Low Fat, Low Cholesterol Diet

Saturated fat intake is at least as closely related to arterial and venous thrombosis as it is to atherosclerosis. Moreover, it is more closely related to the clotting activity of platelets and their response to thrombin than serum cholesterol *(Renaud)*. Crucial to the prevention and treatment of atherosclerosis is the reduction in intake of saturated fat and cholesterol *(Temple)*.

In a double-blind study, 45 patients randomly received either the American Heart Association Hyperlipidemia Diet C or a low-fat, high-fiber, complex carbohydrate diet similar to the Pritikin Maintenance diet. After one year, there was a similar significant increase in walking distance in both groups. As vascular parameters were not significantly different, this improvement was likely due to improved metabolic capacity of the muscles *(Hunchinson)*.

Dietary Fiber and Meat

When 1,592 patients were studied using the ankle brachial pressure index as an indicator of peripheral arterial disease, a high frequency of fiber-containing foods in the diet was associated with greater mean values - although only in males. By contrast, a higher frequency of consumption of meat and meat products was associated with lower mean values in both males and females *(Donnan)*.

Further studies are needed to clarify the meaning of these findings.

Alcohol

Although heavy alcohol intake is contraindicated, moderate alcohol consumption appears to have a protective effect. One study found that low to moderate alcohol intake was associated with a reduced risk of both deep vein thrombosis and pulmonary embolism *(Pahor)*.

Another found that, in men, the consumption of wine (but not beer or spirits) was inversely related to the severity of peripheral arterial disease, although adjustment for age and social class rendered this effect statistically non-significant *(Jepson)*. Yet another study found alcohol intake to be independently, significantly inversely related to vascular disease hospitalizations and deaths *(Gartside)*.

Sugar

In one study, the consumption of sucrose was significantly correlated with both serum insulin levels and platelet adhesiveness in patients with peripheral vascular disease, but not in normals *(Yudkin)*, suggesting that these patients may be more sensitive to the adverse effects of sugar consumption.

HOMOCYSTEINE

Elevated levels of the toxic amino acid homocysteine is now considered to be a major risk factor for atherosclerosis (see Atherosclerosis). Hyperhomocystinemia is believed to be responsible for about 60% of peripheral vascular diseases *(Czeizel)*. Its causal role has been inferred because of consistency across studies by different investigators using different methods in different populations *(Boushey)*.

For example, based on a comparison of 750 patients with vascular disease and 800 control subjects, plasma homocysteine concentrations greater than the 80th percentile for control subjects either fasting (12.1 μmol/L) or after a methionine load (38.0 μmol/L) were associated with an elevated risk of vascular disease independent of all traditional risk factors *(Robinson)*.

Important from a nutritional perspective is the finding that mild hyperhomocystinemia can be reduced to normal in virtually all cases by simple and safe nutritional supplementation *(Boers).*

NUTRITIONAL FACTORS

VITAMINS

Folic Acid

Folate nutriture may be inversely related to the risk of peripheral vascular disease due to the efficacy of folic acid in reducing the concentration of homocysteine. For example, a meta-analysis of 27 studies relating homocysteine to arteriosclerotic vascular disease and 11 studies of folic acid effects on total plasma/serum homocysteine levels concluded that higher folic acid intake, by reducing total homocysteine levels, promises to prevent arteriosclerotic vascular disease *(Boushey).*

An open trial of folate supplementation has found that, when 17 elderly patients with diffuse, chronic arteriosclerosis received daily supplements of folic acid, 15 of them developed increased capillary blood flow and improved vision *(Kopjas).*

The results of controlled clinical trials should be available in the near future.

Vitamin B_6

In a multicenter case-control study, red cell concentrations of vitamin B_6 below the lowest 20th percentile were found to be associated with increased risk of peripheral vascular disease *(Robinson).* Vitamin B_6 nutriture appears to be associated with peripheral vascular disease because of its role in homocysteine metabolism. Specifically, this B vitamin promotes the conversion of homocysteine to the non-toxic cystathionine.

If excessive homocysteine levels are found, supplementation with the vitamin may reduce them *(Boers)*, although it is not clear that vitamin B_6 supplementation adds to the efficacy of folate supplementation *(Van Den Berg).*

Vitamin C

It has been theorized that atherosclerosis is primarily caused by marginal ascorbate deficiency which results in the accumulation of lipoprotein (a) and fibrinogen/fibrin in the vascular wall *(Rath).* In support of this hypothesis vitamin C intake has been inversely associated with the risk of peripheral arterial disease *(Kritchevsky).*

There is evidence from controlled studies that ascorbate supplementation may improve peripheral arterial circulation - possibly by reversing atherosclerosis *(Willis).* Moreover, in hospitalized patients, it may reduce the incidence of deep venous thromboses *(Spittle).*

Vitamin E

The intake of vitamin E has been inversely related to the risk of peripheral vascular disease *(Donnan;Kritchevsky).*

Seven controlled studies, 3 of which were double-blind, have demonstrated the efficacy of vitamin E supplementation. When compared to controls, patients receiving the vitamin exhibited significantly better outcomes in regard to walking distance, exertional leg pain, rate of surgical intervention and survival prognosis. Maximal effectiveness was for patients with femoropopliteal arterial obstruction with poor distal circulation, and least effectiveness was for aortoiliac arterial disease *(Piesse).*

There is also evidence that vitamin E supplementation may prevent post-surgical thromboembolism. In 6 controlled clinical trials, the risk of peripheral venous thrombosis in unsupplemented patients was double that of the supplemented groups, the risk of pulmonary embolism was 6-fold greater, and the chance of fatal pulmonary embolism was 9-fold greater *(Kanofsky).*

MINERALS

Iron

There is evidence that the development of atherosclerosis is linked to the size of body iron stores, possibly due to the role of iron as a catalyst of oxidative reactions and its specific role in macrophage-mediated LDL-oxidation *(Yuan).*

Despite this, a large prospective 10-year follow-up study found that iron intake was independently, inversely correlated with both hospitalization and death from vascular disease *(Gartside).* It appears, therefore, that there may be a U-shaped curve for the relationship between body iron stores and vascular disease, with moderate levels being protective when compared to either low or high levels.

Magnesium Deficiency

Magnesium may be deficient in multiple deep phlebothromboses, deep thrombophlebitis and possible superficial phlebothromboses, as well as in arteritis of the lower limbs. It has been suggested that magnesium deficit should be considered a contributory factor in arterial and arteriolar thrombosis, whether atherosclerotic or diabetic *(Durlach)*. In support of this hypothesis, recent research has found serum magnesium levels to be inversely associated with coronary heart and vascular disease hospitalizations and deaths *(Gartside)*. Similarly, compared to controls, magnesium levels were depressed in 102 out of 138 patients with peripheral vascular disease *(Howard)*.

Supplementation with magnesium (given either intramuscularly or intravenously) has been determined to be helpful for claudication, superficial thrombophlebitis, and deep vein thrombosis *(Browne,1994)*. Oral magnesium may also be beneficial as, 2 months after patients with intermittent claudication received oral magnesium supplements, they were able to walk an average of 82% farther than at baseline *(Neglen)*.

These preliminary open trials still need to be confirmed by controlled clinical studies.

Two elderly men with incipient gangrene and severe pain and swelling of heels and toes rapidly improved on regular intramuscular doses of 4 mmol of magnesium sulfate. Eighteen months later, their feet were much warmer and were free from pain and swelling (Browne,1964).

OTHER NUTRITIONAL FACTORS

L-Carnitine

Patients with severe peripheral vascular disease may have deficient muscle carnitine levels *(Brevetti,1991)*.

Several studies, many of which were double-blind, found that supplementation with either L-carnitine or with propionyl-L-carnitine (a naturally-occurring derivative) was effective in treating intermittent claudication and improving the quality of life *(Brevetti,1997)*, although the evidence suggests that patients with decreased plasma carnitine levels are the best candidates *(Brevetti,1996)*.

Diabetics with peripheral angiopathy have shown an excellent response *(Greco)*. Moreover, in patients with vasospastic disease, L-carnitine decreased the cold-induced blood flow stop duration and increased capillary blood cell velocity after local cooling *(Gasser)*.

Flavonoids

Several flavonoids have shown evidence of efficacy. Daflon 500 mg is a micronized flavonoid mixture with phlebotonic properties consisting of 90% diosmin and 10% hesperidin. In 3 double-blind trials and was found to improve the clinical symptoms of chronic venous insufficiency and to decrease the supra-malleolar circumference. In addition, there were significant decreases in venous capacitance, venous distensibility, and venous emptying time. Only 3 of the 183 treated patients had to withdraw due to side effects *(Geroulakos)*.

Hydroxyethylrutosides is a standardized mixture of semisynthetic flavonoids which acts primarily on the microvascular endothelium to reduce hyperpermeability and edema *(Wadworth)*. Numerous double-blind studies have demonstrated the efficacy of their oral administration in chronic venous insufficiency *(Poynard;Rehn)*.

While much less studied, results of preliminary work suggest that they may also be effective in chronic arterial insufficiency. In an open trial, 3 patients with bilateral arterial insufficiency received the mixture intravenously twice daily. After 3 days, all experienced symptom relief. Moreover, when tested during the second and third hour following its administration, the blood flow in the forefoot was increased by an average of one-third *(Jelnes)*.

In addition, there is evidence from a double-blind study of their efficacy for patients with post-thrombotic syndrome in their legs. Compared to baseline, data from the 4th and 8th week visits showed a mean calf reduction of 8.7 mm in the treated group compared to only 2 mm in the control group, and there was a similar difference in mean ankle circumferences *(de Jongste)*.

Pycnogenol®, a proprietary blend of oligomeric and monomeric procyanidins from the bark of *Pinus maritima* (European coastal pine), has been found to reduce symptoms due to varicose veins under controlled conditions *(Royer)*. Finally, there is evidence from a double-blind study that rutin administration may reduce leg edema in chronic venous insufficiency *(Ihme)*.

Glycosaminoglycans

Heparin is a specific glycosaminoglycan which is the drug of choice most situations that require an anticoagulant. However, it has many side effects, including hemorrhage, thrombocytopenia, eosinophilia and osteoporosis *(Walenga)*; close medical supervision is therefore required.

Mesoglycan is a natural heparin-like extract obtained from the bovine intestinal mucosa whose components include chondroitin, dermatan and heparan sulfates, hyaluronic acid, and related hexosaminoglycans *(Tardieu)*. Patients with peripheral obstructive arterial disease have shown improvement in arterial wall elasticity after only 20 days of supplementation *(Andreozzi)*. While apparently less effective than heparan sulfate (a specific glycosaminoglycan), it significantly increased pain-free walking distance *(Strano)* although, at a lower dosage, it was ineffective in reducing intermittent claudication under double-blind conditions *(Laurora)*.

Mesoglycan has also shown evidence of efficacy in treating venous disease in several open trials *(Petruzzellis;Scondotto)*, although, once again, heparan sulfate may be superior *(Agrati)*.

Hydrolytic Enzymes

Combinations of hydrolytic enzymes have shown evidence of efficacy, although formal well-controlled trials are lacking. When 216 patients with various pathological conditions received Wobenzyme N® (a proprietary mixture of pancreatin, bromelain, papain, lipase, amylase, trypsin, alpha-chymotrypsin and rutin), 30% were cured, while 62% became asymptomatic with substantial improvement in objective measures *(Maehder)*.

Another study compared 245 patients with either superficial or deep thrombophlebitis who were treated with proteolytic enzymes with those treated with conventional anticoagulants and vasoactive substances. It found that the enzyme-treated patients had substantially better outcomes *(Valls-Serra)*.

Inositol Hexanicotinate

This compound is the hexanicotinic acid ester of meso-inositol. It is slowly metabolized over many hours into niacin and inositol, resulting in a sustained increase in the levels of free nicotinic acid. It appears to be free of side effects at doses of up to 4 grams *(Head)*.

Several double-blind studies have found it to be effective in treating intermittent claudication. For example, 120 patients with disease severe enough to limit walking to 500 yards received either inositol nicotinate (Hexopal) 2 grams or placebo twice daily.

After 3 months, the experimental group had significantly larger changes in claudication times and number of free-walking paces than the placebo group. The subjective improvement in smokers was particularly marked. Side-effects were equally distributed between the 2 groups, and were minor and self-limiting *(O'Hara)*.

Omega-3 Essential Fatty Acids

Patients suffering from peripheral arterial disease have been found to have reduced plasma levels of these essential fatty acids *(Leng)*.

The erythrocytes of diabetics tend to exhibit decreased membrane fluidity, a finding that may predispose them to symptoms of peripheral vascular disease by reducing microcapillary blood flow. There is evidence from a controlled trial that dietary sardine oil, a rich source of these fatty acids, restores erythrocyte membrane fluidity to normal in this patient population *(Kamada)*.

Moreover, in patients with peripheral vascular disease, fish oil administration was found to inhibit platelet aggregation and the formation of leukotriene B4. Since platelet hyperactivity and excessive formation of thromboxane B_4 have been implicated in atherogenesis and its manifestations, while leukotriene B_4, when compared to leukotriene B_5, has markedly attenuated chemotactic and aggregating activities for neutrophils, these findings suggest the dietary fish oil exerts beneficial effects on platelet and leukocyte activity in these patients *(Mori)*.

Controlled clinical trials investigating the efficacy of omega-3 fatty acids in reducing the signs and symptoms of peripheral vascular disease have yet to be reported.

Omega-6 Essential Fatty Acids

For a group of patients with intermittent claudication, supplementation with gamma linolenic acid improved exercise tolerance in a double-blind study *(Christie).*

COMBINED NUTRITIONAL TREATMENT

An elderly man with gangrene of 6 toes had no detectable arterial circulation in the feet on arteriograms and was advised to undergo immediate amputation of both legs. He was treated with weekly injections of magnesium along with large oral doses of vitamin C, vitamin E and other nutrients.

He gradually improved and, after many months of treatment, the gangrenous lesions sloughed off, revealing pink, healthy tissue underneath. However, unless he continued to receive magnesium injections twice monthly, the gangrene would start to recur (Gaby).

OTHER RELATED FACTORS

Food Sensitivities

Twenty patients who were disabled due to recurrent nontraumatic thrombophlebitis were divided into 2 matched groups. While the control group was continued on their standard regime (anticoagulants, bed rest and support hose), the experimental group was placed in a specialized ward where all air, food and water could be controlled. They were taken off all medication and not fed until the leg pain and swelling disappeared - a period of 4 to 7 days.

They then demonstrated specific sensitivities to foods and ambient subthreshold doses of inhaled chemicals under controlled double-blind challenges. Eight of the 10 patients had their symptoms reproduced in this manner. Patients in the experimental group were instructed as to how to continue to avoid the substances to which they had demonstrated sensitivity.

At the 5-year follow-up, the experimental group had two 48-hour episodes of phlebitis cleared by home bed rest and food abstinence. In contrast, the control group had more than 60 episodes of phlebitis at home and 41 episodes at the hospital *(Rea).*

Arsenic Toxicity

Arsenic concentrations in the public drinking water in 30 American counties were related to mortality from circulatory diseases. Standard mortality ratios for diseases of the arteries, arterioles and capillaries in counties exceeding 20 mg/L were 1.9 for females and 1.6 for males, suggesting that higher levels of arsenic exposure may make a substantial contribution to the development of peripheral vascular disease *(Engel).*

BIBLIOGRAPHY

Agrati AM et al. [Heparan sulfate: efficacy and safety in patients with chronic venous insufficiency.] Minerva Cardioangiol 39(10):395-400, 1991 (in Italian)

Andreozzi GM et al. Effects of mesoglycan sulfate on the arterial elastic module. Angiology 38(8):593-600, 1987

Boers GH. Hyperhomocysteinaemia: a newly recognized risk factor for vascular disease. Neth J Med 45(1):34-41, 1994

Boushey CJ et al. A quantitative assessment of plasma homocysteine as a risk factor for vascular disease: Probable benefits of increasing folic acid intakes. JAMA 274(13): 1049-57, 1995

Brevetti G et al. Muscle carnitine deficiency in patients with severe peripheral vascular disease. Circulation 84:1490-5, 1991

Brevetti G et al. Carnitine-related alterations in patients with intermittent claudication. Indication for a focused carnitine therapy. Circulation 93:1685-9, 1996

Brevetti G et al. Effect of propionyl-L-carnitine on quality of life in intermittent claudication. Am J Cardiol 79(6):777-80, 1997

Browne SE. Parenteral magnesium sulphate in arterial disease. Practitioner 192:791-7, 1964

Browne SE. The case for intravenous magnesium treatment of arterial disease in general practice: review of 34 years of experience. J Nutr Med 4:169-77, 1994

Christie SBM et al. Observations on the performance of a standard exercise test by claudicants taking gamma-linolenic acid. J Atheroscler Res 8:83-90, 1986

Czeizel E, Matos L. [The role of hyper-homocysteinemia in the etiology of some vascular diseases.] Orv Hetil 139(37):2191-6, 1998 (in Hungarian)

de Jongste AB et al. A double blind three center clinical trial on the short-term efficacy of O-(beta-hydroxyethyl)-rutosides in patients with post-thrombotic syndrome. Thromb Haemost 62(3):826-9, 1989

Donnan PT et al. Diet as a risk factor for peripheral arterial disease in the general population: The Edinburgh Artery Study. Am J Clin Nutr 57:917-21, 1993

Durlach J. Clinical aspects of chronic magnesium deficiency, in MS Seelig, Ed. Magnesium in Health and Disease, New York, Spectrum Publications, 1980

Engel RR, Smith AH. Arsenic in drinking water and mortality from vascular disease: An ecological analysis in 30 counties in the United States. Arch Environ Health 49(5):418-27, 1994

Gaby AR. Treating atherosclerosis: commentary. Nutrition & Healing 4(7), July, 1997

Gartside PS, Glueck CJ. The important role of modifiable dietary and behavioral characteristics in the causation and prevention of coronary heart disease hospitalization and mortality: the prospective NHANES I follow-up study. J Am Coll Nutr 14(1):71-9, 1995

Gasser P et al. Reaction of capillary blood cell velocity in nailfold capillaries to L-carnitine in patients with vasospastic disease. Drugs Exp Clin Res 23(1):39-43, 1997

Geroulakos G, Nicolaides AN. Controlled studies of Daflon 500 mg in chronic venous insufficiency. Angiology 45(6 Pt 2):549-53, 1994

Greco AV et al. Effect of propionyl-L-carnitine in the treatment of diabetic angiopathy: controlled double blind trial versus placebo. Drugs Exp Clin Res 18(2):69-80, 1992

Head KA. Inositol hexaniacinate: a safer alternative to niacin. Altern Med Rev 1(3):176-84, 1996

Howard JMH. Magnesium deficiency in peripheral vascular disease. J Nutr Med 1:39-49, 1990

Hunchinson K et al. Effects of dietary manipulation on vascular status of patients with peripheral vascular disease. JAMA 259(24):3326-30, 1983

Ihme N et al. Leg edema protection from a buckwheat herb tea in patients with chronic venous insufficiency: A single-center, randomized, double-blind, placebo-controlled clinical trial. Eur J Clin Pharmacol 50:443-7, 1995

Jelnes R et al. Improvement of subcutaneous nutritional blood flow in the forefoot by hydroxyethylrutosides in patients with arterial insufficiency: Case studies. Angiology 37(3 Pt 1):198-202, 1986

Jepson RG et al. Alcohol intake as a risk factor for peripheral arterial disease in the general population in the Edinburgh Artery Study. Eur J Epidemiol 11:9-14, 1995

Kamada T et al. Dietary sardine oil increases erythrocyte membrane fluidity in diabetic patients. Diabetes 35:604, 1986

Kanofsky JD, Kanofsky PB. Prevention of thromboembolic disease by vitamin E. Letter. N Engl J Med 305(3):173-4, 1981

Kopjas TL. Effect of folic acid on collateral circulation in diffuse chronic arteriosclersosis. J Am Geriatr Soc 14(11):1187-92, 1966

Kritchevsky SB et al. Dietary antioxidants and carotid artery wall thickness. The ARJC Study. Circulation 92(8):2142-50, 1995

Laurora G et al. Treatment of intermittent claudication with defibrotide or mesoglycan. A double-blind study. Panminerva Med 36(2):83-6, 1994

Leng GC et al. Plasma essential fatty acids, cigarette smoking, and dietary antioxidants in peripheral arterial disease. A population-based case-control study. Arterioscler Thromb 14(3):471-8, 1994

Maehder K. [Enzyme therapy in vascular disorders]. Die Arzipraxis 2:1972 (in German)

Mori TA et al. The effect of fish oil on plasma lipids, platelet and neutrophil function in patients with vascular disease. Adv Prostaglandin Thromboxane Leukotriene Res 21:229-32, 1990

Neglen P et al. Peroral magnesium hydroxide therapy and intermittent claudication. Vasa 14 (3):285-8, 1985

O'Hara J et al. The therapeutic efficacy of inositol nicotinate (Hexopol) in intermittent claudication: a controlled trial. Br J Clin Pract 42(9):377-83, 1988

Pahor M et al. Alcohol consumption and risk of deep venous thrombosis and pulmonary embolism in older persons. J Am Geriatr Soc 44(9):1030-7, 1996

Petruzzellis V, Velon A. [Therapeutic action of oral mesoglycan in the pharmacologic treatment of the varicose syndrome and its complications.] Minerva Med 76(12):543-8, 1985 (in Italian)

Piesse JW. Vitamin E and peripheral vascular disease. Int Clin Nutr Rev 4(4):178-82, 1984

Poynard T, Valterio C. Meta-analysis of hydroxyethylrutosides in the treatment of chronic venous insufficiency. Vasa 23(3):244-50, 1994

Rath M, Pauling L. Solution to the puzzle of human cardiovascular disease: its primary cause is ascorbate deficiency leading to the deposition of lipoprotein (a) and fibrinogen-fibrin in the vascular wall. J Orthomol Med 6(3-4):125-34, 1991

Rea WJ et al. Recurrent Environmentally triggered thrombophlebitis: A five-year follow-up. Ann Allergy 47:338-44, 1981

Rehn D et al. Comparative efficacy and tolerability of oxerutins and horse chestnut extract in patients with chronic venous insufficiency. Arzneimittelforschung 46(5):483-7, 1996

Renaud S. Dietary fatty acids and platelet function. Proc Nutr Soc Aust 10:1-13, 1985

Robinson K et al. Low circulating folate and vitamin B6 concentrations: risk factors for stroke, peripheral vascular disease, and coronary artery disease. European COMAC Group. Circulation 97(5):437-43, 1998

Royer RJ, Schmidt CL. [Evaluation of venotropic drugs by venous gas plethysmography. A study of procyanidolic oligomers.] Sem Hop 57(47-8):2009-13, 1981

Scondotto G et al. [Use of mesoglycan in venous pathology]. Minerva Med 88(12):537-41, 1997 (in Italian)

Spittle CR. Vitamin C and deep-vein thrombosis. Lancet ii:199-201, 1973

Strano A et al. Double-blind controlled study of the efficacy and pharmacological properties of heparan sulfate in patients with occlusive arterial disease of the lower limbs. Drugs Exp Clin Res 16(10):543-50, 1990

Tardieu M et al. Mesoglycan and sulodexide act as stabilizers and protectors of fibroblast growth factors (FGFs). Growth Factors 11(4):291-300, 1994

Temple NJ. Dietary fats and coronary heart disease. Biomed Pharmacother 50(6-7):261-8, 1996

Valls-Serra J. Proteolytische enzyme in der behandlung von thrombophlebitis. Medicina Colinica, 1967 (in German)

Van Den Berg M et al. Hyperhomocysteinemia and endothelial dysfunction in young patients with peripheral arterial occlusive disease. Europ J Clin Invest 25:176-81, 1995

Wadworth AN, Faulds D. Hydroxyethylrutosides. A review of its pharmacology, and therapeutic efficacy in venous insufficiency and related disorders. Drugs 44(6):1013-32, 1992

Walenga JM, Bick RL. Heparin-induced thrombocytopenia, paradoxical thromboembolism, and other side effects of heparin therapy. Med Clin North Am 82(3):635-58, 1998

Willis GC. The reversibility of atherosclerosis. Can Med Assoc J July 15, 1957, pp. 106-9

Yuan XM, Brunk UT. Iron and LDL-oxidation in atherogenesis. APMIS 106(9):825-42, 1998

Yudkin J et al. Sugar intake, serum insulin and platelet adhesiveness in men with and without peripheral vascular disease. Postgrad Med J 45:608, 1969

PREGNANCY-RELATED ILLNESS

See Also: DEPRESSION
DIABETES MELLITUS
HYPERTENSION
MUSCLE CRAMPS (FUNCTIONAL)
ORGANIC MENTAL DISORDERS

NUTRITIONAL TREATMENT GUIDE

✓ = Efficacy generally accepted.
* = Efficacy *demonstrated* by controlled human trials.
[+] = Efficacy *suspected* from uncontrolled human experiments
[-] = Efficacy *suspected* from indirect data
? = Efficacy *challenged* in at least one study of similar design

GENERAL DIET

[-] **Nutritious, Well-balanced, High-protein diet** (70-90 gm protein; 2,300-2,800 kcal)

DIETARY, NUTRITIONAL *AND* RELATED FACTORS

TO PREVENT/TREAT General Complications of Pregnancy and Labor

* **Magnesium deficiency:** ≈ 400 mg daily)
* ? **Zinc deficiency:** ? 20 to 45 mg daily

- -

[-] avoid **Caffeine**

TO PREVENT/TREAT Abnormally Long Labor

[+] **Zinc:** ? 45 mg daily

TO PREVENT/TREAT Anemia of Pregnancy

✓ **Iron deficiency:** 30 mg twice daily until repletion; then minimal possible dosage

TO PREVENT/TREAT Gestational Diabetes

[+] increase **Soluble Fiber** intake (Typical supplements: glucomannan 3 g daily
OR guar 10 g daily

- -

[-] restrict dietary **Fat** intake to less than 35% of total calories
[-] **Chromium deficiency:** 200 µg daily
[-] **Magnesium deficiency:** ≈ 400 mg daily
[-] **Potassium deficiency:** ? 80 to 100 mEq daily total intake, preferably from potassium-rich foods

TO PREVENT/TREAT Leg Cramps

* restrict **Milk** intake to less than 1 pint daily
* avoid dietary sources of **Phosphorus** (such as certain soft beverage)
* **Magnesium:** ? 122 to 400 mg daily
* **Vitamin C:** 1 g twice daily
* ? **Calcium:** 1 g twice daily (not as a phosphate salt)

- -

[+] **Riboflavin:** 5 to 10 mg daily
[+] ? **Pantothenic Acid:** panthenol 100 mg daily (10 day trial)
[+] ? **Thiamine:** ? 50 mg daily

TO PREVENT/TREAT Post-partum Psychosis:

[+] **Folic Acid deficiency:** 800 µg daily
[+] **Vitamin B_{12} deficiency:** 1,000 µg intramuscularly once weekly initially; then once monthly as needed

TO PREVENT/TREAT Toxemias of Pregnancy (General)

* **Magnesium:** *for prevention:* ≈ 400 mg daily
* ? **Calcium:** 1 g twice daily (not as a phosphate salt)

- -

[+] **Vitamin B_6:** ? 10 mg daily

- -

[-] keep dietary **Fiber** intake high

A. ***TO PREVENT/TREAT Preeclampsia and Eclampsia***

✓ **Magnesium:** magnesium sulfate ? 5 g loading dose IM in each buttock and 4 g slowly IV, followed by another 5 g IM every 4 hours

- -

[-] minimize ***Trans* Fatty Acid** intake
[-] **Potassium deficiency:** ? 80 to 100 mEq daily total intake, preferably from potassium-rich foods
[-] **Vitamin A deficiency:** 50,000 IU daily for 6 weeks (100,000 IU during pregnancy)
[-] **Vitamin C deficiency:** 500 mg twice daily
[-] rule out **Lead** toxicity.

B. TO PREVENT/TREAT ***Hyperemesis Gravidarum***

* **Vitamin B_6:** 25 mg every 8 hours

- -

[+] **Vitamin C:** 25 mg daily *AND*
Vitamin K1 (Menadione): 5 mg daily

C. TO PREVENT/TREAT ***Hypertension of Pregnancy***

* ? **Zinc:** ? 20 mg daily

- -

[-] **Omega-6 Fatty Acids:** *example:* evening primrose oil 1 g 3 times daily
[-] **Vitamin C deficiency:** 500 mg twice daily
[-] rule out **Lead** toxicity

TO PREVENT ***Habitual Abortion***

[+] **Vitamin E:** 200 IU daily

- -

[-] avoid **Alcohol**
[-] avoid **Caffeine**
[-] **Selenium deficiency:** 200 μg daily
[-] **Zinc deficiency:** zinc sulfate 220 mg twice daily *AND* **Copper** 2 mg daily
[-] rule out **Lead** toxicity

TO PREVENT ***Premature rupture of fetal membranes***

[+] **Vitamin C deficiency:** 500 mg twice daily

- -

[-] avoid **Caffeine**
[-] rule out **Lead** toxicity

TO PREVENT ***Fetal Malformations and Developmental Problems***

✓ **Folic acid:** 400 μg daily before and during early pregnancy; 4 mg daily for women with a prior history of a fetal neural tube defect
✓ **Vitamin D deficiency:** 10 μg daily for women who avoid milk, eggs and fish; 5 μg daily for women whose consumption of vitamin D-fortified milk is low.

- -

* **Omega-3 Fatty Acid deficiency:** *example:* MaxEPA 1 g caps [180 mg EPA; 120 mg DHA] 10 to 20 daily

- -

[+] **Magnesium:** *to prevent cerebral palsy and mental retardation in low-birth-weight infants:* ≈ 400 mg daily
[+] **Vitamin B_{12} deficiency:** 1,000 μg intramuscularly once weekly initially; then monthly as needed

- -

[-] avoid **Alcohol**

[-] **Copper Deficiency:** 2 mg twice daily for up to 6 weeks *AND* **Zinc** 50 mg daily
[-] **Selenium deficiency:** 200 µg daily
[-] **Vitamin A deficiency:** 10,000 IU daily for 6 weeks

TO PREVENT Hemorrhagic Disease of the Newborn

* **Vitamin K:** 10 mg orally daily for 2 weeks starting at least 10 days before delivery

TO PREVENT Prematurity and Low-birth-weight Infants

* **Magnesium:** 250 to 500 mg daily
* **Omega-3 fatty acids (fish oil):** 2.7 g daily
* ? **Calcium:** 1 g twice daily (not as a phosphate salt)
* ? **Zinc deficiency**: ? 25 mg daily

- -

[+] **Iron deficiency:** 30 mg twice daily until repletion; then minimal possible dosage
[+] **Magnesium deficiency:** ≈ 400 mg daily

- -

[-] avoid **Caffeine**
[-] avoid excessive **Carbohydrate** intake in early pregnancy
[-] avoid excessive **Sugar** intake
[-] avoid ***Trans* Fatty Acid** intake
[-] **Chromium deficiency:** 200 µg daily
[-] **Copper deficiency:** 2 mg twice daily for up to 6 weeks *AND* **Zinc** 50 mg daily
[-] **Niacin deficiency:** 50 to 100 mg daily
[-] **Riboflavin deficiency:** 5 to 10 mg daily
[-] **Thiamine deficiency:** 50 mg daily
[-] **Vitamin A deficiency:** 10,000 IU daily
[-] **Vitamin E deficiency:** D,L-alpha-tocopheryl acetate 200 to 2,000 mg or IU daily for 6 weeks; then maintenance levels as needed
[-] rule out **Cadmium** toxicity
[-] rule out **Lead** toxicity

DIETARY FACTORS

All pregnant women should be on a nutritious, well-balanced diet which includes between 70 and 90 gm of protein and between 2,300 and 2,800 kcal per day. Too high a carbohydrate intake in early pregnancy, especially if combined with a low dairy protein intake in late pregnancy, appears to suppress placental growth and result in low birth weight infants *(Godfrey)*, although protein supplementation later in pregnancy was not found to enhance intrauterine growth *(Viegas)*.

Dietary Fiber

A high intake of dietary fiber has been correlated with a reduced risk of toxemia in a number of studies *(Hipsley)*. Also, vegetable fibers with a high viscosity are known to reduce the levels of basal and post-prandial glycemia in both normal and diabetic subjects. To see their effect during pregnancy, 34 pregnant women received either glucomannan or guar supplements. Compared to baseline, *all* subjects demonstrated reductions in glucose levels both in regard to basal values and values following an oral glucose tolerance test, suggesting that the supplement may reduce the risk of gestational diabetes *(Cesa)*.

Dietary Fats

In order to investigate why women with gestational diabetes mellitus in one pregnancy have a recurrence rate of only 30 to 50 percent in their subsequent pregnancy, a study was conducted to compare the dietary intake of fats in 14 women with a recurrence of gestational diabetes mellitus to 21 women with no recurrence of the disease. The women with the recurrence were found to consume a significantly higher percentage of their total energy intake as fats. The percentage intake of polyunsaturated, monounsaturated, and saturated fatty acids was similar in both groups.

Given the known relationship between saturated fat intake and insulin resistance, these findings suggest that the reduction of dietary fats before and during pregnancy may reduce the recurrence rate of gestational diabetes *(Moses)*.

Trans Fatty Acids

When plasma *trans* fatty acid levels of 23 women who delivered pre-term infants were compared to those of 21 women who delivered at term, an inverse correlation was found both with gestational age and birth weight, suggesting that *trans* isomers of unsaturated fatty acids may impair intrauterine growth *(Jendryczko,1993)*.

The plasma *trans* fatty acid levels of premature infants have also been studied. As in the study of mothers of premature infants, a study of 29 premature infants at day 4 of life found an inverse correlation between the infants' plasma *trans* fatty acid levels and birth weight - although gestational age was unrelated *(Koletzko)*.

Since *trans* fatty acids inhibit the activity of the enzyme delta-6-desaturase, further studies are needed to ascertain whether maternal *trans* fatty acid intake inhibits essential fatty acid metabolism in the infant and interferes with fetal growth and development *(Carlson)*.

Furthermore, mothers with high intakes of *trans* fatty acids may have an increased risk of preeclampsia. When mean erythrocyte fatty acid levels of 22 women with preeclampsia were compared with those of 40 normotensives, mean levels of elaidic acid (one of the most abundant dietary *trans* fatty acids) were 28% higher among preeclamptics. After adjusting for confounding factors, women with the highest levels of elaidic acid were 7.4 times more likely to have their pregnancy complicated by preeclampsia as compared with women with the lowest levels *(Williams,1998)*.

Sugar

In a study of almost 500 nondiabetic, pregnant adolescents, the adjusted odds ratio for the delivery of a small-for-gestational age infant of those in the top 10th percentile of total dietary sugar was double than of the remainder of the group, regardless of their ethnicity *(Lenders)*.

Alcohol

Alcohol is prohibited during pregnancy. It increases the risk of a wide variety of birth abnormalities. The hallmarks of fetal alcohol syndrome are pre- and postnatal growth retardation, central nervous system dysfunction, and characteristic facial dysmorphology. However, its effects can be multi-systemic, encompassing the cardiac, skeletal, and muscular systems, as well as presenting as lack of coordination, hyperactivity, diminished or distorted sense of danger, and lack of ability to function as an independent adult. Children with fetal alcohol effects display fewer of the traits of fetal alcohol syndrome *(Appelbaum)*.

Not surprisingly, alcohol intake also appears to increase the risk of spontaneous abortion. In a prospective study of 5,300 pregnant women, there was a trend of increasing spontaneous abortion rates with increasing alcohol consumption levels during pregnancy. The odds ratio of spontaneous abortion was at least double for women who drank more than 3 drinks a week. Even women who reported only "sips" of alcohol had almost double the risk of spontaneous abortion *(Windham)*

Caffeine

Caffeine intake should be totally avoided. Numerous observational studies have found direct correlations between caffeine intake and spontaneous abortion *(Fernandes;Parazzini)* and fetal loss *(Infante-Rivard)*, intrauterine growth retardation *(Rondo)*, preterm premature membrane rupture *(Williams,1992)*, low-birth-weight infants *(Fernandes)*, and sudden infant death syndrome (SIDS) *(Ford)*.

There is even an association between the average annual national coffee consumption and the age-standardized incidence of insulin-dependent diabetes in the zero to 14-year-old age group *(Tuomilehto)*. Some of these correlations start to be seen with intakes as low as 150 mg day (about one cup of coffee daily) and are notable at 600 mg daily.

Moreover, *all* of a group of 16 women who ingested more than 500 mg daily of caffeine delivered babies with tremors, and one-quarter of the babies had cardiac rhythm disturbances, suggesting that the infants were suffering from symptoms of caffeine withdrawal *(Hadeed)*.

Milk

Excessive phosphate absorption promotes the development of leg cramps of pregnancy (see Phosphorus below). Milk and dairy products appear to cause a fall in diffusible calcium and a rise in inorganic phosphorus in the blood, probably due to an increased efficiency in the intestinal absorption of phosphates during gestation, with a resultant depression of ionized blood calcium. Also, a shift in the acid-base balance to the alkaline side may be contributory *(Page)*.

If the patient is drinking more than 3 pints a day of milk, a reduction of milk intake to less than one pint a day may be adequate to treat the symptom *(Page)*.

HOMOCYSTEINE

Plasma levels of homocysteine, a toxic amino acid, have been related to the risk of to neural tube defects in infants *(Mills,1995)* as well as to preeclampsia *(Powers)*, and abruption and infarction of the placenta *(Goddijn-Wessel)*. The evidence points primarily to a disorder in the remethylation of homocysteine to methionine due to an acquired nutritional or inherited abnormality in folate or vitamin B_{12} metabolism *(Steegers-Theunissen)*.

NUTRITIONAL FACTORS

Nutrient needs are notably increased during pregnancy in order to satisfy the requirements of fetal and placental growth. Limited maternal stores and an often inadequate dietary intake lead to deficiency, the materno-fetal consequences of which are beginning to be understood *(Favier M)*. Multiple nutrient deficiency is therefore common during pregnancy.

For example, in a study of 76 healthy pregnant women, 78% had one or more glaring nutritional deficiencies *(Dostalova)*. There is increasing agreement that nutrient supplements are useful, although the variety of nutrients to be supplemented continues to be debated. Recent studies appear to show that, rather than being selective and seeking out a "high risk" population, supplements should be given routinely to all pregnant women because of their low costs in relation to expected health benefits *(Favier M)*.

VITAMINS

Folic Acid

Folate is the only vitamin whose requirement doubles in pregnancy *(Truswell)*, possibly due to accelerated catabolism *(McPartlin)*. Not only do serum and erythrocyte folate levels decline, but some degree of megaloblastic changes in red blood cells can be found in a substantial minority of women in late pregnancy *(Truswell)*.

Based on current knowledge suggesting the need for a minimum of 400 micrograms daily, the dietary intake of folate during pregnancy is often inadequate *(Herberg; Werler)*. In a prospective study, women with low mean folate intakes at week 28 of gestation had a 2-fold greater risk of preterm delivery and low infant birth weight after controlling for confounding variables *(Scholl,1996)*.

Maternal serum folate levels have also been found to inversely correlate with a greater risk of preterm delivery and low infant birth weight *(Scholl,1996)*. Similarly, in a study of infants with erythroblastosis, the average birth weight was lower than that of controls, and there was a strong correlation between low maternal serum folate and the incidence of small-for-dates babies as well as a strong correlation between maternal and cord blood serum folate values, suggesting that a shortage of folic acid available for fetal growth may be the cause *(Gandy)*.

Supplementation

It is now well accepted that supplementation with folic acid around the time of conception will reduce the risk of neural tube defects *(Morrow)*. While 400 micrograms daily is considered adequate for most women, 10 times that amount has been advocated for women with a prior history of a fetal neural tube defect *(Rayburn)*. There is also evidence that supplementation may reduce the risk of orofacial clefts *(Shaw,1994,1995)*.

Moreover, folate supplementation appears to have favorable effects on birth weight and Apgar scores of newborn infants and may reduce the prevalence of fetal growth retardation *(Tamura,1992)*.

Increasing folate-rich foods in the diet is relatively ineffective compared to providing folate supplementation *(Cuskelly;Neuhouser)*.

The fact that folate deficiency may cause post-partum psychosis is illustrated by a case report:

After giving birth, a woman developed severe depression, confusion, disorientation and hallucinations. Over the next 19 months, trials with numerous medications and electroshock therapy were unsuccessful.

Folic acid deficiency was diagnosed and folate supplementation was started. In 10 days, she was completely cured (Thornton).

Niacin

Maternal niacin intake early in pregnancy may be directly associated with infant birthweight and size. However, in a controlled study, supplementation during the second and third trimesters was ineffective in affecting birth dimensions *(Doyle)*.

Pantothenic Acid

During pregnancy, women appear to require higher intakes of pantothenic acid in order to maintain a similar blood level to that of the nonpregnant state *(Song)*.

In an open trial three-quarters of a group of 32 pregnant women with leg cramps became asymptomatic after receiving panthenol for 10 days *(Dumont)*. However, another observer found the efficacy of pantothenic acid to be equivocal *(Page)*.

A controlled clinical trial (preferably with before and after measures of pantothenic acid nutriture) would help to ascertain the efficacy of the nutrient.

Riboflavin

Riboflavin depletion is common during pregnancy *(Heller,1974;Shaw N;Vir)*.

Its intake was recently found to be directly related to fetal growth *(Bardart-Smook)*, suggesting that improving the diet, or providing supplementation, may reduce the risk of low-birth-weight babies. Also, in open trials, women suffering from leg cramps of pregnancy usually responded to riboflavin supplements *(Kline;Morgan; Thoyer-Rozat)*. This finding is consistent with that of a study of athletes which found that riboflavin supplementation resulted in moderate lowering of neuromuscular irritability *(Haralambie)*.

Thiamine

Thiamine depletion is a common finding *(Icke;Jeffrey)*. There is evidence of a positive correlation between maternal thiamine intake (as measured during one week towards the end of the first trimester) and birth weight, newborn head circumference and newborn length for babies below the median weight *(Doyle)*. While this finding implies that thiamine supplementation may be beneficial, when supplementation was provided after completion of the first trimester, it failed to affect birth dimensions *(Doyle)*.

Also, open trials have suggested that thiamine supplementation may benefit leg cramps of pregnancy *(De Lee)*, although one clinician has reported equivocal results *(Page)*.

Vitamin A

Inadequate intake of vitamin A in early pregnancy may be teratogenic. In one study, babies born to women consuming more than 10,000 IU per day had only about three-quarters the risk of malformations of babies born to women consuming less than 5,000 IU daily *(Mills,1997)*. Another study concluded that the use of moderate doses of the vitamin (less than 10,000 IU daily) during the first trimester appears to protect the fetus against congenital abnormalities *(Czeizel)*.

Results of a study of preterm infants suggest that low vitamin A nutriture promotes prematurity and its associated complications. Sixty-four percent of the 91 preterm infants had low levels of retinol, while retinol-binding proteins were lower on the third day of life in the babies with respiratory distress syndrome. Furthermore, preterm babies who developed bronchopulmonary dysplasia had lower retinol concentrations at birth *(Hustead)*.

In addition to its effects on the fetus, low maternal vitamin A nutriture (as suggested by serum or plasma levels) is associated with an increased risk of preeclampsia *(Jendryczko,1989;Ziari)*.

A Warning

Excessive vitamin A supplementation early in pregnancy appears to be teratogenic. While 10,000 IU of preformed vitamin A daily is usually the maximum recommended safe intake *(Rothman)*, there is considerable evidence suggesting that up to 25,000 or 30,000 IU daily carries only minimal risk, if any *(Miller;Mills,1997)*.

Vitamin B_6

About 50% of pregnant women may be marginally deficient in vitamin B_6, and supplementation with 20 mg pyridoxine daily has been shown in a number of studies to be necessary to keep a laboratory measurement of vitamin B_6 (erythrocyte glutamate-oxaloacetate transaminase) in the normal range during pregnancy *(Heller,1973)*.

Preliminary data suggest that supplementation may prevent pregnancy toxemias *(Brophy)*. The data are more convincing in the specific case of hyperemesis gravidarum (pernicious vomiting of pregnancy). In this instance, there is evidence that serum levels of the vitamin may be low *(Gant)*. Furthermore, double-blind studies have found supplementation to be effective *(Sahakian;Vutyavanich)*.

By impairing pancreatic insulin production, a deficiency of vitamin B_6 may potentiate gestational diabetes *(Jonovic-Peterson)*. Open trials in the 1970s have reported that supplementation with the vitamin has some efficacy in treating this disorder *(Bennink;Gillmer; Spellancy)*. Unfortunately, these preliminary trials have yet to be followed by properly controlled experiments.

A Warning

Higher doses of vitamin B_6 may shut off breast milk. Also, if the mother has been supplementing with large dosages of the vitamin, the baby could have withdrawal seizures if there is inadequate vitamin B_6 in a commercial formula *(Foukas;Marcus)*.

Vitamin B_{12}

There appears to be a relationship between postpartum psychosis and vitamin B_{12} nutriture. Eight cases have been reported, all of which responded dramatically with complete clearing following 2 successive daily doses of intramuscular cyanocobalamin *(Daynes)*.

The risk of neural tube defects is inversely associated with plasma *(Kirke)*, serum *(Wald)* and amnionic fluid *(Steen)* cobalamin concentrations. While adequate folic nutriture appears to be most important in preventing neural tube defects *(Wald)*, adequate nutriture of this vitamin should also be assured.

Lack of vitamin B_{12} in the maternal diet during pregnancy has been shown to cause severe retardation of myelination in the nervous system, usually in the spinal cord. Fortunately, supplementation after birth appears to be beneficial:

A 14 ½ -month-old child of strictly vegetarian parents presented with severe psychomotor retardation. Severely hypotonic, the child had a megaloblastic anemia due to insufficient maternal intake of vitamin B_{12}. An MRI of the brain revealed severe brain atrophy with signs of retarded myelination, the frontal and temporal lobes being most severely affected.

Vitamin B_{12} therapy was instituted and the patient responded well, with improvement of clinical and imaging abnormalities (Daynes).

Vitamin C

Patients with preeclampsia may have low plasma levels of vitamin C *(Mikhail)*. This finding appears to be at least partly due to increased oxidative stress *(Hubel)*.

Ascorbate nutriture also appears to be directly related to the risk of premature rupture of the fetal membranes. Of a group of 80 women, those with preterm rupture of fetal membranes had lower amniotic fluid vitamin C concentrations and lower ratios of amniotic fluid vitamin C to serum vitamin C concentrations *(Barrett,1994a)*. Also, when leukocyte vitamin C levels were followed throughout gestation in another group of women, the levels on week 20 of gestation were inversely associated with the risk of premature rupture *(Casaneuva)*.

In a double-blind study, ascorbic acid supplementation was found to be as effective as calcium for the treatment of leg cramps of pregnancy. For 23% of the total group of 60 women, their symptoms were totally abolished; for 45% symptoms were significantly decreased; for 28%

symptoms were unaffected; and for 3% symptoms increased in frequency *(Hammar,1987)*.

A Warning

There is evidence that infants born to women taking more than 5 grams of vitamin C throughout pregnancy, while born healthy, develop "rebound" scurvy soon thereafter *(Rhead)*. While a subsequent literature review has noted that there is no reliable evidence to support this contention *(Rivers)*, providing vitamin C supplementation to newborn infants of such mothers appears to be a prudent measure.

Vitamin D Deficiency

Maternal vitamin D deficiency during pregnancy may adversely affect fetal growth, bone ossification, tooth enamel formation, and neonatal calcium homeostasis *(Brunvand;Specker)*. Although routine vitamin D supplementation is not necessary, daily supplementation should be considered for selected women whose diets are inadequate in the vitamin *(Committee)*.

Vitamin E

Despite increased plasma tocopherol levels (which reflect elevated blood lipid levels), vitamin E nutriture appears to decline during pregnancy *(Mino)*. Vitamin E levels in red cells of newborns are lower than those of their mothers - and significantly related to their mothers' red cell vitamin E levels. These findings suggest that an increase in vitamin E supplementation to mothers during pregnancy, by increasing vitamin E levels in the newborn, may help to impede the effect of extrauterine oxygen toxicity *(Jain,1996)*.

Furthermore, reduced plasma/serum levels have been repeatedly associated with increased risks of preeclampsia and eclampsia *(Jain,1995;Ziari)*. One study found the opposite correlation, which suggested to the investigators that higher plasma vitamin E concentrations could be a response to increased oxidative stress *(Schiff)*. Data offering some confirmation of this speculation has recently come from a study which found a highly significant fall in vitamin E levels in preeclamptic women as compared to controls, but also found significant increases the levels of serum malonaldehyde (a marker of lipid peroxidation), and a high correlation between the level of serum malonaldehyde and blood pressure *(Kharb)*.

However, when 36 preeclamptic patients received either vitamin E plus conventional therapy or vitamin E alone, fetal mortality was similar, and in both groups proteinuria increased and dosages of antihypertensive drugs had to be increased to control blood pressure *(Stratta)*. Therefore, at least until further controlled trials are conducted, it appears that vitamin E supplementation is ineffective in preeclampsia.

In women whose pregnancies were complicated by fetal complications or maternal risks, the average maternal serum vitamin E levels were lower *(van Mandach)*. A reduced maternal vitamin E status is also associated with premature and low-birth weight-infants *(Shah;van Mandach)*.

The data on habitual abortion are quite different. In this case, plasma vitamin E levels appear to be normal *(Nicotra)*. However, in open trials, supplementation with the vitamin appears to be effective *(Marks;Sutton)*.

A woman with a history of 4 miscarriages was told that any treatment, hormonal or otherwise, would be unlikely to achieve a live birth. She became pregnant again and, as soon as she had missed her first period, she began supplementation with vitamin E ("Ephynal") 50 mg 3 times daily.

At the end of the second month she had a chest infection and, as a result of coughing, she began to bleed vaginally. Treatment with sulfonamides cleared up the chest infection and the bleeding stopped. During the third month she again had a chest infection and threatened abortion, but again antibiotic treatment was successful and the bleeding ceased.

She continued on vitamin E until the 28th week of pregnancy and was confined to home until the delivery of a male child of normal weight (Sutton).

Vitamin K

A subclinical deficiency of vitamin K during pregnancy is common. In one study, one-third of 99 pregnant women were found to have evidence of deficiency *(Anonymous, 1984)*.

Deficiency of vitamin K is well-known to cause hemorrhagic disease of the newborn infant *(von Kries)*. Vitamin K prophylaxis has been recommended for all newborn babies *(McNinch)*. However, since the vitamin crosses that placenta and persists to activate the vitamin K-dependent coagulant factors until at least the fifth day of life, prenatal vitamin K1 (menadione) administration to mothers may replace prophylaxis at birth *(Anai)* - although the efficacy of this approach is still debatable *(Thorp)*.

Supplementation is particularly recommended if mothers are on anticonvulsant therapy or prolonged treatment with certain antibiotics. These medications, if ingested by pregnant women, predispose the neonate to a bleeding tendency caused by vitamin K deficiency *(Thorp)*. It has also been found to be effective in preventing neonatal intraventricular hemorrhage in infants destined to be delivered prematurely *(Morales)*.

Hyperemesis gravidarum is another condition for which supplementation may be effective. In an open trial, the combination of vitamin K1 and vitamin C effectively treated 91% of a group of 70 patients within 72 hours *(Merkel)*.

MINERALS

Calcium

Calcium nutriture is closely related to pregnancy toxemias. Epidemiologic evidence links low calcium intake to an increased risk of eclampsia *(Villar, 1983)*. Hypocalciuria is a feature of pre-eclampsia. Determination of urinary calcium excretion may therefore help to differentiate pre-eclampsia from the more benign forms of gestational hypertension *(Taufield)*. Furthermore, in patients with pregnancy-induced hypertension, both serum and mononuclear cell calcium levels may be decreased *(Qi)*.

Numerous double-blind studies have explored the efficacy of calcium supplementation in treating pre-eclampsia and pregnancy-induced hypertension. A recent meta-analysis in the *Journal of the American Medical Association* reviewed 14 randomized trials involving 2,459 women. The pooled analysis showed significant reductions in systolic BP of -5.40 mm Hg and diastolic BP of -3.44 mm Hg. The odds ratio for preeclampsia in women with calcium supplementation compared to placebo was 0.38 *(Bucher)*.

The following year, however, the *New England Journal of Medicine* published a double-blind study of 4,589 pregnant women which found that calcium supplementation failed to significantly reduce the incidence or severity of pre-eclampsia or delay its onset. Moreover, there was no detectable benefit in women with low baseline 24-hour urinary calcium excretion, or low ratios of urinary calcium to creatinine in the first morning urine, nor was there any benefit among women whose baseline dietary calcium intakes were in the lowest quintile *(Levine)*.

It appears that leg cramps in pregnant women may reflect alterations in calcium metabolism *(Pitkin)*, although one study found similar levels of total serum and ionized calcium in pregnant women with- and without leg cramps *(Hammar, 1981)*. While open trials have reported calcium supplementation to be an effective treatment *(Hammer, 1981)*, controlled studies have failed to confirm its efficacy *(Hammar, 1987; Odendaal)*.

Our knowledge of the efficacy of the third potential application for calcium supplementation is, like the other two, clouded by opposing results of controlled clinical trials. In a study of 189 pregnant female adolescents, supplementation starting by the 23rd week of gestation resulted in a lower incidence of preterm delivery and low birth weight *(Villar, 1990)*. This was followed, however, by a much larger study of 4,589 adult women. Although essentially the same protocol was followed, there were no significant reductions in the numbers of preterm deliveries, small-for-gestational-age births, or fetal and neonatal deaths *(Levine)*.

Chromium Deficiency

Chromium nutriture may decline during pregnancy, suggesting that chromium supplementation may be advisable *(Saner)*. The finding that placental chromium levels are positively correlated with birth weight *(Ward)* is consistent with this suggestion.

Moreover, chromium deficiency, by impairing pancreatic insulin production, could increase the tendency toward hyperglycemia in gestational diabetes *(Jovanovic-Peterson)*. The efficacy of chromium supplementation has yet to be demonstrated, however, in controlled clinical trials.

Copper Deficiency

Placental levels of both cobalt and copper may be positively correlated with birth weight *(Ward)*. Furthermore, when 24 women in their second trimester were studied, it was found that they ingested less than the Recommended Dietary Allowance of copper. Copper retention was 0.02 mg/day. When supplemented with copper, copper retention rose to 0.89 mg/day. These findings caused the investigators to suggest that "adequate copper retention does not appear possible without the use of a supplement *(Taper)*."

It is important to rectify copper deficiency during embryonic and fetal development as a deficiency can cause numerous gross structural and biochemical abnormalities. Changes in free radical defense mechanisms, connective tissue metabolism, and energy production can all contribute to the dysmorphogenesis associated with developmental copper deficiency *(Keen)*.

Iron Deficiency

Although iron absorption is increased during pregnancy *(Barrett, 1994b)*, the requirement for iron is increased, and deficiency occurs in 20 to 40% of pregnancies *(Anonymous, 1996)*. No single test can adequately evaluate iron stores, although serum ferritin is one of the better measures during pregnancy. While low serum ferritin levels during the second trimester indicates absent iron stores *(Carriaga)*, elevated serum ferritin during the second trimester may be predictive of prematurity, possibly related to a subclinical infection *(Tamura, 1996)*.

Iron deficiency may still be present when there is no evidence of anemia *(Tershakovec)*. When iron-deficiency anemia is present, there is an increased risk of low birth weight and preterm delivery *(Scholl, 1994)*, reduced fetal iron status *(Singla)*, and higher maternal mortality *(Allen)*.

Supplementation is often necessary to maintain adequate iron stores during the second and third trimesters *(Anonymous, 1996)*. However, iron supplementation during pregnancy may exacerbate subclinical zinc depletion *(Meadows)* and increase the risk of seizures in the newborn *(Baker)*.

Magnesium Deficiency

On the average, pregnant women only ingest about half of their Recommended Dietary Allowance for magnesium *(Franz)*, while plasma/serum levels, which are lower than those of non-pregnant women *(Stanton)*, fall steadily during pregnancy *(Sheldon)* along with ionized magnesium levels *(Standley)*.

An animal study has shown some of the many possible adverse implications of low magnesium status during pregnancy. Ewes received low magnesium diets with half given magnesium in the water. Plasma and tissue magnesium were significantly lower in the deprived animals. There was a significant elevation of arterial blood pressure, reduction in fetal weight, and pathologic confirmation of placental and renal lesions which were similar to those seen in humans *(Weaver)*.

In humans, maternal magnesium intake during the first trimester has been found to correlate with birth weight, newborn head circumference, and newborn length for babies below the median weight *(Doyle)*. This correlation may be due, at least in part, to the influence of magnesium nutriture on preterm labor. There is evidence suggesting that a low magnesium concentration in the pregnant myometrium may cause premature labor *(Cunze)*. Moreover, regardless of etiology, patients in premature labor may have depressed serum magnesium levels despite the etiology of the labor *(Kurzel)*.

Women with preeclampsia have low serum and urinary magnesium levels *(Standley)*. If, as currently hypothesized, cerebral vasospasm provokes the development of eclampsia, extracellular magnesium may both oppose intracellular calcium-dependent arterial vasoconstriction and antagonize the increase in intracellular calcium caused by the ischemia. (Extracellular calcium has different actions than intracellular calcium; it may even be a "calcium channel blocker" and reduce the transport of the calcium ion into the cell by causing parathyroid hormone secretion to diminish.)

Yet another danger of magnesium deficiency is that, by impairing pancreatic insulin production, it may potentiate the development of gestational diabetes *(Jovanovic-Peterson)*.

Supplementation

Numerous studies, many of which were controlled, have found evidence that magnesium supplementation may reduce the risk of complications of pregnancy and improve the health of the fetus. It has even been argued that, until sufficient research is completed to clarify the situation, the increased need for magnesium in anabolic processes during gestation may justify prophylactic magnesium administration to lower the risk of maternal and infant complications *(Seelig)*.

Based on the results of these studies, parenterally-administered magnesium supplementation has been called the "drug of choice" for the treatment of toxemia, especially for the treatment of eclampsia-associated seizures *(McCombs;Sabai;Skajaa)*. Cerebral vasospasm appears to be involved in the pathogenesis of eclampsia. Magnesium may act by opposing calcium-dependent arterial vasoconstriction; it may also antagonize the increase in intracellular calcium caused by ischemia and thus prevent cell damage and death *(Sadeh)*.

Among very-low-birth-weight children, several observational studies have found a positive association between prenatal magnesium exposure and a reduced risk of cerebral palsy and mental retardation *(Schendel)*. Magnesium has shown itself in double-blind studies to be an effective treatment for leg cramps *(Dahle)*. Finally, although controlled clinical trials are lacking, magnesium supplementation is likely to combat gestational diabetes *(Bardicef;Wibell)*.

Phosphorus: A Warning

There is some evidence that excessive phosphate may promote the development of leg cramps of pregnancy *(Pitkin)* (see Milk above.) A study of 99 pregnant women with this symptom either reduced their milk intake to less than one pint daily (if they had been drinking more than 3 pints a day), substituted calcium lactate for dicalcium phosphate as a source of calcium, or moderately reduced their milk intake and added aluminum hydroxide gel with each meal (to decrease phosphorus absorption). Compared to 21 women who served as controls, there was a highly significant reduction in the number of patients who improved or were asymptomatic in each intervention group *(Page)*.

In an open trial, milk and dairy products were eliminated from the diets of 10 women who were 5 to 8 months pregnant and suffering from leg cramps, and aluminum hydroxide gel was given with each meal. Effective treatment was found to be accompanied by a rise in ionizable calcium and a reduction in blood phosphorus *(Page)*.

Potassium Deficiency

Potassium levels may be reduced during pregnancy, especially in eclampsia *(Sjogren)*. Also, by impairing pancreatic insulin production, potassium deficiency may potentiate the tendency towards hyperglycemia in gestational diabetes *(Jovanovic-Peterson)*.

The benefits of repletion have yet to be studied systematically.

Selenium Deficiency

Selenium deficiency has been linked with increased risks of miscarriage *(Barrington)* and neural tube defects *(Guvenc)*. Controlled clinical trials of selenium supplementation are lacking.

Zinc Deficiency

Pregnant women commonly only ingest about two-thirds of the Recommended Dietary Allowance for zinc *(Hambridge)*. Moreover, plasma/serum zinc declines during pregnancy *(Favier)*. Although some of this decline is merely due to an increase in protein-zinc binding capacity *(Argemi)*, white blood cell and hair zinc also decline *(Favier)*.

Low maternal intake has been related to preterm deliveries and low birth weight *(Scholl,1993)*, and lower serum zinc levels are sometimes found in women who have had a spontaneous abortion *(Breskin)*. Moreover, in an study of pregnant guinea pigs, poor zinc intake resulted in spontaneous abortion and premature delivery in 2 out of 3 experiments *(Apgar)*.

Poor maternal zinc nutriture is strongly associated with various indicators of poor pregnancy outcome *(Caulfield)*. Some, but not all, observational studies have found positive correlations between maternal zinc status and low-birth-weight babies *(Ward)*, fetal distress *(Mukherjee)*, central nervous system malformation *(Buamah)*, prolonged labor *(Lazebnik)*, and toxemias *(Cherry)*.

Supplementation

Despite the intriguing correlations between poor zinc nutriture and poor pregnancy outcome, few clinical trials have found zinc supplementation to be effective. Several controlled trials have investigated the effect of zinc supplementation on pregnancy outcome for mothers at high risk for poor zinc nutriture. The results have been mixed *(Goldenberg;Swanson)*.

Similarly, the majority of controlled trials investigating the efficacy of zinc supplementation in preventing toxemias of pregnancy have failed to substantiate efficacy for the supplement *(Jonsson)*. Results of an open trial suggest that zinc supplementation may reduce the risk of abnormally long labor *(Jameson)*; however, this finding has yet to be confirmed in a controlled clinical trial.

OTHER NUTRITIONAL FACTORS

Essential Fatty Acids

Vitally important structural elements of cell membranes, the essential fatty acids (EFA) are instrumental in the formation of new tissues. While the developing fetus thus has a high EFA requirement, the EFA status of the mother progressively decreases throughout pregnancy *(Hornstra)*.

Omega-3 Fatty Acids

alpha-linolenic acid → EPA → 3 series prostaglandins
↳ DHA

Results of a controlled study suggest that these essential fatty acids are required for the optimal maturation of visual and cortical function in preterm infants. Preterm infants were fed human milk or one of 3 formulas. At both 36 and 57 weeks postconception, infants fed the formula which was deficient in omega-3 essential fatty acids had impaired visual acuity compared to the control groups *(Hoffman)*. Moreover, the fetal status of docosahexaenoic acid (DHA) is positively related to head circumference, birth weight and birth length, implying that supplementation could possibly improve the general prognosis of premature infants *(Hornstra)*.

There is also some evidence suggesting that inadequate omega-3 fatty acid nutriture may foster preterm deliveries. When preterm and control mother-baby dyads were compared, maternal red blood cell eicosapentaenoic acid (EPA) levels and the ratio of omega-3 to omega-6 essential fatty acids were lower in preterm cases, while the levels of DHA, a marker of omega-3 fatty acid deficiency, was higher in the preterm maternal red blood cells and amnion *(Reece)*. Moreover, in a randomized study, fish oil supplementation increased the length of gestation by 4 days on average, suggesting that it may reduce the risk of preterm delivery *(Olsen)*.

Preliminary data from a small observational study suggest that inadequate omega-3 fatty acid nutriture may increase the risk of preeclampsia. After adjusting for confounding variables, women with the lowest erythrocyte level of omega-3 fatty acids were 7.6 times more likely to develop preeclampsia as compared to women with the highest level *(Williams, 1995)*.

However, controlled studies of omega-3 fatty acid supplements have failed to find them to be beneficial in either proteinuric or non-proteinuric *(Bulstra-Ramakers; Onwude; Salvig)* pregnancy-induced hypertension.

Omega-6 Fatty Acids

linoleic acid → GLA → DGLA → 1 series prostaglandins

Pregnancy-induced hypertension is associated with diminished tissue production of the E series prostaglandins and an enhanced pressor response to angiotensin II. Since omega-6 fatty acids are nutritional precursors to prostaglandin E1, normal pregnant subjects were supplemented with two members of this family, linoleic acid and gamma-linolenic acid (GLA), in a controlled study. When compared to unsupplemented controls, supplemented subjects demonstrated a reduced pressor response to angiotensin II, suggesting that supplementation with omega-6 fatty acids may help to prevent pregnancy-induced hypertension *(O'Brien)*.

The efficacy of the omega-6 fatty acids in treating pregnancy-induced hypertension and other toxemias of pregnancy remains to be explored.

OTHER RELATED FACTORS

Heavy Metal Toxicity

Cadmium

The body burden of cadmium has been repeatedly correlated with low birth weight *(Frery; Ward)*.

Lead

Excessive lead exposure may result, not only in low birth weight *(Min; Ward)*, but also in miscarriage, premature membrane rupture, preeclampsia, pregnancy hypertension, and premature delivery *(Winder)*. The developing nervous system appears to be particularly sensitive to lead's adverse effects *(Goyer)*.

As erythrocyte ratios of lead to magnesium and of lead to calcium were higher in a study of preeclamptic patients, an elevated lead body burden may promote preeclampsia by inhibiting calcium and magnesium transport *(Dawson)*.

BIBLIOGRAPHY

Allen LH. Pregnancy and iron deficiency: unresolved issues. Nutr Rev 55(4):91-101, 1997

Anai T et al. Can prenatal vitamin K1 (phylloquinone) supplementation replace prophylaxis at birth? Obstet Gynecol 81(2):251-4, 1993

Anonymous. Family Practice News 14(5):27, 1984

Anonymous. IV iron Works where oral supplementation fails. Family Practice News 26(13):29, July 1, 1996

Apgar J, Everett G. Low zinc intake affects maintenance of pregnancy in guinea pigs. J Nutr 121:192-200, 1991

Appelbaum MG. Fetal alcohol syndrome: diagnosis, management, and prevention. Nurse Pract 20(10):24, 27-8, 31-3 passim, 1995

Argemi J et al. Serum zinc binding capacity in pregnant women. Ann Nutr Metab 32:121-6, 1988

Baker B. Iron exposure in utero may have harsh results. Family Practice News November 15, 1994:2

Badart-Smook A et al. Fetal growth is associated positively with maternal intake of riboflavin and negatively with maternal intake of linoleic acid. J Am Diet Assoc 97(8):867-70, 1997

Bardicef M et al. Extracellular and intracellular magnesium depletion in pregnancy and gestational diabetes. Am J Obstet Gynecol 172(3):1009-13, 1995

Barrett BM et al. Potential role of ascorbic acid and β-carotene in the prevention of preterm rupture of fetal membranes. Int J Vitam Nutr Res 64:192-7, 1994a

Barrett JFR et al. Absorption of non-haem iron from food during normal pregnancy. BMJ 309:79-82, 1994b

Barrington JW et al. Selenium deficiency and miscarriage: a possible link. Br J Obstet Gynecol 103:130-2, 1996

Bennink HJ, Schreurs WH. Improvement of oral glucose tolerance in gestational diabetes by pyridoxine. Br Med J 3(5974):13-5, 1975

Breskin MW et al. First trimester serum zinc concentrations in human pregnancy. Am J Clin Nutr 38(6):943-53, 1983

Brophy MH, Siiteri PK. Pyridoxal phosphate and hypertensive disorders of pregnancy. Am J Obstet Gynecol 121(8):1075-9, 1975

Brunvand L et al. Vitamin D deficiency and fetal growth. Eur Hum Dev 45(1-2):27-33, 1996

Buamah PK et al. Maternal zinc status: A determinant of central nervous system malformation. Br J Obstet Gynaecol 91:788-90, 1984

Bucher HC et al. Effect of calcium supplementation on pregnancy-induced hypertension and preeclampsia. JAMA 275(14):1113-17, 1996

Bulstra-Ramakers MT et al. The effects of 3g eicosapentaenoic acid daily on recurrence of intrauterine growth retardation and pregnancy induced hypertension. Br J Obstet Gynaecol 102(2):123-6, 1995

Carlson SE et al. trans Fatty acids: infant and fetal development. Am J Clin Nutr 66(3):715S-36S, 1997

Carriaga MT et al. Serum transferrin receptor for the detection of iron deficiency in pregnancy. Am J Clin Nutr 54:1077-81, 1991

Casanueva E et al. Vitamin C status, cervico-vaginal infection and premature rupture of amniotic membranes. Arch Med Res 26 Spec No:S149-52, 1995

Caulfield LE et al. Potential contribution of maternal zinc supplementation during pregnancy to maternal and child survival. Am J Clin Nutr 68(2 Suppl):499S-508S, 1998

Cesa F et al. [The use of vegetable fibers in the treatment of pregnancy diabetes and/or excessive weight gain during pregnancy]. Minerva Ginecol 42(6):271-4, 1990 (in Italian)

Cherry FF et al. Plasma zinc in hypertension/toxemia and other reproductive variables in adolescent pregnancy. Am J Clin Nutr 34(11):2367-75, 1981

Committee on Nutritional Status During Pregnancy and Lactation, Food and Nutrition Board, Institute of Medicine, National Academy of Sciences. Nutrition During Pregnancy, Part I: Nutrient Supplements. Washington, DC, National Academy Press, 1992

Cunze T et al. Magnesium and calcium concentration in pregnant and nonpregnant myometrium. Int J Gynecol Obstet 48:9-13, 1995

Cuskelly GJ et al. Effect of increasing dietary folate on red-cell folate: implications for prevention of neural tube defects. Lancet 347:657-9, 1996

Czeizel AE et al. The effect of periconceptional multivitamin-mineral supplement on vertigo, nausea and vomiting in the first semester of pregnancy. Arch Gynecol Obstet 251:181-5, 1992

Dahle LO et al. The effect of oral magnesium substitution on pregnancy-induced leg cramps. Am J Obstet Gynecol 173(1):175-80, 1995

Dawson EB, Kelly R. Calcium, magnesium, and lead relationships in preeclampsia. Abstract. Am J Clin Nutr 51:512, 1990

Daynes G. Cyanocobalamin in postpartum psychosis. Letter. S Afr Med J 49:1373, 1975

De Lee JB, Green Hill JP. Principles and Practice of Obstetrics. 10th Edition. Philadelphia, Saunders, 1951:331

Dostalova L. Correlation of the vitamin status between mother and newborn during delivery. Dev Pharmacol Ther 4 Suppl:45-57, 1982

Doyle W et al. The association between maternal diet and birth dimensions. J Nutr Med 1:9-17, 1990

Dumont M. Action du panthénol sur les crampes musculaires des femmes enceintes. Presse Med 58:3-4, 1950 (in French)

Favier AE. The role of zinc in reproduction: hormonal mechanisms. Biol Trace Elem Res 32:363-82, 1992

Favier M, Faure P. [Supplements during pregnancy: fad or necessity? Rev Fr Gynecol Obstet 89(4):210-5, 1994 (in French)

Fernandes O et al. Moderate to heavy caffeine consumption during pregnancy and relationship to spontaneous abortion and abnormal fetal growth: a meta-analysis. Reprod Toxicol 12(4):435-44, 1998

Ford RP et al. Heavy caffeine intake in pregnancy and sudden infant death syndrome. New Zealand Cot Death Study Group. Arch Dis Child 78(1):9-13, 1998

Foukas MD. An antilactogenic effect of pyridoxine. J Obstet Gynaecol Br Commonw August, 1973, pp. 718-20

Franz KB. Magnesium intake during pregnancy. Magnesium 6:18-27, 1987

Frery N et al. Environmental exposure to cadmium and human birthweight. Toxicology 79(2):109-18, 1993

Gandy G, Jacobson W. Influence of folic acid on birthweight and growth of the erythroblastotic infant. I. Birthweight. Arch Dis Child 52(1):1-6, 1977

Gant H et al. [Vitamin B6 depletion in women with hyperemesis gravidarum.] Wein Klin Wochenschr 87(16):510-13, 1975 (in German)

Gillmer MD, Mazibuko D. Pyridoxine treatment of chemical diabetes in pregnancy. Am J Obstet Gynecol 133(5):499-502, 1979

Goddijn-Wessel TAW, et al. Hyperhomocysteinemia: A Risk Factor for Placental Abruption or Infarction. Eur J Obstet Gynecol Reprod Biol 66:23-9, 1996

Godfrey K et al. Maternal nutrition in early and late pregnancy in relation to placental and fetal growth. BMJ 312:410-5, 1996

Goldenberg RL et al. The effect of zinc supplementation on pregnancy outcome. JAMA 274(6):463-8, 1995

Goyer RA. Results of lead research: prenatal exposure and neurological consequences. Environ Health Perspect 104(10):1050-4, 1996

Guvenc H et al. Low-levels of selenium in mothers and their newborns in pregnancies with a neural-tube defect. Pediatrics 95: 879-82, 1995

Hadeed A Siegel S. Newborn cardiac arrhythmias associated with maternal caffeine use during pregnancy. Clin Pediatr January, 1993:45-7

Hambridge KM et al. Zinc nutritional status during pregnancy. A longitudinal study. Am J Clin Nutr 37:429-42, 1983

Hammar M et al. Calcium treatment of leg cramps in pregnancy. Effect on clinical symptoms and total serum and ionized serum calcium concentrations. Acta Obstet Gynecol Scand 60(4):345-47, 1981

Hammar M et al. Calcium and magnesium status in pregnant women: A comparison between treatment with calcium and vitamin C in pregnant women with leg cramps. Int J Vitam Res 57(2):179- 83, 1987

Haralambie G. Vitamin B2 status in athletes and the influence of riboflavin administration on neuromuscular irritability. Nutr Metab 20(1):1-8, 1976

Heller S et al. Vitamin B6 status in pregnancy. Am J Clin Nutr 26(12):1339-48, 1973

Heller S et al. Riboflavin status in pregnancy. Am J Clin Nutr 27:1225-30, 1974

Herberg S et al. Iron and folacin status of pregnant women: Relationships with dietary intakes. Nutr Rep Int 35(5):915-30, 1987

Hipsley EH. Dietary 'fibre' and pregnancy toxaemia. Br Med J ii:420-2, 1953

Hoffman DR et al. Effects of supplementation with omega 3 long-chain polyunsaturated fatty acids on retinal and cortical development in premature infants. Am J Clin Nutr 57(5 Suppl):807S-812S, 1993

Hornstra G et al. Essential fatty acids in pregnancy and early human development. Eur J Obstet Gynecol Reprod Biol 61(1):57-62, 1995

Hubel CA et al. Increased ascorbate radical formation and ascorbate depletion in plasma from women with preeclampsia: implications for oxidative stress. Free Radic Biol Med 23(4):597-609, 1997

Hustead VA et al. Relationship of vitamin A (retinol) status to lung disease in the preterm infant. J Pediatrics 105(4):610-15, 1984

Icke GC, Nicol DJ. Thiamin status in pregnancy as determined by direct microbiological assay. Int J Vitam Nutr Res 64(1):33-5, 1994

Infante-Rivard C et al. Fetal loss associated with caffeine intake before and during pregnancy. JAMA 270(24):2940-3, 1993

Jain S, Wise R. Relationship between lipid peroxides, vitamin E deficiency and hypertension in preeclampsia. Mol Cell Biochem 151(1):33-8, 1995

Jain SK et al. Vitamin E and vitamin E-quinone levels in red blood cells and plasma of newborn infants and their mothers. J Am Coll Nutr 15(1):44-8, 1996

Jameson S. Zinc Deficiency in Human Subjects. New York Alan R. Liss, 1983:53

Jeffrey HE et al. Thiamine deficiency--a neglected problem of infants and mothers--possible relationships to sudden infant death syndrome. Aust N Z J Obstet Gynaecol 25(3):198-202, 1985

Jendryczko A, Drozdz M. Plasma retinol, beta-carotene and vitamin E levels in relation to the future risk of pre-eclampsia. Zentralbl Gynakol 111(16):1121-3, 1989

Jendryczko A et al. [Unsaturated fatty acids of trans isomers in plasma of pregnant women and birth weight]. Ginekol Pol 64(3):113-6, 1993 (in Polish)

Jonsson B et al. Zinc supplementation during pregnancy: a double-blind, randomized, controlled trial. Acta Obstet Gynecol Scand 75:725-9, 1996

Jovanovic-Peterson L, Peterson CM. Vitamin and mineral deficiencies which may predispose to glucose intolerance of pregnancy. J Am Coll Nutr 15(1):14-20, 1996

Keen CL et al. Effect of copper deficiency on prenatal development and pregnancy outcome. Am J Clin Nutr 67(5 Suppl):1003S-1011S, 1998

Kharb S et al. Lipid peroxidation and vitamin E levels in preeclampsia. Gynecol Obstet Invest 46(4):238-40, 1998

Kirke PN et al. Maternal plasma folate and vitamin B12 are independent risk factors for neural tube defects. Q J Med 86(11):703-8, 1993

Kleine HO. Zentralbl Gynäkol 76:344-56, 1954 (in German)

Koletzko B. Trans fatty acids may impair biosynthesis of long-chain polyunsaturates and growth in man. Acta Paediatr 81:302-6, 1992

Kurzel RB. Serum magnesium levels in pregnancy and preterm labor. Am J Perinatol 8:119-27, 1991

Lazebnik N et al in LS Hurley, Ed. Trace Elements in Man and Animals, Vol. 6, New York, 1988:605

Lenders CM et al. Gestational age and infant size at birth are associated with dietary sugar intake among pregnant adolescents. J Nutr 127(6):1113-7, 1997

Levine RJ et al. Trial of calcium to prevent preeclampsia. N Engl J Med 337(2):69-76, 1997

Marcus RG. Suppression of lactation with high doses of pyridoxine. S Afr Med J December 6, 1975, pp. 2155-6

Marks J. Critical appraisal of the therapeutic value of alpha-tocopherol. Vitam Hormones 20:573-98, 1962

McCombs J. Treatment of preeclampsia and eclampsia. Clin Pharm 11(3):236-45, 1992

McNinch AW, Tripp JH. Haemorrhagic disease of the newborn in the British Isles: two year prospective study. BMJ 303(6810):1105-9, 1991

McPartlin J et al. Accelerated folate breakdown in pregnancy. Lancet 341:148-9, 1993

Meadows NJ et al. Zinc and small babies. Lancet ii:1135-7, 1981

Merkel RL. The use of menadione bisulfite and ascorbic acid in the treatment of nausea and vomiting of pregnancy: A preliminary report. Am J Obstet Gynecol 64(2):416-18, 1952

Mikhail MS et al. Preeclampsia and antioxidant nutrients: decreased plasma levels of reduced ascorbic acid, α-tocopherol, and beta-carotene in women with preeclampsia. Am J Obstet Gynecol 171:150-7, 1994

Miller RK et al. Periconceptional vitamin A use: how much is teratogenic? Reprod Toxicol 12(1):75-88, 1998

Mills JL et al. Homocysteine metabolism in pregnancies complicated by neural-tube defects. Lancet 345:149-51, 1995

Mills JL et al. Vitamin A and birth defects. Am J Obstet Gynecol 177:31-6, 1997

Min YI et al. Parental occupational lead exposure and low birth weight. Am J Ind Med 30(5):569-78, 1996

Mino M, Nagamatu M. An evaluation of nutritional status of vitamin E in pregnant women with respect to red blood cell tocopherol level. Int J Vitam Nutr Res 56:149-53, 1986

Morales WJ et al. The use of antenatal vitamin K in the prevention of early neonatal intraventricular hemorrhage. Am J Obstet Gynecol 159:774-9, 1988

Morgan AA. Treatment of cramp. Letter. J R Soc Med 76(8):712, 1983

Morrow JD, Kelsey K. Folic acid for prevention of neural tube defects: pediatric anticipatory guidance. J Pediatr Health Care 12(2):55-9, 1998

Moses RG et al. The recurrence of gestational diabetes: could dietary differences in fat intake be an explanation? Diabetes Care 20(11):1647-50, 1997

Mukherjee MD et al. Maternal zinc, iron, folic acid, and protein nutriture and outcome of human pregnancy. Am J Clin Nutr 40(3):496-507, 1984

Neuhouser ML et al. Absorption of dietary and supplemental folate in women with prior pregnancies with neural tube defects and controls. J Am Coll Nutr 17(6):625-30, 1998

Nicotra M et al. Blood levels of lipids, lipoperoxides, vitamin E and glutathione peroxidase in women with habitual abortion. Gynecol Obstet Invest 38(4):223-6, 1994

O'Brien PMS et al. The effect of dietary supplementation with linoleic acid and linolenic acid on the pressor response to angiotensin II: A possible role in pregnancy-induced hypertension? Br J Clin Pharmacol 19(3):335-42, 1985

Odendaal HJ. [Calcium for the treatment of leg cramps during pregnancy.] S Afr Med J 48(18):780-1, 1974 (in Afrikaner)

Olsen SF et al. Randomised controlled trial of effect of fish-oil supplementation on pregnancy duration. Lancet 339:1003-7, 1992

Onwude JL et al. A randomised double blind placebo controlled trial of fish oil in high risk pregnancy. Br J Obstet Gynaecol 102(2):95-100, 1995

Page EW, Page EP. Leg cramps in pregnancy: Etiology and treatment. Obstet Gyn 1:94-100, 1953

Parazzini F et al. Coffee consumption and risk of hospitalized miscarriage before 12 weeks of gestation. Hum Reprod 13(8):2286-91, 1998

Pitkin RM. Endocrine regulation of calcium homeostasis during pregnancy. Clin Perinatol 10(3):575-92, 1983

Powers RW et al. Plasma homocysteine concentration is increased in preeclampsia and is associated with evidence of endothelial activation. Am J Obstet Gynecol 179(6 Pt 1):1605-11, 1998

Qi Q et al. [Magnesium and calcium concentration of peripheral serum and mononuclear cells in patients with pregnancy induced hypertension]. Chung Hua Fu Chan Ko Tsa Chih 32(1):15-8, 1997 (in Chinese)

Rayburn WF et al. Periconceptional folate intake and neural tube defects. J Am Coll Nutr 15(2):121-5, 1996

Reece MS et al. Maternal and perinatal long-chain fatty acids: possible roles in preterm birth. Am J Obstet Gynecol 176(4):907-14, 1997

Rhead WJ, Schrauzer GN. Risks of long-term ascorbic acid overdosage. Nutr Rev 29(11):262-3, 1971

Rivers JM. Safety of high level vitamin C ingestion. Ann N Y Acad Sci 498:445-54, 1987

Rondo PH et al. Coffee consumption and intrauterine growth retardation in Brazil. Eur J Clin Nutr 50:705-9, 1996

Rothman KJ et al. Teratogenicity of high vitamin A intake. N Engl J Med 333(21):1369-73, 1995

Sabai BM. Magnesium sulfate is the ideal anticonvulsant in preeclampsia-eclampsia. Am J Obstet Gynecol 162:1141-5, 1990

Sadeh M. Action of magnesium sulfate in the treatment of preeclampsia-eclampsia. Stroke 20(9):1273-5, 1989

Sahakian V et al. Vitamin B6 is effective therapy for nausea and vomiting of pregnancy: A randomized double-blind placebo-controlled study. Obstet Gynecol 78:33-6, 1991

Salvig JD et al. Effects of fish oil supplementation in late pregnancy on blood pressure: a randomized, controlled trial. Br J Obstet Gynaecol 103:529-33, 1996

Saner G. Urinary chromium excretion during pregnancy and its relationship with intravenous glucose loading. Am J Clin Nutr 34(9):1676-9, 1981

Schendel DE et al. Prenatal magnesium sulfate exposure and the risk of cerebral palsy or mental retardation among very low-birth-weight children aged 3 to 5 years. JAMA 276(22):1805-10, 1996

Schiff E et al. Dietary consumption and plasma concentrations of vitamin E in pregnancies complicated by preeclampsia. Am J Obstet Gynecol 175:1024-8, 1996

Scholl TO et al. Low zinc intake during pregnancy: its association with preterm and very preterm delivery. Am J Epidemiol 137:1115-24, 1993

Scholl TO, Hediger ML. Anemia and iron-deficiency anemia: compilation of data on pregnancy outcome. Am J Clin Nutr 59(2 Suppl):492S-500S, 1994

Scholl TO et al. Dietary and serum folate: their influence on the outcome of pregnancy. Am J Clin Nutr 63:520-5, 1996

Seelig MS. Interrelationship of magnesium and estrogen in cardiovascular and bone disorders, eclampsia, migraine and premenstrual syndrome. J Am Coll Nutr 12(4):442-58, 1993

Shah RS et al. Vitamin E status of the newborn in relation to gestational age, birth weight, and maternal vitamin E status. Br J Nutr 58:191-8, 1987

Shaw GM et al. Reduced risk for oral cleft defects associated with periconceptional folic acid vitamin use. Am J Epidemiol 139(11):S3, 1994

Shaw GM et al. Risks of orofacial clefts in children born to women using multivitamins containing folic acid periconceptionally. Lancet 346:393-6, 1995

Shaw N. Riboflavin status in late pregnancy, postpartum and cord blood. Nutr Res 13:147-55, 1993

Sheldon WL et al. The effects of oral iron supplementation on zinc and magnesium levels during pregnancy. Br J Obstet Gynaecol 92:892-8, 1985

Singla P et al. Fetal iron status in maternal anemia. Acta Paediatr 85(11):1327-30, 1996

Sjogren A et al. Reduced concentrations of magnesium, potassium and zinc in skeletal muscle from women during normal pregnancy or eclampsia. Abstract. J Am Coll Nutr 7(5):408, 1988

Skajaa K et al. Established role of magnesium sulfate as prophylactic anticonvulsive agent in preeclampsia-eclampsia. Acta Obstet Gynecol Scand 75:313-15, 1996

Song WO et al. Pantothenic acid status of pregnant and lactating women. J Am Diet Assoc 85(2):192-8, 1985

Specker BL. Do North American women need supplemental vitamin D during pregnancy or lactation? Am J Clin Nutr 59(suppl):484S-91S, 1994

Spellacy WN et al. Vitamin B6 treatment of gestational diabetes mellitus: studies of blood glucose and plasma insulin. Am J Obstet Gynecol 127(6):599-602, 1977

Standley CA et al. Serum ionized magnesium levels in normal and preeclamptic gestation. Obstet Gynecol 89(1):24-7, 1997

Stanton M et al. Serum magnesium in women during pregnancy, while taking contraceptives and after menopause. J Am Coll Nutr 6(4):313-20, 1987

Steegers-Theunissen RPM et al. Maternal hyperhomocysteinemia: a risk factor for neural-tube defects? Metabolism 43(12):1475-80, 1994

Steen MT et al. Neural-tube defects are associated with low concentrations of cobalamin (vitamin B12) in amniotic fluid. Prenat Diagn 18(6):545-55, 1998

Stratta P et al. Vitamin E supplementation in preeclampsia. Gynecol Obstet Invest 37(4):246-9, 1994

Sutton RV. Vitamin E in habitual abortion. Letter to the Editor. Br Med J October 4, 1958, p. 858

Swanson CA, King JC. Zinc and pregnancy outcome. Am J Clin Nutr 46(5):763-71, 1987

Tamura T et al. Maternal folate and zinc concentrations and their relationships to pregnancy outcome. Am J Clin Nutr 56:365-70, 1992

Tamura T et al. Serum ferritin: a predictor of early spontaneous preterm delivery. Obstet Gynecol 87(3):360-5, 1996

Taper LJ et al. Zinc and copper retention during pregnancy: the adequacy of prenatal diets with and without dietary supplementation. Am J Clin Nutr 41(6):1184-92, 1985

Taufield PA et al. Hypocalciuria in preeclampsia. N Engl J Med 316(12):715-18, 1987

Tershakovec AM, Weller SC. Iron status of inner-city elementary school children: lack of correlation between anemia and iron deficiency. Am J Clin Nutr 54:1071-6, 1991

Thornton WE. Folate deficiency in puerperal psychosis. Am J Obstet Gynecol 129(2):222-3, 1977

Thorp JA et al. Current concepts and controversies in the use of vitamin K. Drugs 49(3):376-87, 1995

Thoyer-Rozat J et al. Sem Hop Paris 36:1991-3, 1960 (in French)

Truswell AS. ABC of nutrition. Nutrition for pregnancy. Br Med J 291:263-6, 1985

Tuomilehto J et al. Coffee consumption as trigger for insulin dependent diabetes mellitus in childhood. BMJ 300:642-3, 1990

van Mandach U et al. Maternal and cord serum vitamin E levels in normal and abnormal pregnancy. Int J Vitam Nutr Res 63:26-32, 1994

Viegas OA et al. Dietary protein energy supplementation of pregnant Asian mothers at Sorrento, Birmingham. I: Unselective during second and third trimesters. Br Med J (Clin Res Ed) 285:589-92, 1982

Villar J et al. Epidemiologic observations on the relationship between calcium intake and eclampsia. Int J Gynaecol Obstet 21(4):271-8, 1983

Villar J, Repke JT. Calcium supplementation during pregnancy may reduce preterm delivery in high-risk populations. Am J Obstet Gynecol 163:1124-31, 1990

Vir SC et al. Riboflavin status during pregnancy. Am J Clin Nutr 34(12):2699-705, 1981

von Kries R et al. Vitamin K in infancy. Eur J Pediatr 147(2):106-12, 1988

Vutyavanich T et al. Pyridoxine for nausea and vomiting of pregnancy: a randomized, double-blind, placebo-controlled trial. Am J Obstet Gynecol 173:881-4, 1995

Wald NJ et al. Blood folic acid and vitamin B12 in relation to neural tube defects. Br J Obstet Gynaecol 103(4):319-24, 1996

Ward NI et al. Elemental factors in human fetal development. J Nutr Med 1:19-26, 1990

Weaver K. Pregnancy-induced hypertension and low birth weight in magnesium-deficient ewes. Magnesium 5(3-4):191-200, 1986

Werler M, Mitchell A. Folic acid prevention of neural tube defects (NTDs): Dietary contributions of folate. Am J Epidemiol S4, 1994

Wibell L et al. Magnesium and zinc in diabetic pregnancy. Acta Paediatr Scand Suppl 320:100-6, 1985

Williams MA et al. Cigarettes, coffee and preterm premature rupture of membranes. Am J Epidemiol 135(8):895-903, 1992

Williams MA et al. Omega-3 fatty acids in maternal erythrocytes and risk of preeclampsia. Epidemiology 6(3):232-7, 1995

Williams MA et al. Risk of preeclampsia in relation to elaidic acid (trans fatty acid) in maternal erythrocytes. Gynecol Obstet Invest 46(2):84-7, 1998

Winder C. Lead, reproduction and development. Neurotoxicology 14(2-3):303-17, 1993

Windham GC et al. Moderate alcohol consumption and risk of spontaneous abortion. Am J Epidemiol 139(11):S20, 1994

Ziari SA et al. Serum vitamin A, vitamin E, and beta-carotene levels in preeclamptic women in northern Nigeria. Am J Perinatol 13(5):287-91, 1996

PREMENSTRUAL SYNDROME

See Also: 'HYPOGLYCEMIA' (FUNCTIONAL)

NUTRITIONAL TREATMENT GUIDE

✓ = Efficacy generally accepted.
* = Efficacy *demonstrated* by controlled human trials.
[+] = Efficacy *suspected* from uncontrolled human experiments
[-] = Efficacy *suspected* from indirect data
? = Efficacy *challenged* in at least one study of similar design

DIETARY FACTORS

* **low Fat diet** (cyclical mastopathy)

- -

[+] **low Fat diet** (PMT-H)

- -

[-] **low Fat diet** (PMT-A)
[-] avoid **Alcohol** (PMT-A; PMT-C)
[-] avoid **Caffeine**
[-] increase **dietary Fiber** (PMT-A)
[-] minimize **Salt** (PMT-C)
[-] minimize **refined Sugar** (PMT-A; PMT-C; PMT-H)
[-] **Vegetarian diet** (PMT-A)

NUTRITIONAL FACTORS

* **Calcium:** 1,000 mg daily (PMT-D; PMT-H)
* **Magnesium deficiency:** ≈ 400 mg daily
* **L-Tryptophan:** 1 g daily (PMT-A; PMT-C; PMT-D)
* **Vitamin A:** 200,000 IU daily during the luteal phase
* **Vitamin E:** alpha-tocopherol 300 to 600 IU daily
* ? **Omega-6 Fatty Acids:** evening primrose oil 1.5 g twice daily (3 month trial)
* ? **Vitamin B_6:** 50 mg daily

- -

[+] **Flavonoids:** standardized grape seed oligomeric proanthocyanidins (Endotelon) (PMT-H)
[+] **Potassium deficiency:** potassium 600 to 800 mg daily (rarely, 1200 mg daily) as the gluconate *OR*, preferably, increase the intake of high-potassium foods (4 month trial)

- -

[-] **Zinc deficiency:** repletion

OTHER RELATED FACTORS

[-] rule out **Lead** toxicity

Abraham *(1986)* has suggested dividing premenstrual syndrome into four sub-groups:

PMT-A ('Anxiety'):
- anxiety
- irritability
- insomnia
- depression (late)

Characterized by elevated blood estrogens and low progesterone.

PMT-C ('Craving'):
- craving for sweets
- increased appetite;
- sugar ingestion causes:
  - headache
  - palpitations
  - fatigue or fainting

Characterized by increased carbohydrate tolerance, with a flat curve on glucose tolerance testing.

PMT-D ('Depression'):
- depression
- forgetfulness
- confusion
- lethargy

Mean blood progesterone may be elevated during the mid-luteal phase and elevated adrenal androgens are observed in some patients. Others have evidence of chronic lead intoxication.

PMT-H ('Hyperhydration'):
- weight gain above 1.4 Kg
- breast congestion
- abdominal bloating
- edema of face and extremities

Associated with salt retention and, possibly, with elevated serum aldosterone.

While this grouping, as well as the hypotheses concerning theoretical mechanisms, is badly in need of modification based on newer information, it remains a useful model for appreciating the complexity of the syndrome.

DIETARY FACTORS

Low Fat diet

There is considerable evidence that the intake of dietary fat, and saturated fat in particular, is directly associated with blood estrogen levels *(Goldin,1986)*. Furthermore, experimentally, a low-fat, high-carbohydrate, high-fiber diet reduces blood estrogen levels *(Heber)*, although reducing dietary fat has not been shown to help PMT-A (which is theoretically linked to high estrogen as well as to low progesterone).

There is evidence, however, from an open trial that a low-fat diet (15-20% of calories from fat) may reduce symptoms of PMT-H. Compared to 4 menstrual cycles on a high fat diet, women who subsequently were placed on a low fat diet reported, during both the premenstruum and menses, significant decreases in symptoms associated with water retention such as weight gain, bloating and breast tenderness *(Jones)*.

Moreover, in a controlled study, when 10 women with chronic, severe cyclical mastopathy went on a low-fat diet while increasing complex carbohydrate consumption to maintain calorie intake, 6 had objective evidence of reduced breast swelling, tenderness and nodularity versus only 2 out of 9 women in the control group *(Boyd)*.

Sugar

Premenstrual syndrome is associated with an increased intake of refined sugar *(Rossignol,1991)*. Increased refined sugar intake appears to be particularly related to PMT-D, and may be partly an attempt to enhance serotonin synthesis to improve dysphoria by boosting tryptophan availability *(Brzezinski;Wurtman)*. (See Tryptophan below.)

Perhaps the strongest evidence to confirm this hypothesis comes from a double-blind crossover study in which women with premenstrual syndrome drank a carbohydrate-rich beverage specially formulated to increase the serum ratio of tryptophan to the other large neutral amino acids. As compared to drinking 2 other isocaloric drinks, this beverage decreased self-reported depression, anger, confusion, and carbohydrate craving 90 to 180 minutes after intake. Memory word recognition was also significantly improved *(Sayegh)*.

While refined sugar consumption may reduce the symptoms of PMT-D by increasing tryptophan availability, it appears to promote the other 3 types of premenstrual syndrome. It would theoretically foster the hypoglycemic-like symptoms seen in PMT-C *(Oettle)*. However, although women with premenstrual syndrome often have hypoglycemic symptoms during glucose tolerance testing, these symptoms do not appear to resemble their premenstrual symptoms and are not specific to the luteal phase *(Denicoff)*, and women who complain of premenstrual 'hypoglycemic' symptoms do not appear to have menstrual cycle-related changes in glucose, insulin, or glucagon responses to an oral glucose load *(Reid)*.

Sugar may impair estrogen metabolism in the liver *(Yudkin)*, which could theoretically encourage the development of PMT-A. In fact, one survey found that women with PMT-A consumed two and one-half times the amount of refined sugar consumed by women with or without mild premenstrual tension *(Abraham,1982)*.

A large sugar load stimulates insulin which suppresses ketoacid formation. Since ketoacids help the kidney to clear excess sodium and water, PMT-H could theoretically occur *(Abraham,1986)*.

In addition, refined sugar intake increases urinary magnesium excretion *(Seelig)*, and a marginal magnesium deficiency appears to be an important cause of premenstrual syndrome (see Magnesium below).

Dietary Fiber

Dietary fiber increases estrogen binding and excretion *(Rose)*. Since the estrogen to progesterone ratio is elevated in PMT-A, increasing dietary fiber would theoretically be beneficial; controlled trials are needed to confirm this. Moreover, many of the adverse effects attributed to refined sugar may be due to the lack of dietary fiber in sugary "junk" foods.

Vegetarian diet

When the diets of women with premenstrual syndrome were compared with those without the syndrome, the percent of calories from fats and proteins was similar, but the sources of fats and proteins were predominantly animal in the symptomatic women, and vegetarian in the others *(Abraham,1987)*.

Theoretically, a vegetarian diet may be particularly desirable for women experiencing PMT-A - although this hypothesis has yet to be tested. Vegetarians excrete 2 to 3 times more estrogen in their feces and have 50% lower mean plasma levels of unconjugated estrogens than do omnivores *(Goldin,1982)*. In fact, broccoli, cauliflower and cabbage, member of the Brassica genus, contain a chemical that promotes the inactivation of estrogen *(Michnovicz)*. Animal products, by contrast, are sources of arachidonic acid, precursor to PGF2 which inhibits progesterone synthesis *(Abraham,1984)*.

Salt

PMT-H is associated with a relative deficiency of dopamine at the renal level *(Kuchel)*. Since dopamine is natriuretic and diuretic *(McDonald)*, its reduction promotes sodium and water retention, which suggests that salt restriction would be helpful. However, results of a recent study suggest that the symptoms of PMT-H do not result from sodium retention. While sodium cravings and breast tenderness did increase during the late luteal phase, and bloating increased during early menses, these symptoms were found to be unaccompanied by increased sodium intake. Moreover, sodium restriction failed to decrease symptoms *(Olson)*.

Despite the evidence that sodium restriction is not indicated for PMT-H, it could be of benefit to women with PMT-C. Sodium enhances glucose-induced insulin production by facilitating glucose absorption *(Ferranini)*. As PMT-C may be due to reactive hypoglycemia *(Abraham, 1986)*, salt should theoretically be restricted for women in that sub-group, although this hypothesis remains to be tested.

Alcohol

While the efficacy of alcohol avoidance remains to be shown, women with premenstrual syndrome appear to drink considerably more alcohol than other women in the postmenstrual phase, suggesting that drinking is unlikely to be simply an attempt to cope with premenstrual syndrome *(Caan)*.

Moreover, there are several theoretical reasons why alcohol avoidance may benefit women with premenstrual syndrome. In regard to women with PMT-C, it inhibits gluconeogenesis and promotes a fall in plasma glucose *(Rabin)*. Moreover, the increase in gastric acidity following alcohol ingestion could cause excessive release of gut secretagogues which would stimulate insulin release by augmenting beta-cell responsiveness *(Freinkel)*.

In regard to women with PMT-A, the phytoestrogens in alcohol may be converted to estrogen, thus theoretically exacerbating the syndrome *(Reichman)*.

Caffeine

Caffeine intake has repeatedly been found to correlate with premenstrual syndrome *(Rossignol, 1990)*. To what extent this correlation is due to the stimulatory effects of caffeine is not known, although the anxiety, irritability and insomnia of PMT-A are consistent with these effects *(Clementz)*.

NUTRITIONAL FACTORS

VITAMINS

Vitamin A

Although blood levels of vitamin A are normal *(Chuong, 1990)*, high-dose supplementation has been associated with improvement in several older studies, at least two of which were placebo-controlled. For example, *all* of a group of women who received 200,000 to 300,000 IU of vitamin A premenstrually improved, compared to 25% of placebo controls *(Block)*. Such massive doses of vitamin A must be carefully supervised, however, due to the possibility of side effects.

Vitamin B_6

Most studies have not found evidence of a vitamin B_6 deficiency in premenstrual syndrome. Supplementation with pharmacologic dosages of the vitamin has been effective in numerous double-blind studies, although other studies have failed to find evidence of its efficacy.

In a 1990 review of 12 controlled trials, it was concluded that the evidence of positive effects was weak, mainly because of the small number of patients in the trials *(Kleijnen)*. The vitamin appears to have some efficacy for women with any of the four categories of premenstrual syndrome.

Vitamin B_6 supplementation appears to be able to normalize deficient intracellular magnesium levels *(Abraham, 1981)*. Since intracellular magnesium levels may be decreased in premenstrual syndrome, and the decreased levels may be related to manifestations of the disorder, this effect of the vitamin may explain its efficacy.

Vitamin E

Although serum vitamin E levels are normal *(Chuong, 1990)*, vitamin E supplementation has been shown to be effective in double-blind studies *(London, 1987)*. All sub-groups except PMT-H appear to benefit *(London, 1983)*.

MINERALS

Calcium

Patients with PMT-A consume more calcium than normals *(Goei)* and their dietary ratio of calcium to magnesium is higher than it is for both normals and patients in the other three sub-groups *(Abraham, 1982)*. Moreover, hair calcium levels tend to be elevated *(Abraham, 1983)*, suggesting a metabolic disturbance in calcium regulation.

In a double-blind crossover study, supplementation with calcium was found to reduce premenstrual fluid retention and pain (PMT-H) *(Thys-Jacobs)*, while another similar study also found improvement in fluid retention as well as improvement in mood, concentration and behavior (PMT-D) so long as manganese intake was adequate *(Penland)*.

The efficacy of calcium supplementation suggests that the tendency of patients to consume extra calcium may be an attempt to compensate for a disturbance in calcium metabolism. Since calcium supplementation impairs magnesium absorption *(Spencer)*, and magnesium deficiency may contribute to premenstrual syndrome, magnesium should be supplemented along with calcium.

Magnesium Deficiency

Intracellular (erythrocyte and mononuclear cell) magnesium levels are frequently reduced, while plasma (and serum) levels are normal *(Rosenstein)*. In one study, for example, 45% of 105 patients were found to have erythrocyte magnesium levels which were below the normal range *(Sherwood)*.

Under double-blind conditions, magnesium supplementation has been shown to relieve premenstrual pain and depression (PMT-D) *(Facchinetti)*. In an open trial, nervous tension was relieved in 89% of 192 patients, mastalgia in 96%, weight gain in 95%, and headache in 43% *(Nicholas)*. Moreover, in a controlled study of women with reactive hypoglycemia (PMT-C) and reduced magnesium levels, 50% of 14 women felt better after magnesium supplementation compared to 25% of women on placebo *(Stebbing)*.

Since magnesium has many important functions, the correction of a magnesium deficit could improve premenstrual syndrome through any of several mechanisms. A magnesium deficiency causes adrenal cortical hyperplasia, elevated aldosterone levels and an increased extracellular fluid volume *(Cantin)*; these changes could promote PMT-H. It also causes a depletion of brain dopamine *(Barbeau)*, and PMT-A is believed to be associated with relative dopamine depletion by excess estrogen in the luteal phase *(Redmond)*.

Estrogen excess may, in fact, be promoted by magnesium deficiency, as the hepatic glucuronidation of estrogens in preparation for their excretion requires the enzyme glucuronyl transferase whose activity is fostered by magnesium *(Brown)*. As magnesium may reduce glucose-induced insulin secretion *(Curry)*, a deficiency would favor the development of PMT-C. Finally, a magnesium deficiency may promote lead intoxication (see Lead below).

A 40-year-old woman had a 10-year history of severe premenstrual fluid retention and irritability with a 6 to 7 pound weight gain in the week prior to her menstrual period. Treatment with a diuretic drug was only of temporary benefit. The fluid retention responded to a very-low-salt diet (25 mmol/d) and worsened if she consumed salty foods or ate foods containing wheat.

Her serum magnesium was found to be low at 1.6 mmol/L (normal: 2-3 mmol/L), so she was given magnesium supplementation along with Optivite, a multivitamin/multimineral supplement. As her serum magnesium normalized and her premenstrual fluid retention and irritability decreased, she was able to stop the diuretic. Stopping her oral contraceptive [which tends to antagonize vitamin B_6] helped clear her symptoms completely (Davies).

Potassium Deficiency

An open trial involving 7 women with severe symptoms found that a relatively small amount of potassium supplementation shifted symptoms into the time of menstrual flow in the first cycle. *All* found symptoms to decrease gradually over 3 cycles and were symptom-free by their fourth cycle.

The author theorizes that premenstrual syndrome may be due to a marginal potassium deficiency. She notes that phosphorus-free calcium supplements must be avoided during the first few months and that the potassium supplement must be used daily starting before the fifth or sixth day of the cycle *(Takacs)*.

Her report has yet to be confirmed by controlled clinical trials.

Zinc Deficiency

Plasma *(Posaci)*, serum *(Chuong,1994)*, and sweat *(Stewart)* zinc concentrations may be reduced in PMS patients during the luteal phase. As plasma *(Posaci)* and serum *(Chuong,1994)* copper concentrations tend to rise in PMS patients as zinc decreases, the zinc to copper ratio declines *(Chuong,1994;Posaci)*, possibly because zinc availability is further reduced by elevated copper *(Chuong,1994)*.

While a zinc deficiency may theoretically reduce progesterone and endorphin levels *(Chuong,1991)*, whether the repletion of a zinc deficiency is an effective treatment intervention for premenstrual syndrome is not yet known. However, zinc deficiency is known to cause anorexia, loss of libido and fatigue, all of which suggest depression (PMT-D) *(Tasman-Jones)*; thus supplementation should at least benefit this sub-group of patients.

OTHER NUTRITIONAL FACTORS

Flavonoids

In vitro, flavonoids inhibit estrogen synthesis by competing with estrogen as a substrate; they may have a similar effect *in vivo (Kellis)*.

Of 165 women who received a standardized extract of grape seed oligomeric proanthocyanidins (Endotelon), 61% noted improvement in abdominal swelling, breast symptoms, pelvic pain, weight fluctuations and venous problems after 2 menstrual cycles, while 79% noted improvement after 4 cycles *(Amsellen)*

Omega-6 Fatty Acids

linoleic acid → GLA → DGLA → prostaglandin E_1

A functional deficiency of essential fatty acids, either due to inadequate linoleic acid intake or absorption, or to failure of normal conversion of linoleic acid to gamma-linolenic acid (GLA), has been postulated to cause the features of premenstrual syndrome *(Horrobin,1983)*. Evidence supporting the latter hypothesis comes from 2 studies of women with premenstrual syndrome which found that the levels of linoleic acid were significantly elevated, while the levels of all its metabolites were significantly reduced *(Brush;Horrobin,1991)*.

Several mechanisms have been proposed by which a functional deficiency of essential fatty acids could promote premenstrual symptoms. These include abnormal sensitivity to prolactin *(Horrobin,1983)* and other reproductive hormones *(Brush)*, effects on membrane structures and eicosanoids, actions as second messengers, modification of membrane fluidity and of lipid-associated receptors, and changes in the inositol cycle *(Horrobin,1993)*.

Evening primrose oil, a rich source of gamma-linolenic acid, has been administered under double-blind conditions to women with premenstrual syndrome in several studies. The findings have been mixed, with the most well-controlled studies failing to find evidence of benefit although, because of their small size, a mild treatment effect could have been missed *(Budeiri)*.

One possible explanation for the inconsistent findings is that the treatment only benefits certain of the premenstrual symptom sub-groups. For example, both placebo-controlled studies for women with cyclical mastalgia (PMT-H) reported excellent results *(Pashby;Pye)*. Also, in another placebo-controlled study, depression (PMT-D) was the only symptom which was significantly reduced when compared to placebo *(Puolakka)*.

A woman complained of irritability or depression starting several days prior to menses. Progesterone was ineffective. Evening primrose oil, however, along with vitamin B_6, relieved all her symptoms (Bates).

Tryptophan

Tryptophan is the nutritional precursor of serotonin, and platelet serotonin uptake may be reduced in women with premenstrual dysphoria during the luteal phase of their cycle *(Rojansky)*. Moreover, under placebo-controlled conditions, acute tryptophan depletion aggravated premenstrual symptoms, especially irritability *(Menkes)*.

There is evidence from controlled clinical trials that L-tryptophan supplementation may relieve the symptoms of all the sub-groups of premenstrual syndrome except PMT-H *(Brzezinski;Sayegh)*.

OTHER RELATED FACTORS

Lead Toxicity

Chronic lead intoxication interferes with the binding of estrogen to its receptors *(Young)*. Since decreased peripheral estrogen increases monoamine oxidase levels *(Abraham,1978)*, and increased monoamine oxidase levels are associated with depression *(Van Praag)*, lead toxicity may hypothetically cause depression by increasing monoamine oxidase levels.

In a study of 56 patients and 14 controls, hair lead levels were 34% higher in the patient group. Moreover, two patients with severe PMT-D had hair lead levels which were 11.3 and 14 times the levels of the controls *(Hanson)*.

Magnesium blocks the absorption of lead *(Fine)* and increases its urinary excretion *(Krall)*, so a magnesium deficiency may promote the development of lead intoxication. (See Magnesium above).

BIBLIOGRAPHY

Abraham GE et al. Hormonal and behavioral changes during the menstrual cycle. Senologia 3:33-38, 1978

Abraham GE et al. Effect of vitamin B6 on plasma and red blood cell magnesium levels in premenopausal women. Ann Clin Lab Sci 11(4):333-6, 1981

Abraham GE. Magnesium deficiency in premenstrual tension. Magnesium Bull 1:68-73, 1982

Abraham GE. Nutritional factors in the etiology of the premenstrual syndrome. J Reprod Med 28:446-64, 1983

Abraham GE. Nutrition and the premenstrual tension syndromes. J Appl Nutr 36(2):103-17, 1984

Abraham GE. Management of the premenstrual tension syndrome: rationale for a nutritional approach, in J Bland, Ed. 1986: A Year in Nutritional Medicine. New Canaan, CT, Keats Publishing, Inc., 1986

Abraham GE. Role of nutrition in managing the premenstrual tension syndromes. J Reprod Med 32(6):405-22, 1987

Amsellem M et al. Endotelon in the treatment of venolymphatic problems in premenstrual syndrome: multicenter study on 165 patients. Tempo Med 282, 1987

Barbeau A et al. [Deficiency of magnesium and cerebral dopamine], in J Durlach, Ed. First International Symposium on Magnesium Deficit in Human Pathology. Paris, F. Vitel, 1973, pp. 149-52

Bates C. Essential Fatty Acids and Immunity in Mental Health. Tacoma, WA, Life Sciences Press, 1987, p. 71

Block E. The use of vitamin A in premenstrual tension. Acta Obstet Gynecol Scand 39:586-92, 1960

Boyd NF et al. Effect of a low-fat high-carbohydrate diet on symptoms of cyclical mastopathy. Lancet ii:128-32, 1988

Brown RC, Bidlack WR. Regulation of glucuronyl transferase by intracellular magnesium, in Proceedings of the International Symposium on Magnesium and its Relationship to Cardiovascular, Renal and Metabolic Disorders. Los Angeles, 1985, p. 24

Brush MG et al. Abnormal essential fatty acid levels in plasma of women with premenstrual syndrome. Am J Obstet Gynecol 150(4):363-6, 1984

Brzezinski A. Serotonin and premenstrual dysphoric disorder. Letter. Lancet 347:470-1, 1996

Budeiri D et al. Is evening primrose oil of value in the treatment of premenstrual syndrome? Controlled Clin Trials 17(1):60-8, 1996

Caan B et al. Association between alcoholic and caffeinated beverages and premenstrual syndrome. J Reprod Med 38(8):630-6, 1993

Cantin M. [Hyperaldosteronism secondary to the course of a magnesium deficit.], in J Durlach, Ed. First International Symposium on Magnesium Deficit in Human Pathology. Paris, F. Vitel, 1973, pp. 451-60

Chuong CJ et al. Vitamin A levels in premenstrual syndrome. Fertil Steril 54(4):643-7, 1990

Chuong CJ et al, Baylor College of Medicine, Houston - presented at the 46th Annual Mtg. of the Am. Fertility Society, Washington, DC, 1991

Chuong C, Dawson E. Zinc and copper levels in premenstrual syndrome. Fert Steril 62:313-20, 1994

Clementz GL, Dailey JW. Psychotropic effects of caffeine. Am Fam Physician 37(5):167-72, 1988

Curry DL et al. Magnesium modulation of glucose-induced insulin secretion by the perfused rat pancreas. Endocrinology 101:203, 1977

Davies S, Stewart A. Nutritional Medicine. London, Pan Books, 1987

Denicoff KD et al. Glucose tolerance testing in women with premenstrual syndrome. Am J Psychiatry 147(4):477-80, 1990

Facchinetti F et al. Oral magnesium successfully relieves premenstrual mood changes. Obstet Gynecol 78(2):177-81, 1991

Ferranini E et al. Sodium elevates the plasma glucose response to glucose ingestion in man. J Clin Endocrinol Metab 54:455, 1982

Fine BP et al. Influence of magnesium on the intestinal absorption of lead. Environ Res 12:224, 1976

Freinkel N, Getzer BE. Oral glucose tolerance curve and hypoglycemias in the fed state. N Engl J Med 280:820-8, 1969

Goei GS et al. Dietary patterns of patients with premenstrual tension. J Appl Nutr 34(1):4-11, 1982

Goldin BR et al. Estrogen excretion patterns and plasma levels in vegetarian and omnivorous women. N Engl J Med 307:1542-7, 1982

Goldin BR et al. The relationship between estrogen levels and diets of Caucasian American and Oriental immigrant women. Am J Clin Nutr 44(6):945-53, 1986

Hanson MA et al. Hair tissue concentration of minerals, trace elements, and toxic metals in normal women and patients with premenstrual tension syndromes, in M Abdulla et al, Eds. Health Effects and Interactions of Essential and Toxic Elements. New York, Pergamon Press, 1983, pp. 608-11

Heber D et al. Reduction of serum estradiol in postmenopausal women given free access to low-fat high-carbohydrate diet. Nutrition 7(2):137-9, 1991

Horrobin DF. The role of essential fatty acids and prostaglandins in the premenstrual syndrome. J Reprod Med 28(7):465-8, 1983

Horrobin DF et al. Abnormalities in plasma essential fatty acid levels in women with premenstrual syndrome and with non-malignant breast disease. J Nutr Med 2:259-64, 1991

Horrobin DF. The effects of gamma-linolenic acid in breast pain and diabetic neuropathy: possible non-eicosanoid mechanisms. Prostaglandins Leukot Essent Fatty Acids 48(1):101-4, 1993

Jones DV. Influence of dietary fat on self-reported menstrual symptoms. Physiol Behav 40(4):483-7, 1987

Kellis JT Jr, Vickery LE. Inhibition of human estrogen synthetase (aromatase) by flavones. Science 225:1032-4, 1984

Kleijnen J et al. Vitamin B6 in the treatment of premenstrual syndrome - - a review. Br J Obstet Gynaecol 97(9):847-52, 1990

Krall AR et al. Effects of magnesium infusions on the metabolism of calcium and lead, in M Cantin, MS Seelig, Eds. Magnesium in Health and Disease. Spectrum Publications, 1980, pp. 941-8

Kuchel O et al. Catecholamine excretion in 'idiopathic' edema: decreased dopamine excretion, a pathologic factor? J Clin Endocrinol Metab 44:639-46, 1977

London RS et al. The effect of alpha-tocopherol on premenstrual symptomatology: A double-blind study. J Am Coll Nutr 2(2):115-22, 1983

London RS et al. Efficacy of alpha-tocopherol in the treatment of premenstrual syndrome. J Reprod Med 32(6):400-4, 1987

McDonald RH et al. Effects of dopamine in man: Augmentation of sodium excretion, glomerular filtration rate and renal plasma flow. J Clin Invest 43:1116, 1964

Menkes DB et al. Acute tryptophan depletion aggravates premenstrual syndrome. J Affect Dis 32:37-44, 1994

Michnovicz J, Bradlow HL, Institute for Hormone Research, New York City - reported in Science News, June 16, 1990

Nicholas A. [Treatment of premenstrual syndrome and dysmenorrhea by the magnesium ion], in J Durlach, Ed. First International Symposium on Magnesium Deficiency in Human Pathology. Paris, Springer, Verlag, 1973, pp. 261-3

Oettle GJ et al. Glucose and insulin responses to manufactured and whole-food snacks. Am J Clin Nutr 45:86-91, 1987

Olson BR et al. Relation between sodium balance and menstrual cycle symptoms in normal women. Ann Intern Med 125(7):564-7, 1996

Pashby NL et al. A clinical trial of evening primrose oil in mastalgia. Abstract. Br J Surg 68:801-24, 1981

Penland JG, Johnson PE. Dietary calcium and manganese effects on menstrual cycle symptoms. Am J Obstet Gynecol 168(5):1417-23, 1993

Posaci C et al. Plasma copper, zinc and magnesium levels in patients with premenstrual tension syndrome. Acta Obstet Gynecol Scand 73(6):452-5, 1994

Puolakka J et al. Biochemical and clinical effects of treating the premenstrual syndrome with prostaglandin synthesis precursors. J Reprod Med 39(3):149-53, 1985

Pye JK et al. Clinical experience of drug treatments for mastalgia. Lancet ii:373-77, 1985

Rabin D. Hypoglycemia: Physiologic and diagnostic considerations, in GE Abraham, Ed. Radioassay Systems in Clincal Endocrinology. New York, Marcel Dekker, 1981:609-24

Redmond DE et al. Menstrual cycle and ovarian hormone effects on plasma and platelet monamine oxidase (MAO) and plasma dopamine-hydroxylase activities in the Rhesus monkey. Psychosom Med 37:417, 1975

Reichman ME et al. Effects of alcohol consumption on plasma and urinary hormone concentrations in premenopausal women. J Natl Cancer Inst 85(9):692-3, 1993

Reid RL et al. Oral glucose tolerance during the menstrual cycle in normal women and women with alleged premenstrual "hypoglycemic" attacks: effects of naloxone. J Clin Endocrinol Metab 62(6):1167-72, 1986

Rojansky N et al. Imipramine receptor binding and serotonin uptake in platelets of women with premenstrual changes. Gynecol Obstet Invest 31:146-52, 1991

Rose DP et al. Effects of diet supplementation with wheat bran on serum estrogen levels in the follicular and luteal phases of the menstrual cycle. Nutrition 13(6):535-9, 1997

Rosenstein DL et al. Magnesium measures across the menstrual cycle in premenstrual syndrome. Biol Psychiatry 35:557-61, 1994

Rossignol AM. Caffeine-containing beverages, total fluid consumption, and premenstrual syndrome. Am J Public Health 80(9):1106-10, 1990

Rossignol AM, Bonnlander H. Prevalence and severity of the premenstrual syndrome. Effects of foods and beverages that are sweet or high in sugar content. J Reprod Med 36(2):131-6, 1991

Sayegh R et al. The effect of carbohydrate-rich beverage on mood, appetite, and cognitive function in women with premenstrual syndrome. Obstet Gynecol 86(4 Pt 1):520-8, 1995

Seelig M. Human requirement of magnesium: Factors that increase needs, in J Durlach, Ed. First International Symposium on Magnesium Deficiency in Human Pathol. Paris, Springer, Verlag, 1973, p. 11

Sherwood RA et al. Magnesium and the premenstrual syndrome. Ann Clin Biochem 23(6):667-70, 1986

Spencer H et al. Magnesium in Health and Disease. Jamaica, NY, SP Medical and Scientific Books, 1980, pp. 911-19

Stebbing JB et al. Reactive hypoglycaemia and magnesium. Magnesium Bull 4(2):131-4, 1982

Stewart A. Clinical and biochemical effects of nutritional supplementation on the premenstrual syndrome. J Reprod Med 32:435-41, 1987

Takacs BE. Potassium: a new treatment for premenstrual syndrome. J Orthomol Med 13(4):215-22, 1998

Tasman-Jones C. Zinc deficiency states. Adv Intern Med 26:97-114, 1980

Thys-Jacobs S et al. Calcium supplementation in premenstrual syndrome: a randomized crossover trial. J Gen Intern Med 4(3):183-9, 1989

Van Praag HM. Neuroendocrine disorders in depressions and their significance for the monoamine hypothesis of depression. Acta Psychiatr Scand 57:389-404, 1978

Wurtman JJ et al. Effect of nutrient intake on premenstrual depression. Am J Obstet Gynecol 161(5):1228-34, 1989

Young PCM et al. Effect of metal ions on the binding of 17-beta-estradiol to human endometrial cystol. Fertil Steril 28:312-18, 1972

Yudkin J, Eisa O. Dietary sucrose and oestradiol concentration in young men. Ann Nutr Metabol 32:53-5, 1988

PSORIASIS

NUTRITIONAL TREATMENT GUIDE

✓ = Efficacy generally accepted.
* = Efficacy *demonstrated* by controlled human trials.
[+] = Efficacy *suspected* from uncontrolled human experiments
[-] = Efficacy *suspected* from indirect data
? = Efficacy *challenged* in at least one study of similar design

DIETARY FACTORS

* **consume oily Fish**

- -

[+] **Vegetarian diet**
[+] ? **low Protein diet**

- -

[-] **Minimize Saturated Fat**
[-] **avoid Alcohol**

NUTRITIONAL FACTORS

* **Arachidonic Acid:** topical application of 1% preparation. Apply under occlusion every 1 to 2 days. (2 week trial)
* **Bromine *AND* Nickel:** nickel dibromide (Loma Lux Labs, Tulsa, OK, USA) containing 0.041 mg/kg of bromine and 0.015 mg/kg nickel daily on an empty stomach Adjust dosage for a serum range of 20-40 μg/L nickel. (12 week trial)
* **Fumaric Acid:** *examples:* dimethylfumaric acid ester 240 mg daily, or monoethylfumaric acid ester 720 mg daily (Start at a minimal dosage and increase weekly as tolerated. Take following meals.) May also be used topically and in baths. Combine with the specific diet (see below). (3 month trial)
* **Vitamin A:** etretinate initially 0.75 to 1 mg/kg/d in divided doses. Reduce dosage after response.
* ? **Omega-3 Fatty Acids:** fish oils containing 5 g EPA & DHA daily (2 month trial) *OR* daily IV infusions containing 4.2 g of EPA & DHA (14 day trial)
* ? **Vitamin B_{12}:** 1000 μg IM daily (30 day trial) *OR* intralesional injections

- -

[+] **Chromium deficiency:** chromium chloride 600 μg daily (4 month trial)
[+] **Folic acid:** ? 20 mg 4 times daily *AND*
Vitamin C: 500 mg twice daily (6 month trial)
[+] **Selenium:** topical selenium sulfide 25 mg/ml (Selsun®). Apply for 15 min. daily and wash off. After 1 to 3 weeks, gradually reduce applications as tolerated.
[+] **Vitamin D:** calcitriol initially 0.5 μg/d. Increase by 0.05 μg every 2 wks. to an ave. dose of 2.4 μg (3 month trial) *OR* topical application using a petroleum base (2 month trial)
[+] **Zinc:** topical 10% zinc oxide ointment in a base of soybean oil and white beeswax

OTHER RELATED FACTORS

[+] rule out **Food Sensitivities**
[+] rule out **Hydrochloric Acid deficiency**

DIETARY FACTORS

Vegetarian Diet

Back in 1911, 140 patients were placed on a vegetarian diet. Often the diet was dramatically effective; the eruption steadily faded and actually disappeared with absolutely no internal or local treatment. However, in general, the best results were obtained by combining the diet with other forms of treatment. Sometimes the rash recurred but, as a rule, the outbreak was not be nearly so severe or persistent as previous ones *(Bulkley)*.

Modern clinicians have reported similar results. When patients were placed on a modified fast for 2 weeks followed by a vegan diet for 3 weeks, there were no changes in the rash during the fast. However, some of the patients improved on the vegan diet *(Lithell)*.

Moreover, patients treated with the Kempner rice diet showed a dramatic reduction in, or disappearance of, their skin lesions within 2 to 3 months, and local steroid treatment was able to be discontinued. Many of these patients had previously been treated unsuccessfully for years with systemic and/or local medications, and not a single patient noted worsening of the lesions on the diet *(Newborg)*. (This diet contains no more than 20 grams protein and very little fat with a relatively large percentage of linoleic acid.)

Also consistent with studies suggesting benefits from a vegetarian diet are the findings from a survey which found the risk of psoriasis to be inversely related to the intake of carrots, tomatoes, fresh fruits and, to a lesser extent, green vegetables *(Naldi)*.

The efficacy of a vegetarian diet has yet to be confirmed by controlled clinical trials. Assuming that it is effective, there are many possible reasons for its efficacy that have been poorly explored. For example, psoriasis is associated with high levels of circulating endotoxins, and a diet low in fiber is associated with increased levels of endotoxin-producing bacteria *(Rosenberg)*, while vegetarian diets are usually high in fiber.

Low Protein Diet

In a 1913 study, metabolic studies found patients to have a positive nitrogen balance both on a regular and on a low-protein diet. It was theorized that retained nitrogen was a building source of amino acids from which epidermal protein was synthesized and incorporated into hyperplastic psoriatic plaque; thus a low-protein diet might preferentially "starve" the plaque without significantly harming the body as a whole *(Schamberg,1913)*.

Indeed, when the same investigator placed patients on low-protein diets with an adequate caloric intake, patients experienced a gradual disappearance of the lesions while maintaining their weight, yet the lesions recurred when the diet was stopped. In 18 years of clinical experience, only one patient failed to respond *(Schamberg,1932)*.

However, subsequent studies by other investigators have failed to confirm these optimistic initial reports. Psoriatic patients under strictly controlled metabolic conditions showed no evidence of nitrogen retention *(Block)*. Moreover, when 13 patients were hospitalized and maintained on varying levels of protein intake, all improved during the first 7 weeks, and only 2 subsequently relapsed. There was no significant difference in the degree of rapidity of improvement on the various dietary protein levels, and 3 patients who improved while on a low-protein intake failed to flare when changed to a high-protein diet *(Zackheim)*.

Fish

Given the evidence that supplementation with omega-3 fatty acids may be beneficial (see Omega-3 Fatty Acids below), the efficacy of consuming oily fish has been explored. In a controlled study, it was found that consuming 4 to 6 meals with fish per week, without any other dietary changes, can induce changes in blood lipids similar to those of a fish oil supplement *(Fahrer)*.

Moreover, in a crossover study, patients consumed white fish or oily fish (mackerel, sardine, salmon, pilchard, kipper and herring). While on the white fish diet, patients' conditions deteriorated, but improved on the oily fish diet and deteriorated again when returned to the white fish diet. Both groups improved on the oily fish diet *(Collier)*.

While the oily fish contributed an additional 1 to 2 grams of the omega-3 fatty acid eicosapentaenoic acid (EPA) daily to the diet, they also provided 3 to 4 times the RDI for vitamin D, suggesting that vitamin D could also contribute to their benefits (see Vitamin D below) *(Collier)*.

Dietary Fats

When the frequency of consumption of various foodstuffs by psoriatic patients was compared to that of controls, only the consumption of high-fat foods, and specifically of saturated fats, was significantly greater for patients of both sexes *(Zamboni)*.

The efficacy of reducing saturated fat intake has yet to be investigated.

Alcohol

Alcohol abuse in men increases the risk of psoriasis *(Monk)* and has an adverse effect on treatment outcome *(Gupta)*. While female patients also have a higher alcohol intake than controls *(Zamboni)*, alcohol excess and alcohol-related problems are less common *(Monk)*.

In one survey of men with psoriasis as compared to controls with other skin diseases, the odds ratio for psoriasis at an alcohol intake of 100 grams daily compared to no intake was 2.2. Moreover, while the controls decreased their alcohol intake after disease-onset, the psoriasis patients did not *(Poikolainen)*.

It is not known whether abstention is beneficial. However, the findings of recent *in vitro* studies provide evidence that alcohol has adverse effects on the immune system which gives some confirmation to the suspicion that it promotes the development of the lesions *(Ockenfels;Schopf)*.

NUTRITIONAL FACTORS

VITAMINS

Folic Acid

Several studies have found evidence that patients frequently have a mild folate deficiency *(Fry;Shuster)*. While folate absorption is normal, perhaps one-quarter of patients have low serum folate and hypersegmented polymorphs. This high incidence of deficiency is believed to be due to increased utilization of folate by the disease process as well as by clinically uninvolved skin *(Fry)*.

***AND* Vitamin C**

Large doses of folic acid, when taken in combination with vitamin C, are known to inhibit xanthine oxidase. Allopurinol, an effective drug treatment, is a xanthine oxidase inhibitor.

The combination was tested on 7 patients with longstanding psoriasis. After 3 to 6 months, all 7 patients were markedly improved. However, 2 out of 3 other patients who had previously received treatment with methotrexate (a folate antagonist) became decidedly worse on this regimen *(Oster)*.

This combination has also been tried on a few patients by another investigator who found mixed results, with some patients improving and others showing no change *(Gaby)*, possibly because only the folate-deficient patients responded. Controlled clinical trials, with baseline folate assessments, have yet to be performed.

Vitamin A

While cutaneous retinol levels appear to be normal within the lesions, cutaneous levels of dehydroretinol are increased *(Rollman)*. Moreover, serum retinol levels may be decreased *(Majewski;Marrakchi)*.

Polyamines (putrescine, spermidine and spermine) are increased in psoriasis and, when treatments are successful, both cutaneous and urinary polyamine levels decrease *(Proctor)*. Since vitamin A is an inhibitor of ornithine decarboxylase, the rate-limiting step in endogenous polyamine synthesis *(Haddox)*, supplementation could theoretically be effective by reducing polyamine levels.

Due to the vitamin's potential for serious side effects, long-term administration of vitamin A with full control of other dietary factors has yet to be tested in controlled trials *(Brenner)*. However, etretinate, a synthetic vitamin A analog, has been tested in several studies and was found to be effective for both psoriasis vulgaris *(Committee)* and the associated arthritis *(Hopkins)*. Because it also has the potential for serious side effects, etretinate is only indicated for severe, recalcitrant cases, and its administration requires medical supervision.

Vitamin B_{12}

Open trials of a long series of intramuscular injections of vitamin B_{12} have reported good results *(Cohen; Ruedemann)*. However, a double-blind study failed to find evidence that such injections were better than placebo *(Sneddon)*.

In a placebo-controlled study, the vitamin was injected directly into the lesions with a spring-loaded gun, giving a concentration in the epidermis and penetration into the superficial and middle dermis. While the normal saline control had no effect, lesions injected with B_{12} regressed in 6 out of 8 patients *(Carslaw)*.

Vitamin D

Calcitriol (1,25-dihydroxyvitamin D3), which regulates terminal differentiation of the basal cells of epidermal keratinocytes, may be low in patients' sera *(Staberg)*. Since this metabolite plays a role in epidermal cell proliferation and differentiation, the abnormally low serum level could play a role in the pathogenesis of psoriasis *(Staberg)*. In fact, there is evidence that the efficacy of UV-B phototherapy is due to its ability to dramatically increase calcitriol levels *(Guihou)*.

Both oral supplementation and topical application of calcitriol have been found effective in open trials *(Perez;Gerritsen)*. Vitamin D has also been combined with vitamin A with improvement in roughly 80% of patients *(Dochao;Marron Gasca)*. However, between 2 and 8 percent had side effects, especially headache and gastrointestinal complaints *(Dochao;Marron Gasca)*.

There is concern that excessive intake of the vitamin can produce hypercalcemia, hypercalciuria, soft tissue calcification, kidney stones, and bone resorption *(Lowe)*. A recent 6-month trial found that, while serum calcium and urinary calcium excretion did increase, they remained within the normal range. Even though there was a 22.5% decline in creatinine clearance, the authors concluded that oral calcitriol is reasonably safe *(Perez)*.

Because of concerns over the safety of vitamin D, the administration of vitamin D analogs such as calcipotriol, which is similar in receptor affinity but 200 times less potent than vitamin D, has been investigated and found to be both efficacious and safe in double-blind studies both systemically *(Kragballe)* and topically *(Lowe)*.

A woman first developed psoriasis at age 14 which worsened during her sophomore year in college. She presented with extensive lesions scattered all over her body except her face.

She was treated with 1,25 dihydroxyvitamin D along with supplemental magnesium (to prevent magnesium deficiency) and her serum calcium levels were followed. Two months later, there was no improvement. However, after another 6 months, her psoriasis was nearly gone (Wright).

MINERALS

Bromine

The waters of the Dead Sea are rich in bromine. By bathing in these waters, bromine levels are increased both due to absorption through the skin and inhalation of the bromine aerosol.

Following a 4-week course of bathing in the Dead Sea, patients demonstrated improvement in their clinical condition concurrent with a 2- to 3-fold increase in serum bromine levels *(Shani)*. Whether their improvement was due to the increase in bromine nutriture is not known.

Chromium Deficiency

Psoriasis patients have been reported to be insulin-resistant and prone to diabetes. Because chromium deficiency leads to insulin resistance, and because patients slough tissue, they may be chromium-deficient *(Brewer)*.

Chromium supplementation has been studied in an open trial. At baseline, the mean insulin resistance of patients was significantly greater than that of normals. Following 4 months of supplementation, the lesions improved, but only in the insulin-resistant half of the patient population. These patients also showed a significant improvement in insulin resistance *(Brewer)*.

Iron Deficiency

Psoriatics may be iron-deficient due to the disease process *(Sato)*. While mean iron absorption is similar to that of normals, absorption is pathologically low in some patients. Iron loss is significantly higher in psoriatic men than in normal men, although it is not significantly different in psoriatic women from that of normal menstruating women *(Keszthelyi)*.

Nickel

Plasma/serum nickel levels may be abnormal. One of 2 studies, both using atomic absorption spectrophotometry, found the levels to be significantly lower than those of normals *(Donadini)*, while the other found them to be significantly higher *(Smith,1994)*.

***AND* Bromine**

In an open trial of oral nickel dibromide, 98% of 86 patients had moderate to marked improvement *(Smith S,1997a)*. The same research group then followed up with a double-blind crossover study of 22 age- and sex-matched patients. Those receiving nickel dibromide either stayed the same or improved, while those given placebo steadily worsened. There was no significant carryover effect *(Smith S,1997a)*.

On the basis of experience with another 2,000 patients, the chief investigator has noted that oral nickel sensitivity occurred in fewer than one percent of patients *(Smith,1997b)*.

Selenium

Selenium is required for the activation of glutathione peroxidase, an inhibitor of the 5-lipoxygenase pathway which promotes formation of inflammatory leukotrienes *(White)*. While not all studies agree, patients with psoriasis may have reduced levels of whole blood and plasma selenium *(Michaëlsson)*. Moreover, levels of the selenium-dependent antioxidant enzyme glutathione peroxidase may be low *(Juhlin)*.

Oral selenium administration fails to increase skin selenium levels and is ineffective *(Fairris;Harvima)*, although it may exert a subtle beneficial effect by increasing the number of helper ($CD4^+$) T cells *(Harvima)*.

By contrast, topical selenium applications have shown evidence of efficacy in an open trial using a selenium-containing shampoo *(Broglund)*

A 40 year-old man had suffered from psoriasis for 28 years. In recent years his constant inguinal psoriasis had developed into a lichen simplex-like state with intense pruritus, lichenification and fissuring. Topical corticosteroids had very little effect.

Application of selenium sulfide shampoo every other day relieved the pruritus completely in 6 days. One month later the pruritus had not returned, the lichenification had diminished and the plaques were paler. Since then his improvement has been maintained on once weekly applications of the shampoo (Broglund).

Zinc

Acquired zinc deficiency may produce a psoriasis-like dermatitis that responds rapidly to zinc supplementation *(Gschnait)*.

In psoriatic patients, epidermal zinc levels are reported to be low *(Michaelsson)*, while cutaneous levels may be elevated *(Dreno)*. Plasma/serum levels are inconsistent, possibly because they are decreased in pustular, but not in other forms, of psoriasis *(Dreno)*. Cellular zinc levels as measured in erythrocytes *(Tsambaos)*, leukocytes *(Wasik)*, or neutrophils *(Leung)* may be reduced. Moreover, following zinc loading, peak plasma zinc levels may be reduced *(Linder)*.

Oral zinc supplementation appears to be ineffective in treating psoriatic lesions *(Burrows;Clemmensen; Leibovici)*. There is some evidence of efficacy, however, for zinc supplementation in the treatment of psoriatic arthritis. In a double-blind crossover study, reduction of joint pains as well as increased mobility and decreased swelling of several joints were observed following treatment with zinc sulfate.

Clinical signs of reduced inflammation were accompanied biochemically by a reduction of serum immunoglobulins and an increase of serum albumin, and the need for analgesics was diminished. Psoriatic skin involvement was unchanged, however. There were no severe side effects *(Clemmensen)*.

Topical application of a zinc formulation appears to be more effective. In an open trial, 7 patients were treated successfully with 10% zinc oxide ointment *(Kobota)*. Also, several studies, most of which are unpublished, have explored the use of a patented formulation of pyrithione zinc (Skin Cap™) *(Walker)*.

In an unpublished double-blind study, 20 patients had pyrithione zinc applied to one side of the body and placebo applied to the other side for 4 weeks, and results were assessed in regard to erythema, desquamation, infiltration or thickening, and pruritus. The active ingredient was found to be far superior to placebo and was an effective and reliable treatment, particularly in regard to reducing desquamation and erythema *(Bugnard)*.

This product was withdrawn from the American market, however, after the US Food and Drug Administration found that the formulation contained the potent corticosteroid clobetasol propionate *(Huntley;Smith K)*.

OTHER NUTRITIONAL FACTORS

Essential Fatty Acids

Patients may have abnormal levels of members of both families of essential fatty acids in plasma lipid esters (cholesterol esters, triglycerides and phospholipids) and in adipose tissue *(Grattan;Vahlquist)*.

Omega-3 Fatty Acids

alpha-linolenic acid → EPA → 3 series prostaglandins
↳ DHA

Leukotriene B4, a major proinflammatory metabolite of arachidonic acid, is known to accumulate in psoriatic lesions. Epidermal 15-lipoxygenase, on the other hand, metabolizes arachidonic acid into 15-hydroxy-eicosatetraenoic acid (15-20:4 n-6), presumably serving as a negative feedback to inhibit the local generation of leukotriene B4.

Eicosapentaenoic acid (EPA) is metabolized by epidermal 15-lipoxygenase into monohydroxy acids which are potent *in vitro* inhibitors of leukotriene B4 generation, suggesting that it may suppress cutaneous inflammation *(Ellis;Ziboh)*. Moreover, Greenland Eskimos, with a fishy diet high in omega-3 fatty acids, have a lower incidence of psoriasis than European controls *(Kromann)*.

There have been several double-blind studies of EPA supplementation, and most have found it to be effective. When given orally, its effects appear to be fairly modest *(Bittiner;Kojima;Soyland)*, while intravenous administration appears to produce more impressive results *(Grimminger;Mayser)*.

Fish oil has also been applied topically under placebo-controlled conditions. In a study reported in the *British Journal of Dermatology*, 8 out of 11 patients (73%) had greater improvement in lesions treated with fish oil added to a commercial vehicle than in lesions treated with the vehicle alone *(Dewsbury)*. However, a subsequent randomized double-blind trial found the topical application of preparations of omega-3 fatty acids to be ineffective *(Henneicke-von Zepelin)*.

Omega-6 Fatty Acids

linoleic acid → GLA → DGLA → 1 series prostaglandins

Like EPA, the omega-6 fatty acid gamma-linolenic acid (GLA) is metabolized into *in vitro* inhibitors of leukotriene B4 generation, suggesting that it may also suppress cutaneous inflammation *(Ellis;Ziboh)*.

While there has been little interest in studying the efficacy of oral administration of omega-6 fatty acids, early evidence suggesting modest efficacy comes from a study of patients who received corn oil, an oil that is rich in the omega-6 fatty acid linoleic acid. While, after 4 months, there was no significant change in the Psoriasis Area and Severity Index, scaling was reduced and there was improvement in desquamation and redness *(Soyland)*.

The efficacy of glucocorticoids in treating the lesions appears to be due to their inhibition of skin arachidonic acid release *(Hammarstrom)*. Therefore it is surprising that topical application of arachidonic acid has been shown under double-blind conditions to produce improvement or complete resolution of psoriatic lesions in about 50% of patients. Upon its application, polymorphonuclear cells are drawn to the stratum corneum which is destroyed and the parakeratotic horny layer becomes detached. The granular layer is then restored and an apparently normal stratum corneum develops *(Hebborn)*.

Omega-3 versus Omega-6 Fatty Acids

The results of a double-blind study suggest that a mixture omega-3 fatty acids are far more effective than mixed omega-6 fatty acids. Ten days after patients randomly received daily infusions of either an omega-3 or an omega-6 emulsion, improvements of 45 to 76 percent were seen in the omega-3 group compared to only 16 to 25 percent in the omega-6 group *(Grimminger)*. Another double-blind study compared fish oils with corn oil (which contains mainly omega-6 fatty acids). Each had only modest efficacy *(Soyland)*.

The two families have been combined in two double-blind studies; both failed to find the combination to be effective *(Oliwiecki;Veale)*.

Fumaric Acid

The *trans* isomer of malic acid and an intermediate in the citric acid (Krebs) cycle, fumaric acid is formed in the skin upon exposure to ultraviolet rays. Patients with psoriasis appear to suffer from a biochemical defect in producing adequate amounts.

Controlled studies have reported improvement in patients following the administration of oral dimethylfumaric acid ester (DMFAE) combined with topical fumaric acid *(Nieboer)* or with the administration of any of several salts of monoethylfumaric acid ester (MEFAE) *(Nugteren-Huying)*. Fumaric acid derivatives have also been found to be effective under double-blind conditions *(Altmeyer)*.

Treatment requires the following dietary restrictions:
1. Certain spices (pepper, cloves, nutmeg, mustard, caraway seeds, anisette (licorice), cinnamon, paprika, mixed seasoning, prespiced dishes, mayonnaise).
2. Certain nuts (filberts, peanuts, walnuts).
3. Certain citrus products (skins, artificial or canned citrus juice).
4. Certain alcoholic beverages (wines, brandy, cognac, vermouth, sherry, orange liquor).

Side effects are common, especially initially. Flushing and gastrointestinal symptoms often occur *(Mrowietz)*. Other side effects include malaise, a mild disturbance of liver function, occasional reversible kidney failure and changes in the blood count. Penicillin should be avoided and the treatment is contraindicated during pregnancy.

Because of the possibility of acute toxicity, as well as the question of chronic toxicity, fumaric acid therapy should only be provided under close medical supervision to patients with severe and recalcitrant conditions.

A 28 year-old woman had pustular psoriasis for 3 years during which she was hospitalized 12 times for treatment with limited improvement. Her body was totally covered with lesions and she was in pain from cracking and itching of the skin.

She went to the Clinique Beau Reveil, Leysin, Switzerland for fumaric acid compound therapy and, the morning after starting treatment with fumaric acid pills, ointment and baths and a special diet, her face was 95% cleared; within 3 days it was completely cleared. Within 2 weeks she noted dramatic improvement in the rash covering the rest of her body, and she was 98% cleared after 2½ months when she returned home (Sax).

OTHER RELATED FACTORS

Food Sensitivities

Patients have been found to have increased intestinal permeability, a finding that could be due to alternations in the small intestinal epithelium *(Humbert)*.

In several open trials, excellent improvement has been reported while patients were following various types of food elimination diets. These include the individualized elimination of specific foods *(Douglass)*, a gluten-free diet *(Bazex)* and even fasting *(Lithell)*.

Hydrochloric Acid Deficiency

Older studies have found evidence of baseline hypochlorhydria and achlorhydria in psoriatic patients, and there seemed to be some correlation between the severity of the condition and abnormal hydrochloric acid levels *(Allison;Ayers)*. One author also noted that the severity of the hydrochloric acid deficiency seemed to be associated with signs of B complex deficiency. Conversely, improvement followed the provision of supplemental hydrochloric acid and vitamin B complex *(Allison)*.

Nowadays, baseline gastric acid levels are not considered adequate to judge the stomach's ability to produce hydrochloric acid on demand. Therefore, a potent parietal cell stimulator is used following baseline measurements and gastric acid is remeasured *(Rappaport)*. The results of such testing have yet to be reported for patients with psoriasis.

BIBLIOGRAPHY

Allison JR. The relation of hydrochloric acid and vitamin B complex deficiency in certain skin disorders. South Med J 38:235-241, 1945

Altmeyer PJ et al. Antipsoriatic effect of fumaric acid derivatives. Results of a multicenter double-blind study in 100 patients. J Am Acad Dermatol 30(6):977-81, 1994

Ayers S. Gastric secretion in psoriasis, eczema and dermatitis herpetiformis. Arch Dermatol Syphilol 20:854-7, 1929

Bazex A et al. Diet without gluten and psoriasis. Ann Dermatol Syphiligr (Paris) 103:648, 1976

Bittiner SB et al. A double-blind, randomised, placebo-controlled trial of fish oil in psoriasis. Lancet i:378-80, 1988

Block WD et al. Nitrogen balance and sulfur excretion studies in psoriasis. Arch Klin Exp Derm 227(1):259, 1966

Brenner S, Horwitz C. Possible nutrient mediators in psoriasis and seborrheic dermatitis. Wld Rev Nutr Diet 55:165-82, 1988

Brewer G et al. Chromium supplementation and insulin sensitivity in psoriasis. Abstract. J Am Coll Nutr 12:588, 1993

Broglund E, Enhamre A. Treatment of psoriasis with topical selenium sulphide. Letter. Br J Dermatol 117(5):665-6, 1987

Bugnard A, dermatologist, Finochietto Hospital, Buenos Aires, Argentina, August 1995 - summarized in Walker M. Astonishing healing of psoriasis using the newest Euro-import. Townsend Letter January, 1997:58-64

Bulkley LD. Report of 140 recent cases of psoriasis in private practice under a strictly vegetarian diet. JAMA 58:714, 1911

Burrows NP et al. A trial of oral zinc supplementation in psoriasis. Cutis 54(2):117-8, 1994

Carslaw RW, Neill J. Vitamin B12 in psoriasis. Letter. Br Med J 1:611, 1963

Clemmensen OJ et al. Psoriatic arthritis treated with oral zinc sulphate. Br J Dermatol 103(4):411-5, 1980

Cohen EL. Vitamin B12 in psoriasis. Letter. Br Med J 1:125, 1963

Collier PM et al. Effect of regular consumption of oily fish compared with white fish on chronic plaque psoriasis. Eur J Clin Nutr 47:251-4, 1993

Committee on Drugs. American Academy of Pediatrics. Retinoid therapy for severe dermatological disorders. Pediatrics 90(1):119-20, 1992

Dewsbury CE et al. Topical eicosapentaenoic acid in the treatment of psoriasis. Br J Dermatol 120:581, 1989

Dochao A et al. [Therapeutic effects of vitamin D and vitamin A in psoriasis: A 20-year experiment.] Actas Dermosfiliogr 66(3-4):121-30, 1975

Donadini A et al. [Plasma levels of Zn, Cu and Ni in healthy controls and in psoriatic patients.] Acta Vitaminol Enzymol 2:9-16, 1980 (in Italian)

Douglass JM. Psoriasis and diet. Letter. Calif Med 133(5):450, 1980

Dreno B et al. Plasma zinc is decreased only in generalized pustular psoriasis. Dermatologica 173(5):209-12, 1986

Ellis CN et al. Experimental therapies for psoriasis. Sem Dermatol 4(4):313-19, 1985

Fahrer H et al. Diet and fatty acids: can fish substitute for fish oil? Clin Exp Rheumatol 9(4):403-6, 1991

Fairris GM et al. The effect of supplementation with selenium and vitamin E in psoriasis. Ann Clin Biochem 26(Pt 1):83-8, 1989

Fry L et al. The mechanism of folate deficiency in psoriasis. Br J Dermatol 84:539-44, 1971

Gaby AR. Commentary: Treating psoriasis. Nutrition & Healing 4(12), December, 1997

Gerritsen M et al. Topical treatment of psoriatic plaques with 1, 25 dihydroxyvitamin D3: A cell biological study. Br J Dermatol 128:666-73, 1993

Grattan C et al. Essential-fatty acid metabolites in plasma phospholipids in patients with ichthyosis vulgaris, acne vulgaris and psoriasis. Clin Exp Dermatol 15(3):174-6, 1990

Grimminger F et al. A double-blind, randomized, placebo-controlled trial of n-3 fatty acid based lipid infusion in acute, extended guttate psoriasis. Clin Invest 71:634-43, 1993

Gschnait F et al. [Exogenous zinc deficiency syndrome.] Wien Klin Wochenschr 94(10):475-9, 1982 (in German)

Guilhou JJ et al. Vitamin D metabolism in psoriasis before and after phototherapy. Acta Dermatol Venereol (Stockh) 70(4):351-4, 1990

Gupta MA et al. Alcohol intake and treatment responsiveness of psoriasis: a prospective study. J Am Acad Dermatol 28(5 Pt 1):730-2, 1993

Haddox M et al. Retinol inhibition of ornithine decarboxylase induction and G1 progression in CHD cells. Cancer Res 39:4930-8, 1979

Hammarstrom S et al. Glucocorticoid in inflammatory proliferative skin disease reduces arachidonic and hydroxyeicosatetrenoic acids. Science 197:994-6, 1977

Harvima RJ et al. Screening of effects of selenomethionine-enriched yeast supplementation on various immunological and chemical parameters of skin and blood in psoriatic patients. Acta Derm Venereol 73(2):88-91, 1993

Hebborn P et al. Action of topically applied arachidonic acid on the skin of patients with psoriasis. Arch Dermatol 124:387-91, 1988

Henneicke-von Zepelin HH et al. Highly purified omega-3-polyunsaturated fatty acids for topical treatment of psoriasis. Results of a double-blind, placebo-controlled multicentre study. Br J Dermatol 129(6):613-7, 1993

Hopkins R et al. A double-blind controlled trial of etretinate (Tigason) and ibuprofen in psoriatic arthritis. Ann Rheum Dis 44(3):189-93, 1985

Humbert P et al. Intestinal permeability in patients with psoriasis. J Dermatol Sci 2(4):324-6, 1991

Huntley AC. Dermatol Online J 3(2), December, 1997

Juhlin L et al. Blood glutathione-peroxidase levels in skin diseases: Effect of selenium and vitamin E treatment. Acta Derm Venereol (Stockh) 62:211-14, 1982

Keszthelyi B et al. Iron absorption and loss in psoriasis. Acta Med Acad Sci Hung 33(2):125-31, 1976

Kojima T et al. Long-term administration of highly purified eicosapentaenoic acid provides improvement of psoriasis. Dermatologica 182(4):225-30, 1991

Kragballe K. Vitamin D3 and skin diseases. Arch Dermatol Res 284 Suppl 1:S30-6, 1992

Kromann N, Green A. Epidemiological studies in the Upernavik District, Greenland. Acta Med Scand 208:401-6, 1989

Kubota K et al. [Clinical studies on zinc oxide ointment replacing boric acid and zinc oxide ointment]. Hokkaido Igaku Zasshi 58(4):400-5, 1983 (in Japanese)

Leibovici V et al. Effect of zinc therapy on neutrophil chemotaxis in psoriasis. Is J Med Sci 26(6):306-9, 1990

Leung RS et al. Neutrophil zinc levels in psoriasis and seborrhoeic dermatitis. Br J Dermatol 123(3):319-23, 1990

Linder N et al. An oral zinc loading test in psoriasis. Metabolism 37(9):807-9, 1988

Lithell H et al. A fasting and vegetarian diet treatment trial on chronic inflammatory disorders. Acta Derm Venereol (Stockh) 63(5):397-403, 1983

Lowe K, Normal A. Vitamin D and psoriasis. Nutr Rev 50:138-42, 1992

Majewski S et al. Decreased levels of vitamin A in serum of patients with psoriasis. Arch Dermatol Res 280:499-501, 1989

Marrakchi S et al. Vitamin A and E blood levels in erythrodermic and pustular psoriasis associated with chronic alcoholism. Acta Derm Venereol 74:298-30, 1994

Marron Gasca J et al. [General treatment of psoriasis. Review of our cases.] Actas Dermosifiliogr 65(7-8):295-304, 1974 (in Spanish)

Mayser P et al. Omega-3 fatty acid-based lipid infusion in patients with chronic plaque psoriasis: results of a double-blind, randomized, placebo-controlled, multicenter trial. J Am Acad Dermatol 38(4)539-47, 1998

Michaelsson G, Ljunghall K. Patients with dermatitis herpetiformis, acne, psoriasis and Darier's disease have low epidermal zinc concentrations. Acta Derm Venereol (Stockh) 70(4):304-8, 1990

Monk BE, Neill SM. Alcohol consumption and psoriasis. Dermatologica 173(2):57-60, 1986

Mrowietz U et al. Treatment of psoriasis with fumaric acid esters: results of a prospective multicentre study. German Multicentre Study. Br J Dermatol 138(3):456-60, 1998

Naldi L et al. Dietary factors and the risk of the psoriasis: results of an Italian case-control study. Br J Dermatol 134(1):101-6, 1996

Newborg B. Disappearance of psoriatic lesions on the rice diet. N Carolina Med J 47:253-5, 1986

Nieboer C et al. Systemic therapy with fumaric acid derivatives: new possibilities in the treatment of psoriasis. J Am Acad Dermatol 20(4):601-8, 1989

Nugteren-Huying WM et al. [Fumaric acid therapy in psoriasis: a double-blind, placebo-controlled study.] Ned Tijdschr Geneeskd 134(49):2387-91, 1990 (in Dutch)

Ockenfels HM et al. Ethanol enhances the IFN-gamma, TGF-alpha and IL-6 secretion in psoriatic co-cultures. Br J Dermatol 135(5):746-51, 1996

Oliwiecki S, Burton JL. Evening primrose oil and marine oil in the treatment of psoriasis. Clin Exp Dermatol 19(2):127-9, 1994

Oster KA. A cardiologist considers psoriasis. Cutis 20:39-41, 1977

Perez A et al. Safety and efficacy of oral calcitriol (1,25-dihydroxyvitamin D3) for the treatment of psoriasis. Br J Dermatol 134:1070-8, 1996

Poikolainen K et al. Alcohol intake: a risk factor for psoriasis in young and middle aged men? Br Med J 300:780-3, 1990

Proctor M et al. Lowered cutaneous and urinary levels of polyamines with clinical improvement in treated psoriasis. Arch Dermatol 115:945-9, 1979

Rappaport EM. Achlorhydria: Associated symptoms and response to hydrochloric acid. N Engl J Med 252(19):802-5, 1955

Rollman O, Vahlquist A. Psoriasis and vitamin A. Plasma transport and skin content of retinol, dehydroretinol and carotenoids in adult patients versus healthy controls. Arch Dermatol Res 278(1):17-24, 1985

Rosenberg E, Belew P. Microbial factors in psoriasis. Arch Dermatol 118:1434-44, 1982

Ruedemann R. Treatment of psoriasis with large doses of vitamin B12: 1,000 micrograms per cubic centimeter. Arch Dermatol 69:738-9, 1954

Sato S. Iron deficiency: structural and microchemical changes in hair, nails, and skin. Semin Dermatol 10(4):313-19, 1991

Sax A, Ed. Psoriasis Researcher Newsletter February, 1987

Schamberg JF et al. Protein metabolism in psoriasis. J Cutan Dis 31:892-915, 1913

Schamberg JF. The dietary treatment of psoriasis. JAMA 98:1633, 1932

Schopf RE et al. Ethanol enhances the mitogen-driven lymphocyte proliferation in patients with psoriasis. Acta Derm Venereol 76(4):260-3, 1996

Shani J et al. Serum bromine levels in psoriasis. Pharmacology 25(6):297-307, 1982

Shuster S et al. Folic acid deficiency in patients with skin disease. Br J Dermatol 79:398, 1967

Smith KC. Dermatol Online J 3(2), December, 1997

Smith SA et al. Elevated serum nickel concentration in psoriasis vulgaris. Int J Dermatol 33(11):783-5, 1994

Smith SA et al. Improvement of psoriasis vulgaris with oral nickel dibromide. Letter. Arch Dermatol 133(5):661-3, 1997a

Smith SA - interviewed by Jonathan Wright in Nutrition & Healing June, 1997b

Sneddon JB. Vitamin B12 in psoriasis. Letter. Br Med J 1:328, 1963

Soyland E et al. Effect of dietary supplementation with very-long-chain n-3 fatty acids in patients with psoriasis. N Engl J Med 328:1812-16, 1993

Staberg B et al. Abnormal vitamin D metabolism in patients with psoriasis. Acta Derm Venereol (Stockh) 67:65-8, 1987

Tsambaos D, Orfanos CE. [Zinc distribution disorder in psoriasis.] Arch Dermatol Res 259(1):97-100, 1977

Vahlquist C et al. The fatty-acid spectrum in plasma and adipose tissue in patients with psoriasis. Arch Dermatol Res 278(2):114-19, 1985

Veale DJ et al. A double-blind placebo controlled trial of Efamol Marine on skin and joint symptoms of psoriatic arthritis. Br J Rheumatol 33(10):954-8, 1994

Walker M. Astonishing healing of psoriasis using the newest Euro-import. Townsend Letter January, 1997:58-64

Wasik F et al. [Zinc content of leukocytes and serum in psoriasis patients.] Hautarzt 36(10):573-6, 1985 (in German)

White A et al. Role of lipoxygenase products in the pathogenesis and therapy of psoriasis and other dermatoses. Arch Dermatol 119:541-7, 1983

Wright JV. Psoriasis and 'activated' vitamin D. Let's Live April, 1989

Zackheim HS, Farber EM. Low-protein diet and psoriasis. A hospital study. Arch Dermatol 99(5):580-6, 1969

Zamboni S et al. Dietary behaviour in psoriatic patients. Acta Derm Venereol Suppl (Stockh) 146:182-3, 1989

Ziboh VA. Implications of dietary oils and polyunsaturated fatty acids in the management of cutaneous disorders. Arch Dermatol 125(2):241-5, 1989

RHEUMATOID ARTHRITIS

See Also: PAIN

NUTRITIONAL TREATMENT GUIDE

✓ = Efficacy generally accepted.
* = Efficacy *demonstrated* by controlled human trials.
[+] = Efficacy *suspected* from uncontrolled human experiments
[-] = Efficacy *suspected* from indirect data
? = Efficacy *challenged* in at least one study of similar design

DIETARY FACTORS

* treat **Malnutrition**
* **Vegetarian** or **Vegan diet**

- -

[+] avoid excessive **Saturated Fat** intake

- -

[-] adequate **Fiber** intake
[-] high **Fish** consumption
[-] high **Protein** intake

NUTRITIONAL FACTORS

A. TO REDUCE DISEASE ACTIVITY

* **Copper:** copper salicylate 60 mg twice daily
* **Gold:** intramuscular injections
* **Omega-3 Fatty Acids:** 1.7 to 4.6 g EPA *AND* 0.4 to 2.5 g DHA (1 to 3 month trial)
* **Omega-6 Fatty Acids:** gamma-linolenic acid (GLA) 2.8 g daily (1 to 3 month trial)
* **Pantothenic Acid:** Start with 500 mg daily. Gradually increase to 500 mg 4 times daily by day 10. (2 month trial)
* **Sulfur:** sulfur-containing baths
* **Vitamin E:** alpha-tocopherol 400 mg 3 times daily (3 week trial)
* ? **Selenium:** sodium selenite 200 μg daily (3 month trial)
* ? **Zinc:** 20 to 50 mg 3 times daily (3 month trial)

- -

[+] **Boron:** 6 to 9 mg daily to achieve symptom relief followed by a maintenance dose of 3 mg daily
[+] **Gold:** oral colloidal metallic gold (Aurasol) 60 mg daily for 1 week, then 30 mg daily
[+] **Sulfur:** intravenous injections of colloidal sulfur

- -

[-] **Vitamin C deficiency:** *to protect involved joints from damage:* 500 mg twice daily
[-] **Vitamin D deficiency:** 50,000 to 100,000 IU 2 or 3 times during the first week; then, if needed, either 100,000 IU or ergo- or cholecalciferol every 3 to 6 months *OR* 800 to 1,600 IU daily

B. TO PREVENT/TREAT COMPLICATIONS

* **Calcium** ***AND*** **Vitamin D:** *to prevent bone loss in juvenile patients on corticosteroids*
* **Folic acid:** *to reduce methotrexate toxicity and hyperhomocysteinemia:* 5 mg per week
* **Molybdenum:** *to reduce pain:* 500 µg as amino acid chelate daily. Start with 1 cap with meals and at bedtime. Increase to maximum of 5 caps daily, or decrease to 2 to 3 caps daily, depending upon response. (1 month trial)
* **Vitamin E:** *to reduce pain:* 400 mg 3 times daily

- -

[+] **Iron:** *for iron-deficiency anemia:* 30 mg twice daily until repletion; then minimal possible dosage. (Only supplement if serum ferritin is <60 µg/L.)
[+] **Vitamin C deficiency:** *for spontaneous bruising and cutaneous hemorrhages:* 500 mg twice daily
[+] **Vitamin D deficiency:** *to improve bone metabolism:* 50,000 to 100,000 IU 2 or 3 times during the first week; then, if needed, either 100,000 IU or ergo- or cholecalciferol every 3 to 6 months *OR* 800 to 1,600 IU daily

OTHER RELATED FACTORS

✓ rule out **Food Sensitivities**

- -

[+] **Hydrolytic enzymes:** Wobenzyme® 8 tablets 4 times daily (trial may take weeks to months)
[+] rule out **Hydrochloric Acid deficiency**

DIETARY FACTORS

Malnutrition

Evidence of malnutrition may be found in up to 75% of patients *(McDuffie)*. This is believed to be primarily due to abnormal nutrient absorption and metabolism rather than to inadequate intake as their nutritional status correlates better with the severity of the disease than with dietary intake *(Helliwell)*. However, food habits of patients are often poor, and total energy intake is often too low *(Hansen)*.

Malnutrition is also common among children with juvenile rheumatoid arthritis. Chronic inflammation can cause anorexia, reduced mobility can make eating and preparing foods difficult, drugs to reduce inflammation can cause nausea, and abdominal pain can reduce absorption. Problems caused by malnutrition include growth failure with excessive fat deposits which can result in long-term cardiovascular risks *(Di Toro)*. Even if their calorie and protein intakes are high, they may still have a poor nutritional status *(Haugen)*.

In a single-blind study, patients with active disease were randomly assigned to treatment with or without a specialized diet in which the energy consumption was adjusted to normal standards for body-weight and the intake of fish and antioxidants was increased. After 6 months, those following the diet demonstrated significant improvement in the duration of morning stiffness, the number of swollen joints, and pain status. Moreover, although ratings of their "overall condition" was not significantly improved, the cost of their medicines was significantly decreased *(Hansen)*.

Protein

Protein intake takes to be low. In one group, for example, only 16% of calories were from protein *(Morgan,1997)*. In fact, a relatively high protein intake has been associated with a reduced risk of rheumatoid arthritis *(Shapiro)*.

Dietary Fats

In patients, dietary fats often constitute an excessive percentage of total calories *(Kremer;Morgan,1997)*. This is a relevant finding because dietary fats affect disease activity. For example, patients with active disease experienced long-term remissions of joint symptoms within days of going on a low-calorie, fat-free weight control formula diet, and experienced exacerbations 1 to 2 days after returning to high-fat foods or vegetable oils *(Lucas)*.

Simply reducing dietary fat intake to a very low level is not recommended, however, as it may be deleterious by causing stimulation of lipid peroxidation and eicosanoid formation *(Adam)* as well as because of the lack of essential fatty acids.

Moreover, the effects of dietary fats differ depending upon the degree of saturation of the fatty acids. Saturated fats appear to have a deleterious effect. When a group of patients was compared to healthy controls, the patients had high concentrations of total saturated fatty acids in both serum and adipose tissue, and the severity of this abnormality was associated with disease duration *(Jacobsson)*. By contrast, essential fatty acids appear to be beneficial. (See Essential Fatty Acids below.)

Fish

Fish consumption appears to be beneficial. When female patients were compared to age-matched normals, greater than one serving per week of grilled (broiled) or baked fish (other than tuna) was associated with a decreased risk of rheumatoid arthritis. This association was strengthened when only the patients who were seropositive for rheumatoid factor were included in the analysis *(Shapiro)*.

The beneficial effects of fish have been attributed to their high content of omega-3 essential fatty acids (see Essential Fatty Acids below). In fact, 4 to 6 meals of fish per week induces similar changes in lipids as a supplement of fish oil *(Fahrer)*. Fish may also have additional benefits, as the study alluded to above found that the inverse association between fish consumption and the risk of rheumatoid arthritis was stronger than that for omega-3 fatty acid intake *(Shapiro)*.

Dietary Fiber

Patients with active RA ingest less dietary fiber than the RDA *(Kremer)*. There is no evidence that this has any effect on the disease process, however.

Vegetarian Diet

Several studies, some of which were controlled, have found beneficial effects from a vegetarian or vegan diet. In one study, for example, patients were fasted for 7 to 10 days. They then followed a gluten-free vegan diet for 3 ½ months, and then a lactovegetarian diet for 9 months. Twelve of the 27 patients responded with significant clinical improvement compared to the 27 controls. Moreover, *Proteus mirabilis* in the bacterial flora had a significantly decreased antibody titer during dietary treatment, and changes in the profile of the bacterial wall fatty acids provided evidence of an altered bacterial flora, suggesting that the efficacy of a vegetarian diet may be due to changes in the bacterial flora *(Kjeldsen-Kragh)*.

In another study, patients with class II or III disease randomly received either an uncooked vegan diet or a control diet for 3 months. Those on the vegan diet experienced subjective relief of rheumatic stiffness and joint swellings and an improvement in general well-being. After returning to the omnivorous diet, these symptoms worsened. The Ritchie index of tender joints remained unchanged in controls, but in the diet group their number decreased by more than 2 joints. The health assessment questionnaire also showed improvement *(Nenonen)*.

Objective evidence that a vegan diet results in a rapid decrease in inflammation comes from a study in which patients followed a diet of diluted fruit and vegetable juices. After only 10 days, they showed reduced levels of complement factor 3, orosomucoid and haptoglobin *(Skoldstam)*.

In addition to whatever nutritional benefits this diet may provide, a vegetarian diet may contribute to improvement by removing foods to which particular patients are sensitive (see Food Sensitivities below).

HOMOCYSTEINE

Patients often have elevated levels of the toxic amino acid homocysteine *(Roubenoff, 1997)*. At least in part, these elevated levels are due to the effects of drugs commonly prescribed for the condition, including methotrexate *(van Ede)* and sulfasalazine *(Krogh)*.

Elevated homocysteine levels can usually be normalized by supplementation with folic acid and other specific nutrients (see Atherosclerosis).

NUTRITIONAL FACTORS

VITAMINS

Folic Acid

Patients commonly fail to ingest the RDI for folic acid *(Stone)*, and serum folate levels are often low *(Alter)*. Aspirin, and perhaps the other non-steroidal anti-inflammatory drugs, appears to alter folate transport by competing with binding sites on plasma proteins, although it is unclear whether this results in hypervitaminuria *(Alter)*.

Results of double-blind studies suggest that folate supplementation should be considered for patients receiving methotrexate therapy because it helps to prevent methotrexate toxicity, it prevents or treats folate deficiency, and it prevents hyperhomocysteinemia *(Morgan, 1998)*. However, too high a dosage may exacerbate side-effects related to the drug *(Modesto)*.

Pantothenic Acid

Pantothenic acid is lower in patients than in normals, and the degree of deficiency correlates with disease severity *(Barton-Wright)*.

In a double-blind study by the General Practitioner Research Group, 18 patients who were previously untreated or who had not responded to previous drug treatment randomly received calcium pantothenate or placebo for 2 months. Medication was limited to paracetamol. Supplementation was found to be associated with significant improvements in the duration of morning stiffness, degree of disability and severity of pain which was not seen in those receiving placebo.

Vitamin B_6

Patients commonly ingest less than the recommended intake of vitamin B_6 *(Kremer; Morgan, 1997)*. Not only are plasma levels of the vitamin often reduced, but these levels may be inversely related to the degree of inflammation *(Roubenoff, 1995)*.

However, when patients with low plasma pyridoxal phosphate levels were treated with 50 to 150 mg of pyridoxine hydrochloride for 3 months, there was no clinical improvement despite a large rise in plasma levels *(Schumacher)*.

Vitamin B_{12}

Patients commonly ingest less than the recommended intake of vitamin B_{12} *(Morgan, 1997)*. Moreover, about 4% of patients with severe disease are believed to have low serum levels of the vitamin, a finding that appears to be one of several biochemical signs of gastrointestinal dysfunction *(Pettersson)*.

There is no evidence that vitamin B_{12} supplementation affects the clinical findings.

Vitamin C Deficiency

Leukocyte and plasma/serum levels of vitamin C are frequently decreased *(Mullen; Singh)*, while dehydro-ascorbate, the oxidized form of the vitamin, may be increased, probably due to increase antioxidant and free-radical scavenging activity, especially within inflamed joints *(Lunec)*. The rapid depletion of ascorbic acid in these joints is believed to facilitate proteolytic damage *(Halliwell)*.

Thus, ascorbate repletion will not only erase signs of ascorbate deficiency such as spontaneous bruising and cutaneous hemorrhages *(Oldroyd)*, but may also help to protect involved joints from damage.

Vitamin D Deficiency

Patients commonly fail to ingest the recommended amount of vitamin D *(Hansen; Wordsworth)* and serum levels may be reduced, sometime placing them in the range of osteomalacia due to vitamin D deficiency *(Kroger)*. Among patients who have had the diagnosis for at least 5 years, osteoporosis is common *(Oelzner; Suzuki)*, and those with the severest osteoporosis also have the lowest levels of serum 25-hydroxyvitamin D *(Wordsworth)*.

Moreover, high disease activity has been found to be associated with altered vitamin D metabolism as well as with increased bone resorption. The decrease of 1,25-dihydroxyvitamin D in these patients may contribute to a negative calcium balance and inhibition of bone formation, and may also accelerate the arthritic process *(Oelzner)*

Similar findings have been noted in juvenile rheumatoid arthritis. These patients often have lowered serum levels of osteocalcin, an indicator of bone formation, that normalize when disease activity ceases. Bone formation is reduced *(Falcini; Pepmueller)* leading to reduced bone mineral density which may contribute to their increased frequency of fractures *(Reed)*.

For children with active juvenile rheumatoid arthritis, supplementation may normalize their low osteocalcin levels. However, bone mineral density failed to increase during one year of supplementation; whether it increases when supplementation is continued over a longer period of time is not known *(Reed)*.

Vitamin E

Patients commonly consume less than the recommended intake of vitamin E *(Hansen;Stone)*.

Serum levels of vitamin E may be reduced in adult patients, although the difference may be not be significant *(Comstock)*. Similar findings have been noted in children with juvenile rheumatoid arthritis; in addition, there is evidence that their erythrocyte levels may be increased *(Sklodowska)*.

Both for patients with rheumatoid arthritis *(Wittenborg)*, and for patients with ankylosing spondylitis *(Blankenhorn)*, controlled studies have found vitamin E supplementation to be as effective in reducing pain as a non-steroidal anti-inflammatory drug (NSAID). The vitamin also appears to be effective in reducing pain in patients with rheumatoid arthritis who are under treatment with anti-rheumatic drugs *(Edmonds)*.

Moreover, for patients with rheumatoid arthritis, when vitamin E was compared to a NSAID, patients taking either substance showed similar significant improvements in all assessed clinical parameters *(Wittenborg)*.

MINERALS

Boron

Boron intake has been inversely related to the risk of the disease. In areas of the world where boron intake is routinely less than or equal to 1 mg per day, the estimated incidence of all forms of arthritis is 20 to 70%, yet in areas of the world where boron intake is 3 to 10 mg per day, the estimated incidence is zero to 10% *(Newnham,1994a,)*. Western diets appear to average 1 to 2 mg a day, while an intake of 2 mg or more daily appears to be associated with a reduced incidence of all forms of arthritis *(Newnham,1994b)*.

There is very preliminary evidence that boron supplementation may be beneficial. Rats with induced arthritis benefit from boron when administered either intraperitoneally or orally *(Newnman,1994a)*. In an informal open trial, boron was effective for about 90% of a group of patients with various forms of arthritis, most with complete remission of symptoms. It was especially effective for juvenile arthritis *(Newnham,1991)*.

However, the investigator found that symptomatic relief due to boron supplementation may not occur for 2 to 3 weeks in children, 2 months in adults under age 70, and 4 months for adults of more advanced age. Also, patients with rheumatoid arthritis sometimes experienced an initial aggravation of symptoms (Herxheimer response) for 1 to 3 weeks after onset of supplementation. This subsided, though, with improvements usually becoming apparent by 4 weeks *(Newnham,1994b)*.

Calcium

Patients commonly ingest less than the recommended calcium intake *(Morgan,1997;Stone)*. In juvenile rheumatoid arthritis, bone resorption causes hypercalciuria *(Abrams;Kasapcopur)*, irrespective of the activity of the disease *(Reed)*. However, their bone mineral density has been inversely related to disease activity *(Polito)*, although the primary cause of their decreased bone mineral density appears to be treatment with corticosteroids *(Brik)*.

There is no evidence that calcium supplementation affects the course of the disease, although the danger of osteoporosis should be kept in mind and appropriate preventive and therapeutic measures should be taken. In particular, juvenile patients receiving corticosteroids should be considered for calcium and vitamin D supplementation *(Warady)*. (See Osteoporosis.)

Copper

Patients often fail to ingest the recommended amount of dietary copper *(Kremer;Morgan,1997)*. However, serum copper and ceruloplasmin concentrations tend to be *increased*, both in adults *(Milanino;Zoli)* and in children *(Haugen)*. While plasma copper is correlated with some of the biohumoral markers of the disease, studies have failed to agree on whether it correlates with clinical indices *(Honkanen;Milanino)*.

The rise in serum copper is associated with a fall in liver copper stores, an increased rate of synthesis of ceruloplasmin (a copper-containing protein), and increased ceruloplasmin in the synovial fluid. It does not reflect copper balance in the body *(Sorenson,1982)* and patients do not seem to be copper-deficient *(Milanino)*, although untreated patients have an elevation of urinary copper excretion and bone biopsies may indicate copper deficiency *(Heinitz)*. These changes may reflect a negative change in the oxidative status of the blood *(Banford)*.

Copper supplementation has an anti-inflammatory effect which appears to be related to its ability to form complexes which serve as selective antioxidants; thus reducing the inflammation caused by enhanced oxidant damage *(Sorenson,1980)*. These complexes also appear to activate copper-dependent opioid receptors *(Okuyama)*.

Results of several studies suggest that copper salicylate may be the most effective copper complex to administer. In an open trial, short-term administration of copper salicylate intravenously was followed by normalization of the sedimentation rate along with remission of fever, increased joint mobility and decreased joint swelling in 89% of 1,140 patients for an average of 3 years *(Sorenson,1977)*.

A single-blind crossover study of 240 "arthritis/ rheumatism sufferers" found that topical application of elemental copper by wearing a copper bracelet relieved clinical symptoms. Previous users of copper bracelets deteriorated while wearing the placebo *(Walker)*. This interesting study awaits replication under double-blind conditions with subjects limited to patients with rheumatoid arthritis.

Gold

Rheumatoid arthritis is characterized by increased macrophage activity which produces toxic forms of oxygen that have been suggested as mediators of rheumatoid inflammation. Gold accumulates in lysosomes of the macrophages and stabilizes lysosomal and other cell membranes leading to reduced liberation of toxic oxygen *(Munthe)*.

First introduced in the early part of this century, intramuscular injection of gold (gold salts of monovalent gold with a gold-sulfur ligand; aurothiolates) has become one of the standard treatment options *(Anonymous,1979)*. However, toxicity is not uncommon, and controversy over the efficacy of gold therapy continues *(Anonymous,1991)*.

Recently, an open trial in which colloidal gold was administered orally has reported good results. Ten patients with long-standing erosive bone disease not responding to previous treatment received colloidal metallic gold (Aurasol) orally for 24 weeks. Effects on joint tenderness and swelling were rapid and dramatic, with a significant decrease in both parameters after the first week which then persisted.

By the end of the study, the mean scores were 10 times lower than pretreatment levels. All but one patient were markedly improved. Three patients were in clinical remission and one patient's status improved from totally disabled to full-time work. There was no clinical or lab evidence of toxicity *(Abraham)*.

Even more intriguing is a recent observational study of topical gold application. Ring wearers (patients who had worn a gold ring on the left ring finger throughout most of the time since disease onset) were compared with non-ring wearers. Hand radiographs found less articular erosion at the left ring finger, and perhaps adjacent metacarpophalangeal joints, in the ring wears, suggesting that sufficient gold could be absorbed to reach the nearby joint and delay articular erosion *(Mulherin)*.

Iron

Whether patients consume adequate dietary iron is uncertain. One study found dietary intake to be inadequate *(Morgan,1997)* while another found it to be "largely adequate" and unrelated to the presence of anemia *(Stone)*.

Serum iron may be low *(Niedermeier)*. However, iron may be elevated in both the synovial fluid and the synovial membrane *(Muirden)*, and this accumulation appears to cause inflammatory tissue damage *(Dabbagh)*. As a measure of iron deficiency, serum ferritin levels are superior, not only to serum iron, but also to plasma transferrin, mean corpuscular volume and mean corpuscular hemoglobin capacity. However, as an acute phase reactant, serum ferritin may show some correlation with disease activity *(Rothwell)*.

Although patients often present with a microcytic anemia, iron supplementation should be avoided unless ferritin levels are low, since supplemental iron can increase joint inflammation by forming highly reactive hydroxyl radicals *(Rawley)*.

A 39-year-old female with rheumatoid arthritis developed both subjective and objective worsening of her peripheral synovitis within 48 hours of ingesting ferrous sulfate 200 mg 3 times daily, while placebo caused no change. Serum ferritin rose from 30 to 50 µg/L while her symptoms exacerbated on iron, but returned to 15 µg/L one month after iron was stopped (Blake).

Molybdenum

Molybdenum is required for the synthesis of 4 detoxifying enzymes *(Rajagopalan)*.

In a single-blind crossover study, 14 people with chronic aches and pains due to different forms of arthritis, including 4 with rheumatoid arthritis, graded their pain level and general health for 28 days. They then took either molybdenum or placebo capsules for the next 28 days; then the groups were crossed over for a third 28-day period.

Within one week of starting molybdenum, aches and pains significantly improved, as did their rating of their general health. When discontinued after being taken for 28 days, the effects of the supplement wore off within one week *(Moss)*.

Selenium

In a survey of 48 patients, only 6% achieved the recommended daily intake for selenium *(Stone)*. Several studies have found plasma or serum levels to be low *(Jacobsson;Kose)*.

The administration of selenium in such a form that it incorporates into glutathione peroxidase and increases the efficacy of the enzyme may theoretically lead to accelerated metabolism of toxic oxygen *(Munthe)*. Under double-blind conditions, patients receiving medications and fish oil fatty acids were randomly allocated to supplementation with sodium selenite or placebo for 3 months each. The selenium-supplemented patients were found to have less tender or swollen joints, and less morning stiffness. They also required less non-steroidal anti-inflammatory drugs and cortisone than the placebo controls. Furthermore, laboratory measures showed decreased inflammation *(Heinle)*.

Other double-blind studies have reported both positive *(Peretz,1992)* and negative *(Tarp)* findings following selenium supplementation.

Sulfur

Joint cartilage contains chondroitin-sulphuric acid, which is thought to maintain the suppleness and resistance of the joint, as well as neutral sulfur. Patients' muscle fibers may contain reduced sulfur levels, perhaps because of a decrease in sulfur-rich proteins *(Wroblewski)*. Also, the content of cysteine, a sulfur amino acid, in the nails of "arthritics" may be low *(Sullivan)*.

Sulfur administration, either in the form of sulfur baths or in the form of injections, is an old remedy. An open trial found administration of intravenous colloidal sulfur often reduced effusions as well as pain, while fingernail cysteine levels rose to normal *(Woldenberg)*. Sulfur baths could be of value as sulfur is absorbed through the skin to raise blood sulfur levels, although their efficacy remains to be demonstrated *(Osterberg)*.

In a double-blind study, the effects of diluted mud baths in the presence versus the absence of sulfur compounds were studied. Patients taking sulfur baths experienced a significant lowering in pain sensitivity as measured by changes in pain thresholds in 16 trigger points. The more times patients took the bath, the greater the improvement *(Pratsel)*.

Another study took patients with active disease and gave them either daily mud packs, daily hot sulfur baths, both mud packs and sulfur baths, or no treatment for 2 weeks. Based on the evaluation of a rheumatologist who was blinded as to their treatment, there were statistically significant improvements for a period of up to 3 months in the 3 treatment groups for most of the clinical indices, although the laboratory measures of the disease process were unchanged *(Sukenik)*.

Zinc

Rheumatoid arthritis is characterized by increased macrophage activity causing production of toxic forms of oxygen which may mediate rheumatoid inflammation. Zinc is a component of superoxide dismutase which detoxifies oxygen. In pharmacological doses, it can immobilize macrophages and induce metallothionein-like proteins *(Aaseth;Munthe)*.

Only 10% of a group of 48 patients were found to ingest the recommended daily intake for zinc *(Stone)*. Other studies have found similar results *(Kremer; Morgan,1997)*.

Synovial fluid levels may be elevated *(Niedermeier)*. By contrast, plasma/serum zinc levels may be reduced in both adults *(Naveh;Zoli)* and children *(Haugen)*. This reduction appears to be determined mostly by the activity and extent of the inflammatory process and not by dietary factors *(Honkanen;Milanino)*. Cellular zinc levels may also be reduced *(Svenson)*. Urinary zinc was reduced in one study *(Naveh)* but increased in another *(Pandey)*.

Double-blind studies of zinc supplementation has reported mixed results, however *(Peretz,1993;Rasker; Simkin,1976)*. One author has suggested that the conflicting results may be because zinc is only effective when correcting a zinc deficiency *(Simkin,1981)*. This hypothesis remains to be tested.

OTHER NUTRITIONAL FACTORS

Essential Fatty Acids

Essential fatty acid metabolism appears to be altered in the disease. Reductions in both linoleic acid (omega-6) and alpha-linolenic acid (omega-3) and their metabolites have been reported in the plasma phospholipid fraction and in adipose tissue along with high concentrations of saturated fatty acids *(Jacobsson;Suryaprabha)*. Moreover, the severity of this abnormality is associated with the duration of the disease *(Jacobsson)*.

While omega-3 or omega-6 fatty acids can be supplemented separately (see below), findings from one double-blind study suggest that supplementation with the combination of members of both families of essential fatty acids may be preferable. The combination of *evening primrose oil*, a rich source of the omega-6 fatty acid gamma linolenic acid (GLA), and *fish oil*, rich in the omega-3 fatty acid eicosapentaenoic acid (EPA), was investigated in a double-blind study of 49 patients, all of whom were taking non-steroidal anti-inflammatory drugs. After 3 months, efforts were made to reduce drug use in all patients.

After an additional 9 months, patients on evening primrose oil rated themselves 94% better, those on evening primrose and fish oil rated themselves 100% better, while those on placebo rated themselves only 33% better. Eighty-three percent of patients on evening primrose oil and 94% on evening primrose and fish oils either completely eliminated drugs or cut their dosages in half, while only 34% of patients on placebo were able to reduce their drug intake.

All patients were then placed on placebo. After 3 months, those who had been receiving active treatment had relapsed although, despite the reduction in drugs, measures of disease activity did not worsen *(Belch)*.

Omega-3 Fatty Acids

Patients with active disease appear to have a very low intake of the omega-3 fatty acids *(Hansen)*.

There is consistent evidence from numerous controlled clinical trials that these essential fatty acids have modest beneficial effects. They appear to suppress inflammatory mediators, which include omega-6 eicosanoids and proinflammatory cytokines *(James)*. As their use decreases the long-term requirements for nonsteroidal antiinflammatory drugs, it has been theorized that they may at times provide an alternative to taking these drugs, although studies examining this possibility have yet to be published *(Ariza-Ariza)*.

Omega-6 Fatty Acids

In vitro studies have generally indicated that GLA reduces lymphocyte activation and production of mediators of inflammation. In a small number of clinical studies, treatment with GLA, or with botanical products which are rich in this omega-6 fatty acid (such as evening primrose or borage seed oils), was associated with clinical improvement as measured by duration of morning stiffness, joint pain and swelling, and ability to reduce other medications. However, these studies vary in terms of duration, GLA dosage, whether or not they were placebo-controlled, criteria for evaluation, and the use of concomitant medication *(Rothman)*.

It appears that some of the patients who will improve the most may have a transient worsening in the first 1 to 2 weeks, and that higher dosages of steroids or non-steroidal anti-inflammatory drugs may diminish its effectiveness. However, after 1 to 3 months, drug dosages can often be reduced *(Horrobin)*.

OTHER RELATED FACTORS

Food Sensitivities

Rheumatoid arthritis was absent in prehistory, when cereals and dairy products were not consumed and prolonged cooking was not done. The high frequency of gut mucosal lesions and excessive permeability of the intestinal wall found in patients with rheumatoid arthritis suggests that the enterocyte enzymes may not be well adapted for modern food *(Seignalet)*. Moreover, prolonged treatment with non-steroidal antiinflammatory drugs has been shown to increase intestinal permeability and food antigen absorption *(Bjarnason;Fagiolo)*, while fasting has been shown to decrease intestinal permeability *(Sundquist)* as well as joint inflammation and the erythrocyte sedimentation rate *(Uden)*.

The pernicious influence of food sensitivities on the symptoms, and possibly the progression, of the disease has now been well-documented in scientific studies *(Darlington,1993)*. Besides fasting, various food elimination diets have been utilized, including an elemental diet *(Kavanaghi)*. Reactions to corn, wheat and animal protein are among the most common *(Marshall)*.

Out of a group of 100 patients who underwent dietary manipulation, one-third were still well and controlled on diet alone without any medication up to 7 ½ years after starting dietary treatment. The investigator found cereals to be among the foods most frequently implicated. Corn and wheat provoked symptoms in more than half of the patients *(Darlington,1991)*.

Fifty-three out of another group of 93 unselected patients (57%) were found to have raised IgG antibody levels to milk and/or wheat proteins. Forty-eight patients in this sub-group (90%) also had raised levels of IgA rheumatoid factor compared to only 7 of the 40 antibody negative patients (17%), a significant difference which suggests an association between food sensitivities and disease activity *(O'Farrelly)*.

A woman with a 25-year history of active rheumatoid arthritis was taking azathioprine and soluble aspirin, and had been treated with plasma exchange, but was gradually deteriorating. When challenged, corn (which was the filler in both medications) appeared to be her major food allergen.

She improved dramatically after one week on a corn exclusion diet. However, after 6 weeks she had a severe exacerbation following the inadvertent ingestion of corn as corn flour thickening in gravy.

Afterwards, she improved again and began to regain weight. She was able to discontinue all medications, and now feels and looks better than she has for over 20 years (Williams).

Hydrolytic Enzymes

Patients have been shown to have reduced serum levels of various hydrolytic enzymes *(Aoyagi)*. When animal or plant hydrolytic enzymes are given orally, about 25% are absorbed in a functionally active form. After forming complexes with natural antiproteases, they concentrate in wounds, areas of inflammation and foci of immunopathology *(Nouza)*. Their efficacy in rheumatoid arthritis is believed to be due to their ability to eliminate pathogenic immune complexes which have penetrated the joint cartilage from the synovial fluid by degrading their protective fibrin cloak *(Glenk)*.

In several open trials, oral enzyme mixtures have been reported to be effective. (Wobenzyme®, the product that has been most extensively studied, is an enteric-coated tablet consisting of a mixture of pancreatin, bromelain, papain, lipase, amylase, trypsin and alpha-chymotrypsin combined with rutin.)

In one study, for example, 26 out of 42 patients (62%) were improved after 6 weeks, while only 3 (17%) were worse. Responses were more common among patients who were either negative for immune complexes or who became negative during treatment. There were no side effects *(Steffen)*.

Hydrochloric Acid Deficiency

Both hypochlorhydria and achlorhydria after pentagastrin stimulation are common findings among seropositive patients and are associated with an increased risk of bacterial overgrowth in the small intestine. Among a group of seropositive patients, those with bacterial overgrowth had significantly higher disease activity indices and rheumatoid factor titers *(Henriksson)*.

The efficacy of providing supplemental hydrochloric acid remains to be demonstrated.

COMBINED NUTRITIONAL INTERVENTIONS

A male with increasing foot and shoulder pains was found to have an elevated sedimentation rate and placed on prescription drugs. During the next 6 months, his condition worsened, and he noted increasing pain, stiffness and swelling in his shoulders, elbows, wrists, fingers, knees, feet and ankles. He was unable to tolerate aspirin, and other medications were ineffective. He required two canes to walk, and needed assistance for personal hygiene as well as for sitting and standing.

One year after symptom-onset, he began to avoid white flour and sugar and limited his diet to fresh fruits, vegetables, fish, liver and chicken. He also started supplementation with cod-liver oil (rich in omega-3 fatty acids) 3 teaspoons twice daily. Following meals, he took vitamin C 1 gram and niacin 1 gram. He also drank a blend of one tablespoon each of brewer's yeast and blackstrap molasses daily stirred into 8 ounces of milk.

After a few days, he noted relief of pain and stiffness in his knees. After weeks, he experienced relief in other body areas. Often improvement was followed by exacerbation. By five months after starting nutritional therapy, his feet, knees and ankles began to feel normal. His shoulders, elbows, wrists and hands were still somewhat stiff, but joint pain was limited to overexertion. His sedimentation rate had reduced to only slightly above normal and he had discontinued all medications. By six months, his knees were nearly normal, and the pain and stiffness in his fingers, wrists and shoulders had almost disappeared. His left ankle, however, while improved, continued to be inflamed (Flint).

BIBLIOGRAPHY

Aaseth J et al. Rheumatoid arthritis and metal compounds--perspectives on the role of oxygen radical detoxification. Analyst 123(1):3-6, 1998

Abraham GE, Himmel PB. Management of rheumatoid arthritis: rationale for the use of colloidal metallic gold. J Nutr Environ Med 7:295-305, 1997

Abrams SA et al. Calcium absorption and metabolism in children with juvenile rheumatoid arthritis assessed using stable isotopes. J Rheumatol 20(7):1196-200, 1993

Adam O et al. Low fat diet decreases alpha-tocopherol levels, and stimulates LDL oxidation and eicosanoid biosynthesis in man. Eur J Med Res 1(2):65-71, 1995

Alter HJ et al. Interrelationship of rheumatoid arthritis, folic acid and aspirin. Blood 38:405-16, 1971

Anonymous. Fifty years of gold in rheumatoid arthritis. Br Med J i:289-90, 1979

Anonymous. Editorial: Gold therapy in rheumatoid arthritis. Lancet 338:19-20, 1991

Aoyagi T et al. Decreased serum levels of various hydrolytic enzymes in patients with rheumatoid arthritis. Biochem Int 8(4):529-35, 1984

Ariza-Ariza R et al. Omega-3 fatty acids in rheumatoid arthritis: an overview. Semin Arthritis Rheum 27(6):366-70, 1998

Banford JC et al. Serum copper and erythrocyte superoxide dismutase in rheumatoid arthritis. Ann Rheum Dis 41(5):458-62, 1982

Barton-Wright EC, Elliott WA. The pantothenic acid metabolism of rheumatoid arthritis. Lancet ii:862-3, 1963

Belch JJ et al. Effects of altering dietary essential fatty acids on requirements for non-steroidal anti-inflammatory drugs in patients with rheumatoid arthritis: a double blind placebo controlled study. Ann Rheum Dis 47(2):96-104, 1988

Bjarnason I et al. Intestinal permeability and inflammation in rheumatoid arthritis: Effects of non-steroidal anti-inflammatory drugs. Lancet ii:1171-4, 1984

Blake D, Bacon PA. Iron and rheumatoid disease. Letter. Lancet i:623, 1982

Blankenhorn G. Vitamin E: Clinical research from Europe. Nutr Dietary Consult June, 1988

Brik R et al. Bone mineral density and turnover in children with systemic juvenile chronic arthritis. J Rheumatol 25(5):990-2, 1998

Comstock GW et al. Serum concentrations of alpha-tocopherol, beta-carotene, and retinol preceding the diagnosis of rheumatoid arthritis and systemic lupus erythematosus. Ann Rheum Dis 56:323-5, 1997

Dabbagh AJ et al. Iron in joint inflammation. Ann Rheum Dis 52:67-73, 1993

Darlington LG, Ramsey NW. Diets for rheumatoid arthritis. Letter. Lancet 338:1209, 1991

Darlington LG, Ramsey NW. Review of dietary therapy for rheumatoid arthritis. Br J Rheumatol 32(6):507-14, 1993

Di Toro R, Polito C. Nutrition in juvenile rheumatoid arthritis. Nutr Res 17(4):741-58, 1997

Edmonds SE et al. Putative analgesic activity of repeated oral doses of vitamin E in the treatment of rheumatoid arthritis. Results of a prospective placebo controlled double blind trial. Ann Rheum Dis 56(11):649-55, 1997

Fagiolo U et al. Intestinal permeability and antigen absorption in rheumatoid arthritis. Effects of acetylsalicylic acid and sodium chromoglycate. Int Arch Allergy Appl Immunol 89(1):98-102, 1989

Fahrer H et al. Diet and fatty acids: can fish substitute for fish oil? Clin Exp Rheumatol 9(4):403-6, 1991

Falcini F et al. Bone turnover is reduced in children with juvenile rheumatoid arthritis. J Endocrinol Invest 21(1):31-6, 1998

Flint HJ. Return from arthritis. Prevention March, 1982, pp. 64-67

General Practitioner Research Group. Calcium pantothenate in arthritic conditions. Practitioner 224:208-11, 1980

Glenk W, Neu S. Enzyme Die Bausteine des Lebens Wie Sie Wirken, Helfen und Heilen. Munich, Wilhelm Heyne Verlag, 1990 (in German)

Halliwell B et al. Biologically significant scavenging of the myeloperoxidase-derived oxidant hypochlorous acid by ascorbic acid. Implications for antioxidant protection in the inflamed rheumatoid joint. FEBS Lett 213(11):15-7, 1987

Hansen G et al. [Nutritional status of Danish patients with rheumatoid arthritis and effects of a diet adjusted in energy intake, fish content and antioxidants]. Ugeskr Laeger 160(21):3074-8, 1998 (in Danish)

Haugen M et al. Nutrient intake and nutritional status in children with juvenile chronic arthritis. Scand J Rheumatol 21:165, 1992

Heinle K et al. [Selenium concentration in erythrocytes of patients with rheumatoid arthritis. Clinical and laboratory chemistry infection markers during administration of selenium]. Med Klin 92 Suppl 3:29-31, 1997 (in German)

Heinitz M. Kupfer in der Rheumatologie - ein Rück- und Ausblick. Rheuma 11(2):49-54, 1991 (in German)

Helliwell M et al. Nutritional status in patients with rheumatoid arthritis. Ann Rheum Dis 43(3):386-90, 1984

Henriksson AE et al. Small intestinal bacterial overgrowth in patients with rheumatoid arthritis. Ann Rheum Dis 52(7):503-10, 1993

Honkanen VE et al. Plasma zinc and copper concentrations in rheumatoid arthritis: influence of dietary factors and disease activity. Am J Clin Nutr 54(6):1082-6, 1991

Horrobin DF. The importance of gamma-linolenic acid and prostaglandin E_1 in human nutrition and medicine. J Holistic Med 3:118-39, 1981

Jacobsson L et al. Correlation of fatty acid composition of adipose tissue lipids and serum phosphatidylcholine and serum concentrations of micronutrients with disease duration in rheumatoid arthritis. Ann Rheum Dis 49:901-5, 1990

James MJ, Cleland LG. Dietary n-3 fatty acids and therapy for rheumatoid arthritis. Semin Arthritis Rheum 27(2):85-97, 1997

Kasapcopur O et al. Hypercalciuria and hematuria in juvenile rheumatoid arthritis. J Rheumatol 25(5):993-6, 1998

Kavanaghi R et al. The effects of elemental diet and subsequent food reintroduction on rheumatoid arthritis. Br J Rheumatol 34(3):270-3, 1995

Kjeldsen-Kragh J. Dietary treatment of rheumatoid arthritis. Scand J Rheumatol, 1996

Kose K et al. Plasma selenium levels in rheumatoid arthritis. Biol Trace Elem Res 53:51-6, 1996

Kremer JM, Bigaouette J. Nutrient intake of patients with rheumatoid arthritis is deficient in pyridoxine, zinc, copper, and magnesium. J Rheumatol 23(6):990-4, 1996

Kroger H et al. Low serum vitamin D metabolites in women with rheumatoid arthritis. Scand J Rheumatol 22:172-7, 1993

Krogh Jensen M et al. Folate and homocysteine status and haemolysis in patients treated with sulphasalazine for arthritis. Scand J Clin Lab Invest 56(5):421-9, 1996

Lucas C, Power L. Dietary fat aggravates active rheumatoid arthritis. Clin Res 29(4):754A, 1981

Lunec J, Blake DR. The determination of dehydroascorbic acid and ascorbic acid in the serum and synovial fluid of patients with rheumatoid arthritis (RA). Free Radic Res Commun 1(1):31-9, 1985

Marshall R et al. Food challenge effects on fasted rheumatoid arthritis patients: A multicenter study. Clin Ecol 2:181-90, 1984

McDuffie FC, Arthritis Foundation - reported in Med World News July 22, 1985

Milanino R et al. Copper and zinc status in rheumatoid arthritis: studies of plasma, erythrocytes, and urine, and their relationship to disease activity markers and pharmacological treatment. Clin Exp Rheumatol 11(3):271-81, 1993

Modesto C, Castro L. Folinic acid supplementation in patients with juvenile rheumatoid arthritis treated with methotrexate. J Rheumatol 23(2):403-4, 1996

Morgan SL et al. Supplementation with folic acid during methotrexate therapy for rheumatoid arthritis: a double-blind, placebo-controlled trial. Ann Intern Med 121:833-41, 1994

Morgan SL et al. Nutrient intake patterns, body mass index, and vitamin levels in patients with rheumatoid arthritis. Arthritis Care Res 10(1):9-17, 1997

Morgan SL et al. Folic acid supplementation prevents deficient blood folate levels and hyperhomocysteinemia during longterm, low dose methotrexate therapy for rheumatoid arthritis: implications for cardiovascular disease prevention. J Rheumatol 25(3):441-6, 1998

Moss M. Effects of molybdenum on pain and general health: a pilot study. J Nutr Environ Med 5:55-61, 1995

Muirden KD, Senator GB. Iron in the synovial membrane in rheumatoid arthritis and other joint diseases. Ann Rheum Dis 27:38-48, 1968

Mulherin DM et al. Do gold rings protect against articular erosion in rheumatoid arthritis? Ann Rheum Dis 56(8):497-9, 1997

Mullen A, Wilson CWM. The metabolism of ascorbic acid in rheumatoid arthritis. Proc Nutr Sci 35:8A-9A, 1976

Munthe E et al. Trace elements and rheumatoid arthritis (RA) — pathogenetic and therapeutic aspects. Acta Pharmacol Toxicol (Copenh) 7:365-73, 1986

Naveh Y et al. Zinc metabolism in rheumatoid arthritis: plasma and urinary zinc and relationship to disease activity. J Rheumatol 24(4):643-6, 1997

Nenonen M et al. Effects of uncooked vegan food - 'living food' - on rheumatoid arthritis, a three month controlled and randomized study. Abstract. Am J Clin Nutr 56:762, 1992

Newnham RE. Arthritis or skeletal fluorosis and boron. Letter. Int Clin Nutr Rev 11(2):68-70, 1991

Newnham RE. Essentiality of boron for healthy bones and joints. Environ Health Pespect 102 Suppl 7:83-5, 1994a

Newnham RE. The role of boron in human nutrition. J Appl Nutr 46(3):81-5, 1994b

Niedermeier W, Griggs JH. Trace metal composition of synovial fluid and blood serum of patients with rheumatoid arthritis. J Chron Dis 23:527-36, 1971

Nouza K. Outlooks of systemic enzyme therapy in rheumatoid arthritis and other immunopathological diseases. Acta Univ Carol [Med] (Praha) 40(1-4):101-4, 1994

Oelzner P et al. Relationship between disease activity and serum levels of vitamin D metabolites and PTH in rheumatoid arthritis. Calcif Tissue Int 62(3):193-8, 1998

O'Farrelly C et al. IgA rheumatoid factor and IgG dietary protein antibodies are associated in rheumatoid arthritis. Immunol Invest 18(6):753-64, 1989

Okuyama S et al. Copper complexes of non-steroid antiinflammatory agents: Analgesic activity and possible opioid receptor activation. Agents Actions 21(1-2):130-44, 1987

Oldroyd KG, Dawes PT. Clinically significant vitamin C deficiency in rheumatoid arthritis. Br J Rheumatol 24:362-3, 1985

Osterberg AE et al. Absorption of sulphur compounds during treatment by sulphur baths. Arch Derm Syph 20:156-66, 1929

Pandey SP et al. Zinc in rheumatoid arthritis. Indian J Med Res 81:618-20, 1985

Pepmueller PH et al. Bone mineralization and bone mineral metabolism in children with juvenile rheumatoid arthritis. Arthritis Rheum 39(5):746-57, 1996

Peretz A et al. Adjuvant treatment of recent onset rheumatoid arthritis by selenium supplementation: preliminary observations. Br J Rheumatol 31:281-6, 1992

Peretz A et al. Zinc distribution in blood components, inflammatory status, and clinical indexes of disease activity during zinc supplementation in inflammatory rheumatic diseases. Am J Clin Nutr 57:690-4, 1993

Pettersson T et al. Serum homocysteine and methylmalonic acid in patients with rheumatoid arthritis and cobalaminopenia. J Rheumatol 25(5):859-63, 1998

Polito C et al. Reduced bone mineral content and normal serum osteocalcin in non-steroid-treated patients with juvenile rheumatoid arthritis. Ann Rheum Dis 54(3):193-6, 1995

Pratsel HG et al. [The analgesic efficacy of sulfur mud baths in treating rheumatic diseases of the soft tissues. A study using the double-blind control method]. Vopr Kurortol Fizioter Lech Fiz Kult 3:37-41, 1992 (in Russian)

Rajagopalan KV. Molybdenum: an essential trace element in human nutrition. Ann Rev Nutr 8:401-27, 1988

Rasker JJ, Kardaun SH. Lack of beneficial effect of zinc sulphate in rheumatoid arthritis. Scand J Rheumatol 11:168-70, 1982

Rawley DA, Halliwell B. Formation of hydroxyl radicals from hydrogen peroxide and iron salts by superoxide and ascorbate-dependent mechanisms: Relevance to the pathology of rheumatoid disease. Clin Sci 64:649-53, 1983

Reed A et al. 25-hydroxyvitamin D therapy in children with active juvenile rheumatoid arthritis: short-term effects on serum osteocalcin levels and bone mineral density. J Pediatr 119(4):657-60, 1991

Rothman D et al. Botanical lipids: Effects on inflammation, immune responses, and rheumatoid arthritis. Semin Arth Rheum 25(2):87-96, 1995

Rothwell RS, Davis P. Relationship between serum ferritin, anemia, and disease activity in acute and chronic rheumatoid arthritis. Rheumatol Int 1(2):65-7, 1981

Roubenoff R et al. Abnormal vitamin B6 status in rheumatoid cachexia. Arthritis Rheum 1:105-9, 1995

Roubenoff R et al. Abnormal homocysteine metabolism in rheumatoid arthritis. Arthritis Rheum 40(4):718-22, 1997

Schumacher HR et al. Vitamin B6 levels in rheumatoid arthritis: effect of treatment. Am J Clin Nutr 28(11):1200-3, 1975

Seignalet J. Diet, fasting, and rheumatoid arthritis. Letter. Lancet 339:68-9, 1992

Shapiro JA et al. Diet and rheumatoid arthritis in women: A possible protective effect of fish consumption. Epidemiology 7:256-63, 1996

Simkin PA. Oral zinc sulphate in rheumatoid arthritis. Lancet ii:539-42, 1976

Simkin PA. Treatment of rheumatoid arthritis with oral zinc sulfate. Agents Actions 8:587-96, 1981 (Suppl)

Singh RB et al. Dietary intake and plasma levels of antioxidant vitamins in health and disease: a hospital-based case-control study. J Nutr Environ Med 5:235-42, 1995

Sklodowska M et al. Vitamin E, thiobarbituric acid reactive substance concentrations and superoxide dismutase activity in the blood of children with juvenile rheumatoid arthritis. Clin Exp Rheumatol 14:433-9, 1996

Skoldstam L et al. Specific plasma proteins as indices of inflammation during a modified fast in patients with rheumatoid arthritis. Scand J Rheumatol 12(2):161-5, 1983

Sorenson JR, Hangarter W. Treatment of rheumatoid and degenerative diseases with copper complexes: A review with emphasis on copper-salicylate. Inflammation 2(3):217-38, 1977

Sorenson J. Copper aspirinate: A more potent anti-inflammatory and anti-ulcer agent. J Int Acad Prev Med 1980:7-21

Sorenson J, in The Anti-inflammatory Activities of Copper Complexes. Metal Ions and Biological Systems. Marcel Dekker, 1982:77-125

Steffen C et al. Enzymtherapie im vergleich mit immunokomplex-bestimmungen bei chronischer polyarthritis. Z Rheumatol 44:51-6, 1985 (in German)

Stone J et al. Inadequate calcium, folic acid, vitamin E, zinc, and selenium intake in rheumatoid arthritis patients: results of a dietary survey. Semin Arthritis Rheum 27(3):180-5, 1997

Sukenik S et al. Sulphur bath and mud pack treatment for rheumatoid arthritis at the Dead Sea area. Ann Rheum Dis 49(2):99-102, 1990

Sullivan MX, Hess WC. Cystine content of finger nails in arthritis. J Bone Joint Surg 16:185, 1935

Sundquist T et al. Influence of fasting on intestinal permeability and disease activity in patients with rheumatoid arthritis. Scand J Rheumatol 11(1):33-8, 1982

Suryaprabha P et al. Reactive oxygen species, lipid peroxides and essential fatty acids in patients with rheumatoid arthritis and systemic lupus erythematosus. Prostaglandins Leukot Essent Fatty Acids 43(4):251-5, 1991

Suzuki Y et al. [Osteoporosis in rheumatoid arthritis]. Nippon Rinsho 56(6):1598-603, 1998 (in Japanese)

Svenson KL et al. Reduced zinc in peripheral blood cells from patients with inflammatory connective tissue diseases. Inflammation 9(2):189-99, 1985

Tarp U et al. Selenium treatment in rheumatoid arthritis. Acta Pharmacol Toxicol 59(Suppl 7):382-5, 1986

Uden AM et al. Neutrophil functions and clinical performance after total fasting in patients with rheumatoid arthritis. Ann Rheum Dis 42(1):45-51, 1983

van Ede AE et al. Methotrexate in rheumatoid arthritis: an update with focus on mechanisms involved in toxicity. Semin Arthritis Rheum 27(5):277-92, 1998

Walker WR, Keats DM. An investigation of the therapeutic value of the "copper bracelet:" Dermal assimilation of copper in arthritic/rheumatoid conditions. Agents Actions 6:454, 1976

Warady BD et al. Effects of nutritional supplementation on bone mineral status of children with rheumatic diseases receiving corticosteroid therapy. J Rheumatol 21(3):530-5, 1994

Williams R. Rheumatoid arthritis and food: A case study. Letter to the Editor. Br Med J 283:563, 1981

Wittenborg A et al. [Effectiveness of vitamin E in comparison with diclofenac sodium in treatment of patients with chronic polyarthritis]. Z Rheumatol 57(4):215-21, 1998 (in German)

Woldenberg SC. The treatment of arthritis with colloidal sulphur. J South Med Assoc 28:875-81, 1935

Wordsworth BP et al. Metabolic bone disease among in-patients with rheumatoid arthritis. Br J Rheumatol 23(4):251-7, 1984

Wroblewski R et al. Electron probe X-ray microanalysis of human skeletal muscle involved in rheumatoid arthritis. Histochemistry 57(1):1-8, 1978

Zoli A et al. Serum zinc and copper in active rheumatoid arthritis: correlation with interleukin 1 beta and tumour necrosis factor alpha. Clin Rheumatol 17(5):378-82, 1998

SCHIZOPHRENIA
(including ACUTE AND PARANOID PSYCHOSES and SCHIZOAFFECTIVE DISORDER)

See Also: ORGANIC MENTAL DISORDERS

NUTRITIONAL TREATMENT GUIDE

✓ = Efficacy generally accepted.
* = Efficacy *demonstrated* by controlled human trials.
[+] = Efficacy *suspected* from uncontrolled human experiments
[-] = Efficacy *suspected* from indirect data
? = Efficacy *challenged* in at least one study of similar design

---

DIETARY FACTORS

* avoid **Caffeine**

- -

[+] **high Carbohydrate, low Protein diet:** *to treat a transient, acute, polymorphic psychosis characterized by dysperceptions:* 398 g carbohydrate, 60 g protein, 19 g fat; 2000 calories
[+] avoid **Water intoxication**

- -

[-] **low Saturated Fat diet** (with adequate **Essential Fatty Acids**)

NUTRITIONAL FACTORS

* **Folic acid deficiency:** methylfolate 15 mg daily (6 month trial)
(WARNING: Psychosis may be exacerbated if blood levels become elevated.)
(To treat "histapenics" with the Pfeiffer regimen, also add Niacin 1 g twice daily, Rutin 50 mg each AM, Vitamin B_6 100 mg twice daily, Vitamin B_{12} 1 mg IM weekly, Vitamin C 1 g twice daily, and Vitamin E 200 IU each AM along with a high protein diet and minimal caffeine.)
* **Glycine:** 5 to 25 g daily
* ? **Niacin or Niacinamide:** start with 100 mg 3 times daily after meals and gradually increase as tolerated to at least 1 g 3 times daily after meals (maximum 4 gm 3 times daily). (1 year trial)
* ? **Omega-6 Fatty Acids:** *example:* evening primrose oil 2 g 3 times daily (4 month trial)
* ? **Vitamin C:** ? up to 6 g daily in divided doses (1 month trial)

- -

[+] treat **Copper** toxicity
[+] **Magnesium deficiency:** ≈ 400 mg daily
[+] **Omega-3 Fatty Acids:** *example:* MaxEPA® 5 g twice daily (6 week trial)
[+] **Riboflavin deficiency:** 5 to 10 mg daily

[+] **Vitamin B_6:** 50 to 100 mg daily
(To treat "pyrolurics" with the Pfeiffer regimen, also add **Zinc** 30 mg twice daily and **Manganese** 50 mg twice daily.)

- -

[-] **Selenium deficiency:** 200 µg daily
[-] **Zinc deficiency:** zinc sulfate 220 mg twice daily *AND* **Copper** 2 mg daily

OTHER RELATED FACTORS

* ? rule out **Food Sensitivities** (especially gluten-containing foods and milk)

DIETARY FACTORS

High Carbohydrate, Low Protein Diet

In open trials, a high carbohydrate, low protein diet has seemed to curtail or prevent psychotic episodes in a particular sub-group of schizoaffective patients who fulfill the research diagnostic criteria for Acute Schizo-affective Disorder, Manic Type *(Wunderink;Pepplinkhuizen)*. These patients develop a transient acute polymorphic psychosis characterized by perceptual distortions. There may be sudden mood swings, motility disturbances, states of pananxiety or ecstasy, delusions or visual hallucinations. Psychedelic phenomena are often experienced at the start of the psychosis *(Bruinvels,1986,1988)*.

While the reason for the efficacy for this diet is unknown, the same diet has been suggested for the treatment of porphyria and, indeed, some of these patients have a porphyric disease *(Wunderink)*. Carbohydrate inhibits gamma-aminolevulinate synthetase, the enzyme needed to synthesize porphyrins from glycine and succinate, thus limiting the consumption of glycine for porphyrin synthesis *(Pepplinkhuizen)*. As in porphyria, these patients appear to have an increased demand for glycine which triggers the production of one-carbon units, finally resulting in the endogenous production of beta-carbolines and/or isoquinolines which may act as 'psychotic' substances *(Pepplinkhuizen)*.

Once patients have recovered on the diet, loading tests with glycine or serine often cause the psychosis to reappear *(Wunderink,1986)*.

Dietary Fat

Early research suggests that the intake of fat may have a bearing on the clinical course of the illness. Total fat intake as well as the intake of saturated fat (i.e. fat from land animals and birds) have been found to be positively correlated with both the clinical course and the outcome of schizophrenia *(Christensen)*. Also of note, the same study found a non-significant trend suggesting that a high intake of *unsaturated* fat (i.e. fat from vegetables, fish and seafood) may be associated with a favorable outcome.

Controlled clinical trials of a low-fat diet sufficient in essential fatty acids are needed to ascertain if such a diet is effective in treating schizophrenia.

Caffeine

Hospitalized schizophrenics often have a high intake of caffeine (more than 750 mg daily) *(Rihs)*. Schizophrenia does not reflect primary abnormalities of dopamine transmission, but probably does reflect abnormalities in systems that have an intimate interaction with the dopamine system *(Willner)*. Adenosine plays a role opposite to dopamine in the striatum, and caffeine, an adenosine antagonist, produces effects similar to increased dopaminergic neurotransmission *(Ferre)*.

Under double-blind conditions, caffeine at commonly consumed dosages has been shown to worsen psychosis and mania in schizophrenics *(Lucas)*, although this effect is probably limited to certain sub-groups *(Hyde; Koczapski)*. Often, in the clinical setting, patients markedly increase caffeine consumption when their anxiety increases. This may result in greater anxiety or the onset of overt psychosis *(Mikkelsen)*.

Water intoxication

Twenty percent of chronic schizophrenics ingest excessive amounts of water. Furthermore, one-fifth of this group (4% of the chronic population) experience chronic hyponatremia and episodic water intoxication.

Despite being uncommon, water intoxication is potentially fatal and is believed to be responsible for a considerable amount of the morbidity and excessive clinical expenditures associated with schizophrenia *(Goldman).*

NUTRITIONAL FACTORS

VITAMINS

Folic Acid Deficiency

Folic acid deficiency occurs in 10 to 30 percent of hospitalized psychiatric patients *(Greenblatt).* In addition to psychosis, the deficiency is associated with depression, confusion, disorientation and dementia as well as with neurologic symptoms such as numbness, stiffness, spasticity and weakness, both with and without muscular atrophy.

In a randomized double-blind study reported in the *Lancet*, schizophrenics with low red cell folate levels, but without a deficiency of vitamin B_{12} or significant cognitive impairment, received either methylfolate 15 mg daily or placebo in addition to standard psychotropic drugs. After 6 months, there were significant differences in mean clinical outcome scores between groups in favor of the folate group *(Godfrey).*

Specific mechanisms by which folate deficiency may be implicated are starting to be identified. Folic acid may be an essential cofactor in the conversion of the omega-6 fatty acids to prostaglandins *(Horrobin,1979a)*, and early evidence suggests that impaired prostaglandin metabolism may provoke a schizophrenic picture. (See Omega-6 Fatty Acids below).

Also, hyperhomocysteinemia due to an inborn error of folate metabolism (especially homozygosity for thermolabile methylenetetrahydrofolate reductase) may present as a schizophrenic syndrome sometimes accompanied by neurological signs. (See discussion under Homocysteine in ATHEROSCLEROSIS.)

Case reports suggest that folic acid supplementation, usually along with either vitamin B_6 *(Freeman)* or vitamin B_{12}, *(Regland)* appears to be an effective treatment for this metabolic disorder.

A 15-year-old female with schizophrenic symptoms had homocystinuria due to impaired $N^{5,10}$-tetrahydrofolate reductase activity. Folate and pyridoxine supplementation resulted in substantial improvement (Barber).

A Warning

For schizophrenics, supplementation with as little as 3 mg of folic acid daily can cause an exacerbation of psychotic behavior if blood folate levels become elevated. Thus, blood levels should be followed during a therapeutic trial *(Prakash).*

Niacin

The possible benefit of megadoses of niacin in schizophrenia, advocated by Hoffer and Osmond, launched the orthomolecular psychiatry movement four decades ago *(Hoffer,1962).* Today, such treatment remains controversial as both positive *(Osmond)* and negative *(Wittenborn)* double-blind studies have appeared in the scientific literature. Although the consensus is that niacin therapy is ineffective *(Am. Psychiatric Assn.)*, Hoffer has noted that niacin is primarily effective for early and acute schizophrenics, while it is ineffective, especially when given alone, for the chronic schizophrenics who were included in the negative studies *(Hoffer,1996).*

Patients with sub-clinical pellagra, who may develop perceptual changes and neurasthenia, could be labeled as schizophrenic and would benefit from niacin *(Green).* Blood niacin levels would help to identify such cases. Whether other sub-groups who present with schizophrenic syndromes would benefit from megadoses of niacin remains unknown.

The possibility of adverse side-effects from a therapeutic trial of niacin must also be considered (see discussion under Niacin in Atherosclerosis). While niacinamide could be used as an alternative, it commonly causes sedation, and it may cause depression. Like niacin, it can produce liver toxicity.

Peter, age 9, changed one month earlier from a happy, too quiet, obedient boy to one who was hostile, irritable and fearful. He was terribly worried he might give way to his murderous impulses against his parents or against himself. He was living a life of visions, perceptual illusions and fears, and was on chlorpromazine 50 mg at bedtime.

The chlorpromazine was continued and he was started on niacinamide 1.5 gm and ascorbic acid 1.5 gm daily. His behavior gradually improved over the next three months, but he continued to have auditory and visual hallucinations.

Four months later, he was normal. He was switched from niacinamide to placebo and relapsed in two weeks. After one month he was switched back to niacinamide and the chlorpromazine was discontinued. Within a month he was well again. On follow-up three years later, he had continued to be normal (Hoffer, 1971).

Riboflavin Deficiency

Phenothiazine administration can cause a riboflavin deficiency *(Easlove)*. The deficiency may be manifested as physical complaints, bodily preoccupation, hypersensitivity, emotional shallowness, weakness and lethargy *(Sterner)*.

Vitamin B_6

Pyridoxal-5- phosphate, the activated form of the vitamin, is important for normal brain function. In fact, isoniazid, an antituberculous drug which antagonizes vitamin B_6 activity, produces a variety of neuropsychiatric symptoms which remit with B_6 supplementation.

There have been a few open trials of supplementation with the vitamin which have reported good results. Perhaps the most interesting report concerned a group of female patients who presented with paranoid ideation, emotional lability, irritability, depression and fatigue. These women were taking oral contraceptives, drugs which may foster depletion of the vitamin *(Roe)*. Three-quarters of the group improved following supplementation with pyridoxine *(Baumblatt)*.

The lack of placebo-controlled studies, and the failure of published studies to ascertain vitamin B_6 nutriture at baseline, makes it impossible to reach a conclusion about the efficacy of the vitamin in treating schizophrenia.

Vitamin C Deficiency

There appears to be an inverse correlation between ascorbic acid intake and the risk of schizophrenia *(Singh RB)*. Even when the dietary intake of vitamin C is adequate for normals, schizophrenics may have depressed plasma levels and may demonstrate a greatly reduced urinary excretion of ascorbic acid after an ascorbic acid load *(Suboticanec, 1986, 1990)*. These findings suggest that the utilization of vitamin C in schizophrenics may be enhanced.

Results of an animal study suggest that vitamin C may block the behavioral response to dopamine and enhance the effects of neuroleptic drugs *(Rebec)*. Supplementation with high doses of vitamin C has been shown to produce improvement in mood and paranoid ideation in a randomized double-blind study *(Milner)*, results that have been confirmed in subsequent open trials.

For example, in one study, 21 long-term neuroleptic-refractory hospitalized patients who, nevertheless, were taking neuroleptics, were started on ascorbic acid supplements for at least one month. Two of the patients showed a favorable response on 2 grams daily. One of them, who had been floridly psychotic, went into a full remission within 2 weeks.

Ten of the non-responders were then raised to 6 grams daily. Within one month, 4 of them showed progress. All responders subsequently maintained their progress *(Kanofsky, 1989)*.

MINERALS

Copper

It has also been theorized that excess copper can cause schizophrenia. Wilson's disease is a rare, autosomal recessive disorder of copper metabolism due to low serum ceruloplasmin, resulting in copper deposition, especially in the liver and in the basal ganglia of the brain. A schizophrenia-like disorder may be the initial presentation of the disease *(Muller)*.

With the exception of Wilson's disease, the hypothesis that excess copper can cause schizophrenia has yet to be confirmed. A review of the subject concluded that, although elevated copper seems to be tied to dopamine activity, and although elevated copper may sometimes be found in schizophrenics, elevated copper does *not* cause schizophrenia *(Bowman)*.

Evidence that copper depletion may ameliorate schizophrenic symptoms comes from double-blind studies in which patients received D-penicillamine, a copper chelating drug *(Mattke;Nicholson)*. Whether a nutritional regimen designed to increase copper excretion would be effective is not known. However, Pfeiffer tried various combinations in informal trials and found the combination of zinc 50 mg, manganese 3 mg and pyridoxine 50 mg to be by far the most effective in increasing urinary copper excretion *(Pfeiffer,1983)*.

A 24 year-old Caucasian female diagnosed as a chronic schizophrenic was on perphenazine 8 mg twice daily, lithium carbonate 500 mg three times daily, Deanol 4 drops of 20% daily, and thyroid. In addition, she was supplemented with niacinamide, niacin, vitamin C, vitamin E, manganese and zinc. On this program, blood copper levels were about 150 µg%.

When she was started on oral contraceptives, the blood copper level rose to 329 µg% 6 weeks later. Repeat level after another 6 weeks was 284 µg%. Schizophrenic symptoms exacerbated and she complained of tender breasts and pain while climbing stairs. After oral contraceptives were stopped, schizophrenic symptoms abated and blood copper returned to its former level (Pfeiffer,1987).

Magnesium Deficiency

Brain magnesium levels appear to be normal in schizophrenics *(Kornhuber)*. However, cerebrospinal fluid magnesium levels may be lower in acute schizophrenics versus schizophrenics in remission *(Levine)*.

While, compared to normals, plasma and serum magnesium levels vary widely among schizophrenics, one study found lower plasma levels that increased when the patients went into remission. The authors theorize that these patients developed a marginal magnesium deficiency due to the stress of their illness. The deficiency, in turn, exacerbated certain symptoms such as anxiety, fear, hallucinations, weakness and somatic complaints *(Kirov)*.

While the effects of repleting a magnesium deficiency in schizophrenics have been poorly studied, there is an interesting report of 3 hospitalized chronic schizophrenic patients and hypomagnesemia who were supplemented with oral magnesium. Two of the 3 experienced improvement in their psychiatric condition when their serum magnesium levels normalized *(Kanofsky,1991)*.

Selenium Deficiency

Of all the trace elements, low selenium intake is perhaps most strongly related to the risk of schizophrenia *(Brown;Foster)*. Although blood and serum concentrations appear to be normal *(Alertsen)*, there appears to be a strong correlation between the activity of the selenium-dependent enzyme glutathione peroxidase and computerized tomographic measures of brain atrophy and the ratio of ventricle to brain size. These relationships were not found in a sex- and age-matched group of non-schizophrenic mental patients, suggesting a unique relationship between glutathione peroxidase and the mechanism of tissue damage found in schizophrenic brains *(Buckman)*.

It remains to be established whether selenium supplementation is beneficial.

Zinc Deficiency

At autopsy, the zinc content of the hippocampus and certain other areas of the brains of schizophrenics has been found to be reduced 30 to 50% compared to that of normals *(Kimura;McLardy)*, although this finding was not confirmed in a more recent study *(Kornhuber)*. Similarly while one study found low serum zinc concentrations in 11% of schizophrenics *(Pfeiffer,1972)*, another found normal zinc concentrations in serum, urine, gastric fluid and hair in both acute and chronic patients, and whether or not the subjects were taking various major tranquilizers *(Gillin)*.

A factor which may complicate studies investigating the prevalence of zinc deficiency in schizophrenia is the similarly between the clinical presentation of zinc deficiency to that of schizophrenia. Zinc deficiency is associated with apathy, lethargy, amnesia and mental retardation, often with irritability, depression and paranoia *(Prasad)*. It could therefore be mistakenly diagnosed as schizophrenia.

Zinc deficiency could theoretically promote schizophrenia by inhibiting omega-6 essential fatty acid metabolism either by blocking linoleic acid desaturation or by inhibiting mobilization of DGLA from tissue membrane stores *(Cunnane)*. It could also do so by encouraging copper accumulation and toxicity through increased copper absorption *(Gillin)*.

Unfortunately, controlled intervention trials of zinc supplementation are lacking *(Gillin)*.

OTHER NUTRITIONAL FACTORS

Essential Fatty Acids

Evidence is accumulating that phospholipid metabolism in both the brain and erythrocytes may be disturbed in chronic schizophrenics. This is especially true for patients with the "negative" symptoms of apathy and withdrawal, as their levels of both arachidonic acid (AA) and docosahexaenoic acid (DHA) in erythrocyte membrane phospholipids are seriously depleted while saturated fatty acid levels are high. By contrast, schizophrenics with "positive" symptoms of thought disorder, hallucinations and delusions have the opposite findings *(Glen,1994)*. (As positive symptoms are not unique to schizophrenia, these latter patients may have another psychotic disorder rather than schizophrenia.)

The increased rate of loss of AA and DHA from cell membranes and the resulting abnormalities in neuronal function in schizophrenics with negative symptoms appear to be caused by increased activity of phospholipase A2. This abnormality also results in the absence of a flushing response to a niacin load *(Glen,1996)*, as the response involves prostaglandin-induced vasodilatation. Moreover, conversion from non-flushing to flushing during a 6-month period of essential fatty acid supplementation was predicted by an increase in arachidonic acid levels in erythrocyte membranes *(Glen,1996)*. The flushing response to niacin may therefore be an inexpensive functional diagnostic test for abnormal essential fatty acid metabolism in schizophrenia, and the lack of flushing may suggest the need for corrective supplementation.

It is interesting that, as noted in earlier part of this chapter, there is reason to believe that a deficiency of any of the cofactors involved in essential fatty acid metabolism (folic acid, niacin, vitamin C, vitamin E, magnesium, selenium and zinc) may promote the development of a schizophreniform psychosis. This suggests that the specific nutrient deficiency may act, at least in part, by interfering the essential fatty acid metabolism.

Omega-3 Fatty Acids

alpha-linolenic acid → EPA → 3 series prostaglandins
└→ DHA

When a detailed dietary analysis was performed on 20 patients, none was deficient in fatty acid intake. However, a greater intake of the omega-3 fatty acids, and particularly eicosapentaenoic acid (EPA), was associated with less severe schizophrenic symptoms *(Mellor)*. Moreover, when the plasma membrane phospholipid concentrations were examined in cultured skin fibroblasts from schizophrenics, only total n-3 essential fatty acid contents and DHA were significantly lower in cell lines from the schizophrenic patients as compared to bipolar patients and normals, while arachidonic acid levels were similar *(Mahadik)*.

Rudin believes that some schizophrenics suffer from a form of pellagra due, not to a niacin deficiency, but to a deficiency of the omega-3 fatty acid substrate which is necessary for prostaglandin production. Patients most likely to respond have had a fluctuating clinical course with remissions and exacerbations; they present, he says, with signs and symptoms of an omega-3 fatty acid deficiency such as drying dermatoses, autonomic neuropathies, tinnitus and fatigue *(Rudin)*.

In an open trial, 20 hospitalized chronic schizophrenics showed significant reductions in psychopathology after receiving a fish oil supplement high in EPA and DHA (MaxEPA) for 6 weeks *(Peet)*. Also in an open trial, 5 schizophrenics were treated with linseed oil (which contains 50% alpha-linolenic acid, an omega-3 fatty acid, with the dosage titrated according to individual response. Three showed evidence of clinical improvement, 2 of whom had a history of remissions and relapses. All 3 responding patients had had symptoms suggestive of omega-3 fatty acid deficiency *(Rudin)*.

> *Catherine was a 16-year-old female who had been diagnosed as paranoid schizophrenic 2 years earlier. She was deeply troubled and frightened by voices that told her to kill schoolmates and was taking chlorpromazine. On physical examination, her skin "had the texture of rough sand, visibly peeling from her arms and legs; her hair had the texture of a rusty Brillo."*
>
> *She was started on flaxseed oil 3 tablespoons daily along with a multivitamin/mineral supplement. One month later, her skin and hair were less dry and, instead of being withdrawn, she smiled and made eye contact. She noted that the voices had disappeared and asked to stop taking the neuroleptic.*
>
> *At the next month's appointment, her skin and hair appeared normal. She was no longer taking chlorpromazine and reported that she was attending school daily, doing well in her class work, active in sports, and visiting friends with whom she hadn't spoken for two years. Her intake of flaxseed oil was reduced to one tablespoon daily.*
>
> *On follow-up over the next two years, she had no further evidence of a psychiatric disorder (Galland).*

Omega-6 Fatty Acids

linoleic acid → GLA → DGLA → prostaglandin E_1

There is both direct and indirect evidence of impaired prostaglandin E_1 (PGE_1) metabolism in schizophrenia *(Horrobin, 1992)*, suggesting that the disorder may result from a deficiency of prostaglandin E_1 synthesis or action *(Horrobin, 1979b)*. Specifically, schizophrenics appear to have depressed levels of prostaglandin E_1 and its precursors, while the levels of arachidonic acid and its prostaglandin E_2 series derivatives appear to be elevated in both erythrocyte membranes *(Hitzemann)* and cerebrospinal fluid *(Mathe)*.

Depletion of the omega-6 fatty acids in erythrocyte membranes have been shown to be negatively correlated with plasma thiobarbituric acid reactive substances (TBARS), a marker of lipid peroxidation, suggesting that the cause of the depletion is increased breakdown of essential fatty acids rather than impairment of their incorporation into membranes *(Laugharne)*. The theory that schizophrenia results from PGE_1 deficiency is consistent with the dopamine hypothesis of schizophrenia, as decreased PGE_1 activity appears to be associated with increased dopamine release *(van Kammen)*.

When this theory was tested by giving intravenous infusions of PGE_1 to a group of acute, unmedicated schizophrenics, some appeared to respond *(Kaiya)*. Other studies have administered evening primrose oil, a rich source of GLA. For example, in a double-blind study of hospitalized chronic schizophrenics with tardive dyskinesia, treatment with evening primrose oil for 16 weeks produced highly significant improvements in total psychopathology scores, schizophrenia subscale scores and a significant improvement in memory *(Vaddadi, 1989)*.

Also, 6 schizophrenics inadequately controlled by phenothiazines were able to be withdrawn from all drug therapy after being started on evening primrose oil and penicillin (which stimulates the 1-series prostaglandins). In some of the patients, there was a striking improvement *(Vaddadi, 1979)*. Not all trials have had positive results, however, and properly controlled trials are lacking.

A 31-year-old male was hospitalized after he reported hearing God speaking and claiming to be Jesus Christ. He was treated with ECT and neuroleptics and was discharged 5 months later. In the next 5 years he was admitted 3 more times due to relapses. He was last admitted 7 years earlier and had remained in the hospital since then due to an unchanging psychotic presentation.

At the time that nutritionally-oriented treatment was instituted, he had a severe thought disorder. Spontaneous speech was absent. He would stand in front of a mirror and talk to himself. His affect was markedly incongruous and he complained of hearing voices. All medication was stopped and he was treated with evening primrose oil 2 capsules daily and phenoxymethyl penicillin (to stimulate series-1 prostaglandins) 250 mg daily.

Within the first month he became more cooperative and more spontaneous in speech. Primrose oil was increased to 3 capsules daily. He stopped hallucinating and his thinking became clearer. He gradually became very cooperative and, by the end of the second month, the incongruous affect had clearly almost completely.

After 5 months, his speech was spontaneous and appropriate and affect was almost normal (Vaddadi,1979).

Glycine

Endogenous N-methyl-D-aspartic acid (NMDA) receptor dysfunction may contribute to the pathophysiology of schizophrenia *(Ishimaru;Javitt,1991)*. Since glycine acts at a site on the NMDA-type glutamate receptor, it potentiates NMDA-receptor mediated neurotransmission *(Johnson)*.

Under double-blind conditions, glycine supplementation has been found to be effective for treatment-resistant chronic schizophrenics, especially in reducing negative symptoms, but also in reducing depression and cognitive symptoms. The greatest reductions in negative symptoms was in those patients with the lowest baseline serum glycine levels. Positive symptoms and general psychopathology were unchanged, however *(Heresco-Levy;Javitt,1994)*.

While glycine in these studies was generally well-tolerated in these small studies, elevated brain glycine could theoretically cause adverse side effects due to excitotoxicity of excessive activity of the NMDA receptor complex. Moreover, a sub-population of schizoaffective patients may be especially vulnerable to exacerbation of psychosis from glycine supplementation (see High Carbohydrate, Low Protein Diet above). Therefore, before large-scale application of glycine therapy is undertaken, neurotoxicity needs to be ruled out *(Javitt,1996)*.

OTHER RELATED FACTORS

Food Sensitivities

The results of a number of studies suggest that foods, especially wheat and milk, may provoke schizophrenic-like symptomatology in susceptible people *(Reichelt;Singh MM;Vlissides)*. Endorphin-like proteins ("exorphins") have been identified in pepsin hydrolysates of wheat gluten and casein *(Mycroft;Zioudrou)*.

Moreover, the amino acid sequence in a tripeptide generated by the enzymatic digestion of both alpha-gliadin (a protein in wheat flour) and casein resembles that of melanocyte-stimulating-hormone-release-inhibiting factor (MIF) which enhances CNS dopaminergic activity. Assuming normal intakes of wheat and milk, about 150 mg of the tripeptide might be formed daily. Only 50 mg of MIF produces EEG changes in normals, and 75 mg has induced mood changes in depressed subjects *(Mycroft)*.

A 14 year-old female with a history of gastrointestinal intolerance to milk in childhood was challenged with milk and placebo in a double-blind manner. Milk, but not placebo, produced overt psychotic symptoms (Denman).

The Pfeiffer Hypothesis

In 1961, Irvine reported the discovery of a "mauve factor" in the urine which was frequently present in psychotic patients, but relatively rare in normals *(Irvine, 1961)*. Later, mauve factor, a chromatographic spot found in the urine of psychotic patients, was found to consist of kryptopyrrole (2,4-dimethyl-3-ethylpyrrole) *(Irvine, 1969)*. Kryptopyrrole has been shown in animal studies to affect behavior at a non-toxic level by acting as a depressant *(Somogyi)*; its role in schizophrenia is not established. While there is evidence that its excretion is associated with psychosis, an unusual EEG, and a poor prognosis *(Irvine, 1973)*, a subsequent study of 29 schizophrenics failed to find kryptopyrrole in the urine in a single patient *(Gendler)*.

The excretion of kryptopyrrole is one of the fundamental biochemical findings upon which Carl Pfeiffer has developed a classification of schizophrenia. Based on his evaluation of outpatients, he suggested that about 50% of schizophrenics are low in blood histamine ("histapenic") and high in serum copper, 20% are high in histamine ("histadelic") and normal in copper, and the remaining 30% excrete kryptopyrrole ("pyroluria") *(Pfeiffer, 1975)*. Patients with food sensitivities or porphyria fall into the histapenic group. These patients, he believed, can be differentiated, not only by biochemical measures, but also by signs and symptoms.

Pfeiffer has reported that histapenic schizophrenics have depressed serum folate levels, and suggested a treatment regimen consisting of folic acid along with niacin, vitamin B_{12}, vitamin C and zinc. After 5 to 6 months on this program, he found that patients showed symptomatic improvement coincident with a reduction in serum copper and a rise in blood histamine.

Histadelic schizophrenics, by contrast, were worse following folate supplementation. He found that they responded to mild antifolate drugs (such as phenytoin) and agents that decrease histamine (such as calcium salts and methionine).

Pfeiffer has noted that kryptopyrrole forms a complex with pyridoxal which chelates zinc; the result, he claims, is a relative deficiency of both pyridoxine and zinc in pyroluria. Associated lab findings are lymphocytosis with eosinophilia, increased bilirubin, decreased immunoglobulin A and increased urinary coproporphyrins. Pyrolurics are said to respond "for the most part" to supplementation with pyridoxine, zinc and manganese. Progress, he stated, can be seen within one week, while total recovery may occur in 3 to 4 months. When 2 responding patients were switched to placebos, they developed catatonia, muscle weakness, fever and chills *(Pfeiffer, 1974)*.

Heleniak and Lamola *(1985)* have suggested that histapenic schizophrenics may also be PGE_1-deficient. Blood levels of histamine and prostaglandin E_1 move concurrently in response to various agents and have similar effects on physiological activity, and all the cofactors suggested for the treatment of histapenia are also essential for the production of prostaglandin E_1.

Unfortunately, little has been done outside of Pfeiffer's laboratory to verify his observations. One small study of 10 inpatients failed to find a correlation between pyroluria and the signs and symptoms of B_6 and zinc deficiency *(Cruz)*; the authors suggested that the patients Pfeiffer described may have a form of porphyria, although Pfeiffer had concluded from his studies that only 0.1% of schizophrenics suffer from that disease.

COMBINED NUTRITIONAL TREATMENT

When first seen, a 19-year-old male had been diagnosed as a chronic schizophrenic and his psychiatrist had told his parents that he would never get well, never graduate from high school and never get off of psychotropic drugs. He suffered from severe paranoia and depression. He heard voices of "evil entities" who told him to hurt people, but had not acted on these thoughts. He felt that people were constantly staring at him, he often lost his train of thought, and his memory and concentration were poor.

He was continued on his tranquilizers and started on niacinamide 1 gram after each meal, vitamin C 3 grams daily, and a complete vitamin B complex supplement.

After 4 months, he said the voices in his head were gone and he felt more energy. His drug dosage was decreased by one-third and he was started on vitamin E 400 to 1,200 mg daily both as an antioxidant and to enhance circulation. He continued to improve, and visits were reduced to once a year.

Five years later, he announced that he had graduated from college. He had started a master's degree program, was working nearly full time, and was relating well with others. In addition to the supplements, he was taking a minimal dosage of a major tranquilizer (Hoffer, 1998).

BIBLIOGRAPHY

Alertsen AR et al. Selenium concentrations in blood and serum from patients with mental diseases. Acta Psychiatr Scand 74(2):217-19, 1986

American Psychiatric Association, Task Force on Vitamin Therapy in Psychiatry. Megavitamin and Orthomolecular Therapy in Psychiatry. Washington, DC, American Psychiatric Association, 1973

Barber GW, Spaeth GL. Successful treatment of homocystinuria with pyridoxine. J Pediatr 75:463-78, 1969

Baumblatt MJ, Winston F. Pyridoxine and the pill. Letter to the Editor. Lancet i:832-3, 1970

Bowman MB, Lewis MS. The copper hypothesis of schizophrenia: a review. Neurosci Biobehav Rev 6:321-8, 1982

Brown JS Jr. Role of selenium and other trace elements in the geography of schizophrenia. Schizophr Bull 20(2):387-98, 1994

Bruinvels J, Pepplinkhuizen L. Serine, glycine and carbohydrates in schizoaffective disorders. Bibl Nutr Dieta 38:168-72, 1986

Bruinvels J et al. Derangement of one-carbon metabolism in episodic schizoaffective psychoses. Pharmacopsychiatry 21(1):28-32, 1988

Buckman TD et al. Glutathione peroxidase and CT scan abnormalities in schizophrenia. Biol Psychiatry 22(11):1349-56, 1987

Christensen O, Christensen E. Fat consumption and schizophrenia. Acta Psychiatr Scand 78:587-91, 1988

Cruz R, Vogel WH. Pyroluria: A poor marker in chronic schizophrenia. Am J Psychiatry 135(10):1239-40, 1978

Cunnane SC, Horrobin DF. Parenteral linolenic and gamma-linolenic acids ameliorate the gross effects of zinc deficiency. Proc Soc Exp Biol Med 164:583, 1980

Denman AM. The relevance of immunopathology to research into schizophrenia, in J Hemmings, Ed. Biochemistry of Schizophrenia and Addiction. Lancaster, MTP Press, 1980

Easlove M et al. Severe riboflavin deficiency: A previously undescribed side-effect of phenothiazines. J Orthomol Psychiatry 12(2):113-15, 1983

Ferre S. Adenosine-dopamine interactions in the ventral striatum. Implications for the treatment of schizophrenia. Psychopharmacology (Berl) 133(2):107-20, 1997

Foster HD. Schizophrenia and esophageal cancer: comments on similarities in their spatial distributions. J Orthomol Med 5(3):129-34, 1990

Freeman JM et al. Folate-responsive homocystinuria and schizophrenia. A defect in methylation due to deficient 5,10-methylene-tetrahydrofolate reductase activity. N Engl J Med 292:491-6, 1975

Galland L. The Four Pillars of Healing. New York, Random House, 1997

Gendler PL et al. Hemopyrrole and kryptopyrrole are absent from the urine of schizophrenics and normal persons. Clin Chem 24(2):230-3, 1978

Gillin JC et al. Zinc and copper in patients with schizophrenia. Encephale 8(3):435-44, 1982

Glen AI et al. A red cell membrane abnormality in a subgroup of chronic schizophrenic patients: evidence for two diseases. Schizophr Res 12:53-61, 1994

Glen AI et al. Membrane fatty acids, niacin flushing and clinical parameters. Prostaglandins Leukot Essent Fatty Acids 55(1-2):9-15, 1996

Godfrey PS et al. Enhancement of recovery from psychiatric illness by methylfolate. Lancet 336:392-5, 1990

Goldman MB. Update on treatment and pathophysiology of water imbalance in schizophrenia. Psychiatric Annals 26(2):93-6, 1996

Green RG. Subclinical pellagra: Its diagnosis and treatment. Schizophrenia 2:70-79, 1970

Greenblatt JM et al. Folic acid in neurodevelopment and child psychiatry. Prog Neuropsychopharmacol Biol Psychiatry 18:647-60, 1994

Heleniak EP, Lamola SW. Histamine and prostaglandins in schizophrenia. J Orthomol Psychiatry 14(3):162-77, 1985

Heresco-Levy U et al. Double-blind, placebo-controlled, crossover trial of glycine adjuvant therapy for treatment-resistant schizophrenia. Br J Psychiatry 169:610-17, 1996

Hitzemann RJ, Garver DL. Abnormalities in membrane lipids associated with deficiencies in lithium counterflow. Paper presented to the Society of Biological Psychiatry, New Orleans, June, 1981

Hoffer A. Niacin Therapy in Psychiatry. Springfield, Illinois, Charles C. Thomas, 1962

Hoffer A. Vitamin B3 dependent child. Schizophrenia 3:107-113, 1971

Hoffer A. The vitamin paradigm wars. Townsend Letter for Doctors and Patients, June, 1996:56-60

Hoffer A - reported in Leviton R. Schizophrenia: healing the divided self with nutrients. Alternative Medicine 24:42-9, 1998

Horrobin DF. Interrelationships between folic acid and prostaglandins in epilepsy, schizophrenia, and peripheral neuropathies, in MI Botez & EH Reynolds, Eds. Folic Acid in Neurology, Psychiatry, and Internal Medicine. New York, Raven Press, 1979a

Horrobin DF. Schizophrenia: Reconciliation of the dopamine, prostaglandin, and opioid concepts and the role of the pineal. Lancet 1:529-31, 1979b

Horrobin DF. The relationship between schizophrenia and essential fatty acid and eicosanoid metabolism. Prostaglandins Leukot Essent Fatty Acids 46(1):71-7, 1992

Hyde AP. Response to "Effects of caffeine on behavior of schizophrenic inpatients". Schizophr Bull 16(3):371-2, 1990

Irvine DG. Apparently non-indolic Ehrlich-positive substance related to mental illness. J Neuropsychiatry 2:292, 1961

Irvine DG et al. Identification of kryptopyrrole in human urine and its relation to psychosis. Nature 224:811, 1969

Irvine DG. Kryptopyrrole in molecular psychiatry, in D Hawkins, L Pauling, Eds. Orthomolecular Psychiatry: Treatment of Schizophrenia. San Francisco, W. H. Freeman and Company, 1973

Ishimaru MJ et al. The glutamate hypothesis of schizophrenia: therapeutic implications. CNS Drugs 7(1):47-67, 1997

Javitt DC, Zukin SR. Recent advances in the phencyclidine model of schizophrenia. Am J Psychiatry 148:1301-8, 1991

Javitt DC et al. Amelioration of negative symptoms in schizophrenia by glycine. Am J Psychiatry 151(8):1234-6, 1994

Javitt DC. Glycine therapy of schizophrenia. Biol Psychiatry 40:684-6, 1996

Johnson JW, Ascher P. Glycine potentiates the NMDA response in cultured mouse brain neurons. Nature 325:529-31, 1987

Kaiya H. Prostaglandin E1 treatment of schizophrenia. Biol Psychiatry 19(3):457-63, 1984

Kanofsky JD et al. Ascorbate: An adjunctive treatment for schizophrenia. Abstract. J Am Coll Nutr 8(5):425, 1989

Kanofsky JD et al. Is iatrogenic hypomagnesemia common in schizophrenia? Abstract. J Am Coll Nutr 10(5):537, 1991

Kimura I, Kumura J. Preliminary reports on the metabolism of trace elements in neuropsychiatric diseases. I. Zinc in schizophrenia. Proc Jap Acad Sci 1965, p. 943

Kirov GK, Tsachev KN. Magnesium, schizophrenia and manic-depressive disease. Neuropsychobiology 23(2):79-81, 1990

Koczapski A et al.. Effects of caffeine on behavior of schizophrenic inpatients. Schizophr Bull 15(2):339-44, 1989

Kornhuber J et al. Iron, copper, zinc, magnesium, and calcium in postmortem brain tissue from schizophrenic patients. Biol Psychiatry 36(1):31-4, 1994

Laugharne JD et al. Fatty acids and schizophrenia. Lipids 31 (suppl):S-163-S-165, 1996

Levine J et al. Serum and cerebrospinal levels of calcium and magnesium in acute versus remitted schizophrenic patients. Neuropsychobiology 33(4):169-72, 1996

Lucas PB et al. Effects of the acute administration of caffeine in patients with schizophrenia. Biol Psychiatry 28:35-40, 1990

Mahadik SP et al. Plasma membrane phospholipid fatty acid composition of cultured skin fibroblasts from schizophrenic patients: comparison with bipolar patients and normal subjects. Psychiatry Res 63(2-3):133-42, 1996

Mathe AA. Combined prostaglandin E-1 decrease with PGE-2 increase found in schizophrenics. Clin Psychiatry News, October, 1981

Mattke JD, Adler M. Mode of action of D-penicillamine in chronic schizophrenia. Dis Nerv Sys 32:388, 1971

McLardy T. Hippocampal zinc in chronic alcoholism and schizophrenia. IRCS J Med Sci 2:1010, 1973

Mellor JE et al. Eicosapentaenoic acid and schizophrenia. Abstract. Neuropsychopharmacology 10:256S, 1994

Mikkelsen EJ. Caffeine and schizophrenia. Behavioral Med December, 1980

Milner G. Ascorbic acid in chronic psychiatric patients: A controlled trial. Br J Psychiatry 109:294-9, 1963

Muller J et al. [Schizophrenia-like symptoms in the Westphal-Strumpell variation of Wilson disease]. Nervenarzt 69(3):264-8, 1998 (in German)

Mycroft FJ et al. MIF-like sequences in milk and wheat proteins. Letter to the Editor. N Engl J Med 307(14):895, 1982

Nicholson GA et al. Effect of D-penicillamine on schizophrenic patients. Lancet i:344, 1966

Osmond H, Hoffer A. Massive niacin treatment in schizophrenia: Review of a nine-year study. Lancet i:316-20, 1962

Peet M et al. Essential fatty acid deficiency in erythrocyte membranes form chronic schizophrenic patients, and the clinical effects of dietary supplementation. Prostaglandins Leukot Essent Fatty Acids 55(1&2):71-5, 1996

Pepplinkhuizen L et al. Schizophrenia-like psychosis caused by a metabolic disorder. Lancet i:454-6, 1980

Pfeiffer CC, Illiev V. A study of zinc deficiency and copper excess in the schizophrenias. Int Rev Biol Suppl 1, 1972

Pfeiffer CC et al. Treatment of pyroluric schizophrenia (malvaria) with large doses of pyridoxine and a dietary supplement of zinc. J Orthomol Psychiatry 3(4):292-300, 1974

Pfeiffer CC. Mental and Elemental Nutrients. New Canaan, CT, Keats Publishing, Inc., 1975

Pfeiffer CC, LaMola S. Zinc and manganese in the schizophrenias. J Orthomol Psychiatry 12:215-34, 1983

Pfeiffer CC, Mailloux R. Excess copper as a factor in human diseases. J Orthomol Med 2(3):171-82, 1987

Prakash R, Petric WM. Psychiatric changes associated with an excess of folic acid. Am J Psychiatry 139(9):1192, 1982

Prasad AS et al. Experimental zinc deficiency in humans. Ann Intern Med 89:483, 1978

Rebec GV et al. Ascorbic acid and the behavioral response to haloperidol: Implications for the action of antipsychotic drugs. Science 227:438-40, 1985

Regland B et al. Homocysteinemia and schizophrenia as a case of methylation deficiency. J Neural Transm Gen Sect 98(2):143-52, 1994

Reichelt K-L et al. The effect of gluten-free diet on urinary peptide excretion and clinical state in schizophrenia. J Orthomol Med 5(4):223-9, 1990

Rihs M et al. Caffeine consumption in hospitalized psychiatric patients. Eur Arch Psychiatry Clin Neurosci 246:83-92, 1996

Roe DA. Drug-induced Nutritional Deficiencies. Second Edition. Westport, CT, Avi Publishing, 1985:270-3

Rudin DO. The major psychoses and neuroses as omega-3 essential fatty acid deficiency syndrome: Substrate pellagra. Biol Psychiatry 16(9):837-50, 1981

Singh MM, Kay SR. Wheat gluten as a pathogenic factor in schizophrenia. Science 191:401-2, 1976

Singh RB et al. Dietary intake and plasma levels of antioxidant vitamins in health and disease: a hospital-based case-control study. J Nutr Environ Med 5:235-42, 1995

Somogyi I et al. [The effects of kryptopyrrole on the brain of cats in the quantitative EEG-analysis]. EEG Emg Z Elektroenzepahlogr Verwandte Geg 7(3):151-6, 1976 (in German)

Sterner RT, Price WR. Restricted riboflavin: Within-subject behavioral effects in humans. Am J Clin Nutr 26:150-60, 1973

Suboticanec K. Vitamin C status in schizophrenia. Bibl Nutr Dieta 38:173-81, 1986

Suboticanec K et al. Vitamin C status in chronic schizophrenia. Biol Psychiatry 28(11):959-66, 1990

Vaddadi KS. Penicillin and essential fatty acid supplementation in schizophrenia. Prostaglandins Med 2:77-80, 1979

Vaddadi KS et al. A double-blind trial of essential fatty acid supplementation in patients with tardive dyskinesia. Psychiatry Res 27(3):313-23, 1989

van Kammen DP et al. Polyunsaturated fatty acids, prostaglandins, and schizophrenia. Ann NY Acad Sci 559:411-23, 1989

Vlissides DN et al. A double-blind gluten-free/gluten-load controlled trial in a secure ward population. Br J Psychiatry 148:447-52, 1986

Willner P. The dopamine hypothesis of schizophrenia: current status, future prospects. Int Clin Psychopharmacol 12(6):297-308, 1997

Wittenborn JR et al. Niacin in the long-term treatment of schizophrenia. Arch Gen Psychiatry 28:308-15, 1973

Wunderink A et al. Nutrition and psychoses. Prog Brain Res 65:49-57, 1986

Zioudrou C et al. Opioid peptides derived from food proteins. J Biol Chem 254:2446-49, 1979

SCLERODERMA

NUTRITIONAL TREATMENT GUIDE

✓ = Efficacy generally accepted.
* = Efficacy *demonstrated* by controlled human trials.
[+] = Efficacy *suspected* from uncontrolled human experiments
[-] = Efficacy *suspected* from indirect data
? = Efficacy *challenged* in at least one study of similar design

DIETARY FACTORS

[+] **low Phenylalanine, low Tyrosine** diet (containing roughly 1.1 g/d, the adult minimum requirement for phenylalanine) (30 day trial)

NUTRITIONAL FACTORS

* ? **Para-amino benzoic acid:** 10 to 12.5 g daily of the potassium salt (Potaba®, Glenwood)

- -

[+] **Omega-6 fatty acids:** *example:* evening primrose oil 1 to 2 g 3 times daily (1 year trial)
[+] **Vitamin A:** *to improve cutaneous manifestations:* isotretinoin (3 to 6 month trial)
[+] **Vitamin D:** calcitriol ≈ 1.75 μg daily (6 month trial) *OR* topical application of calcipotriene 0.005% ointment twice daily under an occlusive dressing (3 month trial)
[+] **Vitamin E:** ? 800 IU of D-alpha tocopheryl acetate daily 15 minutes before meals. Increase to 1600 IU if needed, then decrease to minimal maintenance dosage. Avoid taking iron at the same time.

OTHER RELATED FACTORS

[+] rule out **Hydrochloric Acid** deficiency

- -

[-] rule out **Silica** dust exposure

DIETARY FACTORS

Low Phenylalanine, Low Tyrosine Diet

Unfortunately, there is little published research relating diet specifically to scleroderma. There is a report, published in 1959, which described the treatment of 4 hospitalized patients with a low phenylalanine, low tyrosine diet. While on the diet, treatment with steroids and ACTH was avoided.

All 4 patients improved, usually within 30 days, and there were no notable side effects. However, once they went off the diet, symptoms often reappeared *(Nishimura, 1959)*.

The investigators who developed this diet first discovered 2,5-dihydroxyphenylpyruvic acid (DHPP), an intermediary metabolite of phenylalanine and tyrosine, in the urine of patients with generalized autoimmune diseases, but not in the urine of normals. They then tried supplementing these patients with tyrosine, and found that it aggravated the clinical signs of their disease. These findings caused them to investigate the efficacy of the diet *(Nishimura,1958)*. They also suggest that patients being considered for the diet should first be evaluated for the presence of urinary DHPP.

An 18-year-old girl with generalized scleroderma was admitted to the hospital at a late stage with sclerosis of the extremities, face and breast. She complained of dyspnea and difficulty in walking. A low phenylalanine, low tyrosine diet was prescribed.

After 30 days on the diet, there was softening of the skin of her extremities, face, and breast. Dyspnea had disappeared and she no longer had difficulty in walking. Ankylosis of her ankle joints had subsided. Ulcers of her fingers had healed, and she had improved flexibility of her elbow joints. Ankylosis of her wrists and finger joints, however, was unchanged (Nishimura,1959).

NUTRITIONAL FACTORS

VITAMINS

Vitamin A

While the effects of pharmacotherapeutic dosages of vitamin A have not been reported, there is a report of 9 out of an initial group of 13 patients with systemic sclerosis who completed treatment with isotretinoin (13-*cis*-retinoic acid, a stereoisomer of all-*trans*-retinoic acid) for 6 to 14 months. *All* showed an improvement in the cutaneous manifestations of scleroderma. However, the drug did not appear to benefit internal organs affected by the disease, and serum levels of type III procollagen aminopropeptide did not show a consistent decline during treatment *(Maurice)*.

Large dosages of vitamin A may have substantial side effects, and the safety profile of isotretinoin is not significantly better. Teratogenic effects are most important, and mucocutaneous side-effects occur in nearly all patients. Other side-effects include skeletal hyperostoses, problems with dark adaptation, *Staph aureus* infection and aggravation of inflammatory bowel disease *(Leyden)*. Most of the patients in this study experienced side effects, which in 3 cases necessitated withdrawal from the study within 3 months.

Oral isotretinoin does not increase serum levels of retinol, retinol-binding protein, or prealbumin (transthyretin). Following 3 months of treatment, however, a study of patients with acne vulgaris found that epidermal retinol levels significantly increased by an average of 53%, and dehydroretinol levels significantly decreased by 79%, *(Rollman)*. This may explain the finding of improvement specifically in the cutaneous manifestations of scleroderma.

The mode of action of the reported therapeutic effect of isotretinoin in systemic sclerosis is unclear. There may be a preferential suppression of the synthesis of type I collagen, or the drug may be acting by an unrelated mechanism *(Maurice)*.

Vitamin C

While vitamin C intake appears to be similar to that of normals *(Herrick,1996)*, plasma levels are reduced *(Herrick,1994,1996;Lundberg)*, suggesting that the reduced plasma levels are not due to a low intake of the vitamin *(Herrick,1996)*. Moreover, ascorbate absorption appears to be normal, at least in patients with no evidence of bacterial overgrowth *(Teh)*.

The efficacy of vitamin C supplementation has not been reported.

Vitamin D

The bioavailability of vitamin D, as well as most aspects of vitamin D metabolism, appears to be normal *(Matsuoka;Serup)*, although it is suspected that a relative but specific decrease in the renal hydroxylation to 1,25-dihydroxyvitamin D (calcitriol), the active hormone, occurs as the disease progresses and calcinosis occurs *(Serup)*.

Calcitriol is an immunomodulatory hormone which may have a role in controlling collagen deposition and inducing reversal of fibrosis in some tissues *(Humbert,1990)*. *In vitro*, it has been shown to exert an antiproliferative and antisynthetic effect on fibroblasts *(Boelsma)*.

In an open trial, 11 patients with systemic sclerosis were treated with high oral doses of the vitamin for 6 months to 3 years. Compared to baseline, they were significantly improved. No serious side effects were observed *(Humbert,1993)*. However, since pharmacotherapeutic dosages of vitamin D can produce hypercalcemia, hypercalciuria, soft tissue calcification, kidney stones, and bone resorption *(Lowe)*, they should only be given under close medical supervision.

Topical Calcipotriene

Calcipotriene is a synthetic vitamin D analogue. In an open trial, 12 patients with linear scleroderma or active morphea whose condition had failed to respond to topical corticosteroids applied calcipotriene ointment under an occlusive dressing to plaques twice daily for 3 months. All showed statistically significant improvement in the treated lesions, while laboratory studies showed no adverse effects on calcium metabolism *(Cunningham)*.

Vitamin E

Vitamin E intake appears to be similar to that of healthy control subjects *(Herrick,1996)*, yet patients with systemic sclerosis may have reduced blood concentrations of the vitamin *(Lundberg)*.

While controlled clinical trials of vitamin E supplementation have yet to be reported, patients with either systemic sclerosis or localized scleroderma (morphea) appeared to respond to vitamin E supplementation in an informal clinical setting *(Ayres,1973,1978)*. These clinicians suggest that, since vitamin E is a physiologic stabilizer of cellular and lysosomal membranes, and since some autoimmune diseases respond to vitamin E, a relative deficiency of vitamin E damages lysosomal membranes, thus initiating the autoimmune process *(Ayres 1978)*.

MINERALS

Copper

Both serum copper and ceruloplasmin, a copper-containing protein, may be elevated *(Akimov;Jayson)*. In focal scleroderma, there is evidence of a positive correlation between elevated blood copper levels and the cutaneous manifestations of the disease and, in involved skin, the copper concentration may be 7 times the normal value *(Akimov)*.

Ceruloplasmin in an acute phase reactant. It increases as part of a nonspecific response to inflammation, and it is thought that the increase in serum copper is secondary to the increase in ceruloplasmin *(Jayson)*.

There is currently no evidence that decreasing the body copper burden (for example by providing supplemental zinc) is beneficial.

Selenium

While dietary selenium intake appears to be normal *(Herrick,1996)*, serum selenium levels may be low *(Herrick,1996;Lundberg)*.

Whether selenium supplementation is beneficial is not known.

Silica: A Warning

Long-term silica dust exposure can cause systemic sclerosis. The dust is able to activate microvascular endothelial cells, mononuclear cells from peripheral blood, and dermal fibroblasts *in vitro* in a manner similar to the pathophysiological events that occur in idiopathic systemic sclerosis *(Haustein)*.

Zinc

Similar to the findings in rheumatoid arthritis, cellular zinc concentrations as measured in erythrocytes, platelets and granulocytes, are markedly reduced. This finding is unrelated to inflammatory activity or disease duration. Moreover, plasma zinc levels are reduced in the majority of patients, and this measure is negatively correlated with the degree of inflammation as measured by erythrocyte sedimentation rate and orosomucoid, but is unrelated to disease duration *(Svenson)*.

Corticosteroid treatment increases cellular, but not plasma, zinc levels *(Svenson)*. Whether zinc supplementation has positive effects on the clinical course is not known.

OTHER NUTRITIONAL FACTORS

Essential Fatty Acids

In a double-blind study, combined supplementation of both the omega-3 and omega-6 fatty acids showed no objective evidence of benefit in regard to vascular symptoms after 6 months *(Stainforth)*.

Omega-6 Fatty Acids

Patients have very high levels of prostaglandins along with depletion of the prostaglandin precursors, dihomogammalinolenic acid (DGLA) and arachidonic acid (AA), and levels of key arachidonic metabolites which help to maintain cell membrane characteristics are exceptionally low. This suggests that the high levels of prostaglandins may exert a beneficial effect, and that clinical symptoms develop when the prostaglandin precursors start to be depleted *(Horrobin)*.

In a open trial of 4 women who had had systemic sclerosis for 5 to 13 years, supplementation of omega-6 fatty acids in the form of evening primrose oil for one year was followed by clinical improvements. These included relief of pain in the extremities, improvement of telangiectasia and skin texture, and healing of ulcers *(Strong)*.

Para-amino Benzoic Acid

Several studies, some of which were controlled, have found that large doses of Potaba®, the potassium salt of para-amino benzoic acid (PABA), caused softening of affected skin *(Bushnell;Zarafonetis,1961,1964,1988)*. However, a 48-week double-blind study failed to find it effective *(Clegg)*. There is also evidence from a retrospective study that the administration of Potaba® increases 10-year survival *(Zarafonetis,1988)*, and findings from another retrospective study suggest that it slows the decrease in vital capacity, a measure of pulmonary function *(Zarafonetis,1989)*.

Large doses of PABA or Potaba® carry the risk of causing several side effects including skin rash, anorexia, nausea, vitiligo and, rarely, liver toxicity *(Hughes;Kantor; Physicians' Desk Reference)*.

A 45 year-old female had a 10-year history of progressive disease despite a thoracic sympathectomy and most of the accepted therapies. After starting supplementation with potassium para-aminobenzoate (Potaba®, Glenwood) 20 gm daily, she noted a softening of the skin and a wider range of joint motion. This was the first improvement since the disease began. The dosage was reduced to 10 grams daily and continued indefinitely (Grace).

OTHER RELATED FACTORS

Hydrochloric Acid Deficiency

A clinician reports that *all* of his patients were found to have inadequate levels of hydrochloric acid as well as of vitamin B complex. Following supplementation of both, he found that they quickly improved *(Gaier)*.

Controlled clinical trials of hydrochloric acid supplementation have not been reported.

BIBLIOGRAPHY

Akimov VG et al. [The copper content of the blood and skin in children with circumscribed scleroderma]. Vestn Dermatol Venerol (10):9-11, 1990 (in Russian)

Ayres S et al. Raynaud's phenomenon, scleroderma and calcinosis cutis: Response to vitamin E. Cutis 11:54-62, 1973

Ayres S Jr, Mihan R. Is vitamin E involved in the autoimmune mechanism? Cutis 21(3):321-5, 1978

Boelsma E et al. Effects of calcitriol on fibroblasts derived from skin of scleroderma patients. Dermatology 191(3):226-33, 1995

Bushnell WJ et al. The treatment of progressive systemic sclerosis: A comparison of para-aminobenzoate and placebo in a double-blind study. Abstract. Arthritis Rheum 9:493, 1966

Clegg DO et al. Comparison of aminobenzoate potassium and placebo in the treatment of scleroderma. J Rheumatol 21(1):105-10, 1994

Cunningham BB et al. Topical calcipotriene for morphea/linear scleroderma. J Am Acad Dermatol 39(2 Pt 1):211-5, 1998

Gaier H. Alternatives: Scleroderma. What Doctors Don't Tell You 9(11):6, 1999

Grace WJ et al. Therapy of scleroderma and dermatomyositis. N Y State J Med 63(1):140-44, 1963

Haustein UF, Anderegg U. Silica induced scleroderma--clinical and experimental aspects. J Rheumatol 25(10):1917-26, 1998

Herrick A. Micronutrient antioxidant status in patients with primary Raynaud's phenomenon and systemic sclerosis. J Rheumatol 21(8):1477-83, 1994

Herrick AL et al. Dietary intake of micronutrient antioxidants in relation to blood levels in patients with systemic sclerosis. J Rheumatol 23(4):650-3, 1996

Horrobin DF. Essential fatty acid metabolism in diseases of connective tissue with special reference to scleroderma and to Sjogren's syndrome. Med Hypotheses 14(3):233-47, 1984

Hughes CG. Oral PABA and vitiligo. J Am Acad Dermatol 9:770, 1983

Humbert PG et al. Localized scleroderma--response to 1,25-dihydroxyvitamin D3. Clin Exp Dermatol 15(5):396-8, 1990

Humbert P et al. Treatment of scleroderma with oral 1,25-dihydroxyvitamin D3: evaluation of skin involvement using non-invasive techniques. Results of an open prospective trial. Acta Derm Venereol 73(6):449-51, 1993

Jayson MI et al. Serum copper and caeruloplasmin in ankylosing spondylitis, systemic sclerosis, and morphea. Ann Rheum Dis 35(5):443-5, 1975

Kantor GR, Ratz JL. Liver toxicity from potassium para-aminobenzoate. Letter. J Am Acad Dermatol 13(4):671-72, 1985

Leyden JJ. Retinoids and acne. J Am Acad Dermatol 19(1 Pt 2):164-8, 1988

Lowe K, Normal A. Vitamin D and psoriasis. Nutr Rev 50:138-42, 1992

Lundberg AC et al. Dietary intake and nutritional status in patients with systemic sclerosis. Ann Rheum Dis 51(10):1143-8, 1992

Matsuoka LY et al. Cutaneous vitamin D3 formation in progressive systemic sclerosis. J Rheumatol 18(8):1196-8, 1991

Maurice PD et al. Isotretinoin in the treatment of systemic sclerosis. Br J Dermatol 121(3):367-74, 1989

Nishimura N et al. Intermediary metabolism of phenylalanine and tyrosine in diffuse collagen diseases. I. The presence of 2,5-dihydroxyphenylpyruvic acid in the urine of patients with collagen disease. Arch Dermatol 77:255-62, 1958

Nishimura N et al. Intermediary metabolism of phenylalanine and tyrosine in diffuse collagen diseases. II. Influences of the low phenylalanine and tyrosine diet upon patients with collagen disease. Arch Dermatol 80:466-77, 1959

Physicians' Desk Reference. Oradell, NJ, Med. Economics Col, Inc., 1989

Rollman O, Vahlquist A. Oral isotretinoin (13-cis-retinoic acid) therapy in severe acne: Drug and vitamin A concentrations in sebum and skin. J Invest Dermatol 86(4):384-9, 1986

Serup J, Hagdrup H. Vitamin D metabolites in generalized scleroderma. Evidence of a normal cutaneous and intestinal supply with vitamin D. Acta Derm Venereol 65(4):343-5, 1985

Stainforth JM et al. Clinical aspects of the use of gamma linolenic acid in systemic sclerosis. Acta Derm Venerol (Stockh) 76:144-6, 1996

Strong AMM et al. The effect of oral linoleic acid and gamma-linolenic acid (Efamol). Br J Clin Pract Nov/Dec 1985, p. 444

Svenson KL et al. Reduced zinc in peripheral blood cells from patients with inflammatory connective tissue diseases. Inflammation 9(2):189-99, 1985

Teh LS et al. Ascorbic acid absorption in patients with systemic sclerosis. J Rheumatol 24(12):2353-7, 1997

Zarafonetis CJD. The treatment of scleroderma: Results of potassium para-aminobenzoate therapy in 104 cases, in LC Mills & JH Moyer, Eds. Inflammation and Diseases of Connective Tissue. Philadelphia, W.B. Saunders Co., 1961:688-96

Zarafonetis CJD. Antifibrotic therapy with Potaba. Am J Med Sci November, 1964, pp. 350-61

Zarafonetis CJD et al. Retrospective studies in scleroderma: Effect of potassium para-aminobenzoate on survival. J Clin Epidemiol 41:193-204, 1988

Zarafonetis CJ et al. Retrospective studies in scleroderma: pulmonary findings and effect of potassium p-aminobenzoate on vital capacity. Respiration 56:22-33, 1989

ULCERATIVE COLITIS

See Also: CROHN'S DISEASE

NUTRITIONAL TREATMENT GUIDE

✓ = Efficacy generally accepted.
* = Efficacy *demonstrated* by controlled human trials.
[+] = Efficacy *suspected* from uncontrolled human experiments
[-] = Efficacy *suspected* from indirect data
? = Efficacy *challenged* in at least one study of similar design

DIETARY FACTORS

[+] **low Sulfur Amino Acid diet**

- -

[-] **high Fiber, low Refined Carbohydrate diet**
[-] avoid consumption of **"Fast Foods"**
[-] minimize **Fat** intake, especially **Animal Fat**
[-] minimize **Cholesterol** intake
[-] avoid **Margarine**

NUTRITIONAL FACTORS

* **Butyric Acid:** enemas twice daily with 100 ml of 100 mmol/L solution (2 week trial)
* **Folic acid deficiency:** folic acid *OR* folinic acid 15 mg daily
* **Omega-3 Fatty Acids:** example: "MaxEPA" 5 capsules 3 times daily (total of 2.7 g EPA) (8 week trial)
* **Omega-6 fatty acids:** *example:* evening primrose oil ? 2 to 4 g daily

- -

[+] **Glycosaminoglycans:** *example:* calf tracheal cartilage (Catrix-S) sub-cutaneous injections
[+] **Magnesium deficiency:** ≈ 400 mg daily
[+] **Vitamin K deficiency:** phytonadione 10 mg intramuscularly as needed
[+] **Zinc deficiency:** zinc sulfate 220 mg 3 times daily (does not reduce disease activity)
[+] ? **Vitamin E:** alpha-tocopherol 40 IU/kg daily (4 week trial) *OR* alpha-tocopherylquinone (Start at a low dosage and increase gradually to 50 mg/kg daily or greater.) (4 week trial)

- -

[-] **Calcium deficiency:** ≈ 1 g daily
[-] **Iron deficiency:** 30 mg twice daily until repletion; then minimal possible dosage
[-] **Selenium deficiency:** 200 µg daily
[-] **Vitamin A deficiency:** 50,000 IU daily for 6 weeks (10,000 IU during pregnancy)
[-] **Vitamin C deficiency:** 500 mg twice daily
[-] **Vitamin D deficiency:** 50,000 to 100,000 IU 2 or 3 times during the first week; then, if needed, either 100,000 IU of ergo- or cholecalciferol every 3 to 6 months *OR* 800 to 1,600 IU daily

OTHER RELATED FACTORS

* rule out **Food Sensitivities**, especially **Lactose** intolerance
* **Probiotics:** such as selected strains of *Escherichia coli*

DIETARY FACTORS

"Western" diet

In general, research has demonstrated that consumption of a "Western" diet is related to ulcerative colitis risk *(Kono)*. For example, black populations of sub-Saharan Africa, who still consume a largely traditional diet, rarely develop ulcerative colitis *(Segal)*. Several aspects of the modern "Western" diet have been studied:

"Fast Foods"

The most striking finding of a Swedish study which compared food intake over the previous 5 years of 145 patients with that of 305 controls was an increased relative risk related to the consumption of "fast foods." If these food were consumed at least twice a week, the relative risk of ulcerative colitis was increased almost 4-fold *(Persson)*.

Dietary Fat

A high fat intake has been found to be correlated with the risk of disease. Animal fat and cholesterol have the highest risk, with an odds ratio of more than 4 *(Reif)*. However, not all vegetable fat consumption appears to be unrelated, as the consumption of margarine has also been found to be significantly related to risk *(Kono)*, possibly due to its content of unnatural *trans* fatty acids.

Dietary Fiber

In a prospective study of factors associated with the risk of relapse, a fiber-poor diet was the only dietary factor found which was associated with an increased risk, suggesting that a high-fiber diet is protective *(Leo)*. When patients in remission were given ispaghula husk (psyllium), the supplement was found to be safe and effective in relieving gastrointestinal symptoms, and was more effective than placebo *(Hallert)*.

Refined Carbohydrates

A low fiber diet is likely to be contain a high amount of refined carbohydrates. By reducing the physical buffering effect of fecal bulk, refined carbohydrates are believed to allow intense muscle spasm to occur. This increases the pressure in the colonic lumen to facilitate the disease process *(Grimes)*.

Sugar

The intake of refined sugar, and especially of sucrose, has been repeatedly found to be correlated with the risk of ulcerative colitis *(Persson;Reif;Tragnone)*.

Low Sulfur Amino Acid Diet

Compared to normal feces, the release of hydrogen sulfide is increased 3 to 4 fold in the feces of patients *(Levine)*. Recent evidence suggests that excess bacterial formation of sulfide in the colonic lumen, or failure of detoxification of sulfide in the colonic mucosa, could damage colonic epithelial cells by interfering with butyrate-dependent energy metabolism, leading to inflammation *(Roediger,1996)*.

The chief sources of sulfur for colonic fermentation and cellular function are the sulfur amino acids of animal and plant origin, yet patients ingest more protein and thereby more sulfur amino acids than control subjects *(Roediger,1997)*. The value of an exclusion diet was explored in a study of 8 patients, 4 with chronic disease and 4 who, following an acute attack, were starting treatment with salazopyrin and prednisone. They were advised to completely avoid eggs, cheese, whole milk, ice cream, mayonnaise, soya milk, mineral water, and sulfited drinks (wine and cordials) as well as nuts and cruciferous vegetables (cabbage, broccoli, cauliflower, brussel sprouts). They were also advised to decrease the intake of red meat, and to consume chicken, fish, and skimmed milk.

After 56 months of observation, none of the 4 patients who had previously had an acute attack had experienced a relapse - although the expected relapse rate was 22.6%. Moreover, all showed marked histologic improvement.

Of the 4 patients with chronic disease, the average number of daily bowel movements decreased from 6 to 1.5 and their stools were more formed. One ceased steroids and had no further attacks for 18 months compared to 4 attacks in the preceding 18 months.

The other 3 patients all had microscopic improvement of inflammatory changes. Two patients who stopped the diet resumed it when they noted adverse changes in bowel habits *(Roediger, 1998)*.

NUTRITIONAL FACTORS

Nutritional supplies of many nutrients may be low. While poor intestinal absorption is the major cause, inadequate diet as well as drug-induced deficiencies also play a role.

As repleting nutritional deficiencies is important for strengthening the body's defenses and preventing complications due to the deficiencies, an attempt should be made to restore adequate nutriture. Unfortunately, scientific investigation of the effect of nutritional treatment on the course of the disease has been minimal; thus it is not even known whether nutritional deficiencies play a causal role in the progress of the disease.

FAT-SOLUBLE VITAMINS

Low plasma/serum levels of one or more of the 4 fat-soluble vitamins are common.

Vitamin A

There is some evidence that absorption of vitamin A may be impaired. When patients and healthy controls received 100,000 IU of vitamin A orally, plasma vitamin A did not rise as high in the patients as in the controls, suggesting that there may be a reflex mechanism operating from the damaged colon that inhibits absorption from the small intestine with an additional factor of diarrhea often present *(Page)*. Even when absorption is found to be normal, serum retinal levels may be low due to decreased concentrations of retinol-binding proteins as a result of increased protein catabolism *(Janczewska)*.

In one study of serum vitamin levels of children with inflammatory bowel disease, 16% had either hypovitaminosis A or hypovitaminosis E; of the two, hypovitaminosis A was the more common. The severity of disease activity was a better predictor of deficient serum levels than general nutritional status. Whether these low levels represent a true deficiency is not known *(Bousvaros;Ramakrishna)*.

Vitamin D Deficiency

The intake of vitamin D appears to be similar to that of healthy subjects *(Silvennoinen, 1996a)*. Mild deficiency of vitamin D is common *(Bischoff)*, however, especially in patients with active disease *(Dibble)*. Plasma 25-hydroxyvitamin D levels are inversely correlated with both hemoglobin and erythrocyte sedimentation rate, and there may be evidence of secondary hyperparathyroidism, osteomalacia *(Dibble)*, and osteoporosis due to increased bone resorption accompanied by low bone formation *(Schulte)*.

Vitamin E

As mentioned above, one study found that 16% of children with inflammatory bowel disease had either hypovitaminosis A or hypovitaminosis E *(Bousvaros)*. Other studies have found plasma levels of vitamin E to be either normal *(Ramakrishna)* or raised *(Hoffenberg)*.

Three patients have been described who appeared to have experienced a rapid response to alpha-tocopherol supplements. Previously, they had failed to respond to a 12-week program which consisted of a low-carbohydrate, moderately high-protein and fat diet, removal of foods to which they may have been sensitive, nutritional supplementation, stress reduction and spinal manipulation. All therapeutic measures were stopped except for the diet when alpha-tocopherol was started.

Within 2 weeks, all 3 patients experienced a rapid decrease in amount of blood lost per bowel action, and 2 of them reported a substantial and rapid decrease in the amount of mucous present with each evacuation. Tormina and tenesmus eased greatly and were almost gone within 4 weeks. All reported a marked lessening in the number of daily bowel movements and well-formed stools. Proctosigmoid examinations revealed less weeping of blood and less swelling in the rectal and sigmoid mucosa, with a decrease in both the area and amount of capillary seepage. By the 12th week, all 3 patients showed total healing of the rectal and sigmoid mucosa with no evidence of capillary bleeding or inflammation, and bowel actions had returned to normal *(Hood)*.

Another trial which involved 8 patients failed to find evidence of lessened disease activity, or of decreases in luminal concentrations of the proinflammatory mediators prostaglandin E2 and leukotriene B4 following supplementation. The trial only lasted 15 days, however *(Lauritsen)*.

As a result of scavenging reactive oxygen, alpha-tocopherol is converted to an oxidized form, alpha-tocopherylquinone *(Anita)*. A single case has been reported in which supplementation with alpha-tocopherylquinone was followed by dramatic improvement despite the failure of alpha-tocopherol to exert a beneficial effect, possibly by inhibiting vitamin K-dependent colonic bacterial activity *(Bennet, 1986a)*.

Controlled clinical trials are needed to confirm these observations and to elucidate the relationship between vitamin E supplementation and the disease.

The author had a 5-year history of severe, continuously active ulcerative colitis which had failed to respond adequately to medical treatment. Prednisone was beneficial, but symptoms became severe whenever its dosage was reduced below 30 mg/d. A very low fat diet supplemented with vitamin E 3000 IU and ferrous gluconate 1.95 g along with sulfasalazine and intermittent naproxen was found to reduce the symptoms sufficiently for corticosteroids to be discontinued, but symptoms of bloody diarrhea, arthritis, abdominal cramps and skin lesions remained. Colonoscopy revealed severe inflammation in the sigmoid and descending colon.

As vitamin E alone or ferrous gluconate alone had no beneficial effect, the active substance was postulated to be a product of in vivo interaction of vitamin E and iron, most likely alpha-tocopherylquinone (alpha-TQ). Administration of alpha-TQ was started and the dosage was gradually increased to 50 mg/kg/d or greater.

There was dramatic improvement until the only symptom was a mild facial rash. Colonoscopy revealed mild inflammation in the sigmoid and descending colon. Several times, alpha-TQ was discontinued for 1 to 2 days, and each time a recurrence of inflammation was noted until the former dosage of alpha-TQ was restored. There were no side effects (Bennet, 1986b).

Vitamin K Deficiency

Vitamin K deficiency is reported to be common in patients being treated with sulfasalazine or antibiotics *(Krasinski)*.

When patients are vitamin K-deficient, supplementation, is followed by normalization of abnormal prothrombin times *(Krasinski)*.

WATER-SOLUBLE VITAMINS

Folic Acid Deficiency

Serum and red cell folate levels may be low due to insufficient intake, malabsorption, chronic drug-induced low-grade hemolysis *(Elsborg)* or to the antifolate actions of sulfasalazine *(Swinson)*. In one series of 216 patients with chronic inflammatory bowel disease, low serum folate levels were found in 59% and low erythrocyte folate levels in 26% *(Elsborg)*.

Even for patients who remain on sulfasalazine, supplementation with folic or folinic acid can replete folate stores. Of the two, folinic acid is preferable *(Pironi)*.

There appears to be a close relationship between chronic diarrhea and folate deficiency. In a small open trial, 8 patients with chronic diarrhea of diverse etiology received high dosages of folic acid daily. Stools became normal or almost normal in 2 to 5 days, but the diarrhea returned when folate was discontinued *(Carruthers)*.

Folate supplementation may also reduce the risk of colon cancer. Depressed erythrocyte folate is associated with an increased risk of dysplasia and cancer in these patients, and may be a risk factor for neoplastic transformation *(Lashner, 1993)*. For example, a retrospective study found that folate supplementation was associated with a 62% lower incidence of neoplasia as compared to unsupplemented patients *(Lashner, 1989)*.

Moreover, in a placebo-controlled study, patients whose disease was in remission for at least one month received folinic acid or placebo for 3 months. Patients treated with folinic acid demonstrated improvement in an intermediate biomarker for colon cancer, specifically a normalization in the distribution of proliferating cells in the rectal mucosa *(Biasco)*.

Vitamin C Deficiency

Patients have been found to have reduced levels of ascorbic acid in both plasma and leukocytes. Furthermore, ascorbate loading was followed by subnormal urinary excretion of the vitamin *(Dubey)*. This deficiency appears to be secondary to oxidant stress derived from inflammatory cells in the inflamed mucosa, resulting in the loss of roughly half of both total and reduced ascorbate *(Buffinton)*.

The loss of antioxidant buffering capacity would decrease the capacity of the inflamed mucosa to prevent oxidative tissue damage and hinder recovery of the inflamed mucosa *(Buffinton)*. Thus, although we lack controlled clinical trials of ascorbate supplementation, such supplementation should be considered for patients with active disease.

MINERALS

Calcium Deficiency

Patients with inflammatory bowel disease tend to have a lower calcium intake than healthy controls, at least in part because roughly half of them avoid lactose in their diet *(Silvennoinen,1996b)*. Moreover, calcium may be deficient due to malabsorption, increased intestinal losses, vitamin D deficiency or corticosteroid treatment *(Rosenberg)*. In a recent study of 113 patients, calcium was one of the most common nutrients to become deficient during the course of the disease *(Rath)*.

Iron Deficiency

Chronic gastrointestinal bleeding is a major cause for iron deficiency *(Rosenberg)*, one of the most common nutrient deficiencies in this population *(Rath)*. Conversely, mucosal iron levels within inflamed lesions may be elevated *(Lih-Brody;Sturniolo)*.

Magnesium Deficiency

Magnesium intake has been inversely correlated with the risk of ulcerative colitis *(Reif)*. Deficiency is common due to decreased intake, malabsorption and increased intestinal losses *(Galland)*.

While serum magnesium levels are rarely decreased, intracellular levels are frequently low and may be associated with anorexia, hypotension, confusion, hyperirritablity, tetany, convulsions, and EKG or EEG abnormalities *(Rosenberg)*. In a study of 25 patients with severe disease, magnesium depletion as judged by serum and 24-hour urine concentrations was present in 21 of them (16%), 15 of whom required intravenous repletion *(Russell)*.

Selenium Deficiency

Due primarily to impaired intestinal absorption, selenium deficiency is common in patients with severe disease. Among patients who need parenteral supplementation, a low plasma selenium is almost invariably present *(Rannem)*. Even patients with moderately active disease may have reduced plasma selenium and glutathione peroxidase levels as compared to patients in remission or healthy controls *(Sturniolo)*.

Due to the increased risk of carcinoma of the colon in ulcerative colitis, selenium deficiency is of particular concern as it may further increase the risk of developing this cancer *(Mortensen)*.

Sulfur: A Warning

See Low Sulfur Amino Acid Diet above.

Zinc Deficiency

Zinc deficiency is common, even among stable outpatients, due to reduced intake, malabsorption and increased intestinal losses. Depressed serum zinc levels correlate with the degree of hypoalbuminemia. Measurement of immune function, zinc-dependent proteins or enzymes, and the response to a zinc supplement can help confirm zinc deficiency in borderline cases *(Hendricks)*.

Following supplementation, signs and symptoms of zinc deficiency rapidly recede in patients with severe deficiency. The value of supplementation for patients with mild to moderate deficiency is less clear *(Valberg)*. Double-blind studies have failed to find evidence that zinc repletion reduces disease activity *(Dronfield; Mulder)*.

OTHER NUTRITIONAL FACTORS

Butyric Acid

Short chain fatty acids play a vital role in maintenance of colonic integrity and metabolism. They are produced when dietary fibre is fermented by colonic bacteria and are avidly absorbed in the colon where they are used preferentially as fuel for colonic epithelial cells and have trophic effects on the epithelium *(Cook)*.

Butyric acid is the short chain fatty acid which accounts for the major part of the energy needs of colonic epithelial cells *(Roediger, 1980)*. In ulcerative colitis, the colonic mucosa's ability to metabolize butyrate is impaired. The result is a cellular energy deficiency which is believed to contribute to the disease process *(Chapman; Luciano)*.

Four to 6 weeks after excluded segments of the rectosigmoid exhibiting diversion colitis (which is microscopically indistinguishable from ulcerative colitis) were regularly irrigated with sodium n-butyrate along with sodium acetate and sodium propionate (2 other short-chain fatty acids), inflammatory changes and symptoms disappeared, suggesting that the inflammatory changes were due to deficiencies of short-chain fatty acids *(Harig)*.

Butyric acid is primarily derived by the fermentation of dietary fiber as well as starch *(Roediger, 1980)*; thus one method of increasing butyrate formation is by increasing dietary fiber (see Dietary Fiber above). Since the half-life of butyric acid in the body averages less than 15 minutes, the efficacy of oral supplements is limited *(Daniel)*. However, butyrate enemas appear to be effective for patients with distal ulcerative colitis (*Breuer; Scheppach*).

Essential Fatty Acids

Essential fatty acids, which are often deficient in patients with chronic gastrointestinal disorders *(Siguel)*, have anti-inflammatory effects due to their ability to serve as precursors to the prostaglandins.

Omega-3 Fatty Acids

alpha-linolenic acid → EPA → 3 series prostaglandins
↳ DHA

In inflammatory states, eicosapentaenoic acid (EPA) is released to compete with pro-inflammatory arachidonic acid for enzymatic metabolismm, inducing the production of less inflammatory and chemotactic derivatives *(Heller)*. In several double-blind studies, omega-3 fatty acid supplementation in the form of fish oil has been found to be helpful in reducing disease activity *(Almallah; Stenson)*. The results of one study, however, suggested that, while the supplement may increase the time before relapse for patients in remission, the cumulative relapse rate after 2 years may not be reduced *(Loeschke)*.

Omega-6 Fatty Acids

linoleic acid → GLA → DGLA → 1 series prostaglandins

Plasma levels of dihomogammalinolenic acid (DGLA), the immediate precursor to the anti-inflammatory prostaglandin E_1, may be reduced in inflammatory bowel disease *(Esteve-Comas)*.

When evening primrose oil, a rich source of the omega-6 fatty acid gamma linolenic acid (GLA) was compared to fish oil (MaxEPA) and an olive oil placebo in a randomized 6-month study, evening primrose oil significantly improved stool consistency compared to the other 2 substances, a difference that was maintained 3 months after treatment was discontinued. All 3 treatment groups were similar in regard to stool frequency, rectal bleeding, disease relapse, sigmoidoscopic appearance or rectal histology *(Greenfield)*.

Further controlled trials are obviously needed to clarify the picture.

Glycosaminoglycans

Glycosaminoglycans are part of the ground substance of connective tissue and consist of long unbranched chains made up of disaccharide repeating units, usually in combination with protein. Except for hyaluronic acid, they contain sulfate groups.

With intestinal inflammation, changes in vascular and connective tissue glycosaminoglycans may be an important pathogenic mechanism contributing to leakage of protein and fluid, thrombosis, and tissue remodeling *(Murch)*. Specifically, in ulcerative colitis there is some elevation of total glycosaminoglycans in the colonic mucosa as well as of hyaluronic acid and heparan sulfate *(Symonds)*.

The therapeutic value of glycosaminoglycans is thought to be due to the anti-inflammatory effects of the chondroitin sulfates, of which chondroitin-4-sulfate is believed to be the most important. In a small open trial, 6 patients, 5 of whom had inadequate results from traditional treatments, received sub-cutaneous injections of an activated acid-pepsin-digested calf tracheal cartilage preparation ("Catrix-S") rich in glycosaminoglycans. The injections were given over 10 to 35 days followed by booster injections every 3 to 4 weeks. (Oral supplementation causes osmotic diarrhea.)

Three patients had an excellent response; 2 of them went into total remission but later had recurrences, while one showed progressive improvement. Two had a good response; one who had been unable to take sulfasalazine and prednisone due to adverse side effects, and one who, a result, was spared a total colectomy but continued to have 6 bowel movements a day. The final patient had a fair response which was improved with the addition of prednisone *(Prudden).*

A subsequent study involving 9 patients reported equally good results. Not only did repeat sigmoidoscopies reveal marked improvement, but all 6 patients who had been candidates for total colectomy no longer needed surgery *(Brown).*

Assuming that the efficacy of the preparation is due to the presence of the chondroitin sulfates, there is evidence that chondroitin-4-sulfate is well absorbed from the gut intact. However, while Catrix powder did appear to be equally effective, the long-chain glycosaminoglycan molecular caused an osmotic diarrhea *(Prudden).*

In any event, controlled studies with more subjects are needed before any conclusions can be drawn about the efficacy of this treatment.

OTHER RELATED FACTORS

Food Sensitivities

Self-reported food intolerance is common *(Ballegaard).* Although most authorities believe that food sensitivity has yet to be convincingly documented to be of pathogenic importance *(Ballegaard)*, and although there is insufficient research to establish its prevalence, encouraging findings with the use of elimination diets suggest that food sensitivities may be implicated in causing symptoms in some patients *(Candyls;Hodgson; Mishkin).*

Reactions to cow's milk may be the most frequent problem. Both IgG and IgM antibodies to cow's milk proteins may be increased *(Jewell)*, and lactose intolerance is common *(Meryn)*, especially among patients with active disease *(Kochhar)*, older patients, and patients of certain predisposed ethnic backgrounds *(Bernstein).*

A 49-year-old traveling salesman, had a 10-year history of ulcerative colitis with up to 10 bowel movements a day which was unresponsive to medication. Mild iron and zinc deficiencies were treated with supplementation and he was placed on an exclusion diet; however, his diarrhea was only minimally improved.

Since his symptoms were worsened by salicylate-containing medications, he was placed on a low-salicylate diet. Within 3 days has diarrhea was less, and within one week it had completely ceased. He gained over 14 pounds and, as confirmed by the gastroenterologist, went into a full remission (Davies).

Probiotics

In general, patients appear to have normal fecal flora *(Giaffer;Keighley).* However, there is some evidence that patients with active disease may have reductions in total rectal-mucosa-associated flora, obligate anaerobes (including bifidobacteria, eubacteria and clostridia), and facultative organisms and micro-aerobes compared to patients with quiescent disease *(Hartley).*

Recent evidence that decreased epithelial barrier function of the gut mucosa and an exaggerated reaction of the intestinal immune system to even normal intestinal flora suggests that probiotics may help to protect against exacerbations *(von Ritter).* In a double-blind study, 120 patients with inactive disease received either the drug mesalazine or a viable strain of *E. coli* for 12 weeks. The Clinical Activity Index both at baseline and after the 12 weeks revealed no significant difference between the 2 groups, suggesting that probiotic therapy may be as effective as standard drug treatment *(Kruis).*

BIBLIOGRAPHY

Almallah YZ et al. Distal procto-colitis, natural cytotoxicity, and essential fatty acids. Am J Gastroenterol 93(5):804-9, 1998

Anita M et al. Binding of alpha-tocopherylquinone, an oxidized form of alpha-tocopherol, to glutathione-S-transferase in the liver cytosol. FEBS Lett 436(3):424-6, 1998

Ballegaard M et al. Self-reported food intolerance in chronic inflammatory bowel disease. Scand J Gastroenterol 32(6):569-71, 1997

Bennet JD. Ulcerative colitis: The result of an altered bacterial metabolism of bile acids or cholesterol. Med Hypotheses 20(2):125-32, 1986

Bennet JD. Use of alpha-tocopherylquinone in ulcerative colitis. Gut 27(6):695-97, 1986b

Bernstein CN et al. Milk intolerance in adults with ulcerative colitis. Am J Gastroenterol 89(6):872-7, 1994

Biasco G et al. Folic acid supplementation and cell kinetics of rectal mucosa in patients with ulcerative colitis. Cancer Epidemiol Biomarkers Prev 6(6):469-71, 1997

Bischoff SC et al. Altered bone metabolism in inflammatory bowel disease. Am J Gastroenterol 92(7):1157-63, 1997

Bousvaros A et al. Vitamins A and E serum levels in children and young adults with inflammatory bowel disease: effect of disease activity. J Pediatr Gastroenterol Nutr 26(2):129-35, 1998

Breuer RI et al. Short chain fatty acid rectal irrigation for left-sided ulcerative colitis: a randomised, placebo controlled trial. Gut 40(4):485-91, 1997

Brown RA, Weiss JB. Neovascularization and its role in the osteoarthritic process. Ann Rheum Dis 47:881-5, 1988

Buffinton GD, Doe WF. Altered ascorbic acid status in the mucosa from inflammatory bowel disease patients. Free Radic Res 22(2):131-43, 1995

Candyls S et al. The value of an elimination diet in the management of patients with ulcerative colitis. S Afr Med J 85(11):1176-9, 1995

Carruthers LB. Chronic diarrhea treated with folic acid. Lancet i:849-50, 1946

Chapman MAS et al. Butyrate oxidation is impaired in the colonic mucosa of sufferers of quiescent ulcerative colitis. Gut 35(1):73-6, 1994

Cook SI, Sellin JH. Review article: short chain fatty acids in health and disease. Aliment Pharmacol Ther 12(6):499-507, 1998

Daniel P et al. Pharmacokinetic study of butyric acid administered in vivo as sodium and arginine butyrate salts. Clin Chem Acta 181:255-64, 1989

Davies S, Stewart A. Nutritional Medicine. London, Pan Books, 1987

Dibble JB et al. A survey of vitamin D deficiency in gastrointestinal and liver disorders. Quart J Med 53:119-34, 1984

Dronfield MW et al. Zinc in ulcerative colitis: a therapeutic trial and report on plasma levels. Gut 18(1):33-6, 1977

Dubey SS et al. Vitamin C status, glutathione and histamine in gastric carcinoma, tuberculous enteritis and non-specific ulcerative colitis. Indian J Physiol Pharmacol 29(2):111-4, 1985

Elsborg L, Larsen L. Folate deficiency in chronic inflammatory bowel disease. Scand J Gastroenterol 14:1019-24, 1979

Esteve-Comas M et al. Plasma polyunsaturated fatty acid pattern in inflammatory bowel disease. Gut 33(10):1365-9, 1992

Galland L. Magnesium and inflammatory bowel disease. Magnesium 7(2):78-83, 1988

Giaffer MH et al. The assessment of faecal flora in patients with inflammatory bowel disease by a simplified bacteriological technique. J Med Microbiol 35(4):238-43, 1991

Greenfield SM et al. A randomized controlled study of evening primrose oil and fish oil in ulcerative colitis. Aliment Pharmacol Ther 7(2):159-66, 1993

Grimes DS. Refined carbohydrate, smooth-muscle spasm and disease of the colon. Lancet i:395-97, 1976

Hallert C et al. Ispaghula husk may relieve gastrointestinal symptoms in ulcerative colitis in remission. Scand J Gastroenterol 26:747-50, 1991

Harig JM et al. Treatment of diversion colitis with short-chain-fatty acid irrigation. N Engl J Med 320:23-28, 1989

Hartley MG et al. The rectal mucosa-associated microflora in patients with ulcerative colitis. J Med Microbiol 36(2):96-103, 1992

Heller A et al. Lipid mediators in inflammatory disorders. Drugs 55(4):487-96, 1998

Hendricks KM, Walker WA. Zinc deficiency in inflammatory bowel disease. Nutr Rev 46(12):401-8, 1988

Hoffenberg EJ et al. Circulating antioxidant concentrations in children with inflammatory bowel disease. Am J Clin Nutr 65(5):1482-8, 1997

Hodgson HJF. Inflammatory bowel disease and food intolerance. J R Coll Physicians London 20(1):45-8, 1986

Hood RP. Nonspecific ulcerative colitis: successful treatment with D-alpha tocopherol. Digest of Chiropractic Economics Sept.-Oct. 1984

Janczewska I et al. Metabolism of vitamin A in inflammatory bowel disease. Hepatogastroenterology 38(5):391-5, 1991

Jewell DP, Truelove SC. Circulating antibodies to cow's milk in ulcerative colitis. Gut 13:796, 1972

Keighley MR et al. Influence of inflammatory bowel disease on intestinal microflora. Gut 19(12):1099-104, 1978

Kochlar R et al. Lactose intolerance in idiopathic ulcerative colitis in North Americans. Indian J Med Res 98:79-82, 1993

Kono S. Dietary and other risk factors of ulcerative colitis: a case-control study in Japan. J Clin Gastroenterol 19(2):166-71, 1994

Krasinski SD et al. The prevalence of vitamin K deficiency in chronic gastrointestinal disorders. Am J Clin Nutr 41(3):639-43, 1985

Kruis W et al. Double-blind comparison of an oral Escherichia coli preparation and mesalazine in maintaining remission of ulcerative colitis. Aliment Pharmacol Ther 11(5):853-8, 1997

Lashner BA et al. Effect of folate supplementation on the incidence of dysplasia and cancer in chronic ulcerative colitis. A case-control study. Gastroenterology 97(2):255-9, 1989

Lashner BA. Red blood cell folate is associated with the development of dysplasia and cancer in ulcerative colitis. J Cancer Res Clin Oncol 119(9):549-54, 1993

Lauritsen K et al. Does vitamin E supplementation modulate in vivo arachidonate metabolism in human inflammation? Pharmacol Toxicol 61(4):246-9, 1987

Leo S et al. Ulcerative colitis in remission: is it possible to predict the risk of relapse? Digestion 44(4):217-21, 1989

Levine J et al. Fecal hydrogen sulfide production in ulcerative colitis. Am J Gastroenterology 93(1):83-7, 1998

Lih-Brody L et al. Increased oxidative stress and decreased antioxidant defenses in mucosa of inflammatory bowel disease. Dig Dis Sci 41(10):2078-86, 1996

Loeschke K et al. Omega-3 fatty acids only delay early relapse of ulcerative colitis in remission. Dig Dis Sci 41(10):2087-94, 1996

Luciano L et al. Withdrawal of butyrate from the colonic mucosa triggers "mass apoptosis" primarily in the G0/G1 phase of the cell cycle. Cell Tissue Res 286(1):81-92, 1996

Meryn S. [Role of nutrition in acute and long-term therapy of chronic inflammatory bowel diseases.] Wien Klin Wochenschr 98(22):774-9, 1986 (in German)

Mishkin S. Dairy sensitivity, lactose malabsorption, and elimination diets in inflammatory bowel disease. Am J Clin Nutr 65:564-7, 1997

Mortensen PB et al. Serum selenium concentration in patients with ulcerative colitis. Dan Med Bull 36(6):568-70, 1989

Mulder TP et al. Effect of oral zinc supplementation on metallothionein and superoxide dismutase concentrations in patients with inflammatory bowel disease. J Gastroenterol Hepatol 9(5):472-7, 1994

Murch SH et al. Disruption of sulphated glycosaminoglycans in intestinal inflammation. Lancet 341:711-14, 1993

Page RC, Bercovitz Z. The absorption of vitamin A in chronic ulcerative colitis. Am J Dig Dis 10:174-77, 1943

Persson PB et al. Diet and inflammatory bowel disease: a case-control study. Epidemiology 3(1):47-51, 1992

Pironi L et al. Evaluation of oral administration of folic and folinic acid to prevent folate deficiency in patients with inflammatory bowel disease treated with salicylazosulfapyridine. Int J Clin Pharmacol Res 8(2):143-8, 1988

Prudden JF, Balassa LL. The biological activity of bovine cartilage preparations. Sem Arthritis Rheum 3(4):287-321, 1974

Ramakrishna BS et al. Circulating antioxidants in ulcerative colitis and their relationship to disease severity and activity. J Gastroenterol Hepatol 12(7):490-4, 1997

Rannem T et al. Selenium depletion in patients with gastrointestinal diseases: are there any predictive factors? Scand J Gastroenterol 33(10):1057-61, 1998

Rath HC et al. [Nutritional deficiencies and complications in chronic inflammatory bowel diseases]. Med Klin 93(1):6-10, 1998 (in German)

Reif S et al. Pre-illness dietary factors in inflammatory bowel disease. Gut 40(6):754-60, 1997

Roediger WE. Role of anaerobic bacteria in the metabolic welfare of the colonic mucosa in man. Gut 21:793-98, 1980a

Roediger WE et al. Colonic sulfide in pathogenesis and treatment of ulcerative colitis. Dig Dis Sci 42(8):1571-9, 1997

Roediger WEW. Decreased sulphur aminoacid intake in ulcerative colitis. Lancet 351:1555, 1998

Rosenberg IH et al. Nutritional aspects of inflammatory bowel disease. Ann Rev Nutr 5:463-84, 1985

Russell RI. Magnesium requirements in patients with chronic inflammatory disease receiving intravenous nutrition. J Am Coll Nutr 4(5):553-8, 1985

Scheppach W et al. Effect of butyrate enemas on the colonic mucosa in distal ulcerative colitis. Gastroenterology 103(1):51-6, 1992

Schulte C et al. Reduced bone mineral density and unbalanced bone metabolism in patients with inflammatory bowel disease. Inflamm Bowel Dis 4(4):268-75, 1998

Segal I et al. The rarity of ulcerative colitis in South African blacks. Am J Gastroenterol 74(4):332-6, 1980

Siguel E, Lerman R. Prevalence of essential fatty acid deficiency in patients with chronic gastrointestinal disorders. Metabolism 45(1):12-23, 1996

Silvennoinen J. Relationships between vitamin D, parathyroid hormone and bone mineral density in inflammatory bowel disease. J Intern Med 239(2):131-7, 1996a

Silvennoinen J et al. Dietary calcium intake and its relation to bone mineral density in patients with inflammatory bowel disease. J Intern Med 240:285-92, 1996b

Stenson WF et al. Dietary supplementation with fish oil in ulcerative colitis. Ann Intern Med 116:609-14, 1992

Sturniolo GC et al. Altered plasma and mucosal concentrations of trace elements and antioxidants in active ulcerative colitis. Scand J Gastroenterol 3(6):644-9, 1998

Swinson CM et al. Role of sulphasalazine in the aetiology of folate deficiency in ulcerative colitis. Gut 22(6):456-61, 1981

Symonds DA. The glycosaminoglycans of the human colon in inflammatory and neoplastic conditions. Arch Pathol Lab Med 102(3):146-9, 1978

Tragnone A et al. Dietary habits as risk factors for inflammatory bowel disease. Eur J Gastroenterol Hepatol 7(1):47-51, 1995

Valberg LS et al. Zinc absorption in inflammatory bowel disease. Dig Dis Sci 31(7):724-31, 1986

von Ritter C. [Chronic inflammatory bowel diseases. Pathophysiology and drug therapy]. Radiologe 38(1):3-7, 1998 (in German)

PART THREE

APPENDICES

ELEMENTAL MINERAL CONTENT OF COMMON MINERAL SALTS

	MINERAL SALT	MILLIGRAMS OF ELEMENTAL MINERAL PER 100 mg OF MINERAL SALT	REFERENCE
Boron			
	Sodium Borate	21 mg	(1)
Calcium			
	Carbonate	40 mg	(1)
	Ascorbate	10 mg	(1)
	Chloride	36 mg	(1)
	Citrate	24 mg	(1)
	Gluconate	9 mg	(1)
	Glycerophosphate	19 mg	(1)
	Lactate	18 mg	(1)
	Pantothenate	8 mg	(1)
	Phosphate	29 mg	(1)
Chromium (per 100 μg)			
	Chloride	33 μg	(2)
	Picolinate	12 μg	(3)
Copper			
	Gluconate	14 mg	(1)
	Glycinate	30 mg	(1)
	Oxide	79 mg	(1)
Iodine			
	Potassium	76 mg	(1)
	Kelp	0.1 mg	(4)
Iron			
	Gluconate	12 mg	(1)
	Lactate	24 mg	(1)
	Sulfate	37 mg	(1)

Magnesium			
	Chloride	25 mg	(1)
	Citrate	16 mg	(1)
	Gluconate	5 mg	(5)
	Lactate	12 mg	(1)
	Oxide	60 mg	(1)
	Phosphate	27 mg	(1)
	Sulfate	20 mg	(1)
Manganese			
	Gluconate	11 mg	(5)
	Sulfate	36 mg	(1)
Molybdenum			
	Sodium molybdate	47 mg	(1)
Potassium			
	Chloride	52 mg	(1)
	Citrate	38 mg	(1)
	Gluconate	17 mg	(1)
	Iodine	24 mg	(1)
Selenium (per 100 µg)			
	Selenomethionine	40 µg	(1)
	Selenite	46 µg	(1)
Vanadium			
	Sulfate	31 mg	(1)
Zinc			
	Citrate	34 mg	(1)
	Gluconate	14 mg	(5)
	Oxide	80 mg	(1)
	Sulfate	41 mg	(1)

REFERENCES

1. Windholz M et al, eds., The Merck Index, Tenth Edition. Merck & Co., Inc., Rahway, NJ, 1983
2. Budavari S et al, eds., The Merck Index, Twelfth Edition. Merck & Co., Inc., Rahway, NJ 1996
3. U.S. Patent 4,315, 927
4. Food Codex
5. United States Pharmacopeia

IDEAL DIETARY NUTRIENT RATIOS

Calcium to Magnesium: 2-2.5 to 1

(*Mildred Seelig, M.D., Ph.D. - interviewed by Zucker M in* Let's Live, *April, 1996:36-8*).

Review Article: "It is important to emphasize the maintenance of a Ca/Mg ratio close to 2 in the intake" (*Durlach J. Recommended dietary amounts of magnesium: Mg RDA.* Magnes Res *2(3):195-203, 1989*).

Calcium to Phosphorus: 1 to 1

Review Article: For many people, the calcium-to-phosphorus ratio is reduced to somewhere between 1 to 2 and 1 to 4 (*Worthington-Roberts B.* Contemporary Developments in Nutrition. *St. Lewis, MO, C.V. Mosby Co., 1981:240-53*).

Zinc to Copper: 7.5 to 1 (range: 5-14 to 1)

Review Article: In published studies, nearly 16% of 51 subjects who appeared to have normal cardiac status at baseline displayed cardiac abnormalities that were associated with a dietary zinc to copper ratio of 16 as compared to a ratio of 5-14 in the diets consumed by many Americans (8-12 mg Zn; 0.8-1.5 mg Cu). However, prior copper status was unknown (*Sandstead HH. Requirements and toxicity of essential trace elements, illustrated by zinc and copper.* Am J Clin Nutr *61(suppl):621S-4S, 1995*).

Observational Study: Compared to 27 age- and sex-matched controls, the diets of 27 chronic juvenile offenders (juveniles adjudicated for 3 or more offenses including a felony) had an elevated zinc/copper ratio (11.2 to 1; optimum 7.5 to 1) (*Schauss AG et al. A critical analysis of the diets of chronic juvenile offenders, Part II.* J Orthomol Psychiatry *8(4): 222-6, 1979*).

Omega-3 to Omega-6 essential fatty acids: 1 to 4 **(range: 1-6 to 1)**

(*Erasmus U. Fats that are essential.* Int J Altern Comp Med *February, 1997:9-10*)

Review Article: In adult humans the optimal omega-3 to omega-6 ratio is considered to be 6 to 1 (*Billeaud C, Bougle D, Sarda P, et al. Effects of preterm infant formula supplementation with a-linolenic acid with a-linoleate/a-linolenate ratio of 6: a multicentric study.* Eur J Clin Nutr *51:520-6, 1997*).

Experimental Study: 26 nonsmoking, atopic, asthmatic pts. (mean age 22 yrs.) were supplemented for 4 wks. with an omega-3 to omega-6 fatty acid ratio of 1:10, followed by 4 wks. of a higher ratio of omega-3 to omega-6 fatty acids of 1:5. There was a diminishing of the respiratory capacity in pts. in the low omega-3 fatty acid gp. but a significant respiratory benefit after methacholine challenge in >40% of those with the higher ratio of omega-3 to omega-6 fatty acid supplementation. The ave. low and high dose of fish oil provided was approximately 0.7 and 3.3 g of EPA and DHA daily, respectively (*Broughton KS et al. Reduced asthma symptoms with n-3 fatty acid ingestion are related to 5- series leukotriene production.* Am J Clin Nutr *65:1011-17, 1997*).

Review Article: The omega-3 to omega-6 fatty acid ratio should be about 1:1. Since, however, the Western diet is very low in omega-3 fatty acids, it is 1:10 to 1:20-25 (*Labadarios D, Walker ARP. Dietary avoidance of coronary heart disease - How practicable is the Mediterranean Diet? Cardiovasc J So Afr Cardiovascular Suppl. 1:C30-C36, 1996*).

Oleic acid to Linoleic Acid (or to cholesterol-raising fatty acids): 1:1 to 3:1

(*Grundy SM. What is the desirable ratio of saturated, polyunsaturated, and monounsaturated fatty acids in the diet? Am J Clin Nutr 988S-90S, 1997*)

MEASURES OF NUTRIENT POTENCY

<u>Beta-Carotene</u>

1 mg all-*trans* beta-carotene = 1667 IU of vitamin A activity

(*Sauberlich HE, Hodges HE, Wallace DL, et al. Vitamin A metabolism and requirements in the human studied with the use of labeled retinol. <u>Vitam Horm</u> 32:251-75, 1974*)

> ***Note:*** *Since international units are based on vitamin A activity, many carotenoids, including most xanthophylls and lycopene, which have no vitamin A activity, have no international units.*

1 μg <u>dietary</u> beta-carotene = 0.167 μg retinol

(*National Research Council. <u>Recommended Dietary Allowances</u>. 9th Edition. Washington, DC, National Academy Press, 1980*)

<u>Enzymes</u>

<u>Pancreatin</u>

The enzyme activity (i.e. digestive capacity) of pancreatic material is rated using a comparative system established by the US Pharmacopeia. By definition, pancreas material (1X) provides the following minimal activity:

<u>amylase</u>: no less than 25 USP units/mg
<u>lipase</u>: no less than 2 USP units/mg
<u>protease</u>: no less than 25 USP units/mg

Higher levels of activities are described in multiples of these numbers. For example, 6X pancreas material provides six times the activity for each of these three enzymes.

(*United States Pharmacopeia*).

<u>Plant enzymes</u>

Fungal or 'plant enzyme' products, although they have industry activity standards, have no recognized activity units that are used consistently throughout the industry.

In their purest forms, plant enzymes typically have the following minimal activity:

<u>amylase</u>: 100,000 SKB/gram = 89 USP units/mg
<u>cellulase</u>: 6,500 GD (Guar)/gram
<u>lactase</u>: 95,000 LU/gram
<u>lipase</u>: 100,000 LU/gram = 80 USP units/mg
<u>protease</u>: 500,000 LU/gram = 197 USP units/mg

(*Thorne Research Product Book. Sandpoint, Idaho, Thorne Research, Inc., 1995*)

Vitamin A (retinol)

1 μg retinol = 3.34 IU of vitamin A activity

(*Sauberlich HE, Hodges HE, Wallace DL, et al. Vitamin A metabolism and requirements in the human studied with the use of labeled retinol. Vitam Horm 32:251-75, 1974*)

Retinol equivalents (RE): the vitamin A activity in foods

1 RE = 1 μg all-*trans* retinol
= 6 μg all-*trans*-beta-carotene
= 12 μg other provitamin A carotenoids

(*Bieri JG, McKenna MC. Expressing dietary values for fat-soluble vitamins; changes in concepts and terminology. Am J Clin Nutr 34:289-95, 1981; National Research Council. Recommended Dietary Allowances. 9th Edition. Washington, DC, National Academy Press, 1980*)

Vitamin D

1 IU = the biological activity of 0.025 μg cholecalciferol (vitamin D_3) in bioassays with rats and chicks.
1 μg vitamin D (cholecalciferol) = 40 IU
1 μg 25-hydroxyvitamin D = 80 IU
1 μg 1,25-dihydroxyvitamin D = 200 IU

(*National Research Council. Recommended Dietary Allowances. 10th Edition. Washington, DC, National Academy Press, 1989*)

Vitamin E

1 mg = 1.49 IU d-alpha-tocopherol (natural vitamin E; RRR-alpha-tocopherol)
1 mg = 1.10 IU dl-alpha-tocopherol (synthetic vitamin E; all-*rac*-alpha-tocopherol)

Synthetic vitamin E (dl-alpha-tocopherol; all-*rac*-alpha-tocopherol) is a mixture of 8 stereoisomers, one of which (12.5%) is d-alpha-tocopherol. The other 7 isomers have lower biological activities, ranging from 21% to 90% of the biological activity of d-alpha-tocopherol (*Weiser H, Vecchi M. Stereoisomers of α-tocopheryl acetate. II. Biopotencies of all eight stereoisomers, individually or in mixtures, as determined by rat resorption-Gestation Tests. Int J Vitam Nutr Res 52:351-70, 1982*).

> ***Note:*** *While, based on earlier animal studies using the rat resorption assay, natural-source vitamin E is officially recognized as having 36% greater potency than synthetic vitamin E, recent human and animal studies suggest that natural-source vitamin E is almost twice as effective as synthetic vitamin E (Acuff RV, Thedford SS, Hidiroglou NN, et al. Relative bioavailability of RRR- and all-rac-α-tocopheryl acetate in humans: studies using deuterated compounds. Am J Clin Nutr 60:397-402, 1994; Vitamin E Fact Book. La Grange, IL, Vitamin E Research and Information Service, 1994).*

1 α-TE (RRR-alpha-tocopherol therapeutic equivalents) = the activity of 1 mg of RRR-alpha-tocopherol

INDEX

ORDERING INFORMATION

The following books and CD-ROM by Melvyn R. Werbach, M.D. are available by mail directly from *Third Line Press*:

(USE THE HANDY ORDER FORM ON THE NEXT PAGE.)

1. **Textbook of Nutritional Medicine** (*with* Jeffrey Moss, DDS, CNS, CCN) ISBN 0-9618550-9-6
   740 pages 8 ½" x 11" 1999 hard cover ***Price:*** $74.95

2. **Nutritional Influences on Mental Illness.** *Second* Edition ISBN 0-9618550-8-8
   454 pages 8 ½" x 11" 1999 hard cover ***Price:*** $59.95

   "This is a book that deserves to be on every professional's shelf within easy reach." Russell M. Jaffe, M.D., Ph.D., **International Clinical Nutritional Review**

3. **Foundations of Nutritional Medicine** ISBN 0-9618550-6-1
   330 pages 8 ½" x 11" 1997 hard cover ***Price:*** $49.95

   "Packed with useful and easy-to-access information that is essential for . . . anyone who integrates nutritional medicine into their daily practice." Shari Lieberman, Ph.D., C.N.S., **Townsend Letter**

4. **Nutritional Influences on Illness CD-ROM (*including* Nutritional Influences on Mental Illness)**
   approx. 4200 pages multi-platform (Adobe Acrobat) 1998 with *hypertext* links ***Price:*** $395.00 (single user)

5. **Nutritional Influences on Illness.** *Second* Edition ISBN 0-9618550-3-7
   700 pages 8 ½" x 11" 1993 hard cover ***Price:*** $64.95

   "I cannot imagine a health care provider who would not gain from appropriating the information in this book . . . ." James Heffley, Ph.D. Editor, **Journal of Applied Nutrition**

6. **Botanical Influences on Illness** (Michael T. Murray, N.D., co-author) ISBN 0-9618550-4-5
   344 pages 7" x 10" 1994 hard cover ***Price:*** $39.95

   "This will become a standard reference for practitioners utilizing botanicals, and should be a required reference for those who don't." Steven Foster, **Quarterly Review of Natural Medicine**

7. **Third Line Medicine: Modern Treatment for Persistent Symptoms** ISBN 0-14-19063-5
   215 pages 5" x 7 ½" 1986 soft cover ***Price:*** $10.95

   "For this clear exposition of what has happened and where we are going, all doctors . . . ought to be grateful." Abram Hoffer, M.D., Ph.D., Editor-in-Chief, **Journal of Orthomolecular Medicine**

THIRD LINE PRESS, INC.
4751 Viviana Drive, Suite 102
Tarzana, California 91356
USA

Phones: (800) 916-0076; (818) 996-0076
FAX: (818) 774-1575
e-mail: tlp@third-line.com
internet: www.third-line.com

✔ **Please send:**

___ copies of **Textbook of Nutritional Medicine** @ $ 74.95 $ ___________

___ copies of **Nutritional Influences on Mental Illness**, ***Second*** Edition @ $ 59.95 $ ___________

___ copies of **Foundations of Nutritional Medicine** @ $49.95 $ ___________

___ copies of **Nutritional Influences on Illness**, ***Second*** Edition @ $64.95 $ ___________

___ copies of **Nutritional Influences on Illness CD-ROM** @ $395.00 $ ___________

___ copies of **Botanical Influences on Illness** @ $39.95 $ ___________

___ copies of **Third Line Medicine** @ $10.95 $ ___________

_ ***A free brochure with further information about your publications.***

* **SHIPPING CHARGES**
(add $4.00 for orders outside the US)

1 book	$7.00
2 books:	$8.00
3 books:	$9.50
4-6 books:	$11.00

Subtotal $ ___________

8.25% tax (California only) $ ___________

* Shipping $ ___________

TOTAL $ ___________

QUANTITY PRICES ON REQUEST
Prices subject to change without notice

✔ **If a check is *not* enclosed, please charge my:** **Visa** ___ **MasterCard** ___

Card #: __________ - __________ - __________ - __________ **Expiring:** _______

Signature: ____

OUTSIDE OF THE UNITED STATES

* Beyond North America, shipping charges are for surface shipping (up to 3 months).
* Air mail rates are available on request.
* If payment is *not* made by Visa or MasterCard, your check must be in US dollars and drawn on a US bank.

NAME: ____

ADDRESS: ____

____

____

PHONE: ____________________ **FAX:** ____________________ **E-MAIL:** ____________________